NCLEX-RN Review

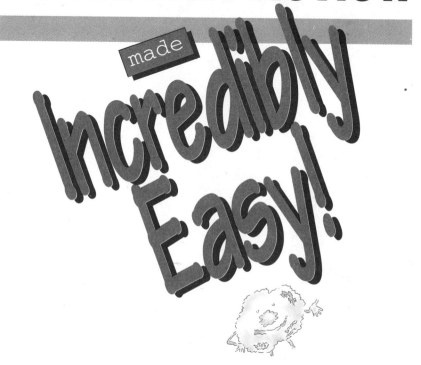

made Incredibly Easy!

NCLEX-RN Review

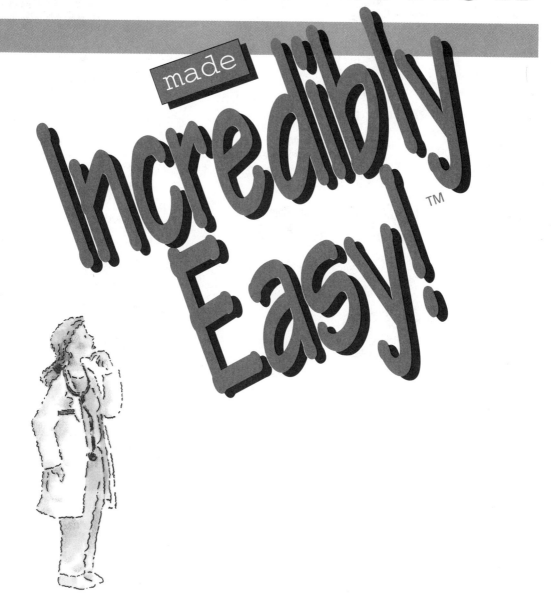

made **Incredibly Easy!** ™

Springhouse Corporation
Springhouse, Pennsylvania

Staff

Vice President
Matthew Cahill

Clinical Director
Judith A. Schilling McCann, RN, MSN

Art Director
John Hubbard

Director, Electronic Publishing
Andrew Nusbickel

Executive Editor
Michael Shaw

Managing Editor
Andrew T. McPhee, RN, BSN

Editors
Kevin Haworth, David Moreau, Kirk
Robinson, Patricia Wittig

Clinical Project Manager
Collette Bishop Hendler, RN, CCRN

Clinical Editors
Clare Brabson, RN, BSN; Jill M. Curry, RN,
BSN, CCRN; Kate McGovern, RN, BSN,
CCRN; Lori Musolf Neri, RN, MSN, CCRN;
Joan M. Robinson, RN, MSN, CCRN; Carla
Roy, RN, BSN, CCRN; Beverly Ann
Tscheschlog, RN

Manager, Electronic Products
Don Saul

Electronic Products Editor
Karen Diamond

Copy Editors
Brenna H. Mayer (manager), Priscilla
DeWitt, Mary T. Durkin, Jaime Stockslager,
Kathryn M. Tevelson, Patricia Turkington,
Pamela Wingrod

Designers
Arlene Putterman (associate art director),
Mary Ludwicki (book designer), Joseph
John Clark, Jacalyn B. Facciolo, Donna S.
Morris, Susan Sheridan

Illustrator
Bot Roda

Typography
Diane Paluba (manager), Joyce Rossi
Biletz, Valerie Molettiere

Manufacturing
Deborah Meiris (director), Patricia K.
Dorshaw (manager), Otto Mezei (book
production manager)

Editorial Assistants
Beverly Lane, Liz Schaeffer

Indexer
Judith Schaeffer Young

© 2000 by Springhouse Corporation. All rights reserved. No part of this publication may be used or reproduced in any manner whatsoever without written permission, except for brief quotations embodied in critical articles and reviews. For information, write Springhouse Corporation, 1111 Bethlehem Pike, P.O. Box 908, Springhouse, PA 19477-0908. Authorization to photocopy items for internal or personal use, or for the internal or personal use of specific clients, is granted by Springhouse Corporation for users registered with the Copyright Clearance Center (CCC) Transactional Reporting Service, provided that the fee of $.75 per page is paid directly to CCC, 222 Rosewood Dr., Danvers, MA 01923. For those organizations that have been granted a photocopy license by CCC, a separate system of payment has been arranged. The fee code for users of the Transactional Reporting Service is 1582550166/2000 $00.00 + .75.

Printed in the United States of America.

IEREV- D N O S A J J M A M
02 01 00   10 9 8 7 6 5 4 3 2

Ⓡ A member of the Reed Elsevier plc group

Library of Congress Cataloging-in-Publication Data

NCLEX-RN Review made incredibly easy
    p.   cm.
    Includes index.
    1. Nursing—Examinations, questions, etc. I.
Springhouse Corporation
    [DNLM: 1. Nursing Care. 2. Nursing. WY 18.2
N3576 1999]
RT55.N74 1999
610.73'076—dc21
DNLM/DLC   99-040804
ISBN 1-58255-016-6 (alk. paper)   CIP

Contents

Part V

Care of the child

Appendices

Contributors and consultants

Joanne M. Bartelmo, RN, MSN, CCRN
Clinical Educator
Pottstown (Pa.) Memorial Medical Center

Marcy Caplin, RN, MSN, CS
Independent Consultant
Hudson, Ohio

Joseph T. Catalano, RN, PhD
Professor of Nursing
East Central University
Ada, Okla.

Marlene Ciranowicz, RN, MSN, CDE
Independent Nurse Consultant
Dresher, Pa.

Karen L. Cobb, RN, EdD
Assistant Professor
Indiana University
Indianapolis

Jean Sheerin Coffey, RN, MSN
Pediatric Trauma Outreach Coordinator
Fletcher Allen Health Care
University of Vermont
Burlington

Patricia Davies, RN, MSN
Instructor
School of Nursing
University of Pittsburgh

Diane M. Ellis, RN, MSN, CCRN, CS
Critical Care Educator
Graduate Hospital
Philadelphia

Sandra A. Faux, RN, PhD
Associate Professor
Rush University College of Nursing
Chicago

Ann Boyle Grant, RN, PhD
Dean of Instruction
Cuesta College
San Louis Obispo, Calif.
Instructor, Division of Nursing
California State University Dominguez Hills
Carson

Bonnie Handerhan, RN, MSN, CCRN
Nurse Manager
Intensive Coronary Care Unit
North Penn Hospital
Lansdale, Pa.

Virginia Richardson, RN, DNS, CPNP
Assistant Dean for Student Affairs
Indiana University School of Nursing
Indianapolis

Karin K. Roberts, RN, PhD
Associate Professor
Research College of Nursing
Kansas City, Mo.

Alean Royes, RN, MSN, CNS
Faculty-Specialist
School of Nursing
The University of Texas at Arlington

June Schneberger, RN, MSN, CS
Instructor
Baptist Health System
School of Professional Nursing
San Antonio, Tex.

Bruce Austin Scott, RN, MSN, CS
Nursing Instructor
San Joaquin Delta College
Staff Nurse
St. Joseph's Medical Center
Stockton, Calif.

Cynthia Miller Taylor, RN, MS, CNAA
Independent Nurse Consultant
Rockville, Md.

Foreword

You're well on your way to becoming a licensed registered nurse. First, though, you've got to prove yourself by passing the NCLEX-RN. Face it — that's enough to make anybody a little uneasy.

This is where we come in. The book you're holding is the brainchild of experienced nurses who once stood where you stand now, nervous about taking the NCLEX yet eager to begin their professional lives. These nurses passed the NCLEX, just as each day, they pass a much more difficult test — providing safe, effective, expert nursing care to all kinds of patients. Now they pass their knowledge to you.

Flip through a few pages of *NCLEX-RN Review Made Incredibly Easy*. You'll see right away that our approach to preparation for NCLEX-RN is revolutionary. First, we promise never to waste your valuable study time with minutia, dense prose, or impenetrable jargon. You'll find page after page of solid clinical information in an easy-to-read outline format. Nurse Joy, your *Incredibly Easy* guide and mentor, points out critical facts. She also reminds you that it's okay to laugh and take time for yourself; indeed, it will help you succeed on the NCLEX. Unlike many other NCLEX guides, *NCLEX-RN Review Made Incredibly Easy* provides a clear, concise rationale for every nursing intervention. Like you, we believe that understanding *why* an answer is correct is just as important as knowing the correct answer.

As you approach the day of your examination, *NCLEX-RN Review Made Incredibly Easy* will be with you every step: getting you ready and easing your anxieties. It will help you devise an effective study plan, set realistic goals, and let you know what to expect on the day of the test — and will keep you entertained all the while.

In addition to superb clinical and nursing information, you'll find tons of test-taking tips taught by the best teacher ever — experience.

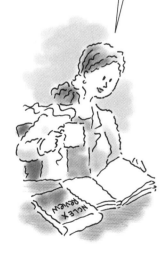

Passing the NCLEX is important but don't let it distract you from what's REALLY important — becoming a skilled, caring nurse.

Taking it one chapter at a time

Each chapter provides features you won't find in any other NCLEX review book. Each feature is designed with your NCLEX success in mind.

- **Brush up on key concepts** helps you review the most important information, including respiratory care, cardiovascular, neurologic, maternal-neonatal, psychiatric, and pediatric care, and much, much more.
- **Memory joggers** give you helpful, effective ways to remember key information.
- **Keep abreast of diagnostic tests** helps you review relevant diagnostic and laboratory tests and provides easy-to-understand nursing care guidelines.

- **Polish up on patient care** focuses on the care you give your patients, a topic at the heart of the NCLEX. It's organized logically, beginning with a clear description of a key disorder (including myocardial infarction, acquired immunodeficiency syndrome, asthma, tuberculosis, cerebrovascular accident, spinal cord injury, and many more) followed by causes, assessment findings, diagnostic test results, nursing diagnoses, treatment (including drug therapy) and, finally, interventions and rationales.
- **Cheat sheets** present all crucial data from each chapter in an easy-to-read format, ideal for quick study and review.
- **Pump up on practice questions** gives you an opportunity to test your understanding with 10 NCLEX-RN–style questions, all accompanied by answers with clear, detailed rationales. In addition, at the end of each unit are 30 more NCLEX-RN–style questions accompanied by answers and rationales. You'll reinforce what you learn right away.

Putting it all together

There's more: Turn to the inside back cover and find your free CD-ROM. Use it and discover 750 *more* practice questions in an easy-to-use program that lets you design your own tests. You can select questions by subject or take a random test. You can receive immediate feedback on your answers or simulate the conditions of an actual NCLEX examination.

All in all, *NCLEX-RN Review Made Incredibly Easy* will serve as your faithful guide as you journey toward NCLEX success. Study hard and take care of yourself. Believe in your heart that you'll succeed, and you *will*. Good luck on the NCLEX and best wishes as you become the best nurse you can be.

Ann Boyle Grant, RN, PhD
Dean of Instruction, Cuesta College
San Louis Obispo, California
Instructor, Division of Nursing
California State University Dominguez Hills
Carson, California

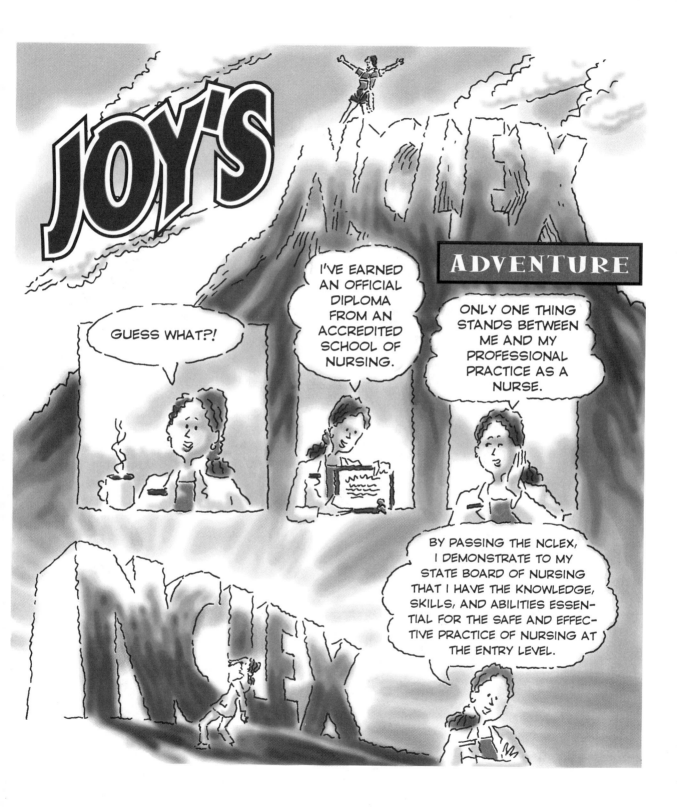

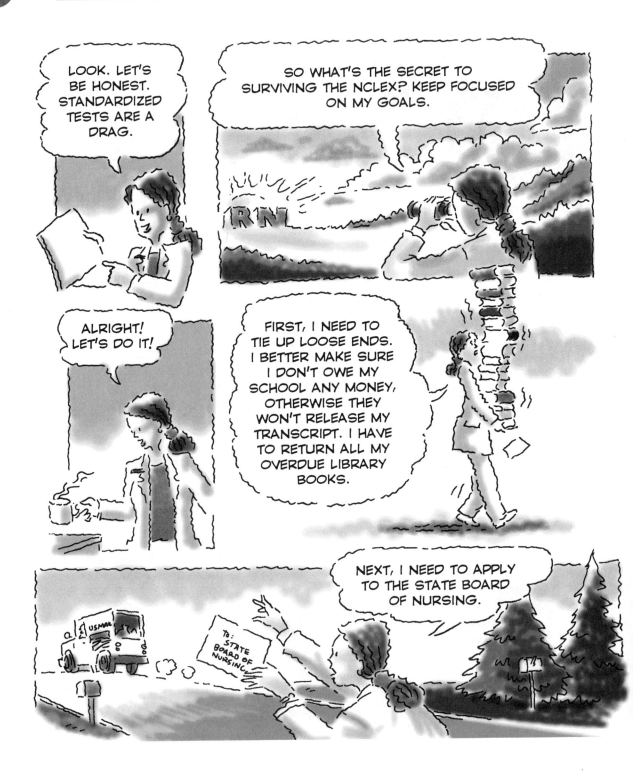

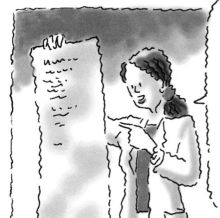

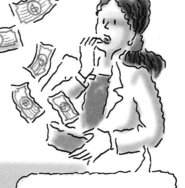

I MUST BE SURE OF THE LICENSURE REQUIREMENTS OF THE STATE WHERE I PLAN TO PRACTICE. MY SCHOOL'S NURSING DEPARTMENT OR THE APPROPRIATE STATE BOARD OF NURSING CAN PROVIDE THE INFORMATION I NEED.

ALSO, I NEED TO REGISTER TO TAKE THE NCLEX.

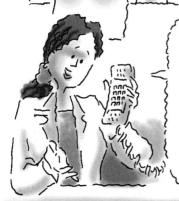

MOST NCLEX CANDIDATES REGISTER WITH THE CHAUNCEY GROUP, A SUBSIDIARY OF THE EDUCATIONAL TESTING SERVICE. I CAN CALL THE CHAUNCEY GROUP AT 1-800-551-1912 FOR MORE INFORMATION.

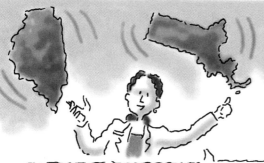

I CAN'T FORGET TO PAY THE REQUIRED FEE. IT COSTS MORE TO REGISTER OVER THE PHONE USING A CREDIT CARD.

HOWEVER, IN ILLINOIS OR MASSACHUSETTS, I MUST REGISTER FOR THE NCLEX THROUGH THE STATE BOARD OF NURSING AS PART OF MY APPLICATION FOR LICENSURE.

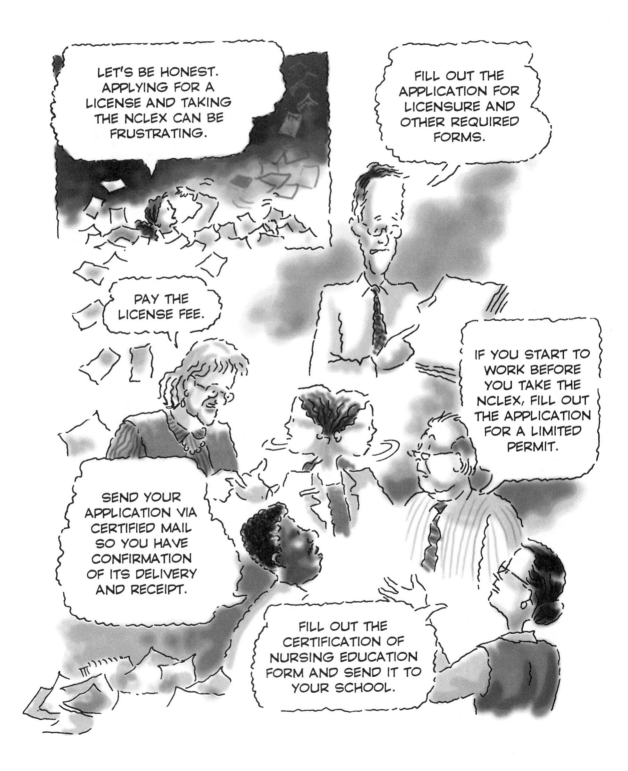

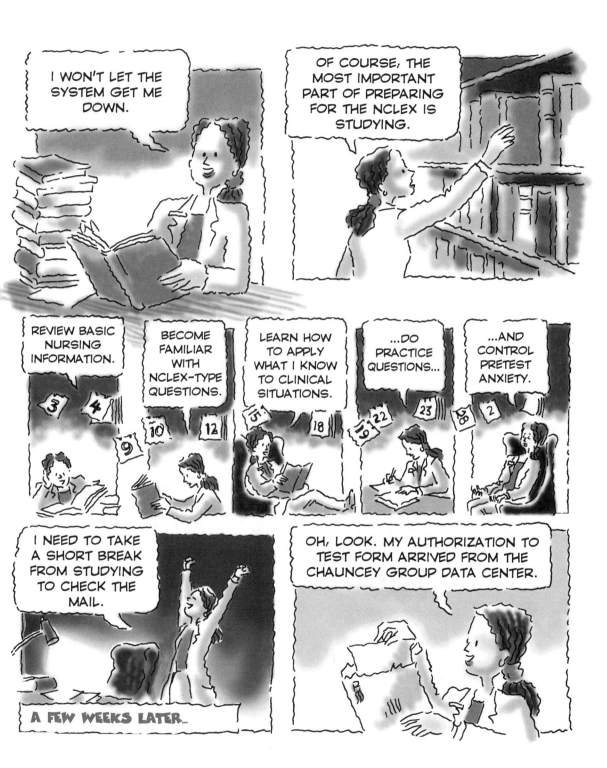

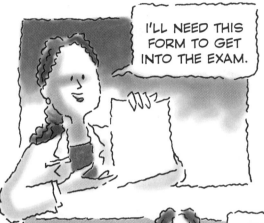

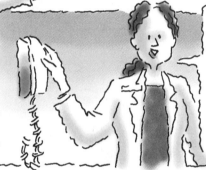

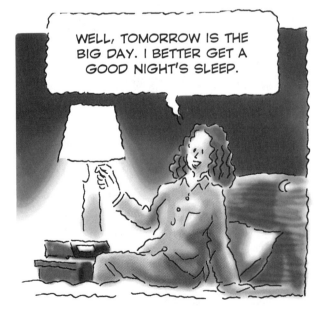

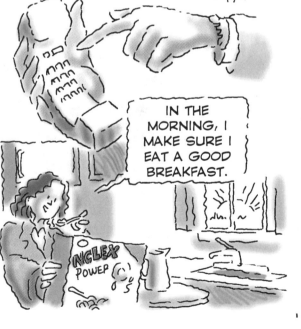

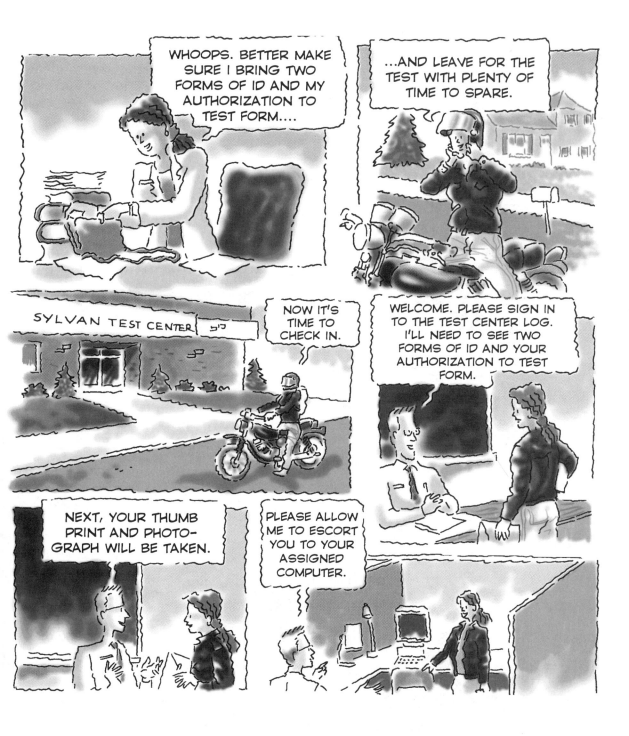

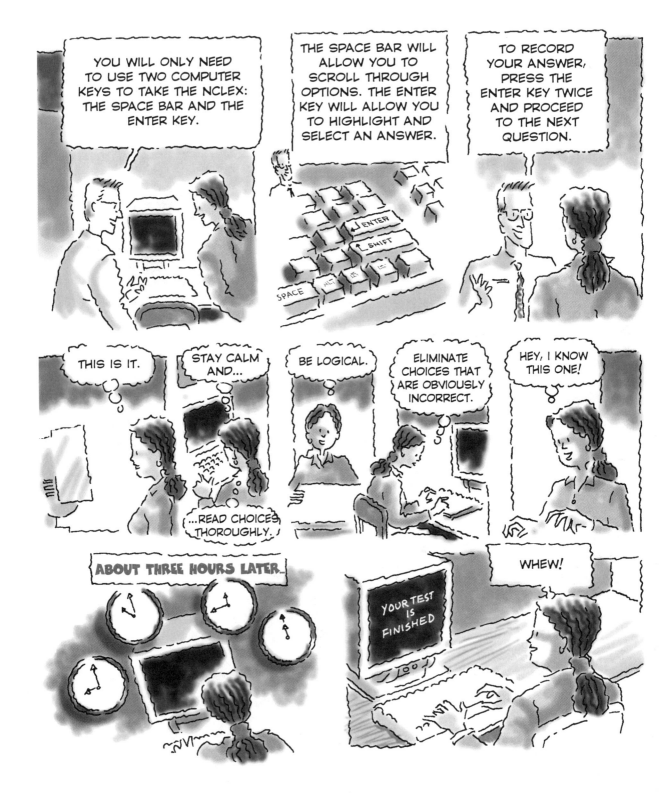

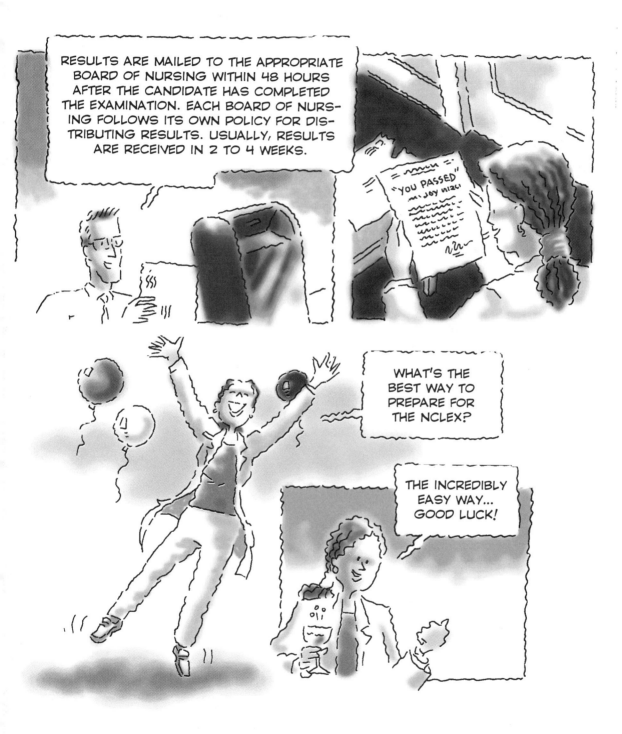

Part I Getting ready

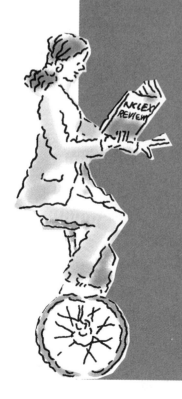

Understanding the NCLEX

Passing the National Council Licensure Examination (NCLEX) is a vital step in your career as a nurse. The first step on your way to passing the NCLEX is to understand what the NCLEX is and how it's administered.

NCLEX structure

The NCLEX is a multiple-choice test written by nurses who, like most of your nursing instructors, have master's degrees and clinical expertise in particular areas. Only one small difference distinguishes nurses who write NCLEX questions: They're trained to write questions in a style particular to the NCLEX.

If you've completed an accredited nursing program, you've already taken numerous tests written by nurses with backgrounds and experiences similar to those of the nurses who write for the NCLEX. The test-taking experience you've gained will help you pass the NCLEX. So your NCLEX review should be just that — a review.

The point of it all
The NCLEX is designed for one purpose: To determine whether it's appropriate for you to receive a license to practice as a nurse. By passing the NCLEX, you demonstrate that you possess the minimum level of knowledge necessary to practice nursing safely.

An integrated exam
In nursing school, you probably took courses organized by the medical model. Courses were separated into such subjects as medical-surgical, pediatric, and psychiatric nursing. By contrast, the NCLEX is integrated, meaning that different subjects are mixed together. As you answer NCLEX questions, you may encounter patients in any stage of life, from neonatal to geriatric. These patients — clients, in NCLEX lingo — may be of any background and may be completely well or extremely ill and have any of a variety of disorders.

What you need to know about client needs
The NCLEX draws questions from four categories of client needs that were developed by the National Council of State Boards of Nursing, the organization that sponsors and manages the NCLEX. Client needs categories ensure that a wide variety of topics appear on every NCLEX examination.

The National Council of State Boards of Nursing developed client needs categories after conducting a work-study analysis of new nurses. All aspects of nursing care observed in the study were broken down into categories. Categories were broken down further into subcategories. (See *Client needs categories,* page 4.)

The categories and subcategories are used to develop the NCLEX test plan, the content guidelines for the distribution of test questions. Question-writers and the people who put the NCLEX examination together use the test plan and client needs categories to make sure that a full spectrum of nursing activities are covered in the NCLEX. Client needs categories appear in most NCLEX review and question-and-answer books, including this one. The truth is, however, that as a test-taker you don't have to concern yourself with client needs categories. You'll see those categories for each question and answer in this book but they'll be invisible on the actual NCLEX.

Testing by computer

The NCLEX, like many standardized tests today, is administered by computer. That means you won't be filling in empty circles, sharpening pencils, or erasing frantically. It also

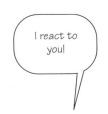

I react to you!

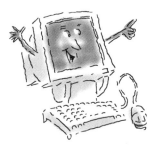

means that you must become familiar with computer tests, if you aren't already. Fortunately, the skills required to take the NCLEX on a computer are simple enough to allow you to focus on the questions, not the keyboard.

Two keys
The only keys you need to take the NCLEX are the SPACE and the ENTER keys. When you take the test, you'll be presented with a question and four possible answers, called options. (See *A sample NCLEX question*.) Follow these steps:

Use the SPACE bar to move the cursor among the four possible answers.

When you've highlighted the option you want, press ENTER.

Check again to make sure that the option you highlighted is the answer you want. If you

want to change options, you'll need to do it now.

Press ENTER again to register your answer.

Computer-adaptive testing
The NCLEX is a computer-adaptive test, meaning that the computer reacts to the answers you give, supplying more difficult questions if you answer correctly and slightly easier questions if you answer incorrectly. Each test is thus uniquely adapted to the individual test-taker.

A matter of time
You have a great deal of flexibility with the amount of time you can spend on individual questions. The examination lasts a maximum of 5 hours, however, so don't waste time. If you fail to answer a set number of questions

Now I get it!

Client needs categories

The NCLEX assigns each question a certain category based on client needs. This chart lists client needs categories and subcategories and the percentages of each type of question that appear on an NCLEX examination.

Category	Subcategories	Percentage of NCLEX questions
Safe, effective care environment	Management of care	7% to 13%
	Safety and infection control	5% to 11%
Health promotion and maintenance	Growth and development through the life span	7% to 13%
	Prevention and early detection of disease	5% to 11%
Psychosocial integrity	Coping and adaptation	5% to 11%
	Psychosocial adaptation	5% to 11%
Physiological integrity	Basic care and comfort	7% to 13%
	Pharmacological and parenteral therapies	5% to 11%
	Reduction of risk potential	12% to 18%
	Physiological adaptation	12% to 18%

A sample NCLEX question

NCLEX examinations, given on a computer, present a question and four options. Many questions present a clinical scenario. Here is an example of a typical NCLEX question.

42. A client is being evaluated for a possible renal tumor. Which of the following assessment findings would most likely indicate a renal tumor?

1. Intermittent hematuria
2. Polyuria
3. Frothy, dark amber urine
4. Cloudy, foul-smelling urine

(Correct answer: 1. Intermittent hematuria)

within 5 hours, the computer will determine that you lack minimum competency.

Most students have plenty of time to complete the test, so take as much time as you need to get the question right without wasting time. Keep moving at a decent pace to help you maintain concentration.

Difficult items = Good news

If you find as you progress through the test that the questions seem to be increasingly difficult, it's a good sign. The more questions you answer correctly, the more difficult the questions become.

Some students, though, knowing that questions get progressively harder, focus on the degree of difficulty of subsequent questions to try to figure out if they're answering questions correctly. Avoid the temptation to do this. Stay focused on selecting the best answer for each question put before you.

Finished

The computer test finishes when one of the following events occurs:
• You demonstrate minimum competency, according to the computer program.
• You demonstrate a lack of minimum competency, according to the computer program.
• You've answered the maximum number of questions (265 total questions).
• You've used the maximum time allowed (5 hours).

Answering NCLEX questions

NCLEX questions are commonly long. As a result, it's easy to become overloaded with information. (See *Anatomy of an NCLEX question,* page 6.) To focus on the question and avoid becoming overwhelmed, apply proven strategies for answering NCLEX questions, including:
• determining what the question asks
• determining relevant facts about the client
• rephrasing the question
• choosing the best option.

What is the question asking?

Read the question twice. If the answer isn't apparent, rephrase the question in simpler, more personal terms. Breaking down the question into easier, less intimidating terms may help you to focus more accurately on the correct answer.

Sample question

For example, a question might be, "A 74-year-old client with a history of heart failure is admitted to the coronary care unit with pulmonary edema. He is intubated and placed on a mechanical ventilator. Which of the follow-

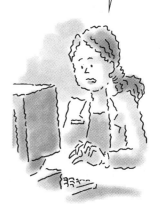

The harder it gets, the better I'm doing.

ing parameters should the nurse monitor closely to assess the client's response to a bolus dose of furosemide (Lasix) I.V.?"

The options for this question — each numbered from 1 to 4 — might include:
1. Daily weight
2. 24-hour intake and output
3. Serum sodium levels
4. Hourly intake and output

Hocus, focus on the question
Read the question again, ignoring all details except what is being asked. Focus on the last line of the question. It asks you to select the appropriate assessment for monitoring a client who received a bolus of furosemide I.V.

What facts about the client are relevant?

Next, sort out the relevant client information. Start by asking whether any of the information provided about the client isn't relevant.

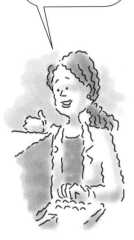

Say it again. Rephrase a confusing question to make it clear.

For instance, do you need to know that the client has been admitted to the coronary care unit? Probably not; his reaction to I.V. furosemide won't be affected by his location in the hospital.

Determine what you do know about the client. In the example, you know that:
• he just received an I.V. bolus of furosemide, a crucial fact
• he has pulmonary edema, the most fundamental aspect of the client's underlying condition
• he's intubated and placed on a mechanical ventilator, suggesting that his pulmonary edema is serious
• he's 74 years old and has a history of heart failure, a fact that may or may not be relevant.

Rephrase the question

After you've determined relevant information about the client and the question being asked, consider rephrasing the question to make it more clear. Eliminate jargon and put the ques-

---

Now I get it!

Anatomy of an NCLEX question

When taking the NCLEX, you may note that the structure and tone of questions is repetitive. That is no accident. NCLEX questions are constructed according to strict standards. As shown below, each question has a stem and four options: a key (correct answer) and three distractors (incorrect answers). A brief case study may precede the question.

Case study
A 48-year-old client comes to the hospital complaining of severe substernal chest pain that radiates down his left arm. He's admitted to the coronary care unit with a diagnosis of myocardial infarction (MI).

Stem	Options
Which of the following nursing assessment activities is a priority on admission to coronary care?	1. Begin telemetry monitoring. (key)
	2. Obtain information about family history of heart disease. (distractor)
	3. Auscultate lung fields. (distractor)
	4. Determine if the client smokes. (distractor)

tion in simpler, more personal terms. Here's how you might rephrase the question in the example: "My client has pulmonary edema. He requires intubation and mechanical ventilation. He's 74 years old and has a history of heart failure. He received an I.V. bolus of furosemide. What assessment parameter should I monitor?"

Choose the best option

Armed with all the information you now have, it's time to select an option. You know that the client received an I.V. bolus of furosemide, a diuretic. You know that monitoring fluid intake and output is a key nursing intervention for a client taking a diuretic, a fact that eliminates options 1 and 3 (daily weight and serum sodium levels), narrowing the answer down to options 2 or 4 (24-hour intake and output or hourly urine output).

You also know that the drug was administered by I.V. bolus, suggesting a rapid effect. (In fact, furosemide administered by I.V. bolus takes effect almost immediately.) Monitoring the client's 24-hour intake and output would be appropriate for assessing the effects of repeated doses of furosemide. Hourly urine output, however, is most appropriate in this situation because it monitors the immediate effect of this rapid-acting drug.

When more than one option seems correct

What if you encounter a question for which two or more options appear correct? You're most likely facing a common NCLEX question, one for which there may be two or more appropriate options. NCLEX questions commonly include phrases such as:
- most appropriate
- best
- first
- last
- next
- most helpful
- most suitable.

Such questions ask you to determine priority. Determining priority means deciding which answer is best, is most appropriate, or should be implemented first.

Key strategies

Regardless of the type of question or the number of seemingly correct options, four key strategies will help you determine the correct answer for each question. (See *Strategies for success,* page 8.) These strategies are:
- considering the nursing process
- referring to Maslow's hierarchy of needs
- reviewing patient safety
- reflecting on principles of therapeutic communication.

Nursing process

One of the ways to determine which answer takes priority is to apply the nursing process. Steps in the nursing process include:
- assessment
- analysis
- planning
- implementation
- evaluation.

First things first
The nursing process may provide insights to help you analyze a question and eliminate incorrect options. According to the nursing process, assessment comes before analysis, which comes before planning, which comes before implementation, which comes before evaluation.

You're halfway to the correct answer when you encounter a question that asks you to assess the situation and then provides two assessment options and two implementation options. You can immediately eliminate the implementation options, which then gives you, at worst, a 50-50 chance of selecting the correct answer. Use the following sample question to apply the nursing process.

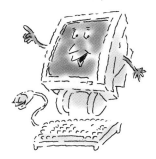

I can be ambivalent. More than one answer may be correct.

A client returns from an endoscopic procedure during which he was sedated. Before offering the client food, which of the following actions should the nurse take?

1. Assess the client's respiratory status.
2. Check the client's gag reflex.
3. Place the client in a side-lying position.
4. Have the client drink a few sips of water.

Assess before intervening

According to the nursing process, the nurse must assess a client before performing an intervention. Does the question indicate that the client has been properly assessed? No, it doesn't. Therefore, you can eliminate options 3 and 4 because they're both interventions.

That leaves options 1 and 2, both of which are assessments. Your nursing knowledge should tell you the correct answer — in this case, option 2. The sedation required for an endoscopic procedure may impair the client's gag reflex, so you would assess the gag reflex before giving food to the client to reduce the risk of aspiration and airway obstruction.

Final elimination

Why not select option 1, assessing the client's respiratory status? You might select this option but the question is specifically asking about offering the client food, an action that wouldn't be taken if the client's respiratory status was at all compromised. In this case, you're making a judgment based on the phrase, "Before offering the client food." If the question was trying to test your knowledge of respiratory depression following an endoscopic procedure, it probably wouldn't mention a function — such as giving food to a client — that so clearly occurs only after the client's respiratory status has been stabilized.

Maslow's hierarchy

Knowledge of Maslow's hierarchy of needs can be a vital tool for establishing priorities on the NCLEX examination. Maslow's theory states that physiologic needs are the most basic human needs of all. Only after physiologic needs have been met can safety concerns be addressed. Only after safety concerns are met can concerns involving love and belonging be addressed, and so forth. (See *Maslow's hierarchy of needs.*) Apply the principles of Maslow's hierarchy of needs to the following sample question:

A client complains of severe pain 2 days after surgery. Which of the following actions should the nurse perform first?

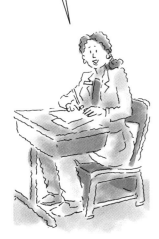

Say it 1,000 times: Studying for the NCLEX is fun..studying for the NCLEX is fun...

Advice from the experts

Strategies for success

Keeping a few main strategies in mind as you answer each NCLEX question can help ensure greater success. These four strategies are critical for answering NCLEX questions correctly:
• If the question asks what you should do in a situation, use the nursing process to determine which step in the process would be next.
• If the question asks what the client needs, use Maslow's hierarchy to determine which need to address first.
• If the question indicates that the client doesn't have an urgent physiologic need, focus on the patient's safety.
• If the question involves communicating with a patient, use the principles of therapeutic communication.

Now I get it!

Maslow's hierarchy of needs

Maslow's hierarchy of needs is a vital tool for establishing priorities on the NCLEX examination. These illustrations show Maslow's hierarchy of needs and a definition for each stage in the hierarchy. The stages, from most basic to most complex, are physiologic needs, safety and security, love and belonging, self-esteem, and self-actualization.

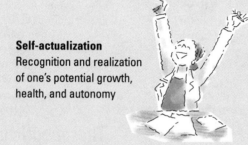

Self-actualization
Recognition and realization of one's potential growth, health, and autonomy

Self-esteem
Sense of self-worth, self-respect, independence, dignity, privacy, and self-reliance

Love and belonging
Affiliation, affection, intimacy, support, and reassurance

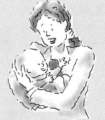

Safety and security
Safety from physiologic and psychological threat, protection, continuity, stability, and lack of danger

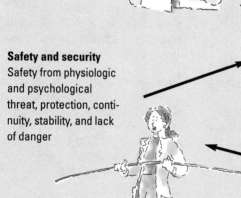

Physiologic needs
Oxygen, food, elimination, temperature control, sex, movement, rest, and comfort

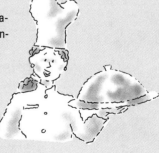

1. Offer reassurance to the client that he will feel less pain tomorrow.
2. Allow the client time to verbalize his feelings.
3. Check the client's vital signs.
4. Administer an analgesic.

Phys before psych

In this example, two of the options — 3 and 4 — address physiological needs. The other two answer choices — 1 and 2 — address psychosocial concerns. According to Maslow, physiologic needs must be met before psychosocial needs, so you can eliminate options 1 and 2.

Final elimination

Now use your nursing knowledge to choose the best answer from the two remaining options. In this case, 3 is correct because the client's vital signs should be checked before administering an analgesic (assessment before intervention). When prioritizing according to Maslow's hierarchy, remember your ABCs — airway, breathing, circulation — to help you further prioritize. Check for a patent airway before addressing breathing. Check breathing before checking the health of the cardiovascular system.

One caveat...

Just because an option appears on the NCLEX doesn't mean it's a viable choice for the client referred to in the question. Always examine your choice in light of your knowledge and experience. Ask yourself, "Does this choice make sense for this client?" Allow yourself to eliminate choices — even ones that might normally take priority — if they don't make sense for a particular client's situation.

Patient safety

As you might expect, patient safety takes high priority on the NCLEX. You'll encounter many questions that can be answered by asking yourself, "Which answer will best ensure the safety of this client?" Use patient safety criteria for situations involving laboratory values,

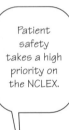

Patient safety takes a high priority on the NCLEX.

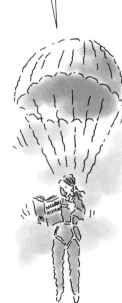

drug administration, or nursing care procedures.

Client 1st, equipment 2nd

You may encounter a question in which some options address the client and others address the equipment. When in doubt, select an option relating to the client; never place equipment before a client.

For instance, suppose a question asks what the nurse should do first when entering a client's room where an infusion pump alarm is sounding. If two options deal with the infusion pump, one with the infusion tubing, and another with the client's catheter insertion site, select the one relating to the client's catheter insertion site. Always check the client first; the equipment can wait.

Therapeutic communication

Some NCLEX questions focus on the nurse's ability to communicate effectively with the client. Therapeutic communication incorporates verbal or nonverbal responses and involves:
• listening to the client
• understanding the client's needs
• promoting clarification and insight about the client's condition.

Poor therapeutic communication

Like other NCLEX questions, questions dealing with therapeutic communication commonly require choosing the best response from among the four options. First, eliminate options that indicate the use of poor therapeutic communication techniques, such as those in which the nurse:
• tells the client what to do without regard to the client's feelings or desires (the "do this" response)
• asks a question that can be answered "yes" or "no" or with another one-syllable response
• seeks reasons for the client's behavior
• implies disapproval of the client's behavior
• offers false reassurances
• attempts to interpret the client's behavior rather than allowing the client to verbalize his own feelings

• offers a response that focuses on the nurse, not the client.

Good therapeutic communication

When answering NCLEX questions, look for responses that:
• allow the client time to think and reflect
• encourage the client to talk
• encourage the client to describe a particular experience
• reflect that the nurse has listened to the client, such as through paraphrasing the client's response.

Avoiding pitfalls

Even the most knowledgeable students can get tripped up on certain NCLEX questions. (See *A tricky question*.) Students commonly cite three areas that can be difficult for unwary test takers:

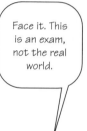 knowing the difference between the NCLEX and the "real world"

delegating care

knowing laboratory values.

NCLEX versus the real world

Some students who take the NCLEX have extensive practical experience in health care. For example, many test takers have worked as licensed practical nurses or nurse's assistants. In one of those capacities, test takers might have been exposed to less than optimum clinical practice and may carry those experiences over to the NCLEX.

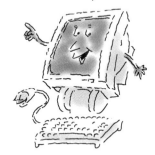

Face it. This is an exam, not the real world.

Advice from the experts

A tricky question

The NCLEX occasionally asks a particular kind of question called the "further teaching" question, which involves patient-teaching situations. These questions can be tricky. You'll have to choose the response that suggests that the patient has *not* learned the correct information. Here is an example:

37. A client undergoes a total hip replacement. Which statement by the client indicates that she requires further teaching?

1. "I'll need to keep several pillows between my legs at night."
2. "I'll need to remember not to cross my legs. It's such a bad habit."
3. "The occupational therapist is showing me how to use a 'sock puller' to help me get dressed."
4. "I don't know if I'll be able to get off that low toilet seat at home by myself."

The answer you should choose is 4 because it indicates the client has a poor understanding of the precautions required after a total hip replacement and needs further teaching. *Remember:* If you see the phrase *further teaching* or *further instruction*, you're looking for a wrong answer by the patient.

Normal laboratory values

- Blood urea nitrogen: 8 to 25 mg/dl
- Creatinine: 0.6 to 1.5 mg/dl
- Sodium: 135 to 145 mmol/L
- Potassium: 3.5 to 5.5 mEq/L
- Chloride: 97 to 110 mmol/L
- Glucose (fasting plasma): 65 to 115 mg/dl
- Hemoglobin
  Male: 13.8 to 17.2 g/dl
  Female: 12.1 to 15.1 g/dl
- Hematocrit
  Male: 40.7 to 50.3%
  Female: 36.1 to 44.3%

However, the NCLEX is a textbook examination — not a test of clinical skills. Take the NCLEX with the understanding that what happens in the real world may differ from what the NCLEX and your nursing school say should happen.

Don't take shortcuts

If you've had practical experience in health care, you may know a quicker way to perform a procedure or tricks to get by when you don't have the right equipment. Situations such as staff shortages may force you to improvise. On the NCLEX, such scenarios can lead to trouble. Always check your practical experiences against textbook nursing care, taking care to select the response that follows the textbook.

Delegating care

On the NCLEX, you may encounter questions that assess your ability to delegate care. Delegating care involves coordinating the efforts of other health care workers to provide effective care for your client. On the NCLEX, you may be asked to assign duties to:
- licensed practical nurses or licensed vocational nurses
- nursing assistants
- other support staff.

In addition, you'll be asked to decide when to notify a physician, social worker, or other hospital staff member. In each case, you'll have to decide when, where, and how to delegate.

Shoulds and shouldn'ts

As a general rule, it's okay to delegate actions that involve stable clients or standard, unchanging procedures. Bathing, feeding, dressing, and transferring clients are examples of procedures that can be delegated.

Be careful not to delegate complicated or complex activities. In addition, don't delegate activities that involve assessment, evaluation, or your own nursing judgment. On the NCLEX and in the real world, these duties fall squarely on your shoulders. Make sure that you take primary responsibility for assessing

and evaluating the client and for making decisions about the client's care. Never hand off those responsibilities to someone with less training.

Calling in reinforcements

Deciding when to notify a physician, social worker, or other hospital staff comprises an important element of nursing care. On the NCLEX, however, choices that involve notifying the physician are usually incorrect. Remember that the NCLEX wants to see you, the nurse, at work.

If you're sure the correct answer is to notify the physician, however, make sure the client's safety has been addressed before notifying a physician or other staff member. On the NCLEX, the client's safety has a higher priority than notifying other health care providers.

Knowing laboratory values

Some NCLEX questions supply laboratory results without indicating normal levels. As a result, answering questions involving laboratory values requires you to have the normal range of the most common laboratory values memorized to make an informed decision (See *Normal laboratory values*.)

2 Strategies for success

Study preparations

If you're like most people preparing to take the test, you're probably feeling nervous, anxious, or concerned. Keep in mind that most test-takers pass the NCLEX the first time around.

Passing the test won't happen by accident, though; you'll need to prepare carefully and efficiently. To help jump-start your preparations:

- determine your strengths and weaknesses
- create a study schedule
- set realistic goals
- find an effective study space
- think positively
- start studying sooner rather than later.

Strengths and weaknesses

Most students recognize that, even at the end of their nursing studies, they know more about some topics than others. Because the NCLEX covers a broad range of material, you should make some decisions about how intensively you'll review each topic.

Make a list

Base those decisions on a list. Divide a sheet of paper in half vertically. On one side, list topics you think you know well. On the other side, list topics you feel less secure about. Pay no attention if one side is longer than the other. When you're done studying, you'll feel strong in every area.

Where the list comes from

To make sure your list reflects a comprehensive view of all the areas you studied in school, look at the contents page in the front of this book. For each topic listed, place it in the "know well" column or "needs review" column. Separating content areas this way shows immediately which topics need less study time and which need more time.

Scheduling study time

Study when you're most alert. Most people can identify a period of the day when they feel most alert. If you feel most alert and energized in the morning, for example, set aside sections of time in the morning for topics that need a lot of review. Then you can use the evening, a time of lesser alertness, for topics that need some refreshing. The opposite is true as well; if you're more alert in the evening, study difficult topics at that time.

What you'll do, when

Set up a basic schedule for studying. Using a calendar or organizer, determine how much time remains before you'll take the NCLEX. (See *2 to 3 months before the NCLEX,* page 14.) Fill in the remaining days with specific times and topics to be studied. For example, you might schedule the respiratory system on a Tuesday morning and the GI system that afternoon. Remember to schedule difficult topics during your most alert times.

Keep in mind that you shouldn't fill each day with studying. Be realistic and set aside time for normal activities. Try to create ample study time before the NCLEX and then stick to the schedule.

Set goals you can meet

Part of creating a schedule means setting goals you can accomplish. You no doubt studied a great deal in nursing school, and by now you have a sense of your own capabilities. Ask yourself, "How much can I cover in a day?" Set that amount of time aside and then stay on task. You'll feel better about yourself — and

To-do list

2 to 3 months before the NCLEX

With 2 to 3 months remaining before you plan to take the examination, take these steps:
• Establish a study schedule. Set aside ample time to study but also leave time for social activities, exercise, family or personal responsibilities, and other matters.
• Become knowledgeable about the NCLEX-RN, its content, the types of questions it asks, and the testing format.
• Begin studying your notes, texts, and other study materials.
• Take some NCLEX practice questions to help you diagnose strengths and weaknesses as well as to become familiar with NCLEX-style questions.

your chances of passing the NCLEX — when you meet your goals regularly.

Study space

Find a space conducive to effective learning and then study there. Whatever you do, don't study with a television on in the room. Instead, find a quiet, inviting study space that:
• is located in a quiet, convenient place, away from normal traffic patterns
• contains a solid chair that encourages good posture (Avoid studying in bed; you'll be more likely to fall asleep and not accomplish your goals.)
• uses comfortable, soft lighting with which you can see clearly without eye strain
• has a temperature between 65° and 70° F
• contains flowers or green plants, familiar photos or paintings, and easy access to soft, instrumental background music.

Accentuate the positive
Consider taping positive messages around your study space. Make signs with words of encouragement, such as, "You can do it!" "Keep studying!" and "Remember the goal!" These upbeat messages can help keep you going when your attention begins to waver.

Maintaining concentration

When you're faced with reviewing the amount of information covered by the NCLEX, it's easy to become distracted and lose your concentration. When you lose concentration, you make less effective use of valuable study time. To help stay focused, keep these tips in mind:
• Alternate the order of the subjects you study during the day to add variety to your study. Try alternating between topics you find most interesting and those you find least interesting.
• Approach your studying with enthusiasm, sincerity, and determination.
• Once you've decided to study, begin immediately. Don't let anything interfere with your thought processes once you've begun.
• Concentrate on accomplishing one task at a time, to the exclusion of everything else.
• Don't try to do two things at once, such as studying and watching television or conversing with friends.
• Work continuously without interruption for a while, but don't study for such a long period that the whole experience becomes grueling or boring.
• Allow time for periodic breaks to give yourself a change of pace. Use these breaks to ease your transition into studying a new topic.

Approach your studying with enthusiasm, sincerity, and determination.

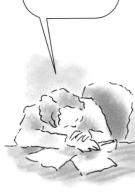

• When studying in the evening, wind down from your studies slowly. Don't progress directly from studying to sleeping.

Taking care of yourself

Never neglect your physical and mental well-being in favor of longer study hours. Maintaining physical and mental health are critical for success in taking the NCLEX. (See *4 to 6 weeks before the NCLEX*.)

A few simple rules
You can increase your likelihood of passing the test by following these simple health rules:
• Get plenty of rest. You can't think deeply or concentrate for long periods when you're tired.
• Eat nutritious meals. Maintaining your energy level is impossible when you're undernourished.
• Exercise regularly. Regular exercise helps you work harder and think more clearly. As a result, you'll study more efficiently and increase the likelihood of success on the all-important NCLEX.

Memory powers, activate!
If you're having trouble concentrating but would rather push through than take a break, try making your studying more active by reading out loud. Active studying can renew your powers of concentration. By reading review material out loud to yourself, you're engaging your ears as well as your eyes — and making your studying a more active process. Hearing the material out loud also fosters memory and subsequent recall.

You can also rewrite in your own words a few of the more difficult concepts you're reviewing. Explaining these concepts in writing forces you to think through the material and can jump-start your memory.

Study schedule

When you were creating your schedule, you might have asked yourself, "How long should I study? One hour at a stretch? Two hours? Three?" To make the best use of your study time, you'll need to answer those questions.

Optimum study time

Experts are divided about the optimum length of study time. Some say you should study no more than 1 hour at a time several times per day. Their reasoning: You remember the material you study at the beginning and end of a session best and tend to remember less material studied in the middle of the session.

Other experts say you should hold longer study sessions because you lose time in the beginning, when you're just getting warmed

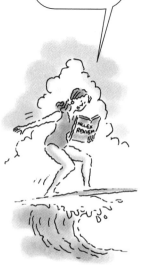

Kowabonga! Regular exercise helps you work harder and think more clearly.

To-do list

4 to 6 weeks before the NCLEX

With 4 to 6 weeks remaining before you plan to take the examination, take these steps:
• Focus on your areas of weakness. That way, you'll have time to review these areas again before the test date.
• Find a study partner or form a study group.
• Take a practice test to gauge your skill level early.
• Take time to eat, sleep, exercise, and socialize to avoid burnout.

To-do list

1 week before the NCLEX

With 1 week remaining before the NCLEX examination, take these steps:
- Take a review test to measure your progress.
- Record key ideas and principles on note cards or audiotapes.
- Rest, eat well, and avoid thinking about the examination during nonstudy times.
- Treat yourself to one special event. You've been working hard, and you deserve it!

Studying getting dull? Get creative and liven it up.

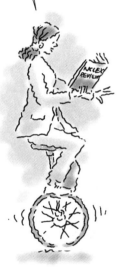

up, and again at the end, when you're cooling down. Therefore, say those experts, a long, concentrated study period will allow you to cover more material.

To thine own self be true
So what's the answer? It doesn't matter as long as you determine what's best for you. At the beginning of your NCLEX study schedule, try study periods of varying lengths. Pay close attention to those that seem more successful.

Remember that you're a trained nurse who is competent at assessment. Think of yourself as a patient, and assess your own progress. Then implement the strategy that works best for you.

Finding time to study

So does that mean that short sections of time are useless? Not at all. We all have spaces in our day that might otherwise be dead time. (See *1 week before the NCLEX.*) These are perfect times to review for the NCLEX but not to cover new material because, by the time you get deep into new material, your time will be over. Always keep some flashcards or a small notebook handy for situations when you have a few extra minutes.

You'll be amazed how many short sessions you can find in a day and how much reviewing you can do in 5 minutes. The following places offer short stretches of time you can use:
- eating breakfast
- waiting for, or riding on, a train or bus
- waiting in line at the bank, post office, bookstore, or other places.

Creative studying

Even when you study in a perfect study space and concentrate better than ever, studying for the NCLEX can get a little, well, dull. Even people with terrific study habits occasionally feel bored or sluggish. That is why it's important to have some creative tricks in your study bag to liven up your studying during those down times.

Creative studying doesn't have to be hard work. It involves making efforts to alter your study habits a bit. Some techniques that might help include studying with a partner or group and creating flashcards or other audiovisual study tools.

Study partners

Studying with a partner or group of students can be an excellent way to energize your studying. Working with a partner allows you to test each other on the material you've reviewed. Your partner can give you encouragement and motivation. Perhaps most important, working with a partner can provide a welcome break from solitary studying.

What to look for in a partner

Exercise some care when choosing a study partner or assembling a study group. A partner who doesn't fit your needs won't help you make the most of your study time. Look for a partner who:

• possesses similar goals to yours. For example, someone taking the NCLEX at approximately the same date who feels the same sense of urgency as you do might make an excellent partner.

• possesses about the same level of knowledge as you. Tutoring someone can sometimes help you learn, but partnering should be give-and-take so both partners can gain knowledge.

• can study without excess chatting or interruptions. Socializing is an important part of creative study but, remember, you still have to pass the NCLEX — so stay serious!

Audiovisual tools

Using flash cards and other audiovisual tools fosters retention and makes learning and reviewing fun.

Flash Gordon? No, it's Flash Card!

Flash cards can provide you with an excellent study tool. The process of writing material on a flash card will help you remember it. In addition, flash cards are small and easily portable, perfect for those 5-minute slivers of time that show up during the day.

Creating a flash card should be fun. Use magic markers, highlighters, and other colorful tools to make them visually stimulating. The more effort you put into creating your flash cards, the better you'll remember the material contained on the cards.

Other visual tools

Flowcharts, drawings, diagrams, and other image-oriented study aids can also help you learn material more effectively. Substituting images for text can be a great way to give your eyes a break and recharge your brain. Remember to use vivid colors to make your creations visually engaging.

Hear's the thing

If you learn more effectively when you hear information rather than see it, consider recording key ideas using a handheld tape recorder. Recording information helps promote memory because you say the information aloud when taping and then listen to it when playing it back. Like flash cards, tapes are portable and perfect for those short study periods during the day. (See *The day before the NCLEX*.)

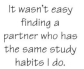

It wasn't easy finding a partner who has the same study habits I do.

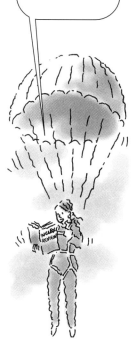

To-do list

The day before the NCLEX

With one day before the NCLEX examination, take these steps:

• Drive to the test site, review traffic patterns, and find out where to park. If your route to the test site occurs during heavy traffic or if you're expecting bad weather, set aside extra time to ensure prompt arrival.

• Do something relaxing during the day.

• Avoid concentrating on the test.

• Rest, eat well, and avoid dwelling on the NCLEX during nonstudy periods.

• Call a supportive friend or relative for some last-minute words of encouragement.

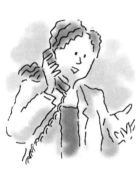

Not tonight. I have to practice for the NCLEX.

Practice questions

Practice questions should be an important part of your NCLEX study strategy. Practice questions can improve your studying by helping you review material and familiarizing yourself with the exact style of questions you'll encounter on the NCLEX.

Practice at the beginning

Consider working through some practice questions as soon as you begin studying for the NCLEX. For example, you might try a few of the questions that appear at the end of each chapter in this book.

If you do well, you probably know the material contained in that chapter fairly well and can spend less time reviewing that particular topic. If you have trouble with the questions, spend extra study time on that topic.

I'm getting there

Practice questions can also provide an excellent means of marking your progress. Don't worry if you have trouble answering the first few practice questions you take; you'll need time to adjust to the way the questions are asked. Eventually you'll become accustomed to the question format and begin to focus more on the questions themselves.

If you make practice questions a regular part of your study regimen, you'll be able to notice areas in which you're improving. You can then adjust your study time accordingly.

Practice makes perfect

As you near the examination date, you should increase the number of NCLEX practice questions you answer at one sitting. This will enable you to approximate the experience of taking the actual NCLEX examination. Using your CD-ROM found at the back of *NCLEX-RN Review Made Incredibly Easy,* you can take practice tests of 10, 25, 50, or 75 questions. Note that 75 questions is the minimum number of questions you will be asked on the actual NCLEX examination. By gradually tackling larger practice tests, you will increase your confidence, build test-taking endurance, and strengthen the concentration skills that enable you to succeed on the NCLEX. (See *The day of the NCLEX.*)

Part II Care of the adult

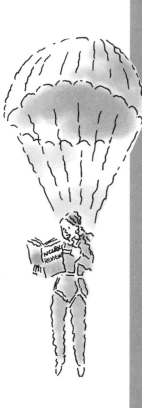

3 Cardiovascular System

Brush up on key concepts

The heart, arteries, and veins make up the cardiovascular system. These structures:
• transport life-supporting oxygen and nutrients to cells
• remove metabolic waste products
• carry hormones from one part of the body to another.

At the center of the system, the heart propels blood through the body by continuous rhythmic contractions.

At any time, you can review the major points of this chapter by consulting the *Cheat sheet* on pages 22 to 30.

2 atria & 2 ventricles
The heart is a muscular organ composed of two **atria** and two **ventricles.**

A sac
The heart is surrounded by a **pericardial sac** that consists of two layers: the **visceral** (inner) layer and the **parietal** (outer) layer.

3 layers
The heart wall has three layers. They are:
• **epicardium** (visceral pericardium), the outer layer
• **myocardium,** the thick, muscular middle layer
• **endocardium,** the inner layer.

4 valves
Inside the heart are four valves. The **tricuspid valve** and **mitral valve** lie between the atria and ventricles; because of their location, they're also called atrioventricular (AV) valves. These valves prevent backflow of blood during systole. The **pulmonic semilu-**nar valve lies between the right ventricle and the pulmonary artery. The **aortic semilunar valve** lies between the left ventricle and the aorta. These valves prevent backflow of blood during diastole.

Pumping it in
The heart itself is nourished by blood from two main arteries, the **left coronary artery** and the **right coronary artery**. As it branches off the aorta, the left coronary artery branches into the left anterior descending (LAD) artery and the circumflex artery. The LAD artery then supplies blood to the anterior wall of the left ventricle, the anterior ventricular septum, and the apex of the left ventricle, while the circumflex artery supplies blood to the left atrium, the lateral and posterior portions of the left ventricle.

The right coronary artery (RCA) fills the groove between the atria and ventricles and gives rise to the acute marginal artery, which becomes the posterior descending artery. The RCA sends blood to the sinoatrial (SA) and AV nodes and to the right atrium. The posterior descending artery supplies the posterior and inferior wall of the left ventricle and the posterior portion of the right ventricle.

Pumping it through (and out)
Blood circulates through the heart following this pathway:
• From the inferior and superior venae cavae to the right atrium
• Through the tricuspid valve to the right ventricle
• Through the pulmonic valve to the pulmonary artery, to the lungs where blood is oxygenated, through the pulmonary veins to the left atrium
• Through the mitral valve to the left ventricle
• Through the aortic valve to the aorta and throughout the body.

(Text continues on page 30.)

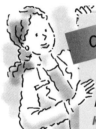

Cheat sheet

Cardiovascular refresher

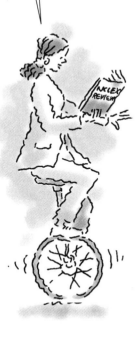

Want a quick overview of this chapter? Check out the Cheat sheet.

ABDOMINAL AORTIC ANEURYSM

Key signs and symptoms
• Commonly asymptomatic

Key test results
• Chest X-ray shows aneurysm.

Key treatments
• Abdominal aortic aneurysm resection

Key interventions
• Assess cardiovascular status and monitor and record vital signs.
• Monitor intake and output and laboratory studies.
• Observe the patient for signs of hypovolemic shock from aneurysm rupture, such as anxiety, restlessness, severe back pain, decreased pulse pressure, increased thready pulse, and pale, cool, moist, clammy skin.

ANGINA

Key signs and symptoms
• Pain: may be substernal, crushing, or compressing; may radiate to the arms, jaw, or back; usually lasts 3 to 5 minutes. It usually occurs after exertion, emotional excitement, or exposure to cold but can also develop when the patient is at rest.

Key test results
• Electrocardiogram (ECG) shows ST-segment depression and T-wave inversion during anginal pain.

Key treatments
• Percutaneous transluminal coronary angioplasty (PTCA)

Key interventions
• Administer medications, as prescribed. Hold nitrates and notify physician for systolic blood pressure less than 90 mm Hg. Hold beta-blocker and notify physician for heart rate less than 60 beats per minute.
• Assess for chest pain and evaluate its characteristics.
• Obtain 12-lead ECG during an acute attack.

ARRHYTHMIAS

Key signs and symptoms
Atrial fibrillation
• Often asymptomatic
• Irregular pulse with no pattern to the irregularity
Asystole
• Apnea
• Cyanosis
• No palpable blood pressure
• Pulselessness
Ventricular fibrillation
• Apnea
• No palpable blood pressure
• Pulselessness
Ventricular tachycardia
• Diaphoresis
• Hypotension
• Weak pulse
• Dizziness

Key test results
Atrial fibrillation
• ECG shows irregular atrial rhythm, atrial rate greater than 400 beats/minute, irregular ventricular rhythm, QRS complexes of uniform configuration and duration, indiscernible PR interval, and no P waves or P waves that appear as erratic, irregular baseline fibrillation waves.
Asystole
• ECG shows no atrial or ventricular rate or rhythm and no discernible P waves, QRS complexes, or T waves.
Ventricular fibrillation
• ECG shows rapid and chaotic ventricular rhythm, wide and irregular QRS complexes, and no visible P waves.
Ventricular tachycardia
• ECG shows ventricular rate of 140 to 220 beats/minute, wide and bizarre QRS complexes, and no discernible P waves. Ventricular tachycardia may start or stop suddenly.

Cardiovascular refresher *(continued)*

ARRHYTHMIAS *(continued)*

Key treatments
Atrial fibrillation
- Antiarrhythmics (if patient is stable): propranolol (Inderal), digoxin (Lanoxin), diltiazem (Cardizem), procainamide (Pronestyl), quinidine (Quinamm), verapamil (Calan)
- Synchronized cardioversion (if patient is unstable)

Asystole
- Advanced cardiac life support (ACLS) protocol for endotracheal intubation and possible transcutaneous pacing
- Antiarrhythmics: atropine, epinephrine (Adrenalin) per ACLS protocol
- Cardiopulmonary resuscitation

Ventricular fibrillation
- ACLS protocol for endotracheal intubation
- Antiarrhythmics: bretylium (Bretylol), epinephrine (Adrenalin), lidocaine (Xylocaine), magnesium sulfate, procainamide (Pronestyl) per ACLS protocol
- Cardiopulmonary resuscitation
- Defibrillation

Ventricular tachycardia
- ACLS protocol for endotracheal intubation, if pulseless
- Antiarrhythmics: bretylium (Bretylol), epinephrine (Adrenalin), lidocaine (Xylocaine), magnesium sulfate, procainamide (Pronestyl)
- Cardiopulmonary resuscitation, if pulseless
- Synchronized cardioversion, if symptomatic

Key interventions
- If the patient's pulse is abnormally rapid, slow, or irregular, watch for signs of hypoperfusion, such as hypotension and diminished urine output.
- When life-threatening arrhythmias develop, rapidly assess the level of consciousness, respirations, and pulse.
- Initiate cardiopulmonary resuscitation, if indicated.
- If trained, perform defibrillation early for ventricular tachycardia and ventricular fibrillation.
- Administer medications as needed, and prepare for medical procedures (for example, cardioversion) if indicated.
- Provide adequate oxygen and reduce the heart's workload, while carefully maintaining metabolic, neurologic, respiratory, and hemodynamic status.

ARTERIAL OCCLUSIVE DISEASE

Key signs and symptoms
Femoral, popliteal, or innominate arteries
- Mottling of the extremity
- Pallor

- Paralysis and paresthesia in the affected arm or leg
- Pulselessness distal to the occlusion
- Sudden and localized pain in the affected arm or leg (most common symptom)
- Temperature change that occurs distal to the occlusion

Internal and external carotid arteries
- Transient ischemic attacks (TIAs), which produce transient monocular blindness, dysarthria, hemiparesis, possible aphasia, confusion, decreased mentation, headache

Subclavian artery
- Subclavian steel syndrome (characterized by the backflow of blood from the brain through the vertebral artery on the same side as the occlusion, into the subclavian artery distal to the occlusion; clinical effects of vertebrobasilar occlusion and exercise-induced arm claudication)

Vertebral and basilar arteries
- TIAs, which produce binocular vision disturbances, vertigo, dysarthria, and falling down without loss of consciousness

Key test results
- Arteriography demonstrates the type (thrombus or embolus), location, and degree of obstruction, and collateral circulation.
- Doppler ultrasonography shows decreased blood flow distal to the occlusion.

Key treatments
- Surgery (for acute arterial occlusive disease): atherectomy, balloon angioplasty, bypass graft, embolectomy, laser angioplasty, patch grafting, stent placement, thromboendarterectomy, amputation
- Thrombolytic agents: alteplase (Activase), streptokinase (Streptase), urokinase (Abbokinase)

Key interventions
Preoperatively (during an acute episode)
- Assess the patient's circulatory status by checking for the most distal pulses and by inspecting his skin color and temperature.
- Provide pain relief as needed.
- Administer heparin by continuous I.V. drip, as needed, using an infusion monitor or pump.
- Watch for signs of fluid and electrolyte imbalance, and monitor intake and output for signs of renal failure (urine output less than 30 ml/hour).

Postoperatively
- Monitor the patient's vital signs. Continuously assess his circulatory function by inspecting skin color and temperature and by checking for distal pulses. In charting, compare earlier assessments and observations. Watch closely for signs of hemorrhage

(continued)

Cardiovascular refresher (continued)

ARTERIAL OCCLUSIVE DISEASE (continued)

(tachycardia, hypotension), and check dressings for excessive bleeding.

• In carotid, innominate, vertebral, or subclavian artery occlusion, assess neurologic status frequently for changes in level of consciousness or muscle strength and pupil size.

• In mesenteric artery occlusion, connect a nasogastric tube to low intermittent suction. Monitor intake and output. (Low urine output may indicate damage to renal arteries during surgery.) Assess abdominal status.

• In saddle block occlusion, check distal pulses for adequate circulation. Watch for signs of renal failure and mesenteric artery occlusion (severe abdominal pain) and cardiac arrhythmias, which may precipitate embolus formation.

• In iliac artery occlusion, monitor urine output for signs of renal failure from decreased perfusion to the kidneys as a result of surgery. Provide meticulous catheter care.

• In both femoral and popliteal artery occlusions, assist with early ambulation but discourage prolonged sitting.

CARDIAC TAMPONADE

Key signs and symptoms

• Muffled heart sounds on auscultation
• Narrow pulse pressure
• Neck vein distention
• Pulsus paradoxus (an abnormal inspiratory drop in systemic blood pressure greater than 15 mm Hg)
• Restlessness
• Upright, leaning forward posture

Key test results

• Chest X-ray shows slightly widened mediastinum and cardiomegaly.
• Echocardiography records pericardial effusion with signs of right ventricular and atrial compression.
• ECG may reveal changes produced by acute pericarditis. This test rarely reveals tamponade but is useful to rule out other cardiac disorders.

Key treatments

• Surgery: pericardiocentesis (needle aspiration of the pericardial cavity) or surgical creation of an opening to drain fluid, thoracotomy
• Inotropics: dopamine (Intropin), isoproterenol (Isupril)

Key interventions

If the patient needs pericardiocentesis
• Keep a pericardial aspiration needle attached to a 50-ml syringe by a three-way stopcock, an ECG machine, and an emergency cart with a defibrillator at the bedside. Make sure the equipment is turned on and ready for immediate use.

• Position the patient at a 45- to 60-degree angle. Connect the precordial ECG lead to the hub of the aspiration needle with an alligator clamp and connecting wire. When the needle touches the myocardium during fluid aspiration, an ST-segment elevation or premature ventricular contractions will be seen.

• Monitor blood pressure and central venous pressure (CVP) during and after pericardiocentesis to monitor for complications such as hypotension, which may indicate cardiac chamber puncture.

• Watch for complications of pericardiocentesis, such as ventricular fibrillation, vasovagal response, or coronary artery or cardiac chamber puncture.

If the patient needs thoracotomy
• Explain the procedure to him. Tell him what to expect postoperatively (chest tubes, drainage bottles, administration of oxygen). Teach him how to turn, deep-breathe, and cough.
• Maintain the chest drainage system and be alert for complications, such as hemorrhage and arrhythmias.

CARDIOGENIC SHOCK

Key signs and symptoms

• Cold, clammy skin
• Hypotension (systolic pressure below 90 mm Hg), narrow pulse pressure
• Oliguria (urine output of less than 30 ml/hour)
• Tachycardia or other arrhythmias

Key test results

• ECG shows MI (enlarged Q wave, elevated ST segment).

Key treatments

• Intra-aortic balloon pump (IABP)
• Adrenergic agent: epinephrine hydrochloride (Adrenalin chloride)
• Cardiac glycoside: digoxin (Lanoxin)
• Cardiac inotropes: dopamine hydrochloride (Intropin), dobutamine (Dobutrex), amrinone lactate (Inocor), milrinone (Primacor)
• Diuretics: furosemide (Lasix), bumetanide (Bumex), metolazone (Zaroxolyn)
• Vasodilator: nitroprusside sodium (Nitropress)
• Vasopressor: norepinephrine (Levophed)

Key interventions

• Assess cardiovascular status including hemodynamic variables, vital signs, heart sounds, capillary refill, skin temperature, and peripheral pulses.
• Assess respiratory status including breath sounds and ABGs.
• Administer I.V. fluids, oxygen, and medications, as prescribed.

Cardiovascular refresher (continued)

CARDIOMYOPATHY

Key signs and symptoms
- Murmur and S_3 and S_4 heart sounds

Key test results
- ECG shows left ventricular hypertrophy and nonspecific changes.

Key treatments
- Dual chamber pacing (for hypertrophic cardiomyopathy)
- Beta-adrenergic blockers: propranolol (Inderal), nadolol (Corgard), metoprolol (Lopressor) for hypertrophic cardiomyopathy
- Calcium channel blockers: particularly, verapamil (Calan) and diltiazem (Cardizem) for hypertrophic cardiomyopathy
- Diuretics: furosemide (Lasix), bumetanide (Bumex), metolazone (Zaroxolyn) for dilated cardiomyopathy
- Inotropic drugs: dobutamine (Dobutrex), milrinone (Primacor), digoxin for dilated cardiomyopathy
- Oral anticoagulant: warfarin (Coumadin) for dilated and hypertrophic cardiomyopathy

Key interventions
- Monitor ECG.
- Assess cardiovascular status, vital signs, and hemodynamic variables.
- Administer oxygen and medications, as prescribed.

CORONARY ARTERY DISEASE

Key signs and symptoms
- Angina: Pain may be substernal, crushing, or compressing; may radiate to the arms, jaw, or back; usually lasts 3 to 5 minutes. It usually occurs after exertion, emotional excitement, or exposure to cold but can also develop when the patient is at rest.

Key test results
- Blood chemistry tests show increased cholesterol (decreased high-density lipoproteins, increased low-density lipoproteins).
- ECG or Holter monitoring shows ST-segment depression and T-wave inversion during an anginal episode.

Key treatments
- Activity changes include weight loss, if necessary
- Dietary changes include establishing a low-sodium, low-cholesterol, low-fat diet involving increased dietary fiber (low-calorie only if appropriate)
- Estrogen replacement for postmenopausal women
- Antilipemic agents: cholestyramine (Questran), lovastatin (Mevacor), simvastatin (Zocor), nicotinic acid (Niacor), gemfibrozil (Lopid), colestipol hydrochloride (Colestid)
- Low-dose aspirin therapy

Key interventions
- Assess cardiovascular status, including vital signs and hemodynamic variables.
- Obtain ECG during anginal episodes.
- Monitor laboratory studies.
- Monitor intake and output.
- Administer nitroglycerin for anginal episodes.

ENDOCARDITIS

Key signs and symptoms
- Chills
- Fatigue
- Loud, regurgitant murmur

Key test results
- Echocardiography may identify valvular damage.
- ECG may show atrial fibrillation and other arrhythmias that accompany valvular disease.
- Three or more blood cultures in a 24- to 48-hour period identify the causative organism in up to 90% of patients.

Key treatments
- Maintaining sufficient fluid intake
- Antibiotics: based on infecting organism
- Aspirin

Key interventions
- Watch for signs of embolization (hematuria, pleuritic chest pain, left upper quadrant pain, and paresis), a common occurrence during the first 3 months of treatment.
- Monitor the patient's renal status (blood urea nitrogen [BUN] levels, creatinine clearance, and urine output).
- Observe for signs of heart failure, such as dyspnea, tachypnea, tachycardia, crackles, neck vein distention, edema, and weight gain.
- Make sure a susceptible patient understands the need for prophylactic antibiotics before, during, and after dental work, childbirth, and genitourinary, GI, or gynecologic procedures.

HEART FAILURE

Key signs and symptoms
For left-sided failure:
- crackles
- dyspnea
- gallop rhythm: S_3, S_4
  For right-sided failure:
- dependent edema
- jugular vein distention
- weight gain.

(continued)

Cardiovascular refresher (continued)

HEART FAILURE (continued)

Key test results

For left-sided failure:
• Chest X-ray shows increased pulmonary congestion and left ventricular hypertrophy.
  For right-sided failure:
• Chest X-ray reveals pulmonary congestion, cardiomegaly, and pleural effusions.

Key treatments
• Angiotensin-converting enzyme (ACE) inhibitors: captopril (Capoten), enalapril (Vasotec), lisinopril (Prinivil)
• Cardiac glycoside: digoxin (Lanoxin)
• Inotropic agents: dopamine hydrochloride (Intropin), dobutamine hydrochloride (Dobutrex), amrinone lactate (Inocor)
• Diuretics: furosemide (Lasix), bumetanide (Bumex), metolazone (Zaroxolyn)
• Nitrates: isosorbide dinitrate (Isordil), nitroglycerin (Nitro-Bid)
• Vasodilator: nitroprusside sodium (Nitropress)

Key interventions
• Assess cardiovascular status including vital signs and hemodynamic variables.
• Assess respiratory status.
• Keep the patient in semi-Fowler's position.
• Administer oxygen.
• Weigh the patient daily.

HYPERTENSION

Key signs and symptoms
• Asymptomatic

Key test results
• Blood pressure measurements result in sustained readings greater than 140/90 mm Hg.

Key treatments
• ACE inhibitors: captopril (Capoten), enalapril (Vasotec), lisinopril (Prinivil)

Key interventions
• Take an average of two or more blood pressure readings rather than relying on a single, possibly abnormal reading.

HYPOVOLEMIC SHOCK

Key signs and symptoms
• Cold, pale, clammy skin
• Decreased sensorium
• Hypotension with narrowing pulse pressure
• Reduced urine output (less than 25 ml/hour)
• Tachycardia

Key test results
• Blood tests show elevated potassium, elevated serum lactate, elevated BUN levels, increased urine specific gravity (greater than 1.020) and increased urine osmolality, decreased blood pH, decreased partial pressure of arterial oxygen, and increased partial pressure of arterial carbon dioxide.
• Arterial blood gas (ABG) analysis reveals metabolic acidosis.

Key treatments
• Blood and fluid replacement
• Control of bleeding

Key interventions
• Record blood pressure, pulse rate, peripheral pulses, respiratory rate, and other vital signs every 15 minutes and monitor the ECG continuously. A systolic blood pressure lower than 80 mm Hg usually results in inadequate coronary artery blood flow, cardiac ischemia, arrhythmias, and further complications of low cardiac output. When blood pressure drops below 80 mm Hg, increase the oxygen flow rate and notify the doctor immediately.
• Start I.V. lines with normal saline or lactated Ringer's solution, using a large-bore catheter (14G), which allows easier administration of later blood transfusions.
• An indwelling urinary catheter may be inserted to measure hourly urine output. If output is less than 30 ml/hour in adults, increase the fluid infusion rate but watch for signs of fluid overload such as an increase in pulmonary artery wedge pressure (PAWP). Notify the doctor if urine output doesn't improve. An osmotic diuretic such as mannitol (Osmitrol) may be ordered.
• Check blood pressure, urine output, CVP, or PAWP.
• During therapy, assess skin color and temperature and note any changes. Cold, clammy skin may be a sign of continuing peripheral vascular constriction, indicating progressive shock.

MYOCARDIAL INFARCTION

Key signs and symptoms
• Crushing substernal chest pain: may radiate to the jaw, back, and arms; lasts longer than anginal pain; unrelieved by rest or nitroglycerin; may not be present (in asymptomatic or silent MI)

Key test results
• ECG: enlarged Q wave, elevated or depressed ST segment, T-wave inversion

Key treatments
• Thrombolytic therapy: tissue plasminogen activator (tPA) (Activase), streptokinase (Steptase), anistreplase (Eminase); thrombolytics (given within 6 hours of onset of symptoms but most effective when started within 3 hours).

Cardiovascular refresher *(continued)*

MYOCARDIAL INFARCTION *(continued)*

Key interventions
- Assess cardiovascular and respiratory status.
- Obtain an ECG reading during acute pain.

MYOCARDITIS

Key signs and symptoms
- Arrhythmias (S_3 and S_4 gallops, faint S_1)
- Dyspnea
- Fatigue
- Fever

Key test results
- ECG typically shows diffuse ST-segment and T-wave abnormalities (as in pericarditis), conduction defects (prolonged PR interval), and other supraventricular arrhythmias.
- Endomyocardial biopsy confirms the diagnosis, but a negative biopsy doesn't exclude the diagnosis. A repeat biopsy may be needed.

Key treatments
- Bed rest
- Antiarrhythmics: quinidine (Quinora), procainamide (Pronestyl)
- Antibiotics according to sensitivity of infecting organism
- Digitalis glycosides: digoxin (Lanoxin) to increase myocardial contractility
- Diuretics: furosemide (Lasix)

Key interventions
- Assess cardiovascular status frequently to monitor for signs of heart failure, such as dyspnea, hypotension, and tachycardia. Check for changes in cardiac rhythm or conduction.
- Stress the importance of bed rest. Assist with bathing as necessary; provide a bedside commode. Reassure the patient that activity limitations are temporary.

PERICARDITIS

Key signs and symptoms
Acute pericarditis
- Pericardial friction rub (grating sound heard as the heart moves)
- Sharp and commonly sudden pain that usually starts over the sternum and radiates to the neck, shoulders, back, and arms (Unlike the pain of MI, pericardial pain is often pleuritic, increasing with deep inspiration and decreasing when the patient sits up and leans forward, pulling the heart away from the diaphragmatic pleurae of the lungs.)

Chronic pericarditis
- Pericardial friction rub
- Symptoms similar to those of chronic right-sided heart failure (fluid retention, ascites, hepatomegaly)

Key test results
- Echocardiography confirms the diagnosis when it shows an echo-free space between the ventricular wall and the pericardium (in cases of pleural effusion).
- ECG shows the following changes in acute pericarditis: elevation of ST segments in the standard limb leads and most precordial leads without significant changes in QRS morphology that occur with MI, atrial ectopic rhythms such as atrial fibrillation, and diminished QRS voltage in pericardial effusion.

Key treatments
- Bed rest
- Surgery: pericardiocentesis (in cases of cardiac tamponade), partial pericardectomy (for recurrent pericarditis), total pericardectomy (for constrictive pericarditis)
- Antibiotics: according to sensitivity of infecting organism

Key interventions
- Provide complete bed rest.
- Assess pain in relation to respiration and body position.
- Place the patient in an upright position.
- Provide analgesics and oxygen, and reassure the patient with acute pericarditis that his condition is temporary and treatable.

PULMONARY EDEMA

Key signs and symptoms
- Dyspnea, orthopnea, tachypnea

Key test results
- Hemodynamic monitoring shows increases in PAP, PAWP, and CVP as well as decreased cardiac output.

Key treatments
- Cardiac glycoside: digoxin (Lanoxin)
- Cardiac inotropics: dobutamine (Dobutrex), amrinone lactate (Inocor), milrinone (Primacor)
- Diuretics: furosemide (Lasix), bumetanide (Bumex), metolazone (Zaroxolyn)
- Nitrates: isosorbide dinitrate (Isordil), nitroglycerin (Nitro-Bid)
- Vasodilator: nitroprusside sodium (Nitropress)

Key interventions
- Assess cardiovascular and respiratory status and hemodynamic variables.
- Keep the patient in high Fowler's position if blood pressure tolerates; if hypotensive, maintain in a semi-Fowler's position if tolerated.

(continued)

Cardiovascular refresher (continued)

RAYNAUD'S DISEASE

Key signs and symptoms
- Numbness and tingling relieved by warmth
- Typically, blanching of the skin on the fingers, which then becomes cyanotic before changing to red (after exposure to cold or stress)

Key test results
- Arteriography reveals vasospasm.

Key treatments
- Activity changes: avoidance of cold
- Smoking cessation (if appropriate)
- Surgery (used in fewer than one-quarter of patients): sympathectomy
- Calcium channel blockers: diltiazem (Cardizem)

Key interventions
- Warn against exposure to the cold. Tell the patient to wear mittens or gloves in cold weather or when handling cold items or defrosting the freezer.

RHEUMATIC FEVER AND RHEUMATIC HEART DISEASE

Key signs and symptoms
- Carditis
- Temperature of at least 100.4° F (38° C)
- Migratory joint pain or polyarthritis

Key test results
- Blood tests show: elevated white blood cell count and erythrocyte sedimentation rate; slight anemia during inflammation.
- Cardiac enzyme levels may be increased in severe carditis.
- C-reactive protein is positive (especially during the acute phase).

Key treatments
- Bed rest (in severe cases)
- Surgery: corrective valvular surgery (in cases of persistent heart failure)
- Antibiotics: erythromycin (Erythrocin), penicillin (Pfizerpen)
- NSAID: aspirin, indomethacin (Indocin)

Key interventions
- Before giving penicillin, ask the patient if he's ever had a hypersensitivity reaction to it. Even if the patient has never had a reaction to penicillin, warn that such a reaction is possible.
- Instruct the patient to watch for and report early signs of heart failure, such as dyspnea and a hacking, nonproductive cough.

- Warn the patient to watch for and immediately report signs of recurrent streptococcal infection — sudden sore throat, diffuse throat redness and oropharyngeal exudate, swollen and tender cervical lymph glands, pain on swallowing, a temperature of 101° to 104° F (38.3° to 40° C), headache, and nausea. Urge the patient to keep away from people with respiratory tract infections.

THORACIC AORTIC ANEURYSM

Key signs and symptoms
Ascending aneurysm
- Pain (described as severe, boring, and ripping and extending to the neck, shoulders, lower back, or abdomen)
- Unequal intensities of the right carotid and left radial pulses
Descending aneurysm
- Pain (described as sharp and tearing, usually starting suddenly between the shoulder blades and possibly radiating to the chest)
Transverse aneurysm
- Dyspnea
- Pain (described as sharp and tearing and radiating to the shoulders)

Key test results
- Aortography, the definitive test, shows the lumen of the aneurysm, its size and location, and the false lumen in a dissecting aneurysm.
- Chest X-ray shows widening of the aorta.
- Computed tomography scan can confirm and locate the aneurysm and may be used to monitor its progression.

Key treatments
- Surgery: resection of aneurysm through a Dacron or Teflon graft replacement, possible replacement of aortic valve
- Analgesics
- Antihypertensive: nitroprusside (Nitropress)
- Negative inotropic: propranolol (Inderal)

Key interventions
- Monitor the patient's blood pressure, PAWP, and CVP. Also evaluate pain, breathing, and carotid, radial, and femoral pulses.
- Review laboratory test results, which must include a complete blood count, differential, electrolytes, typing and crossmatching for whole blood, ABG studies, and urinalysis.
- Insert an indwelling urinary catheter. Administer dextrose 5% in water or lactated Ringer's solution and antibiotics as needed. Carefully monitor nitroprusside I.V. infusion rate; use a separate I.V. line for infusion. Adjust the dose by slowly increasing the in-

Cardiovascular refresher (continued)

THORACIC AORTIC ANEURYSM (continued)

fusion rate. Meanwhile, check blood pressure every 5 minutes until it stabilizes.

• With suspected bleeding from an aneurysm, give a whole-blood transfusion.

After repair of a thoracic aneurysm:

• Evaluate the patient's level of consciousness. Monitor vital signs; pulmonary artery pressure, PAWP, and CVP; pulse rate; urine output; and pain.

• Check respiratory function. Carefully observe and record type and amount of chest tube drainage, and frequently assess heart and breath sounds.

• Monitor I.V. therapy to prevent fluid excess, which may occur with rapid fluid replacement.

• Give medications as appropriate to help improve the patient's condition.

THROMBOPHLEBITIS

Key signs and symptoms

In deep vein thrombophlebitis:

• cramping pain
• edema
• positive Homans' sign
• tenderness to touch.

Key test results

• Photoplethysmography shows venous-filling defects.
• Ultrasound reveals decreased blood flow.

Key treatments

• Activity changes: maintaining bed rest and elevating the affected extremity
• Anticoagulants: warfarin sodium (Coumadin), heparin sodium (Liquaemin Sodium)
• Anti-inflammatory agent: aspirin
• Fibrinolytic agents: streptokinase (Streptase)

Key interventions

• Assess pulmonary status.
• Keep the patient in bed, and elevate the affected extremity.
• Apply warm, moist compresses to improve circulation.
• Perform neurovascular checks.
• Monitor laboratory values.

VALVULAR HEART DISEASE

Key signs and symptoms

Aortic insufficiency

• Angina
• Cough
• Dyspnea
• Fatigue
• Palpitations

Mitral insufficiency

• Angina
• Dyspnea
• Fatigue
• Orthopnea
• Peripheral edema

Mitral stenosis

• Dyspnea on exertion
• Fatigue
• Orthopnea
• Palpitations
• Peripheral edema
• Weakness

Mitral valve prolapse

• Possibly asymptomatic
• Palpitations

Tricuspid insufficiency

• Dyspnea
• Fatigue

Key test results

Aortic insufficiency

• Echocardiography shows left ventricular enlargement.
• X-ray shows left ventricular enlargement and pulmonary vein congestion.

Mitral insufficiency

• Cardiac catheterization shows mitral regurgitation and elevated atrial and pulmonary artery wedge pressures.

Mitral stenosis

• Cardiac catheterization shows diastolic pressure gradient across valve, and elevated left atrial and pulmonary artery wedge pressures.
• Echocardiography shows thickened mitral valve leaflets.
• ECG shows left atrial hypertrophy.
• X-ray shows left atrial and ventricular enlargement.

Mitral valve prolapse

• ECG shows prolapse of the mitral valve into the left atrium.

Tricuspid insufficiency

• Echocardiography shows systolic prolapse of the tricuspid valve.
• ECG shows right atrial or right ventricular hypertrophy.
• X-ray shows right atrial dilation and right ventricular enlargement.

(continued)

Cardiovascular refresher (continued)

VALVULAR HEART DISEASE (continued)

Key treatments
• Surgery: open-heart surgery using cardiopulmonary bypass for valve replacement (in severe cases)
• Anticoagulants: warfarin (Coumadin) to prevent thrombus formation around diseased or replaced valves

Key interventions
• Watch closely for signs of heart failure or pulmonary edema and for adverse effects of drug therapy.
• Place the patient in an upright position.

• Maintain bed rest and provide assistance with bathing, if necessary.
• If the patient undergoes surgery, watch for hypotension, arrhythmias, and thrombus formation. Monitor vital signs, ABG levels, intake, output, daily weight, blood chemistries, chest X-rays, and pulmonary artery catheter readings.

The body electric

The system that conducts electrical impulses and coordinates the heart's contractions consists of the SA node, internodal tracts, AV node, bundle of His, right and left bundle branches, and Purkinje fibers.

A normal electrical impulse is initiated at the **SA node,** the heart's intrinsic pacemaker, which results in the following chain of events:
• atrial depolarization
• atrial contraction
• impulse transmission to the AV node
• impulse transmission to the bundle of His, bundle branches, and Purkinje fibers
• ventricular depolarization
• ventricular contraction
• ventricular repolarization.

How's it working?

Cardiac function can be assessed by measuring the following parameters:
• **Cardiac output** is the total amount of blood ejected from a ventricle per minute. Cardiac output equals stroke volume multiplied by heart rate (CO = SV × HR).
• **Stroke volume** is the amount of blood ejected from a ventricle with each beat.
• **Ejection fraction** is the percent of left ventricular end-diastolic volume ejected during systole (60% to 70% normally).

A system of canals

Blood flows throughout the body via arteries and veins, as well as through smaller vessels such as arterioles, capillaries, and venules. Think of them as a series of large and small canals forming an interlocking system of blood flow.
• **Arteries** are three-layered vessels (intima, media, adventitia) that carry oxygenated blood from the heart to the tissues.
• **Arterioles** are small-resistance vessels that feed into capillaries.
• **Capillaries** join arterioles to venules (larger, lower-pressured vessels than arterioles), where nutrients and wastes are exchanged.
• **Venules** join capillaries to veins.
• **Veins** are large-capacity, low-pressure vessels that return unoxygenated blood to the heart.

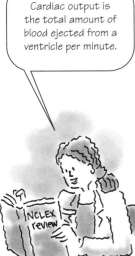

Cardiac output is the total amount of blood ejected from a ventricle per minute.

NCLEX review

Keep abreast of diagnostic tests

Here are the most important tests used to diagnose cardiovascular disorders, along with common nursing interventions associated with each test.

Graphing the heart's electrical activity

Electrocardiography (ECG) is a noninvasive test that gives a graphic representation of the heart's electrical activity.

Nursing actions
- Determine the patient's ability to lie still for several minutes.
- Reassure the patient that electrical shock won't occur.
- Interpret the ECG for changes, such as life-threatening arrhythmias or ischemia.

24-hour record of the heart

Ambulatory ECG, also known as Holter monitoring, is a noninvasive test that records the heart's electrical activity and cardiac events over a 24-hour period.

Nursing actions
- Instruct the patient to keep an activity diary.
- Advise the patient not to bathe or shower, operate machinery, or use a microwave oven or an electric shaver while wearing the monitor.

View through a catheter

Cardiac catheterization and arteriography (also called angiography) involve an injection of radiopaque dye through a catheter, after which a fluoroscope is used to examine the coronary arteries and intracardiac structures. The procedure also monitors major pressures, oxygenation, and cardiac output.

Nursing actions
Before the procedure, you should:
- withhold the patient's food and fluids after midnight
- discuss any anxiety the patient may have about the procedure
- assess and record baseline vital signs and peripheral pulses
- make sure that written, informed consent has been obtained
- inform the patient about possible nausea, chest pain, flushing of the face, or a sudden urge to urinate from the injection of radiopaque dye
- note the patient's allergies to seafood, iodine, or radiopaque dyes.

After the procedure, you should:
- monitor vital signs, peripheral pulses, and the injection site for bleeding
- maintain a pressure dressing and bed rest for 8 hours after the procedure
- keep the patient's left leg straight for 6 to 8 hours if the femoral approach was used; if the antecubital fossa was used, keep the arm extended for 3 hours
- encourage fluids unless contraindicated
- monitor for complaints of chest pain, and report any complaints immediately.

Echoing heart structures

Echocardiography is a noninvasive examination of the heart that uses echoes from sound waves to visualize intracardiac structures and monitor the direction of blood flow.

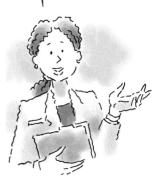

Cardiac catheterization is an invasive procedure. Be aware of the complications that may occur.

Memory jogger

To remember how blood flows from the heart, think **Arteries away.**

Arteries away — arteries carry oxygenated blood **away** from the heart to the tissues. Veins, by contrast, carry blood to the heart. To remember the flow of blood in the veins, think **veto**, for **veins to.**

Nursing actions
• Determine the patient's ability to lie still for 30 to 60 minutes.
• Explain the procedure to the patient.

Jog and monitor
An **exercise ECG,** also known as a stress test, is a noninvasive test that studies the heart's electrical activity and monitors for ischemic events during levels of increasing exercise.

Nursing actions
• Explain the procedure to the patient.
• Withhold food and fluids for 2 to 4 hours before the test.
• Instruct the patient to wear loose-fitting clothing and supportive shoes.
• Perform a cardiopulmonary assessment.
• Tell the patient to report chest discomfort, shortness of breath, fatigue, leg cramps, or dizziness immediately if it occurs during the test.

No fallout here
Nuclear cardiology examines the heart using radioisotopes. After I.V. injection of the isotopes, a monitor is used to read images of myocardial perfusion and contractility.

Nursing actions
Before the procedure:
• Explain the procedure.
• Determine the patient's ability to lie still during the procedure.
    After the procedure:
• Examine the injection site for bleeding.

A complete picture of arterial blood supply
Digital subtraction angiography (DSA) is an invasive procedure involving fluoroscopy with an image intensifier. This test allows complete visualization of the arterial blood supply to a specific area.

Nursing actions
Before the procedure:
• Determine the patient's ability to lie still during the test.

• Make sure that written, informed consent has been obtained.
    After the procedure:
• Monitor the patient's vital signs.
• Check the insertion site for bleeding.
• Instruct the patient to drink at least 1 L of fluid after the procedure.

Balloon and blood flow
Hemodynamic monitoring, also known as single procedure monitoring or continuous monitoring, uses a balloon-tipped, flow-directed pulmonary artery catheter to measure intracardiac pressures and cardiac output.

Nursing actions
• Assess for complications such as hemorrhage, clot formation and air embolus.
• Make sure that written, informed consent has been obtained.
• Explain the procedure to the patient.
• Check the insertion site for signs of infection.
• Monitor the pressure tracings and record readings.

One for the photo album
A **chest X-ray** supplies a radiographic picture that determines the size and position of the heart. It can also detect the presence of fluid in the lungs.

Nursing actions
• Determine the patient's ability to hold his breath.
• Ensure that the patient removes jewelry before the X-ray is taken.

Blood to the lab, part 1
Blood chemistry tests use blood samples to measure blood urea nitrogen (BUN), creatinine, sodium, potassium, bicarbonate, glucose, magnesium, calcium, phosphorus, cholesterol, triglycerides, creatine kinase (CK), CK isoenzymes, aspartate aminotransferase (AST), cardiac troponin levels, lactate dehydrogenase (LD) and LD isoenzymes.

Nursing actions
• Note any drugs that may alter test results.

• Restrict the patient's exercise before the blood sample is drawn.
• Withhold I.M. injections or note the time of the injection on the laboratory slip (after CK levels).
• Withhold food and fluids, as ordered.
• Assess the venipuncture site for bleeding.

Blood to the lab, part 2

Hematologic studies use blood samples to analyze and measure red blood cells, white blood cells (WBCs), erythrocyte sedimentation rate (ESR), prothrombin time, international normalized ratio, partial thromboplastin time, platelets, hemoglobin (Hb), and hematocrit.

Nursing actions
• Note any drugs that might alter test results before the procedure.
• Assess the venipuncture site for bleeding after the procedure.

ABCs of ABGs

An **arterial blood gas (ABG) analysis** assesses arterial blood for tissue oxygenation, ventilation, and acid-base status.

Nursing actions
Before the procedure, you should:
• document the patient's temperature
• note whether the patient is receiving supplemental oxygen and the amount or mechanical ventilation along with the ventilator settings.
  After the procedure, you should:
• apply continuous pressure to the puncture site for at least 5 minutes, then apply a pressure dressing for at least 30 minutes
• check the site for bleeding, periodically.

Hear that sound? It's blood flow

A **Doppler ultrasound** transforms echoes from sound waves into audible sounds, allowing examination of blood flow in peripheral circulation.

Nursing actions
• Determine the patient's ability to lie still.
• Explain the procedure.

Visualize the veins

In a **venogram,** a dye is injected to allow visualization of the veins. This picture is then used to diagnose deep vein thrombosis or incompetent valves.

Nursing actions
Before the procedure:
• Withhold food and fluids after midnight.
• Assess and record the patient's baseline vital signs and peripheral pulses.
• Make sure that written, informed consent has been obtained.
• Note the patient's allergies to seafood, iodine, or radiopaque dyes.
• Inform the patient about possible flushing of the face or throat irritation from the injection of the dye.
  After the procedure:
• Check the injection site for bleeding, infection, and hematoma.
• Encourage fluids unless contraindicated.

Oxygen in arterial blood

Pulse oximetry uses infrared light to measure arterial oxygen saturation in the blood. This test helps assess a patient's pulmonary status.
  To distinguish it from oxygen saturation obtained by ABGs, oxygen saturation obtained by pulse oximetry is abbreviated Spo_2.

Nursing actions
• Protect the sensor from bright light.
• Don't place the sensor on an extremity that has impeded blood flow.
• Attach the monitoring sensor to a fingertip, ear lobe, bridge of the nose, or toe.
• Remove artificial nails, nail tips and nail polish, which may interfere with light transmission if a fingertip is used.

Polish up on patient care

Major cardiovascular disorders include abdominal aortic aneurysm, angina, arrhythmias, arterial occlusive disease, cardiac tam-

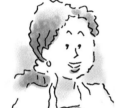

For all cardiac disorders, the goal of nursing care is to decrease cardiac workload and increase myocardial blood supply.

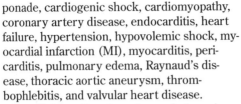

ponade, cardiogenic shock, cardiomyopathy, coronary artery disease, endocarditis, heart failure, hypertension, hypovolemic shock, myocardial infarction (MI), myocarditis, pericarditis, pulmonary edema, Raynaud's disease, thoracic aortic aneurysm, thrombophlebitis, and valvular heart disease.

For all these disorders, the goal of nursing management is to decrease cardiac workload and increase myocardial blood supply. These steps increase oxygenation to the tissues and reduce overall damage to the heart.

Abdominal aortic aneurysm

An abdominal aortic aneurysm results from damage to the medial layer of the abdominal portion of the aorta. Aneurysm commonly results from atherosclerosis, which over time causes a weakening in the medial layer of the artery. Continued weakening from the force of blood flow results in outpouching of the artery and formation of the aneurysm. The aneurysm may then cause a rupture, leading to hemorrhage, hypovolemic shock, and even death.

There are four types of abdominal aneurysms:

dissecting (the vessel wall ruptures, and a blood clot is retained in an outpouching of tissue)

false (bilateral outpouching in which layers of the vessel wall separate from creating a cavity)

fusiform (bilateral outpouching)

saccular (unilateral outpouching).

CAUSES
• Atherosclerosis
• Congenital defect
• Hypertension
• Infection
• Marfan syndrome
• Syphilis
• Trauma

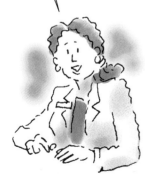

Look for signs of shock when caring for patients with abdominal aortic aneurysm.

ASSESSMENT FINDINGS
• Abdominal mass to the left of the midline
• Abdominal pulsations
• Bruits over the site of the aneurysm
• Commonly asymptomatic
• Diminished femoral pulses
• Lower abdominal pain, low back pain
• Systolic blood pressure in the legs lower than that in the arms

DIAGNOSTIC TEST RESULTS
• Abdominal computed tomography scan shows aneurysm.
• Abdominal ultrasound shows aneurysm.
• Arteriography shows aneurysm.
• Chest X-ray shows aneurysm.
• ECG differentiates aneurysm from MI.

NURSING DIAGNOSES
• Pain
• Risk for altered peripheral tissue perfusion
• Risk for fluid volume deficit

TREATMENT
• Abdominal aortic aneurysm resection
• Maintaining bed rest

Drug therapy
• Analgesic: oxycodone (Oxycontin)
• Antihypertensives: hydralazine (Apresoline), prazosin (Minipress), nitroprusside (Nitropress)
• Beta-adrenergic blocker: propranolol (Inderal)

INTERVENTIONS AND RATIONALES
• Assess cardiovascular status and monitor and record vital signs. *Tachycardia, dyspnea or hypotension may indicate fluid volume deficit caused by rupture of aneurysm.*
• Monitor intake and output and laboratory studies. *Low urine output and high specific gravity indicate hypovolemia.*
• Observe the patient for signs of hypovolemic shock from aneurysm rupture, such as anxiety, restlessness, severe back pain, decreased pulse pressure, increased thready pulse, and pale, cool, moist, clammy skin *to detect early signs of compromise.*

- Gently palpate the abdomen for distention. *Increasing distention may signify impending rupture.*
- Check peripheral circulation: pulses, temperature, color, and complaints of abnormal sensations *to detect poor arterial blood flow.*
- Assess pain *to detect enlarging aneurysm or rupture.*
- Administer medications, as prescribed, *to reduce hypertension and control pain.*
- Encourage the patient to express feelings such as a fear of dying *to reduce anxiety.*
- Maintain a quiet environment *to control blood pressure and reduce risk of rupture.*

Teaching topics
- Signs and symptoms of decreased peripheral circulation, such as change in skin color or temperature, complaints of numbness or tingling, and absent pulses
- Activity limitations, including alternating rest periods with activity, and adhering to prescribed exercise and diet regimen

Angina

Angina is chest pain caused by inadequate myocardial oxygen supply. It's usually caused by narrowing of the coronary arteries, which results from plaque accumulation in the intimal lining.

  Angina is generally categorized as one of three main forms: stable, unstable, or Prinzmetal.
- In stable angina, symptoms are consistent and pain is relieved by rest.
- In unstable angina, pain is marked by increasing severity, duration, and frequency. Pain from unstable angina responds slowly to nitroglycerin.
- In Prinzmetal angina, pain is unpredictable and may occur at rest.

CAUSES
- Activity or disease that increases metabolic demands
- Aortic stenosis
- Atherosclerosis
- Pulmonary stenosis

- Small-vessel disease (associated with rheumatoid arthritis, radiation injury, or lupus erythematosus)
- Thromboembolism
- Vasospasm

ASSESSMENT FINDINGS
- Anxiety
- Diaphoresis
- Dyspnea
- Epigastric distress
- Palpitations
- Pain: may be substernal, crushing, or compressing; may radiate to the arms, jaw, or back; usually lasts 3 to 5 minutes. It usually occurs after exertion, emotional excitement, or exposure to cold but can also develop when the patient is at rest.
- Tachycardia

DIAGNOSTIC TEST RESULTS
- Blood chemistry shows increased cholesterol levels.
- Cardiac enzymes are within normal limits.
- Coronary arteriography shows plaque accumulation.
- ECG shows ST-segment depression and T-wave inversion during anginal pain.
- Holter monitoring reveals ST-segment depression and T-wave inversion.
- Stress test results include abnormal ECG findings and chest pain.

NURSING DIAGNOSES
- Pain
- Anxiety
- Decreased cardiac output

TREATMENT
- Diet: low fat, low sodium, and low cholesterol (low calorie if necessary)
- Coronary artery bypass grafting
- Oxygen therapy
- Percutaneous transluminal coronary angioplasty (PTCA)
- Semi-Fowler's position

Drug therapy
- Anticoagulant: heparin

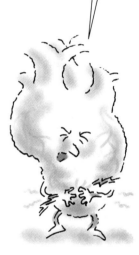

That's not hard to understand. If I don't get enough oxygen, it hurts.

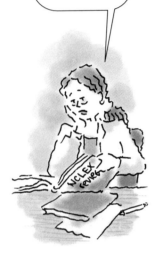

Anginal pain can be difficult to identify. It's usually shorter in duration than pain from MI.

• Beta-adrenergic blockers: propranolol (Inderal), nadolol (Corgard), atenolol (Tenormin), metoprolol (Lopressor)
• Calcium channel blockers: verapamil (Calan), diltiazem (Cardizem), nifedipine (Procardia), nicardipine (Cardene)
• Low-dose aspirin therapy
• Nitrates: nitroglycerin (Nitrostat), isosorbide dinitrate (Isordil), topical nitroglycerin (Nitrol), transdermal nitroglycerin (Transderm-Nitro)

INTERVENTIONS AND RATIONALES
• Assess cardiovascular status, hemodynamic variables, and vital signs *to detect evidence of cardiac compromise and response to treatment.*
• Monitor and record intake and output *to monitor fluid status.*
• Administer medications, as prescribed, *to increase oxygenation and to reduce cardiac workload.* Hold nitrates and notify physician for systolic blood pressure less than 90 mm Hg. Hold beta-blocker and notify physician for heart rate less than 60 beats per minute *to prevent complications that can occur as a result of therapy.*
• Assess for chest pain and evaluate its characteristics. *Assessment allows for care plan modification as necessary.*
• Advise the patient to rest if pain begins *to reduce cardiac workload.*
• Obtain 12-lead ECG during an acute attack *to assess for ischemic changes.*
• Keep the patient in semi-Fowler's position *to promote chest expansion and ventilation.*
• Maintain the patient's prescribed diet (low fat, low sodium, and low cholesterol; low calorie, if necessary) *to reduce risk of coronary artery disease.*
• Encourage weight reduction, if necessary, *to reduce risk of coronary artery disease.*
• Encourage the patient to express anxiety, fears, or concerns *since anxiety can increase oxygen demands.*
• Administer oxygen *to increase oxygenation supply.*

Teaching topics
• Taking sublingual nitroglycerin for acute attacks and prophylactically to prevent anginal episodes
• Reducing risk factors through diet, exercise, weight loss, smoking cessation, and stress reduction
• Avoiding activities or situations that cause angina, such as exertion, heavy meals, emotional upsets, and exposure to cold
• Seeking medical attention if pain lasts more than 20 minutes
• Differentiating between symptoms of angina and symptoms of MI
• Contacting the American Heart Association

Arrhythmias

In cardiac arrhythmias, abnormal electrical conduction or automaticity changes heart rate and rhythm. Arrhythmias vary in severity, from mild and asymptomatic ones that require no treatment (such as sinus arrhythmia, in which heart rate increases and decreases with respirations) to catastrophic ventricular fibrillation (VF), which necessitates immediate resuscitation.

Arrhythmias are generally classified according to their origin (atrial or ventricular). Their effect on cardiac output and blood pressure, partially influenced by the site of origin, determines their clinical significance. The most common arrhythmias include atrial fibrillation (AF), asystole, VF, and ventricular tachycardia (VT).

CAUSES
• Congenital
• Degeneration of conductive tissue
• Drug toxicity
• Heart disease
• MI
• Myocardial ischemia

ASSESSMENT FINDINGS
Atrial fibrillation
• Often asymptomatic
• Palpitations
• Complaints of feeling faint
• Irregular pulse with no pattern to the irregularity

Asystole
- Apnea
- Cyanosis
- No palpable blood pressure
- Pulselessness

Ventricular fibrillation
- Apnea
- No palpable blood pressure
- Pulselessness

Ventricular tachycardia
- Chest pain
- Diaphoresis
- Hypotension
- Weak pulse
- Dizziness
- Possible loss of consciousness

DIAGNOSTIC TEST RESULTS
Atrial fibrillation
- ECG shows irregular atrial rhythm, atrial rate greater than 400 beats/minute, irregular ventricular rhythm, QRS complexes of uniform configuration and duration, indiscernible PR interval, and no P waves or P waves that appear as erratic, irregular baseline fibrillation waves.

Asystole
- ECG shows no atrial or ventricular rate or rhythm, and no discernible P waves, QRS complexes, or T waves.

Ventricular fibrillation
- ECG shows rapid and chaotic ventricular rhythm, wide and irregular QRS complexes, and no visible P waves.

Ventricular tachycardia
- ECG shows ventricular rate of 140 to 220 beats/minute, wide and bizarre QRS complexes, and no discernible P waves. VT may start or stop suddenly.

NURSING DIAGNOSES
- Altered tissue perfusion: cardiopulmonary
- Decreased cardiac output
- Impaired gas exchange

TREATMENT
Atrial fibrillation
- Antiarrhythmics (if patient is stable): propranolol (Inderal), digoxin (Lanoxin), diltiazem (Cardizem), procainamide (Pronestyl), quinidine (Quinalan), verapamil (Calan)
- Permanent pacemaker
- Radiofrequency catheter ablation
- Synchronized cardioversion (if patient is unstable)

Asystole
- Advanced cardiac life support (ACLS) protocol for endotracheal intubation and possible transcutaneous pacing
- Antiarrhythmics: atropine, epinephrine (Adrenalin) per ACLS protocol
- Cardiopulmonary resuscitation

Ventricular fibrillation
- ACLS protocol for endotracheal intubation
- Antiarrhythmics: bretylium (Bretylol), epinephrine (Adrenalin), lidocaine (Xylocaine), magnesium sulfate, procainamide (Pronestyl) per ACLS protocol
- Cardiopulmonary resuscitation
- Defibrillation
- Implantable cardiac defibrillator

Ventricular tachycardia
- ACLS protocol for endotracheal intubation, if pulseless
- Antiarrhythmics: bretylium (Bretylol), epinephrine (Adrenalin), lidocaine (Xylocaine), magnesium sulfate, procainamide (Pronestyl)
- Cardiopulmonary resuscitation, if pulseless
- Implantable cardiac defibrillator
- Synchronized cardioversion, if symptomatic

INTERVENTIONS AND RATIONALES
- Assess an unmonitored patient for rhythm disturbances *to promptly identify and treat life-threatening arrhythmias.*
- If the patient's pulse is abnormally rapid, slow, or irregular, watch for signs of hypoperfusion, such as hypotension and diminished urine output *to prevent complications, such as renal failure and cerebral anoxia.*

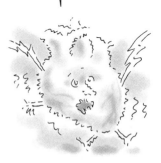

What a shock! A change in electrical conduction breaks my rhythm.

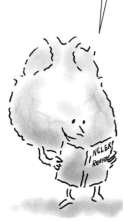

Whatta ya know? Fluid and electrolyte imbalances can pre-dispose me to arrhythmias.

• Document any arrhythmias in a monitored patient *to create a record of their occurrence.* Asess for possible causes and effects *so proper treatment can be instituted.*
• When life-threatening arrhythmias develop, rapidly assess the level of consciousness, respirations, and pulse *to avoid crisis.*
• Initiate cardiopulmonary resuscitation, if indicated, *to maintain cerebral perfusion until other ACLS measures are successful.*
• Evaluate the patient for altered cardiac output resulting from arrhythmias. *Decreased cardiac output may cause inadequate perfusion of major organs leading to irreversible damage.*
• If trained, perform defibrillation early for VT and VF. *Studies show that early intervention with defibrillation improves the patient's chance of survival.*
• Administer medications as needed, and prepare for medical procedures (for example, cardioversion) if indicated *to ensure prompt treatment of life-threatening arrhythmias.*
• Monitor for predisposing factors — such as fluid and electrolyte imbalance — and signs of drug toxicity, especially with digoxin. Drug toxicity may require withholding the next dose. *Alleviating predisposing factors decreases the risk for arrhythmias.*
• Provide adequate oxygen and reduce the heart's workload, while carefully maintaining metabolic, neurologic, respiratory, and hemodynamic status *to prevent arrhythmias in a cardiac patient.*
• Install a fresh pacemaker battery before each insertion. Carefully secure the external catheter wires and the pacemaker box. Assess the threshold daily. Watch closely for premature contractions, a sign of myocardial irritation. *These measures are necessary to avoid temporary pacemaker malfunction.*
• Restrict the patient's activity after permanent pacemaker insertion. Monitor the pulse rate regularly, and watch for signs of decreased cardiac output. *These measures avert permanent pacemaker malfunction.*
• If the patient has a permanent pacemaker, warn him about environmental hazards as indicated by the pacemaker manufacturer *to avoid pacemaker malfunction.*

Teaching topics
• Reporting light-headedness or syncope
• Coming in for regular checkups
• Environmental hazards for patients with permanent pacemakers
• Follow-up permanent pacemaker function tests

Arterial occlusive disease

In arterial occlusive disease, the obstruction or narrowing of the lumen of the aorta and its major branches causes an interruption of blood flow, usually to the legs and feet. Arterial occlusive disease may affect the carotid, vertebral, innominate, subclavian, mesenteric, and celiac arteries. Occlusions may be acute or chronic, and often cause severe ischemia, skin ulceration, and gangrene.

Arterial occlusive disease is more common in males than in females. The prognosis depends on the location of the occlusion, the development of collateral circulation to counteract reduced blood flow and, in acute disease, the time elapsed between occlusion and its removal.

CAUSES
• Atherosclerosis
• Emboli formation
• Thrombosis
• Trauma or fracture

Risk factors
• Age
• Diabetes
• Family history of vascular disorders, MI, or cerebrovascular accident (CVA)
• Hyperlipemia
• Hypertension
• Smoking

ASSESSMENT FINDINGS
Assessment findings depend on the site of the occlusion.

Femoral, popliteal, or innominate arteries
• Mottling of the extremity
• Pallor

• Paralysis and paresthesia in the affected arm or leg
• Pulselessness distal to the occlusion
• Sudden and localized pain in the affected arm or leg (most common symptom)
• Temperature change that occurs distal to the occlusion

Internal and external carotid arteries
• Absent or decreased pulsation with an auscultatory bruit over affected vessels
• CVA
• Transient ischemic attacks (TIAs), which produce transient monocular blindness, dysarthria, hemiparesis, possible aphasia, confusion, decreased mentation, headache

Subclavian artery
• Subclavian steel syndrome (characterized by the backflow of blood from the brain through the vertebral artery on the same side as the occlusion, into the subclavian artery distal to the occlusion; clinical effects of vertebrobasilar occlusion and exercise-induced arm claudication)

Vertebral and basilar arteries
• TIAs, which produce binocular vision disturbances, vertigo, dysarthria, and falling down without loss of consciousness

DIAGNOSTIC TEST RESULTS
• Arteriography demonstrates the type (thrombus or embolus), location, and degree of obstruction, and collateral circulation.
• Doppler ultrasonography shows decreased blood flow distal to the occlusion.
• EEG and a computed tomography scan may be necessary to rule out brain lesions.
• Ophthalmodynamometry helps determine the degree of obstruction in the internal carotid artery by comparing ophthalmic artery pressure to brachial artery pressure on the affected side. A more than 20% difference between pressures suggests insufficiency.

NURSING DIAGNOSES
• Altered tissue perfusion (type depends on the location of the occlusion)
• Fear
• Risk for injury

TREATMENT
• Light exercise such as walking
• Surgery (for acute arterial occlusive disease): atherectomy, balloon angioplasty, bypass graft, embolectomy, laser angioplasty, patch grafting, stent placement, thromboendarterectomy, or amputation

Drug therapy
• Anticoagulants: heparin (Liquaemin), warfarin (Coumadin)
• Antiplatelet: aspirin, pentoxifylline (Trental)
• Thrombolytic agents: alteplase (Activase), streptokinase (Streptase), urokinase (Abbokinase)

INTERVENTIONS AND RATIONALES
• Advise the patient to stop smoking and to follow the prescribed medical regimen *to modify risk factors and promote compliance.*

Preoperatively (during an acute episode)
• Assess the patient's circulatory status by checking for the most distal pulses and by inspecting his skin color and temperature. *Decreased tissue perfusion causes mottling; skin also becomes cooler and skin texture changes.*
• Provide pain relief as needed *to help decrease ischemic pain.*
• Administer heparin by continuous I.V. drip as needed *to prevent thrombi.* Use an infusion monitor or pump *to ensure the proper flow rate.*
• Wrap the patient's affected foot in soft cotton batting, and reposition it frequently *to prevent pressure on any one area.* Strictly avoid elevating or applying heat to the affected leg. *Directly heating extremities causes increased tissue metabolism; if arteries don't dilate normally, tissue perfusion decreases and ischemia may occur.*
• Watch for signs of fluid and electrolyte imbalance, and monitor intake and output for signs of renal failure (urine output < 30 ml/ hour). *Electrolyte imbalances and renal failure are complications that may occur as a result of arterial occlusion and tissue damage.*
• If the patient has a carotid, innominate, vertebral, or subclavian artery occlusion, moni-

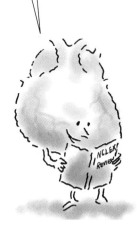

Tickle my toes. Everyone depends on me. If my aorta is obstructed, the feet feel it.

tor him for signs of CVA, such as numbness in an arm or leg and intermittent blindness, *to detect early signs of decreased cerebral perfusion.*

Postoperatively

• Monitor the patient's vital signs. Continuously assess his circulatory function by inspecting skin color and temperature and by checking for distal pulses. In charting, compare earlier assessments and observations. Watch closely for signs of hemorrhage (tachycardia, hypotension) and check dressings for excessive bleeding *to prevent or detect postoperative complications.*
• In carotid, innominate, vertebral, or subclavian artery occlusion, assess neurologic status frequently for changes in level of consciousness or muscle strength and pupil size *to ensure prompt treatment of deteriorating neurologic status.*
• In mesenteric artery occlusion, connect a nasogastric tube to low intermittent suction. Monitor intake and output. (Low urine output may indicate damage to renal arteries during surgery.) Assess abdominal status. *Increasing abdominal distention and tenderness may indicate extension of bowel ischemia with resulting gangrene, necessitating further excision, or peritonitis.*
• In saddle block occlusion, check distal pulses for adequate circulation. Watch for signs of renal failure and mesenteric artery occlusion (severe abdominal pain) and cardiac arrhythmias, which may precipitate embolus formation, *to ensure prompt recognition and treatment of complications.*
• In iliac artery occlusion, monitor urine output for signs of renal failure from decreased perfusion to the kidneys as a result of surgery. Provide meticulous catheter care *to prevent complications.*
• In both femoral and popliteal artery occlusions, assist with early ambulation but discourage prolonged sitting *to encourage circulation to the extremities.*
• After amputation, check the patient's stump carefully for drainage and record its color and amount and the time *to detect hemorrhage.* Elevate the stump, and administer adequate analgesic medication *to treat edema and pain.*

Because phantom limb pain is common, explain this phenomenon to the patient *to reduce the patient's anxiety.*
• When preparing the patient for discharge, instruct him to watch for signs of recurrence (pain, pallor, numbness, paralysis, absence of pulse) that can result from graft occlusion or occlusion at another site. Warn him against wearing constrictive clothing. *These measures enable the patient to join actively in his care, and allow him to make more informed decisions about his health status.*

Teaching topics
• Performing proper foot care
• Recognizing signs of arterial occlusion
• Modifying risk factors

Cardiac tamponade

In cardiac tamponade, a rapid, unchecked rise in intrapericardial pressure impairs diastolic filling of the heart. The rise in pressure usually results from blood or fluid accumulation in the pericardial sac.

If fluid accumulates rapidly, this condition is commonly fatal and necessitates emergency lifesaving measures. Slow accumulation and rise in pressure, as in pericardial effusion associated with cancer, may not produce immediate symptoms because the fibrous wall of the pericardial sac can gradually stretch to accommodate as much as 1 to 2 L of fluid.

CAUSES
• Dressler's syndrome
• Effusion (in cancer, bacterial infections, tuberculosis and, rarely, acute rheumatic fever)
• Hemorrhage from nontraumatic causes (such as rupture of the heart or great vessels or anticoagulant therapy in a patient with pericarditis)
• Hemorrhage from trauma (such as gunshot or stab wounds of the chest and perforation by a catheter during cardiac or central venous catheterization or after cardiac surgery)
• MI
• Uremia

ASSESSMENT FINDINGS
- Anxiety
- Diaphoresis
- Dyspnea
- Hepatomegaly
- Increased venous pressure
- Muffled heart sounds on auscultation
- Narrow pulse pressure
- Neck vein distention
- Pallor or cyanosis
- Pulsus paradoxus (an abnormal inspiratory drop in systemic blood pressure greater than 15 mm Hg)
- Reduced arterial blood pressure
- Restlessness
- Tachycardia
- Upright, leaning forward posture

DIAGNOSTIC TEST RESULTS
- Chest X-ray shows slightly widened mediastinum and cardiomegaly.
- Echocardiography records pericardial effusion with signs of right ventricular and atrial compression.
- ECG may reveal changes produced by acute pericarditis. This test rarely reveals tamponade but is useful to rule out other cardiac disorders.
- Pulmonary artery catheterization detects increased right atrial pressure, right ventricular diastolic pressure, and central venous pressure (CVP).

NURSING DIAGNOSES
- Altered tissue perfusion: cardiopulmonary
- Anxiety
- Decreased cardiac output

TREATMENT
- Surgery: pericardiocentesis (needle aspiration of the pericardial cavity), surgical creation of an opening to drain fluid, or thoracotomy

Drug therapy
- Heparin antagonist: protamine sulfate in heparin-induced tamponade
- Inotropic agents: dopamine (Intropin), isoproterenol (Isuprel)
- Vitamins: vitamin K (AquaMEPHYTON) in warfarin-induced cardiac tamponade

INTERVENTIONS AND RATIONALES
If the patient needs pericardiocentesis
- Explain the procedure to the patient *to alleviate anxiety.*
- Keep a pericardial aspiration needle attached to a 50-ml syringe by a three-way stopcock, an ECG machine, and an emergency cart with a defibrillator at the bedside. Make sure the equipment is turned on and ready for immediate use *to avoid treatment delay.*
- Position the patient at a 45- to 60-degree angle. Connect the precordial ECG lead to the hub of the aspiration needle with an alligator clamp and connecting wire. When the needle touches the myocardium during fluid aspiration, an ST-segment elevation or premature ventricular contractions will be seen. *Monitoring the patient's ECG ensures accuracy of the procedure and helps prevent complications.*
- Monitor blood pressure and CVP during and after pericardiocentesis to monitor for complications such as hypotension, which may indicate cardiac chamber puncture.
- Infuse I.V. solutions *to maintain blood pressure.* Watch for a decrease in CVP and a concomitant rise in blood pressure, *which indicate relief of cardiac compression.*
- Watch for complications of pericardiocentesis, such as VF, vasovagal response, and coronary artery or cardiac chamber puncture *to prevent crisis.*
- Closely monitor ECG changes, blood pressure, pulse rate, level of consciousness, and urinary output *to detect signs of decreased cardiac output.*

If the patient needs thoracotomy
- Explain the procedure to him. Tell him what to expect postoperatively (chest tubes, drainage bottles, administration of oxygen). Teach him how to turn, deep-breathe, and cough *to prevent postoperative complications and relieve patient's anxiety.*
- Give antibiotics *to prevent or treat infection* and protamine sulfate or vitamin K (AquaMEPHYTON) as needed *to prevent hemorrhage.*
- Postoperatively, monitor critical parameters, such as vital signs and ABG levels, and assess heart and breath sounds *to detect early signs of complications such as reaccumulation of fluid.*

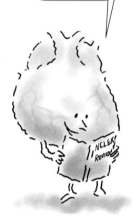

You think the NCLEX creates pressure? In cardiac tamponade, excess fluid puts so much pressure on me, I may need emergency treatment.

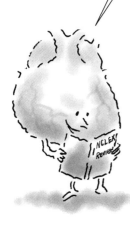

Hmm. In cardiogenic shock, the heart fails to pump adequately.

• Give pain medication as needed *to alleviate pain and promote comfort.*
• Maintain the chest drainage system and be alert for complications, such as hemorrhage and arrhythmias, *to prevent further decompensation.*

Teaching topics
• Alerting the nurse if condition worsens

Cardiogenic shock

Cardiogenic shock occurs when the heart fails to pump adequately, thereby reducing cardiac output and compromising tissue perfusion.

Here's how cardiogenic shock progresses:
• decreased stroke volume results in increased left ventricular volume
• blood pooling in the left ventricle backs up into the lungs, causing pulmonary edema
• to compensate for a falling cardiac output, heart rate and contractility increase
• these compensating mechanisms increase the demand for myocardial oxygen
• an imbalance between oxygen supply and demand results, increasing myocardial ischemia and further compromising the heart's pumping action.

CAUSES
• Advanced heart block
• Cardiomyopathy
• Heart failure
• MI
• Myocarditis
• Papillary muscle rupture

ASSESSMENT FINDINGS
• Anxiety, restlessness, disorientation, and confusion
• Cold, clammy skin
• Crackles in lungs
• Hypotension (systolic pressure below 90 mm Hg), narrow pulse pressure
• Jugular venous distention
• Oliguria (urine output of less than 30 ml/hour)
• S_3 and S_4 heart sounds
• Tachycardia or other arrhythmias

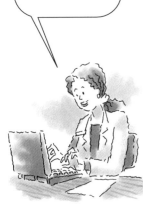

A post-MI patient exhibits cold, clammy skin; hypotension; oliguria; and tachycardia. Hmmmm. Probably adds up to cardiogenic shock.

• Tachypnea, hypoxia
• Weak, thready pulse

DIAGNOSTIC TEST RESULTS
• ABG levels show respiratory alkalosis initially. As shock progresses, metabolic acidosis develops.
• Blood chemistry tests show increased BUN and creatinine levels.
• ECG shows MI (enlarged Q wave, elevated ST segment).
• Hemodynamic monitoring reveals decreased stroke volume and decreased cardiac output; it also shows increased pulmonary artery pressure (PAP), increased pulmonary artery wedge pressure (PAWP), and increased CVP.

NURSING DIAGNOSES
• Decreased cardiac output
• Altered tissue perfusion (cardiopulmonary)
• Altered tissue perfusion (renal)

TREATMENT
• Intra-aortic balloon pump (IAPB) (See *IABP action.*)
• Activity changes, including maintaining bed rest and implementing passive range-of-motion and isometric exercises
• Oxygen therapy: intubation and mechanical ventilation, if necessary
• Continuous arterial venous hemofiltration or continuous arterial venous hemodialysis
• Dietary changes, including withholding food and oral fluids

Drug therapy
• Adrenergic agent: epinephrine hydrochloride (Adrenalin chloride)
• Cardiac glycoside: digoxin (Lanoxin)
• Cardiac inotropes: dopamine hydrochloride (Intropin), dobutamine (Dobutrex), amrinone lactate (Inocor), milrinone (Primacor)
• Diuretics: furosemide (Lasix), bumetanide (Bumex), metolazone (Zaroxolyn)
• Vasodilator: nitroprusside sodium (Nitropress)
• Vasopressor: norepinephrine (Levophed)

INTERVENTIONS AND RATIONALES

• Assess cardiovascular status including hemodynamic variables, vital signs, heart sounds, capillary refill, skin temperature, and peripheral pulses *to monitor effects of drug therapy and detect cardiac decompensation.*
• Assess respiratory status including breath sounds and ABGs. *Tachypnea, crackles, and hypoxemia may indicate pulmonary edema.*
• Monitor fluid balance, including intake and output, *to monitor kidney function and detect fluid overload leading to pulmonary edema.*
• Monitor level of consciousness *to detect cerebral hypoxia caused by reduced cardiac output.*
• Monitor laboratory studies *to detect evidence of MI, evaluate renal function, and assess oxygen-carrying capacity of the blood.*
• Withhold food and fluids, as directed, *to reduce risk of aspiration with a reduced level of consciousness.*
• Administer I.V. fluids, oxygen, and medications, as prescribed, *to maximize cardiac, pulmonary, and renal functioning.*
• Provide suctioning *to aid in the removal of secretions and reduce risk of aspiration.*
• Encourage the patient *to express feelings such as a fear of dying to reduce patient's anxiety.*

Teaching topics
• Recognizing early signs and symptoms of fluid overload
• Maintaining activity limitations, including alternating rest periods with activity
• Maintaining a low-fat, low-sodium diet

Cardiomyopathy

In cardiomyopathy, the myocardium (middle muscular layer) around the left ventricle becomes flabby, altering cardiac function and resulting in decreased cardiac output. Increased heart rate and increased muscle mass compensate in early stages, but in later stages heart failure develops.

The three types of cardiomyopathy are:
• dilated (congestive), the most common form, in which dilated heart chambers contract poorly, causing blood to pool and reducing cardiac output
• hypertrophic (obstructive), in which a hypertrophied left ventricle is unable to relax and fill properly
• restrictive (obliterative), a rare form, characterized by stiff ventricles resistant to ventricular filling.

CAUSES
For dilated cardiomyopathy:
• chronic alcoholism
• infection
• metabolic and immunologic disorders
• pregnancy and postpartum disorders.
  For hypertrophic cardiomyopathy:
• congenital
• hypertension.
  For restrictive cardiomyopathy:
• amyloidosis
• cancer and other infiltrative diseases.

ASSESSMENT FINDINGS
• Cough
• Crackles on lung auscultation

In dilated cardiomyopathy, the muscles around my left ventricle become flabby.

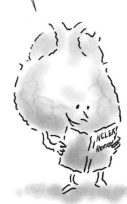

Battling illness

IABP action

With an intra-aortic balloon pump (IAPB), an inflatable balloon is inserted through the femoral artery into the descending aorta. The balloon inflates during diastole, when the aortic valve is closed, to increase coronary artery perfusion. It also deflates during systole, when the aortic valve opens, to reduce resistance to ejection (afterload) and to reduce cardiac workload.

- Dependent pitting edema
- Dyspnea, paroxysmal nocturnal dyspnea
- Enlarged liver
- Fatigue
- Jugular vein distention
- Murmur, S_3 and S_4 heart sounds

DIAGNOSTIC TEST RESULTS
- Cardiac catheterization excludes the diagnosis of coronary artery disease.
- Chest X-ray shows cardiomegaly and pulmonary congestion.
- ECG findings indicate left ventricular hypertrophy and nonspecific changes.
- Echocardiogram shows decreased myocardial function.

NURSING DIAGNOSES
- Decreased cardiac output
- Impaired gas exchange
- Activity intolerance

TREATMENT
- Dietary changes: establishing a low-sodium diet with vitamin supplements
- Dual-chamber pacing (for hypertrophic cardiomyopathy)
- Surgery (when medication fails): heart transplantation or cardiomyoplasty (for dilated cardiomyopathy); ventricular myotomy (for hypertrophic cardiomyopathy)

Drug therapy
- Beta-adrenergic blockers: propranolol (Inderal), nadolol (Corgard), metoprolol (Lopressor) for hypertrophic cardiomyopathy
- Calcium channel blockers: particularly, verapamil (Calan), and diltiazem (Cardizem) for hypertrophic cardiomyopathy
- Diuretics: furosemide (Lasix), bumetanide (Bumex), metolazone (Zaroxolyn) for dilated cardiomyopathy
- Inotropic drugs: dobutamine (Dobutrex), milrinone (Primacor), digoxin, for dilated cardiomyopathy
- Oral anticoagulant: warfarin (Coumadin) for dilated and hypertrophic cardiomyopathy

INTERVENTIONS AND RATIONALES
- Monitor ECG *to detect arrhythmias and ischemia.*
- Monitor laboratory results *to detect abnormalities such as hypokalemia from the use of diuretics.*
- Monitor respiratory status *to detect evidence of heart failure such as dyspnea and crackles.*
- Assess cardiovascular status, vital signs, and hemodynamic variables *to detect heart failure.*
- Monitor and record intake and output *to detect fluid volume overload.*
- Keep the patient in semi-Fowler's position *to enhance gas exchange.*
- Maintain bed rest *to reduce oxygen demands on the heart.*
- Administer oxygen and medications, as prescribed, *to improve oxygenation and cardiac output.*
- Maintain the patient's prescribed diet. *A low-sodium diet reduces fluid retention.*

Teaching topics
- Early signs and symptoms of heart failure
- Monitoring pulses and blood pressure
- Measuring weight daily and reporting increases over 3 lb (1.36 kg)
- Exercises to increase cardiac output, such as raising arms
- Avoiding straining during bowel movements
- Refraining from smoking and drinking alcohol
- Contacting the American Heart Association

Coronary artery disease

Coronary artery disease (CAD) results from the buildup of atherosclerotic plaque in the arteries of the heart. This causes a narrowing of the arterial lumen, reducing blood flow to the myocardium.

CAUSES
- Aging
- Arteriosclerosis
- Atherosclerosis
- Depletion of estrogen post-menopause

- Diabetes
- Genetics
- High-fat, high-cholesterol diet
- Hyperlipidemia
- Hypertension
- Obesity
- Sedentary lifestyle
- Smoking
- Stress

ASSESSMENT FINDINGS
- Angina: pain may be substernal, crushing, or compressing; may radiate to the arms, jaw, or back; usually lasts 3 to 5 minutes. It usually occurs after exertion, emotional excitement, or exposure to cold but can also develop when the patient is at rest.

DIAGNOSTIC TEST RESULTS
- Blood chemistry tests show increased cholesterol levels (decreased high-density lipoproteins, increased low-density lipoproteins).
- Coronary arteriography shows plaque formation.
- ECG or Holter monitoring shows ST-segment depression and T-wave inversion during anginal episode.
- Stress test reveals ST-segment changes, multiple premature ventricular contractions, and chest pain.

NURSING DIAGNOSES
- Activity intolerance
- Impaired gas exchange
- Pain

TREATMENT
- Activity changes, including weight loss, if necessary
- Atherectomy
- Coronary artery bypass surgery
- Coronary artery stent placement
- Dietary changes, including establishing a low-sodium, low-cholesterol, and low-fat diet involving increased dietary fiber (low-calorie only if appropriate)
- Estrogen replacement for postmenopausal women
- Laser angioplasty
- PTCA

Drug therapy
- Analgesic: morphine sulfate (I.V.)
- Anticoagulant: heparin
- Antilipemic agents: cholestyramine (Questran), lovastatin (Mevacor), simvastatin (Zocor), nicotinic acid (Niacor), gemfibrozil (Lopid), colestipol hydrochloride (Colestid)
- Beta-adrenergic blockers: metoprolol (Lopressor), propranolol (Inderal), nadolol (Corgard)
- Calcium channel blockers: nifedipine (Procardia), verapamil (Calan), diltiazem (Cardizem)
- Low-dose aspirin therapy
- Nitrates: nitroglycerin (Nitro-Bid), isosorbide dinitrate (Isordil)

INTERVENTIONS AND RATIONALES
- Obtain ECG during anginal episodes *to detect evidence of ischemia.*
- Monitor laboratory studies. *Evaluate cardiac enzymes to rule out MI. Obtain lipid panel to determine need for diet changes and lipid-lowering drugs.*
- Assess cardiovascular status, vital signs, and hemodynamic variables *to detect evidence of compromise.*
- Monitor intake and output *to detect changes in fluid status.*
- Encourage the patient to express anxiety, fears, or concerns *to help cope with illness.*
- Administer nitroglycerin sublingual for anginal episodes *to provide pain relief.*

Teaching topics
- Limiting activity, alcohol intake, and dietary fat
- Smoking cessation, if appropriate
- Taking nitroglycerin for chest pain
- Contacting the American Heart Association

Endocarditis

Endocarditis is an infection of the endocardium, heart valves, or a cardiac prosthesis resulting from bacterial or fungal invasion. This invasion produces vegetative growths on the heart valves, the endocardial lining of a heart chamber, or the endothelium of a blood vessel that may embolize to the spleen, kidneys, cen-

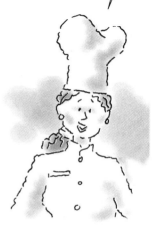

Dietary changes are a key for patients with CAD. Try something from our low-sodium, low-fat, and low-cholesterol menu.

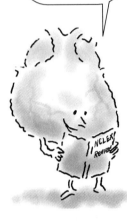

I never promised you a rose garden. Vegetative growths on my valves lead to endocarditis.

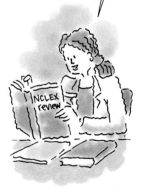

Antibiotics are a key treatment for endocarditis. Make sure to administer antibiotics on time to maintain consistent antibiotic blood levels.

tral nervous system, and lungs. This disorder may also be called infective endocarditis and bacterial endocarditis.

In endocarditis, fibrin and platelets aggregate on the valve tissue and engulf circulating bacteria or fungi that flourish and produce friable verrucous vegetations. Such vegetations may cover the valve surfaces, causing ulceration and necrosis; they may also extend to the chordae tendineae, leading to their rupture and subsequent valvular insufficiency.

Untreated endocarditis is usually fatal, but with proper treatment, about 70% of patients recover. The prognosis is worst when endocarditis causes severe valvular damage, leading to insufficiency and heart failure, or when it involves a prosthetic valve.

CAUSES
- Enterococci
- I.V. drug abuse
- Mitral valve prolapse
- Prosthetic heart valve
- Rheumatic heart disease
- Streptococci (especially *Streptococcus viridans*)
- Staphylococci (especially *Staphylococcus aureus*)

Risk factors
- Coarctation of the aorta
- Degenerative heart disease
- Marfan's syndrome
- Pulmonary stenosis
- Subaortic and valvular aortic stenosis
- Tetralogy of Fallot
- Ventricular septal defects

ASSESSMENT FINDINGS
- Anorexia
- Arthralgia
- Chills
- Fatigue
- Intermittent, recurring fever
- Loud, regurgitant murmur
- Malaise
- Night sweats
- Signs of cerebral, pulmonary, renal, or splenic infarction
- Valvular insufficiency

- Weakness
- Weight loss

DIAGNOSTIC TEST RESULTS
- Blood test results may include normal or elevated WBC count, abnormal histiocytes (macrophages), elevated ESR, normocytic normochromic anemia (in 70% to 90% of endocarditis cases), and positive serum rheumatoid factor (in about one-half of all patients with endocarditis after the disease is present for 3 to 6 weeks).
- Echocardiography may identify valvular damage.
- ECG may show AF and other arrhythmias that accompany valvular disease.
- Three or more blood cultures in a 24- to 48-hour period identify the causative organism in up to 90% of patients.

NURSING DIAGNOSES
- Activity intolerance
- Decreased cardiac output
- Risk for injury

TREATMENT
- Bed rest
- Maintaining sufficient fluid intake
- Surgery (in cases of severe valvular damage) to replace defective valve

Drug therapy
- Antibiotics: based on infecting organism
- Aspirin

INTERVENTIONS AND RATIONALES
- Before giving antibiotics, obtain a patient history of allergies *to prevent anaphylaxis.*
- Observe for signs of infiltration and inflammation, possible complications of long-term I.V. drug administration, at the venipuncture site. Rotate venous access sites *to reduce the risk of these complications.*
- Watch for signs of embolization (hematuria, pleuritic chest pain, left upper quadrant pain, and paresis), a common occurrence during the first 3 months of treatment. *These signs may indicate impending peripheral vascular occlusion or splenic, renal, cerebral, or pulmonary infarction.*

• Monitor the patient's renal status (BUN levels, creatinine clearance, and urine output) *to check for signs of renal emboli or evidence of drug toxicity.*

• Observe for signs of heart failure, such as dyspnea, tachypnea, tachycardia, crackles, neck vein distention, edema, and weight gain. *Detecting heart failure early ensures prompt intervention and treatment and decreases the risk of heart failure progressing to pulmonary edema.*

• Provide reassurance by teaching the patient and his family about this disease and the need for prolonged treatment. Tell them to watch closely for fever, anorexia, and other signs of relapse about 2 weeks after treatment stops. Suggest quiet diversionary activities to prevent excessive physical exertion. *Having the patient and his family involved in care gives them a feeling of control and promotes compliance with long-term therapy.*

• Make sure a susceptible patient understands the need for prophylactic antibiotics before, during, and after dental work, childbirth, and genitourinary, GI, or gynecologic procedures *to prevent further episodes of endocarditis.*

Teaching topics
• Recognizing symptoms of endocarditis; notifying the doctor immediately if symptoms occur
• Need for prophylactic antibiotics before, during, and after dental work, child birth, and genitourinary, GI, or gynecologic procedures

Heart failure

Heart failure occurs when the heart can't pump enough blood to meet the body's metabolic needs.

Heart failure can occur as left-sided failure or right-sided failure. Left-sided heart failure causes mostly pulmonary symptoms, such as shortness of breath, dyspnea on exertion, and a moist cough.

Right-sided heart failure causes systemic symptoms, such as edema and swelling, jugular vein distention, and hepatomegaly.

CAUSES
• Atherosclerosis
• Cardiac conduction defects (in left-sided failure)
• Chronic obstructive pulmonary disease (in right-sided failure)
• Fluid overload
• Hypertension (in left-sided failure)
• Left-sided heart failure (in right-sided failure)
• MI
• Pulmonary hypertension (in right-sided failure)
• Valvular insufficiency
• Valvular stenosis

ASSESSMENT FINDINGS
Left-sided failure
• Anxiety
• Arrhythmias
• Cough
• Crackles
• Dyspnea
• Fatigue
• Gallop rhythm: S_3 and S_4
• Orthopnea
• Paroxysmal nocturnal dyspnea
• Tachycardia
• Tachypnea

Right-sided failure
• Anorexia
• Ascites
• Dependent edema
• Fatigue
• Gallop rhythm: S_3 and S_4
• Hepatomegaly
• Jugular vein distention
• Nausea
• Signs of left-sided heart failure
• Tachycardia
• Weight gain

DIAGNOSTIC TEST RESULTS
Left-sided failure
• ABG levels indicate hypoxemia and hypercapnia.
• Blood chemistry tests reveal decreased potassium and sodium levels and increased BUN and creatinine levels.

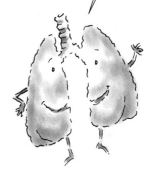

Left-sided heart failure causes pulmonary symptoms.

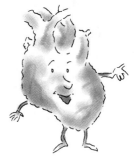

Right-sided failure causes systemic symptoms.

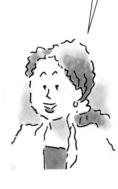

In left-sided heart failure, fluid in the lungs interferes with breathing and the transfer of oxygen to the blood...

...this causes coughing, shortness of breath, and fatigue.

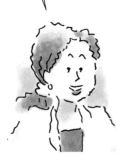

• Chest X-ray shows increased pulmonary congestion and left ventricular hypertrophy.
• ECG shows left ventricular hypertrophy.
• Echocardiography shows increased size of cardiac chambers and decreased wall motion.
• Hemodynamic monitoring reveals increased PAP and PAWP and decreased cardiac output.

Right-sided failure
• ABG levels indicate hypoxemia.
• Blood chemistry tests show decreased sodium and potassium levels and increased BUN and creatinine levels.
• Chest X-ray reveals pulmonary congestion, cardiomegaly, and pleural effusions.
• ECG shows left and right ventricular hypertrophy.
• Echocardiogram shows increased size of chambers and decrease in wall motion.
• Hemodynamic monitoring shows increased right atrial pressure, CVP, and right ventricular pressure and decreased cardiac output.

NURSING DIAGNOSES
• Decreased cardiac output
• Fluid volume excess
• Impaired gas exchange

TREATMENT
• Establishing a low-sodium diet and limiting fluids
• IABP
• Oxygen therapy: may require intubation and mechanical ventilation
• Left ventricular assist device (for left-sided failure)
• Paracentesis (for right-sided failure)
• Thoracentesis (for right-sided failure)

Drug therapy
• Angiotensin-converting enzyme (ACE) inhibitors: captopril (Capoten), enalapril (Vasotec), lisinopril (Prinivil)
• Analgesic: morphine sulfate (I.V.)
• Cardiac glycoside: digoxin (Lanoxin)
• Inotropic agents: dopamine hydrochloride (Intropin), dobutamine hydrochloride (Dobutrex), amrinone lactate (Inocor)
• Diuretics: furosemide (Lasix), bumetanide (Bumex), metolazone (Zaroxolyn)

• Nitrates: isosorbide dinitrate (Isordil), nitroglycerin (Nitro-Bid)
• Vasodilator: nitroprusside sodium (Nitropress)

INTERVENTIONS AND RATIONALES
• Assess cardiovascular status, vital signs, and hemodynamic variables *to detect signs of reduced cardiac output.*
• Assess respiratory status *to detect increasing fluid in the lungs and respiratory failure.*
• Keep the patient in semi-Fowler's position *to increase chest expansion and improve ventilation.*
• Administer medications, as prescribed, *to enhance cardiac performance and reduce excess fluids.*
• Administer oxygen *to enhance arterial oxygenation.*
• Measure and record intake and output. *Intake greater than output may indicate fluid retention.*
• Monitor laboratory studies *to detect electrolyte imbalances, renal failure, and impaired cardiac circulation.*
• Provide suctioning, if necessary, and assist with turning, coughing, and deep breathing *to prevent pulmonary complications.*
• Restrict oral fluids *since excess fluids can worsen heart failure.*
• Weigh the patient daily. *A weight gain of 0.5 to 1 kg/day indicates fluid gain.*
• Measure and record patient's abdominal girth. *An increase in abdominal girth suggests worsening fluid retention and right-sided heart failure.*
• Maintain the patient's prescribed diet (low sodium) *to reduce fluid accumulation.*
• Encourage the patient to express feelings, such as a fear of dying, *to reduce anxiety.*

Teaching topics
• Limiting sodium intake and supplementing diet with foods high in potassium
• Recognizing signs and symptoms of fluid overload
• Elevating legs when seated
• Contacting the American Heart Association

Hypertension

Persistent elevation of systolic or diastolic blood pressure (systolic pressure higher than 140 mm Hg, diastolic pressure higher than 90 mm Hg) indicates hypertension. Hypertension results from a narrowing of the arterioles, which increases peripheral resistance, necessitating increased force to circulate blood through the body.

There are two major types of hypertension. Essential hypertension, the most common, has no known cause, though many factors play a role in its development. Secondary hypertension is caused by renal disease or other systemic diseases.

Mild to very severe

Hypertension is classified according to four stages:

 stage 1: 140 to 159/90 to 99 mm Hg

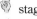 stage 2: 160 to 179/100 to 109 mm Hg

 stage 3: 180 to 209/110 to 119 mm Hg

 stage 4: ≥210/≥120 mm Hg.

CAUSES
- Coarctation of the aorta
- Cushing's disease
- Neurological disorders
- No known cause (essential hypertension)
- Oral contraceptive use
- Pheochromocytoma
- Pregnancy
- Primary hyperaldosteronism
- Renovascular disease
- Thyroid, pituitary, or parathyroid disease
- Use of drugs such as cocaine, epoetin alfa, and cyclosporine

Risk factors for essential hypertension
- Aging
- Atherosclerosis
- Diet (sodium and caffeine)
- Family history
- Obesity
- Race (higher in blacks)
- Sex (more common in males over age 40)
- Smoking
- Stress

ASSESSMENT FINDINGS
- Asymptomatic
- Cerebral ischemia
- Dizziness
- Elevated blood pressure
- Headache
- Heart failure
- Left ventricular hypertrophy
- Papilledema
- Renal failure
- Visual disturbances, including blindness

DIAGNOSTIC TEST RESULTS
- Blood chemistry tests show elevated sodium, BUN, creatinine, and cholesterol levels.
- Blood pressure measurements result in sustained readings higher than 140/90 mm Hg.
- Chest X-ray reveals cardiomegaly.
- ECG shows left ventricular hypertrophy.
- Ophthalmoscopic examination shows retinal changes, such as severe arteriolar narrowing, papilledema, and hemorrhage.
- Urinalysis shows proteinuria, RBCs, and WBCs.

NURSING DIAGNOSES
- Fluid volume excess
- Knowledge deficit
- Altered nutrition: More than body requirements

TREATMENT
- Activity changes: regular exercise to reduce weight, if appropriate
- Dietary changes: establishing a low-sodium diet and limiting alcohol intake (See *Treating hypertension: Step-by-step,* page 50.)

Drug therapy
- ACE inhibitors: captopril (Capoten), enalapril (Vasotec), lisinopril (Prinivil)
- Antihypertensives: methyldopa (Aldomet), hydralazine (Apresoline), prazosin (Minipress), doxazosin mesylate (Cardura)
- Beta-adrenergic blockers: propranolol (Inderal), metoprolol (Lopressor), carteolol hy-

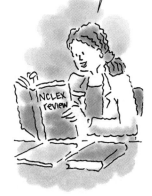

In hypertension, the blood exerts too much pressure on the arteries.

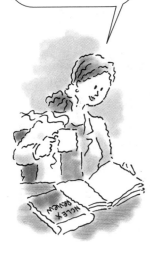

Understanding risk factors for hypertension is important. After all, some of these risk factors can be modified, eliminating the need for drug therapy.

drochloride (Cartrol), penbutolol sulfate (Levatol)
• Calcium channel blockers: nifedipine (Procardia), verapamil (Calan), diltiazem (Cardizem), nicardipine (Cardene)
• Diuretics: furosemide (Lasix), spironolactone (Aldactone), hydrochlorothiazide (HydroDIURIL), bumetanide (Bumex)
• Vasodilators: nitroprusside sodium (Nitropress)

INTERVENTIONS AND RATIONALES
• Assess cardiovascular status including vital signs *to detect cardiac compromise.*
• Take an average of two or more blood pressure readings rather than relying on one single abnormal reading *to establish hypertension.*
• Assess blood pressure reading in the lying, sitting and standing positions *to monitor for orthostatic hypotension* (observe for pallor, diaphoresis, or vertigo).
• Assess neurologic status and observe *for changes that may indicate an alteration in cerebral perfusion* (CVA or hemorrhage).
• Monitor and record intake and output and daily weight *to detect fluid volume overload.*
• Administer medications as prescribed *to lower blood pressure.*

• Maintain the patient's prescribed diet *since a high-sodium, high-cholesterol diet may contribute to hypertension.*
• Encourage the patient to express feelings about daily stress *to reduce anxiety.*
• Maintain a quiet environment *to reduce stress.*

Teaching topics
• Taking blood pressure daily and starting an exercise program
• Beginning a smoking cessation program
• Reducing alcohol intake to moderate levels
• Following a low-cholesterol, low-sodium diet
• Following a program of regular exercise
• Losing weight, if appropriate
• Contacting the American Heart Association

Hypovolemic shock

In hypovolemic shock, reduced intravascular blood volume causes circulatory dysfunction and inadequate tissue perfusion. Without sufficient blood or fluid replacement, hypovolemic shock syndrome may lead to irreversible cerebral and renal damage, cardiac arrest and, ultimately, death.

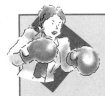

Battling illness

Treating hypertension: Step-by-step

The National Institutes of Health recommends a stepped-care approach for treating primary hypertension.

STEP 1
The first step involves lifestyle modifications, including weight reduction, moderation of alcohol intake, reduction of sodium intake, and smoking cessation.

STEP 2
If the patient fails to achieve the desired blood pressure, continue lifestyle modifications and begin drug therapy. Preferred drugs include diuretics or beta-adrenergic blockers. If diuretics or beta-blockers aren't effective or acceptable, angiotensin-converting enzyme (ACE) inhibitors or calcium channel blockers may be used.

STEP 3
If desired blood pressure still isn't achieved, drug dosage is increased, another drug is substituted for the first drug, or a drug from a different class is added.

STEP 4
If the patient fails to achieve the desired blood pressure or make significant progress, add a second or third agent or a diuretic (if one isn't already prescribed). Second or third agents may include vasodilators, alpha$_1$-antagonists, peripherally acting adrenergic neuron antagonists, ACE inhibitors, and calcium channel blockers.

Hypovolemic shock requires early recognition of signs and symptoms and prompt, aggressive treatment to improve the prognosis.

CAUSES
• Acute blood loss (approximately one-fifth of total volume)
• Acute pancreatitis
• Dehydration from excessive perspiration
• Diabetes insipidus
• Diuresis
• Inadequate fluid intake
• Intestinal obstruction
• Peritonitis
• Severe diarrhea or protracted vomiting

ASSESSMENT FINDINGS
• Cold, pale, clammy skin
• Decreased sensorium
• Hypotension with narrowing pulse pressure
• Rapid, shallow respirations
• Reduced urine output (less than 25 ml/hour)
• Tachycardia

DIAGNOSTIC TEST RESULTS
• Blood tests show elevated potassium, elevated serum lactate, elevated BUN levels, increased urine specific gravity (greater than 1.020) and urine osmolality, decreased blood pH, decreased partial pressure of arterial oxygen, and increased partial pressure of arterial carbon dioxide.
• Gastroscopy, aspiration of gastric contents through a nasogastric tube, and X-rays identify internal bleeding sites.
• ABG analysis reveals metabolic acidosis.

NURSING DIAGNOSES
• Altered tissue perfusion: cardiopulmonary, cerebral, or renal
• Decreased cardiac output
• Fluid volume deficit

TREATMENT
• Blood and fluid replacement
• Control of bleeding
• Pneumatic antishock garment

INTERVENTIONS AND RATIONALES
Management of hypovolemic shock necessitates prompt, aggressive supportive measures and careful assessment and monitoring of vital signs. Follow these priorities:
• Check for a patent airway and adequate circulation. If blood pressure and heart rate are absent, start cardiopulmonary resuscitation *to prevent irreversible organ damage and death.*
• Record blood pressure, pulse rate, peripheral pulses, respiratory rate, and other vital signs every 15 minutes and monitor the ECG continuously. A systolic blood pressure lower than 80 mm Hg usually results in inadequate coronary artery blood flow, cardiac ischemia, arrhythmias, and further complications of low cardiac output. When blood pressure drops below 80 mm Hg, increase the oxygen flow rate and notify the doctor immediately. *A progressive drop in blood pressure accompanied by a thready pulse generally signals inadequate cardiac output from reduced intravascular volume.*
• Start I.V. lines with normal saline or lactated Ringer's solution, using a large-bore catheter (14G), which allows easier administration of later blood transfusions *to correct fluid volume deficit.*
• An indwelling urinary catheter may be inserted to measure hourly urine output. If output is less than 30 ml/hour in adults, increase the fluid infusion rate but watch for signs of fluid overload, such as an increase in PAWP. Notify the doctor if urine output doesn't improve. An osmotic diuretic such as mannitol (Osmitrol) may be ordered *to increase renal blood flow and urine output.*
• Check blood pressure, urine output, CVP, or PAWP *to determine how much fluid to give.*
• Draw an arterial blood sample to measure ABG values. Administer oxygen by face mask and adjust the oxygen flow rate to a higher or lower level as ABG measurements indicate *to ensure adequate oxygenation of tissues.*
• Draw venous blood for complete blood count and electrolyte, type and crossmatch, and coagulation studies *to guide the treatment regimen.*

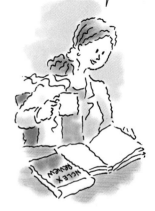

I'd better study assessment findings again. Early recognition of signs and symptoms of hypovolemic shock are necessary to prevent irreversible damage.

• During therapy, assess skin color and temperature and note any changes. Cold, clammy skin may be a sign of continuing peripheral vascular constriction, indicating progressive shock.

• Explain all procedures and their purpose. Throughout these emergency measures, provide emotional support to the patient and his family *to help them cope with the overwhelming situation.*

Teaching topics

• Cause of hypovolemia and treatment options

Myocardial infarction

In MI, reduced blood flow in one of the coronary arteries leads to myocardial ischemia, injury, and necrosis.

In transmural (Q wave) MI, tissue damage extends through all myocardial layers. In subendocardial (non-Q wave) MI, usually only the innermost layer is damaged.

CAUSES

• Aging
• Decreased serum high-density lipoprotein levels
• Diabetes mellitus
• Elevated serum triglyceride, low-density lipoprotein, and cholesterol levels
• Excessive intake of saturated fats, carbohydrates, or salt
• Hypertension
• Obesity
• Positive family history of coronary artery disease
• Sedentary lifestyle
• Smoking
• Stress
• Use of amphetamines or cocaine
• Postmenopausal women

ASSESSMENT FINDINGS

• Anxiety
• Arrhythmias
• Crushing substernal chest pain: may radiate to the jaw, back, and arms; lasts longer than anginal pain; unrelieved by rest or nitroglycerin; may not be present (in asymptomatic or silent MI)
• Diaphoresis
• Dyspnea
• Elevated temperature
• Nausea and vomiting
• Pallor

DIAGNOSTIC TEST RESULTS

• ECG shows an enlarged Q wave, elevated or depressed ST segment, and T-wave inversion.
• Blood chemistry studies show increased CK, LD, AST, and lipids; positive CK-MB fraction; flipped LD_1 (LD_1 levels exceed LD_2 levels, the reversal of their normal patterns) and increased Troponin T.
• Blood studies show increased WBC count.

NURSING DIAGNOSES

• Decreased cardiac output
• Denial
• Altered tissue perfusion (cardiopulmonary, peripheral, renal)

TREATMENT

• Bed rest with bedside commode
• Coronary artery bypass graft
• IABP
• Left ventricular assist device
• Low-calorie, low-cholesterol, low-fat diet
• Monitoring vital signs, urine output, ECG, and hemodynamic status
• Ongoing laboratory studies: ABG levels, CK with isoenzymes, electrolyte levels, cardiac troponins
• Oxygen therapy
• PTCA
• Pulmonary artery catheterization (to detect left- or right-sided heart failure)

Drug therapy

• Analgesics: morphine sulfate (I.V.)
• ACE inhibitors: captopril (Capoten), enalapril (Vasotec)
• Antiarrhythmics: lidocaine (Xylocaine), procainamide (Pronestyl)
• Anticoagulants: aspirin; heparin I.V. (Liquamin sodium) after thrombolytic therapy
• Antihypertensive: hydralazine (Apresoline)
• Beta-adrenergic blockers: propranolol (Inderal), nadolol (Corgard), metoprolol tartrate

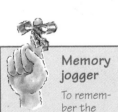

Memory jogger

To remember the signs and symptoms of MI, think DANCE PAD:

Dyspnea

Anxiety

Nausea and vomiting

Crushing substernal chest pain

Elevated temperature

Pallor

Arrhythmias

Diaphoresis

(Lopressor); beta blockers contraindicated if patient also has hypotension or bronchospasm
• Calcium channel blockers: nifedipine (Procardia), verapamil (Calan), diltiazem (Cardizem)
• I.V. atropine or pacemaker for symptomatic bradycardia or heart block
• Nitrates: nitroglycerin I.V. (Nitro-bid)
• Morphine sulfate for pain and sedation.
• Thrombolytic therapy: tissue plasminogen activator (tPA) (Activase), streptokinase (Steptase), anistreplase (Eminase); thrombolytics are given within 6 hours of onset of symptoms but are most effective when started within 3 hours.

INTERVENTIONS AND RATIONALES
• Monitor ECG *to detect ischemia, injury, new or extended infarction, arrhythmias, conduction defects.*
• Monitor and record vital signs and hemodynamic variables *to monitor response to therapy and detect complications.*
• Monitor and record intake and output *to assess renal perfusion and possible fluid retention.*
• Follow laboratory values *to detect myocardial damage, electrolyte abnormalities, drug levels, renal function, and coagulation.*
• Assess cardiovascular and respiratory status *to watch for signs of heart failure, such as an S_3 or S_4 gallop, crackles, cough, tachypnea, and edema.*
• Maintain bed rest *to reduce oxygen demands on the heart.*
• Administer oxygen, as prescribed, *to improve oxygen supply to heart muscle.*
• Obtain an ECG reading during acute pain *to detect myocardial ischemia, injury or infarction.*
• Maintain the patient's prescribed diet *to reduce fluid retention and cholesterol levels.*
• Provide postoperative care, if necessary, *to avoid postoperative complications and help the patient achieve a full recovery.*
• Allay the patient's anxiety *because anxiety increases oxygen demands.*

Teaching topics
• Undergoing cardiac rehabilitation
• Maintaining activity limitations
• Maintaining a low-cholesterol, low-fat, low-sodium diet
• Differentiating between the pain of angina and MI
• Contacting the American Heart Association

Myocarditis

Myocarditis is focal or diffuse inflammation of the cardiac muscle (myocardium). It may be acute or chronic and can occur at any age. Frequently, myocarditis fails to produce specific cardiovascular symptoms or ECG abnormalities, and recovery is usually spontaneous, without residual defects. Occasionally, myocarditis is complicated by heart failure; rarely, it may lead to cardiomyopathy.

CAUSES
• Bacterial infections: diphtheria, tuberculosis, typhoid fever, tetanus, and staphylococcal, pneumococcal, and gonococcal infections
• Chemical poisons such as chronic alcoholism
• Helminthic infections such as trichinosis
• Hypersensitive immune reactions, such as acute rheumatic fever and postcardiotomy syndrome
• Parasitic infections, especially South American trypanosomiasis (Chagas' disease) in infants and immunosuppressed adults; also, toxoplasmosis
• Radiation therapy: large doses of radiation to the chest in treating lung or breast cancer
• Viral infections (most common cause in the United States and western Europe): coxsackievirus A and B strains and, possibly, poliomyelitis, influenza, rubeola, rubella, and adenoviruses and echoviruses

ASSESSMENT FINDINGS
• Arrhythmias (S_3 and S_4 gallops, faint S_1)
• Cardiomyopathy
• Chronic valvulitis (when myocarditis results from rheumatic fever)
• Dyspnea
• Fatigue
• Fever

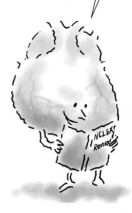

My oh my. In myocarditis my middle muscular layer becomes inflamed.

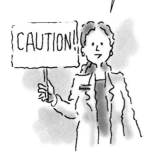

Administer digitalis glycosides carefully. Some patients with myocarditis show a paradoxical sensitivity to even small doses.

CAUTION!

• Mild, continuous pressure or soreness in the chest (unlike the recurring, stress-related pain of angina pectoris)
• Palpitations
• Thromboembolism

DIAGNOSTIC TEST RESULTS
• Blood tests show elevated cardiac enzyme levels (CK, the CK-MB isoenzyme, AST, and LD), increased WBC count and ESR, and elevated antibody titers (such as antistreptolysin O titer in rheumatic fever).
• ECG typically shows diffuse ST-segment and T-wave abnormalities (as in pericarditis), conduction defects (prolonged PR interval), and other supraventricular arrhythmias.
• Endomyocardial biopsy confirms the diagnosis, but a negative biopsy doesn't exclude the diagnosis. A repeat biopsy may be needed.
• Stool and throat cultures may identify the causative bacteria.

NURSING DIAGNOSES
• Activity intolerance
• Decreased cardiac output
• Hyperthermia

TREATMENT
• Bed rest
• Diet: sodium restriction

Drug therapy
• Antiarrhythmics: quinidine (Quinora), procainamide (Pronestyl)
• Antibiotics according to sensitivity of infecting organism
• Anticoagulants: warfarin (Coumadin), heparin (Liquaemin)
• Digitalis glycosides: digoxin (Lanoxin) to increase myocardial contractility
• Diuretics: furosemide (Lasix)

INTERVENTIONS AND RATIONALES
• Assess cardiovascular status frequently to monitor for signs of heart failure, such as dyspnea, hypotension, and tachycardia. Check for changes in cardiac rhythm or conduction. *Rhythm disturbances may indicate early cardiac decompensation.*

• Observe for signs of digitalis toxicity (anorexia, nausea, vomiting, blurred vision, cardiac arrhythmias) and for complicating factors that may potentiate toxicity, such as electrolyte imbalances or hypoxia, *to prevent further complications.*
• Stress the importance of bed rest *to decrease oxygen demands on the heart.* Assist with bathing as necessary; provide a bedside commode, *which puts less stress on the heart than using a bedpan.* Reassure the patient that activity limitations are temporary.
• Offer diversional activities that are physically undemanding *to decrease anxiety.*

Teaching topics
• Restricting activities for as long as the doctor prescribes
• If taking digoxin (Lanoxin) at home, checking pulse for 1 full minute before taking the dose and withholding the dose and notifying the doctor if pulse rate falls below the predetermined rate (usually 60 beats/minute)
• Resuming normal activities slowly, when appropriate, and avoiding competitive sports

Pericarditis

Pericarditis is an inflammation of the pericardium, the fibroserous sac that envelops, supports, and protects the heart. It occurs in both acute and chronic forms. Acute pericarditis can be fibrinous or effusive, with purulent, serous, or hemorrhagic exudate; chronic constrictive pericarditis is characterized by dense fibrous pericardial thickening. The prognosis depends on the underlying cause but is generally good in acute pericarditis, unless constriction occurs.

CAUSES
• Bacterial, fungal, or viral infection (infectious pericarditis)
• Drugs, such as hydralazine or procainamide
• High dose radiation to the chest
• Hypersensitivity or autoimmune disease, such as acute rheumatic fever (most common cause of pericarditis in children), systemic lupus erythematosus, and rheumatoid arthritis

• Idiopathic factors (most common in acute pericarditis)
• Neoplasms (primary, or metastases from lungs, breasts, or other organs)
• Postcardiac injury, such as MI (which later causes an autoimmune reaction [Dressler's syndrome] in the pericardium), trauma, or surgery that leaves the pericardium intact but causes blood to leak into the pericardial cavity
• Uremia

ASSESSMENT FINDINGS

Acute pericarditis
• Pericardial friction rub (grating sound heard as the heart moves)
• Sharp and commonly sudden pain that usually starts over the sternum and radiates to the neck, shoulders, back, and arms (Unlike the pain of MI, pericardial pain is often pleuritic, increasing with deep inspiration and decreasing when the patient sits up and leans forward, pulling the heart away from the diaphragmatic pleurae of the lungs.)
• Symptoms of cardiac tamponade (pallor, clammy skin, hypotension, pulsus paradoxus, neck vein distention)
• Symptoms of heart failure (dyspnea, orthopnea, tachycardia, ill-defined substernal chest pain, feeling of fullness in the chest)

Chronic pericarditis
• Gradual increase in systemic venous pressure
• Pericardial friction rub
• Symptoms similar to those of chronic right-sided heart failure (fluid retention, ascites, hepatomegaly)

DIAGNOSTIC TEST RESULTS
• Blood tests reflect inflammation and may show normal or elevated WBC count, especially in infectious pericarditis; elevated ESR; and slightly elevated cardiac enzyme levels with associated myocarditis.
• Culture of pericardial fluid obtained by open surgical drainage or cardiocentesis sometimes identifies a causative organism in bacterial or fungal pericarditis.

• Echocardiography confirms the diagnosis when it shows an echo-free space between the ventricular wall and the pericardium (in cases of pleural effusion).
• ECG shows the following changes in acute pericarditis: elevation of ST segments in the standard limb leads and most precordial leads without significant changes in QRS morphology that occur with MI, atrial ectopic rhythms such as AF, and diminished QRS voltage in pericardial effusion.

NURSING DIAGNOSES
• Decreased cardiac output
• Diversional activity deficit
• Pain

TREATMENT
• Bed rest
• Surgery: pericardiocentesis (in cases of cardiac tamponade), partial pericardectomy (for recurrent pericarditis), total pericardectomy (for constrictive pericarditis)

Drug therapy
• Antibiotics: according to sensitivity of infecting organism
• Corticosteroids: methylprednisolone (Solu-Medrol)
• Nonsteroidal anti-inflammatory drugs (NSAIDs): aspirin, indomethacin (Indocin)

INTERVENTIONS AND RATIONALES
• Provide complete bed rest *to decrease oxygen demands on the heart.*
• Assess pain in relation to respiration and body position *to distinguish pericardial pain from myocardial ischemic pain.*
• Place the patient in an upright position *to relieve dyspnea and chest pain.* Provide analgesics and oxygen, and reassure the patient with acute pericarditis that his condition is temporary and treatable *to promote patient comfort and allay anxiety.*
• Monitor the patient for signs of cardiac compression or cardiac tamponade, possible complications of pericardial effusion. Signs include decreased blood pressure, increased CVP, and pulsus paradoxus. Keep a pericardiocentesis set handy whenever pericardial ef-

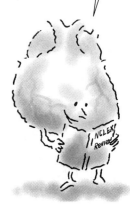

Oh, the perils of the pericardium. It becomes inflamed and, presto, pericarditis.

fusion is suspected *because cardiac tamponade requires immediate treatment.*
• Explain tests and treatments to the patient. If surgery is necessary, he should learn deep breathing and coughing exercises beforehand *to alleviate fear and anxiety and promote compliance with the postoperative treatment regimen.* Postoperative care is similar to that given after cardiothoracic surgery.

Teaching topics
• Explanation of all tests and treatments
• Coughing and deep breathing exercises
• Slow resumption of daily activities and scheduled rest periods in daily routine

Pulmonary edema

Pulmonary edema is a complication of left-sided heart failure. It occurs when pulmonary capillary pressure exceeds intravascular osmotic pressure, and results in increased pressure in the capillaries of the lungs and acute transudation of fluid. This leads to impaired oxygenation and hypoxia.

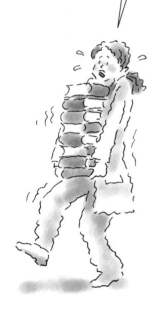

Face it. Cardiovascular care is a huge topic. Feeling weighed down by information? Take a break to clear your head.

CAUSES
• Adult respiratory distress syndrome
• Atherosclerosis
• Drug overdose: heroin, barbiturates, morphine sulfate
• Heart failure
• Hypertension
• MI
• Myocarditis
• Overload of I.V. fluids
• Smoke inhalation
• Valvular disease

ASSESSMENT FINDINGS
• Agitation, restlessness, intense fear
• Blood-tinged, frothy sputum, and paroxysmal cough
• Cold, clammy skin
• Crackles auscultated over lung fields
• Dyspnea, orthopnea, tachypnea
• Jugular vein distention
• Syncope
• Tachycardia, S_3 and S_4, chest pain

DIAGNOSTIC TEST RESULTS
• ABGs show respiratory alkalosis or acidosis and hypoxemia.
• ECG reveals tachycardia and ventricular enlargement.
• Hemodynamic monitoring shows increases in PAP, PAWP, and CVP as well as decreased cardiac output.
• Pulse oximetry reveals hypoxia.

NURSING DIAGNOSES
• Anxiety
• Fluid volume excess
• Impaired gas exchange

TREATMENT
• Activity changes: maintaining bed rest and implementing range-of-motion and isometric exercises
• Dietary changes: establishing a low-sodium diet and limiting oral fluids
• Oxygen therapy: may include intubation and mechanical ventilation
• Hemodialysis and ultrafiltration, if available

Drug therapy
• Analgesic: morphine sulfate I.V.
• Cardiac glycoside: digoxin (Lanoxin)
• Inotropic agents: dobutamine hydrochloride(Dobutrex), amrinone lactate (Inocor), milrinone (Primacor)
• Diuretics: furosemide (Lasix), bumetanide (Bumex), metolazone (Zaroxolyn)
• Nitrates: isosorbide dinitrate (Isordil), nitroglycerin (Nitro-Bid)
• Vasodilator: nitroprusside sodium (Nitropress)

INTERVENTIONS AND RATIONALES
• Assess cardiovascular status, hemodynamic variables, and respiratory status *to detect changes in fluid balance. Tachycardia, S_3 heart sound, hypotension, increased respiratory rate and crackles indicate increased fluid volume.*
• Monitor and record intake and output. *Intake greater than output and elevated specific gravity suggest fluid retention.*
• Weigh patient daily to detect fluid retention. *Weight gain of 0.5 to 1 kg per day suggests a fluid gain.*

• Track laboratory values. *BUN and creatinine indicate renal function. Electrolytes, hemoglobin and hematocrit indicate fluid status.*
• Keep the patient in high Fowler's position if blood pressure tolerates; if hypotensive, maintain in a semi-Fowler's position if tolerated. *Elevating the head of the bed reduces venous return to the heart and promotes chest expansion.*
• Administer oxygen, as prescribed, *to increase alveolar oxygen concentration and enhance arterial blood oxygenation.*
• Administer medications *to improve gas exchange, improve myocardial function, and reduce anxiety.*
• Note the color, amount, and consistency of sputum. *Sputum amount and consistency may indicate hydration status. A change in color or foul-smelling sputum may indicate a respiratory infection.*
• Withhold food and fluids, as directed, *to prevent aspiration.*
• Encourage the patient to express feelings such as a fear of suffocation *to reduce anxiety and lessen oxygen demands.*

Teaching topics
• Elevating the head of the bed while sleeping
• Eating foods high in potassium
• Recognizing the early signs of fluid overload
• Recognizing the signs and symptoms of respiratory distress
• Taking medications exactly as prescribed
• Recording weight daily

Raynaud's disease

Raynaud's disease is characterized by episodic vasospasm in the small peripheral arteries and arterioles, precipitated by exposure to cold or stress. This condition occurs bilaterally and usually affects the hands or, less often, the feet.

Raynaud's disease is most prevalent in women, particularly between puberty and age 40. A benign condition, it requires no specific treatment and has no serious sequelae.

Raynaud's phenomenon, however, a condition often associated with several connective tissue disorders — such as scleroderma, systemic lupus erythematosus, and polymyositis — has a progressive course, leading to ischemia, gangrene, and amputation. Differentiating the two disorders is difficult because some patients who experience mild symptoms of Raynaud's disease for several years may later develop overt connective tissue disease — most commonly scleroderma.

CAUSES
• Unknown (most probable theory involves an antigen antibody immune response)

ASSESSMENT FINDINGS
• Numbness and tingling relieved by warmth
• Sclerodactyly, ulcerations, or chronic paronychia (in longstanding disease)
• Typically, blanching of skin on the fingers, which then becomes cyanotic before changing to red (after exposure to cold or stress)

DIAGNOSTIC TEST RESULTS
• Arteriography reveals vasospasm.
• Plethysmography reveals intermittent vessel occlusion.

NURSING DIAGNOSES
• Altered tissue perfusion: peripheral
• Risk for injury
• Risk for peripheral neurovascular dysfunction

TREATMENT
• Activity changes: avoidance of cold
• Smoking cessation (if appropriate)
• Surgery (used in fewer than one-quarter of patients): sympathectomy

Drug therapy
• Calcium channel blockers: diltiazem (Cardizem)
• Vasodilators: phenoxybenzamine (Dibenzyline), reserpine (Diupres)

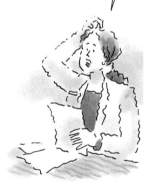

Hmmm. Because adverse effects of vasodilators may be more bothersome than the disease itself, they're typically used only in severe cases of Raynaud's disease.

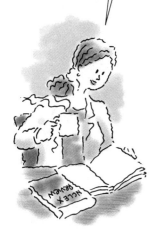

Fever vs. disease. Rheumatic fever follows a group A beta-hemolytic streptococcal infection. Rheumatic heart disease refers to the cardiac manifestations of rheumatic fever,

INTERVENTIONS AND RATIONALES

• Warn against exposure to the cold. Tell the patient to wear mittens or gloves in cold weather or when handling cold items or defrosting the freezer *to prevent vasospasm, which causes onset of symptoms.*
• Advise the patient to avoid stressful situations and to stop smoking *to prevent exacerbation of symptoms.*
• Instruct the patient to inspect the skin frequently and to seek immediate care for signs of skin breakdown or infection *to prevent complications.*
• Teach the patient about drugs, their use, and their adverse effects *to prevent further complications.*
• Provide psychological support and reassurance *to allay the patient's fear of amputation and disfigurement.*

Teaching topics

• Modifying risk factors, such as quitting smoking
• Preventive measures such as avoiding cold and stress

Rheumatic fever and rheumatic heart disease

Often recurrent, acute rheumatic fever is a systemic inflammatory disease of childhood that follows a group A beta-hemolytic streptococcal infection. Rheumatic heart disease refers to the cardiac manifestations of rheumatic fever and includes pancarditis (myocarditis, pericarditis, and endocarditis) during the early acute phase and chronic valvular disease later.

Long-term antibiotic therapy can minimize recurrence of rheumatic fever, reducing the risk of permanent cardiac damage and eventual valvular deformity. However, severe pancarditis occasionally produces fatal heart failure during the acute phase. Of the patients who survive this complication, about 20% die within 10 years.

This disease strikes most often during cool, damp weather in the winter and early spring.

In the United States, it's most common in the northern states.

CAUSES

• Hypersensitivity reaction to a group A beta-hemolytic streptococcal infection

ASSESSMENT FINDINGS

• Carditis
• Temperature of at least 100.4° F (38° C)
• Migratory joint pain or polyarthritis
• Skin lesions such as erythema marginatum (in only 5% of patients)
• Transient chorea (can develop up to 6 months after the original streptococcal infection)

DIAGNOSTIC TEST RESULTS

• Blood tests show elevated WBC count and ESR; slight anemia during inflammation.
• Cardiac catheterization evaluates valvular damage and left ventricular function in severe cardiac dysfunction.
• Cardiac enzyme levels may be increased in severe carditis.
• Chest X-rays show normal heart size (except with myocarditis, heart failure, or pericardial effusion).
• C-reactive protein is positive (especially during the acute phase).
• Echocardiography helps evaluate valvular damage, chamber size, and ventricular function.
• ECG shows prolonged PR interval in 20% of patients.

NURSING DIAGNOSES

• Activity intolerance
• Decreased cardiac output
• Risk for infection

TREATMENT

• Bed rest (in severe cases)
• Surgery: corrective valvular surgery (in cases of persistent heart failure)

Drug therapy

• Antibiotics: erythromycin (Erythrocin), penicillin (Pfizerpen)
• NSAID: aspirin, indomethacin (Indocin)

INTERVENTIONS AND RATIONALES

• Before giving penicillin, ask the patient if he's ever had a hypersensitivity reaction to it. Even if the patient has never had a reaction to penicillin, warn that such a reaction is possible *to adequately inform the patient about possible treatment complications.*

• Tell the patient to stop taking the drug and immediately report the development of a rash, fever, chills, or other signs of allergy at any time during penicillin therapy *to prevent anaphylaxis.*

• Instruct the patient to watch for and report early signs of heart failure, such as dyspnea and a hacking, nonproductive cough, *to prevent further cardiac decompensation.*

• Stress the need for bed rest during the acute phase and suggest appropriate, physically undemanding diversions. *These measures decrease oxygen demands of the heart.*

• After the acute phase, encourage family and friends to spend as much time as possible with the patient *to minimize boredom.*

• If the patient has severe carditis, help him prepare for permanent changes in his lifestyle *to promote positive coping strategies.*

• Warn the patient to watch for and immediately report signs of recurrent streptococcal infection — sudden sore throat, diffuse throat redness and oropharyngeal exudate, swollen and tender cervical lymph glands, pain on swallowing, a temperature of 101° to 104° F (38.3° to 40° C), headache, and nausea *to prevent complications associated with delayed treatment such as heart valve damage.* Urge the patient to keep away from people with respiratory tract infections *to prevent reinfection.*

• Make sure the patient understands the need to comply with prolonged antibiotic therapy and follow-up care and the need for additional antibiotics during dental surgery *to prevent reinfection.*

• Arrange for a visiting nurse to oversee home care if necessary *to promote compliance.*

Teaching topics

• Watching for and reporting signs of heart failure
• Starting normal activities slowly
• Taking prophylactic antibiotics during dental surgery
• Importance of good dental hygiene to prevent gingival infection

Thoracic aortic aneurysm

Thoracic aortic aneurysm is characterized by an abnormal widening of the ascending, transverse, or descending part of the aorta. Aneurysm of the ascending aorta is most common and most commonly fatal.

The aneurysm may be *dissecting,* a hemorrhagic separation in the aortic wall, usually within the medial layer; *saccular,* an outpouching of the arterial wall, with a narrow neck; or *fusiform,* a spindle-shaped enlargement encompassing the entire aortic circumference.

Some aneurysms progress to serious and, eventually, lethal complications such as rupture of an untreated thoracic dissecting aneurysm into the pericardium, with resulting tamponade.

CAUSES

• Atherosclerosis
• Congenital disorders, such as coarctation of the aorta
• Fungal infection (infected aneurysm) of the aortic arch and descending segments
• Hypertension
• Syphilis, usually of the ascending aorta (uncommon because of antibiotics)
• Trauma, usually of the descending thoracic aorta, from an accident that shears the aorta transversely (acceleration-deceleration injuries)

ASSESSMENT FINDINGS

Ascending aneurysm

• Bradycardia
• Pain (described as severe, boring, and ripping and extending to the neck, shoulders, lower back, or abdomen)
• Pericardial friction rub caused by a hemopericardium
• Unequal intensities of the right carotid and left radial pulses

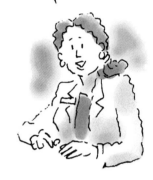

For patients with rheumatic fever, good dental hygiene is necessary to prevent gingival infection.

Descending aneurysm
• Pain (described as sharp and tearing, usually starting suddenly between the shoulder blades and possibly radiating to the chest)

Transverse aneurysm
• Dry cough
• Dyspnea
• Dysphagia
• Hoarseness
• Pain (described as sharp and tearing and radiating to the shoulders)

DIAGNOSTIC TEST RESULTS
• Aortography, the definitive test, shows the lumen of the aneurysm, its size and location, and the false lumen in a dissecting aneurysm.
• Blood tests may show low hemoglobin because of blood loss from a leaking aneurysm.
• Chest X-ray shows widening of the aorta.
• Computed tomography scan can confirm and locate the aneurysm and may be used to monitor its progression.
• Echocardiography may help identify a dissecting aneurysm of the aortic root.
• ECG helps distinguish a thoracic aneurysm from MI.
• Transesophageal echocardiography is used to measure the aneurysm in the ascending and descending aorta.

NURSING DIAGNOSES
• Decreased cardiac output
• Ineffective breathing pattern
• Pain

TREATMENT
• Surgery: resection of aneurysm through a Dacron or Teflon graft replacement, possible replacement of aortic valve

Drug therapy
• Analgesics
• Antihypertensive: nitroprusside (Nitropress)
• Negative inotropic: propranolol (Inderal)

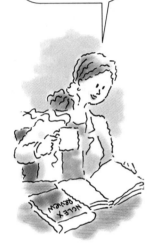

> Pain is the key assessment finding with thoracic aortic aneurysm, but the kind of pain depends on the type of aneurysm.

INTERVENTIONS AND RATIONALES
• Monitor the patient's blood pressure, PAWP, and CVP *to detect fluid volume deficit.* Also evaluate pain, breathing, and carotid, radial, and femoral pulses *to detect early signs of aneurysm rupture.*
• Review laboratory test results, which must include a complete blood count, differential, electrolytes, typing and crossmatching for whole blood, ABG studies, and urinalysis, *to note hemoglobin levels and ensure that the patient can tolerate surgery.*
• Insert an indwelling urinary catheter. Administer dextrose 5% in water or lactated Ringer's solution and antibiotics as needed. Carefully monitor nitroprusside I.V. infusion rate; use a separate I.V. line for infusion. Adjust the dose by slowly increasing the infusion rate. Meanwhile, check blood pressure every 5 minutes until it stabilizes *to note effectiveness of treatment and prevent hypotension from large dose nitroprusside.*
• With suspected bleeding from an aneurysm, give a whole-blood transfusion *to adequately replace fluid volume deficit.*
• Explain diagnostic tests. If surgery is scheduled, explain the procedure and expected postoperative care (I.V. lines, endotracheal and drainage tubes, cardiac monitoring, ventilation) *to alleviate the patient's anxiety.*
  After repair of a thoracic aneurysm:
• Evaluate the patient's level of consciousness. Monitor vital signs; PAP, PAWP, and CVP; pulse rate; urine output; and pain *to guide treatment regimen and evaluate its effectiveness.*
• Check respiratory function. Carefully observe and record type and amount of chest tube drainage and frequently assess heart and breath sounds *to detect early signs of compromise.*
• Monitor I.V. therapy to prevent fluid excess, which may occur with rapid fluid replacement.
• Give medications as appropriate to help improve the patient's condition.
• Watch for signs of infection, especially fever, and excessive wound drainage *to initiate treatment promptly and prevent complications such as sepsis.*

• Assist with range-of-motion exercises of legs *to prevent thromboembolism due to venostasis during prolonged bed rest.*
• After stabilization of vital signs and respiration, encourage and assist the patient in turning, coughing, and deep breathing. If necessary, provide intermittent positive pressure breathing *to promote lung expansion.*
• Help the patient walk as soon as he's able *to prevent complications of immobility such as pneumonia and thromboembolism formation.*
• Before discharge, ensure adherence to antihypertensive therapy by explaining the need for such drugs and the expected adverse effects. Teach the patient how to monitor his blood pressure *to prevent complications associated with ineffective blood pressure management such as CVA.*
• Throughout hospitalization, offer the patient and family psychological support *to relieve anxiety and feelings of helplessness.*

Teaching topics
• Monitoring blood pressure and reducing hypertension
• Quitting smoking

Thrombophlebitis

Thrombophlebitis is marked by inflammation of the venous wall and thrombus formation. It may affect deep veins or superficial veins. The thrombus may occlude a vein or detach and embolize to the lungs.

CAUSES
• Hypercoagulability (from cancer, blood dyscrasias, oral contraceptives)
• Injury to the venous wall (from I.V. injections, fractures, antibiotics)
• Venous stasis (from varicose veins, pregnancy, heart failure, prolonged bed rest)

ASSESSMENT FINDINGS

Deep vein thrombophlebitis
• Cramping pain
• Edema
• Positive Homans' sign
• Tenderness to touch

Superficial vein thrombophlebitis
• Redness along the vein
• Warmth and tenderness along the vein

DIAGNOSTIC TEST RESULTS
• Hematology reveals increased WBC count.
• Photoplethysmography shows venous-filling defects.
• Ultrasound reveals decreased blood flow.
• Venography shows venous-filling defects.

NURSING DIAGNOSES
• Pain
• Impaired skin integrity
• Altered tissue perfusion (peripheral)

TREATMENT
• Activity changes: maintaining bed rest and elevating the affected extremity
• Embolectomy and insertion of a vena cava umbrella or filter
• Antiembolism stockings
• Warm, moist compresses

Drug therapy
• Anticoagulants: warfarin sodium (Coumadin), heparin sodium (Liquaemin Sodium)
• Anti-inflammatory agent: aspirin
• Fibrinolytic agents: streptokinase (Streptase)

INTERVENTIONS AND RATIONALES
• Assess pulmonary status. *Crackles, dyspnea, tachypnea, hemoptysis and chest pain suggest pulmonary embolism.*
• Assess cardiovascular status. *Tachycardia and chest pain may indicate pulmonary embolism.*
• Assess for Homans' sign. *Although it suggests deep vein thrombosis, it may be unreliable since it's not specific to this condition.*
• Assess for bleeding *due to anticoagulant therapy.*

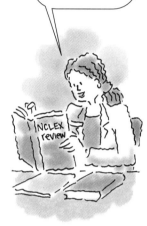

Homans' sign is positive when there is pain on passive dorsiflexion of the foot.

A clot is typically caused by venous stasis, endothelial damage, and hypercoagulability. This is called Virchow's triad.

• Monitor and record vital signs, such as hypotension, tachycardia, tachypnea, and restlessness. Observe for bruising, epistaxis, blood in stool, bleeding gums, and painful joints. *Tachypnea and tachycardia may suggest pulmonary embolism or hemorrhage.*

• Perform neurovascular checks *to detect nerve or vascular damage.*

• Monitor laboratory values. *Partial thromboplastin time (PTT) in a patient on heparin and prothrombin time (PT) in a patient receiving warfarin should be one and a half to two times the control. International normalized ratio (INR) should be 2 to 3 for the patient receiving warfarin. A falling hemoglobin and hematocrit indicate blood loss.*

• Keep the patient in bed and elevate the affected extremity *to promote venous return and reduce swelling.*

• Administer medications, as prescribed, *to control or dissolve blood clots.*

• Apply warm, moist compresses to improve circulation *to the affected area and relieve pain and inflammation.*

• Measure and record the circumference of thighs and calves. Compare measurement to unaffected leg *to assess for worsening inflammation.*

Teaching topics

• Recognizing signs and symptoms of bleeding and clot formation

• Avoiding prolonged sitting or standing, constrictive clothing, or crossing the legs when seated

• Avoiding oral contraceptives

Valvular heart disease

In valvular heart disease, three types of mechanical disruption can occur: stenosis, or narrowing, of the valve opening; incomplete closure of the valve; or prolapse of the valve. These conditions can result from such disorders as endocarditis (most common), congenital defects, and inflammation, and they can lead to heart failure.

Valvular heart disease occurs in several forms. The most common include:

• aortic insufficiency, in which blood flows back into the left ventricle during diastole, causing fluid overload in the ventricle, which dilates and hypertrophies (The excess volume causes fluid overload in the left atrium and, finally, the pulmonary system. Left ventricular failure and pulmonary edema eventually result.)

• mitral insufficiency, in which blood from the left ventricle flows back into the left atrium during systole, causing the atrium to enlarge to accommodate the backflow (As a result, the left ventricle also dilates to accommodate the increased volume of blood from the atrium and to compensate for diminishing cardiac output.)

• mitral stenosis, in which narrowing of the valve by valvular abnormalities, fibrosis, or calcification obstructs blood flow from the left atrium to the left ventricle (Consequently, left atrial volume and pressure rise and the chamber dilates.)

• mitral valve prolapse (MVP), in which one or both valve leaflets protrude into the left atrium (MVP syndrome is the term used when the anatomic prolapse is accompanied by assessment findings unrelated to the valvular abnormality.)

• tricuspid insufficiency, in which blood flows back into the right atrium during systole, decreasing blood flow to the lungs and left side of the heart (Cardiac output also lessens. Fluid overload in the right side of the heart can eventually lead to right-sided heart failure.)

CAUSES
Aortic insufficiency
• Endocarditis
• Hypertension
• Idiopathic origin
• Rheumatic fever
• Syphilis

Mitral insufficiency
• Hypertrophic cardiomyopathy
• Left ventricular failure
• Mitral valve prolapse
• Rheumatic fever

Three types of mechanical disruption can affect heart valves: stenosis, or narrowing, of the valve opening; incomplete closure of the valve; and prolapse of the valve.

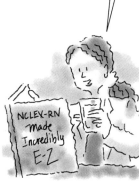

NCLEX-RN made Incredibly E-Z

Mitral stenosis
- Rheumatic fever

Mitral valve prolapse
- Unknown

Tricuspid insufficiency
- Endocarditis
- Rheumatic fever
- Right-sided heart failure
- Trauma

ASSESSMENT FINDINGS
Aortic insufficiency
- Angina
- Cough
- Dyspnea
- Fatigue
- Palpitations
- Pulmonary vein congestion
- Rapidly rising and collapsing pulses

Mitral insufficiency
- Angina
- Dyspnea
- Fatigue
- Orthopnea
- Peripheral edema

Mitral stenosis
- Dyspnea on exertion
- Fatigue
- Orthopnea
- Palpitations
- Peripheral edema
- Weakness

Mitral valve prolapse
- Chest pain
- Fatigue
- Headache
- Possibly asymptomatic
- Palpitations

Tricuspid insufficiency
- Dyspnea
- Fatigue
- Peripheral edema

DIAGNOSTIC TEST RESULTS
Aortic insufficiency
- Cardiac catheterization shows reduction in arterial diastolic pressures.
- Echocardiography shows left ventricular enlargement.
- ECG shows sinus tachycardia and left ventricular hypertrophy.
- X-ray shows left ventricular enlargement and pulmonary vein congestion.

Mitral insufficiency
- Cardiac catheterization shows mitral regurgitation and elevated atrial and pulmonary artery wedge pressures.
- Echocardiography shows abnormal valve leaflet motion.
- ECG may show left atrial and ventricular hypertrophy.
- X-ray shows left atrial and ventricular enlargement.

Mitral stenosis
- Cardiac catheterization shows diastolic pressure gradient across the valve and elevated left atrial and pulmonary artery wedge pressures.
- Echocardiography shows thickened mitral valve leaflets.
- ECG shows left atrial hypertrophy.
- X-ray shows left atrial and ventricular enlargement.

Mitral valve prolapse
- Color-flow Doppler studies show mitral insufficiency.
- ECG shows prolapse of the mitral valve into the left atrium.

Tricuspid insufficiency
- Echocardiography shows systolic prolapse of the tricuspid valve.
- ECG shows right atrial or right ventricular hypertrophy.
- X-ray shows right atrial dilation and right ventricular enlargement.

NURSING DIAGNOSES
- Activity intolerance
- Anxiety
- Decreased cardiac output

TREATMENT
- Diet: sodium restrictions (in cases of heart failure)
- Surgery: open-heart surgery using cardiopulmonary bypass for valve replacement (in severe cases)

Drug therapy
- Anticoagulants: warfarin (Coumadin) to prevent thrombus formation around diseased or replaced valves

INTERVENTIONS AND RATIONALES
- Watch closely for signs of heart failure or pulmonary edema and for adverse effects of drug therapy *to prevent cardiac decompensation.*
- Place the patient in an upright position *to relieve dyspnea.*
- Maintain bed rest and provide assistance with bathing, if necessary, *to decrease oxygen demands on the heart.*

- If the patient undergoes surgery, watch for hypotension, arrhythmias, and thrombus formation. Monitor vital signs, ABG levels, intake, output, daily weight, blood chemistries, chest X-rays, and pulmonary artery catheter readings *to detect early signs of postoperative complications and ensure early intervention and treatment.*
- Allow the patient to verbalize concerns over being unable to meet life demands because of activity restrictions *to reduce anxiety.*

Teaching topics
- Following diet restrictions and medication schedule
- Need for consistent follow-up care
- Incorporating rest into the daily routine

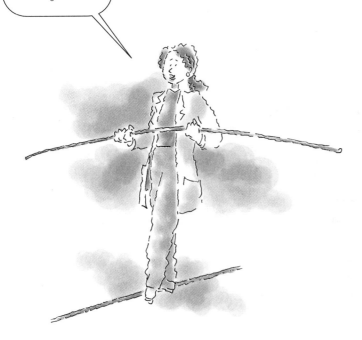

Don't lose your motivation in the middle of your NCLEX preparation. It's important to keep a positive attitude for the long haul.

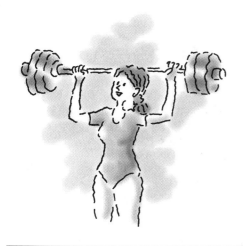

Answer: D. The client has likely developed a hematoma from bleeding at the femoral puncture site. The bleeding must be stopped so the nurse should apply pressure to the site and notify the physician. At some point, a heavier sandbag may be indicated but not in lieu of direct pressure. The leg should be neutral and not elevated. Monitoring coagulation is a later concern.

➡ *NCLEX keys*
Nursing process step: Implementation
Client needs category: Physiological integrity
Client needs subcategory: Reduction of risk potential
Taxonomic level: Application

Pump up on practice questions

1. After undergoing cardiac catheterization, a client has a 10-lb sandbag resting over the left femoral insertion site. When the nurse removes the sandbag, she observes a swelling at the site, about 2″ (5 cm) in diameter. The nurse should initially:

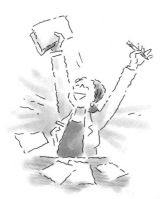

A. replace the 10-lb bag with a 15-lb sandbag for additional pressure.
B. place a pressure dressing over the site and elevate the left leg at least 45 degrees.
C. draw a stat partial thromboplastin time and stop any heparin infusions.
D. apply firm pressure to the site and instruct another staff member to notify the physician.

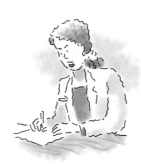

2. A client is prescribed diltiazem (Cardiazem) to manage his hypertension. The nurse should tell the client the diltiazem will:
A. lower his blood pressure only.
B. lower his heart rate and blood pressure.
C. lower his blood pressure and increase his urine output.
D. lower his heart rate and blood pressure and increase his urine output.
Answer: B. Diltiazem (Cardiazem), a calcium channel blocker, will reduce both the heart rate and blood pressure. It doesn't directly affect urine output.

➡ *NCLEX keys*
Nursing process step: Implementation
Client needs category: Physiological integrity
Client needs subcategory: Pharmacological and parenteral therapies
Taxonomic level: Comprehension

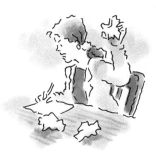

3. A client reports substernal chest pain. Test results show electrocardiographic changes and an elevated cardiac troponin level. What should be the focus of nursing care?

A. Improving myocardial oxygenation and reducing cardiac workload
B. Confirming a suspected diagnosis and preventing complications
C. Reducing anxiety and relieving pain
D. Eliminating stressors and providing a nondemanding environment

Answer: A. The client is exhibiting clinical signs and symptoms of a myocardial infarction (MI); therefore, nursing care should focus on improving myocardial oxygenation and reducing cardiac workload. Confirming the diagnosis of MI and preventing complications, reducing anxiety and relieving pain, and providing a nondemanding environment are secondary to improving myocardial oxygenation and reducing workload. Stressors can't be eliminated, only reduced.

➡ *NCLEX keys*
Nursing process step: Planning
Client needs category: Physiological integrity
Client needs subcategory: Reduction of risk potential
Taxonomic level: Analysis

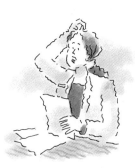

4. A client with a myocardial infarction and cardiogenic shock is placed on an intra-aortic balloon pump (IAPB). If the device is functioning properly, the balloon inflates when the:

A. tricuspid valve is closed.
B. pulmonic valve is open.
C. aortic valve is closed.
D. mitral valve is closed.

Answer: C. An intra-aortic balloon pump (IAPB) inflates during diastole when the tricuspid and mitral valves are open and the aortic and pulmonic valves are closed.

➡ *NCLEX keys*
Nursing process step: Implementation
Client needs category: Physiological integrity
Client needs subcategory: Physiological adaptation
Taxonomic level: Comprehension

5. A client with unstable angina receives routine applications of nitroglycerin ointment. The nurse should delay the next dose if the client has:

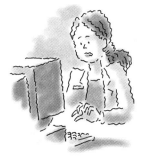

A. atrial fibrillation.
B. a systolic blood pressure below 90 mm Hg.
C. a headache.
D. skin redness at the current site.

Answer: B. Nitroglycerin is a vasodilator and can lower arterial blood pressure. As a rule, when the client's systolic blood pressure is below 90 mm Hg, the nurse should delay the dose and notify the physician. Nitroglycerin isn't contraindicated in a client with atrial fibrillation. Headache, a common occurrence with nitroglycerin, can be treated with an analgesic and isn't a cause for withholding a dose. Sites should be changed with each dose, especially if skin irritation occurs.

➡ NCLEX keys
Nursing process step: Implementation
Client needs category: Physiological integrity
Client needs subcategory: Pharmacological and parenteral therapies
Taxonomic level: Application

6. A client experiences acute myocardial ischemia. The nurse administers oxygen and sublingual nitroglycerin. When assessing an

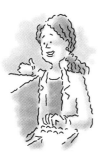

electrocardiogram (ECG) for evidence that blood flow to the myocardium has improved, the nurse should focus on the:
  A. widening of the QRS complex.
  B. frequency of ectopic beats.
  C. return of the ST segment from baseline.
  D. presence of a significant Q wave.
Answer: C. During episodes of myocardial ischemia, an ECG may show ST-segment elevation or depression. With successful treatment, the ST segment should return to baseline. Other changes — widening QRS complex, presence of a Q wave, and frequent ectopic beats — aren't directly indicative of myocardial ischemia.

➡ NCLEX keys
Nursing process step: Assessment
Client needs category: Physiological integrity
Client needs subcategory: Pharmacological and parenteral therapies
Taxonomic level: Application

7. Following a left anterior myocardial infarction, a client undergoes insertion of a pulmonary artery catheter. Which finding most strongly suggests left-sided heart failure?
  A. A drop in the central venous pressure
  B. An increase in the cardiac index
  C. A rise in pulmonary artery diastolic pressure
  D. A decline in the mean pulmonary artery pressure
Answer: C. A rise in pulmonary artery diastolic pressure suggests left-sided heart failure. Central venous pressure would rise in heart failure. The cardiac index would decline in heart failure. The mean pulmonary artery pressure would increase in heart failure.

➡ NCLEX keys
Nursing process step: Assessment
Client needs category: Physiological integrity
Client needs subcategory: Physiological adaptation
Taxonomic level: Application

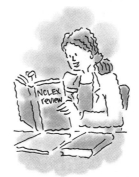

8. A client with dilated cardiomyopathy, pulmonary edema, and severe dyspnea is placed on dobutamine. Which assessment finding indicates that the drug is effective?
  A. Increased activity tolerance
  B. Absence of arrhythmias
  C. Negative Homans' sign
  D. Blood pressure of 160/90 mm Hg
Answer: A. Dobutamine should improve the client's symptoms and the client should experience an increased tolerance for activity. Ar-

rhythmias and hypertension are adverse effects associated with dobutamine. A negative Homans' sign indicates absence of blood clots, which is not a therapeutic effect of dobutamine.

➡ NCLEX keys
Nursing process step: Evaluation
Client needs category: Physiological integrity
Client needs subcategory: Pharmacological and parenteral therapies
Taxonomic level: Analysis

9. The nurse administers warfarin (Coumadin) to a client with deep vein thrombophlebitis. Which of the following laboratory values indicates that the client has a therapeutic level of warfarin?

- A: Partial thromboplastin time (PTT) 1½ to 2 times the control
- B: Prothrombin time (PT) 1½ to 2 times the control
- C: International normalized ratio (INR) of 3 to 4
- D: Hematocrit of 32%

Answer: B. Warfarin is at a therapeutic level when the prothrombin time is 1½ to 2 times the control. Values greater than this increase the risk of bleeding and hemorrhage, while lower values increase the risk of blood clot formation. Heparin, not warfarin, prolongs the partial thromboplastin time. The international normalized ratio may also be used to determine whether warfarin is at a therapeutic level; a therapeutic international normalized ratio of 2 to 3 is considered therapeutic. Hematocrit does not provide information on the effectiveness of warfarin. However, a falling hematocrit in a client taking warfarin may be a sign of hemorrhage.

➡ NCLEX keys
Nursing process step: Evaluation
Client needs category: Physiological integrity
Client needs subcategory: Pharmacological and parenteral therapies
Taxonomic level: Application

10. A client comes into the emergency room with a dissecting aortic aneurysm. The client is at greatest risk for:

- A. septic shock.
- B. anaphylactic shock.
- C. cardiogenic shock.
- D. hypovolemic shock.

Answer: D. A dissecting aortic aneurysm is a precursor to aortic rupture, which will lead to hemorrhage and hypovolemic shock.

➡ NCLEX keys
Nursing process step: Assessment
Client needs category: Physiological integrity
Client needs subcategory: Reduction of risk potential
Taxonomic level: Comprehension

Congrats! You finished the chapter. My advice: Take an exercise break.

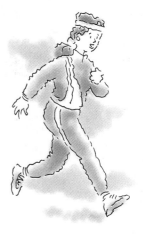

4 Respiratory System

Brush up on key concepts

In this chapter, you'll review:

- components of the respiratory system and their function
- tests used to diagnose respiratory disorders
- common respiratory disorders.

The major function of the respiratory system is gas exchange. During gas exchange, air is taken into the body through inhalation and travels through respiratory passages to the lungs. In the lungs, oxygen (O_2) takes the place of carbon dioxide (CO_2) in the blood, and the CO_2 is then expelled from the body through exhalation.

At any time, you can review the major points of this chapter by consulting the *Cheat sheet* on pages 70 to 77.

Enter here

The **nose** and **mouth** allow air flow into and out of the body. They also humidify inhaled air, which reduces irritation of the mucous membranes. Within the nose, the **nares** (nostrils) contain olfactory receptor sites, providing for the body's sense of smell.

Keep out!

The **paranasal sinuses** are air-filled, cilia-lined cavities within the nose. Their function is to trap particles of foreign matter that might interfere with the workings of the respiratory system.

Going down

The **pharynx** serves as a passageway to the digestive and respiratory tracts. The pharynx maintains air pressure in the middle ear and also contains a mucosal lining. This lining continues the process of humidifying and warming inhaled air, as well as the trapping of foreign particles.

If you can read this aloud and cough, thank your larynx

The **larynx,** known as the voice box, connects the upper and lower airways. It contains vocal cords that produce sounds. The larynx also initiates the cough reflex, which is part of the respiratory system's defense mechanisms.

C-shaped connector

The **trachea** contains C-shaped cartilaginous rings composed of smooth muscle. It connects the larynx to the bronchi.

Branching into bronchi

The trachea branches into the right and left **bronchi,** the large air passages which lead to the right and left lungs. The right main bronchus is slightly larger and more vertical than the left.

As they pass into the lungs, the bronchi form smaller branches called **bronchioles,** which themselves branch into terminal bronchioles and alveoli.

Gas exchange center

Alveoli are clustered microscopic sacs enveloped by capillaries. It is over the millions of alveoli in the lungs that gas exchange occurs, as gases diffuse across the alveolar-capillary membrane. The alveoli also contain a coating of surfactant, which reduces surface tension and keeps them from collapsing.

Lobes: 3 and 2

As a unit, the lungs are composed of three **lobes** on the right side and two lobes on the left side. The lungs regulate air exchange by a concentration gradient. In the alveoli, gases move from an area of high concentration to an area of low concentration. Because the concentration of CO_2 is greater in the alveoli, it diffuses out into the lungs and is exhaled. Because the lungs contain a greater concentra-

(Text continues on page 77.)

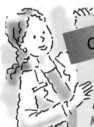

Cheat sheet

Respiratory refresher

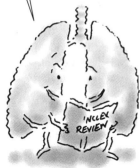

Because the major function of the respiratory system is gas exchange, focus on keeping airways clear and facilitating breathing.

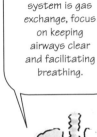

ACUTE RESPIRATORY FAILURE

Key signs and symptoms

- Decreased respiratory excursion, accessory muscle use, retractions
- Difficulty breathing, shortness of breath, dyspnea, tachypnea, orthopnea
- Fatigue

Key test results

- Arterial blood gas (ABG) levels show hypoxemia, acidosis, alkalosis, and hypercapnia.

Key treatments

- Oxygen (O_2) therapy, intubation, and mechanical ventilation (possibly with positive end-expiratory pressure [PEEP]).
- Analgesic: morphine sulfate
- Antianxiety agent: lorazepam (Ativan)
- Bronchodilators: terbutaline (Brethine), aminophylline (Aminophyllin), theophylline (Theo-Dur); via nebulizer: albuterol (Proventil), ipratropium bromide (Atrovent), metaproterenol sulfate (Alupent)
- Neuromuscular blocking agents: pancuronium bromide (Pavulon), vecuronium bromide (Norcuron), atracurium besylate (Tracrium)
- Steroids: hydrocortisone sodium succinate (Solu-Cortef), methylprednisolone sodium succinate (Solu-Medrol)

Key interventions

- Assess respiratory status.
- Administer O_2.
- Provide suctioning; assist with turning, coughing, and deep breathing; and perform chest physiotherapy and postural drainage.
- Maintain bed rest.

ADULT RESPIRATORY DISTRESS SYNDROME

Key signs and symptoms

- Anxiety, restlessness
- Crackles, rhonchi, decreased breath sounds
- Dyspnea, tachypnea

Key test results

- ABG levels show respiratory acidosis, metabolic acidosis, hypoxemia that doesn't respond to increased fraction of oxygen (F_{IO_2}).

- Chest X-ray shows bilateral infiltrates (in early stages) and lung fields with a ground-glass appearance and, with irreversible hypoxemia, massive consolidation of both lung fields (in later stages).

Key treatments

- Intubation and mechanical ventilation using PEEP or pressure-controlled inverse ratio ventilation
- Antibiotics, according to infectious organism
- Analgesic: morphine sulfate
- Neuromuscular blocking agents: pancuronium bromide (Pavulon), vecuronium bromide (Norcuron)
- Steroids: hydrocortisone (Solu-Cortef), methylprednisolone sodium succinate (Solu-Medrol)

Key interventions

- Assess respiratory, cardiovascular, and neurologic status.
- Maintain bed rest, with prone positioning if possible.
- Provide turning, chest physiotherapy, and postural drainage.

ASBESTOSIS

Key signs and symptoms

- Dry crackles at lung bases
- Dry cough
- Dyspnea on exertion (usually first symptom)
- Pleuritic chest pain

Key test results

- Chest X-rays show fine, irregular, and linear diffuse infiltrates; extensive fibrosis results in a "honeycomb" or "ground-glass" appearance. X-rays may also show pleural thickening and pleural calcification, with bilateral obliteration of costophrenic angles and, in later stages, an enlarged heart with a classic "shaggy" heart border.

Key treatments

- Chest physiotherapy
- Fluid intake: at least 3 L/day
- O_2 therapy or mechanical ventilator (in advanced cases)

Respiratory refresher *(continued)*

ASBESTOSIS *(continued)*
- Antibiotic therapy according to susceptibility of infecting organism (for treatment of respiratory tract infections)
- Mucolytic inhalation therapy: acetylcysteine (Mucomyst)

Key interventions
- Perform chest physiotherapy techniques, such as controlled coughing and segmental bronchial drainage, with chest percussion and vibration.
- Administer O_2 by cannula or mask (1 to 2 L/minute), or by mechanical ventilation if arterial oxygen can't be maintained above 40 mm Hg.

ASPHYXIA

Key signs and symptoms
- Agitation
- Altered respiratory rate (apnea, bradypnea, occasional tachypnea)
- Anxiety
- Central and peripheral cyanosis (cherry-red mucous membranes in late-stage carbon monoxide poisoning)
- Confusion leading to coma
- Decreased breath sounds
- Dyspnea

Key test results
- ABG measurement indicates decreased partial pressure of arterial oxygen (Pao_2) < 60 mm Hg) and increased partial pressure of arterial CO_2 ($Paco_2$) > 50 mm Hg.
- Pulse oximetry reveals decreased hemoglobin (Hb) saturation with oxygen.

Key treatments
- Bronchoscopy (for extraction of a foreign body)
- O_2 therapy, which may include endotracheal intubation and mechanical ventilation
- Narcotic antagonist: naloxone (for narcotic overdose)

Key interventions
- Assess cardiac and respiratory status.
- Position the patient upright, if patient's condition tolerates.
- Suction carefully, as needed, and encourage deep breathing.

ASTHMA

Key signs and symptoms
- Usually asymptomatic between attacks
- Wheezing, primarily on expiration but also sometimes on inspiration

Key test results
- Pulmonary function tests (PFTs) during attacks show decreased forced expiratory volumes that improve with therapy, and increased residual volume and total lung capacity.

Key treatments
- Fluids to 3,000 ml/day as tolerated
- Beta-adrenergic drugs: epinephrine hydrochloride (Adrenalin), salmeterol (Serevent)
- Bronchodilators: terbutaline (Brethine), aminophylline (Aminophyllin), theophylline (Theo-Dur); via nebulizer: albuterol (Proventil), ipratropium bromide (Atrovent), metaproterenol sulfate (Alupent)
- Respiratory inhalant: cromolyn sodium (Intal)

Key interventions
- Administer low-flow humidified O_2.
- Assess respiratory status.
- Keep the patient in high-Fowler's position.

ATELECTASIS

Key signs and symptoms
- Diminished or bronchial breath sounds
- Dyspnea
In severe cases
- Anxiety
- Cyanosis
- Diaphoresis
- Severe dyspnea
- Substernal or intercostal retraction
- Tachycardia

Key test results
- Chest X-ray shows characteristic horizontal lines in the lower lung zones and, with segmental or lobar collapse, characteristic dense shadows often associated with hyperinflation of neighboring lung zones (in widespread atelectasis).

Key treatments
- Bronchoscopy
- Chest physiotherapy
- Bronchodilators: albuterol (Proventil)
- Mucolytic inhalation therapy: acetylcysteine (Mucomyst)

Key interventions
- Encourage postoperative and other high-risk patients to cough and deep-breathe every 1 to 2 hours.
- Hold a pillow tightly over the incision; teach the patient this technique as well. Gently reposition these patients often and help them walk as soon as possible.
- Administer adequate analgesics.

(continued)

Respiratory refresher (continued)

ATELECTASIS (continued)

• Use an incentive spirometer. Teach the patient how to use the spirometer and encourage him to use it every 1 to 2 hours.
• Humidify inspired air and encourage adequate fluid intake. Use postural drainage and chest percussion.
• Assess breath sounds and ventilatory status frequently and be alert for any changes.

BRONCHIECTASIS

Key signs and symptoms

• Chronic cough that produces copious, foul-smelling, mucopurulent secretions, possibly totaling several cupfuls daily
• Coarse crackles during inspiration over involved lobes or segments
• Dyspnea
• Weight loss

Key test results

• Chest X-rays show peribronchial thickening, areas of atelectasis, and scattered cystic changes.
• Sputum culture and Gram stain identify predominant organisms.

Key treatments

• Bronchoscopy (to mobilize secretions)
• Chest physiotherapy
• O_2 therapy
• Antibiotics according to sensitivity of causative organism
• Bronchodilators such as albuterol (Proventil)

Key interventions

• Assess respiratory status.
• Provide supportive care and help the patient adjust to the permanent changes in lifestyle that irreversible lung damage necessitates.
• Perform chest physiotherapy, including postural drainage and chest percussion designed for involved lobes, several times a day. The best times to do this are early morning and just before bedtime. Instruct the patient to maintain each position for 10 minutes; then perform percussion and tell him to cough.

CHRONIC BRONCHITIS

Key signs and symptoms

• Dyspnea
• Increased sputum production
• Productive cough

Key test results

• Chest X-ray shows hyperinflation and increased bronchovascular markings.

• PFTs may reveal increased residual volume, decreased vital capacity and forced expiratory volumes, normal static compliance and diffusion capacity.

Key treatments

• Fluid intake up to 3,000 ml/day, if not contraindicated
• Intubation and mechanical ventilation if respiratory status deteriorates
• Antibiotics: according to sensitivity of infective organism
• Bronchodilators: terbutaline (Brethine), aminophylline (Aminophyllin), theophylline (Theo-Dur); via nebulizer: albuterol (Proventil), ipratropium bromide (Atrovent), metaproterenol sulfate (Alupent)
• Influenza and Pneumovax vaccine
• Steroids: hydrocortisone (Solu-Cortef), methylprednisolone sodium succinate (Solu-Medrol)
• Steroids (via nebulizer): beclomethasone (Vanceril), triamcinolone (Azmacort)

Key interventions

• Administer low-flow O_2.
• Assess respiratory status, ABGs, and pulse oximetry.
• Assist with diaphragmatic and pursed-lip breathing.
• Monitor and record the color, amount, and consistency of sputum.
• Provide chest physiotherapy, postural drainage, incentive spirometry, and suction.

COR PULMONALE

Key signs and symptoms

• Dyspnea on exertion
• Edema
• Fatigue
• Orthopnea
• Tachypnea
• Weakness

Key test results

• ABG analysis shows decreased $Pao_2 < 70$ mm Hg.
• Chest X-ray shows large central pulmonary arteries and suggests right ventricular enlargement by rightward enlargement of cardiac silhouette on an anterior chest film.
• Pulmonary artery pressure measurements show increased right ventricular and pulmonary artery pressures as a result of increased pulmonary vascular resistance.

Key treatments

• O_2 therapy by mask or cannula in concentrations ranging from 24% to 40%, depending on Pao_2, as necessary, and, in acute cases, mechanical ventilation

Respiratory refresher *(continued)*

COR PULMONALE *(continued)*
- Digitalis glycosides: digoxin (Lanoxin)
- Diuretic (to reduce edema): furosemide (Lasix)
- Vasodilators: diazoxide, hydralazine, nitroprusside, prostaglandins (in primary pulmonary hypertension)
- Calcium channel blockers such as diltiazem (Cardizem)
- Angiotensin-converting enzyme inhibitor, such as captopril (Capoten)

Key interventions
- Limit the patient's fluid intake to 1,000 to 2,000 ml/day and provide a low-sodium diet.
- Reposition bedridden patients often.
- Provide meticulous respiratory care, including O_2 therapy and, for patients with chronic obstructive pulmonary disease, pursed-lip breathing exercises.
- Periodically measure ABG levels and watch for signs of respiratory failure such as a change in pulse rate; deep, labored respirations; and increased fatigue produced by exertion.

EMPHYSEMA
Key signs and symptoms
- Barrel chest
- Dyspnea
- Pursed-lip breathing

Key test results
- Chest X-ray in advanced disease reveals a flattened diaphragm, reduced vascular markings in the lung periphery, enlarged anteroposterior chest diameter, and a vertical heart.
- PFTs show increased residual volume, total lung capacity, and compliance, as well as decreased vital capacity, diffusing capacity, and expiratory volumes.

Key treatments
- Chest physiotherapy, postural drainage, and incentive spirometry
- Fluid intake up to 3,000 ml/day, if not contraindicated by heart failure
- O_2 therapy at 2 to 3 L/minute, transtracheal therapy for home O_2 therapy
- Antibiotics: according to sensitivity of infective organism
- Bronchodilators: terbutaline (Brethine), aminophylline (Aminophyllin), theophylline (Theo-Dur); via nebulizer: albuterol (Proventil), ipratropium bromide (Atrovent), metaproterenol sulfate (Alupent)
- Influenza and Pneumovax vaccine

- Steroids: hydrocortisone (Solu-Cortef), methylprednisolone sodium succinate (Solu-Medrol)
- Steroids (via nebulizer): beclomethasone (Vanceril), triamcinolone (Azmacort)

Key interventions
- Assess respiratory status, ABGs, and pulse oximetry.
- Assist with diaphragmatic and pursed-lip breathing.
- Monitor and record the color, amount, and consistency of sputum.
- Provide chest physiotherapy, postural drainage, incentive spirometry, and suction.

LEGIONNAIRES' DISEASE
Key signs and symptoms
- Cough, initially nonproductive, that eventually produces grayish, nonpurulent, blood-streaked sputum
- Fever
- Generalized weakness
- Malaise
- Recurrent chills

Key test results
- Chest X-ray shows patchy, localized infiltration, which progresses to multilobar consolidation (usually involving the lower lobes), pleural effusion and, in fulminant disease, opacification of the entire lung.
- Direct immunofluorescence of *Legionella pneumophila* and indirect fluorescent serum antibody testing compares findings from initial blood studies with findings from those done at least 3 weeks later. A convalescent serum sample showing a fourfold or greater rise in antibody titer for *L. pneumophila* confirms the diagnosis.

Key treatments
- Antibiotic: erythromycin (Erythrocin), rifampin (Rifadin), tetracycline (Achromycin V)
- Antipyretics: acetaminophen (Tylenol), aspirin

Key interventions
- Closely monitor the patient's respiratory status. Evaluate chest wall expansion, depth and pattern of respirations, cough, and chest pain.
- Continually monitor the patient's vital signs, pulse oximetry or arterial blood gas values, level of consciousness, and dryness and color of the lips and mucous membranes. Watch for signs of shock (decreased blood pressure, thready pulse, diaphoresis, clammy skin).
- Replace fluid and electrolytes as needed. The patient with renal failure may require dialysis.

(continued)

Respiratory refresher (continued)

LEGIONNAIRES' DISEASE (continued)

• Provide mechanical ventilation and other respiratory therapy as needed.
• Give antibiotics as necessary, and observe carefully for adverse effects.

LUNG CANCER

Key signs and symptoms

• Cough, hemoptysis
• Weight loss, anorexia

Key test results

• Chest X-ray shows lesion or mass.

Key treatments

• Resection of the affected lobe (lobectomy) or lung (pneumonectomy)
• Antineoplastics: cyclophosphamide (Cytoxan), doxorubicin hydrochloride (Adriamycin), cisplatin (Platinol), vincristine (Oncovin)

Key interventions

• Assess the patient's pain and administer analgesics, as prescribed.
• Provide suctioning and assist with turning, coughing, and deep breathing.
• Monitor for bleeding, infection, and electrolyte imbalance due to effects of chemotherapy.

PLEURAL EFFUSION AND EMPYEMA

Key signs and symptoms

• Decreased breath sounds
• Dyspnea
• Fever
• Pleuritic chest pain

Key test results

• Chest X-ray shows radiopaque fluid in dependent regions.
• Thoracentesis shows lactate dehydrogenase (LD) levels less than 200 IU and protein levels less than 3 g/dl (in transudative effusions); ratio of protein in pleural fluid to serum greater than or equal to 0.5, LD in pleural fluid greater than or equal to 200 IU, and ratio of LD in pleural fluid to LD in serum greater than 0.6 (in exudative effusions); and acute inflammatory white blood cells and microorganisms (in empyema).

Key treatments

• Thoracentesis (to remove fluid)
• Thoracotomy if thoracentesis isn't effective
• Antibiotics (for empyema) according to sensitivity of causative organism

Key interventions

• Explain thoracentesis to the patient. Before the procedure, tell the patient to expect a stinging sensation from the local anesthetic and a feeling of pressure when the needle is inserted.
• Instruct the patient to tell you immediately if he feels uncomfortable or has trouble breathing during the procedure.
• Administer O_2.
• Administer antibiotics.
• Provide meticulous chest tube care, and use aseptic technique for changing dressings around the tube insertion site in empyema.
• Ensure chest tube patency by watching for bubbles in the underwater seal chamber.
• Record the amount, color, and consistency of any tube drainage.

PLEURISY

Key signs and symptoms

• Pleural friction rub (a coarse, creaky sound heard during late inspiration and early expiration)
• Sharp, stabbing pain that increases with respiration

Key test results

• Although diagnosis generally rests on the patient's history and the nurse's respiratory assessment, diagnostic tests help rule out other causes and pinpoint the underlying disorder.

Key treatments

• Bed rest
• Analgesics such as acetaminophen with oxycodone (Percocet)
• Anti-inflammatories such as indomethacin (Indocin)

Key interventions

• Stress the importance of bed rest and plan care to allow the patient as much uninterrupted rest as possible.
• Administer antitussives and pain medication as necessary.
• Encourage the patient to cough. Apply firm pressure at the pain site during coughing exercises.

PNEUMOCYSTIS CARINII PNEUMONIA

Key signs and symptoms

• Generalized fatigue
• Low-grade, intermittent fever
• Nonproductive cough
• Shortness of breath
• Weight loss

Respiratory refresher (continued)

PNEUMOCYSTIS CARINII PNEUMONIA *(continued)*

Key test results

- Chest X-ray may show slowly progressing, fluffy infiltrates and occasionally nodular lesions or a spontaneous pneumothorax, but these findings must be differentiated from findings in other types of pneumonia or adult respiratory distress syndrome.
- Histologic studies confirm *P. carinii.* In patients with human immunodeficincy virus (HIV) infection, initial examination of a first morning sputum specimen (induced by inhaling an ultrasonically dispersed saline mist) may be sufficient; however, this technique is usually ineffective in patients without HIV infection.

Key treatments

- O_2 therapy, which may include endotracheal intubation and mechanical ventilation

Key interventions

- Frequently assess the patient's respiratory status, and monitor ABG levels every 4 hours.
- Administer O_2 therapy as necessary. Encourage the patient to ambulate and to perform deep-breathing exercises and incentive spirometry.
- Administer antipyretics, as required.
- Monitor intake and output and daily weight. Replace fluids as necessary.
- Give antimicrobial drugs as required. Never give pentamidine I.V. Administer the I.V. drug form slowly over 60 minutes.
- Monitor the patient for adverse reactions to antimicrobial drugs. If he's receiving cotrimoxazole, watch for nausea, vomiting, rash, bone marrow suppression, thrush, fever, hepatotoxicity, and anaphylaxis. If he's receiving pentamidine, watch for cardiac arrhythmias, hypotension, dizziness, azotemia, hypocalcemia, and hepatic disturbances.
- Supply nutritional supplements as needed. Encourage the patient to eat a high-calorie, protein-rich diet. Offer small, frequent meals if the patient can't tolerate large amounts of food.

PNEUMONIA

Key signs and symptoms

- Chills, fever
- Crackles, rhonchi, pleural friction rub on auscultation
- Shortness of breath, dyspnea, tachypnea, accessory muscle use
- Sputum production that is rusty, green, or bloody with pneumococcal pneumonia; yellow-green with bronchopneumonia

Key test results

- Chest X-ray shows pulmonary infiltrates.
- Sputum study identifies organism.

Key treatments

- Antibiotics: according to organism sensitivity

Key interventions

- Monitor and record intake and output.
- Monitor laboratory studies.
- Monitor pulse oximetry.
- Assess respiratory status.
- Force fluids to 3 to 4 L/day and administer I.V. fluids.

PNEUMOTHORAX AND HEMOTHORAX

Key signs and symptoms

- Diminished or absent breath sounds unilaterally
- Dyspnea, tachypnea, subcutaneous emphysema, cough
- Sharp pain that increases with exertion

Key test results

- Chest X-ray reveals pneumothorax or hemothorax.

Key treatments

- Chest tube to water-seal drainage

Key interventions

- Monitor and record vital signs.
- Assess respiratory status.
- Monitor chest tube drainage.
- Assess cardiovascular status.
- Maintain chest tube to water-seal drainage. The water seal chamber prevents air from entering the chest tube when the patient inhales.

PULMONARY EMBOLISM

Key signs and symptoms

- Sudden onset of dyspnea, tachypnea, crackles

Key test results

- ABG levels show respiratory alkalosis and hypoxemia.
- Lung scan shows $\dot{V}/\dot{Q}$ mismatch.

Key treatments

- Vena cava filter insertion
- Anticoagulants: heparin (Liquaemin Sodium), warfarin (Coumadin)
- Fibrinolytics: streptokinase (Streptase), urokinase (Abbokinase)

Key interventions

- Assess respiratory status.
- Assess cardiovascular status.
- Administer O_2.

(continued)

Respiratory refresher (continued)

RESPIRATORY ACIDOSIS

Key signs and symptoms
• Cardiovascular abnormalities such as tachycardia, hypertension, atrial and ventricular arrhythmias and, in severe acidosis, hypotension with vasodilation

Key test results
• ABG measurements confirm respiratory acidosis. $Paco_2$ exceeds the normal level of 45 mm Hg and pH is usually below the normal range of 7.35 to 7.45. The patient's bicarbonate level is normal in the acute stage and elevated in the chronic stage.

Key treatments
• Sodium bicarbonate in severe cases

Key interventions
• Closely monitor the patient's blood pH level.
• Be alert for critical changes in the patient's respiratory, central nervous system (CNS), and cardiovascular functions. Also watch closely for variations in ABG values and electrolyte status. Maintain adequate hydration.
• If acidosis requires mechanical ventilation, maintain a patent airway and provide adequate humidification. Perform tracheal suctioning regularly and vigorous chest physiotherapy if needed. Continuously monitor ventilator settings and respiratory status.

RESPIRATORY ALKALOSIS

Key signs and symptoms
• Agitation
• Cardiac arrhythmias that fail to respond to conventional treatment (severe respiratory alkalosis)
• Circumoral or peripheral paresthesias (a prickling sensation around the mouth or extremities)
• Deep, rapid breathing, possibly exceeding 40 breaths/minute (cardinal sign)
• Light-headedness or dizziness (from decreased cerebral blood flow)

Key test results
• ABG analysis confirms respiratory alkalosis and rules out respiratory compensation for metabolic acidosis. $Paco_2$ is below 35 mm Hg and pH is elevated in proportion to the fall in $Paco_2$ in the acute stage but drops toward normal in the chronic stage. Bicarbonate level is normal in the acute stage but below normal in the chronic stage.

Key treatments
• Having the patient breathe into a paper bag, which helps relieve acute anxiety and increases CO_2 levels (for severe respiratory alkalosis)

Key interventions
• Watch for and report any changes in neurologic, neuromuscular, or cardiovascular functions.
• Remember that twitching and cardiac arrhythmias may be associated with alkalemia and electrolyte imbalances. Monitor ABG and serum electrolyte levels closely, watching for any variations.

SARCOIDOSIS

Key signs and symptoms
Initial signs
• Arthralgia (in the wrists, ankles, and elbows)
• Fatigue
• Malaise
• Weight loss
Respiratory
• Breathlessness
• Substernal pain
Cutaneous
• Erythema nodosum
• Subcutaneous skin nodules with maculopapular eruptions
Ophthalmic
• Anterior uveitis (common)
Musculoskeletal
• Muscle weakness
• Pain
Hepatic
• Granulomatous hepatitis (usually asymptomatic)
Genitourinary
• Hypercalciuria (excessive calcium in the urine)
Cardiovascular
• Arrhythmias (premature beats, bundle branch block, or complete heart block)
Central nervous system
• Cranial or peripheral nerve palsies
• Basilar meningitis (inflammation of the meninges at the base of the brain)

Key test results
• A positive Kveim-Siltzbach skin test supports the diagnosis. In this test, the patient receives an intradermal injection of an antigen prepared from human sarcoidal spleen or lymph nodes from patients with sarcoidosis. If the patient has active sarcoidosis, granuloma develops at the injection site in 2 to 6 weeks. This reaction is considered positive when a biopsy of the skin at the injection site shows discrete epithelioid cell granuloma.

Respiratory refresher (continued)

SARCOIDOSIS (continued)

Key treatments

• A low-calcium diet and avoiding direct exposure to sunlight (in patients with hypercalcemia)
• O_2 therapy
• Systemic or topical steroid, if sarcoidosis causes ocular, respiratory, CNS, cardiac, or systemic symptoms (such as fever and weight loss), hypercalcemia, or destructive skin lesions

Key interventions

• Provide a nutritious, high-calorie diet and plenty of fluids. If the patient has hypercalcemia, suggest a low-calcium diet. Weigh the patient regularly.

TUBERCULOSIS

Key signs and symptoms

• Fever
• Night sweats

Key test results

• Mantoux skin test is positive.
• Sputum study is positive for acid-fast bacillus and *Mycobacterium tuberculosis*.

Key treatments

• Standard and airborne precautions (While the patient is contagious, everyone entering the patient's room must wear a respirator with a high-efficiency particulate air filter.)
• Antituberculars: isoniazid (INH), ethambutol (Myambutol), rifampin (Rifadin), pyrazinamide (Pyrazinamide)

Key interventions

• Maintain infection control precautions.
• Instruct the patient to cover nose and mouth when sneezing.
• Provide a negative pressure room.

---

tion of O_2, O_2 diffuses out of the lungs and into the alveoli, to be carried to the rest of the body.

A pleur-ality of coverings

Pleura refers to the membrane covering the lungs and lining the thoracic cavity. The pleura covering the lungs is known as the visceral pleura, while the parietal pleura lines the thoracic cavity. Pleural fluid lubricates the pleura to reduce friction during respiration.

Keep abreast of diagnostic tests

Here are the most important tests used to diagnose respiratory disorders, along with common nursing interventions associated with each test.

Deep, direct visualization

In **bronchoscopy,** a doctor uses a bronchoscope to directly visualize the trachea and bronchial tree. During a bronchoscopy, the doctor may take biopsies and perform deep tracheal suctioning.

Nursing actions

Before the procedure:
• withhold food and fluids for 6 to 12 hours, if possible
• make sure that a written, informed consent has been obtained.
   After the procedure:
• check cough and gag reflex to minimize the risk of aspiration
• assess sputum
• assess respiratory status
• withhold food and fluids until gag reflex returns
• monitor during and after the procedure for bradycardia, which may be caused by a vasovagal response.

Looking in from the outside

A **chest X-ray** produces a radiographic picture of lung tissue. It can detect tumors, inflammation, air, and fluid in and around the

After any invasive test involving the airway — like bronchoscopy — assess respiratory status to ensure the patient's safety.

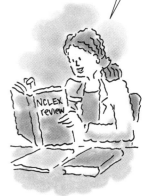

lung. It can also be used to monitor equipment such as catheters and chest tubes.

Nursing actions
• Determine the patient's ability to inhale and hold his breath.
• Make sure that the patient removes jewelry before the X-ray is taken.

Dye-ing to see the lungs
In **pulmonary angiography,** the patient receives an injection of a radiopaque dye through a catheter. This provides a radiographic picture of pulmonary circulation.

Nursing actions
Before the procedure:
• note the patient's allergies to iodine, seafood, and radiopaque dyes
• withhold food and fluids for 8 hours
• make sure that a written, informed consent has been obtained
• instruct the patient about possible flushing of the face or burning in the throat after dye is injected.
  After the procedure:
• assess peripheral neurovascular status
• check the insertion site for bleeding
• avoid taking blood pressure measurements in the extremity used for dye injection for 24 hours after the procedure.

Sensitive about sputum
A **sputum study** is a laboratory test that provides a microscopic evaluation of sputum, evaluating it for culture and sensitivity, Gram stain, and acid-fast bacillus.

Nursing actions
• Obtain an early-morning sterile specimen from suctioning or expectoration.
• Make sure that the specimen is truly sputum and not saliva before sending the specimen to the laboratory.

Focusing on intrapleural fluid
Thoracentesis uses a needle to obtain a sample of intrapleural fluid to determine the cause of infection or empyema. It's performed using local anesthesia.

Patients allergic to iodine and seafood are at risk for reactions in any test involving radiopaque dyes.

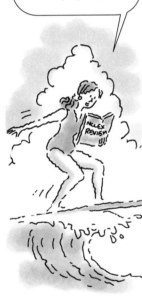

Nursing actions
Before the procedure:
• make sure that a written, informed consent has been obtained
• reassure the patient
• place the patient in the proper position (either sitting on the edge of the bed or, if the patient is unable to sit up, on his unaffected side with the arm of his affected side raised above his head; elevate the head of the bed 30 to 45 degrees, if possible).
  After the procedure:
• assess the patient's respiratory status
• monitor vital signs frequently
• position the patient on the affected side, as ordered, for at least 1 hour to seal the puncture site
• check the puncture site for fluid leakage.

Finding out about lung function
Pulmonary function tests (PFTs) are non-invasive tests that measure lung volume, ventilation, and diffusing capacity using a spirometer. The client is asked to breathe through a mouthpiece following specific directions. A computer then calculates the volumes.

Nursing actions
• Instruct the patient to refrain from smoking or eating a heavy meal 4 to 6 hours before testing.
• Document bronchodilators or narcotics used before testing.

From the artery to the lab
Arterial blood gas (ABG) analysis is a laboratory test that assesses the arterial blood for tissue oxygenation, ventilation, and acid-base status.

Nursing actions
Before the procedure:
• note the patient's temperature
• document O_2 and assisted mechanical ventilation used.
  After the procedure:
• apply pressure to the site for at least 5 minutes
• assess the puncture site for bleeding

• maintain a pressure dressing for at least 30 minutes.

Image through inhalation or injection

A **lung scan,** or ventilation/perfusion scan (V̇/Q̇ scan), uses visual inhalation or I.V. injection of radioisotopes to create an image of blood flow in the lungs.

Nursing actions
• Make sure that a written, informed consent has been obtained.
• Instruct the patient to remove all metal objects before the procedure.
• Determine the patient's ability to lie still for about 1 hour during procedure.
• Check the catheter insertion site for bleeding after the procedure.

TB or not TB?

In the **Mantoux intradermal skin test,** the patient receives an injection of tuberculin to detect tuberculosis (TB) antibodies.

Nursing actions
• Document current dermatitis or rashes.
• Document history of positive results in past skin testing or exposure to bacille Calmette-Guérin immunization.
• Circle and record test site.
• Note date for follow-up reading (48 to 72 hours after injection).

Let's look at the larynx

Laryngoscopy uses a laryngoscope to directly visualize the larynx.

Nursing actions
Before the procedure:
• make sure that a written, informed consent has been obtained
• withhold food or fluids for 6 to 8 hours
• explain that the patient will receive a sedative to promote relaxation.
   After the procedure:
• assess respiratory status
• allay the patient's anxiety
• withhold food and fluids until gag reflex returns.

Little bit of lung tissue

A **lung biopsy** involves the removal of a small amount of lung tissue for histologic evaluation. Lung biopsy may be done by surgical exposure of the lung (open biopsy) or with endoscopy using a needle designed to remove a core of lung tissue.

Nursing actions
Before the procedure:
• withhold food and fluids for 8 hours
• make sure that a written, informed consent has been obtained.
   After the procedure:
• monitor and record vital signs
• assess respiratory status (checking for signs of pneumothorax, air embolism, hemoptysis, and hemorrhage)
• check the incision site for bleeding.

Analyzing blood, part A

A **hematologic study** uses a blood sample to analyze red blood cells (RBCs), white blood cells (WBCs), prothrombin time (PT), international normalized ratio (INR), partial thromboplastin time (PTT), erythrocyte sedimentation rate (ESR), platelets, hemoglobin (Hb), and hematocrit (HCT).

Nursing actions
• Note current drug therapy before the procedure.
• Check the venipuncture site for bleeding after the procedure.

Analyzing blood, part B

A **blood chemistry test** assesses a blood sample for potassium, sodium, calcium, phosphorus, glucose, bicarbonate, blood urea nitrogen, creatinine, protein, albumin, osmolality, and alpha$_1$-antitrypsin.

Nursing actions
• Withhold food and fluids before the procedure, as directed.
• Check the site for bleeding after the procedure.

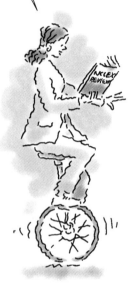

Time to switch gears. Now that you're familiar with diagnostic tests, get ready to review common disorders.

Polish up on patient care

Major respiratory disorders include acute respiratory failure, adult respiratory distress syndrome, asbestosis, asphyxia, asthma, atelectasis, bronchiectasis, chronic bronchitis, cor pulmonale, emphysema, Legionnaires' disease, lung cancer, pleural effusion and empyema, pleurisy, *Pneumocystis carinii* pneumonia, pneumonia, pneumothorax and hemothorax, pulmonary embolism, respiratory acidosis, respiratory alkalosis, sarcoidosis, and tuberculosis.

Acute respiratory failure

In acute respiratory failure, the respiratory system can't adequately supply the body with the O_2 it needs or adequately remove CO_2. A patient is considered to be in respiratory failure when the partial pressure of arterial oxygen (Pao_2) is less than or equal to 50 mm Hg or the partial pressure of arterial carbon dioxide ($Paco_2$) is greater than or equal to 50 mm Hg with a pH of less than or equal to 7.25.

Acute respiratory failure can be classified as ventilatory failure or oxygenation failure. Ventilatory failure is characterized by alveolar hypoventilation. Oxygenation failure is characterized by ventilation-perfusion mismatching (blood flow to areas of the lung with reduced ventilation, or ventilation to lung tissue that's experiencing reduced blood flow) or physiologic shunting (blood moving from the right side of the heart to the left without being oxygenated).

CAUSES
- Abdominal or thoracic surgery
- Adult respiratory distress syndrome
- Anesthesia
- Atelectasis
- Brain tumors
- Cerebrovascular accidents
- Chronic obstructive pulmonary disease
- Drug overdose
- Encephalitis

- Flail chest
- Guillain-Barré syndrome
- Head trauma
- Hemothorax
- Meningitis
- Multiple sclerosis
- Muscular dystrophy
- Myasthenia gravis
- Pleural effusion
- Pneumonia
- Pneumothorax
- Poliomyelitis
- Polyneuritis
- Pulmonary edema
- Pulmonary embolism

ASSESSMENT FINDINGS
- Adventitious breath sounds (crackles, rhonchi, wheezing, and pleural friction rub)
- Change in mentation, anxiety
- Chest pain
- Cough, sputum production, hemoptysis
- Cyanosis, diaphoresis
- Decreased respiratory excursion, accessory muscle use, retractions
- Difficulty breathing, shortness of breath, dyspnea, tachypnea, orthopnea
- Fatigue
- Nasal flaring
- Tachycardia

DIAGNOSTIC TEST RESULTS
- ABG levels show hypoxemia, acidosis, alkalosis, and hypercapnia.
- Chest X-ray shows pulmonary infiltrates, interstitial edema, and atelectasis.
- Hematology reveals increased WBCs and ESR.
- Lung scan shows $\dot{V}/\dot{Q}$ ratio mismatches.
- Sputum study identifies organism.

NURSING DIAGNOSES
- Ineffective airway clearance
- Anxiety
- Ineffective breathing pattern

TREATMENT
- Chest physiotherapy, postural drainage (position the patient prone or supine with the foot of the bed elevated higher than the head for postural drainage), incentive spirometry

• Chest tube insertion if pneumothorax develops from high positive end-expiratory pressure (PEEP) administration
• Dietary changes including establishing a high-calorie, high-protein diet, and restricting or forcing fluids depending on cause of disorder
• O_2 therapy, intubation, and mechanical ventilation (possibly with PEEP)

Drug therapy
• Analgesic: morphine sulfate
• Antianxiety agent: lorazepam (Ativan)
• Antibiotics: according to sensitivity of causative organism
• Anticoagulants: heparin sodium (Liquaemin Sodium), warfarin (Coumadin)
• Bronchodilators: terbutaline (Brethine), aminophylline (Aminophyllin), theophylline (Theo-Dur); via nebulizer: albuterol (Proventil), ipratropium bromide (Atrovent), metaproterenol sulfate (Alupent)
• Diuretics such as furosemide (Lasix) if fluid overload is the cause
• Histamine-2 blockers: famotidine (Pepcid), ranitidine (Zantac), cimetidine (Tagamet), nizatidine (Axid)
• Neuromuscular blocking agents: pancuronium bromide (Pavulon), vecuronium bromide (Norcuron), atracurium besylate (Tracrium)
• Steroids: hydrocortisone sodium succinate (Solu-Cortef), methylprednisolone sodium succinate (Solu-Medrol)

INTERVENTIONS AND RATIONALES
• Assess respiratory status *to detect early signs of compromise and hypoxemia.*
• Monitor and record intake and output *to detect fluid volume excess, which may lead to pulmonary edema.*
• Track laboratory values. Report deteriorating ABGs, such as a fall in Pao_2 levels and rise in $Paco_2$ levels. *Low Hb and HCT levels reduce oxygen-carrying capacity of the blood. Electrolyte abnormalities may result from use of diuretics.*
• Monitor pulse oximetry *to detect a drop in arterial oxygen saturation (Sao_2).*
• Monitor and record vital signs. *Tachycardia and tachypnea may indicate hypoxemia.*

• Monitor and record color, consistency, and amount of sputum *to determine hydration status, effectiveness of therapy, and presence of infection.*
• Administer O_2 *to reduce hypoxemia and relieve respiratory distress.*
• Monitor mechanical ventilation *to prevent complications and optimize Pao_2.*
• Provide suctioning; assist with turning, coughing, and deep breathing; and perform chest physiotherapy and postural drainage *to facilitate removal of secretions.*
• Maintain bed rest *to reduce O_2 requirement.*
• Keep the patient in semi- or high-Fowler's position *to promote chest expansion and ventilation.*
• Maintain diet restrictions. *Fluid restrictions and a low-sodium diet may be necessary to avoid fluid overload.*
• Administer medications, as prescribed, *to treat infection, dilate airways, and reduce inflammation.*
• Monitor chest tube system *to assess for lung re-expansion.*

Teaching topics
• Recognizing the early signs and symptoms of respiratory difficulty
• Performing deep-breathing and coughing exercises

Adult respiratory distress syndrome

In adult respiratory distress syndrome (ARDS), fluid builds up in the lungs and causes them to stiffen. This impairs breathing, thereby reducing the amount of O_2 in the capillaries that supply the lungs. When severe, the syndrome can cause an unmanageable and ultimately fatal lack of O_2. However, people who recover may have little or no permanent lung damage.

CAUSES
• Aspiration
• Decreased surfactant production
• Fat emboli
• Fluid overload

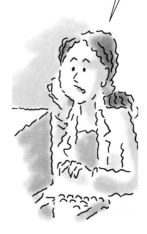

The patient exhibits adventitious breath sounds and reports feeling "tired of breathing." It could be acute respiratory failure.

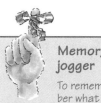

Memory jogger

To remember what happens in ARDS, use this mnemonic.

Assault to the pulmonary system

Respiratory distress

Decreased lung compliance

Severe respiratory failure

- Neurologic injuries
- O_2 toxicity
- Respiratory infection
- Sepsis
- Shock
- Trauma

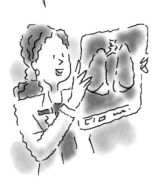

Chest X-ray reveals the different stages of ARDS.

ASSESSMENT FINDINGS
- Anxiety, restlessness
- Cough
- Crackles, rhonchi, decreased breath sounds
- Cyanosis
- Dyspnea, tachypnea

DIAGNOSTIC TEST RESULTS
- ABG levels show respiratory acidosis, metabolic acidosis, and hypoxemia that doesn't respond to increased fraction of inspired oxygen (FIO_2).
- Blood culture shows infectious organism.
- Chest X-ray shows bilateral infiltrates (in early stages) and lung fields with a ground-glass appearance and, with irreversible hypoxemia, massive consolidation of both lung fields (in later stages).
- Sputum study reveals the infectious organism.

NURSING DIAGNOSES
- Impaired gas exchange
- Ineffective breathing pattern
- Altered tissue perfusion (cardiopulmonary)

TREATMENT
- Bed rest with prone positioning, if possible; passive range-of-motion exercises
- Chest physiotherapy, postural drainage, and suction
- Dietary changes including restricting fluid intake or, if intubated, nothing by mouth
- Extracorporeal membrane oxygenation, if available

Patients with ARDS should be kept in a prone position.

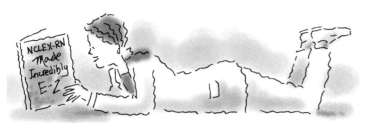

- Intubation and mechanical ventilation using PEEP or pressure-controlled inverse ratio ventilation
- O_2 therapy
- Transfusion therapy: platelets, packed RBCs

Drug therapy
- Analgesic: morphine sulfate
- Antacid: aluminum hydroxide gel (AlternaGEL)
- Antibiotics: according to infectious organism sensitivity
- Anticoagulant: heparin sodium (Liquaemin Sodium)
- Diuretics: furosemide (Lasix), ethacrynic acid (Edecrin)
- Exogenous surfactant: beractant (Survanta)
- Mucosal barrier fortifier: sucralfate (Carafate)
- Neuromuscular blocking agents: pancuronium bromide (Pavulon), vecuronium bromide (Norcuron)
- Steroids: hydrocortisone (Solu-Cortef), methylprednisolone sodium succinate (Solu-Medrol)

INTERVENTIONS AND RATIONALES
- Assess respiratory, cardiovascular, and neurologic status *to detect evidence of hypoxemia, such as tachycardia, tachypnea, and irritability.*
- Monitor pulse oximetry continuously *to determine the effectiveness of therapy.*
- Monitor laboratory studies. *A drop in Hb and HCT affects oxygen-carrying capacity of the blood. An increase in WBC count suggests an infection such as pneumonia. To detect disseminated intravascular coagulation (DIC), a complication of ARDS, monitor platelets, fibrinogen level, PT, and PTT.*
- Monitor and record intake and output and central venous pressure (CVP) *to determine fluid status and hemodynamic variables.*
- Monitor mechanical ventilation (high PEEP leaves the patient at risk for pneumothorax) *to increase PaO_2 without raising FIO_2, thereby reducing risk of O_2 toxicity* and provide suction, as necessary, *to aid in removal of secretions.*
- Maintain bed rest, with prone positioning, if possible, *to promote oxygenation.*

- Maintain fluid restrictions *to reduce fluid volume overload.*
- Provide turning, chest physiotherapy, and postural drainage *to promote drainage and keep airways clear.*
- Keep the patient in high-Fowler's position *to promote chest expansion.*
- Administer total parenteral nutrition or enteral feedings, as appropriate, *to prevent respiratory muscle impairment and maintain nutritional status.*
- Administer medications, as prescribed, *to optimize respiratory and hemodynamic status.*
- Organize nursing care *to allow rest periods to conserve energy, and avoid overexertion and fatigue.*
- Weigh the patient daily *to detect fluid retention.*
- Encourage the patient to express feelings about fear of suffocation *to reduce anxiety and, therefore, O_2 demands.*

Teaching topics
- Recognizing the signs and symptoms of respiratory distress
- Performing deep-breathing and coughing exercises
- Avoiding exposure to chemical irritants and pollutants

Asbestosis

Asbestosis is characterized by widespread filling and inflammation of lung spaces with asbestos fibers.

In asbestosis, asbestos fibers assume a longitudinal orientation in the airway, move in the direction of airflow, and penetrate respiratory bronchioles and alveolar walls. This causes diffuse interstitial fibrosis (tissue is filled with fibers).

Asbestosis can develop as long as 15 to 20 years after regular exposure to asbestos has ended. It increases the risk of lung cancer in cigarette smokers.

CAUSES
- Inhalation of asbestos fibers

ASSESSMENT FINDINGS
- Cor pulmonale
- Dry crackles at lung bases
- Dry cough
- Dyspnea on exertion (usually first symptom)
- Dyspnea at rest (in advanced disease)
- Finger clubbing
- Pleuritic chest pain
- Pulmonary hypertension
- Recurrent respiratory infections
- Right ventricular hypertrophy
- Tachypnea

DIAGNOSTIC TEST RESULTS
- ABG gas analysis reveals decreased Pao_2 and low $Paco_2$.
- Chest X-rays show fine, irregular, and linear diffuse infiltrates; extensive fibrosis results in a "honeycomb" or "ground-glass" appearance. X-rays may also show pleural thickening and pleural calcification, with bilateral obliteration of costophrenic angles and, in later stages, an enlarged heart with a classic "shaggy" heart border.
- PFTs show decreased vital capacity, forced vital capacity, and total lung capacity and reduced diffusing capacity of the lungs.

NURSING DIAGNOSES
- Altered nutrition: Less than body requirements
- Fatigue
- Impaired gas exchange

TREATMENT
- Chest physiotherapy
- Fluid intake: at least 3 L/day
- O_2 therapy or mechanical ventilation (in advanced cases)

Drug therapy
- Antibiotics: according to susceptibility of infecting organism (for treatment of respiratory tract infections)
- Digitalis glycoside: digoxin (Lanoxin)
- Diuretic: furosemide (Lasix)
- Mucolytic inhalation therapy: acetylcysteine (Mucomyst)

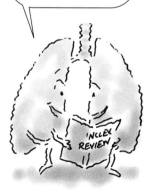

Filled and inflamed with asbestos fibers!

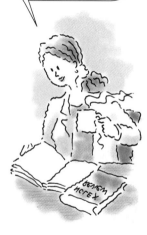

Because asbestosis can't be cured, patient care focuses on relieving respiratory symptoms and controlling complications.

INTERVENTIONS AND RATIONALES

• Chest physiotherapy techniques, such as controlled coughing and segmental bronchial drainage, with chest percussion and vibration *to relieve respiratory symptoms*. Aerosol therapy, inhaled mucolytics, and increased fluid intake (at least 3 qt [3 L] daily) *may also help relieve respiratory symptoms*.

• Administer diuretics and digitalis glycoside preparations for patients with cor pulmonale *to treat dyspnea, tachycardia, and dependent edema*.

• Administer O_2 by cannula or mask (1 to 2 L/minute), or by mechanical ventilation if Pao_2 can't be maintained above 40 mm Hg *to prevent complications of hypoxemia*.

• Prompt administration of antibiotics is required for respiratory infections *to prevent complications such as sepsis*.

Teaching topics

• Preventing infections by avoiding crowds, avoiding persons with infections, and receiving influenza and pneumococcal vaccines

Asphyxia

In asphyxia, interference with respiration leads to insufficient O_2 and accumulating CO_2 in the blood and tissues. Asphyxia leads to cardiopulmonary arrest and is fatal without prompt treatment.

CAUSES

• Extrapulmonary obstruction, such as tracheal compression from a tumor, strangulation, trauma, or suffocation

• Hypoventilation as a result of narcotic abuse, medullary disease, hemorrhage, pneumothorax, respiratory muscle paralysis, or cardiopulmonary arrest

• Inhalation of toxic agents, such as carbon monoxide poisoning, smoke inhalation, and excessive O_2 inhalation

• Intrapulmonary obstruction, such as airway obstruction, severe asthma, foreign body aspiration, pulmonary edema, pneumonia, and near-drowning

ASSESSMENT FINDINGS

• Agitation

• Altered respiratory rate (apnea, bradypnea, occasional tachypnea)

• Anxiety

• Central and peripheral cyanosis (cherry-red mucous membranes in late-stage carbon monoxide poisoning)

• Confusion leading to coma

• Decreased breath sounds

• Dyspnea

• Fast, slow, or absent pulse

• Seizures

DIAGNOSTIC TEST RESULTS

• ABG measurement indicates decreased Pao_2 (< 60 mm Hg) and increased $Paco_2$ (> 50 mm Hg).

• Chest X-rays may show a foreign body, pulmonary edema, or atelectasis.

• PFTs may indicate respiratory muscle weakness.

• Pulse oximetry reveals decreased Hb saturation of O_2.

• Toxicology tests may show drugs, chemicals, or abnormal Hb.

NURSING DIAGNOSES

• Impaired gas exchange

• Inability to sustain spontaneous ventilation

• Risk for suffocation

TREATMENT

• Bronchoscopy (for extraction of a foreign body)

• Gastric lavage (for poisoning)

• O_2 therapy, which may include endotracheal intubation and mechanical ventilation

Drug therapy

• Narcotic antagonist: naloxone (for narcotic overdose)

INTERVENTIONS AND RATIONALES

• Assess cardiac and respiratory status *to detect early signs of compromise*.

• Position the patient upright, if patient's condition tolerates, *to promote lung expansion and improve oxygenation*.

Gasp. In asphyxia, patient care focuses on treating the cause and providing me with oxygen.

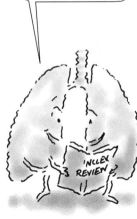

• Reassure the patient during treatment *to ease anxiety associated with respiratory distress.*
• Give prescribed medications *to promote ventilation and oxygenation.*
• Suction carefully, as needed, and encourage deep breathing *to mobilize secretions and maintain patent airway.*
• Closely monitor vital signs and laboratory test results *to guide treatment plan.*

Teaching topics
• Need for follow-up medical care
• Avoiding a combination of alcohol with other central nervous system (CNS) depressants

Asthma

Asthma is a form of chronic obstructive airway disease in which the bronchial linings overreact to various stimuli, causing episodic spasms and inflammation that severely restrict the airways. Symptoms range from mild wheezing and labored breathing to life-threatening respiratory failure.

Asthma can be extrinsic or intrinsic (or a person may have both). Extrinsic (atopic) asthma is caused by sensitivity to specific external allergens. Intrinsic (nonatopic) asthma is caused by a reaction to internal, nonallergic factors.

CAUSES
Extrinsic asthma
• Allergens (pollen, dander, dust, sulfite food additives)

Intrinsic asthma
• Endocrine changes
• Noxious fumes
• Respiratory infection
• Stress
• Temperature and humidity

ASSESSMENT FINDINGS
• Absent or diminished breath sounds during severe obstruction
• Chest tightness
• Dyspnea
• Productive cough with thick mucus

• Prolonged expiration
• Tachypnea, tachycardia
• Use of accessory muscles
• Usually asymptomatic between attacks
• Wheezing, primarily on expiration but also sometimes on inspiration

DIAGNOSTIC TEST RESULTS
• ABGs in acute severe asthma show decreased PaO_2 and decreased, normal, or increased $PaCO_2$.
• Blood tests: Serum immunoglobulin E may increase from an allergic reaction; complete blood count (CBC) may reveal increased eosinophil count.
• Chest X-ray shows hyperinflated lungs with air trapping during an attack.
• PFTs during attacks show decreased forced expiratory volumes that improve with therapy, and increased residual volume and total lung capacity.
• Skin tests may identify allergens.

NURSING DIAGNOSES
• Ineffective airway clearance
• Impaired gas exchange
• Ineffective management of therapeutic regimen

TREATMENT
• Desensitization to allergens
• Intubation and mechanical ventilation if respiratory status worsens
• Oxygen therapy at 2 L/minute
• Fluids to 3,000 ml/day as tolerated

Drug therapy
• Antacid: aluminum hydroxide gel (AlternaGEL)
• Antibiotics: according to sensitivity of infective organism
• Antileukotrienes: zileuton (Zyflo), zafirlokast (Accolate)
• Beta-adrenergic drugs: epinephrine hydrochloride (Adrenalin), salmeterol (Serevent)
• Bronchodilators: terbutaline (Brethine), aminophylline (Aminophyllin), theophylline (Theo-Dur); via nebulizer: albuterol (Proventil), ipratropium bromide (Atrovent), metaproterenol sulfate (Alupent)

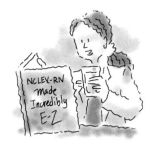

Here's to ya! Patients with asthma should receive 3,000 ml of fluids a day.

• Respiratory inhalant: cromolyn sodium (Intal)
• Steroids: hydrocortisone (Solu-Cortef), methylprednisolone sodium succinate (Solu-Medrol)
• Steroids (via nebulizer): beclomethasone (Vanceril), triamcinolone (Azmacort)

INTERVENTIONS AND RATIONALES

• Administer low-flow humidified O_2 *to reduce inflammation of the airways, ease breathing, and increase SaO_2.*
• Administer medications, as prescribed, *to reduce inflammation and obstruction of airways.* Auscultate lungs for improved breath sounds. Observe for complications of drug therapy.
• Encourage patient to express feelings about fear of suffocation *to reduce anxiety. As breathlessness and hypoxemia are relieved, anxiety should be reduced.*
• Allow activity, as tolerated, with rest periods *to reduce work of breathing and reduce O_2 demands.*
• Assess respiratory status *to determine effectiveness of therapy, such as clear breath sounds and improved airflow, PFTs, SaO_2, and ease of breathing.* Louder wheezing may be heard as airways respond to therapy and open up. As condition improves and airflow increases, wheezing should diminish and breath sounds improve.
• Assist with turning, coughing, deep breathing, and breathing retraining *to mobilize and clear secretions. Pursed-lip and diaphragmatic breathing promote more effective ventilation.*
• Keep the patient in high-Fowler's position *to improve ventilation.*
• Maintain the patient's diet and administer small, frequent feedings *to reduce pressure on the diaphragm and increase caloric intake.*
• Encourage fluids *to treat dehydration and liquefy secretions to facilitate their removal.*
• Monitor and record the color, amount, and consistency of sputum. *Changes in sputum characteristics may signal a respiratory infection.*
• Monitor and record vital signs. *Tachycardia may indicate worsening asthma or drug toxicity. Hypertension may indicate hypoxemia. Fever may signal infection.*

• Monitor laboratory studies. *An increase in WBC count may signal infection. Eosinophilia may indicate an allergic response. Drug levels may reveal toxicity.*
• Provide chest physiotherapy, postural drainage, incentive spirometry, and suction *to aid in the removal of secretions.*

Teaching topics

• Recognizing the early signs and symptoms of respiratory infection and hypoxia
• Taking medications properly and using a metered dose inhaler
• Using a peak flow meter
• Performing pursed-lip, diaphragmatic breathing and coughing and deep breathing exercises
• Avoiding exposure to chemical irritants and pollutants
• Avoiding gas-producing foods, spicy foods, and extremely hot or cold foods
• Smoking cessation
• Increasing fluid intake to 3,000 ml/day
• Contacting the American Lung Association

Atelectasis

Atelectasis is marked by incomplete expansion of lobules (clusters of alveoli) or lung segments, which may result in partial or complete lung collapse. The collapsed areas are unavailable for gas exchange; blood that lacks O_2 passes through unchanged, thereby producing hypoxia.

Atelectasis may be chronic or acute. It occurs to some degree in many patients undergoing upper abdominal or thoracic surgery. The prognosis depends on prompt removal of any airway obstruction, relief of hypoxia, and re-expansion of the collapsed lung.

CAUSES

• Bronchial occlusion by mucus plugs, as in patients with chronic obstructive pulmonary disease (COPD), bronchiectasis, or cystic fibrosis or those who smoke heavily
• CNS depression
• External compression, such as from upper abdominal surgical incisions, rib fractures,

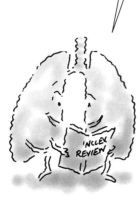

Atelectasis is the incomplete expansion of a lung, which may result in its partial or complete collapse.

pleuritic chest pain, tight dressings around the chest, or obesity
• Occlusion by foreign bodies, bronchogenic carcinoma, and inflammatory lung disease
• Prolonged immobility

ASSESSMENT FINDINGS
• Diminished or bronchial breath sounds
• Dyspnea

In severe cases
• Anxiety
• Cyanosis
• Diaphoresis
• Hyperinflation of unaffected areas of the lung
• Peripheral circulatory collapse
• Severe dyspnea
• Substernal or intercostal retraction
• Tachycardia

DIAGNOSTIC TEST RESULTS
• Chest X-ray shows characteristic horizontal lines in the lower lung zones and, with segmental or lobar collapse, characteristic dense shadows often associated with hyperinflation of neighboring lung zones (in widespread atelectasis).

NURSING DIAGNOSES
• Impaired gas exchange
• Ineffective breathing pattern
• Risk for infection

TREATMENT
• Bronchoscopy
• Chest physiotherapy
• Surgery or radiation therapy to remove an obstructing neoplasm

Drug therapy
• Analgesics: morphine
• Bronchodilators: albuterol (Proventil)
• Mucolytic inhalation therapy: acetylcysteine (Mucomyst)

INTERVENTIONS AND RATIONALES
• Encourage postoperative and other high-risk patients to cough and deep-breathe every 1 to 2 hours *to prevent atelectasis.*

• Hold a pillow tightly over the incision; teach the patient this technique as well *to minimize pain during coughing exercises in postoperative patients.* Gently reposition these patients often and help them walk as soon as possible *to prevent atelectasis.*
• Administer adequate analgesics *to control pain. Pain may prevent the patient from taking deep breaths, which leads to atelectasis.*
• During mechanical ventilation, maintain tidal volume at 10 to 15 ml/kg of the patient's body weight *to ensure adequate lung expansion.* Use the sigh mechanism on the ventilator, if appropriate, *to intermittently increase tidal volume at the rate of 10 to 15 sighs/hour.*
• Use an incentive spirometer *to encourage deep inspiration through positive reinforcement.* Teach the patient how to use the spirometer and encourage him to use it every 1 to 2 hours.
• Humidify inspired air and encourage adequate fluid intake *to mobilize secretions.* Use postural drainage and chest percussion *to promote loosening and clearance of secretions.*
• If the patient is intubated or uncooperative, provide suctioning as needed. Use sedatives with discretion *because they depress respirations and the cough reflex and suppress sighing.*
• Assess breath sounds and ventilatory status frequently and be alert for any changes *to prevent respiratory compromise.*
• Encourage the patient to stop smoking, lose weight, or both, as needed. Refer him to appropriate support groups for help *to modify risk factors.*
• Provide reassurance and emotional support *because the patient may be frightened by his limited breathing capacity.*

Teaching topics
• Performing respiratory care such as postural drainage, coughing, and deep breathing
• Stopping smoking and losing weight if appropriate
• Relaxation techniques

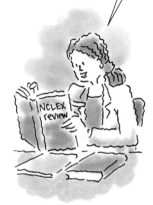

Using an incentive spirometer can help patients become involved in their own care.

NCLEX review

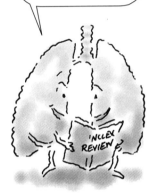

The bad news: bronchiectasis is irreversible when established. The good news: antibiotics have drastically reduced the incidence of this disorder.

Bronchiectasis

Bronchiectasis is marked by chronic abnormal dilation of bronchi (large air passages of the lungs) and destruction of bronchial walls.

Bronchiectasis has three forms: cylindrical (fusiform), varicose, and saccular (cystic). It can occur throughout the tracheobronchial tree or can be confined to one segment or lobe. However, it's usually bilateral and involves the basilar segments of the lower lobes.

The disorder affects people of both sexes and all ages and, once established, is irreversible. Because of the availability of antibiotics to treat acute respiratory tract infections, the incidence of bronchiectasis has dramatically decreased in the past 20 years.

CAUSES
• Inhalation of corrosive gas or repeated aspiration of gastric juices into the lungs
• Immunologic disorders such as agammaglobulinemia
• Mucoviscidosis (in cases of cystic fibrosis)
• Obstruction (by a foreign body, tumor, or stenosis) in association with recurrent infection
• Recurrent, inadequately treated bacterial respiratory tract infections, such as TB and complications of measles, pneumonia, pertussis, or influenza

ASSESSMENT FINDINGS
• Chronic cough that produces copious, foul-smelling, mucopurulent secretions, possibly totaling several cupfuls daily
• Coarse crackles during inspiration over involved lobes or segments
• Dyspnea
• Occasional wheezes
• Sinusitis
• Weight loss

DIAGNOSTIC TEST RESULTS
• Bronchoscopy helps to identify the source of secretions or the bleeding site in hemoptysis
• Chest X-rays show peribronchial thickening, areas of atelectasis, and scattered cystic changes.

• CBC detects anemia and leukocytosis.
• PFTs detect decreased vital capacity, expiratory flow, and hypoxemia.
• Sputum culture and Gram stain identify predominant organisms.

NURSING DIAGNOSES
• Altered nutrition: Less than body requirements
• Impaired gas exchange
• Ineffective airway clearance

TREATMENT
• Bronchoscopy (to mobilize secretions)
• Chest physiotherapy
• O_2 therapy

Drug therapy
• Antibiotics according to sensitivity of causative organism
• Bronchodilators such as albuterol (Proventil)

INTERVENTIONS AND RATIONALES
• Assess respiratory status *to detect early signs of decompensation.*
• Provide supportive care and help the patient adjust to the permanent changes in lifestyle that irreversible lung damage necessitates *to facilitate positive coping.*
• Administer antibiotics as needed *to eradicate infection.*
• Explain all diagnostic tests to the patient *to decrease anxiety.*
• Perform chest physiotherapy, including postural drainage and chest percussion designed for involved lobes, several times per day. The best times to do this are early morning and just before bedtime. Instruct the patient to maintain each position for 10 minutes; then perform percussion and tell him to cough. *These measures mobilize secretions.*

Teaching topics
• Home O_2 therapy
• Instruction for family members on how to perform chest physiotherapy
• Importance of quitting smoking
• Dietary considerations such as avoiding mild products because milk increases the viscosity of secretions

• Proper disposal of secretions to prevent spread of infection to others

Chronic bronchitis

Chronic bronchitis, a form of COPD, results from irritants and infections that increase mucus production, impair airway clearance, and cause irreversible narrowing of the small airways. This causes a severe $\dot{V}/\dot{Q}$ imbalance, leading to hypoxemia and CO_2 retention.

CAUSES
• Airborne irritants and pollutants
• Chronic respiratory infections
• Smoking

ASSESSMENT FINDINGS
• Dyspnea
• Finger clubbing, later in the disease
• Increased sputum production
• Productive cough
• Prolonged expiration
• Rhonchi, wheezes
• Use of accessory muscles
• Weight gain, edema, jugular venous distention

DIAGNOSTIC TEST RESULTS
• ABGs show decreased Pao_2 and normal or increased $Paco_2$.
• Chest X-ray shows hyperinflation and increased bronchovascular markings.
• Electrocardiography (ECG) shows atrial arrhythmias, peaked P waves in leads II, III, and aV_F and, occasionally, right ventricular hypertrophy.
• PFTs may reveal increased residual volume, decreased vital capacity and forced expiratory volumes, and normal static compliance and diffusion capacity.
• Sputum culture may reveal many microorganisms and neutrophils.

NURSING DIAGNOSES
• Activity intolerance
• Ineffective airway clearance
• Ineffective breathing pattern

TREATMENT
• Chest physiotherapy, postural drainage, and incentive spirometry
• Dietary changes, including establishing a diet high in protein, vitamin C, calories, and nitrogen
• Fluid intake up to 3,000 ml/day, if not contraindicated
• Intubation and mechanical ventilation if respiratory status deteriorates
• O_2 therapy at 2 to 3 L/minute
• Ultrasonic or mechanical nebulizer treatments

Drug therapy
• Antacid: aluminum hydroxide gel (AlternaGEL)
• Antibiotics: according to sensitivity of infective organism
• Bronchodilators: terbutaline (Brethine), aminophylline (Aminophyllin), theophylline (Theo-Dur); via nebulizer: albuterol (Proventil), ipratropium bromide (Atrovent), metaproterenol sulfate (Alupent)
• Diuretics such as furosemide (Lasix) for edema
• Expectorant: guaifenesin (Robitussin)
• Influenza and Pneumovax vaccine
• Steroids: hydrocortisone (Solu-Cortef), methylprednisolone sodium succinate (Solu-Medrol)
• Steroids (via nebulizer): beclomethasone (Vanceril), triamcinolone (Azmacort)

INTERVENTIONS AND RATIONALES
• Administer low-flow O_2. *Because patients with chronic bronchitis have chronic hypercapnia, they have a hypoxic respiratory drive. Higher flow rates may eliminate this hypoxic respiratory drive.*
• Administer medications, as prescribed, *to relieve symptoms and prevent complications.*
• Allow activity, as tolerated, *to avoid fatigue and reduce O_2 demands.*
• Assess respiratory status, ABGs, and pulse oximetry *to detect respiratory compromise, severe hypoxemia, and hypercapnia.*
• Assist with turning, coughing, and deep breathing *to mobilize secretions and facilitate removal.*

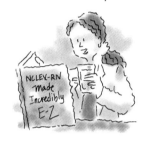

You should encourage patients with chronic bronchitis to drink 3,000 ml of fluids a day — unless it's contraindicated.

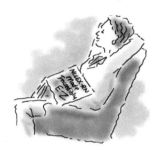

You've read about your patient's breathing — now it's time to do some breathing of your own. Take a deep breath and relax — and then get back to studying.

• Assist with diaphragmatic and pursed-lip breathing *to strengthen respiratory muscles.*
• Keep the patient in high-Fowler's position *to improve ventilation.*
• Maintain the patient's diet and administer small, frequent feedings *to avoid fatigue when eating and reduce pressure on the diaphragm from a full stomach.*
• Monitor and record the color, amount, and consistency of sputum. *Changes in sputum characteristics may signal a respiratory infection.*
• Monitor and record cardiovascular status and vital signs. *Edema, jugular venous distention, tachycardia, and an elevated CVP suggest right-sided heart failure. An irregular pulse may indicate an arrhythmia caused by altered ABGs. Tachycardia and tachypnea may indicate hypoxemia.*
• Monitor laboratory studies. *Follow drug levels for evidence of toxicity. Electrolyte imbalances may occur with the use of diuretics. Reduced Hb and HCT affect the oxygen-carrying capacity of the blood.*
• Monitor intake and output and daily weights *to detect fluid overload associated with right-sided heart failure. Dehydration impairs the removal of secretions.*
• Provide chest physiotherapy, postural drainage, incentive spirometry, and suction *to aid in removal of secretions.*
• Weigh the patient daily *to detect edema caused by right-sided heart failure.*

Teaching topics
• Pulmonary rehabilitation
• Recognizing the early signs and symptoms of respiratory infection and hypoxia
• Using home O_2 and nebulizer equipment properly
• Performing pursed-lip, diaphragmatic breathing, and coughing and deep breathing exercises
• Avoiding exposure to chemical irritants and pollutants
• Avoiding gas-producing foods, spicy foods, and extremely hot or cold foods
• Smoking cessation
• Increasing fluid intake to 3,000 ml/day, if not contraindicated
• Contacting the American Lung Association

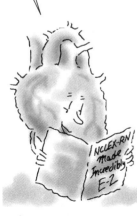

Pulmonary peril. In cor pulmonale, my right ventricle enlarges because of diseases that affect the lungs.

Cor pulmonale

A chronic heart condition, cor pulmonale is hypertrophy (enlargement) of the heart's right ventricle that results from diseases affecting the function or the structure of the lungs. To compensate for the extra work needed to force blood through the lungs, the right ventricle dilates and enlarges.

Invariably, cor pulmonale follows some disorder of the lungs, pulmonary vessels, chest wall, or respiratory control center. For instance, COPD produces pulmonary hypertension, which leads to right ventricular hypertrophy and right-sided heart failure. Because cor pulmonale generally occurs late during the course of COPD and other irreversible diseases, the prognosis is generally poor.

CAUSES
• COPD (about 25% of patients with COPD eventually develop cor pulmonale)
• Living at high altitudes (chronic mountain sickness)
• Loss of lung tissue after extensive lung surgery
• Obesity hypoventilation syndrome (pickwickian syndrome) and upper airway obstruction
• Obstructive lung diseases such as bronchiectasis and cystic fibrosis
• Pulmonary vascular diseases, such as recurrent thromboembolism, primary pulmonary hypertension, schistosomiasis, and pulmonary vasculitis
• Respiratory insufficiency without pulmonary disease, as seen in chest wall disorders, such as kyphoscoliosis, neuromuscular incompetence resulting from muscular dystrophy and amyotrophic lateral sclerosis, polymyositis, and spinal cord lesions above C6
• Restrictive lung diseases, such as pneumoconiosis, interstitial pneumonitis, scleroderma, and sarcoidosis

ASSESSMENT FINDINGS
• Chronic productive cough
• Dyspnea on exertion
• Edema
• Fatigue

- Orthopnea
- Tachypnea
- Weakness
- Wheezing respirations

DIAGNOSTIC TEST RESULTS
- ABG analysis shows decreased PaO_2 (< 70 mm Hg).
- Blood tests show HCT greater than 50%.
- Chest X-ray shows large central pulmonary arteries and suggests right ventricular enlargement by rightward enlargement of cardiac silhouette on an anterior chest film.
- Echocardiography or angiography indicates right ventricular enlargement, and echocardiography can estimate pulmonary artery pressure (PAP).
- ECG commonly shows arrhythmias, such as premature atrial and ventricular contractions and atrial fibrillation during severe hypoxia. It may also show right bundle-branch block, right axis deviation, prominent P waves and an inverted T wave in right precordial leads, and right ventricular hypertrophy.
- PAP measurements show increased right ventricular pressure as a result of increased pulmonary vascular resistance.
- PFTs show results consistent with the underlying pulmonary disease.

NURSING DIAGNOSES
- Activity intolerance
- Fluid volume excess
- Impaired gas exchange

TREATMENT
- Diet: low-salt, with restricted fluid intake
- O_2 therapy by mask or cannula in concentrations ranging from 24% to 40%, depending on PaO_2, as necessary, and, in acute cases, mechanical ventilation

Drug therapy
- Angiotensin-converting enzyme inhibitor such as captopril (Capoten)
- Antibiotics (when respiratory infection is present)
- Anticoagulant: heparin
- Calcium channel blockers such as diltiazem (Cardizem)
- Digitalis glycoside: digoxin (Lanoxin)

- Diuretic (to reduce edema): furosemide (Lasix)
- Vasodilators: diazoxide, hydralazine, nitroprusside, prostaglandins (in primary pulmonary hypertension)

INTERVENTIONS AND RATIONALES
- The patient will need a diet carefully planned in consultation with the staff dietitian. Provide small, frequent feedings rather than three heavy meals *because the patient may lack energy and tire easily when eating.*
- Limit the patient's fluid intake to 1,000 to 2,000 ml/day, and provide a low-sodium diet *to prevent fluid retention.*
- Monitor serum potassium levels closely if the patient is receiving diuretics. *Low serum potassium levels can potentiate the risk of arrhythmias associated with digitalis glycosides.*
- Monitor digoxin level *to prevent symptoms of digitalis toxicity, such as anorexia, nausea, vomiting, and yellow halos around visual images.*
- Teach the patient to check his radial pulse before taking digoxin or any digitalis glycoside and to report any changes in pulse rate *to avoid complications of digoxin therapy.*
- Reposition bedridden patients often *to prevent atelectasis.*
- Provide meticulous respiratory care, including O_2 therapy and, for COPD patients, pursed-lip breathing exercises, *to improve oxygenation.*
- Periodically measure ABG levels and watch for signs of respiratory failure such as a change in pulse rate; deep, labored respirations; and increased fatigue produced by exertion. *Monitoring these parameters helps detect early signs of worsening respiratory status.*

Teaching topics
- Importance of follow-up examinations.
- Home O_2 therapy

Emphysema

Emphysema is a form of COPD in which recurrent pulmonary inflammation damages and eventually destroys the alveolar walls, creating large air spaces. This breakdown

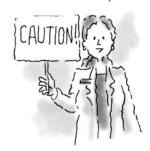

Cor pulmonale patients with underlying COPD shouldn't receive high concentrations of oxygen. It could lead to subsequent respiratory depression.

CAUTION!

leaves the alveoli unable to recoil normally after expanding, and, upon expiration, results in bronchiolar collapse. This traps air in the lungs, leading to overdistention and reduced gas exchange.

CAUSES
- Deficiency of alpha$_1$-antitrypsin
- Smoking

ASSESSMENT FINDINGS
- Anorexia, weight loss
- Barrel chest
- Decreased breath sounds
- Dyspnea
- Finger clubbing, late in the disease
- Prolonged expiration
- Pursed-lip breathing
- Use of accessory muscles for breathing

DIAGNOSTIC TEST RESULTS
- ABGs show reduced Pao_2, with normal Paco_2 until late in the disease.
- Chest X-ray in advanced disease reveals a flattened diaphragm, reduced vascular markings in the lung periphery, enlarged anteroposterior chest diameter, and a vertical heart.
- CBC shows increased Hb late in disease when patient has severe persistent hypoxia.
- ECG shows tall, symmetrical P waves in leads II, III, and aV$_F$, vertical QRS axis, and signs of right ventricular hypertrophy late in disease.
- PFTs show increased residual volume, total lung capacity, and compliance, as well as decreased vital capacity, diffusing capacity, and expiratory volumes.

NURSING DIAGNOSES
- Fatigue
- Impaired gas exchange
- Risk for infection

TREATMENT
- Chest physiotherapy, postural drainage, and incentive spirometry
- Dietary changes, including establishing a diet high in protein, vitamin C, calories, and nitrogen

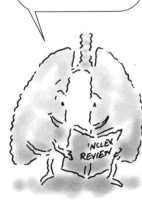

Check it out. With emphysema, PFTs show an increase in my residual volume, total capacity, and compliance.

- Fluid intake up to 3,000 ml/day, if not contraindicated by heart failure
- Intubation and mechanical ventilation if respiratory status deteriorates
- O$_2$ therapy at 2 to 3 L/minute, transtracheal therapy for home O$_2$ therapy
- Ultrasonic or mechanical nebulizer treatments
- Lung volume reduction surgery

Drug therapy
- Alpha$_1$-antitrypsin therapy
- Antacid: aluminum hydroxide gel (AlternaGEL)
- Antibiotics: according to sensitivity of infective organism
- Bronchodilators: terbutaline (Brethine), aminophylline (Aminophyllin), theophylline (Theo-Dur); via nebulizer: albuterol (Proventil), ipratropium bromide (Atrovent), metaproterenol sulfate (Alupent)
- Diuretics such as furosemide (Lasix) for edema
- Expectorant: guaifenesin (Robitussin)
- Influenza and Pneumovax vaccine
- Steroids: hydrocortisone (Solu-Cortef), methylprednisolone sodium succinate (Solu-Medrol)
- Steroids (via nebulizer): beclomethasone (Vanceril), triamcinolone (Azmacort)

INTERVENTIONS AND RATIONALES
- Administer low-flow O$_2$ *because emphysema patients have chronic hypercapnia, so they have a hypoxic respiratory drive. Higher flow rates may eliminate this hypoxic respiratory drive.*
- Administer medications, as prescribed, *to relieve symptoms and prevent complications.*
- Allow activity, as tolerated, *to avoid fatigue and reduce O$_2$ demands.*
- Assess respiratory status, ABGs, and pulse oximetry *to detect respiratory compromise, severe hypoxemia, and hypercapnia.*
- Monitor and record cardiovascular status and vital signs. *An irregular pulse may indicate an arrhythmia caused by altered ABGs. Tachycardia and tachypnea may indicate hypoxemia. Late in the disease, pulmonary hypertension may lead to right ventricular hypertrophy and right-sided heart failure. Jugular ve-*

nous distention, edema, hypotension, tachycardia, S₃ heart sound, a loud pulmonic component of S₂, heart murmurs, and hepatojugular reflux may be present.

- Assist with turning, coughing, and deep breathing *to mobilize secretions and facilitate removal.*
- Assist with diaphragmatic and pursed-lip breathing *to strengthen respiratory muscles.*
- Keep the patient in high-Fowler's position *to improve ventilation.*
- Maintain the patient's diet and administer small, frequent feedings *to avoid fatigue when eating. Small meals relieve pressure on the diaphragm and allow fuller lung movement.*
- Monitor and record the color, amount, and consistency of sputum. *Changes in sputum may signal a respiratory infection.*
- Monitor laboratory studies. *Follow drug levels for evidence of toxicity. Electrolyte imbalances may occur with the use of diuretics. Reduced Hb and HCT affect the oxygen-carrying capacity of the blood.*
- Monitor intake and output and daily weights *to detect fluid overload associated with right-sided heart failure. Dehydration may impair the removal of secretions.*
- Encourage fluids, unless contraindicated, *to liquefy secretions.*
- Provide chest physiotherapy, postural drainage, incentive spirometry, and suction *to aid in removal of secretions.*
- Weigh the patient daily *to detect edema caused by right-sided heart failure.*

Teaching topics
- Pulmonary rehabilitation
- Recognizing the early signs and symptoms of respiratory infection and hypoxia
- Using home O₂ and nebulizer equipment properly
- Performing pursed-lip, diaphragmatic breathing, and coughing and deep breathing exercises
- Avoiding exposure to chemical irritants and pollutants
- Avoiding gas-producing foods, spicy foods, and extremely hot or cold foods
- Smoking cessation
- Increasing fluid intake to 3,000 ml/day, if not contraindicated

- Avoiding people with respiratory infections
- Receiving vaccinations
- Contacting the American Lung Association

Legionnaires' disease

Legionnaires' disease is an acute bronchopneumonia, an inflammation of the lungs that begins in the terminal bronchioles. It's produced by a fastidious, gram-negative bacillus (rod-shaped bacterium).

Legionnaires' disease derives its name from the peculiar, highly publicized disease that struck 182 people (29 of whom died) at an American Legion convention in Philadelphia in July 1976.

This disease may occur epidemically or sporadically, usually in late summer or early fall. Its severity ranges from a mild illness, with or without pneumonitis, to multilobar pneumonia, with a mortality as high as 15%. A milder, self-limiting form (Pontiac syndrome) subsides within a few days but leaves the patient fatigued for several weeks; this form mimics Legionnaires' disease but produces few or no respiratory symptoms, no pneumonia, and no fatalities.

CAUSE
- *Legionella pneumophila*

ASSESSMENT FINDINGS
- Amnesia
- Anorexia
- Bradycardia
- Cough that is initially nonproductive but that can eventually produce grayish, nonpurulent, blood-streaked sputum
- Diarrhea
- Diffuse myalgias
- Fever
- Generalized weakness
- Headache
- Malaise
- Mental sluggishness
- Recurrent chills

DIAGNOSTIC TEST RESULTS
- Blood tests show leukocytosis, increased ESR, increased liver enzyme levels (alanine

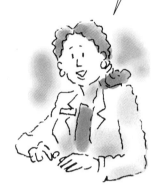

Legionnaires' disease is produced by a fastidious, gram-negative bacterium.

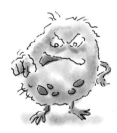

A fastidious bacterium has complex requirements for growth. Gram-negative refers to how the bacterium reacts in Gram's method of staining.

aminotransferase, aspartate aminotransferase, alkaline phosphatase), and hyponatremia.

• Chest X-ray shows patchy, localized infiltration, which progresses to multilobar consolidation (usually involving the lower lobes), pleural effusion and, in fulminant disease, opacification of the entire lung.

• Direct immunofluorescence of *L. pneumophila* and indirect fluorescent serum antibody testing compare findings from initial blood studies with findings from those done at least 3 weeks later. A convalescent serum sample showing a fourfold or greater rise in antibody titer for *L. pneumophila* confirms the diagnosis.

• Sputum test eliminates other organisms.

NURSING DIAGNOSES
• Hyperthermia
• Impaired gas exchange
• Risk for injury

TREATMENT
• O₂ therapy, which may require intubation and mechanical ventilation

Drug therapy
• Antibiotics: erythromycin (Erythrocin), rifampin (Rifadin), tetracycline (Achromycin V)
• Antipyretics: acetaminophen (Tylenol), aspirin
• Inotropic agents: dopamine (Intropin)

INTERVENTIONS AND RATIONALES
• Closely monitor the patient's respiratory status. Evaluate chest wall expansion, depth and pattern of respirations, cough, and chest pain *to detect respiratory decompensation.*
• Continually monitor the patient's vital signs, pulse oximetry or ABG values, level of consciousness, and dryness and color of the lips and mucous membranes. Watch for signs of shock (decreased blood pressure, thready pulse, diaphoresis, clammy skin) *to avoid crisis.*
• Keep the patient comfortable; avoid chills and exposure to drafts, *which increase metabolic demands.* Provide mouth care frequently. If necessary, apply soothing cream to the nos-

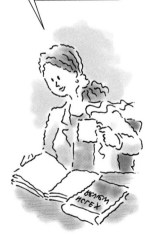

Erythromycin is the antibiotic of choice for Legionnaires' disease. If it's contraindicated, rifampin is used, sometimes with tetracycline.

trils *to promote comfort and prevent skin breakdown.*
• Replace fluid and electrolytes as needed. The patient with renal failure may require dialysis.
• Provide mechanical ventilation and other respiratory therapy as needed *to promote oxygenation.*
• Give antibiotics as necessary *to eradicate infection*, and observe carefully for adverse effects *to prevent complications.*

Teaching topics
• Coughing and deep breathing exercises
• Importance of continuing treatment until recovery is complete

Lung cancer

In lung cancer, unregulated cell growth and uncontrolled cell division result in the development of a neoplasm. Cancer may also reach the lungs due to metastasis from other organs, mainly the liver, brain, bone, kidneys, and adrenal glands.

Four histologic types of lung cancer include:

☝ squamous cell (epidermoid), a slow-growing cancer that originates from bronchial epithelium. It metastasizes late to the surrounding area, but may cause bronchial obstruction.

✌ adenocarcinoma, a moderately growing cancer located in peripheral areas of the lung. It metastasizes through the bloodstream to other organs.

🖐 large-cell anaplastic, a very fast-growing cancer associated with early and extensive metastasis. It's more common in peripheral lung tissue.

🖐 small-cell (oat cell cancer), a very fast-growing cancer that metastasizes very early through lymph vessels and the bloodstream to other organs.

CAUSES
• Cigarette smoking

- Exposure to environmental pollutants
- Exposure to occupational pollutants

ASSESSMENT FINDINGS
- Chest pain
- Chills, fever
- Cough, hemoptysis
- Dyspnea, wheezing
- Weakness, fatigue
- Weight loss, anorexia

DIAGNOSTIC TEST RESULTS
- Bronchoscopy reveals a positive biopsy.
- Chest X-ray shows lesion or mass.
- Lung scan shows a mass.
- Open lung biopsy reveals a positive biopsy.
- Sputum study reveals positive cytology for cancer cells.

NURSING DIAGNOSES
- Activity intolerance
- Anxiety
- Impaired gas exchange

TREATMENT
- Dietary changes, including establishing a high-protein, high-calorie diet and providing small, frequent meals
- Incentive spirometry
- Laser photocoagulation
- O_2 therapy, intubation and, if the condition deteriorates, mechanical ventilation
- Radiation therapy
- Resection of the affected lobe (lobectomy) or lung (pneumonectomy)

Drug therapy
- Analgesics: morphine sulfate, fentanyl (Sublimaze)
- Antiemetics: prochlorperazine (Compazine), ondansetron hydrochloride (Zofran)
- Antineoplastics: cyclophosphamide (Cytoxan), doxorubicin hydrochloride (Adriamycin), cisplatin (Platinol), vincristine (Oncovin)
- Diuretics: furosemide (Lasix), ethacrynic acid (Edecrin)

INTERVENTIONS AND RATIONALES
- Assess respiratory status to detect respiratory complications. *Cyanosis may suggest re-*

spiratory failure while an increase in sputum production may suggest an infection.
- Assess the patient's pain and administer analgesics, as prescribed, *to control pain. Assessment allows for care plan modification as needed.*
- Monitor and record vital signs. *Tachycardia and tachypnea may indicate hypoxemia. An elevated temperature suggests an infection.*
- Monitor and record intake and output *to assess fluid status.*
- Track laboratory values, and monitor for bleeding, infection, and electrolyte imbalance due to effects of chemotherapy. *A low WBC count increases the risk of infection. Low platelets increase the risk of bleeding. Electrolyte abnormalities, especially hypercalcemia, may also occur.*
- Monitor pulse oximetry values and report a drop in O_2 saturation, *which suggests hypoxemia.*
- Administer O_2 *to maintain tissue oxygenation.*
- Encourage fluids and administer I.V. fluids *to provide hydration and liquefy secretions to facilitate removal. Drinking moistens mucous membranes.*
- Provide suctioning, and assist with turning, coughing, and deep breathing *to facilitate removal of secretions.*
- Keep the patient in semi-Fowler's position *to maximize ventilation.*
- Administer total parenteral nutrition or enteral feeding, as indicated, *to optimize nutrition and bolster immune system.*
- Administer medications, as prescribed, *to treat the cancer and provide pain relief.*
- Encourage the patient to express feelings about changes in body image and a fear of dying *to reduce anxiety.*
- Provide mouth care *to improve comfort and reduce risk of stomatitis (with chemotherapy).* Provide skin care *to minimize adverse effects of radiation therapy.*
- Provide rest periods *to enhance tissue oxygenation.*

Teaching topics
- Performing deep-breathing and coughing exercises
- Alternating rest periods with activity

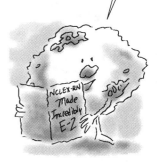

In lung cancer, unregulated cell growth and uncontrolled cell division result in the development of a neoplasm.

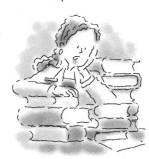

Say it 100 times: Studying for the NCLEX is fun, studying for the NCLEX is fun, studying for the NCLEX is fun…

• Following dietary recommendations and restrictions
• Measures to prevent infection, such as avoiding crowds and infected individuals, especially children with communicable disease
• Contacting the American Cancer Society

Pleural effusion and empyema

Pleural effusion is an excess of fluid in the pleural space (the thin space between the lung tissue and the membranous sac that protects it). Normally, the pleural space contains a small amount of extracellular fluid that lubricates the pleural surfaces. Increased production or inadequate removal of this fluid results in pleural effusion.

Empyema is the accumulation of pus and necrotic tissue in the pleural space. Blood (hemothorax) and chyle (chylothorax) may also collect in this space.

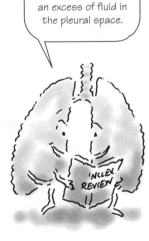

I need my space. Pleural effusion is an excess of fluid in the pleural space.

CAUSES
• Bacterial or fungal pneumonitis or empyema
• Chest trauma
• Collagen disease (lupus erythematosus and rheumatoid arthritis)
• Heart failure
• Hepatic disease with ascites
• Hypoalbuminemia
• Infection in the pleural space
• Malignancy
• Myxedema
• Pancreatitis
• Peritoneal dialysis
• Pulmonary embolism with or without infarction
• Subphrenic abscess
• TB

ASSESSMENT FINDINGS
• Decreased breath sounds
• Dyspnea
• Fever
• Malaise
• Pleuritic chest pain

DIAGNOSTIC TEST RESULTS
• Chest X-ray shows radiopaque fluid in dependent regions.
• Thoracentesis shows lactate dehydrogenase (LD) levels less than 200 IU and protein levels less than 3 g/dl (in transudative effusions); ratio of protein in pleural fluid to serum greater than or equal to 0.5, LD in pleural fluid greater than or equal to 200 IU, and ratio of LD in pleural fluid to LD in serum greater than 0.6 (in exudative effusions); and acute inflammatory WBCs and microorganisms (in empyema).
• Tuberculin skin test rules out TB as the cause.

NURSING DIAGNOSES
• Hyperthermia
• Impaired gas exchange
• Risk for infection

TREATMENT
• Thoracentesis (to remove fluid)
• Thoracotomy if thoracentesis isn't effective

Drug therapy
• Antibiotics (for empyema) according to sensitivity of causative organism

INTERVENTIONS AND RATIONALES
• Explain thoracentesis to the patient. Before the procedure, tell the patient to expect a stinging sensation from the local anesthetic and a feeling of pressure when the needle is inserted *to allay the patient's anxiety.*
• Instruct the patient to tell you immediately if he feels uncomfortable or has trouble breathing during the procedure. *Difficulty breathing may indicate pneumothorax, which requires immediate chest tube insertion.*
• Reassure the patient during thoracentesis *to allay anxiety.* Remind him to breathe normally and to avoid sudden movements, such as coughing and sighing, *to prevent improper placement of needle.* Monitor vital signs and watch for syncope *to prevent injury.*
• Watch for respiratory distress or pneumothorax (sudden onset of dyspnea, cyanosis) after thoracentesis *to detect complications of thoracentesis.*
• Administer O_2 *to improve oxygenation.*

- Administer antibiotics *to treat empyema*.
- Encourage the patient to do deep breathing exercises *to promote lung expansion*. Use an incentive spirometer *to promote deep breathing*.
- Provide meticulous chest tube care, and use aseptic technique for changing dressings around the tube insertion site in empyema *to prevent infection at insertion site*.
- Ensure chest tube patency by watching for bubbles in the underwater seal chamber *to prevent respiratory distress resulting from chest tube obstruction*.
- Record the amount, color, and consistency of any tube drainage *to monitor effectiveness of treatment*.
- Make visiting nurse referrals for patients who will be discharged with the tube in place *because weeks of such drainage are usually necessary to obliterate the space*.

Teaching topics
- Seeking prompt medical attention for chest colds (if pleural effusion was a complication of pneumonia or influenza)
- Importance of continuing antibiotic therapy for the duration prescribed
- Chest tube care, if necessary, after discharge

Pleurisy

Also known as pleuritis, pleurisy is inflammation of the visceral and parietal pleurae, the serous membranes that line the inside of the thoracic cage and envelop the lungs.

CAUSES
- Cancer
- Chest trauma
- Dressler's syndrome
- Pneumonia
- Pulmonary infarction
- Rheumatoid arthritis
- Systemic lupus erythematosus
- TB
- Uremia
- Viruses

ASSESSMENT FINDINGS
- Dyspnea
- Pleural friction rub (a coarse, creaky sound heard during late inspiration and early expiration)
- Sharp, stabbing pain that increases with respiration

DIAGNOSTIC TEST RESULTS
Although diagnosis generally rests on the patient's history and the nurse's respiratory assessment, diagnostic tests help rule out other causes and pinpoint the underlying disorder.
- ECG rules out coronary artery disease as the source of the patient's pain.
- Chest X-rays can identify pneumonia.

NURSING DIAGNOSES
- Activity intolerance
- Ineffective breathing pattern
- Pain

TREATMENT
- Bed rest
- Thoracentesis (for pleurisy with pleural effusion)

Drug therapy
- Analgesics such as acetaminophen with oxycodone (Percocet)
- Anti-inflammatories such as indomethacin (Indocin)

INTERVENTIONS AND RATIONALES
- Stress the importance of bed rest and plan your care *to allow the patient as much uninterrupted rest as possible*.
- Administer antitussives and pain medication as necessary *to relieve cough and pain*.
- If the pain requires a narcotic analgesic, warn the patient about to be discharged *to avoid overuse because such medication depresses coughing and respiration*.
- Encourage the patient to cough. Apply firm pressure at the pain site during coughing exercises *to minimize pain*.

Teaching topics
- Coughing and deep breathing exercises
- All procedures including thoracentesis if appropriate

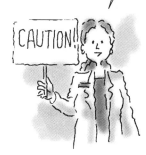

If fluid is removed too quickly during thoracentesis, the patient may suffer bradycardia, hypotension, pain, pulmonary edema, or even cardiac arrest.

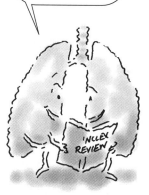

Pleurisy is an inflammation of the membranes that line the inside of the rib cage and envelop the lungs.

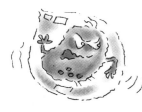

P. carinii is part of the normal flora in most healthy people. However, in the immunocompromised patient, it becomes an aggressive pathogen.

• Importance of regular rest periods

Pneumocystis carinii pneumonia

The microorganism *Pneumocystis carinii* is part of the normal flora in most healthy people. However, in the immunocompromised patient, *P. carinii* becomes an aggressive pathogen. *Pneumocystis carinii* pneumonia (PCP) is an opportunistic infection strongly associated with human immunodeficiency virus (HIV) infection.

PCP occurs in up to 90% of HIV-infected patients in the United States at some point during their lifetime. It's the leading cause of death in these patients. Disseminated infection doesn't occur.

PCP is also associated with other immunocompromised conditions, including organ transplantation, leukemia, and lymphoma.

CAUSES
• *Pneumocystis carinii*

ASSESSMENT FINDINGS
• Anorexia
• Dyspnea
• Generalized fatigue
• Low-grade, intermittent fever
• Nonproductive cough
• Shortness of breath
• Tachypnea
• Weight loss

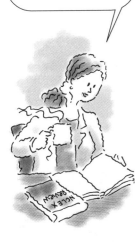

Watch out! Because of immune system impairment due to HIV, many PCP patients experience serious adverse drug reactions.

DIAGNOSTIC TEST RESULTS
• ABG studies detect hypoxia and an increased alveolar-arterial gradient.
• Chest X-ray may show slowly progressing, fluffy infiltrates and occasionally nodular lesions or a spontaneous pneumothorax, but these findings must be differentiated from findings in other types of pneumonia or adult respiratory distress syndrome.
• Fiberoptic bronchoscopy confirms PCP.
• Gallium scan may show increased uptake over the lungs even when the chest X-ray appears relatively normal.
• Histologic studies confirm *P. carinii*. In patients with HIV infection, initial examination of a first morning sputum specimen (induced by inhaling an ultrasonically dispersed saline mist) may be sufficient; however, this technique is usually ineffective in patients without HIV infection.

NURSING DIAGNOSES
• Altered protection
• Impaired gas exchange
• Risk for infection

TREATMENT
• Diet: maintaining adequate nutrition
• O_2 therapy, which may include endotracheal intubation and mechanical ventilation

Drug therapy
• Antibiotics: cotrimoxazole (Bactrim), pentamidine (Nebupent)

INTERVENTIONS AND RATIONALES
• Frequently assess the patient's respiratory status, and monitor ABG levels every 4 hours *to detect early signs of hypoxemia.*
• Administer O_2 therapy as necessary. Encourage the patient to ambulate and to perform deep-breathing exercises and incentive spirometry *to facilitate effective gas exchange.*
• Administer antipyretics, as required, *to relieve fever.*
• Monitor intake and output and daily weight *to evaluate fluid balance.* Replace fluids as necessary *to correct fluid volume deficit.*
• Give antimicrobial drugs as required. Never give pentamidine I.M. *because it can cause pain and sterile abscesses.* Administer the I.V. drug form slowly over 60 minutes *to reduce the risk of hypotension.*
• Monitor the patient for adverse reactions to antimicrobial drugs. If he's receiving co-trimoxazole, watch for nausea, vomiting, rash, bone marrow suppression, thrush, fever, hepatotoxicity, and anaphylaxis. If he's receiving pentamidine, watch for cardiac arrhythmias, hypotension, dizziness, azotemia, hypocalcemia, and hepatic disturbances. *These measures detect problems early to avoid crisis.*
• Provide diversional activities and coordinate health care team activities *to allow adequate rest periods between procedures.*

• Supply nutritional supplements as needed. Encourage the patient to eat a high-calorie, protein-rich diet. Offer small, frequent meals if the patient can't tolerate large amounts of food. *These measures ensure that the patient's nutritional intake meets metabolic needs.*
• Provide a relaxing environment, eliminate excessive environmental stimuli, and allow ample time for meals *to reduce anxiety.*
• Give emotional support and help the patient identify and use meaningful support systems *to promote emotional well-being.*

Teaching topics
• Practicing energy conservation techniques.
• Home O_2 therapy
• Recognizing adverse reactions to medications

Pneumonia

Pneumonia refers to a bacterial, viral, parasitic, or fungal infection that causes inflammation of the alveolar spaces. In pneumonia, microorganisms enter alveolar spaces through droplet inhalation, resulting in inflammation and an increase in alveolar fluid. Ventilation decreases as secretions thicken.

CAUSES
• Aspiration
• Chemical irritants
• Organisms such as *Escherichia coli, Haemophilus influenzae, Staphylococcus aureus, Pneumocystis carinii, Streptococcus pneumoniae,* and *Pseudomonas*

ASSESSMENT FINDINGS
• Chills, fever
• Cough
• Crackles, rhonchi, pleural friction rub on auscultation
• Malaise
• Pleuritic pain
• Restlessness, confusion
• Shortness of breath, dyspnea, tachypnea, accessory muscle use
• Sputum production that is rusty, green, or bloody with pneumococcal pneumonia and yellow-green with bronchopneumonia

DIAGNOSTIC TEST RESULTS
• ABG levels show hypoxemia and respiratory alkalosis.
• Chest X-ray shows pulmonary infiltrates.
• Hematology study shows increased WBCs and ESR.
• Sputum study identifies organism.

NURSING DIAGNOSES
• Ineffective airway clearance
• Risk for aspiration
• Inability to sustain spontaneous ventilation

TREATMENT
• Chest physiotherapy, postural drainage, and incentive spirometry
• Dietary changes, including establishing a high-calorie, high-protein diet and forcing fluids
• Intubation and mechanical ventilation if condition deteriorates
• Nutritional support, including enteral nutrition if patient requires intubation

Drug therapy
• Antibiotics: according to organism sensitivity
• Antipyretics: aspirin, acetaminophen (Tylenol)
• Bronchodilators: metaproterenol sulfate (Alupent), isoetharine hydrochloride (Bronkosol), albuterol (Proventil)

INTERVENTIONS AND RATIONALES
• Monitor and record intake and output. *Insensible water loss secondary to fever may cause dehydration.*
• Monitor laboratory studies. *An elevated WBC count suggests infection. Blood and sputum cultures may identify the causative agent.*
• Monitor pulse oximetry *to detect respiratory compromise.*
• Assess respiratory status *to detect early signs of compromise.*
• Monitor and record vital signs. *An elevated temperature increases O_2 demands. Hypotension and tachycardia may suggest hypovolemic shock.*
• Monitor and record color, consistency, and amount of sputum. *Sputum amount and consistency may indicate hydration status and ef-*

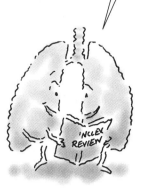

In pneumonia, microorganisms enter alveolar spaces through droplet inhalation. Sounds dreadful.

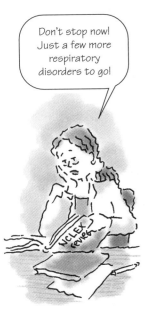

Don't stop now! Just a few more respiratory disorders to go!

fectiveness of therapy. *Foul-smelling sputum suggests respiratory infection.*
• Administer O_2 *to help relieve respiratory distress.*
• Maintain the patient's diet *to offset hypermetabolic state due to infection.*
• Force fluids to 3,000 ml/day and administer I.V. fluids *to help liquefy secretions to aid in their removal.*
• Provide suction and assist with turning, coughing, and deep breathing *to promote mobilization and removal of secretions.*
• Administer chest physiotherapy *to facilitate removal of secretions.*
• Administer medications, as prescribed, *to treat infection and improve ventilation.*
• Encourage the patient to express feelings about fear of suffocation *to reduce anxiety.*
• Provide tissues and a bag for hygienic sputum disposal *to prevent spread of infection.*
• Provide oral hygiene *to promote comfort and improve nutrition.*

Teaching topics
• Recognizing the early signs and symptoms of respiratory infections
• Avoiding exposure to people with infections
• Increasing fluid intake to 3,000 ml/day

Pneumothorax and hemothorax

In pneumothorax, loss of negative intrapleural pressure results in the collapse of the lung. Pneumothorax may be described as spontaneous, open, or tension:
• Spontaneous pneumothorax results from the rupture of a bleb.
• Open pneumothorax occurs when an opening through the chest wall allows air to flow between the pleural space and the outside of the body.
• Tension pneumothorax results from a buildup of air in the pleural space that can't escape.
    In all cases, the surface area for gas exchange is reduced, resulting in hypoxia and hypercapnia.

In hemothorax, blood accumulates in the pleural space when a rib lacerates lung tissue or an intercostal artery. This compresses the lung and limits respiratory capacity. Hemothorax can also result from rupture of large or small pulmonary vessels.

CAUSES
• Blunt chest trauma
• Central venous catheter insertion
• Penetrating chest injuries
• Rupture of a bleb
• Thoracentesis
• Thoracic surgeries

ASSESSMENT FINDINGS
• Anxiety
• Diaphoresis, pallor
• Diminished or absent breath sounds unilaterally
• Dullness on chest percussion (in the case of hemothorax and tension pneumothorax)
• Dyspnea, tachypnea, subcutaneous emphysema, cough
• Hypotension (in the case of hemothorax)
• Sharp pain that increases with exertion
• Tachycardia
• Tracheal shift, decreased chest expansion unilaterally

DIAGNOSTIC TEST RESULTS
• ABG levels show respiratory and hypoxemia.
• Chest X-ray reveals pneumothorax or hemothorax.
• Ventilation-perfusion scintigraphy is decreased.
• Lung scan shows $\dot{V}/\dot{Q}$ ratio mismatches.

NURSING DIAGNOSES
• Ineffective breathing pattern
• Impaired gas exchange
• Pain

TREATMENT
• Active range-of-motion exercises to affected arm
• Blood transfusions for hemothorax, as indicated
• Chest tube to water-seal drainage (see *Checking in on chest tubes,* page 102)

- Incentive spirometry
- Occlusive dressing (for open pneumothorax)
- O_2 therapy

Drug therapy
- Analgesic: morphine

INTERVENTIONS AND RATIONALES
- Monitor and record vital signs. *Hypotension, tachycardia, and tachypnea suggest tension pneumothorax.*
- Check the chest drainage system for air leaks *that can impair lung expansion.*
- Assess respiratory status. *Dyspnea, tachypnea, diminished breath sounds, subcutaneous emphysema, and use of accessory muscles suggest accumulation of air in pleural space.*
- Monitor chest tube drainage. *An increase in the amount of bloody drainage suggests new bleeding or an increase in bleeding. Check tubing for kinks if there is a sudden reduction in drainage.*
- Monitor and record vital signs. *Hypotension, tachycardia, and tachypnea suggest tension pneumothorax.*
- Assess cardiovascular status. *Tachycardia, hypotension, and jugular venous distention suggest tension pneumothorax.*
- Assess the patient's pain and administer medications, as prescribed, *to control pain.*
- Administer O_2 *to relieve respiratory distress caused by hypoxemia.*
- Assist with turning, coughing, deep breathing, and incentive spirometry *to enhance mobilization of secretions and prevent atelectasis.*
- Maintain chest tube to water-seal drainage. *The water-seal chamber prevents air from entering the chest tube when the patient inhales.*
- Keep the patient in high Fowler's position *to enhance chest expansion.*

Teaching topics
- Recognizing the early signs and symptoms of pneumothorax and respiratory infection
- Avoiding heavy lifting

Pulmonary embolism

Pulmonary embolism results from an undissolved substance (such as fat, air, or thrombus) in the pulmonary vessels that obstructs blood flow. The embolus travels from the venous circulation to the right side of the heart and pulmonary artery, obstructing blood flow and resulting in pulmonary hypertension and possible infarction.

CAUSES
- Abdominal, pelvic, or thoracic surgery
- Central venous catheter insertion
- Flat, long bone fractures
- Heart failure
- Hypercoagulability
- Malignant tumors
- Obesity
- Oral contraceptives
- Polycythemia vera
- Pregnancy
- Prolonged bed rest
- Sickle cell anemia
- Thrombophlebitis
- Venous stasis

ASSESSMENT FINDINGS
- Anxiety
- Chest pain
- Cough, hemoptysis
- Fever
- Hypotension
- Sudden onset of dyspnea, tachypnea, crackles
- Tachycardia, arrhythmias

DIAGNOSTIC TEST RESULTS
- ABG levels show respiratory alkalosis and hypoxemia.
- Blood chemistry tests reveal increased LD level.
- Chest X-ray shows dilated pulmonary arteries, pneumoconstriction, and diaphragm elevation on the affected side.
- ECG shows tachycardia, nonspecific ST-segment changes, and right axis deviation.
- Pulmonary angiography shows location of embolism and filling defect of pulmonary artery.
- Lung scan shows $\dot{V}/\dot{Q}$ mismatch.

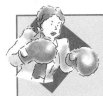

Battling illness

Checking in on chest tubes

Caring for a patient with a chest tube is a common subject on the NCLEX. Here are some typical nursing actions regarding chest tubes, beginning when the chest tube is in place.

- First, have the patient take several deep breaths to fully inflate his lungs and help push pleural air out through the tube.
- Next, palpate his chest around the tube for subcutaneous emphysema and notify the doctor of any increase.
- Routinely assess the function of the chest tube. Describe and record the amount of drainage on the intake and output sheet.
- When most of the air has been removed, the water seal chamber should bubble only during forced expiration unless the patient has a bronchopleural fistula.
- Constant bubbling in the water-seal chamber may indicate a loose connection or that the tube has come slightly out of the patient's chest. Promptly correct any loose connections.

IF THE TUBE BECOMES DISLODGED
- Cover the opening immediately with petroleum gauze and apply pressure to prevent negative inspiratory pressure from sucking into the patient's chest. Call the doctor and continue to keep the opening closed. Then get ready to start the chest tube process all over again.
- If the chest tube becomes cracked, place the distal end of the tube in sterile water and call the doctor.

NURSING DIAGNOSES
- Anxiety
- Impaired gas exchange
- Altered tissue perfusion (cardiopulmonary)

TREATMENT
- Bed rest with active and passive range-of-motion and isometric exercises
- Vena cava filter insertion
- O_2 therapy, intubation, and mechanical ventilation, if necessary

Drug therapy
- Analgesic: morphine
- Anticoagulants: heparin (Liquaemin Sodium), followed by warfarin (Coumadin)
- Diuretic: furosemide (Lasix) if right ventricular failure develops
- Fibrinolytics: streptokinase (Streptase), urokinase (Abbokinase)

INTERVENTIONS AND RATIONALES
- Assess respiratory status *to detect respiratory distress.*
- Assess cardiovascular status. *An irregular pulse may signal arrhythmia caused by hypoxemia. If pulmonary embolism is caused by thrombophlebitis, temperature may be elevated.*

- Monitor laboratory studies. *Maintain PTT at 1½ to 2 times control in patient receiving heparin. Maintain PT at 1½ to 2 times control or INR at 2 to 3 in patient receiving warfarin. Monitor ABGs for evidence of pulmonary compromise.*
- Monitor and record CVP. *CVP may rise if right-sided heart failure develops.*
- Monitor and record intake and output *to detect fluid volume overload and renal perfusion.*
- Assess for positive Homans' sign *to detect thromboembolism as a cause of pulmonary embolus.*
- Administer O_2 *to enhance arterial oxygenation.*
- Assist with turning, coughing, and deep breathing *to mobilize secretions and clear airways.*
- Keep the patient in high-Fowler's position *to enhance ventilation.*
- Provide suctioning and monitor and record color, consistency, and amount of sputum. *A productive cough and blood-tinged sputum may be present with pulmonary embolism.*
- Administer I.V. fluids, as ordered, *to maintain hydration.*
- Administer medications, as prescribed, *to enhance tissue oxygenation.*

> The patient has a pulmonary embolism. Interventions are likely to include administering an anticoagulant such as heparin.

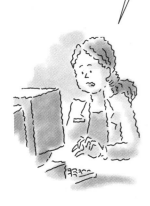

Teaching topics
• Recognizing the early signs and symptoms of respiratory distress
• Avoiding activities that promote venous thrombosis (prolonged sitting and standing, wearing constrictive clothing, crossing legs when seated, using oral contraceptives)
• Reporting signs of bleeding from excessive anticoagulant therapy

Respiratory acidosis

Respiratory acidosis is an acid-base disturbance characterized by excess of CO_2 in the blood (hypercapnia), indicated by a Pa_{CO_2} greater than 45 mm Hg. It results from reduced alveolar ventilation. It can be acute (from a sudden failure in ventilation) or chronic (as in long-term pulmonary disease).

CAUSES
• Airway obstruction or parenchymal lung disease
• CNS trauma
• Chronic metabolic alkalosis
• Drugs such as narcotics, anesthetics, hypnotics, and sedatives
• Neuromuscular disease such as myasthenia gravis, Guillain-Barré syndrome, and poliomyelitis

ASSESSMENT FINDINGS
• Cardiovascular abnormalities such as tachycardia, hypertension, atrial and ventricular arrhythmias and, in severe acidosis, hypotension with vasodilation
• Coma
• Confusion
• Dyspnea and tachypnea with papilledema and depressed reflexes
• Fine or flapping tremor (asterixis)
• Headaches
• Hypoxemia
• Restlessness

DIAGNOSTIC TEST RESULTS
• ABG measurements confirm respiratory acidosis. Pa_{CO_2} exceeds the normal level of 45 mm Hg and pH is usually below the normal range of 7.35 to 7.45. The patient's bicarbonate level is normal in the acute stage and elevated in the chronic stage.

NURSING DIAGNOSES
• Fear
• Impaired gas exchange
• Ineffective breathing pattern

TREATMENT
Treatment of respiratory acidosis is designed to correct the underlying source of alveolar hypoventilation. It may include:
• endotracheal intubation and mechanical ventilation
• dialysis to remove toxic drugs
• removal of foreign body, if appropriate.

Drug therapy
• Antibiotics if pneumonia is present
• Bronchodilators
• Sodium bicarbonate in severe cases

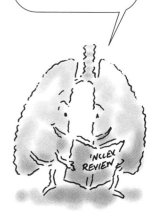

INTERVENTIONS AND RATIONALES
• Closely monitor the patient's blood pH level *to guide the treatment plan.*
• Be alert for critical changes in the patient's respiratory, CNS, and cardiovascular functions. Also watch closely for variations in ABG values and electrolyte status. Maintain adequate hydration. *These measures help detect life-threatening complications.*
• If acidosis requires mechanical ventilation, maintain a patent airway and provide adequate humidification. Perform tracheal suctioning regularly and vigorous chest physiotherapy if needed. Continuously monitor ventilator settings and respiratory status *to ensure adequate oxygenation.*
• Closely monitor patients with COPD and chronic CO_2 retention for signs of acidosis. Also, administer O_2 at low flow rates and closely monitor all patients who receive narcotics and sedatives *to prevent respiratory acidosis.*
• Instruct the patient who has received a general anesthetic to turn, cough, and perform deep-breathing exercises frequently *to prevent the onset of respiratory acidosis.*

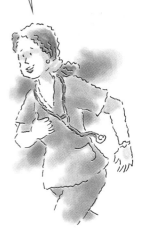

Teaching topics
• Home O_2 use

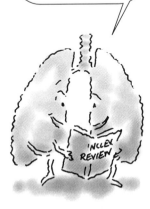

I overdo it sometimes. When I eliminate CO_2 faster than it's produced at the cellular level, it leads to deficiency of CO_2 in the blood, a loss of hydrogen ions, and an increase in pH.

• Coughing and deep breathing exercises
• Medication regimen and possible adverse reactions

Respiratory alkalosis

Respiratory alkalosis is characterized by a deficiency of CO_2 in the blood (hypocapnia), as indicated by a decrease in $Paco_2$. $Paco_2$ is below 35 mm Hg (normal level is 45 mm Hg).

This condition is caused by alveolar hyperventilation. Elimination of CO_2 by the lungs exceeds the production of CO_2 at the cellular level, leading to deficiency of CO_2 in the blood.

Uncomplicated respiratory alkalosis leads to a decrease in hydrogen ion concentration, which causes elevated blood pH.

CAUSES
Respiratory alkalosis can result from pulmonary or nonpulmonary causes.

Pulmonary causes
• Acute asthma
• Interstitial lung disease
• Pneumonia
• Pulmonary vascular disease

Nonpulmonary causes
• Anxiety
• Aspirin toxicity
• CNS disease (inflammation or tumor)
• Fever
• Hepatic failure
• Metabolic acidosis
• Pregnancy
• Sepsis

ASSESSMENT FINDINGS
• Agitation
• Cardiac arrhythmias that fail to respond to conventional treatment (severe respiratory alkalosis)
• Carpopedal spasms (spasms affecting the wrist and the foot)
• Circumoral or peripheral paresthesias (a prickling sensation around the mouth or extremities)
• Deep, rapid breathing, possibly exceeding 40 breaths/minute (cardinal sign)
• Light-headedness or dizziness (from decreased cerebral blood flow)
• Muscle weakness
• Seizures (severe respiratory alkalosis)
• Twitching (possibly progressing to tetany)

DIAGNOSTIC TEST RESULTS
• ABG analysis confirms respiratory alkalosis and rules out respiratory compensation for metabolic acidosis. In the acute stage, $Paco_2$ is below 35 mm Hg and pH is elevated in proportion to the fall in $Paco_2$, but pH drops toward normal in the chronic stage. Bicarbonate level is normal in the acute stage but below normal in the chronic stage.

NURSING DIAGNOSES
• Anxiety
• Impaired gas exchange
• Ineffective breathing pattern

TREATMENT
Treatment seeks to eradicate the underlying condition. It may include:
• removal of ingested toxins
• treatment of CNS disease
• treatment of fever or sepsis.

Memory jogger

To remember the significance of pH, think "percentage hydrogen," recalling that H is the symbol for hydrogen. pH refers to the balance of hydrogen ions (acids) and bicarbonate ions (base) in a solution.

When H goes up, pH goes down. Normal arterial pH is 7.35 to 7.45. In acidosis, hydrogen ions (acids) accumulate and pH goes down. In alkalosis, hydrogen ions decrease and pH goes up.

In severe respiratory alkalosis
• Having the patient breathe into a paper bag, which helps relieve acute anxiety and increases CO_2 levels

INTERVENTIONS AND RATIONALES
• Watch for and report any changes in neurologic, neuromuscular, or cardiovascular functions *to ensure prompt recognition and treatment.*
• Remember that twitching and cardiac arrhythmias may be associated with alkalemia and electrolyte imbalances. Monitor ABG and serum electrolyte levels closely, watching for any variations *to detect early changes and prevent complications.*

Teaching topics
• Relaxation techniques
• Breathing into a paper bag during an acute anxiety attack

Sarcoidosis

Sarcoidosis is a multisystemic, granulomatous disorder (this means it affects many body systems and produces nodules of chronically inflamed tissue). Sarcoidosis may lead to lymphadenopathy (disease of the lymph nodes), pulmonary infiltration, and skeletal, liver, eye, or skin lesions.

Sarcoidosis occurs most often in young adults (ages 20 to 40). In the United States, sarcoidosis occurs predominantly among blacks and affects twice as many women as men.

Acute sarcoidosis usually resolves within 2 years. Chronic, progressive sarcoidosis, which is uncommon, is associated with pulmonary fibrosis and progressive pulmonary disability.

CAUSES
Although the cause of sarcoidosis is unknown, the following explanations are possible:
• hypersensitivity response (possibly from a T-cell imbalance) to such agents as mycobacteria, fungi, and pine pollen

• genetic predisposition (suggested by a slightly higher incidence of sarcoidosis within the same family)
• chemicals, such as zirconium or beryllium, which can lead to illnesses resembling sarcoidosis.

ASSESSMENT FINDINGS
Initial signs
• Arthralgia (in the wrists, ankles, and elbows)
• Fatigue
• Malaise
• Weight loss

Respiratory
• Breathlessness
• Cor pulmonale (in advanced pulmonary disease)
• Cough (usually nonproductive)
• Pulmonary hypertension (in advanced pulmonary disease)
• Substernal pain

Cutaneous
• Erythema nodosum
• Subcutaneous skin nodules with maculopapular eruptions
• Extensive nasal mucosal lesions

Ophthalmic
• Anterior uveitis (common)
• Glaucoma and blindness (rare)

Lymphatic
• Lymphadenopathy
• Splenomegaly (enlarged spleen)

Musculoskeletal
• Muscle weakness
• Polyarthralgia (pain affecting many joints)
• Pain
• Punched-out lesions on phalanges

Hepatic
• Granulomatous hepatitis (usually asymptomatic)

Genitourinary
• Hypercalciuria (excessive calcium in the urine)

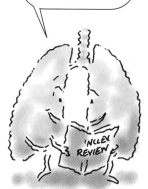

Yes, sarcoidosis is a pulmonary disorder, but it affects many body systems.

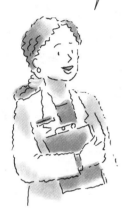

Remember that the patient on long-term or high-dose steroid therapy is vulnerable to infection.

Cardiovascular
- Arrhythmias (premature beats, bundle branch block, or complete heart block)
- Cardiomyopathy (rare)

Central nervous system
- Cranial or peripheral nerve palsies
- Basilar meningitis (inflammation of the meninges at the base of the brain)
- Seizures
- Pituitary and hypothalamic lesions producing diabetes insipidus

DIAGNOSTIC TEST RESULTS
- A positive Kveim-Siltzbach skin test supports the diagnosis. In this test, the patient receives an intradermal injection of an antigen prepared from human sarcoidal spleen or lymph nodes from patients with sarcoidosis. If the patient has active sarcoidosis, granuloma develops at the injection site in 2 to 6 weeks. This reaction is considered positive when a biopsy of the skin at the injection site shows discrete epitheloid cell granuloma.
- ABG analysis shows decreased Pao_2.
- Chest X-ray shows bilateral hilar and right paratracheal adenopathy with or without diffuse interstitial infiltrates; occasionally large nodular lesions are present in lung parenchyma.
- Lymph node, skin, or lung biopsy reveals noncaseating granulomas with negative cultures for mycobacteria and fungi.
- Negative tuberculin skin test, fungal serologies, and sputum cultures for mycobacteria and fungi, as well as negative biopsy cultures, help rule out infection.
- Other laboratory data infrequently reveal increased serum calcium, mild anemia, leukocytosis, or hyperglobulinemia.
- PFTs show decreased total lung capacity and compliance and decreased diffusing capacity.

NURSING DIAGNOSES
- Anxiety
- Impaired gas exchange
- Risk for injury

TREATMENT
- Low-calcium diet and avoidance of direct exposure to sunlight (in patients with hypercalcemia)
- O_2 therapy
- No treatment (for asymptomatic sarcoidosis)

Drug therapy
- Systemic or topical steroid, if sarcoidosis causes ocular, respiratory, CNS, cardiac, or systemic symptoms (such as fever and weight loss), hypercalcemia, or destructive skin lesions

INTERVENTIONS AND RATIONALES
- Watch for and report any complications. Be aware of any abnormal laboratory results (anemia, for example) *that could alter patient care.*
- For the patient with arthralgia, administer analgesics as needed *to promote patient comfort.* Record signs of progressive muscle weakness *to detect deterioration in the patient's condition.*
- Provide a nutritious, high-calorie diet and plenty of fluids *to ensure that nutritional intake meets the patient's metabolic needs.* If the patient has hypercalcemia, suggest a low-calcium diet *to prevent complications of hypercalcemia, such as muscle weakness, heart block, hypertension, and cardiac arrest.* Weigh the patient regularly *to detect weight loss.*
- Monitor respiratory function. Check chest X-rays for the extent of lung involvement; note and record any bloody sputum or increase in sputum. If the patient has pulmonary hypertension or end-stage cor pulmonale, check ABG values, watch for arrhythmias, and administer O_2 as needed. *These measures promptly detect deterioration in patient's condition.*
- Perform fingerstick glucose tests at least every 12 hours at the beginning of steroid therapy, *because steroids may induce or worsen diabetes mellitus.*
- Assess for fluid retention, electrolyte imbalance (especially hypokalemia), moon face, hypertension, and personality change, *which are adverse effects of steroids.*

Teaching topics
• Need for compliance with prescribed steroid therapy and regular, careful follow-up examinations and treatment
• Information on community support and resource groups and the American Foundation for the Blind, if necessary

Tuberculosis

TB is an airborne, infectious, communicable disease that can occur acutely or chronically. In TB, alveoli become the focus of infection from inhaled droplets containing bacteria. Tubercle bacilli multiply, spread through the lymphatics, and drain into the systemic circulation. Cell-mediated immunity to the mycobacteria, which develops 3 to 6 weeks later, usually contains the infection and arrests the disease.

If the infection reactivates, the body's response characteristically leads to caseation — the conversion of necrotic tissue to a cheese-like material. The caseum may localize, undergo fibrosis, or excavate and form cavities, the walls of which are studded with multiplying tubercle bacilli. If this occurs, infected caseous debris may spread throughout the lungs by the tracheobronchial tree.

CAUSES
• *Mycobacterium tuberculosis*

ASSESSMENT FINDINGS
• Anorexia, weight loss
• Cough, yellow and mucoid sputum, hemoptysis
• Crackles
• Dyspnea
• Fatigue, malaise, irritability
• Fever
• Night sweats
• Tachycardia

NURSING DIAGNOSES
• Ineffective airway clearance
• Fatigue
• Social isolation

DIAGNOSTIC TEST RESULTS
• Chest X-ray shows active or calcified lesions.
• Hematology shows increased WBCs and ESR.
• Mantoux skin test is positive.
• Sputum study is positive for acid-fast bacillus and *M. tuberculosis.*

TREATMENT
• Chest physiotherapy, postural drainage, and incentive spirometry
• Dietary changes, including establishing a diet high in carbohydrates, protein, vitamins B_6 and C, and calories
• Standard and airborne precautions (While the patient is contagious, everyone entering the patient's room must wear a respirator with a high-efficiency particulate air filter.)

Drug therapy
• Antibiotic: streptomycin
• Antituberculars: isoniazid (INH), ethambutol (Myambutol), rifampin (Rifadin), pyrazinamide (Pyrazinamide)

INTERVENTIONS AND RATIONALES
• Assess respiratory status *to detect respiratory complications such as pleural effusion.*
• Monitor and record vital signs and laboratory studies *to detect signs of compromise.*
• Maintain the patient's diet and provide small, frequent meals *to increase caloric intake.*
• Perform chest physiotherapy and postural drainage *to facilitate mobilization of secretions.*
• Assist with turning, coughing, and deep-breathing and provide suction, if necessary, *to mobilize and remove secretions.*
• Administer medications, as prescribed, *to avoid development of drug-resistant organisms.*
• Maintain infection-control precautions *to reduce the spread of infectious organisms.*
• Instruct the patient to cover nose and mouth when sneezing *to reduce transmission by droplet.*
• Encourage fluids *to liquefy secretions.*
• Provide frequent oral hygiene *to promote comfort and improve appetite.*
• Provide a negative pressure room *to prevent the spread of infection.*

• Monitor vital signs. *Fever, tachycardia, and tachypnea may be present with tuberculosis.*
• Monitor and record intake and output *to assess hydration. Adequate hydration is necessary to facilitate removal of secretions.*
• Monitor laboratory studies *to detect adverse effects of drug therapy.*

Teaching topics
• Preventing spread of droplets of sputum
• Finishing the entire course of medication (6 to 18 months)
• Contacting the American Lung Association

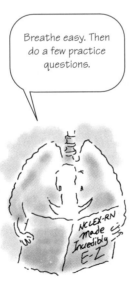

Breathe easy. Then do a few practice questions.

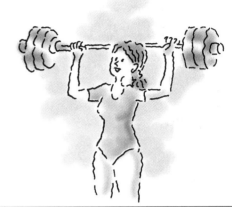

Pump up on practice questions

1. During the insertion of a rigid scope for bronchoscopy, a client experiences a vasovagal response. The nurse should expect:
   A. the client's pupils to become dilated.
   B. the client to experience bronchodilation.
   C. a decrease in gastric secretions.
   D. a drop in the client's heart rate.
Answer: D. During a bronchoscopy, a vasovagal response may be caused by stimulating the pharynx, which, in turn, may cause stimulation of the vagus nerve. The client may experience a sudden drop in the heart rate leading to syncope. Stimulation of the vagus nerve doesn't lead to mydriasis (pupillary dilation) or bronchodilation. Stimulation of the vagus nerve increases gastric secretions.

➡ *NCLEX keys*
Nursing process step: Assessment
Client needs category: Physiological integrity
Client needs subcategory: Reduction of risk potential
Taxonomic level: Comprehension

2. A client with right lower lobe pneumonia is prescribed percussion and postural drainage. When performing percussion and postural drainage, the nurse should position the client:

A. in semi-Fowler's position with the knees bent.
B. right side-lying with the foot of the bed elevated.
C. prone or supine with the foot of the bed elevated higher than the head.
D. bent at the waist leaning slightly forward.

Answer: C. The aim of percussion and postural drainage is to mobilize pulmonary secretions so they can be effectively expectorated. In right lower lobe bronchopneumonia, the nurse should position the client with the right side up or lower lobes elevated above the upper lobes. This would employ gravity in mobilizing pulmonary secretions. Semi-Fowler's position and being bent at the waist would hamper mobilization of secretions from the right lower lobe.

➡ *NCLEX keys*
Nursing process step: Implementation
Client needs category: Physiological integrity
Client needs subcategory: Physiological adaptation
Taxonomic level: Application

3. A client with acquired immunodeficiency syndrome (AIDS) develops *Pneumocystis carinii* pneumonia. Which nursing diagnosis has the highest priority for this client?
A. Impaired gas exchange
B. Altered oral mucous membranes
C. Altered nutrition: less than body requirements
D. Activity intolerance

Answer: A. While all these nursing diagnoses are appropriate for the client with AIDS, impaired gas exchange is the priority nursing diagnosis for the client with *P. carinii* pneumonia. Airway, breathing, and circulation take top priority for any client.

➡ *NCLEX keys*
Nursing process step: Analysis
Client needs category: Physiological integrity
Client needs subcategory: Physiological adaptation
Taxonomic level: Analysis

4. A client has chronic bronchitis. The nurse is teaching him breathing exercises. Which should the nurse include in the teaching?
A. Make inhalation longer than exhalation.
B. Exhale through an open mouth.
C. Use diaphragmatic breathing.
D. Use chest breathing.

Answer: C. In chronic bronchitis the diaphragm is flat and weak. Diaphragmatic breathing helps to strengthen the diaphragm and maximizes ventilation. Exhalation should be no longer than inhalation to prevent collapse of the bronchioles. The client with chronic bronchitis should exhale through pursed lips to prolong exhalation, keep the bronchioles from collapsing, and prevent air trapping. Diaphragmatic breathing, not chest breathing, increases lung expansion.

➡ *NCLEX keys*
Nursing process step: Planning
Client needs category: Physiological integrity
Client needs subcategory: Reduction of risk potential
Taxonomic level: Application

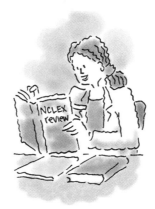

5. In a client with emphysema, the initiative to breathe is triggered by:
A. high carbon dioxide (CO_2) levels.
B. low CO_2 levels.
C. high oxygen (O_2) levels.
D. low O_2 levels.

Answer: D. Because of long-standing hypercapnia, breathing in a client with emphysema is triggered by low O_2 levels. In a client with a normal respiratory drive, the initiative to breathe is triggered by increased CO_2 levels.

➡ NCLEX keys
Nursing process step: Analysis
Client needs category: Physiological integrity
Client needs subcategory: Physiological adaptation
Taxonomic level: Knowledge

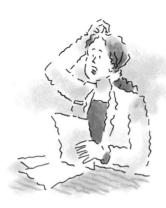

6. A client experiencing acute respiratory failure will most likely demonstrate:
   A. hypocapnia, hypoventilation, hyperoxemia.
   B. hypocapnia, hyperventilation, hyperoxemia.
   C. hypercapnia, hyperventilation, hypoxemia.
   D. hypercapnia, hypoventilation, hypoxemia.
Answer: D. Acute respiratory failure is marked by hypercapnia (elevated arterial carbon dioxide), hypoventilation, and hypoxemia (subnormal oxygen).

➡ NCLEX keys
Nursing process step: Assessment
Client needs category: Physiological integrity
Client needs subcategory: Physiological adaptation
Taxonomic level: Comprehension

7. During an asthmatic episode, a client receives a beta$_2$-adrenergic agonist. What is the best evidence that the drug is effective?
   A. Normal drug serum levels
   B. Productive cough
   C. Clear breath sounds
   D. Improved heart rate
Answer: C. Beta$_2$-adrenergic agonists cause bronchodilation, which is the opening up of narrowed airways. In an asthmatic episode, the client exhibits wheezes. Treating the client with a beta$_2$-adrenergic agonist should cause a diminution or disappearance of the wheezes. Beta$_2$-adrenergic agonists aren't monitored for serum levels. Beta$_2$-adrenergic agonists aren't expectorants so a productive cough wouldn't indicate the drug is effective. Beta$_2$-adrenergic agonists are cardiac stimulants and cause tachycardia, which in itself isn't evidence of bronchodilation.

➡ NCLEX keys
Nursing process step: Evaluation
Client needs category: Physiological integrity
Client needs subcategory: Pharmacological and parenteral therapies
Taxonomic level: Comprehension

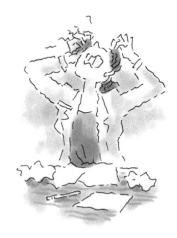

8. A client with adult respiratory distress syndrome (ARDS) is intubated and placed on mechanical ventilation. His partial pressure of arterial oxygen (PaO_2) is 60 mm Hg on 100% fraction of inspired oxygen (FIO_2). To increase his Pao_2 without raising the Fio_2, the client will most likely be placed on:

A. time-cycled ventilation.
B. volume-cycled ventilation.
C. pressure support.
D. positive end-expiratory pressure (PEEP).

Answer: D. PEEP is widely used during mechanical ventilation of the client with ARDS. It improves gas exchange over the alveolar capillary membrane. Time- or volume-cycled ventilation is less likely to be used in ARDS than pressure-cycled ventilation. Pressure support is dependent on the client's inspiratory effort and not as effective as PEEP in the treatment of ARDS.

➡ *NCLEX keys*

Nursing process step: Implementation
Client needs category: Physiological integrity
Client needs subcategory: Physiological adaptation
Taxonomic level: Application

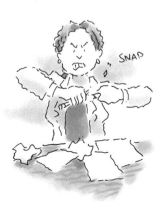

9. A client with clinically active pulmonary tuberculosis is prescribed isoniazid, rifampin, pyrazinamide, and ethambutol. Which findings best indicate effectiveness of drug therapy?

A. Cavities are no longer evident on chest X-ray.
B. Tuberculin skin test is negative.
C. The client is afebrile and no longer coughing.
D. The sputum culture converts to negative.

Answer: D. A change in sputum culture from positive to negative is the best indication of the effectiveness of antitubercular medication. Cavities disappearing from the chest X-ray aren't a reliable indicator of drug effectiveness. Tuberculin skin tests don't convert from positive to negative. Disappearance of symptoms isn't the best indicator of the treatment's effectiveness.

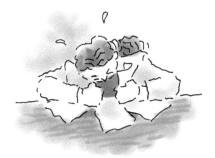

➡ *NCLEX keys*

Nursing process step: Evaluation
Client needs category: Physiological integrity
Client needs subcategory: Pharmacological and parenteral therapies
Taxonomic level: Application

10. Following a pneumothorax, a client receives a chest tube attached to a three-chamber chest drainage system. During the night, the client becomes disoriented, gets out of bed, and steps on the drainage device, causing it to crack open and lose its seal. The nurse should immediately:

A. clamp the chest tube close to the client's thorax.
B. attach the chest tube directly to low wall suction.
C. place the device on a sterile field and call the physician.
D. place the end of the chest tube in a container of sterile water.

Answer: D. When a chest drainage system cracks open, the closed system between the pleural space and the device is broken. This will allow air to move through the tubing into the pleural space, exacerbating the pneumothorax. The nurse should immediately place the distal end of the tube in sterile water, closing the system again. The tube shouldn't be clamped because it increases pressure against the pleural space. It's inappropriate to attach the drain directly to wall suction. Calling the physician should occur after correcting the problem.

➡ NCLEX keys

Nursing process step: Implementation
Client needs category: Physiological integrity
Client needs subcategory: Physiological adaptation
Taxonomic level: Application

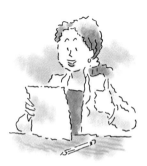

Hematologic & Immune Systems

Brush up on key concepts

The immune system and hematologic system are closely related. The immune system consists of specialized cells and structures that defend the body against invasion by harmful organisms or chemical toxins. The hematologic system also functions as an important part of the body's defenses. The blood transports the components of the immune system throughout the body. In addition, the blood delivers oxygen and nutrients to all tissues and removes wastes. Both immune system cells and blood cells originate in the bone marrow.

The key components of the immune system are the lymph nodes, thymus, spleen, and tonsils. The key components of the hematologic system are blood and bone marrow. Blood components play a vital role in transporting electrolytes and regulating acid-base balance.

At any time, you can review the major points of this chapter by consulting the *Cheat Sheet* on pages 114 to 123.

Fluid movers

Lymphatic vessels consist of capillary-like structures that are permeable to large molecules. Lymphatic vessels prevent edema by moving fluid and proteins from interstitial spaces to venous circulation. They also reabsorb fats from the small intestine.

Bacteria filters

Lymph nodes are tissues that filter out bacteria and other foreign cells. They are grouped by region. Here are the groups of lymph nodes:
• cervicofacial
• supraclavicular
• axillary
• epitrochlear
• inguinal
• femoral.

Water plus

Lymph is the fluid found in interstitial spaces. Lymph is composed of water and the end products of cell metabolism.

Body guard

The **tonsils** are located at the back of the mouth in the oropharynx and fight off pathogens entering the mouth and nose. They are made of lymphatic tissue and produce lymphocytes.

Filters blood, kills bacteria

The **spleen** is a major lymphatic organ. Here's what it does:
• destroys bacteria
• filters blood
• serves as blood reservoir
• forms lymphocytes and monocytes
• traps formed particles.

Home of hematopoiesis

Bone marrow may be described as either red or yellow.

Hematopoiesis is carried out by red marrow. Hematopoiesis produces erythrocytes, leukocytes, and thrombocytes. Red bone marrow is a source of lymphocytes and macrophages.

Yellow bone marrow is red bone marrow that has changed to fat.

Getting down to the marrow

Bone marrow contains **stem cells,** which may develop into several different cell types during hematopoiesis.
• Some stem cells evolve into lymphocytes; lymphocytes may become B cells or T cells.
• Other stem cells evolve into phagocytes.

(Text continues on page 123.)

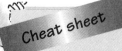

Hematologic and immunologic refresher

ACQUIRED IMMUNODEFICIENCY SYNDROME

Key signs and symptoms
- Anorexia, weight loss, recurrent diarrhea
- Disorientation, confusion, dementia
- Night sweats
- Opportunistic infections

Key test results
- CD4+ T-cell level is less than 200 cells/µl
- ELISA shows positive HIV antibody titer.
- Western blot is positive.

Key treatments
- Transfusion therapy: fresh frozen plasma, platelets, and packed red blood cells (RBCs)
- Antibiotics: trimethoprim and sulfamethoxazole (Bactrim)
- Antivirals: dapsone, didanosine (Videx), ganciclovir (Cytovene), zidovudine (Retrovir, AZT), acyclovir (Zovirax), pentamidine (Pentam), aerosolized pentamidine (NebuPent)

Combination therapy
- Nonnucleoside reverse transcriptase inhibitors: delavirdine (Rescriptor), nevirapine (Viramune)
- Nucleoside reverse transcriptase inhibitors such as lamivudine (Epivir), zalcitabine (Dideoxycytidine, ddC), zidovudine (Retrovir, AZT)
- Protease inhibitors: indinavir (Crixivan), nelfinavir (Viracept), ritonavir (Norvir), saquinavir (Invirase)

Key interventions
- Monitor for opportunistic infections.
- Maintain the patient's diet.
- Provide mouth care.
- Maintain standard precautions.
- Make referrals to community agencies for support.
- Assess respiratory status.
- Monitor laboratory values.

ANAPHYLAXIS

Key signs and symptoms
- Cardiovascular symptoms (hypotension, shock, cardiac arrhythmias) that may precipitate circulatory collapse if untreated
- Sudden physical distress within seconds or minutes after exposure to an allergen (may include feeling of impending doom or fright, weakness, sweating, sneezing, shortness of breath, nasal pruritus, urticaria, and angioedema, followed rapidly by symptoms in one or more target organs)

Key test results
- Anaphylaxis can be diagnosed by the rapid onset of severe respiratory or cardiovascular symptoms after ingestion or injection of a drug, vaccine, diagnostic agent, food or food additive, or after an insect sting.

Key treatments
- Immediate injection of epinephrine 1:1,000 aqueous solution, 0.1 to 0.5 ml, repeated every 5 to 20 minutes as necessary

Key interventions
- In the early stages of anaphylaxis, when the patient hasn't yet lost consciousness and is still normotensive, give epinephrine I.M. or subcutaneously (S.C.), and help it move into the circulation faster by massaging the injection site. In severe reactions, when the patient has lost consciousness and is hypotensive, give epinephrine I.V.
- Maintain airway patency. Observe for early signs of laryngeal edema (stridor, hoarseness, and dyspnea), and prepare for endotracheal tube insertion or a tracheotomy and oxygen therapy.
- Watch for hypotension and shock, and maintain circulatory volume with volume expanders (plasma, plasma expanders, saline solution, and albumin) as needed. Stabilize blood pressure with the I.V. vasopressors norepinephrine (Levophed) and dopamine (Intropin). Monitor blood pressure, central venous pressure, and urine output.

ANKYLOSING SPONDYLITIS

Key signs and symptoms
- Intermittent low back pain (the first indication), usually most severe in morning or after period of inactivity
- Mild fatigue, fever, anorexia, or loss of weight; unilateral acute anterior uveitis; aortic insuffi-

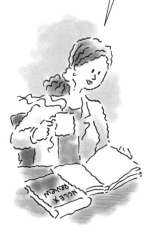

No time to study a long chapter? Then skip straight to the cheat sheet.

Hematologic and immunologic refresher *(continued)*

ANKYLOSING SPONDYLITIS *(continued)*

ciency and cardiomegaly; upper lobe pulmonary fibrosis (mimics tuberculosis)
- Stiffness and limited motion of the lumbar spine
- Symptoms progress unpredictably; disease can go into remission, exacerbation, or arrest at any stage

Key test results
- Confirmation requires characteristic X-ray findings: blurring of the bony margins of joints in the early stage, bilateral sacroiliac involvement, patchy sclerosis with superficial bony erosions, eventual squaring of vertebral bodies, and "bamboo spine" with complete ankylosis.
- Typical symptoms, a family history, and the presence of HLA-B27 strongly suggest ankylosing spondylitis.

Key treatments
- Anti-inflammatory agents: aspirin, indomethacin (Indocin), sulfasalazine (Azulfidine), and sulindac (Clinoril) to control pain and inflammation
- Good posture, stretching and deep-breathing exercises and, in some patients, braces and lightweight supports to delay further deformity (because ankylosing spondylitis progression can't be stopped)

Key interventions
- Offer support and reassurance. Keep in mind that the patient's limited range of motion makes simple tasks difficult.
- Administer medications as needed.
- Apply local heat and provide massage. Assess mobility and degree of discomfort frequently.

APLASTIC ANEMIA

Key signs and symptoms
- Dyspnea, tachypnea
- Epistaxis
- Melena
- Palpitations, tachycardia
- Purpura, petechiae, ecchymosis, pallor

Key test results
- Bone marrow biopsy shows fatty marrow with reduction of stem cells.

Key treatments
- Transfusion of platelets and packed RBCs
- Antithymocyte globulin (Atgam)
- Hematopoietic growth factor: epoetin alfa (Epogen)

Key interventions
- Monitor for infection, bleeding, and bruising.
- Administer oxygen.

- Administer transfusion therapy, as prescribed.
- Maintain protective precautions.
- Avoid giving the patient I.M. injections.

CALCIUM IMBALANCE

Key signs and symptoms
Hypocalcemia
- Cardiac arrhythmias
- Chvostek's sign
- Tetany
- Trousseau's sign

Hypercalcemia
- Anorexia
- Decreased muscle tone
- Lethargy
- Muscle weakness
- Nausea
- Polydipsia
- Polyuria

Key test results
- A serum calcium level less than 4.5 mEq/L confirms hypocalcemia; a level greater than 5.5 mEq/L confirms hypercalcemia. (Because approximately one-half of serum calcium is bound to albumin, changes in serum protein must be considered when interpreting serum calcium levels.)
- Electrocardiogram (ECG) reveals a lengthened QT interval, a prolonged ST segment, and arrhythmias in hypocalcemia; in hypercalcemia, a shortened QT interval and heart block.

Key treatments
Hypocalcemia
- Diet: adequate intake of calcium, vitamin D, and protein
- Ergocalciferol (vitamin D_2), cholecalciferol (vitamin D_3), calcitriol, dihydrotachysterol (synthetic form of vitamin D_2) for severe deficiency
- Immediate correction by I.V. calcium gluconate or calcium chloride for acute hypocalcemia (an emergency)

Hypercalcemia
- Calcitonin (Calcimar)
- Loop diuretics, such as ethacrynic acid (Edecrin) and furosemide (Lasix), to promote calcium excretion (thiazide diuretics contraindicated in hypercalcemia because they inhibit calcium excretion)

Key interventions
Hypocalcemia
- Monitor serum calcium levels every 12 to 24 hours. When giving calcium supplements, frequently check the pH level. Check for Trousseau's and Chvostek's signs.

(continued)

Hematologic and immunologic refresher (continued)

CALCIUM IMBALANCE (continued)

Hypercalcemia
• Monitor serum calcium levels frequently. Watch for cardiac arrhythmias if the serum calcium level exceeds 5.7 mEq/L. Increase fluid intake.

CHLORIDE IMBALANCE

Key signs and symptoms

Hypochloremia
• Muscle hypertonicity (in conditions related to loss of gastric secretions)
• Muscle weakness
• Shallow, depressed breathing
• Twitching

Hyperchloremia
• Agitation
• Deep, rapid breathing
• Diminished cognitive ability
• Hypertension
• Pitting edema
• Tachycardia
• Weakness

Key test results
• Serum chloride level that's less than 98 mEq/L confirms hypochloremia; supportive values with metabolic alkalosis include a serum pH greater than 7.45 and a serum carbon dioxide level greater than 32 mEq/L.
• Serum chloride level greater than 108 mEq/L confirms hyperchloremia; with metabolic acidosis, serum pH is less than 7.35 and the serum carbon dioxide level is less than 22 mEq/L.

Key treatments

Hypochloremia
• Acidifying agent: ammonium chloride
• Diet: salty broth
• Saline solution I.V.

Hyperchloremia
• Alkalinizing agent: sodium bicarbonate I.V.
• Lactated Ringer's solution

DISSEMINATED INTRAVASCULAR COAGULATION

Key signs and symptoms
• Abnormal bleeding without an accompanying history of serious hemorrhagic disorder
• Oliguria
• Shock

Key test results
• Blood tests show prolonged prothrombin time (PT) greater than 15 seconds; prolonged partial thromboplastin time (PTT) greater than 60 to 80 seconds; fibrinogen levels less than 150 mg/dl; platelets less than 100,000/µl; fibrin degradation products often greater than 100 µg/ml; and a positive D-dimer test specific for disseminated intravascular coagulation.

Key treatments
• Anticoagulant: Heparin I.V.
• Bed rest
• Transfusion therapy: fresh frozen plasma, platelets, packed RBCs

Key interventions
• Enforce complete bed rest during bleeding episodes. If the patient is very agitated, pad the side rails.
• Check all I.V. and venipuncture sites frequently for bleeding. Apply pressure to injection sites for at least 10 minutes. Alert other personnel to the patient's tendency to hemorrhage. These measures prevent hemorrhage.
• Watch for transfusion reactions and signs of fluid overload. Weigh dressings and linen and record drainage. Weigh the patient daily, particularly in renal involvement.
• Monitor the results of serial blood studies (particularly hematocrit [HCT], hemoglobin [Hb], and coagulation times).

HEMOPHILIA

Key signs and symptoms
• Hematuria (for all hemophilias)
• Joint tenderness
• Pain and swelling in a weight-bearing joint (for all hemophilias)
• Prolonged bleeding after major trauma or surgery (in mild hemophilia)
• Spontaneous or severe bleeding after minor trauma (in severe hemophilia)
• S.C. and I.M. hematomas (in moderate hemophilia)
• Tarry stools (for all hemophilias)

Key test results
• Factor VII assay reveals 0% to 25% of normal factor VIII (hemophilia A).
• Factor IX assay shows deficiency (hemophilia B).

Key treatments
• Administration of cryoprecipitate antihemophilic factor (AHF) and lyophilized (dehydrated) AHF to encourage normal hemostasis (for hemophilia A)
• Administration of recombinant factor VIII and purified factor IX to promote hemostasis (for hemophilia B)
• Administration of analgesics to control joint pain (for both types)

Hematologic and immunologic refresher *(continued)*

HEMOPHILIA *(continued)*

Key interventions

• During bleeding episodes, give sufficient clotting factor or plasma, as ordered. Also administer analgesics. Avoid I.M. injections because they may cause hematomas at the injection site. Aspirin and aspirin-containing medications are contraindicated because they decrease platelet adherence and may increase bleeding.
• If the patient has bled into a joint, immediately elevate the joint.

IRON DEFICIENCY ANEMIA

Key signs and symptoms

• Pallor
• Sensitivity to cold
• Weakness and fatigue

Key test results

• Hematology shows decreased Hb, HCT, iron, ferritin, reticulocytes, red cell indices, transferrin, and saturation; absent hemosiderin; and increased iron-binding capacity.

Key treatments

• Diet: establish a diet high in iron, roughage, and protein with increased fluids; avoid teas and coffee, which reduce absorption of iron
• Vitamins: pyridoxine hydrochloride (vitamin B_6), ascorbic acid (vitamin C)
• Antianemics: ferrous sulfate (Feosol), iron dextran (DexFerrum)

Key interventions

• Assess cardiovascular and respiratory status.
• Monitor stool, urine, and emesis for occult blood.
• Administer medications, as prescribed. Administer iron injection deep into muscle using Z-track technique to avoid subcutaneous irritation and discoloration from leaking drug.
• Provide mouth, skin, and foot care.

KAPOSI'S SARCOMA

Key signs and symptoms

• One or more obvious lesions in various shapes, sizes, and colors (ranging from red-brown to dark purple) appearing most commonly on the skin, buccal mucosa, hard and soft palates, lips, gums, tongue, tonsils, conjunctiva, and sclera
• Pain (if the sarcoma advances beyond the early stages or if a lesion breaks down or impinges on nerves or organs)

Key test results

• Tissue biopsy identifies the lesion's type and stage.

Key treatments

• High-calorie, high-protein diet
• Radiation therapy

• Chemotherapy: doxorubicin (Adriamycin), etoposide (VePesid), vinblastine (Velban), vincristine (Oncovin)
• Antiemetic: trimethobenzamide (Tigan)

Key interventions

• Inspect the patient's skin every shift. Look for new lesions and skin breakdown. If the patient has painful lesions, help him into a more comfortable position.
• Administer pain medications. Suggest distractions, and help the patient with relaxation techniques.
• Urge the patient to share his feelings, and provide encouragement.
• Supply the patient with high-calorie, high-protein meals. If he can't tolerate regular meals, provide him with frequent smaller meals. Consult with the dietitian, and plan meals around the patient's treatment.
• Be alert for adverse reactions to radiation therapy or chemotherapy — such as anorexia, nausea, vomiting, and diarrhea — and take steps to prevent or alleviate them.
• Explain infection-prevention techniques and, if necessary, demonstrate basic hygiene measures. Advise the patient not to share his toothbrush, razor, or other items that may be contaminated with blood. These measures are especially important if the patient also has AIDS.

LEUKEMIA

Key signs and symptoms

• Enlarged lymph nodes, spleen, and liver
• Frequent infections
• Weakness and fatigue

Key test results

• Bone marrow biopsy shows large numbers of immature leukocytes.

Key treatments

• Antimetabolites: fluorouracil, methotrexate sodium
• Alkylating agents: busulfan, chlorambucil
• Antineoplastics: vinblastine, vincristine sulfate
• Antibiotics: doxorubicin (Adriamycin), plicamycin (Mithracin)
• Hematopoietic growth factor: epoetin alfa (Epogen)

Key interventions

• Monitor laboratory studies.
• Monitor for bleeding. Place patient with epistaxis in an upright position, leaning slightly forward to reduce vascular pressure to prevent aspiration.
• Monitor for infection. Promptly report fever over 101° F, and decreased white blood cell (WBC) counts so that antibiotic therapy may be initiated.

(continued)

Hematologic and immunologic refresher *(continued)*

LEUKEMIA *(continued)*
• Administer transfusion therapy as prescribed and monitor for adverse reactions.
• Provide gentle mouth and skin care.

LYMPHOMA

Key signs and symptoms
• A predictable pattern of spread (Hodgkin's disease)
• Enlarged, nontender, firm, and movable lymph nodes in lower cervical regions (Hodgkin's disease)
• Less predictable pattern of spread (malignant lymphoma)
• Prominent, painless, generalized lymphadenopathy (malignant lymphoma)

Key test results
• Bone marrow aspiration and biopsy reveals small, diffuse lymphocytic or large, follicular-type cells (malignant lymphoma).
• Lymph node biopsy is positive for Reed-Sternberg cells (Hodgkin's disease).

Key treatments
• Radiation therapy
• Transfusion of packed RBCs
• Chemotherapy for Hodgkin's disease: mechlorethamine (Mustargen), vincristine sulfate (Oncovin), procarbazine (Matulane), doxorubicin (Adriamycin), bleomycin (Blenoxane), vinblastine (Velban), dacarbazine (DTIC-Dome)
• Chemotherapy for malignant lymphoma: cyclophosphamide (Cytoxan), vincristine sulfate (Oncovin), doxorubicin (Adriamycin)

Key interventions
• Monitor for bleeding, infection, jaundice, and electrolyte imbalance.
• Provide mouth and skin care.
• Encourage fluids.
• Administer medications, as prescribed, and monitor for adverse effects.
• Administer transfusion therapy, as prescribed, and monitor for adverse reactions.

MAGNESIUM IMBALANCE

Key signs and symptoms
Hypomagnesemia
• Arrhythmias
• Neuromuscular irritability
• Chvostek's sign
• Mood changes
• Confusion

Hypermagnesemia
• Diminished deep tendon reflexes
• Weakness
• Confusion
• Heart block
• Nausea
• Vomiting

Key test results
• Blood test that shows decreased serum magnesium levels (less than 1.5 mEq/L) confirms hypomagnesemia.
• Blood test that shows increased serum magnesium levels (greater than 2.5 mEq/L) confirms hypermagnesemia.

Key treatments
Hypomagnesemia
• Daily magnesium supplements I.M. or by mouth
• High-magnesium diet
• Magnesium sulfate I.V. (10 to 40 mEq/L diluted in I.V. fluid) for severe cases

Hypermagnesemia
• Diet: low magnesium with increased fluid intake
• Loop diuretic: furosemide (Lasix)
• Magnesium antagonist: calcium gluconate (10%)
• Peritoneal dialysis or hemodialysis if renal function fails or if excess magnesium can't be eliminated

Key interventions
For patients with hypomagnesemia
• Monitor serum electrolyte levels (including magnesium, calcium, and potassium) daily for mild deficits and every 6 to 12 hours during replacement therapy.
• Measure intake and output frequently. (Urine output shouldn't fall below 25 ml/hour or 600 ml/day.)
• Monitor vital signs during I.V. therapy. Infuse magnesium replacement slowly, and watch for bradycardia, heart block, and decreased respiratory rate.
• Have calcium gluconate I.V. available to reverse hypermagnesemia from overcorrection.

For patients with hypermagnesemia
• Frequently assess level of consciousness, muscle activity, and vital signs.
• Keep accurate intake and output records. Provide sufficient fluids.
• Correct abnormal serum electrolyte levels immediately.
• Monitor the patient receiving digitalis glycosides and calcium gluconate simultaneously.

Hematologic and immunologic refresher (continued)

METABOLIC ACIDOSIS

Key signs and symptoms
- Central nervous system depression
- Kussmaul's respirations
- Lethargy

Key test results
- Arterial blood gas (ABG) analysis reveals pH below 7.35 and bicarbonate level less than 24 mEq/L.

Key treatments
- Sodium bicarbonate I.V., or orally for chronic metabolic acidosis

Key interventions
- Keep sodium bicarbonate ampules handy. Frequently monitor vital signs, laboratory results, and level of consciousness.
- Record intake and output accurately.

METABOLIC ALKALOSIS

Key signs and symptoms
- Atrial tachycardia
- Confusion
- Diarrhea
- Hypoventilation
- Twitching
- Vomiting

Key test results
- ABG analysis reveals pH greater than 7.45 and a bicarbonate level above 29 mEq/L.

Key treatments
- Acidifying agent: ammonium chloride I.V.

Key interventions
- When administering ammonium chloride 0.9%, limit the infusion rate to 1¼ hours. Avoid overdosage. Don't give ammonium chloride to a patient with signs of hepatic or renal disease.

MULTIPLE MYELOMA

Key signs and symptoms
- Anemia, thrombocytopenia, hemorrhage
- Constant, severe bone pain
- Pathologic fractures, skeletal deformities of sternum and ribs, loss of height

Key test results
- X-ray shows diffuse, round, punched out bone lesions; osteoporosis; osteolytic lesions of the skull; and widespread demineralization.

Key treatments
- Orthopedic devices: braces, splints, casts
- Alkylating agents: melphalan (Alkeran), cyclophosphamide (Cytoxan)
- Androgen: fluoxymesterone (Halotestin)
- Antibiotics: doxorubicin (Adriamycin), plicamycin (Mithracin)
- Antigout: allopurinol (Zyloprim)
- Antineoplastics: vinblastine (Velban), vincristine sulfate (Oncovin)
- Glucocorticoid: prednisone (Deltasone)

Key interventions
- Assess renal status.
- Assess bone pain.
- Administer I.V. fluids.

PERNICIOUS ANEMIA

Key signs and symptoms
- Tingling and paresthesia of hands and feet
- Weight loss, anorexia, dyspepsia

Key test results
- Bone marrow shows increased megaloblasts, few maturing erythrocytes, and defective leukocyte maturation.
- Peripheral blood smear reveals oval, macrocytic, hyperchromic erythrocytes.

Key treatments
- Vitamins: pyridoxine hydrochloride (vitamin B_6), ascorbic acid (vitamin C), cyanocobalamin (vitamin B_{12}), folic acid (vitamin A)

Key interventions
- Assess cardiovascular status.
- Administer medications, as prescribed.
- Provide mouth care before and after meals.
- Prevent the patient from falling.

PHOSPHORUS IMBALANCE

Key signs and symptoms
Hypophosphatemia
- Anorexia
- Muscle weakness
- Paresthesia
- Tremor

Hyperphosphatemia
- Usually asymptomatic

Key test results
- Serum phosphorus level less than 1.7 mEq/L (or 2.5 mg/dl) confirms hypophosphatemia. A urine phosphorus level more than 1.3 g/24 hours supports this diagnosis.

(continued)

Hematologic and immunologic refresher *(continued)*

PHOSPHORUS IMBALANCE *(continued)*

• Serum phosphorus level exceeding 2.6 mEq/L (or 4.5 mg/dl) confirms hyperphosphatemia. Supportive values include decreased levels of serum calcium (less than 9 mg/dl) and urine phosphorus (less than 0.9 g/24 hours).

Key treatments

Hypophosphatemia

• Diet: high-phosphorus diet
• Phosphate supplements

Hyperphosphatemia

• Low-phosphorus diet
• Calcium supplement: calcium acetate (PhosLo)

Key interventions

For patients with hypophosphatemia

• Record intake and output accurately. Administer potassium phosphate slow I.V.. Assess renal function, and be alert for hypocalcemia when giving phosphate supplements. If phosphate salt tablets cause nausea, use capsules instead.
• Advise the patient to follow a high-phosphorus diet containing milk and milk products, kidney, liver, turkey, and dried fruits.

For patients with hyperphosphatemia

• Monitor intake and output. If urine output falls below 25 ml/hour or 600 ml/day, notify the doctor immediately.
• Watch for signs of hypocalcemia, such as muscle twitching and tetany, which often accompany hyperphosphatemia.
• Advise the patient to eat foods low in phosphorus, such as vegetables. Obtain dietary consultation if the condition results from chronic renal insufficiency.

POLYCYTHEMIA VERA

Key signs and symptoms

• Clubbing of the digits
• Dizziness
• Headache
• Hypertension
• Ruddy cyanosis of the nose
• Thrombosis of smaller vessels
• Visual disturbances (blurring, diplopia, engorged veins of fundus and retina)

Key test results

• Blood tests show increased RBC mass and normal arterial oxygen saturation in association with splenomegaly or two of the following: thrombocytosis, leukocytosis, elevated leukocyte alkaline phosphatase level, or elevated serum vitamin B_{12} or unbound B_{12} binding capacity.

Key treatments

• Phlebotomy (typically, 350 to 500 ml of blood is removed every other day until the patient's HCT is reduced to the low-normal range)
• Plasmapheresis
• Chemotherapy: busulfan (Myleran), chlorambucil (Leukeran), melphalan (Alkeran)
• Antigout agent: allopurinol (Zyloprim)

Key interventions

• Check blood pressure, pulse rate, and respirations prior to and during phlebotomy.
• During phlebotomy, make sure the patient is lying down comfortably.
• Stay alert for tachycardia, clamminess, or complaints of vertigo. If these effects occur, the procedure should be stopped.
• Immediately after phlebotomy, check blood pressure and pulse rate. Have the patient sit up for about 5 minutes before allowing him to walk. Also, administer 24 oz (720 ml) of juice or water.
• Tell the patient to watch for and report any symptoms of iron deficiency (pallor, weight loss, weakness, glossitis).
• Give additional fluids, administer allopurinol, and alkalinize the urine.
• Monitor complete blood count and platelet count before and during therapy. Warn an outpatient who develops leukopenia that his resistance to infection is low; advise him to avoid crowds and watch for the symptoms of infection.
• Tell the patient about possible adverse effects (nausea, vomiting, and risk of infection) of alkylating agents.
• Have the patient lie down during I.V. administration to facilitate the procedure and prevent extravasation and for 15 to 20 minutes afterward.

RHEUMATOID ARTHRITIS

Key signs and symptoms

• Painful, swollen joints, crepitus, morning stiffness
• Symmetrical joint swelling (mirror image of affected joints)

Key test results

• Antinuclear antibody test is positive.
• Rheumatoid factor test is positive.

Key treatments

• Cold therapy during acute episodes
• Heat therapy to relax muscles and relieve pain for chronic disease
• Antirheumatic: hydroxychloroquine (Plaquenil)
• Glucocorticoids: prednisone (Deltasone), hydrocortisone (Hydrocortone)

Hematologic and immunologic refresher *(continued)*

RHEUMATOID ARTHRITIS *(continued)*

• Nonsteroidal anti-inflammatory drugs (NSAIDs): indomethacin (Indocin), ibuprofen (Advil, Motrin), sulindac (Clinoril), piroxicam (Feldene), flurbiprofen (Ansaid), diclofenac sodium (Voltaren), naproxen (Naprosyn), diflunisal (Dolobid)

Key interventions

• Check joints for swelling, pain, and redness.
• Monitor laboratory studies.
• Splint inflamed joints.
• Provide warm or cold therapy, as prescribed.

SCLERODERMA

Key signs and symptoms

• Pain
• Signs and symptoms of Raynaud's phenomenon, such as blanching, cyanosis, and erythema of the fingers and toes in response to stress or exposure to cold
• Stiffness
• Swelling of fingers and joints
• Taut, shiny skin over the entire hand and forearm
• Tight and inelastic facial skin, causing a masklike appearance and "pinching" of the mouth
• Renal involvement, usually accompanied by malignant hypertension, the main cause of death

Key test results

• Blood studies show slightly elevated erythrocyte sedimentation rate (ESR), positive rheumatoid factor in 25% to 35% of patients, and positive antinuclear antibody test.
• Skin biopsy may show changes consistent with the progress of the disease, such as marked thickening of the dermis and occlusive vessel changes.

Key treatments

• Palliative measures: use of immunosuppressants such as cyclosporine (Sandimmune) or chlorambucil (Leukeran) and physical therapy to maintain function and promote muscle strength (currently, no cure exists for scleroderma)

Key interventions

• Assess motion restrictions, pain, vital signs, intake and output, respiratory function, and daily weight.
• Teach the patient to monitor blood pressure at home and report any increases above baseline.
• Whenever possible, let the patient participate in treatment by measuring his own intake and output, planning his own diet, assisting in dialysis, giving himself heat therapy, and doing prescribed exercises.

SEPTIC SHOCK

Key signs and symptoms

Early stage
• Chills
• Oliguria
• Sudden fever (over 101° F [38.3° C])

Late stage
• Altered level of consciousness
• Anuria
• Hyperventilation
• Hypotension
• Hypothermia
• Restlessness
• Tachycardia
• Tachypnea

Key test results

• Blood cultures isolate the organism.
• Blood tests show decreased platelet count and leukocytosis (15,000 to 30,000/µl), increased blood urea nitrogen and creatinine levels, decreased creatinine clearance, and abnormal PT and PTT.

Key treatments

• Removing and replacing any I.V., intra-arterial, or urinary drainage catheters that may be the source of infection
• Oxygen therapy (may require endotracheal intubation and mechanical ventilation)
• Colloid or crystalloid infusion to increase intravascular volume
• Diuretics such as furosemide (Lasix) after sufficient fluid volume has been replaced to maintain urine output above 20 ml/hour.
• Antibiotics: according to sensitivity of causative organism.
• Vasopressors: dopamine (Intropin) if fluid resuscitation fails to increase blood pressure

Key interventions

• Remove any I.V., intra-arterial, or urinary drainage catheters and send them to the laboratory. New catheters can be reinserted.
• Start an I.V. infusion with normal saline solution or lactated Ringer's solution, usually a large-bore (14G to 18G) catheter.
• If the patient's blood pressure drops below 80 mm Hg, increase oxygen flow rate and call the doctor immediately.
• Keep accurate intake and output records. Maintain adequate urine output (0.5 to 1 ml/kg/hour) and systolic pressure.
• Administer antibiotics I.V. and monitor drug levels.

(continued)

Hematologic and immunologic refresher *(continued)*

SICKLE CELL ANEMIA

Key signs and symptoms

- Aching bones
- Jaundice, pallor (jaundice worsens during painful crisis)
- Unexplained dyspnea or dyspnea on exertion
- Tachycardia
- Severe pain (during sickle cell crisis)

Key test results

- Blood tests show low RBC counts, elevated WBC and platelet counts, decreased ESR, increased serum iron levels, decreased RBC survival, and reticulocytosis.
- Hb electrophoresis shows Hb S.

Key treatments

- Iron and folic acid supplements to prevent anemia
- I.V. fluid therapy to prevent dehydration and vessel occlusion
- Analgesics: meperidine or morphine (to relieve pain from vaso-occlusive crises)

Key interventions

- Apply warm compresses to painful areas and cover patient with a blanket.
- Maintain bed rest.
- Encourage fluid intake.
- Administer prescribed I.V. fluids.

SODIUM IMBALANCE

Key signs and symptoms

Hyponatremia

- Abdominal cramps
- Cold, clammy skin
- Cyanosis
- Hypotension
- Oliguria or anuria
- Seizures
- Tachycardia

Hypernatremia

- Dry, sticky mucous membranes
- Excessive weight gain
- Flushed skin
- Hypertension
- Intense thirst
- Oliguria
- Pitting edema
- Rough, dry tongue
- Tachycardia

Key test results

- Serum sodium level less than 135 mEq/L indicates hyponatremia.
- Serum sodium level greater than 145 mEq/L indicates hypernatremia.

Key treatments

Hyponatremia

- I.V. infusion of saline solution
- Potassium supplements: Potassium chloride (K-Lor)

Hypernatremia

- Diet: sodium restrictions
- Salt-free solution (such as dextrose in water), followed by infusion of 0.45% sodium chloride to prevent hyponatremia

Key interventions

For hyponatremia

- Watch for extremely low serum sodium and accompanying serum chloride levels. Monitor urine specific gravity and other laboratory results. Record fluid intake and output accurately, and weigh the patient daily.
- During administration of isosmolar or hyperosmolar saline solution, watch closely for signs of hypervolemia (dyspnea, crackles, engorged neck or hand veins).

For hypernatremia

- Measure serum sodium levels every 6 hours or at least daily. Monitor vital signs for changes, especially for rising pulse rate. Watch for signs of hypervolemia, especially in the patient receiving I.V. fluids.
- Record fluid intake and output accurately, checking for body fluid loss. Weigh the patient daily.

SYSTEMIC LUPUS ERYTHEMATOSUS

Key signs and symptoms

- Butterfly rash on face (rash may vary in severity from malar erythema to discoid lesions)
- Fatigue
- Migratory pain, stiffness, and joint swelling

Key test results

- Lupus erythematosus cell preparation is positive.

Key treatments

- Cytotoxic drugs: azathioprine (Imuran), methotrexate (Folex); these drugs may delay or prevent deteriorating renal status
- Immunosuppressants: azathioprine (Imuran), cyclophosphamide (Cytoxan)
- NSAIDs: indomethacin (Indocin), ibuprofen (Motrin), sulindac (Clinoril), piroxicam (Feldene), flurbiprofen (Ansaid), diclofenac sodium (Voltaren), naproxen (Naprosyn), diflunisal (Dolobid)

Hematologic and immunologic refresher *(continued)*

SYSTEMIC LUPUS ERYTHEMATOSUS *(continued)*

Key interventions

- Assess musculoskeletal status.
- Monitor renal status.
- Provide prophylactic skin, mouth, and perineal care.
- Maintain seizure precaution.
- Minimize environmental stress and provide rests periods.

VASCULITIS

Key signs and symptoms

Wegener's granulomatosis
- Cough
- Fever
- Malaise
- Pulmonary congestion
- Weight loss

Temporal arteritis
- Fever
- Headache (associated with polymyalgia rheumatica syndrome)
- Jaw claudication
- Myalgia
- Visual changes

Takayasu's arteritis
- Arthralgias
- Bruits
- Loss of distal pulses
- Malaise
- Pain or paresthesia distal to affected area

- Syncope
- Weight loss

Key test results

Wegener's granulomatosis
- Tissue biopsy shows necrotizing vasculitis with granulomatous inflammation.

Temporal arteritis
- Tissue biopsy shows panarteritis with infiltration of mononuclear cells, giant cells within vessel wall, fragmentation of internal elastic lamina, and proliferation of intima.

Takayasu's arteritis
- Arteriography shows calcification and obstruction of affected vessels.
- Tissue biopsy shows inflammation of adventitia and intima of vessels and thickening of vessel walls.

Key treatments

- Removal of identified environmental antigen
- Diet: elimination of antigenic food, if identifiable
- Corticosteroid: prednisone (Deltasone)
- Antineoplastic: Cyclophosphamide (Cytoxan)

Key interventions

- Regulate environmental temperature.
- Monitor vital signs. Use a Doppler ultrasonic flowmeter, if possible.
- Monitor intake and output. Check daily for edema. Keep the patient well hydrated (3 L daily).
- Monitor the patient's WBC count during cyclophosphamide therapy.

Oxygen carriers

Erythrocytes (also called **red blood cells** or **RBCs**) are formed in the bone marrow and contain hemoglobin (Hb). Oxygen binds with Hb to form oxyhemoglobin, which is then carried by erythrocytes throughout the body.

Clotting contributors

Thrombocytes (also called **platelets**) are formed in the bone marrow and function in the coagulation of blood.

Infection fighters

Leukocytes (also called **white blood cells** or **WBCs**) are formed in the bone marrow and lymphatic tissue and include granulocytes and agranulocytes. WBCs provide immunity and protection from infection by phagocytosis (engulfing, digesting, destroying microorganisms).

Liquid partner

Plasma is the liquid portion of the blood, and its composition is water, protein (albumin and globulin), glucose, and electrolytes.

Of donors and recipients

A person's **blood type** is determined by a system of antigens located on the surface of RBCs. The four blood types are:
- A antigen
- B antigen
- AB (both A and B) antigens
- O (no antigens).

Because group O blood lacks both A and B antigens, it can be transfused in limited

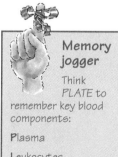

Memory jogger

Think PLATE to remember key blood components:

Plasma

Leukocytes

AB antigens

Thrombocytes

Erythrocytes

amounts in an emergency to any patient, regardless of the recipient's blood type, with little risk of adverse reaction. That's why people with group O blood are called universal donors. A person with AB blood type has neither anti-A nor anti-B antibodies. This person may receive A, B, AB, or O blood, which makes him a universal recipient.

In addition, the antigen Rh factor is found on the RBCs of approximately 85% of people. A person with the Rh factor is Rh positive. A person without the factor is Rh negative. A person may only receive blood from a person with the same Rh factor.

Now, some more about the immune system

In cell-mediated immunity, T cells respond directly to antigens (foreign substances such as bacteria or toxins that induce antibody formation). This response involves destruction of target cells — such as virus-infected cells and cancer cells — through secretion of lymphokines (lymph proteins). Examples of cell-mediated immunity are rejection of transplanted organs and delayed immune responses that fight disease.

About 80% of blood cells are T cells. They probably originate from stem cells in the bone marrow; the thymus gland controls their maturity. In the process, a large number of antigen-specific cells are produced.

Killer, helper, or suppressor

T cells can be killer, helper, or suppressor T cells.
• Killer cells bind to the surface of the invading cell, disrupt the membrane, and destroy it by altering its internal environment.
• Helper cells stimulate B cells to mature into plasma cells, which begin to synthesize and secrete immunoglobulin (proteins with known antibody activity).
• Suppressor cells reduce the humoral response.

Don't forget B cells

B cells act in a different way than T cells to recognize and destroy antigens. B cells are responsible for humoral or immunoglobulin-me-

diated immunity. B cells originate in the bone marrow and mature into plasma cells that produce antibodies (immunoglobulin molecules that interact with a specific antigen). Antibodies destroy bacteria and viruses, thereby preventing them from entering host cells.

A word about immunoglobulins

Five major classes of immunoglobulin exist:
• Immunoglobulin G (IgG) makes up about 80% of plasma antibodies. It appears in all body fluids and is the major antibacterial and antiviral antibody.
• Immunoglobulin M (IgM) is the first immunoglobulin produced during an immune response. It's too large to easily cross membrane barriers and is usually present only in the vascular system.
• Immunoglobulin A (IgA) is found mainly in body secretions, such as saliva, sweat, tears, mucus, bile, and colostrum. It defends against pathogens on body surfaces, especially those that enter the respiratory and GI tracts.
• Immunoglobulin D (IgD) is present in plasma and is easily broken down. It's the predominant antibody on the surface of B cells and is mainly an antigen receptor.
• Immunoglobulin E (IgE) is the antibody involved in immediate hypersensitivity reactions, or allergic reactions that develop within minutes of exposure to an antigen. IgE stimulates the release of mast cell granules, which contain histamine and heparin.

Keep abreast of diagnostic tests

Here are the most important tests used to diagnose hematologic and immune disorders, along with common nursing actions associated with each test.

Blood sample study #1

A **blood chemistry test** uses a blood sample to measure potassium, sodium, calcium, blood urea nitrogen (BUN), creatinine, protein, albumin, and bilirubin levels.

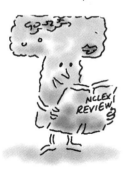

Wow! I can be a killer, helper, or suppressor!

Nursing actions
• Before the procedure, withhold food and fluids, as directed.
• After the procedure, check the venipuncture site for bleeding.

Blood sample study #2
A **hematologic study** uses a blood sample to analyze WBCs, RBCs, erythrocyte sedimentation rate (ESR), Hb, and hematocrit (HCT), red cell indices, hemoglobin electrophoresis, iron and total iron binding capacity, sickle cell test, and CD4 cell count.

Nursing actions
Before the procedure:
• note the patient's current drug therapy.
  After the procedure:
• check the venipuncture site for bleeding
• handle the specimen gently to prevent hemolysis.

Check on immune status
Immunologic studies use a small sample of blood to analyze rheumatoid factor, lupus erythematosus cell preparation, antinuclear antibodies, and serum protein electrophoresis.

Nursing actions
• Before the procedure, note the patient's current drug therapy.
• After the procedure, check the venipuncture site for bleeding.

HIV detector
Enzyme-linked immunosorbent assay (ELISA) uses a blood sample to detect the human immunodeficiency virus (HIV) antibody.

Nursing actions
• Verify that informed consent has been obtained and documented.
• Provide the patient with appropriate pretest counseling.
• After the procedure, check the venipuncture site for bleeding.

Confirming the diagnosis
A **Western blot test** uses a blood sample to detect the presence of specific viral proteins to confirm HIV infection.

Nursing actions
• Verify that informed consent has been obtained and documented.
• After the procedure, check the venipuncture site for bleeding.

Small sample
A **urine test** uses a small sample of urine to analyze hemosiderin and Hb.

Nursing actions
• Collect a random urine specimen of about 30 ml.

Radiographic snapshot
A **lymphangiography** involves an injection of radiopaque dye through a catheter, which provides a radiographic picture of the lymphatic system and the dissection of lymph vessels.

Nursing actions
Before the procedure, you should:
• note the patient's allergies to iodine, seafood, and radiopaque dyes
• tell the patient of possible throat irritation and flushing of his face after injection of the dye
• make sure that a written, informed consent has been obtained
• withhold food and fluids, as directed.
  After the procedure, you should:
• assess vital signs and peripheral pulses
• check catheter insertion site for bleeding
• force fluids
• advise the patient that skin, stool, and urine will have a blue discoloration for about 48 hours following the procedure.

Marrow removal
A **bone marrow examination,** also called aspiration or biopsy, involves the percutaneous removal of bone marrow and an examination of erythrocytes, leukocytes, thrombocytes, and precursor cells.

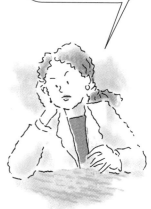

Hmmm. Postdiagnostic test monitoring, such as checking the venipuncture site, the catheter insertion site, or the site of bone marrow aspiration, is a key nursing responsibility.

Nursing actions

Before the procedure, you should:
• make sure that a written, informed consent has been obtained
• determine the patient's ability to lie still during aspiration
• tell the patient that he may experience a burning sensation as the bone marrow is aspirated.

After the procedure, you should:
• maintain pressure dressing
• check the aspiration site for bleeding and infection.
• maintain bed rest, as ordered.

Swallow this and wait

A **Schilling test** involves the administration of an oral radioactive cyanocobalamin and an intramuscular cyanocobalamin. Following this is microscopic examination of a 24-hour urine sample for cyanocobalamin (vitamin B_{12}).

Nursing actions

• Withhold food and fluids for 12 hours before the test.
• Withhold laxatives during the test.
• After the test, instruct the patient to save all voided urine for 24 hours and keep the urine at room temperature.

What's in the stomach?

Gastric analysis involves the aspiration of stomach contents through a nasogastric tube. A fasting analysis of gastric secretions is then performed to measure acidity and to diagnose pernicious anemia.

Nursing actions

Before the procedure, you should:
• withhold food and fluids for 12 hours
• instruct the patient not to smoke or chew gum for at least 8 hours before the test
• withhold medications that can affect gastric secretions.

After the procedure, you should:
• obtain vital signs
• assess for reactions to gastric acid stimulant, if used.

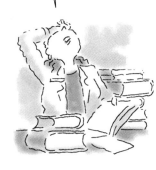

Say it 10 times. Studying for the NCLEX is fun, studying for the NCLEX is fun....

No red meats or turnips

A **fecal occult blood test** involves a microscopic analysis of hemoglobin to detect occult blood in stool.

Nursing actions

• Before the test, instruct the patient to maintain a high-fiber diet and to refrain from eating red meats, turnips, and horseradish for 48 to 72 hours.
• Tell the patient the test requires collection of 3 stool specimens.
• Withhold iron preparations, iodides, rauwolfia derivatives, indomethacin, colchicine, salicylates, phenylbutazone, steroids, and ascorbic acid for 48 hours before the test and throughout the collection period.

RBC longevity measure

Erythrocyte life span determination involves a reinjection of the patient's blood that has been tagged with chromium 51. Its purpose is to measure the life span of circulating RBCs.

Nursing actions

• Inform the patient that frequent blood samples will be drawn over a 2-week period.
• Check the venipuncture site for bleeding.
• Apply a pressure dressing after the procedure.

Balancing act

The **Romberg test** is a physical test in which the patient stands with his feet together, his eyes open, and his arms at either side, while the examiner stands and protects the patient from falling. The patient is then asked to close his eyes. If he loses his balance or sways to one side, the Romberg test is positive. This is done to assess loss of balance in pernicious anemia.

Nursing actions

• Explain the procedure to the patient.
• Monitor the patient for imbalance.
• Prevent the patient from falling.

How fast does it burst?

In the **erythrocyte fragility test,** a blood sample is used to measure the rate at which RBCs burst in varied hypotonic solutions.

Nursing actions

- Explain the procedure to the patient.
- Send the specimen to the laboratory.

Bone picture

A **bone scan** is an I.V. injection of radioisotope, which creates a visual image of bone metabolism.

Nursing actions

Before the procedure, you should:
- determine the patient's ability to lie still for approximately 1 hour
- advise the patient to drink lots of fluids to maintain hydration and reduce the radiation dose to the bladder. (Have the patient do this during the interval between the injection of the tracer and the actual scanning.)

After the procedure, you should:
- check the injection site for redness or swelling
- avoid scheduling any other radionuclide test for 24 to 48 hours
- tell the patient to drink lots of fluids and to empty his bladder frequently for 24 to 48 hours
- provide analgesics for pain resulting from positioning on the scanning table, as needed.

Clot measure

A **coagulation study** tests a blood sample to analyze platelet function, platelet count, prothrombin time (PT), international normalized ratio, partial thromboplastin time (PTT), coagulation time, and bleeding time.

Nursing actions

- Note the patient's current drug therapy before the procedure.
- Check the venipuncture site for bleeding after the procedure.

Polish up on patient care

Major hematologic and immune disorders include acquired immunodeficiency syndrome, anaphylaxis, ankylosing spondylitis, aplastic anemia, calcium imbalance, chloride imbalance, disseminated intravascular coagulation, hemophilia, iron deficiency anemia, Kaposi's sarcoma, leukemia, lymphoma, magnesium imbalance, metabolic acidosis, metabolic alkalosis, multiple myeloma, pernicious anemia, phosphorus imbalance, polycythemia vera, rheumatoid arthritis, scleroderma, septic shock, sickle cell anemia, sodium imbalance, systemic lupus erythematosus, and vasculitis.

Acquired immunodeficiency syndrome

Acquired immunodeficiency syndrome (AIDS) is a defect in T-cell–mediated immunity caused by the human immunodeficiency virus (HIV). AIDS places a patient at significant risk for the development of potentially fatal opportunistic infections. A diagnosis of AIDS is based on laboratory evidence of HIV infection coexisting with one or more indicator diseases, such as herpes simplex virus, cytomegalovirus, mycobacteria, candidal infection, *Pneumocystis carinii* pneumonia, Kaposi's sarcoma, wasting syndrome, or dementia.

CAUSES

- Exposure to blood containing HIV: transfusions, contaminated needles, handling of blood, in utero
- Exposure to semen and vaginal secretions containing HIV: sexual intercourse, handling of semen and vaginal secretions

ASSESSMENT FINDINGS

- Anorexia, weight loss, recurrent diarrhea
- Disorientation, confusion, dementia
- Fatigue and weakness
- Fever
- Lymphadenopathy

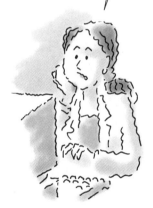

Most NCLEX questions focus on what a nurse should do in a specific situation. Always look for the patient care angle.

- Malnutrition
- Night sweats
- Opportunistic infections
- Pallor

DIAGNOSTIC TEST RESULTS
- Blood chemistry shows increased transaminase, alkaline phosphatase, and gamma globulin levels and a decreased albumin level.
- CD4+ T-cell level is less than 200 cells/µl
- ELISA shows positive HIV antibody titer.
- Hematology shows decreased WBCs, RBCs, and platelets.
- Western blot is positive.

NURSING DIAGNOSES
- Altered protection
- Hopelessness
- Social isolation

TREATMENT
- Activity: as tolerated, active and passive range-of-motion exercises
- Diet: high calorie, high protein in small, frequent feedings
- Nutritional support: total parenteral nutrition (TPN), enteral feedings if necessary
- Plasmapheresis
- Respiratory treatments: chest physiotherapy, postural drainage, and incentive spirometry
- Specialized bed: air therapy bed
- Standard precautions
- Transfusion therapy: fresh frozen plasma, platelets, and packed RBCs

Drug therapy
- Antibiotics: trimethoprim and sulfamethoxazole (Bactrim)
- Antiemetic: prochlorperazine (Compazine)
- Antifungals: fluconazole (Diflucan), amphotericin B (Fungizone)
- Antivirals: dapsone, didanosine (Videx), ganciclovir (Cytovene), zidovudine (Retrovir, AZT), acyclovir (Zovirax), pentamidine (Pentam 300), aerosolized pentamidine (NebuPent)
- Interferon alfa-2a, recombinant (Roferon-A)

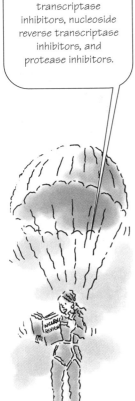

Combination therapy to treat HIV-AIDS usually includes nonnucleoside reverse transcriptase inhibitors, nucleoside reverse transcriptase inhibitors, and protease inhibitors.

Medications used in combination to fight HIV
- Nonnucleoside reverse transcriptase inhibitors: delavirdine (Rescriptor), nevirapine (Viramune)
- Nucleoside reverse transcriptase inhibitors such as lamivudine (Epivir), zalcitabine (Dideoxycytidine, ddC), zidovudine (Retrovir, AZT)
- Protease inhibitors: indinavir (Crixivan), nelfinavir (Viracept), ritonavir (Norvir), saquinavir (Inivirase)

INTERVENTIONS AND RATIONALES
- Assess respiratory and neurologic systems *to detect AIDS-related dementia. Other factors such as anemia, fever, hypoxemia, and fluid balance can affect neurologic status.*
- Monitor and record vital signs *to detect evidence of compromise.*
- Monitor for opportunistic infections *because early treatment may limit complications.*
- Administer oxygen *to enhance oxygenation.*
- Provide incentive spirometry and assist with turning, coughing, and deep breathing *to mobilize and remove secretions.*
- Encourage fluids or administer I.V. fluids *to prevent dehydration.*
- Maintain the patient's diet *to fight opportunistic infection and maintain weight.*
- Administer TPN and enteral feedings if necessary *to bolster nutritional reserves and immune system.*
- Administer medications, as prescribed, *to reduce the risk of complications and halt reproduction of HIV.*
- Maintain activity, as tolerated, *to encourage independence.*
- Provide rest periods *to reduce oxygen demands and prevent fatigue.*
- Provide mouth care *to prevent infection, provide comfort, and enhance taste of meals.*
- Maintain standard precautions *to avoid exposure to blood, body fluids, and secretions.*
- Encourage the patient to express feelings about changes in body image, a fear of dying, and social isolation *to help cope with chronic illness and reduce anxiety.*
- Make referrals to community agencies for support *to enhance quality of life and independence.*

• Monitor intake and output, daily weight, and urine specific gravity *for early recognition and treatment of dehydration.*
• Assess respiratory status *to detect complications such as pneumonia or malignancies.*
• Monitor laboratory values *for early detection and complications. Thrombocytopenia requires precautions to prevent bleeding. Leukopenia requires precautions to protect patient from infection.*

Teaching topics
• Refraining from donating blood
• Avoiding use of alcohol and recreational drugs
• Using condoms during sexual intercourse
• Avoiding anal sex
• If using I.V. drugs, cleaning drug paraphernalia with bleach

Anaphylaxis

Anaphylaxis is a dramatic and widespread acute atopic reaction. It's marked by the sudden onset of rapidly progressive urticaria and respiratory distress. A severe anaphylactic reaction may cause vascular collapse, leading to systemic shock and, sometimes, death.

CAUSES
Systemic exposure to or ingestion of sensitizing drugs or other substances such as:
• allergen extracts
• diagnostic chemicals (sulfobromophthalein, sodium dehydrocholate, and radiographic contrast media)
• enzymes (such as L-asparaginase)
• foods (legumes, nuts, berries, seafood, and egg albumin) and sulfite-containing food additives
• hormones
• insect venom (honeybees, wasps, hornets, yellow jackets, fire ants, mosquitoes, and certain spiders)
• local anesthetics
• penicillin and other antibiotics
• polysaccharides
• ruptured hydatid cyst (rarely)
• salicylates
• serums (usually horse serum)

• sulfonamides
• vaccines.

ASSESSMENT FINDINGS
• Cardiovascular symptoms (hypotension, shock, cardiac arrhythmias) that may precipitate circulatory collapse if untreated
• Sudden physical distress within seconds or minutes after exposure to an allergen (may include feeling of impending doom or fright, weakness, sweating, sneezing, shortness of breath, nasal pruritus, urticaria, and angioedema, followed rapidly by symptoms in one or more target organs)
• GI and genitourinary symptoms (severe stomach cramps, nausea, diarrhea, urinary urgency and incontinence)
• Persistent or delayed reaction (may occur up to 24 hours after exposure to allergen)
• Respiratory symptoms (nasal mucosal edema, profuse watery rhinorrhea, itching, nasal congestion, sudden sneezing attacks; edema of upper respiratory tract that causes hoarseness, stridor, and dyspnea is early sign of acute respiratory failure)
• Severity of reaction inversely related to interval between exposure to an allergen and onset of symptoms — the longer the interval, the less severe the reaction

DIAGNOSTIC TEST RESULTS
• Anaphylaxis can be diagnosed by the rapid onset of severe respiratory or cardiovascular symptoms after ingestion or injection of a drug, vaccine, diagnostic agent, food, or food additive, or after an insect sting.
• If symptoms occur without a known allergic stimulus, other possible causes of shock (such as acute myocardial infarction, status asthmaticus, or heart failure) need to be ruled out.

NURSING DIAGNOSES
• Risk for suffocation
• Decreased cardiac output
• Anxiety

TREATMENT
• Cardiopulmonary resuscitation in case of cardiac arrest

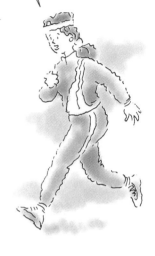

Yikes! Anaphylaxis may cause vascular collapse and lead to systemic shock and, sometimes, death.

• Endotracheal tube insertion or a tracheotomy and oxygen therapy in case of laryngeal edema
• Other therapy as indicated by clinical response

Drug therapy

• Immediate injection of epinephrine 1:1,000 aqueous solution, 0.1 to 0.5 ml, repeated every 5 to 20 minutes as necessary
• Other medications given after initial emergency (may include subcutaneous [S.C.] epinephrine, longer-acting epinephrine, corticosteroids, diphenhydramine [Benadryl] I.V. for long-term management)
• Vasopressors: norepinephrine (Levophed) and dopamine (Intropin), if hypotensive

INTERVENTIONS AND RATIONALES

• In the early stages of anaphylaxis, when the patient hasn't yet lost consciousness and is still normotensive, give epinephrine I.M. or S.C., and help it move into the circulation faster by massaging the injection site. In severe reactions, when the patient has lost consciousness and is hypotensive, give epinephrine I.V *to prevent crisis.*
• Maintain airway patency. Observe for early signs of laryngeal edema (stridor, hoarseness, and dyspnea), and prepare for endotracheal tube insertion or a tracheotomy and oxygen therapy *to prevent cerebral anoxia.*
• In case of cardiac arrest, begin cardiopulmonary resuscitation, including closed-chest heart massage, assisted ventilation, and sodium bicarbonate; other therapy is indicated by clinical response. *These measures are necessary to prevent irreversible organ damage.*
• Watch for hypotension and shock, and maintain circulatory volume with volume expanders (plasma, plasma expanders, saline solution, and albumin) as needed. Stabilize blood pressure with the I.V. vasopressors norepinephrine and dopamine *to prevent altered tissue perfusion.* Monitor blood pressure, central venous pressure, and urine output *to monitor response to treatment.*
• After the initial emergency, administer other medications, such as S.C. epinephrine, longer-acting epinephrine, corticosteroids,

and diphenhydramine I.V. for long-term management *to prevent recurrence of symptoms.*
• If a patient must receive a drug to which he's allergic, make sure he receives careful desensitization with gradually increasing doses of the antigen or advance administration of steroids *to prevent a severe reaction.*
• A person with a known history of allergies should receive a drug with a high anaphylactic potential only after cautious pretesting for sensitivity. Closely monitor the patient during testing, and make sure that resuscitative equipment and epinephrine are ready *to prevent a severe reaction that may lead to cardiopulmonary arrest.*
• When any patient needs a drug with high anaphylactic potential (particularly parenteral drugs), make sure he receives each dose under close medical observation *to prevent a severe reaction.*
• Closely monitor a patient undergoing diagnostic tests that use radiographic contrast dyes, such as cardiac catheterization, excretory urography, and angiography *to detect early signs of anaphylaxis.*

Teaching topics

• Risks of delayed symptoms and need to report any recurrence of shortness of breath, chest tightness, sweating, angioedema, or other symptoms
• Preventing anaphylaxis (avoiding exposure to known allergens, including all forms of the offending food or drug, avoiding open fields and wooded areas during the insect season in case of reaction to insect bite or sting, carrying an anaphylaxis kit containing epinephrine, an antihistamine, and a tourniquet)
• Wearing a medical identification bracelet identifying the patient's allergies

Ankylosing spondylitis

Ankylosing spondylitis is a chronic, usually progressive inflammatory disease that primarily affects the spine and adjacent soft tissue. Generally, the disease begins in the sacroiliac joints (between the sacrum and the ileum) and gradually progresses to the lumbar, tho-

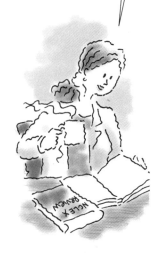

Immediately after exposure to an allergen, the patient may report a feeling of impending doom or fright.

racic, and cervical regions of the spine. Deterioration of bone and cartilage can lead to fibrous tissue formation and eventual fusion of the spine or peripheral joints.

Ankylosing spondylitis affects five times as many males as females. Progressive disease is well recognized in men, but the diagnosis is often overlooked in women, who tend to have more peripheral joint involvement.

CAUSES
• Familial tendency strongly suggested
• Possible link to underlying infection
• Presence of histocompatibility antigen HLA-B27 and circulating immune complexes suggests immunologic activity
• Secondary ankylosing spondylitis may be associated with reactive arthritis (Reiter's syndrome), psoriatic arthritis, or inflammatory bowel disease

ASSESSMENT FINDINGS
• Intermittent low back pain (the first indication) usually most severe in morning or after period of inactivity
• Kyphosis in advanced stages, caused by chronic stooping to relieve symptoms, and hip deformity and associated limited range of motion (ROM)
• Mild fatigue, fever, anorexia, or loss of weight; unilateral acute anterior uveitis; aortic insufficiency and cardiomegaly; upper lobe pulmonary fibrosis (mimics tuberculosis)
• Pain and limited expansion of the chest due to involvement of the costovertebral joints
• Pain or tenderness at tendon insertion sites (enthesitis), especially the Achilles or patellar tendon
• Peripheral arthritis involving shoulders, hips, and knees
• Severe neurologic complications, such as cauda equina syndrome or paralysis, secondary to fracture of a rigid cervical spine or C1-C2 subluxation
• Stiffness and limited motion of the lumbar spine
• Symptoms that progress unpredictably; disease can go into remission, exacerbation, or arrest at any stage
• Tenderness over the site of inflammation

DIAGNOSTIC TEST RESULTS
• Confirmation requires characteristic X-ray findings: blurring of the bony margins of joints in the early stage, bilateral sacroiliac involvement, patchy sclerosis with superficial bony erosions, eventual squaring of vertebral bodies, and "bamboo spine" with complete ankylosis.
• ESR and alkaline phosphatase and creatine kinase levels may be slightly elevated. A negative rheumatoid factor helps rule out rheumatoid arthritis, which produces similar symptoms.
• Typical symptoms, a family history, and the presence of HLA-B27 strongly suggest ankylosing spondylitis.

NURSING DIAGNOSES
• Pain
• Impaired physical mobility
• Activity intolerance

TREATMENT
• Good posture, stretching and deep-breathing exercises and, in some patients, braces and lightweight supports to delay further deformity (because ankylosing spondylitis progression can't be stopped)
• Long-term daily exercise program (essential to delay loss of function)
• Spinal wedge osteotomy to separate and reposition vertebrae in case of severe spinal involvement (performed only on selected patients because of risk of spinal cord damage and long convalescence)
• Surgical hip replacement in case of severe hip involvement

Drug therapy
• Anti-inflammatory agents: aspirin, indomethacin (Indocin), sulfasalazine (Azulfidine), sulindac (Clinoril) to control pain and inflammation

INTERVENTIONS AND RATIONALES
• Offer support and reassurance. *Ankylosing spondylitis can be an extremely painful and crippling disease; the caregiver's main responsibility is to promote the patient's comfort while preserving as much mobility as possible.* Keep

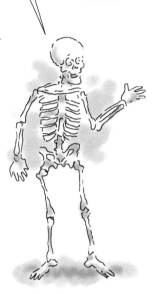

Typically, ankylosing spondylitis begins in the lower back and progresses up the spine to the neck.

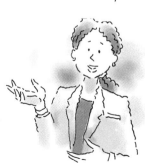

Ankylosing spondylitis can be an extremely painful and debilitating disease. Promote the patient's comfort while preserving as much mobility as possible.

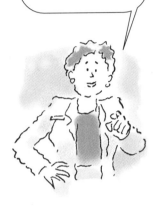

The fact that you're studying for the NCLEX shows that you have the ability to set a goal for yourself. Give yourself credit for setting achievable goals.

in mind that the patient's limited ROM makes simple tasks difficult.

• Administer medications as needed *to decrease inflammation and pain.*

• Apply local heat and provide massage *to relieve pain.* Assess mobility and degree of discomfort frequently *to monitor for disease progression.*

• Teach and assist with daily exercises as needed *to maintain strength and function.* Stress the importance of maintaining good posture *to prevent kyphosis.*

• If treatment includes surgery, provide good postoperative care *to prevent postoperative complications such as wound infection, thrombophlebitis, and pneumonia.*

• Comprehensive treatment should also reflect counsel from a social worker, visiting nurse, and dietitian *because ankylosing spondylitis is a chronic, progressively crippling condition.*

Teaching topics

• Avoiding any physical activity that places undue stress on the back, such as lifting heavy objects

• Standing upright; sitting upright in a high, straight chair; and avoiding leaning over a desk

• Sleeping in a prone position on a hard mattress and avoiding use of pillows under neck or knees

• Avoiding prolonged walking, standing, sitting, or driving

• Performing regular stretching and deep-breathing exercises and swimming regularly, if possible

• Having height measured every 3 to 4 months to detect any tendency toward kyphosis

• Seeking vocational counseling if the patient's work requires standing or prolonged sitting at a desk

• Contacting the local Arthritis Foundation chapter for a support group

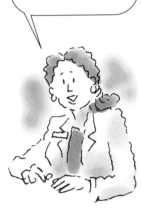

Aplastic anemia results from injury or destruction to stem cells, which are located in the bone marrow and function to produce new blood cells.

Aplastic anemia

Aplastic anemia, also known as pancytopenia, results from suppression, destruction, or aplasia of the bone marrow. This damage to the bone marrow causes an inability to produce adequate amounts of erythrocytes, leukocytes, and platelets.

CAUSES
• Chemotherapy
• Drug-induced from chloramphenicol (Chloromycetin), phenylbutazone (Butazolidin), phenytoin (Dilantin)
• Exposure to chemicals
• Idiopathic
• Radiation
• Viral hepatitis

ASSESSMENT FINDINGS
• Anorexia
• Dyspnea, tachypnea
• Epistaxis
• Fatigue, weakness
• Gingivitis
• Headache
• Melena
• Multiple infections, fever
• Palpitations, tachycardia
• Purpura, petechiae, ecchymosis, pallor

DIAGNOSTIC TEST RESULTS
• Bone marrow biopsy shows fatty marrow with reduction of stem cells.
• Fecal occult blood test is positive.
• Hematology shows decreased granulocytes, thrombocytes, and RBCs.
• Peripheral blood smear shows pancytopenia.
• Urine chemistry reveals hematuria.

NURSING DIAGNOSES
• Activity intolerance
• Risk for fluid volume deficit
• Risk for infection

TREATMENT
• Dietary changes including establishing a high-protein, high-calorie, high-vitamin diet
• Tepid sponge baths, cooling blankets
• Transfusion of platelets and packed RBCs

Drug therapy
- Analgesics: ibuprofen (Motrin), acetaminophen (Tylenol)
- Androgens: fluoxymesterone (Halotestin), oxymetholone (Anadrol-50)
- Antibiotics: according to the sensitivity of the infecting organism
- Antithymocyte globulin (Atgam)
- Hematopoietic growth factor: epoetin alfa (Epogen)
- Human granulocyte colony-stimulating factor: filgastim (Neupogen)

INTERVENTIONS AND RATIONALES
- Assess respiratory status *to detect hypoxemia caused by low hemoglobin levels.*
- Assess vital signs *for signs of hemorrhage, infection, and activity intolerance.*
- Assess cardiovascular status *to detect arrhythmias or myocardial ischemia.*
- Monitor and record intake and output and urine specific gravity *to determine fluid balance.*
- Monitor laboratory values *to determine effectiveness of therapy.*
- Assess stool, urine, and emesis *for occult blood loss caused by reduced platelet levels.*
- Monitor for infection, bleeding, and bruising *caused by reduced levels of WBCs and platelets.*
- Encourage fluids and administer I.V. fluids *to replace fluids lost by fever and bleeding.*
- Administer oxygen *to improve tissue oxygen because low hemoglobin levels reduce oxygen-carrying capacity of the blood.*
- Assist with turning, coughing, and deep breathing t*o mobilize and remove secretions.*
- Administer transfusion therapy, as prescribed, *to replace low blood components.*
- Administer medications, as prescribed, *to treat disorder and prevent complications.*
- Maintain the patient's diet *to promote red blood cell production and fight infection.*
- Encourage verbalization of concerns and fears *to allay the patient's anxiety.*
- Alternate rest periods with activity *to conserve energy and reduce weakness caused by anemia.*

- Provide cooling blankets and tepid sponge baths for fever *to promote comfort and reduce metabolic demands.*
- Maintain protective precautions *to prevent infection and hemorrhage.*
- Provide mouth care before and after meals *to enhance the taste of meals.*
- Provide skin care *to prevent skin breakdown due to bed rest, dehydration, and fever.*
- Protect the patient from falls *to reduce risk of hemorrhage.*
- Avoid giving the patient I.M. injections *to reduce risk of hemorrhage.*
- Avoid using hard toothbrushes and straight razors on the patient *to reduce risk of hemorrhage.*

Teaching topics
- Recognizing the early signs and symptoms of bleeding and infection
- Avoiding contact sports
- Wearing a medical identification bracelet
- Refraining from using over-the-counter medications
- Monitoring stool for occult blood
- Using an electric razor to avoid bleeding
- Refraining from taking aspirin

Calcium imbalance

Calcium plays an indispensable role in cell permeability, formation of bones and teeth, blood coagulation, transmission of nerve impulses, and normal muscle contraction.

Nearly all (99%) of the body's calcium is found in the bones. The remaining 1% exists in ionized form in serum; maintaining ionized calcium in the serum is critical to healthy neurologic function.

The parathyroid glands regulate ionized calcium and determine its resorption into bone, absorption from the GI mucosa, and excretion in urine and stool. Severe calcium imbalance requires emergency treatment, because a deficiency (hypocalcemia) can lead to tetany and seizures; an excess (hypercalcemia), to cardiac arrhythmias and coma.

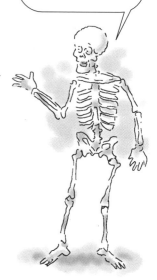

Together with phosphorus, calcium is responsible for the formation and structure of bones and teeth.

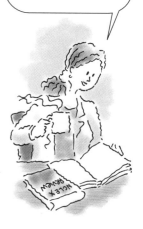

Hypocalcemia can occur when the body doesn't take in enough calcium, doesn't absorb the mineral properly, or loses excessive amounts of calcium.

Hypercalcemia occurs when the rate of calcium entry into the extracellular fluid exceeds the rate of calcium excretion by the kidneys.

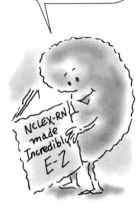

Because nearly half of all calcium is bound to the protein albumin, serum protein abnormalities can influence total serum calcium levels.

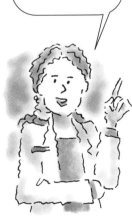

CAUSES
Hypocalcemia
- Hypomagnesemia
- Hypoparathyroidism
- Inadequate intake of calcium and vitamin D
- Malabsorption or loss of calcium from the GI tract
- Overcorrection of acidosis
- Pancreatic insufficiency
- Renal failure
- Severe infections or burns

Hypercalcemia
- Hyperparathyroidism
- Hypervitaminosis D
- Multiple fractures and prolonged immobilization
- Multiple myeloma
- Other causes (milk-alkali syndrome, sarcoidosis, hyperthyroidism, adrenal insufficiency, and thiazide diuretics)
- Tumors

ASSESSMENT FINDINGS
Hypocalcemia
- Cardiac arrhythmias
- Carpopedal spasm
- Chvostek's sign
- Perioral paresthesia
- Seizures
- Tetany
- Trousseau's sign
- Twitching

Hypercalcemia
- Anorexia
- Cardiac arrhythmias and eventual coma with severe hypercalcemia (serum levels greater than 5.7 mEq/L)
- Constipation
- Decreased muscle tone
- Dehydration
- Lethargy
- Muscle weakness
- Nausea
- Polydipsia
- Polyuria
- Vomiting

DIAGNOSTIC TEST RESULTS
- A serum calcium level less than 4.5 mEq/L confirms hypocalcemia; a level greater than 5.5 mEq/L confirms hypercalcemia. (Because approximately one-half of serum calcium is bound to albumin, changes in serum protein must be considered when interpreting serum calcium levels.)
- Sulkowitch urine test shows increased urine calcium precipitation in hypercalcemia.
- Electrocardiogram (ECG) reveals a lengthened QT interval, a prolonged ST segment, and arrhythmias in hypocalcemia; in hypercalcemia, a shortened QT interval and heart block.

NURSING DIAGNOSES
Hypocalcemia
- Altered nutrition: Less than body requirements
- Pain

Hypercalcemia
- Impaired physical mobility
- Altered urinary elimination

TREATMENT
Hypocalcemia
- Diet: adequate intake of calcium, vitamin D, and protein

Drug therapy
- Ergocalciferol (vitamin D_2), cholecalciferol (vitamin D_3), calcitriol, dihydrotachysterol (synthetic form of vitamin D_2) for severe deficiency
- Immediate correction by I.V. calcium gluconate or calcium chloride for acute hypocalcemia (an emergency)
- Vitamin D in multivitamin preparation for mild hypocalcemia
- Vitamin D supplements to facilitate GI absorption of calcium to treat chronic hypocalcemia

Hypercalcemia
- Hydration with normal saline solution to eliminate excess serum calcium through urine excretion

• Diet: Low calcium with increased oral fluid intake

Drug therapy
• Calcitonin (Calcimar)
• Corticosteroids, such as prednisone (Deltasone) and hydrocortisone (Solu-Cortef), for treating sarcoidosis, hypervitaminosis D, and certain tumors
• Loop diuretics, such as ethacrynic acid (Edecrin) and furosemide (Lasix), to promote calcium excretion (thiazide diuretics contraindicated in hypercalcemia because they inhibit calcium excretion)
• Plicamycin (Mithracin) to lower serum calcium level (especially against hypercalcemia secondary to certain tumors)
• Sodium phosphate solution administered by mouth or by retention enema (promotes calcium deposits in bone and inhibits absorption from GI tract)

INTERVENTIONS AND RATIONALES
• Watch for hypocalcemia in patients receiving massive transfusions of citrated blood and in those with chronic diarrhea, severe infections, and insufficient dietary intake of calcium and protein (especially elderly patients). *Identifying patients at risk can ensure early treatment intervention.*

For the patient with hypocalcemia
• Monitor serum calcium levels every 12 to 24 hours; *a calcium level below 4.5 mEq/L requires immediate attention.* When giving calcium supplements, frequently check the pH level; *an alkalotic state that exceeds 7.45 pH inhibits calcium ionization.* Check for Trousseau's and Chvostek's signs, *which indicate hypocalcemia.*
• Administer calcium gluconate slow I.V. in dextrose 5% in water (*never in saline solution, which encourages renal calcium loss*). Don't add calcium gluconate I.V. to solutions containing bicarbonate *to avoid precipitation.*
• When administering calcium solutions, watch for anorexia, nausea, and vomiting, *which are possible signs of overcorrection to hypercalcemia.*

• Monitor the patient closely for a possible drug interaction if he's receiving digitalis glycosides with large doses of oral calcium supplements. *Administration of digoxin concomitantly with calcium supplements may cause synergistic effects of digoxin that precipitate arrhythmias.* Watch for signs of digitalis toxicity (anorexia, nausea, vomiting, yellow vision, and cardiac arrhythmias). Administer oral calcium supplements 1 to 1½ hours after meals or with milk *to promote absorption.*
• Provide a quiet, stress-free environment for the patient with tetany *to prevent seizure activity.* Observe seizure precautions for patients with severe hypocalcemia that may lead to seizures *to prevent patient injury.*

For the patient with hypercalcemia
• Monitor serum calcium levels frequently. Watch for cardiac arrhythmias if the serum calcium level exceeds 5.7 mEq/L. Increase fluid intake *to dilute calcium in serum and urine and to prevent renal damage and dehydration.*
• Watch for signs of heart failure in patients receiving normal saline solution diuresis therapy. *Infusion of large volumes of normal saline may cause fluid volume excess, leading to heart failure.*
• Administer loop diuretics (not thiazide diuretics) *to promote diuresis and rid the body of excess calcium.* Monitor intake and output, and check the urine for renal calculi and acidity. Provide acid-ash drinks, such as cranberry or prune juice, *because calcium salts are more soluble in acid than in alkali.*
• Check the patient's ECG and vital signs frequently. In the patient receiving digitalis glycosides, watch for signs of toxicity, such as anorexia, nausea, vomiting, and bradycardia (often with arrhythmia). *Fatal arrhythmias may result when digoxin is administered in hypercalcemia.*
• Help the patient walk as soon as possible. Handle the patient with chronic hypercalcemia gently *to prevent pathologic fractures.*
• If the patient is bedridden, reposition him frequently, and encourage ROM exercises *to promote circulation and prevent urinary stasis and calcium loss from bone.*

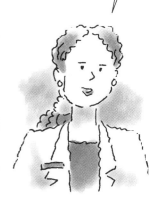

When calcium levels are too high, the thyroid releases calcitonin. High levels of calcitonin inhibit bone resorption, which causes a decrease in the amount of calcium available from bone, thereby decreasing serum calcium levels. Calcitonin may also be administered as a drug to treat hypercalcemia.

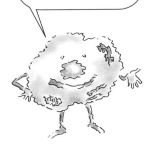

Chloride is quite an anion. It helps maintain acid-base balance and assists in carbon dioxide transport in red blood cells.

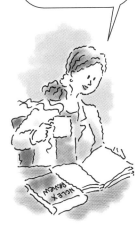

Sodium imbalance? Or chloride imbalance? These two conditions often produce similar assessment findings, such as muscle twitching, weakness, or dyspnea.

Teaching topics

• The importance of calcium for normal bone formation and blood coagulation
• Eating foods rich in calcium, vitamin D, and protein, such as fortified milk and cheese, to prevent hypocalcemia
• Avoiding chronic laxative use and overuse of antacids to prevent hypocalcemia
• Eating a low-calcium diet and increasing fluid intake to prevent recurrence of hypercalcemia

Chloride imbalance

Hypochloremia and hyperchloremia are, respectively, conditions of deficient or excessive serum levels of the anion chloride (an anion is a negatively charged ion). Chloride appears predominantly in extracellular fluid (fluid outside the cells) and accounts for two-thirds of all serum anions.

Secreted by stomach mucosa as hydrochloric acid, chloride provides an acid medium conducive to digestion and activation of enzymes. It also participates in maintaining acid-base and body water balances, influences the osmolality or tonicity of extracellular fluid, plays a role in the exchange of oxygen and carbon dioxide in red blood cells, and helps activate salivary amylase (which, in turn, activates the digestive process).

CAUSES
Hypochloremia
• Administration of dextrose I.V. without electrolytes
• Loss of hydrochloric acid in gastric secretions from vomiting, gastric suctioning, or gastric surgery
• Low dietary sodium intake
• Metabolic alkalosis
• Potassium deficiency
• Prolonged diarrhea or diaphoresis
• Sodium deficiency

Hyperchloremia
• Hyperingestion of ammonium chloride
• Ureterointestinal anastomosis, which can lead to hyperchloremia by allowing reabsorption of chloride by the bowel

ASSESSMENT FINDINGS
Hypochloremia
• Muscle hypertonicity (in conditions related to loss of gastric secretions)
• Muscle weakness
• Shallow, depressed breathing
• Tetany
• Twitching

Hyperchloremia
• Agitation
• Coma
• Deep, rapid breathing
• Diminished cognitive ability
• Dyspnea
• Hypertension
• Pitting edema
• Tachycardia
• Weakness

DIAGNOSTIC TEST RESULTS
• Serum chloride level that is less than 98 mEq/L confirms hypochloremia; supportive values with metabolic alkalosis include a serum pH greater than 7.45 and a serum carbon dioxide level greater than 32 mEq/L.
• Serum chloride level greater than 108 mEq/L confirms hyperchloremia; with metabolic acidosis, serum pH is less than 7.35 and the serum carbon dioxide level is less than 22 mEq/L.

NURSING DIAGNOSES
Hypochloremia
• Ineffective breathing pattern
• Risk for injury

Hyperchloremia
• Fluid volume excess
• Altered thought processes

TREATMENT
Hypochloremia
• Diet: salty broth
• Saline solution I.V.

Drug therapy
• Acidifying agent: ammonium chloride

Hyperchloremia
• Lactated Ringer's solution

Drug therapy
• Alkalinizing agent: Sodium bicarbonate I.V.

INTERVENTIONS AND RATIONALES
• Monitor serum chloride levels frequently, particularly during I.V. therapy, *to guide the treatment plan.*
• Watch for signs of hyperchloremia or hypochloremia. Be alert for respiratory difficulty *to prevent respiratory distress.*

For the patient with hypochloremia
• Monitor laboratory results (serum electrolyte and arterial blood gas [ABG] levels) and fluid intake and output of patients who are vulnerable to chloride imbalance, particularly those recovering from gastric surgery *to prevent hypochloremia.*
• Watch for excessive or continuous loss of gastric secretions, as well as prolonged infusion of dextrose in water without saline, *to prevent chloride imbalance.*

For the patient with hyperchloremia
• Check serum electrolyte levels every 3 to 6 hours. If the patient is receiving high doses of sodium bicarbonate, watch for signs of overcorrection (metabolic alkalosis, respiratory depression) or lingering signs of hyperchloremia, which indicate inadequate treatment. *Frequent monitoring of electrolyte levels helps guide the treatment plan and avoids complications of chloride imbalance.*
• Check laboratory results for elevated serum chloride or potassium imbalance if the patient is receiving I.V. solutions containing sodium chloride, and monitor fluid intake and output *to prevent hyperchloremia.*

Teaching topics
• Explanation of all tests and procedures
• Dietary sources of sodium, potassium, and chloride in the patient experiencing hypochloremia

Disseminated intravascular coagulation

Disseminated intravascular coagulation (DIC), also called consumption coagulopathy and defibrination syndrome, occurs as a complication of diseases and conditions that accelerate clotting. This accelerated clotting process causes small blood vessel occlusion, organ necrosis, depletion of circulating clotting factors and platelets, and activation of the fibrinolytic system—which, in turn, can provoke severe hemorrhage.

Clotting in the microcirculation usually affects the kidneys and extremities but may occur in the brain, lungs, pituitary and adrenal glands, and GI mucosa. Other conditions, such as vitamin K deficiency, hepatic disease, and anticoagulant therapy, may cause a similar hemorrhage.

DIC is generally an acute condition but may be chronic in cancer patients. The prognosis depends on early detection and treatment, the severity of the hemorrhage, and treatment of the underlying disease or condition.

CAUSES
• Disorders that produce necrosis, such as extensive burns and trauma, brain tissue destruction, transplant rejection, and hepatic necrosis
• Infection (the most common cause of DIC), including gram-negative or gram-positive septicemia; viral, fungal, or rickettsial infection; and protozoal infection (falciparum malaria)
• Neoplastic disease, including acute leukemia and metastatic carcinoma
• Obstetric complications, such as abruptio placentae, amniotic fluid embolism, and retained dead fetus

ASSESSMENT FINDINGS
• Abnormal bleeding without an accompanying history of a serious hemorrhagic disorder (petechiae, hematomas, ecchymosis, cutaneous oozing)
• Coma
• Dyspnea
• Nausea
• Oliguria

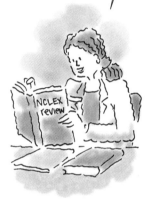

DIC causes blockages in the small blood vessels, depletes the body's supply of clotting factors and platelets, and destroys fibrin.

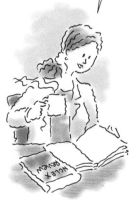

Abnormal bleeding? With no accompanying hemorrhagic disorder? That sounds like DIC.

- Seizures
- Severe muscle, back, and abdominal pain
- Shock
- Vomiting

DIAGNOSTIC TEST RESULTS
- Blood tests show prolonged PT greater than 15 seconds; prolonged PTT greater than 60 to 80 seconds; fibrinogen levels less than 150 mg/dl; platelets less than 100,000/µl; fibrin degradation products often greater than 100 µg/ml; and a positive D-dimer test specific for DIC.

NURSING DIAGNOSES
- Risk for fluid volume deficit
- Altered peripheral tissue perfusion
- Fatigue

TREATMENT
- Bed rest
- Transfusion therapy: fresh frozen plasma, platelets, packed RBCs

Drug therapy
- Anticoagulant: Heparin I.V.

INTERVENTIONS AND RATIONALES
- Don't scrub bleeding areas *to prevent clots from dislodging and causing fresh bleeding.* Use pressure, cold compresses, and topical hemostatic agents *to control bleeding.*
- Enforce complete bed rest during bleeding episodes. If the patient is very agitated, pad the side rails *to protect the patient from injury.*
- Check all I.V. and venipuncture sites frequently for bleeding. Apply pressure to injection sites for at least 10 minutes. Alert other personnel to the patient's tendency to hemorrhage. *These measures prevent hemorrhage.*
- Monitor intake and output hourly in acute DIC, especially when administering blood products, *to monitor effectiveness of volume replacement.*
- Watch for transfusion reactions and signs of fluid overload. Weigh dressings and linen and record drainage *to measure the amount of blood lost.* Weigh the patient daily, particularly in renal involvement, *to monitor for fluid volume excess.*

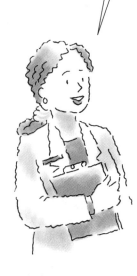

Some key signs of DIC: oozing from the skin, red or purple skin spots, and hematomas caused by bleeding into the skin.

- Watch for bleeding from the GI and genitourinary tracts *to detect early signs of hemorrhage.* Measure the patient's abdominal girth at least every 4 hours, and monitor closely for signs of shock *to detect intra-abdominal bleeding.*
- Monitor the results of serial blood studies (particularly HCT, Hb, and coagulation times) *to guide the treatment plan.*
- Inform the family of the patient's progress. Prepare them for his appearance (I.V. lines, nasogastric tubes, bruises, dried blood). Provide emotional support for the patient and family. As needed, enlist the aid of a social worker, chaplain, and other members of the health care team in providing such support. *Providing support in a crisis situation reduces the family's anxiety.*

Teaching topics
- Explaining the disorder and treatment options to the patient and family
- Bleeding prevention

Hemophilia

A hereditary bleeding disorder that affects only males, hemophilia produces mild to severe abnormal bleeding. After a platelet plug develops at a bleeding site, the lack of clotting factor prevents a stable fibrin clot from forming. Although hemorrhaging doesn't usually happen immediately, delayed bleeding is common. Two types of hemophilia exist:
- hemophilia A or classic hemophilia (deficiency or nonfunction of factor VIII)
- hemophilia B or Christmas disease (deficiency or nonfunction of factor IX).

Severity and prognosis of hemophilia vary with the degree of deficiency and the site of bleeding.

CAUSES
- Genetic inheritance: Both types of hemophilia are inherited as X-linked recessive traits.

ASSESSMENT FINDINGS
Severe hemophilia
- Excessive bleeding following circumcision (often the first sign of the disease)
- Large subcutaneous and deep intramuscular hematomas
- Spontaneous or severe bleeding after minor trauma

Moderate hemophilia
- Occasional spontaneous bleeding
- Subcutaneous and intramuscular hematomas

Mild hemophilia
- No spontaneous bleeding
- Prolonged bleeding after major trauma or surgery (blood may ooze slowly or intermittently for up to 8 days following surgery)

For all degrees of severity
- Hematemesis (bloody vomit)
- Hematomas on the extremities, torso, or both
- Hematuria (bloody urine)
- History of prolonged bleeding after surgery, dental extractions, or trauma
- Joint tenderness
- Limited ROM
- Pain and swelling in a weight-bearing joint (such as the hip, knee, or ankle)
- Signs of decreased tissue perfusion: chest pain, confusion, cool and clammy skin, decreased urine output, hypotension, pallor, restlessness, anxiety, tachycardia
- Signs of internal bleeding, such as abdominal, chest, or flank pain
- Tarry stools

DIAGNOSTIC TEST RESULTS
Hemophilia A
- Activated PTT is prolonged.
- Factor VIII assay reveals 0% to 25% of normal factor VIII.
- Platelet count and function, bleeding time, and PT are normal.

Hemophilia B
- Baseline coagulation result is similar to that of hemophilia A, with normal factor VIII.
- Factor IX assay shows deficiency.

NURSING DIAGNOSES
- Impaired gas exchange
- Pain
- Parental role conflict

TREATMENTS
Hemophilia A
- Administration of cryoprecipitate antihemophilic factor (AHF) and lyophilized (dehydrated) AHF to encourage normal hemostasis (arrest of bleeding)
- Immediate notification of doctor following injury, especially to the head, neck, or abdomen

Hemophilia B
- Administration of recombinant factor VIII and purified factor IX to promote hemostasis
- Immediate notification of doctor following injury, especially to the head, neck, or abdomen

Drug therapy (both types)
- Administration of analgesics to control joint pain

INTERVENTIONS AND RATIONALES
- Provide emotional support *because hemophilia is a chronic disorder.*
- Refer new patients to a hemophilia treatment center *for education, evaluation, and development of a treatment plan.*
- Refer patients and carriers for genetic counseling *to determine risk of passing the disease to offspring.*

During bleeding episodes
- Apply pressure to cuts and during epistaxis *to stop bleeding. Pressure is often the only treatment needed for surface cuts.*
- Apply cold compresses or ice bags and elevate the injured part *to control bleeding.*
- Give sufficient clotting factor or plasma, as ordered, *to promote hemostasis.* The body uses AHF in 48 to 72 hours, so repeat infusions may be necessary.
- Administer analgesics *to control pain.* Avoid I.M. injections because they may cause hematomas at the injection site. Aspirin and aspirin-containing medications are contraindi-

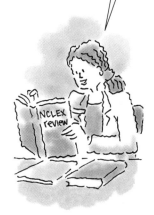

Hemophilia is inherited as an X-linked recessive trait...

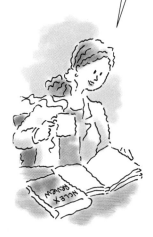

...this means that female carriers have a 50% chance of transmitting the gene to a daughter, making her a carrier, and a 50% chance of transmitting the gene to a son, who would be born with the disease.

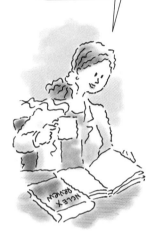

Creating NCLEX question scenarios while you study can help you remember important info...

cated because they decrease platelet adherence and may increase bleeding.

If the patient has bled into a joint

• Immediately elevate the joint *to control bleeding.*
• Begin range-of-motion exercises, if ordered, at least 48 hours after the bleeding has been controlled *to restore joint mobility.*
• Don't allow patient to bear weight on the affected joint until bleeding stops and swelling subsides *to prevent deformities due to hemarthrosis.*

After bleeding episodes and surgery

• Watch for signs of further bleeding *to detect and control bleeding as soon as possible.*
• Closely monitor PTT. *Prolonged times increase risk of bleeding.*

Teaching topics

• Signs of severe internal bleeding
• When to notify primary care provider; for example, after even a minor injury
• Wearing medical identification bracelet
• Protecting a child from injury
• Importance of medical follow-up
• Risk of infection such as hepatitis from blood component administration
• Caring for injuries
• Home administration of blood factor components, as appropriate

Iron deficiency anemia

Iron deficiency anemia is a chronic, slowly progressing disease involving circulating RBCs. Iron deficiency results when an individual either absorbs inadequate amounts of iron or loses excessive amounts (such as through chronic bleeding). This decreased iron affects formation of hemoglobin and RBCs, which, in turn, decreases the capacity of the blood to transport oxygen.

CAUSES

• Acute and chronic bleeding
• Alcohol abuse
• Drug-induced

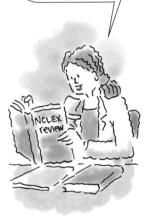

...For example, imagine that you're teaching a patient with iron deficiency anemia about dietary changes. What would you teach?

• Gastrectomy
• Inadequate intake of iron-rich foods
• Malabsorption syndrome
• Menstruation
• Pregnancy
• Vitamin B_6 deficiency

ASSESSMENT FINDINGS

• Cheilosis (scalp and fissures of the lips)
• Dizziness
• Dyspnea
• Koilonychia (spoon-shaped nails)
• Pale, dry mucous membranes
• Pallor
• Palpitations
• Papillae atrophy of the tongue
• Sensitivity to cold
• Stomatitis
• Weakness and fatigue

DIAGNOSTIC TEST RESULTS

• Hematology shows decreased Hb, HCT, iron, ferritin, reticulocytes, red cell indices, transferrin, and saturation; absent hemosiderin; and increased iron-binding capacity.
• Peripheral blood smear reveals microcytic and hypochromic RBCs.

NURSING DIAGNOSES

• Activity intolerance
• Altered nutrition: Less than body requirements
• Impaired gas exchange

TREATMENT

• Diet: establish a diet high in iron, roughage, and protein with increased fluids; avoid teas and coffee, which reduce absorption of iron
• Transfusion therapy with packed RBCs, if necessary
• Vitamins: pyridoxine hydrochloride (vitamin B_6), ascorbic acid (vitamin C)

Drug therapy

• Antianemics: ferrous sulfate (Feosol), iron dextran (DexFerrum)

INTERVENTIONS AND RATIONALES

• Monitor intake and output *to detect fluid imbalances.*

• Monitor laboratory studies *to determine therapeutic effect of therapy.*
• Assess cardiovascular and respiratory status *to detect decreased activity intolerance and dyspnea on exertion.*
• Monitor and record vital signs *to determine activity intolerance.*
• Monitor stool, urine, and emesis for occult blood *to identify cause of anemia.*
• Administer oxygen, as necessary, *to treat hypoxemia caused by reduced hemoglobin.*
• Provide a diet high in iron *to replace iron stores in body.*
• Administer medications, as prescribed, *to replace iron stores in body.* Administer iron injection deep into muscle using Z-track technique *to avoid subcutaneous irritation and discoloration from leaking drug.*
• Encourage fluids *to avoid dehydration.*
• Provide rest periods *to avoid fatigue and reduce oxygen demands.*
• Provide mouth, skin, and foot care *because the tongue or lips may be dry or inflamed and nails may be brittle.*
• Protect the patient from falls caused by weakness and fatigue. *Falls may result in bleeding and bruising.*
• Keep the patient warm *to enhance comfort.*

Teaching topics
• Eating foods rich in iron
• Recognizing signs and symptoms of bleeding
• Monitoring stools for occult blood
• Refraining from using hot pads and hot water bottles

Kaposi's sarcoma

Once, this cancer of the lymphatic cell wall was rare, occurring mostly in elderly Italian and Jewish men. The incidence of Kaposi's sarcoma has risen dramatically along with the incidence of AIDS. Currently, it's the most common AIDS-related cancer.

Kaposi's sarcoma causes structural and functional damage. When associated with AIDS, it progresses aggressively, involving the lymph nodes, the viscera and, possibly, GI structures.

CAUSES
• Unknown, possibly related to immunosuppression

ASSESSMENT FINDINGS
• Dyspnea (in cases of pulmonary involvement), wheezing, hypoventilation, and respiratory distress from bronchial blockage
• Edema from lymphatic obstruction
• One or more obvious lesions in various shapes, sizes, and colors (ranging from red-brown to dark purple) appearing most commonly on the skin, buccal mucosa, hard and soft palates, lips, gums, tongue, tonsils, conjunctiva, and sclera
• Pain (if the sarcoma advances beyond the early stages or if a lesion breaks down or impinges on nerves or organs)

DIAGNOSTIC TEST RESULTS
• Computed tomography scan detects and evaluates possible metastasis.
• Tissue biopsy identifies the lesion's type and stage.

NURSING DIAGNOSES
• Altered protection
• Risk for infection
• Body image disturbance

TREATMENT
• High-calorie, high-protein diet
• Radiation therapy
• I.V. fluid therapy

Drug therapy
• Chemotherapy: doxorubicin (Adriamycin), etoposide (VePesid), vinblastine (Velban), vincristine (Oncovin)
• Biological response modifier: interferon alfa-2b (ineffective in advanced disease)
• Antiemetic: trimethobenzamide (Tigan)

INTERVENTIONS AND RATIONALES
• Provide a referral for psychological counseling *to assist the patient who's coping poorly.* Family members may also need help in coping with the patient's disease and with any associated demands that the disorder places upon them.

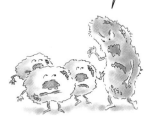

Kaposi's sarcoma is aggressive. It involves the lymph nodes, internal organs and, possibly, the digestive tract.

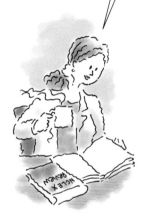

One or more obvious lesions, in conjunction with an AIDS diagnosis, indicate Kaposi's sarcoma.

• As appropriate, allow the patient to participate in self-care decisions whenever possible, and encourage him to participate in self-care measures as much as he can. *Involving the patient in the treatment plan helps him gain some sense of control over his situation.*
• Inspect the patient's skin every shift. Look for new lesions and skin breakdown. If the patient has painful lesions, help him into a more comfortable position *to alleviate pain and promote patient comfort.*
• Administer pain medications. Suggest distractions, and help the patient with relaxation techniques *to divert the patient from his pain and promote comfort.*
• Urge the patient to share his feelings, and provide encouragement *to help him adjust to changes in his appearance.*
• Monitor the patient's weight daily *to evaluate if nutritional needs are being met.*
• Supply the patient with high-calorie, high-protein meals. If he can't tolerate regular meals, provide him with frequent smaller meals. Consult with the dietitian, and plan meals around the patient's treatment. *Adverse reactions to medications and the disease itself may make it difficult for the patient's nutritional intake to meet his metabolic needs.*
• If the patient can't take food by mouth, administer I.V. fluids *to maintain hydration.* Also provide antiemetics *to combat nausea and encourage nutritional intake.*
• Be alert for adverse reactions to radiation therapy or chemotherapy — such as anorexia, nausea, vomiting, and diarrhea — and take steps to prevent or alleviate them. *Adverse reactions are common and can further compromise the patient's condition.*
• Reinforce the explanation of treatments. Make sure the patient understands which adverse reactions to expect and how to manage them *to ensure prompt intervention and treatment.* For example, during radiation therapy, instruct the patient to keep irradiated skin dry *to avoid possible breakdown and subsequent infection.*
• Explain all prescribed medications, including any possible adverse effects and drug interactions, *to promote compliance with the medication regimen.*

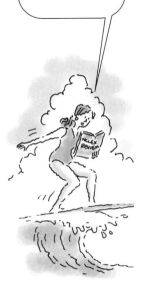

You're more than halfway through this chapter. Take a break if you need to refresh your mind.

• Explain infection-prevention techniques and, if necessary, demonstrate basic hygiene measures *to prevent infection.* Advise the patient not to share his toothbrush, razor, or other items that may be contaminated with blood. These measures are especially important if the patient also has AIDS. *These measures prevent the spread of infection to others.*
• Encourage the patient to set priorities, accept the help of others, and delegate nonessential tasks. Help the patient plan daily periods of alternating activity and rest *to help him cope with fatigue.*
• Explain the proper use of assistive devices, when appropriate, *to ease ambulation and promote independence.*
• As appropriate, refer the patient to support groups offered by the social services department *to promote emotional well-being.*
• If the patient's prognosis is poor (less than 6 months to live), suggest immediate hospice care. *Hospice care provides much needed support to caregivers and helps the patient through the dying process.*

Teaching topics
• Energy-conservation techniques
• High-calorie, high-protein diet, consumed in small, frequent amounts if necessary
• Infection control measures
• Ongoing treatment and care
• Benefits of initiating and executing advance directives and a durable power of attorney

Leukemia

Leukemia is characterized by an uncontrolled proliferation of WBC precursors that fail to mature. Leukemia occurs when normal hemopoietic cells are replaced by leukemic cells in bone marrow. Immature forms of WBCs circulate in the blood, infiltrating the liver, spleen, and lymph nodes. Types of leukemia include:
• acute lymphocytic
• acute myelogenous
• chronic lymphocytic
• chronic myelocytic.

CAUSES
- Altered immune system
- Exposure to chemicals
- Genetics
- Radiation
- Virus

ASSESSMENT FINDINGS
- Enlarged lymph nodes, spleen, and liver
- Epistaxis
- Fever
- Frequent infections
- Generalized pain
- Gingivitis and stomatitis
- Hematemesis
- Hypotension
- Jaundice
- Joint, abdominal, and bone pain
- Melena
- Night sweats
- Petechiae and ecchymoses
- Prolonged menses
- Tachycardia
- Weakness and fatigue

DIAGNOSTIC TEST RESULTS
- Bone marrow biopsy reveals a large number of immature leukocytes.
- Hematology shows decreased HCT, Hb, RBCs, and platelets and increased ESR, immature WBCs, and prolonged bleeding time.

NURSING DIAGNOSES
- Altered nutrition: Less than body requirements
- Pain
- Risk for infection

TREATMENT
- Diet: establish a high-protein, high-vitamin and high-mineral diet, involving soft, bland foods in small, frequent feedings
- Stem cell transplant
- Transfusion of platelets, packed RBCs, and whole blood

Drug therapy
- Alkylating agents: busulfan (Myleran), chlorambucil (Leukeran)
- Antibiotics: doxorubicin (Adriamycin), plicamycin (Mithracin)
- Antimetabolites: fluorouracil (Adrucil), methotrexate sodium (Folex)
- Antineoplastics: vinblastine (Velban), vincristine sulfate (Oncovin)
- Hematopoietic growth factor: epoetin alfa (Epogen)

INTERVENTIONS AND RATIONALES
- Monitor and record vital signs *to promptly detect deterioration in patient's condition.*
- Monitor intake, output, and daily weight *because body weight may decrease as a result of fluid loss.*
- Monitor laboratory studies *to help establish blood replacement needs, assess fluid status, and detect possible infection.*
- Monitor for bleeding. *Regular assessment may help anticipate or alleviate problems.*
- Place patient with epistaxis in an upright position leaning slightly forward *to reduce vascular pressure and prevent aspiration.*
- Monitor for infection. *Damage to bone marrow may suppress WBC formation.* Promptly report fever over 101° F and decreased WBC counts so that antibiotic therapy may be initiated.
- Monitor oxygen therapy. *Oxygen therapy increases alveolar oxygen concentration and enhances arterial blood oxygenation.*
- Force fluids *to maintain adequate hydration.*
- Administer I.V. fluids *to replace fluid loss.*
- Encourage turning every 2 hours *to prevent venous stasis and skin breakdown.*
- Encourage coughing and deep breathing *to help remove secretions and prevent pulmonary complications.*
- Keep the patient in semi-Fowler's position when in bed *to promote chest expansion and ventilation of basilar lung fields.*
- Maintain the patient's diet *to provide necessary nutrition.*
- Administer TPN, if needed, *to provide the patient with electrolytes, amino acids, and other nutrients tailored to his needs.*
- Administer transfusion therapy as prescribed and monitor for adverse reactions. *Transfusion reactions may occur during blood administration and may further compromise the patient's condition.*
- Administer medications as prescribed *to combat disease and promote wellness.*

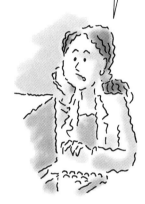

Frequent infections and easy bruising are key signs of leukemia.

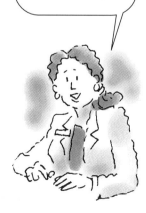

Think about therapeutic communication. A patient with leukemia might want to talk about body image changes. Allow the patient to express his feelings.

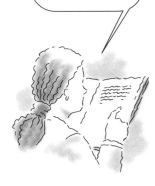

Remember that in Hodgkin's disease, tumors follow a pattern. In malignant lymphoma, tumors occur more randomly.

• Provide gentle mouth and skin care *to prevent oral mucous membrane or skin breakdown.*
• Encourage the patient to express his feelings about changes in his body image and fear of dying *to reduce anxiety.*
• Avoid giving the patient I.M. injections and enemas and taking rectal temperature *to prevent bleeding.*

Teaching topics
• Recognizing the signs and symptoms of occult bleeding
• Preventing constipation
• Using an electric razor
• Refraining from using over-the-counter (OTC) medications (unless cleared by the patient's doctor)
• Increasing fluid intake
• Contacting the American Cancer Society

Lymphoma

Lymphoma can be classified as either Hodgkin's disease or malignant lymphoma (also called non-Hodgkin's lymphoma).

In Hodgkin's disease, Reed-Sternberg cells proliferate in a single lymph node and travel contiguously through the lymphatic system to other lymphatic nodes and organs. (See *Hodgkin's progress.*)

In malignant lymphoma, tumors occur throughout lymph nodes and lymphatic organs in unpredictable patterns. Malignant lymphoma may be categorized as:
• lymphocytic
• histiocytic
• mixed cell types.

Keeping the lymphoma patient in semi-Fowler's position promotes ventilation and chest expansion.

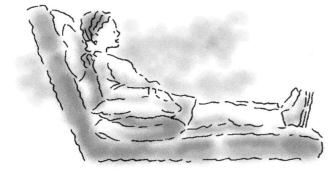

CAUSES
• Environmental (Hodgkin's disease)
• Genetic (Hodgkin's disease)
• Immunologic
• Viral

ASSESSMENT FINDINGS

Hodgkin's disease
• Bone pain
• Dysphagia
• Dyspnea
• Edema and cyanosis of face and neck
• Enlarged, nontender, firm, and movable lymph nodes in lower cervical regions
• Predictable pattern of spread

Malignant lymphoma
• Less predictable pattern of spread
• Prominent, painless, generalized lymphadenopathy

For both lymphomas
• Anorexia and weight loss
• Cough
• Hepatomegaly
• Malaise and lethargy
• Night sweats
• Recurrent infection
• Recurrent, intermittent fever
• Severe pruritus
• Splenomegaly

DIAGNOSTIC TEST RESULTS
• Bone marrow aspiration and biopsy reveals small, diffuse lymphocytic or large, follicular-type cells (malignant lymphoma).
• Blood chemistry shows increased alkaline phosphatase (Hodgkin's disease).
• Chest X-ray reveals lymphadenopathy.
• Hematology shows decreased Hb, HCT, and platelets and increased ESR, increased immature leukocytes, and increased gammaglobulin (Hodgkin's disease).
• Lymph node biopsy is positive for Reed-Sternberg cells (Hodgkin's disease).
• Lymphangiogram shows positive lymph node involvement (Hodgkin's disease).

NURSING DIAGNOSES
• Altered protection

Hodgkin's progress

Hodgkin's disease occurs in four stages.

 Stage I: Disease occurs in a single lymph node region or single extralymphatic organ.

Stage II: Disease occurs in two or more nodes on same side of diaphragm or in an extralymphatic organ.

Stage III: Disease spreads to both sides of diaphragm and perhaps to an extralymphatic organ, the spleen, or both.

Stage IV: Disease disseminates.

• Impaired tissue integrity
• Risk for infection

TREATMENT
• Establishing a diet high in protein, calories, vitamins, minerals, iron, and calcium that should consist of bland, soft foods
• Radiation therapy
• Transfusion of packed RBCs

Chemotherapy
• Hodgkin's disease: mechlorethamine (Mustargen), vincristine sulfate (Oncovin), procarbazine (Matulane), doxorubicin (Adriamycin), bleomycin (Blenoxane), vinblastine (Velban), dacarbazine (DTIC-Dome)
• Malignant lymphoma: cyclophosphamide (Cytoxan), vincristine sulfate (Oncovin), doxorubicin (Adriamycin)

INTERVENTIONS AND RATIONALES
• Monitor and record vital signs *to allow for early detection of complications.*
• Monitor intake and output and specific gravity. *Low urine output and high specific gravity indicate hypovolemia.*
• Monitor laboratory studies. *Electrolytes, Hb, and HCT help indicate fluid status; WBC measurement may indicate bone marrow suppression.*
• Monitor for bleeding, infection, jaundice, and electrolyte imbalance *to detect complications associated with lymphoma.*
• Keep the patient in semi-Fowler's position when in bed *to promote chest expansion and ventilation of basilar lung fields.*

• Administer oxygen. *Supplemental oxygen helps reduce hypoxemia.*
• Encourage turning every 2 hours *to prevent skin breakdown* and coughing and deep breathing *to help remove secretions and prevent pulmonary complications.*
• Provide mouth and skin care *to prevent breakdown of oral mucous membrane and skin.*
• Help the patient maintain his diet *to ensure nutritional requirements are met.*
• Encourage fluids *to prevent dehydration and complications associated with chemotherapy drugs.*
• Administer I.V. fluids as prescribed *to replace fluid loss.*
• Administer medications as prescribed, and monitor for adverse effects *to prevent further complications.*
• Administer transfusion therapy as prescribed, and monitor for adverse reactions. *Transfusion reactions during blood administration may further compromise the patient's condition.*
• Provide rest periods *to enhance immune function and decrease weakness caused by anemia.*
• Encourage the patient to express his feelings about changes in his body image and a fear of dying *to allay the patient's anxiety.*

Teaching topics
• Recognizing early signs and symptoms of motor and sensory deficits
• Increasing fluid intake
• Using an electric razor only

> Monitor the patient with lymphoma for bleeding, infection, jaundice, and electrolyte imbalance. Provide mouth and skin care. Encourage fluids.

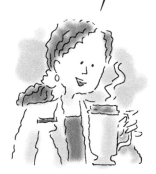

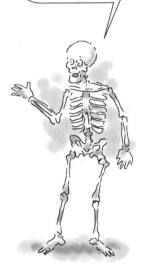

By acting on the myoneural junctions (the site where nerve and muscle fibers meet), magnesium affects the irritability and contractility of skeletal muscles...

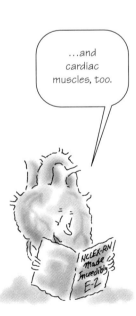

...and cardiac muscles, too.

• Refraining from using OTC medications (unless cleared by the patient's doctor)
• Contacting the American Cancer Society

Magnesium imbalance

Magnesium is the second most common cation in intracellular fluid (a cation is a positively charged ion). Its major function is to enhance neuromuscular integration. Magnesium regulates muscle contractions. By acting on the myoneural junctions (the sites where nerve and muscle fibers meet), magnesium affects the irritability and contractility of skeletal and cardiac muscles.

Magnesium also stimulates parathyroid hormone (PTH) secretion, thus regulating intracellular fluid calcium levels. Therefore, magnesium deficiency (hypomagnesemia) may result in transient hypoparathyroidism and may interfere with the peripheral action of PTH.

In addition, magnesium activates many enzymes for proper carbohydrate and protein metabolism, aids in cell metabolism and the transport of sodium and potassium across cell membranes, and influences sodium, potassium, calcium, and protein levels.

Approximately one-third of the magnesium taken into the body is absorbed through the small intestine and is eventually excreted in urine; the remaining unabsorbed magnesium is excreted in stool.

Because many common foods contain magnesium, a dietary deficiency is rare. Hypomagnesemia generally follows impaired absorption, too-rapid excretion, or inadequate intake during TPN. It frequently coexists with other electrolyte imbalances, especially low calcium and potassium levels. Magnesium excess (hypermagnesemia) is common in patients with renal failure and excessive intake of magnesium-containing antacids.

CAUSES
Hypomagnesemia usually results from impaired absorption of magnesium in the intestines or excessive excretion in the urine or stools. Hypermagnesemia results from the kidneys' inability to excrete magnesium that was either absorbed from the intestines or was infused.

Hypomagnesemia
• Chronic alcoholism
• Excessive loss of magnesium, as in severe dehydration and diabetic acidosis
• Decreased magnesium intake or absorption, as in malabsorption syndrome, chronic diarrhea, or postoperative complications after bowel resection
• Hyperaldosteronism and hypoparathyroidism, which result in hypokalemia and hypocalcemia
• Hyperparathyroidism and hypercalcemia; excessive release of adrenocortical hormones; diuretic therapy
• Prolonged diuretic therapy, nasogastric suctioning, or administration of parenteral fluids without magnesium salts; starvation or malnutrition

Hypermagnesemia
• Chronic renal insufficiency
• Overcorrection of hypomagnesemia
• Overuse of magnesium-containing antacids
• Severe dehydration (resulting oliguria can cause magnesium retention)
• Use of laxatives (magnesium sulfate, milk of magnesia, and magnesium citrate solutions), especially with renal insufficiency

ASSESSMENT FINDINGS
Hypomagnesemia
• Arrhythmias
• Neuromuscular irritability
• Leg and foot cramps
• Chvostek's sign
• Mood changes
• Confusion
• Delusions
• Hallucinations
• Seizures

Hypermagnesemia
• Diminished deep tendon reflexes
• Weakness
• Flaccid paralysis
• Respiratory muscle paralysis (severe hypermagnesemia)
• Drowsiness

- Confusion
- Diminished sensorium may progress to coma
- Bradycardia
- Weak pulse
- Hypotension
- Heart block
- Cardiac arrest (severe hypermagnesemia)
- Nausea
- Vomiting

DIAGNOSTIC TEST RESULTS
- Blood test that shows decreased serum magnesium levels (less than 1.5 mEq/L) confirms hypomagnesemia.
- Blood test that shows increased serum magnesium levels (greater than 2.5 mEq/L) confirms hypermagnesemia.

NURSING DIAGNOSES
- Risk for injury
- Decreased cardiac output
- Impaired gas exchange

TREATMENT
Hypomagnesemia
- Daily magnesium supplements I.M. or by mouth
- High-magnesium diet
- I.V. fluid therapy
- Magnesium sulfate I.V. (10 to 40 mEq/L diluted in I.V. fluid) for severe cases

Hypermagnesemia
- Diet: Low magnesium with increased fluid intake
- Loop diuretic: furosemide (Lasix)
- Magnesium antagonist: calcium gluconate (10%)
- Peritoneal dialysis or hemodialysis if renal function fails or if excess magnesium can't be eliminated

INTERVENTIONS AND RATIONALES
For patients with hypomagnesemia
- Monitor serum electrolyte levels (including magnesium, calcium, and potassium) daily for mild deficits and every 6 to 12 hours during replacement therapy *to guide the treatment plan*.
- Measure intake and output frequently. (Urine output shouldn't fall below 25 ml/hour or 600 ml/day.) *The kidneys excrete excess magnesium, and hypermagnesemia could occur with renal insufficiency.*
- Monitor vital signs during I.V. therapy. Infuse magnesium replacement slowly, and watch for bradycardia, heart block, and decreased respiratory rate *to prevent complications that may occur with rapid infusion.*
- Have calcium gluconate I.V. available *to reverse hypermagnesemia from overcorrection.*
- Advise patients to eat foods high in magnesium, such as fish and green vegetables, *to help raise magnesium level with dietary sources.*
- Watch for and report signs of hypomagnesemia in patients with predisposing diseases or conditions, especially those not permitted anything by mouth or who receive I.V. fluids without magnesium *to prevent complications associated with magnesium deficiency.*

For patients with hypermagnesemia
- Frequently assess level of consciousness, muscle activity, and vital signs *to detect complications of magnesium excess.*
- Keep accurate intake and output records. Provide sufficient fluids *for adequate hydration and maintenance of renal function.*
- Correct abnormal serum electrolyte levels immediately *to prevent complications of magnesium excess.*
- Monitor the patient receiving digitalis glycosides and calcium gluconate simultaneously *because excessive calcium enhances digitalis glycoside action, predisposing the patient to digitalis toxicity.*
- Watch for signs of hypermagnesemia in predisposed patients. Observe closely for respiratory distress if serum magnesium levels exceed 10 mEq/L *to prevent respiratory decompensation.*

Teaching topics for hypomagnesemia
- Consuming foods high in magnesium, such as seed grains, nuts, and legumes (fresh meat, fish, and fresh fruits usually contain small amounts of magnesium)
- Avoiding laxative and diuretic abuse (this practice may result in loss of magnesium)

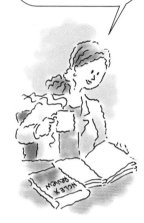

Here are the key numbers: serum magnesium under 1.5 mEq/L confirms hypomagnesemia; over 2.5 mEq/L confirms hypermagnesemia.

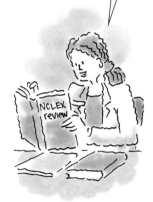

The best treatment for hypomagnesemia is prevention. Keep a watchful eye on patients at risk for this imbalance, such as those who can't tolerate oral intake.

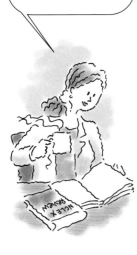

You win some, you lose some. Metabolic acidosis is characterized by a gain in acid and a loss of bicarbonate (base) in the plasma.

ABG analysis is the key diagnostic test for detecting metabolic acidosis.

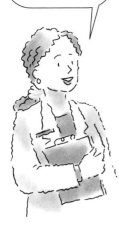

Teaching topics for hypermagnesemia
• In patients with renal failure, checking with the doctor before taking any OTC medications.
• Avoiding abuse of laxatives and antacids containing magnesium, particularly if the patient is elderly or has impaired renal function

Metabolic acidosis

Metabolic acidosis refers to a state of excess acid accumulation and deficient base bicarbonate. It is produced by an underlying pathologic disorder. Symptoms result from the body's attempts to correct the acidotic condition through compensatory mechanisms in the lungs, kidneys, and cells.

Metabolic acidosis is more prevalent among children, who are vulnerable to acid-base imbalance because their metabolic rates are faster and their ratios of water to total-body weight are lower. Severe or untreated metabolic acidosis can be fatal.

CAUSES
• Anaerobic carbohydrate metabolism
• Chronic alcoholism
• Diabetic ketoacidosis
• Diarrhea or intestinal malabsorption
• Low-carbohydrate, high-fat diet
• Malnutrition
• Renal insufficiency and failure

ASSESSMENT FINDINGS
• Central nervous system depression
• Drowsiness
• Headache
• Kussmaul's respirations
• Lethargy
• Stupor

DIAGNOSTIC TEST RESULTS
• ABG analysis reveals pH below 7.35 and bicarbonate level less than 24 mEq/L.

NURSING DIAGNOSES
• Ineffective breathing pattern
• Altered thought processes
• Decreased cardiac output

TREATMENT
Correcting the underlying cause is the goal of treatment
• Endotracheal intubation and mechanical ventilation to ensure adequate respiratory compensation (in severe cases)

Drug therapy
• Sodium bicarbonate I.V., or orally for chronic metabolic acidosis
• Insulin administration and I.V. fluid administration if diabetic ketoacidosis is the cause

INTERVENTIONS AND RATIONALES
• Keep sodium bicarbonate ampules handy *for emergency administration*. Frequently monitor vital signs, laboratory results, and level of consciousness *because changes can occur rapidly.*
• In diabetic acidosis, watch for secondary changes due to hypovolemia, such as decreasing blood pressure, *to prevent complications of hypoperfusion.*
• Record intake and output accurately *to monitor renal function.*
• Watch for signs of excessive serum potassium — weakness, flaccid paralysis, and arrhythmias, possibly leading to cardiac arrest. After treatment, check for overcorrection to hypokalemia *to prevent complications of potassium imbalance.*
• Prepare for possible seizures with seizure precautions *to prevent injury.*
• Provide good oral hygiene. Use sodium bicarbonate washes *to neutralize mouth acids,* and lubricate the patient's lips *to prevent skin breakdown.*
• Carefully observe patients receiving I.V. therapy or who have intestinal tubes in place, as well as those suffering from shock, hyperthyroidism, hepatic disease, circulatory failure, or dehydration, *to prevent metabolic acidosis.*

Teaching topics
• Testing urine for sugar and acetone
• Encouraging strict adherence to insulin or oral antidiabetic therapy
• Medication therapy and possible adverse reactions

Metabolic alkalosis

Metabolic alkalosis is a clinical state marked by decreased amounts of acid or increased amounts of base bicarbonate. It causes metabolic, respiratory, and renal responses, producing characteristic symptoms — most notably, hypoventilation. This condition always occurs secondary to an underlying cause. With early diagnosis and prompt treatment, the prognosis is good; however, untreated metabolic alkalosis may lead to coma and death.

CAUSES
• Loss of acid from vomiting, nasogastric tube drainage, or lavage without adequate electrolyte replacement, fistulas, the use of steroids and certain diuretics (furosemide, thiazides, and ethacrynic acid), or hyperadrenocorticism
• Retention of base from excessive intake of bicarbonate of soda or other antacids (usually for treatment of gastritis or peptic ulcer), excessive intake of absorbable alkali (as in milk-alkali syndrome), administration of excessive amounts of I.V. fluids with high concentrations of bicarbonate or lactate, or respiratory insufficiency

ASSESSMENT FINDINGS
• Apnea
• Atrial tachycardia
• Confusion
• Cyanosis
• Diarrhea
• Hypoventilation
• Irritability
• Nausea
• Picking at bedclothes (carphology)
• Twitching
• Vomiting

DIAGNOSTIC TEST RESULTS
• ABG analysis reveals pH greater than 7.45 and a bicarbonate level above 29 mEq/L

NURSING DIAGNOSES
• Altered thought processes
• Decreased cardiac output
• Risk for injury

TREATMENT
Goal of treatment is treating the underlying cause

Drug therapy
• Acidifying agent: ammonium chloride I.V.
• Potassium supplement: Potassium chloride I.V.

INTERVENTIONS AND RATIONALES
• When administering ammonium chloride 0.9%, limit the infusion rate to 1¼ hours; *faster administration may cause hemolysis of RBCs.* Avoid overdosage *because it may cause over-correction to metabolic acidosis.* Don't give ammonium chloride to a patient with signs of hepatic or renal disease *to avoid toxicity.*
• Monitor vital signs frequently, and record intake and output *to evaluate respiratory, fluid, and electrolyte status. Respiratory rate usually decreases in an effort to compensate for alkalosis. Hypotension and tachycardia may indicate electrolyte imbalance, especially hypokalemia.*
• Irrigate nasogastric tubes with isotonic saline solution instead of plain water *to prevent loss of gastric electrolytes.* Monitor I.V. fluid concentrations of bicarbonate or lactate *to prevent acid base imbalance.*

Teaching topics
• For patients with ulcers, recognizing signs of milk-alkali syndrome: a distaste for milk, anorexia, weakness, and lethargy
• Avoiding overuse of alkaline agents

Multiple myeloma

Multiple myeloma involves the abnormal proliferation of plasma cells. These plasma cells are immature and malignant and invade the bone marrow, lymph nodes, liver, spleen, and kidneys, triggering osteoblastic activity and leading to bone destruction throughout the body.

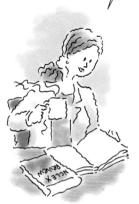

You lose some, you win some. Metabolic alkalosis is characterized by a loss of acid, a gain in bicarbonate (base), or both.

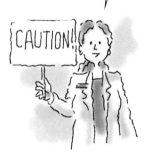

Dilute potassium when administering potassium chloride I.V. to a patient with metabolic alkalosis. Also monitor the infusion rate.

CAUSES
- Environmental
- Genetic
- Unknown

ASSESSMENT FINDINGS
- Anemia, thrombocytopenia, hemorrhage
- Constant, severe bone pain
- Headaches
- Hepatomegaly
- Multiple infections
- Pathologic fractures, skeletal deformities of sternum and ribs, loss of height
- Renal calculi
- Splenomegaly
- Vascular insufficiency

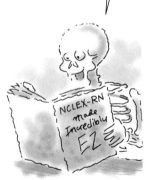

Because multiple myeloma causes bone destruction, bone pain and fractures are assessment findings to remember for this disorder.

DIAGNOSTIC TEST RESULTS
- Bence Jones protein assay is positive.
- Blood chemistry tests show increased calcium, uric acid, BUN, and creatinine.
- Bone marrow biopsy shows increased number of immature plasma cells.
- Bone scan reveals increased uptake.
- Hematology shows decreased HCT, WBCs, and platelets and increased ESR.
- Immunoelectrophoresis shows monoclonal spike.
- Urine chemistry shows increased calcium and uric acid.
- X-rays show diffuse, round, punched-out bone lesions; osteoporosis; osteolytic lesions of the skull; and widespread demineralization.

NURSING DIAGNOSES
- Pain
- Impaired physical mobility
- Risk for infection

TREATMENT
- Allogenic bone marrow transplantation
- Diet: high protein, high carbohydrate, high vitamin and high mineral in small, frequent feedings
- Orthopedic devices: braces, splints, casts
- Peritoneal dialysis and hemodialysis
- Radiation therapy
- Transfusion therapy: packed RBCs

Drug therapy
- Alkylating agents: melphalan (Alkeran), cyclophosphamide (Cytoxan)
- Analgesic: morphine
- Androgen: fluoxymesterone (Halotestin)
- Antacids: magnesium hydroxide and aluminum hydroxide (Maalox), aluminum hydroxide (AlternaGEL)
- Antibiotics: doxorubicin (Adriamycin), plicamycin (Mithracin)
- Antiemetic: prochlorperazine (Compazine)
- Antigout: allopurinol (Zyloprim)
- Antineoplastics: vinblastine (Velban), vincristine sulfate (Oncovin)
- Diuretic: furosemide (Lasix)
- Glucocorticoid: prednisone (Deltasone)

INTERVENTIONS AND RATIONALES
- Assess renal status *to detect renal stones and renal failure secondary to hypercalcemia.*
- Monitor and record vital signs *to allow for early detection of complications.*
- Monitor intake and output, urine specific gravity, and daily weight *to identify fluid volume excess or deficit.*
- Monitor laboratory studies. *RBCs, WBCs, Hb, HCT, and platelets may be affected by chemotherapy.*
- Assess cardiovascular, and respiratory status *to detect signs of compromise.*
- Assess bone pain *to determine patient's response to analgesics.*
- Monitor for infection and bruising *to detect complications.*
- Maintain the patient's diet *to ensure nutritional requirements are met.*
- Encourage fluids *to prevent dehydration and dilute calcium.*
- Administer I.V. fluids *to replace fluid loss, dilute calcium, and prevent renal protein precipitation.*
- Assist with turning, coughing, and deep breathing *to mobilize and remove secretions.*
- Administer transfusion therapy as prescribed *to replace blood components.*
- Administer medications, as prescribed, and monitor for adverse effects *to prevent complications.*
- Maintain seizure precautions *to prevent injury.*

- Provide skin and mouth care *to prevent breakdown of oral mucous membrane and skin.*
- Alternate rest periods with activity *to prevent fatigue.*
- Prevent the patient from falling *because he is vulnerable to fractures.*
- Move the patient gently, keeping body in alignment, *to prevent injury.*
- Apply and maintain braces, splints, and casts *to prevent injury and reduce pain.*

Teaching topics
- Exercising regularly, with particular attention to muscle-strengthening exercises
- Recognizing signs and symptoms of renal calculi, fractures, and seizures
- Avoiding lifting, constipation, and OTC medications
- Monitoring stool for occult blood
- Using braces, splints, and casts
- Contacting the American Cancer Society

Pernicious anemia

Pernicious anemia is a chronic, progressive, macrocytic anemia caused by a deficiency of intrinsic factor, a substance normally secreted by the stomach. Without intrinsic factor, dietary vitamin B_{12} can't by absorbed by the ileum, inhibiting normal deoxyribonucleic acid (DNA) synthesis and resulting in defective maturation of RBCs.

CAUSES
- Autoimmune disease
- Bacterial or parasitic infections
- Deficiency of intrinsic factor
- Gastric mucosal atrophy
- Genetics
- Lack of administration of vitamin B_{12} after small-bowel resection or total gastrectomy
- Malabsorption
- Prolonged iron deficiency

ASSESSMENT FINDINGS
- Constipation or diarrhea
- Depression, delirium
- Dyspnea
- Glossitis, sore mouth
- Mild jaundice of sclera
- Pallor
- Paralysis, gait disturbances
- Tachycardia, palpitations
- Tingling and paresthesia of hands and feet
- Weakness, fatigue
- Weight loss, anorexia, dyspepsia

DIAGNOSTIC TEST RESULTS
- Blood chemistry tests reveal increased bilirubin and lactate dehydrogenase levels.
- Bone marrow aspiration shows increased megaloblasts, few maturing erythrocytes, and defective leukocyte maturation.
- Gastric analysis shows hypochlorhydria.
- Hematology shows decreased HCT and Hb.
- Peripheral blood smear reveals oval, macrocytic, hyperchromic erythrocytes.
- Romberg test is positive.
- Schilling test is positive.
- Upper GI series shows atrophy of gastric mucosa.

NURSING DIAGNOSES
- Altered nutrition: Less than body requirements
- Impaired gas exchange
- Risk for injury

TREATMENT
- Establishing a diet high in iron and protein and restricting highly seasoned, coarse, or extremely hot foods
- Transfusion therapy with packed RBCs
- Vitamins: pyridoxine hydrochloride (vitamin B_6), ascorbic acid (vitamin C), cyanocobalamin (vitamin B_{12}), folic acid (vitamin B_C)

Drug therapy
- Antianemics: ferrous sulfate (Feosol), iron dextran (DexFerrum)

INTERVENTIONS AND RATIONALES
- Assess cardiovascular status *to detect signs of compromise as the heart works harder to compensate for the reduced oxygen-carrying capacity of the blood.*
- Monitor and record vital signs *to allow for early detection of compromise.*

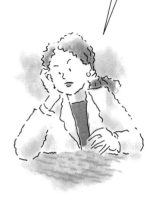

If you remember that pernicious anemia results from a lack of B_{12} absorption, then it's easy to recall that vitamins are a big part of treating this disorder.

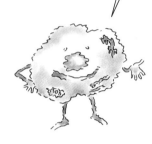

Phosphorus plays a crucial role in cell membrane integrity...

• Monitor and record amount, consistency, and color of stools *to allow for early detection and treatment of diarrhea and constipation.*
• Maintain the patient's diet *to ensure adequate intake of vitamins, iron, and protein.*
• Administer medications as prescribed. *Vitamin B_{12} injections are given monthly and are lifelong.*
• Maintain activity, as tolerated, *to avoid fatigue.*
• Provide mouth care before and after meals, *for comfort and to reduce risk of oral mucous membrane breakdown.*
• Use soft toothbrushes *to avoid injuring mucous membranes.*
• Maintain warm environment *for patient comfort.*
• Provide foot and skin care *because sensation to feet may be reduced.*
• Prevent the patient from falling *due to reduced coordination, paresthesia of feet, and reduced thought processes*
• Assess neurologic status *because poor memory and confusion increase the risk of injury.*
• Monitor laboratory studies *to detect effectiveness of therapy.*

Teaching topics
• Recognizing the signs and symptoms of skin breakdown
• Altering activities of daily living (ADLs) to compensate for paresthesia
• Complying with lifelong, monthly injections of vitamin B_{12}
• Avoiding the use of heating pads and electric blankets

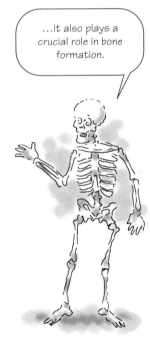

...it also plays a crucial role in bone formation.

Phosphorus imbalance

Phosphorus exists primarily in inorganic combination with calcium in teeth and bones. In extracellular fluid, the phosphate ion supports several metabolic functions: utilization of B vitamins, acid-base homeostasis, bone formation, nerve and muscle activity, cell membrane integrity, transmission of hereditary traits, and metabolism of carbohydrates, proteins, and fats.

Renal tubular reabsorption of phosphate is inversely regulated by calcium levels — an increase in phosphorus causes a decrease in calcium. An imbalance causes hypophosphatemia or hyperphosphatemia. Incidence of hypophosphatemia varies with the underlying cause; hyperphosphatemia occurs most often in patients who tend to consume large amounts of phosphorus-rich foods and beverages and in those with renal insufficiency.

CAUSES
Hypophosphatemia
• Chronic diarrhea
• Deficiency of vitamin D
• Hyperparathyroidism with resultant hypercalcemia
• Hypomagnesemia
• Inadequate dietary intake, such as from malnutrition resulting from a prolonged catabolic state or chronic alcoholism
• Intestinal malabsorption

Hyperphosphatemia
• Hypervitaminosis D
• Hypocalcemia
• Hypoparathyroidism
• Overuse of phosphate enemas or laxatives with phosphates
• Renal failure

ASSESSMENT FINDINGS
Hypophosphatemia
• Anorexia
• Muscle weakness
• Osteomalacia (inadequate mineralization of bone)
• Paresthesia
• Peripheral hypoxia
• Tremor

Hyperphosphatemia
• Tetany and seizures (with hypocalcemia)
• Usually asymptomatic

DIAGNOSTIC TEST RESULTS
• Serum phosphorus level less than 1.7 mEq/L (or 2.5 mg/dl) confirms hypophosphatemia. A urine phosphorus level more than 1.3 g/ 24 hours supports this diagnosis.

• Serum phosphorus level exceeding 2.6 mEq/L (or 4.5 mg/dl) confirms hyperphosphatemia. Supportive values include decreased levels of serum calcium (less than 9 mg/dl) and urine phosphorus (less than 0.9 g/24 hours).

NURSING DIAGNOSES
• Altered nutrition: Less than or more than body requirements
• Risk for injury
• Knowledge deficit

TREATMENT
Hypophosphatemia
• Diet: high-phosphorus diet

Drug therapy
• Phosphate supplements
• Potassium phosphate I.V. (in severe deficiency)

Hyperphosphatemia
• Low-phosphorus diet
• Peritoneal dialysis or hemodialysis (in severe cases)

Drug therapy
• Calcium supplement: calcium acetate (PhosLo)

INTERVENTIONS AND RATIONALES
• Carefully monitor serum electrolyte, calcium, magnesium, and phosphorus levels. Report any changes immediately *to guide treatment plan.*

For patients with hypophosphatemia
• Record intake and output accurately. Administer potassium phosphate slow I.V. *to prevent overcorrection to hyperphosphatemia.* Assess renal function, and be alert for hypocalcemia when giving phosphate supplements. If phosphate salt tablets cause nausea, use capsules instead *to encourage compliance with treatment regimen.*
• Advise the patient to follow a high-phosphorus diet containing milk and milk products, kidney, liver, turkey, and dried fruits *to prevent recurrence.*

For patients with hyperphosphatemia
• Monitor intake and output. If urine output falls below 25 ml/hour or 600 ml/day, notify the doctor immediately *because decreased output can seriously affect renal clearance of excess serum phosphorus.*
• Watch for signs of hypocalcemia, such as muscle twitching and tetany, which often accompany hyperphosphatemia *to ensure timely intervention.*
• Advise the patient to eat foods with low phosphorus content, such as vegetables, *to prevent recurrence.* Obtain dietary consultation if the condition results from chronic renal insufficiency *to aid the patient in making sound nutritional choices that help prevent hyperphosphatemia.*

Teaching topics for hypophosphatemia
• High-phosphorus diet
• Taking phosphate supplements

Teaching topics for hyperphosphatemia
• Medication regimen and possible adverse reactions
• Avoiding OTC drugs that contain phosphorus, such as laxatives and enemas.

Polycythemia vera

Polycythemia vera is a chronic myeloproliferative disorder characterized by increased RBC mass, leukocytosis, thrombocytosis, and increased Hb concentration, with normal or increased plasma volume. It usually occurs between the ages of 40 and 60, most commonly among males of Jewish ancestry; it rarely affects children or blacks and doesn't appear to be familial. It may also be known as primary polycythemia, erythremia, polycythemia rubra vera, splenomegalic polycythemia, or Vaquez Osler disease.

The prognosis depends on age at diagnosis, the treatment used, and complications. Mortality is high if polycythemia is untreated or is associated with leukemia or myeloid metaplasia.

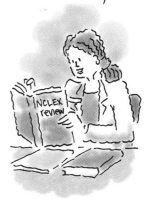

A myeloproliferative disorder, such as polycythemia vera, is characterized by proliferation of bone marrow constituents.

CAUSES
• Unknown (possibly due to a multipotential stem cell defect)

ASSESSMENT FINDINGS
• Clubbing of the digits
• Congestion of the conjunctiva, retina, and retinal veins
• Dizziness
• Dyspnea
• Feeling of fullness in the head
• Headache
• Hemorrhage
• Hypertension
• Ruddy cyanosis of the nose
• Thrombosis of smaller vessels
• Visual disturbances (blurring, diplopia, engorged veins of fundus and retina)
• Weight loss

DIAGNOSTIC TEST RESULTS
• Blood tests show increased RBC mass and normal arterial oxygen saturation in association with splenomegaly or two of the following: thrombocytosis, leukocytosis, elevated leukocyte alkaline phosphatase level, or elevated serum vitamin B_{12} or unbound B_{12} binding capacity.

NURSING DIAGNOSES
• Altered cardiovascular tissue perfusion
• Altered nutrition: Less than body requirements
• Sensory or perceptual alteration (visual)

TREATMENT
• Phlebotomy (typically, 350 to 500 ml of blood is removed every other day until the patient's HCT is reduced to the low-normal range)
• Plasmapheresis

Drug therapy
• Chemotherapy: busulfan (Myleran), chlorambucil (Leukeran), melphalan (Alkeran)
• Myelosuppressive drugs: hydroxyurea (Hydrea), radioactive phosphorus (^{32}P)
• Antigout agent: allopurinol (Zyloprim)

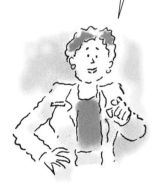

Phlebotomy is usually the first treatment for polycythemia vera. The patient may have 350 to 500 ml of blood removed every other day.

INTERVENTIONS AND RATIONALES
• Check blood pressure, pulse rate, and respirations prior to and during phlebotomy *to monitor patient's tolerance to the procedure.*
• During phlebotomy, make sure the patient is lying down comfortably *to prevent vertigo and syncope.*
• Stay alert for tachycardia, clamminess, or complaints of vertigo. If these effects occur, the procedure should be stopped. *These signs and symptoms indicate hypovolemia.*
• Immediately after phlebotomy, check blood pressure and pulse rate. Have the patient sit up for about 5 minutes before allowing him to walk *to prevent vasovagal attack or orthostatic hypotension.* Also, administer 24 oz (720 ml) of juice or water *to replace fluid volume lost during the procedure.*
• Tell the patient to watch for and report any symptoms of iron deficiency (pallor, weight loss, weakness, glossitis). *After repeated phlebotomies, the patient will develop iron deficiency, which stabilizes RBC production and reduces the need for phlebotomy.*
• Keep the patient active and ambulatory *to prevent thrombosis.* If bed rest is absolutely necessary, prescribe a daily program of both active and passive range-of-motion exercises *to prevent thrombosis and maintain joint mobility.*
• Watch for complications: hypervolemia, thrombocytosis, and signs of an impending cerebrovascular accident (decreased sensation, numbness, transitory paralysis, fleeting blindness, headache, and epistaxis) *to ensure early treatment intervention.*
• Regularly examine the patient closely for bleeding. Tell him which bleeding sites are most common (such as the nose, gingiva, and skin) so he can check for bleeding. Advise him to report any abnormal bleeding promptly. *These measures decrease the risk of hemorrhage.*
• Give additional fluids, administer allopurinol, and alkalinize the urine *to compensate for increased uric acid production and prevent uric acid calculi.*
• If the patient has symptomatic splenomegaly, suggest or provide small, frequent meals, followed by a rest period, *to prevent nausea and vomiting.*

• Report acute abdominal pain immediately *to avoid treatment delay.* Acute pain may signal splenic infarction, renal calculi, or abdominal organ thrombosis.

During myelosuppressive treatment:
• Monitor complete blood count (CBC) and platelet count before and during therapy. Warn an outpatient who develops leukopenia that his resistance to infection is low; advise him to avoid crowds and watch for the symptoms of infection. *These measures protect the patient from developing life-threatening infection.*
• If leukopenia develops in a hospitalized patient who needs reverse isolation, follow facility guidelines. If thrombocytopenia develops, tell the patient to watch for signs of bleeding (blood in urine, nosebleeds, black stools) *to prevent hemorrhage.*
• Tell the patient about possible adverse effects (nausea, vomiting, and risk of infection) of alkylating agents *to allay the patient's anxiety and ensure early treatment.*
• Watch for adverse reactions. If nausea and vomiting occur, begin antiemetic therapy and adjust the patient's diet *to promote patient comfort.*
• Take a blood sample for CBC and platelet count before beginning treatment with ^{32}P. Use of ^{32}P requires radiation precautions *to prevent contamination.*
• Have the patient lie down during I.V. administration *to facilitate the procedure and prevent extravasation* and for 15 to 20 minutes afterward *to monitor patient's tolerance to the procedure.*

Teaching topics
• Disease process and treatment options
• Importance of remaining as active as possible
• Avoiding infection
• Keeping the environment free of hazards that could cause falls
• Using safety razor to prevent bleeding
• Measures to prevent adverse reaction to treatment such as using antiemetics to prevent nausea and vomiting
• Available community resources

Rheumatoid arthritis

Believed to be an autoimmune disorder, rheumatoid arthritis is a systemic inflammatory disease that affects the synovial lining of the joints. Antibodies first attack the synovium of the joint, causing it to become inflamed and swollen. Eventually, the articular cartilage and surrounding tendons and ligaments are affected.

Inflammation of the synovial membranes is followed by formation of pannus (granulation tissue) and destruction of cartilage, bone, and ligaments. Pannus is replaced by fibrotic tissue and calcification, which causes subluxation of the joint. The joint becomes ankylosed — or fused — leaving a very painful joint and limited ROM.

CAUSES
• Autoimmune disease
• Genetic transmission

ASSESSMENT FINDINGS
• Anorexia and weight loss
• Dry eyes and mucous membranes
• Enlarged lymph nodes
• Fatigue
• Fever
• Leukopenia and anemia
• Limited range of motion
• Malaise
• Painful, swollen joints; crepitus; and morning stiffness
• Paresthesia of the hands and the feet
• Pericarditis
• Raynaud's phenomenon
• Splenomegaly
• Subcutaneous nodules
• Symmetrical joint swelling (mirror image of affected joints)

DIAGNOSTIC TEST RESULTS
• Antinuclear antibody (ANA) test is positive.
• Hematology shows increased ESR, WBC, platelets, and anemia.
• Rheumatoid factor test is positive.
• Serum protein electrophoresis shows elevated serum globulins.

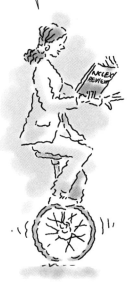

In rheumatoid arthritis, antibodies attack the synovial lining of the joints, the membrane that lines the joint space between the bones and allows bones to move against one another.

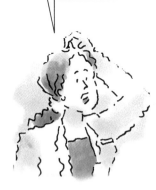

Cold therapy for acute episodes, heat therapy for chronic aches and pains.

• Synovial fluid analysis shows increased WBCs, increased volume and turbidity, but decreased viscosity and complement (C_3 and C_4 levels).
• X-rays reveal bone demineralization and soft-tissue swelling in early stages; in later stages, X-rays reveal a loss of cartilage, a narrowing of joint spaces, cartilage and bone destruction, and erosion, subluxations, and deformity.

NURSING DIAGNOSES
• Activity intolerance
• Body image disturbance
• Pain

TREATMENT
• Cold therapy during acute episodes
• Heat therapy to relax muscles and relieve pain for chronic disease
• Physical therapy (to forestall loss of joint function), passive ROM exercises, and observance of rest periods
• Weight control because obesity adds stress to joints
• Well-balanced diet

Drug therapy
• Analgesic: aspirin
• Antacids: magnesium hydroxide and aluminum hydroxide (Maalox), aluminum hydroxide (Amphogel)
• Antimetabolite: methotrexate (Rheumatrex)
• Antirheumatic: hydroxychloroquine (Plaquenil)
• Glucocorticoids: prednisone (Deltasone) and hydrocortisone (Hydrocortone)
• Gold therapy: gold sodium thiomalate (Myochrysine)
• Nonsteroidal anti-inflammatory drugs (NSAIDs): indomethacin (Indocin), ibuprofen (Advil, Motrin), sulindac (Clinoril), piroxicam (Feldene), flurbiprofen (Ansaid), diclofenac sodium (Voltaren), naproxen (Naprosyn), diflunisal (Dolobid)

INTERVENTIONS AND RATIONALES
• Monitor vital signs *to allow for early detection of complications.*
• Monitor neuromuscular status *to determine patient's capabilities.*

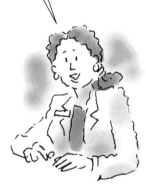

Help the patient understand that rheumatoid arthritis is a chronic disorder that requires major lifestyle changes.

• Check joints for swelling, pain, and redness *to determine the extent of disease and effectiveness of treatment.*
• Monitor laboratory studies *to detect remissions and exacerbations.*
• Administer medications as prescribed *to enhance the treatment regimen.* Administer medications such as misprostol (Cytotec) *to treat and prevent NSAID-induced gastric ulcers.*
• Provide passive ROM exercises *to prevent joint contractures and muscle atrophy.*
• Splint inflamed joints *to maintain joints in a functional position and prevent musculoskeletal deformities.*
• Provide warm or cold therapy as prescribed *to help alleviate pain.*
• Provide skin care *to prevent skin breakdown.*
• Minimize environmental stress and plan rest periods *to help the patient cope with the disease.*
• Encourage the patient to express his feelings about changes in his body image *to help the patient express doubts and resolve concerns.*

Teaching topics
• Ways to reduce stress
• The need for 8 to 10 hours of sleep every night
• Avoiding cold, stress, and infection
• Performing complete skin and foot care daily
• Contacting groups such as the Arthritis Foundation

Scleroderma

Scleroderma is a diffuse connective tissue disease characterized by inflammatory and then degenerative and fibrotic changes in skin, blood vessels, synovial membranes, skeletal muscles, and internal organs (especially the esophagus, intestinal tract, thyroid, heart, lungs, and kidneys). The disease, also known as progressive systemic sclerosis, affects more women than men, especially between ages 30 and 50.

CAUSES
• Unknown

ASSESSMENT FINDINGS
• Pain
• Signs and symptoms of Raynaud's phenomenon, such as blanching, cyanosis, and erythema of the fingers and toes in response to stress or exposure to cold
• Slowly healing ulcerations on the tips of the fingers or toes that may lead to gangrene
• Stiffness
• Swelling of fingers and joints
• Taut, shiny skin over the entire hand and forearm
• Tight and inelastic facial skin, causing a masklike appearance and "pinching" of the mouth
• Cardiac and pulmonary fibrosis (in advanced disease)
• Renal involvement is usually accompanied by malignant hypertension, the main cause of death

DIAGNOSTIC TEST RESULTS
• Blood studies show slightly elevated ESR, positive rheumatoid factor in 25% to 35% of patients, and positive antinuclear antibody test.
• Chest X-rays show bilateral basilar pulmonary fibrosis.
• ECG reveals possible nonspecific abnormalities related to myocardial fibrosis.
• GI X-rays show distal esophageal hypomotility and stricture, duodenal loop dilation, small-bowel malabsorption pattern, and large diverticula.
• Hand X-rays show terminal phalangeal tuft resorption, subcutaneous calcification, and joint space narrowing and erosion.
• Pulmonary function studies show decreased diffusion and vital capacity.
• Skin biopsy may show changes consistent with the progress of the disease, such as marked thickening of the dermis and occlusive vessel changes.
• Urinalysis reveals proteinuria, microscopic hematuria, and casts (with renal involvement).

NURSING DIAGNOSES
• Impaired physical mobility
• Pain
• Impaired skin integrity

TREATMENT
• Palliative measures: immunosuppressants such as cyclosporine (Sandimmune) or chlorambucil (Leukeran) and physical therapy to maintain function and promote muscle strength (currently, no cure exists for scleroderma)

INTERVENTIONS AND RATIONALES
• Assess motion restrictions, pain, vital signs, intake and output, respiratory function, and daily weight *to monitor disease progression and guide the treatment plan.*
• Teach the patient to monitor blood pressure at home and report any increases above baseline. *Malignant hypertension is the main cause of death in patients diagnosed with scleroderma.*
• Warn against finger-stick blood tests *because of compromised circulation.*
• Help the patient and family adjust to the patient's new body image and to the limitations and dependence that these changes cause. *Patients and their families need time to adjust to the overwhelming effects of illness.*
• Help the patient and family accept the fact that this condition is incurable. Encourage them to express their feelings, and help them cope with their fears and frustrations by offering information about the disease, its treatment, and relevant diagnostic tests. *Providing information helps alleviate anxiety and provides the patient with knowledge necessary for informed decision making.*
• Whenever possible, let the patient participate in treatment by measuring his own intake and output, planning his own diet, assisting in dialysis, giving himself heat therapy, and doing prescribed exercises *to help the patient gain a sense of control over his condition.*
• Involve the patient's family in treatment *to help the family overcome feelings of helplessness.*

Teaching topics
• Ways to recognize an impending relapse
• Methods to manage symptoms such as tension, nervousness, insomnia, decreased ability to concentrate, and apathy
• Avoiding air conditioning and tobacco use, which may aggravate Raynaud's phenomenon
• Avoiding fatigue by pacing activities and organizing schedules to include necessary rest

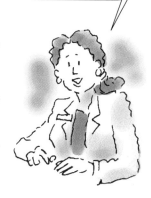

Fibrotic changes to the skin are usually the first clue to diagnosis in scleroderma.

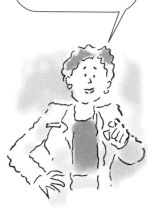

Treatment for scleroderma aims to preserve normal body functions and minimize complications.

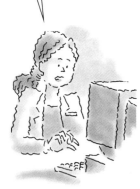

What a shock! Septic shock causes inadequate blood perfusion and circulatory collapse. Without prompt treatment, it may rapidly progress to death.

Hypotension, altered level of consciousness, and hyperventilation may be the only signs of septic shock among infants and elderly people.

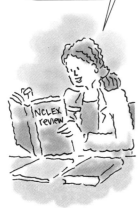

• Importance of complying with the medication regimen; reporting any adverse reactions instead of discontinuing the drug
• Follow-up visit for drug dosing if the patient takes a slow-release formulation

Septic shock

Septic shock is usually the result of bacterial infection. It causes inadequate blood perfusion and circulatory collapse.

Septic shock occurs most often among hospitalized patients, especially men over age 40 and women ages 25 to 45. It is second only to cardiogenic shock as the leading cause of shock death. About 25% of patients who develop gram-negative bacteremia go into shock. Unless vigorous treatment begins promptly, preferably before symptoms fully develop, septic shock rapidly progresses to death (often within a few hours) in up to 80% of these patients.

CAUSES
• Infection with gram-negative bacteria (in two-thirds of patients): *Escherichia coli, Klebsiella, Enterobacter, Proteus, Pseudomonas,* and *Bacteroides*
• Infection from gram-positive bacteria: *Streptococcus pneumoniae, S. pyogenes,* and *Actinomyces*

ASSESSMENT FINDINGS
Indications of septic shock vary according to the stage of the shock, the organism causing it, and the age of the patient.

Early stage
• Chills
• Diarrhea
• Nausea
• Oliguria
• Prostration
• Sudden fever (over 101° F [38.3° C])
• Vomiting

Late stage
• Altered level of consciousness
• Anuria
• Apprehension

• Hyperventilation
• Hypotension
• Hypothermia
• Irritability
• Restlessness
• Tachycardia
• Tachypnea
• Thirst from decreased cerebral tissue perfusion

DIAGNOSTIC TEST RESULTS
• ABG analysis indicates respiratory alkalosis (low partial pressure of carbon dioxide [Pco_2], low or normal bicarbonate [HCO_3^-] level, and high pH).
• Blood cultures isolate the organism.
• Blood tests show decreased platelet count and leukocytosis (15,000 to 30,000/µl), increased BUN and creatinine levels, decreased creatinine clearance, and abnormal PT and PTT.
• ECG shows ST-segment depression, inverted T waves, and arrhythmias resembling myocardial infarction.

NURSING DIAGNOSES
• Decreased cardiac output
• Fluid volume deficit
• Risk for injury

TREATMENT
• Removing and replacing any I.V., intra-arterial, or urinary drainage catheters that may be the source of infection
• Oxygen therapy (may require endotracheal intubation and mechanical ventilation)
• Colloid or crystalloid infusion to increase intravascular volume
• Diuretics such as furosemide (Lasix) after sufficient fluid volume has been replaced to maintain urine output above 20 ml/hour.
• Blood transfusion, if anemia is present
• Surgery to drain abscesses, if present

Drug therapy
• Antibiotics: according to sensitivity of causative organism
• Vasopressor: dopamine (Intropin) if fluid resuscitation fails to increase blood pressure

INTERVENTIONS AND RATIONALES

• Remove any I.V., intra-arterial, or urinary drainage catheters and send them to the laboratory *to culture the causative organism.* New catheters can be reinserted *to provide access for fluid resuscitation and to ensure accurate measurement of urine output.*

• Start an I.V. infusion with normal saline solution or lactated Ringer's solution, usually a large-bore (14G to 18G) catheter *to allow easier infusion.*

• When the patient's blood pressure drops below 80 mm Hg, increase oxygen flow rate and call the doctor immediately. *A progressive drop in blood pressure accompanied by a thready pulse generally signifies inadequate cardiac output from reduced vascular volume.*

• Carefully maintain the pulmonary artery catheter *to monitor fluid volume status and cardiac output.* Check ABG values for adequate oxygenation or gas exchange, watching for any changes *to prevent hypoxemia.*

• Keep accurate intake and output records. Maintain adequate urine output (0.5 to 1 ml/kg/hour) and systolic pressure *to prevent kidney damage and fluid overload.*

• Administer antibiotics I.V. *to achieve effective blood levels quickly* and monitor drug levels *to prevent toxicity.*

• Watch closely for complications of septic shock: DIC (abnormal bleeding), renal failure (oliguria, increased specific gravity), heart failure (dyspnea, edema, tachycardia, distended neck veins), GI ulcers (hematemesis, melena), and hepatic abnormalities (jaundice, hypoprothrombinemia, and hypoalbuminemia) *to prevent crisis.*

Teaching topics
• Risk associated with blood transfusion
• Disease process and treatment options

Sickle cell anemia

Sickle cell anemia is a congenital hematologic disease that causes impaired circulation, chronic ill health, and premature death. Although it's most common in tropical Africa and in people of African descent, it also occurs in people from Puerto Rico, Turkey, India, the Middle East, and the Mediterranean.

In patients with sickle cell anemia, a change in the gene that encodes the beta chain of Hb results in a defect in HbS. When hypoxia (oxygen deficiency) occurs, the HbS in the RBCs becomes insoluble. The cells become rigid and rough, forming an elongated sickle shape and impairing circulation. Infection, stress, dehydration, and conditions that provoke hypoxia — strenuous exercise, high altitude, unpressurized aircraft, cold, and vasoconstrictive drugs — may all provoke periodic crisis. Crises can occur in different forms, including painful crisis, aplastic crisis, and acute sequestration crisis.

CAUSES
• Genetic inheritance: The disease results from homozygous inheritance of an autosomal recessive gene that produces a defective Hb molecule (HbS). Heterozygous inheritance results in sickle cell trait; people with this trait are carriers who can then pass the gene to their offspring.

ASSESSMENT FINDINGS
• Aching bones
• Chronic fatigue
• Family history of the disease
• Frequent infections
• Jaundice, pallor
• Joint swelling
• Leg ulcers (especially on ankles)
• Severe localized and generalized pain
• Tachycardia
• Unexplained dyspnea or dyspnea on exertion
• Unexplained, painful erections (priapism)

Sickle cell crisis (general symptoms)
• Hematuria
• Irritability
• Lethargy
• Pale lips, tongue, palms, and nail beds
• Severe pain

Painful crisis (vaso-occlusive crisis, which appears periodically after age 5)
• Dark urine
• Low-grade fever

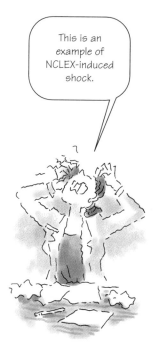

This is an example of NCLEX-induced shock.

• Severe abdominal, thoracic, muscle, or bone pain
• Tissue anoxia and necrosis, caused by blood vessel obstruction by tangled sickle cells
• Worsening of jaundice

Aplastic crisis (generally associated with viral infection)
• Dyspnea
• Lethargy, sleepiness
• Markedly decreased bone marrow activity
• Pallor
• Possible coma
• RBC hemolysis (destruction)

Acute sequestration crisis (rare; occurs in infants ages 8 months to 2 years)
• Hypovolemic shock caused by entrapment of RBCs in spleen and liver
• Lethargy
• Liver congestion and enlargement
• Pallor
• Worsened chronic jaundice

DIAGNOSTIC TEST RESULTS
• Blood tests show low RBC counts, elevated WBC and platelet counts, decreased ESR, increased serum iron levels, decreased RBC survival, and reticulocytosis.
• Hb electrophoresis shows HbS.
• Hb levels may be low or normal.
• Stained blood smear shows sickle cells.

NURSING DIAGNOSES
• Impaired gas exchange
• Pain
• Altered tissue perfusion (peripheral, renal)

TREATMENT
• Application of warm compresses for pain relief
• Blood transfusion therapy if Hb levels drop

• Iron and folic acid supplements to prevent anemia
• I.V. fluid therapy to prevent dehydration and vessel occlusion

Drug therapy
• Analgesics: meperidine (Demerol) or morphine (to relieve pain from vaso-occlusive crises)

INTERVENTIONS AND RATIONALES
• Provide emotional support *to allay the patient's anxiety.*
• Refer for genetic counseling *to decrease anxiety and help the patient to understand the chances of passing the disease to offspring.*
• Refer patient and family to community support groups *to help the patient and his family cope with his illness.*

During a crisis
• Apply warm compresses to painful areas and cover patient with a blanket. *Cold compresses and temperature can aggravate condition.*
• Administer an analgesic-antipyretic such as aspirin or acetaminophen *for pain relief.* (Additional pain relief may be necessary during an acute crisis.)
• Maintain bed rest *to reduce workload on the heart and to reduce pain.*
• Administer blood components (packed RBCs), as ordered, *for aplastic crisis caused by bone marrow suppression.*
• Administer oxygen *to enhance oxygenation and reduce sickling.*
• Encourage fluid intake *to prevent dehydration, which can precipitate a crisis.*
• Administer prescribed I.V. fluids *to ensure fluid balance and renal perfusion.*
• Give antibiotics as ordered *to treat infections and avoid precipitating a crisis.*

Teaching topics
• How to avoid restricting circulation
• Importance of normal childhood immunizations
• Importance of prompt treatment for infections
• Maintaining increased fluid intake to prevent dehydration
• How to prevent hypoxia

In the autosomal recessive inheritance pattern, if two carriers have offspring, each child has a one-in-four chance of developing the disease.

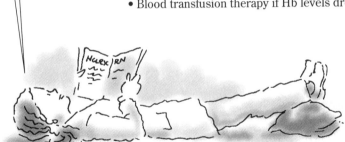

Sodium imbalance

Sodium is the major cation (positively charged ion) in extracellular fluid. Its functions include maintaining tonicity and concentration of extracellular fluid, acid-base balance (reabsorption of sodium ions and excretion of hydrogen ions), nerve conduction and neuromuscular function, glandular secretion, and water balance.

A sodium-potassium pump is constantly at work in every body cell. Potassium is the major cation in intracellular fluid. According to the laws of diffusion, a substance moves from an area of high concentration to an area of lower concentration. Sodium ions, normally most abundant outside the cells, want to diffuse inward. Potassium ions, normally outside the cells, want to diffuse outward. The sodium-potassium pump works to combat this ionic diffusion and maintain normal sodium-potassium balance.

During repolarization, the sodium-potassium pump continually shifts sodium into the cells and potassium out of the cells; during depolarization, it does the reverse.

The body requires only 2 to 4 g of sodium daily. However, most Americans consume 6 to 10 g daily (mostly sodium chloride, as table salt), excreting excess sodium through the kidneys and skin.

A low-sodium diet or excessive use of diuretics may induce hyponatremia (decreased serum sodium concentration); dehydration may induce hypernatremia (increased serum sodium concentration).

CAUSES
Hyponatremia
- Diarrhea
- Excessive perspiration or fever
- Excessive water intake
- Low-sodium diet
- Malnutrition
- Potent diuretics
- Starvation
- Suctioning
- Trauma, wound drainage, or burns
- Vomiting

Hypernatremia
- Decreased water intake
- Diabetes insipidus
- Excess adrenocortical hormones, as in Cushing's syndrome
- Severe vomiting and diarrhea with water loss that exceeds sodium loss

ASSESSMENT FINDINGS
Hyponatremia
- Abdominal cramps
- Anxiety
- Cold, clammy skin
- Cyanosis
- Headaches
- Hypotension
- Muscle twitching and weakness
- Nausea and vomiting
- Oliguria or anuria
- Renal dysfunction
- Seizures
- Tachycardia

Hypernatremia
- Agitation and restlessness
- Circulatory disorders
- Decreased level of consciousness
- Dry, sticky mucous membranes
- Dyspnea
- Excessive weight gain
- Fever
- Flushed skin
- Hypertension
- Intense thirst
- Oliguria
- Pitting edema
- Pulmonary edema
- Rough, dry tongue
- Seizures
- Tachycardia

DIAGNOSTIC TEST RESULTS
- Serum sodium level less than 135 mEq/L indicates hyponatremia.
- Serum sodium level greater than 145 mEq/L indicates hypernatremia.

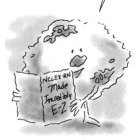

Pass the salt. The body needs sodium to maintain proper extracellular fluid osmolality, the proper concentration of fluid outside cells.

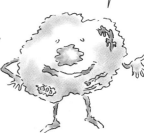

Pump it up. A sodium-potassium pump is constantly at work in every body cell to maintain normal sodium-potassium balance.

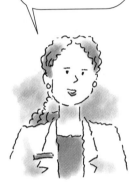

Too little sodium can cause kidney dysfunction and, in severe cases, seizures. Too much sodium can produce fluid in the lungs, circulatory disorders, and decreased level of consciousness.

NURSING DIAGNOSES
Hyponatremia
- Fluid volume deficit
- Risk for injury

Hypernatremia
- Fluid volume excess
- Altered thought processes

TREATMENT
Hyponatremia
- Antibiotic: demeclocycline (Declomycin)
- I.V. infusion of saline solution
- Potassium supplements: Potassium chloride (K-Lor)

Hypernatremia
- Diet: sodium restrictions
- Salt-free solution (such as dextrose in water), followed by infusion of 0.45% sodium chloride to prevent hyponatremia

INTERVENTIONS AND RATIONALES
For hyponatremia
- Watch for extremely low serum sodium and accompanying serum chloride levels. Monitor urine specific gravity and other laboratory results. Record fluid intake and output accurately, and weigh the patient daily *to guide the treatment plan.*
- During administration of isosmolar or hyperosmolar saline solution, watch closely for signs of hypervolemia (dyspnea, crackles, engorged neck or hand veins) *to prevent respiratory distress.*
- Note conditions that may cause excessive sodium loss — diaphoresis, prolonged diarrhea or vomiting, or severe burns *to prevent hyponatremia.*
- Refer the patient receiving a maintenance dosage of diuretics to a dietitian for instruction about dietary sodium intake *to increase dietary intake of sodium and decrease the risk for hyponatremia.*

For hypernatremia
- Measure serum sodium levels every 6 hours or at least daily. Monitor vital signs for changes, especially for rising pulse rate. Watch for signs of hypervolemia, especially in

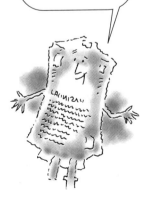

Don't overdo it. During administration of isosmolar or hyperosmolar saline solution to a patient with hyponatremia, watch closely for signs of hypervolemia.

the patient receiving I.V. fluids, *to guide the treatment regimen.*
- Record fluid intake and output accurately, checking for body fluid loss *to prevent dehydration and accompanying hypernatremia.* Weigh the patient daily *to monitor fluid volume status.*
- Obtain a drug history *to check for drugs that promote sodium retention.*

Teaching topics for hyponatremia
- Rationale for fluid restriction, if necessary
- Increasing dietary intake of sodium
- Medication regimen and possible adverse reactions

Teaching topics for hypernatremia
- Importance of sodium restriction and how to plan a low-sodium diet

Systemic lupus erythematosus

Systemic lupus erythematosus (SLE) is an autoimmune disorder that involves most organ systems. It is chronic in nature and characterized by periods of exacerbation and remission.

In SLE, there is a depression of T-cell activity and an increase in the production of antibodies, specifically antibodies to DNA and ribonucleic acid and anti-erythrocyte, antinuclear, and antiplatelet antibodies. The immune response results in an inflammatory process involving the veins and arteries (vasculitis), which causes pain, swelling, and tissue damage in any area of the body.

CAUSES
- Autoimmune disease
- Drug-induced: procainamide (Pronestyl), hydralazine (Apresoline), and phenytoin (Dilantin)
- Genetic
- Unknown
- Viral

ASSESSMENT FINDINGS
- Alopecia
- Anorexia and weight loss
- Anemia, leukopenia, and thrombocytopenia
- Butterfly rash on face (rash may vary in severity from malar erythema to discoid lesions)
- Erythema on palms
- Fatigue
- Glomerulonephritis, renal dysfunction and failure (renal involvement)
- Impaired cognitive function, psychosis, depression, seizures, peripheral neuropathies, cerebrovascular accidents, and organic brain syndrome (central nervous system involvement)
- Low-grade fever
- Lymphadenopathy, splenomegaly, and hepatomegaly
- Migratory pain, stiffness, and joint swelling
- Oral and nasopharyngeal ulcerations
- Photosensitivity
- Pleurisy, pericarditis, myocarditis, noninfectious endocarditis, and hypertension (cardiac involvement)
- Raynaud's phenomenon

DIAGNOSTIC TEST RESULTS
- ANA test is positive.
- Blood chemistry shows decreased complement fixation.
- Hematology shows decreased Hb, HCT, WBC, and platelets and an increased ESR.
- Lupus erythematosus cell preparation is positive.
- Rheumatoid factor is positive.
- Urine chemistry shows proteinuria and hematuria.

NURSING DIAGNOSES
- Impaired mobility
- Ineffective breathing pattern
- Risk for infection

TREATMENT
- Diet high in iron, protein, and vitamins (especially vitamin C)
- Hemodialysis or kidney transplant if renal failure occurs
- Limited exertion and maintenance of adequate rest
- Plasmapheresis

Drug therapy
- Analgesic: aspirin
- Antianemics: ferrous sulfate (Feosol), ferrous gluconate (Fergon)
- Antirheumatic: hydroxychloroquine (Plaquenil)
- Cytotoxic drugs: azathioprine (Imuran), methotrexate (Folex); these drugs may delay or prevent deteriorating renal status
- Glucocorticoid: prednisone (Deltasone)
- Immunosuppressants: azathioprine (Imuran), cyclophosphamide (Cytoxan)
- NSAIDs: indomethacin (Indocin), ibuprofen (Motrin), sulindac (Clinoril), piroxicam (Feldene), flurbiprofen (Ansaid), diclofenac sodium (Voltaren), naproxen (Naprosyn), diflunisal (Dolobid)

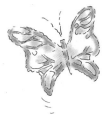

INTERVENTIONS AND RATIONALES
- Assess musculoskeletal status *to determine the patient's baseline functional abilities.*
- Monitor renal status. *Decreased urine output without lowered fluid intake may indicate decreased renal perfusion, a possible indication of decreased cardiac output.*
- Monitor vital signs *to promptly determine if the patient's condition is deteriorating and evaluate the effectiveness of treatment.* Fever can signal an exacerbation.
- Provide prophylactic skin, mouth, and perineal care *to prevent skin and oral mucous membrane breakdown.*
- Administer medications as prescribed *to enhance the treatment regimen.*
- Maintain seizure precautions *to prevent patient injury.*
- Monitor dietary intake *to help ensure adequate nutritional intake.*
- Minimize environmental stress and provide rest periods *to avoid fatigue and help the patient to cope with illness.*
- Promote independence in ADLs *to help the patient develop self-esteem.*
- Administer antiemetics *to alleviate nausea and vomiting.*
- Administer antidiarrheals, as prescribed, *to alleviate diarrhea.*

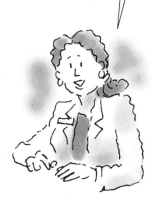

SLE can affect many different organs, but note that a butterfly rash is the signature finding.

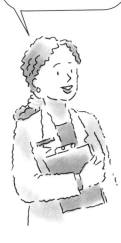

One name, many disorders. Vasculitis refers to a variety of disorders characterized by inflammation and necrosis of blood vessels.

• Encourage the patient to express feelings about changes in his body image and the chronic nature of the disease *to help the patient ventilate doubts and resolve concerns.*

Teaching topics
• Smoking cessation (if appropriate)
• Ways to reduce stress
• Recognizing early signs and symptoms of renal failure
• Avoiding exposure to people with infections
• Monitoring for infection, fatigue, and joint pain
• Performing daily, complete mouth care
• Avoiding OTC medications
• Avoiding exposure to sunlight
• Avoiding hair spray or hair coloring
• Avoiding oral contraceptives
• Using liquid cosmetics to cover rashes
• Contacting groups such as the Lupus Foundation of America

Vasculitis

Vasculitis is a broad spectrum of disorders characterized by inflammation and necrosis of blood vessels. Its clinical effects depend on the vessels involved and reflect tissue ischemia caused by blood flow obstruction.

Prognosis is also variable. For example, hypersensitivity vasculitis is usually a benign disorder limited to the skin, but more extensive polyarteritis nodosa can be rapidly fatal.

Vasculitis can occur at any age, except for mucocutaneous lymph node syndrome, which occurs only during childhood. Vasculitis may be a primary disorder or secondary to other disorders, such as rheumatoid arthritis or SLE.

CAUSES
• Excessive levels of antigen
• High-dose antibiotic therapy
• Often associated with serious infectious disease such as hepatitis B or bacterial endocarditis

ASSESSMENT FINDINGS
A few examples of vasculitis and their specific assessment findings are listed below.

Wegener's granulomatosis
This form of vasculitis affects medium- to large-sized vessels of the upper and lower respiratory tract and kidney; may also involve small arteries and veins. Assessment findings include:
• anorexia
• cough
• fever
• malaise
• mild to severe hematuria
• pulmonary congestion
• weight loss.

Temporal arteritis
This type of vasculitis affects medium- to large-sized arteries, most commonly branches of the carotid artery; involvement may skip segments. Assessment findings include:
• fever
• headache (associated with polymyalgia rheumatica syndrome)
• jaw claudication
• myalgia
• visual changes.

Takayasu's arteritis
Also known as aortic arch syndrome, Takayasu's arteritis affects medium- to large-sized arteries, particularly the aortic arch and its branches and, possibly, the pulmonary artery. Assessment findings include:
• anorexia
• arthralgias
• bruits
• cerebrovascular accident (with disease progression)
• diplopia and transient blindness if carotid artery is involved
• heart failure (with disease progression)
• loss of distal pulses
• malaise
• nausea
• night sweats
• pain or paresthesia distal to affected area
• pallor
• syncope
• weight loss.

DIAGNOSTIC TEST RESULTS
Wegener's granulomatosis
• Tissue biopsy shows necrotizing vasculitis with granulomatous inflammation.

• Blood studies show leukocytosis, elevated ESR, IgA, and IgG; low titer rheumatoid factor; circulating immune complexes: antineutrophil cytoplasmic antibody in more than 90% of patients.
• Renal biopsy shows focal segmental glomerulonephritis.

Temporal arteritis
• Blood studies show decreased Hb; elevated ESR
• Tissue biopsy shows panarteritis with infiltration of mononuclear cells, giant cells within vessel wall (seen in 50%), fragmentation of internal elastic lamina, and proliferation of intima.

Takayasu's arteritis
• Blood studies show decreased Hb, leukocytosis, positive lupus erythematosus cell preparation, and elevated ESR.
• Arteriography shows calcification and obstruction of affected vessels.
• Tissue biopsy shows inflammation of adventitia and intima of vessels and thickening of vessel walls.

NURSING DIAGNOSES
• Altered peripheral tissue perfusion
• Risk for injury
• Sensory or perceptual alterations (tactile)

TREATMENT
• Removal of identified environmental antigen
• Diet: elimination of antigenic food, if identifiable

Drug therapy
• Corticosteroid: prednisone (Deltasone)
• Antineoplastic: Cyclophosphamide (Cytoxan)

INTERVENTIONS AND RATIONALES
• Assess for dry nasal mucosa in patients with Wegener's granulomatosis. Instill nose drops *to lubricate the mucosa and help diminish crusting.* Or irrigate the nasal passages with warm normal saline solution *to combat drying.*
• Regulate environmental temperature *to prevent additional vasoconstriction caused by cold.*
• Monitor vital signs. Use a Doppler ultrasonic flowmeter, if available, *to auscultate blood*

pressure in patients with Takayasu's arteritis, whose peripheral pulses are frequently difficult to palpate.
• Monitor intake and output. Check daily for edema. Keep the patient well-hydrated (3 L daily) *to reduce the risk of hemorrhagic cystitis associated with cyclophosphamide therapy.*
• Provide emotional support to help the patient and his family cope with an altered body image — the result of the disorder or its therapy. (For example, Wegener's granulomatosis may be associated with saddle nose, steroids may cause weight gain, and cyclophosphamide may cause alopecia.)
• Monitor the patient's WBC count during cyclophosphamide therapy *to prevent severe leukopenia.*

Teaching topics
• Recognizing adverse reactions to medication
• Importance of increasing fluids during cyclophosphamide therapy

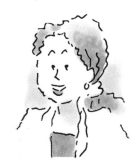

Treatment for vasculitis aims to minimize tissue damage associated with decreased blood flow.

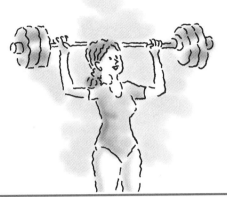

Pump up on practice questions

1. A client with major abdominal trauma needs an emergency blood transfusion. The client's blood type is AB negative. Of the blood types available, the safest type for the nurse to administer is:

A. AB positive.
B. A positive.
C. B negative.
D. O positive.

Answer: C. Individuals with AB negative blood (AB type, Rh negative) can receive A negative, B negative, and AB negative blood. It's unsafe to give Rh-positive blood to an Rh-negative person.

➡ *NCLEX keys*

Nursing process step: Implementation
Client needs category: Physiological integrity
Client needs subcategory: Pharmacological and parenteral therapies
Taxonomic level: Application

2. The nurse is preparing a client with systemic lupus erythematosus for discharge. Which instructions should the nurse include in the teaching plan?

A. Exposure to sunlight will help control skin rashes.
B. There are no activity limitations between flare-ups.
C. Monitor body temperature.
D. Corticosteroids may be stopped when symptoms are relieved.

Answer: C. The client should monitor his temperature, because fever can signal an exacerbation and should be reported to the physician. Sunlight and other sources of ultraviolet light may precipitate severe skin reactions and exacerbate the disease. Fatigue can cause a flare-up of systemic lupus erythematosus, and clients should be encouraged to pace activities and plan for rest periods. Corticosteroids must be gradually tapered because they can suppress the function of the adrenal gland. Abruptly stopping corticosteroids can cause adrenal insufficiency, a potentially life-threatening situation.

➡ *NCLEX keys*

Nursing process step: Planning
Client needs category: Physiological integrity
Client needs subcategory: Reduction of risk potential
Taxonomic level: Application

3. A client with rheumatoid arthritis has a history of long-term nonsteroidal anti-inflammatory drug (NSAID) use and has developed peptic ulcer disease. To prevent and treat this adverse effect, the nurse wound administer:

A. cyanocobalamin (vitamin B_{12}).
B. ticlopidine (Ticlid).
C. prednisone (Deltasone).
D. misoprostol (Cytotec).

Answer: D. NSAIDs decrease prostaglandin synthesis. Misoprostol (Cytotec), a synthetic analog of prostaglandin, is used to treat and prevent NSAID-induced gastric ulcers. Cyanocobalamin is used to treat vitamin B_{12} deficiency. Ticlopidine is an antiplatelet agent used to reduce the risk of stroke. Prednisone is a glucocorticoid used to treat several inflammatory disorders and may promote gastric ulcer development.

➡ *NCLEX keys*

Nursing process step: Implementation
Client needs category: Physiological integrity
Client needs subcategory: Pharmacological and parenteral therapies
Taxonomic level: Comprehension

4. A client with thrombocytopenia, secondary to leukemia, develops epistaxis. The nurse should instruct the client to:

    A. lie supine with his neck extended.

    B. sit upright, leaning slightly forward.

    C. blow his nose and then put lateral pressure on his nose.

    D. hold his nose while bending forward at the waist.

Answer: B. The upright position, leaning slightly forward, avoids increasing the vascular pressure in the nose and helps the client avoid aspirating blood. Lying supine won't prevent aspiration of the blood. Nose blowing can dislodge any clotting that has occurred. Bending at the waist increases vascular pressure in the nose and promotes bleeding rather than halting it.

➡ *NCLEX keys*

Nursing process step: Implementation
Client needs category: Physiological integrity
Client needs subcategory: Physiological adaptation
Taxonomic level: Application

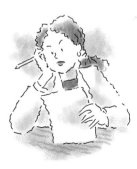

5. A client with leukemia is scheduled to get chemotherapy, including vincristine. To prevent extravasation of the drug into peripheral tissue, the nurse should avoid placing the I.V. access device in the:

    A. antebrachial vein.

    B. cephalic vein.

    C. antecubital vein.

    D. basilic vein.

Answer: C. The antecubital vein is positioned at the bend of the arm. Arm flexion could dislodge the I.V. access device, causing an extravasation. The veins of the forearm, including the cephalic, basilic, and antebrachial, are the preferred sites.

➡ *NCLEX keys*

Nursing process step: Planning
Client needs category: Physiological integrity
Client needs subcategory: Pharmacological and parenteral therapies
Taxonomic level: Comprehension

6. The nurse is reviewing the laboratory report of a client who underwent a bone marrow biopsy. The finding that would most strongly support a diagnosis of acute leukemia is the existence of a large number of immature:

    A. lymphocytes.

    B. thrombocytes.

    C. reticulocytes.

    D. leukocytes.

Answer: D. Leukemia is manifested by an abnormal overproduction of immature leukocytes in the bone marrow.

➡ *NCLEX keys*

Nursing process step: Analysis
Client needs category: Physiological integrity
Client needs subcategory: Reduction of risk potential
Taxonomic level: Comprehension

7. The nurse is reviewing assessment data for a client diagnosed with stage III lymphoma. This diagnosis is most strongly supported by lymphatic involvement in both sides of the:

    A. blood-brain barrier.

    B. diaphragm.

    C. descending aorta.

    D. spinal column.

Answer: B. In stage III lymphoma, there are malignant cells widely disseminated to lymph nodes on both sides of the diaphragm.

➡ *NCLEX keys*

Nursing process step: Analysis
Client needs category: Physiological integrity
Client needs subcategory: Physiological adaptation
Taxonomic level: Comprehension

8. The nurse is providing care for a client with acquired immunodeficiency syndrome (AIDS) and *Pneumocystis carinii* pneumonia. The client is receiving aerosolized pentamidine isethionate (NebuPent). What is the best evidence that the therapy is succeeding?

A. A sudden gain in lost body weight
B. Whitening of lung fields on the chest X-ray
C. Improving client vitality and activity tolerance
D. Afebrile body temperature and development of leukocytosis

Answer: C. *Pneumocystis carinii* pneumonia is a protozoal infection of the lungs. Pentamidine isethionate is one of the agents used to treat this infection. Because a common manifestation of the infection is activity intolerance and loss of vitality, improvements in these areas would suggest success of the therapy. Sudden weight gain, whitening of the lung fields on chest X-ray, and development of leukocytosis aren't evidence of therapeutic success.

➡ NCLEX keys
Nursing process step: Evaluation
Client needs category: Physiological integrity
Client needs subcategory: Pharmacological and parenteral therapies
Taxonomic level: Application

9. The nurse is documenting her care for a client with iron deficiency anemia. Which of the following nursing diagnoses is most appropriate?

A. Impaired gas exchange
B. Fluid volume deficit
C. Ineffective airway clearance
D. Impaired breathing pattern

Answer: A. Iron is necessary for hemoglobin synthesis. Hemoglobin is responsible for oxygen transport in the body. Iron deficiency anemia causes subnormal hemoglobin levels, which impair tissue oxygenation and bring about a nursing diagnosis of impaired gas exchange. Iron deficiency anemia doesn't cause fluid volume deficit and is less directly related to ineffective airway clearance and impaired breathing pattern than it is to ineffective gas exchange.

➡ NCLEX keys
Nursing process step: Analysis
Client needs category: Physiological integrity
Client needs subcategory: Physiological adaptation
Taxonomic level: Comprehension

10. The nurse is administering cyanocobalamin (vitamin B_{12}) to a client with pernicious anemia, secondary to gastrectomy. Which route should the nurse use to most effectively administer the vitamin?

A. Topical route
B. Transdermal route
C. Enteral route
D. Parenteral route

Answer: D. Following a gastrectomy, the client no longer has the intrinsic factor available to promote vitamin B_{12} absorption in his GI tract. Vitamin B_{12} is administered parenterally (I.M. or deep subcutaneous). Topical and transdermal administrations aren't available, and the enteral route is inappropriate in a gastrectomy.

➡ NCLEX keys
Nursing process step: Implementation
Client needs category: Physiological integrity
Client needs subcategory: Pharmacological and parenteral therapies
Taxonomic level: Application

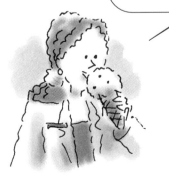

Now it's time to reward yourself. Remember, it's an important part of an effective study program.

6 Neurosensory System

Brush up on key concepts

In this chapter, you'll review:

✐ components of the neurosensory system and their function

✐ tests used to diagnose neurosensory disorders

✐ common neurosensory disorders.

The neurosensory system serves as the body's communication network. It processes information from the outside world (through the sensory portion) and coordinates and organizes the functions of all other body systems. Major parts of the neurosensory system include the brain, the spinal cord, the peripheral nerves, the eyes, and the ears.

At any time, you can review the major points of the disorders in this chapter by consulting the *Cheat sheet* on pages 170 to 177.

The little conductor that could

The **neuron,** or nerve cell, is the basic functional unit of the neurosensory system. This highly specialized conductor cell receives and transmits electrochemical nerve impulses. From its cell body, delicate, threadlike nerve fibers called axons and dendrites extend and transmit signals. Axons carry impulses away from the cell body; dendrites carry impulses toward the cell body.

A covering called a myelin sheath protects the entire neuron. Substances known as neurotransmitters (acetylcholine, serotonin, dopamine, endorphins, gamma-aminobutyric acid, and norepinephrine) help conduct impulses across a synapse and into the next neuron.

House of intelligence

The **central nervous system (CNS)** includes the brain and spinal cord. These fragile structures are protected by the skull and vertebrae, cerebrospinal fluid (CSF), and three membranes: the dura mater, the pia mater, and the arachnoid membrane.

The **cerebrum,** the largest part of the brain, houses the nerve center that controls motor and sensory functions and intelligence. It's divided into hemispheres. Because motor impulses descending from the brain cross in the medulla, the right hemisphere controls the left side of the body and the left hemisphere controls the right side of the body. Several fissures divide the cerebrum into four lobes:

• frontal lobe — the site of personality; memory, reasoning, concentration, and motor control of speech

• parietal lobe — the site of sensation, integration of sensory information, and spatial relationships

• temporal lobe — the site of hearing, speech, memory, and emotion

• occipital lobe — the site of vision and involuntary eye movements.

Brain networking

The **thalamus** is a structure located deep within the brain that consists of two oval-shaped parts, one located in each hemisphere. The thalamus is referred to as the relay station of the brain because it receives input from all of the senses except olfaction (smell), analyzes that input, and then transmits that information to other parts of the brain.

The **hypothalamus,** located beneath the thalamus, controls sleep and wakefulness, temperature, respiration, blood pressure, sexual arousal, fluid balance, and emotional response.

Movement, balance, and posture

The **cerebellum,** at the base of the brain, coordinates muscle movements, maintains balance, and controls posture.

Conjunction junction

The **brain stem** provides the connection between the spinal cord and the brain. It contains three sections:

(Text continues on page 177.)

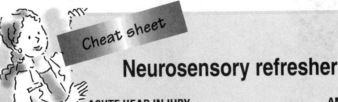

Neurosensory refresher

ACUTE HEAD INJURY

Key signs and symptoms
- Disorientation to time, place, or person
- Unequal pupil size, loss of pupillary reaction (if edema is present)

Key test results
- Computed tomography (CT) scan shows hemorrhage, cerebral edema, or shift of midline structures.
- Magnetic resonance imaging (MRI) shows hemorrhage, cerebral edema, or shift of midline structures.

Key treatments
- Cervical collar (until neck injury is ruled out)
- Anticonvulsant: phenytoin (Dilantin)
- Barbiturate: pentobarbital (Nembutal), if unable to control intracranial pressure (ICP) with diuresis
- Diuretics: mannitol (Osmitrol), furosemide (Lasix) to combat cerebral edema
- Dopamine (Intropin) to maintain cerebral perfusion pressure above 50 mm Hg (if blood pressure is low and ICP is elevated)
- Glucocorticoid: dexamethasone (Decadron) to reduce cerebral edema
- Histamine$_2$ (H$_2$)-receptor antagonists: ranitidine (Zantac), famotidine (Pepcid), nizatidine (Axid)
- Mucosal barrier fortifier: sucralfate (Carafate)
- Posterior pituitary hormone: vasopressin (Pitressin) if patient develops diabetes insipidus

Key interventions
- Assess neurologic and respiratory status.
- Observe for signs of increasing ICP (greater than 20 mm Hg for more than 10 minutes).
- Monitor and record vital signs and intake and output, hemodynamic variables, ICP, cerebral perfusion pressure, specific gravity, laboratory studies, and pulse oximetry.
- Check for signs of diabetes insipidus (low urine specific gravity, high urine output).
- Allow a rest period between nursing activities.

AMYOTROPHIC LATERAL SCLEROSIS

Key signs and symptoms
- Awkwardness of fine finger movements
- Dysphagia
- Fatigue
- Muscle weakness of hands and feet

Key test results
- Creatinine kinase level is elevated.
- Electromyography (EMG) shows decreased amplitude of evoked potentials.

Key treatments
- Symptomatic relief
- Neuroprotective agent: riluzole (Rilutek)

Key interventions
- Assess neurologic and respiratory status.
- Assess swallow and gag reflexes.
- Monitor and record vital signs and intake and output.
- Devise an alternate method of communication, when necessary.
- Suction oral pharynx, as necessary.

BELL'S PALSY

Key signs and symptoms
- Inability to close eye completely on the affected side
- Pain around the jaw or ear
- Unilateral facial weakness

Key test results
- EMG helps predict the level of expected recovery by distinguishing temporary conduction defects from a pathologic interruption of nerve fibers.

Key treatments
- Moist heat
- Corticosteroid: prednisone (Deltasone) to reduce facial nerve edema and improve nerve conduction and blood flow

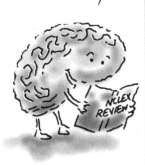

When I'm on overload, I skip directly to the Cheat sheet.

NCLEX REVIEW

Neurosensory refresher *(continued)*

BELL'S PALSY *(continued)*

Key interventions

• During treatment with prednisone, watch for adverse reactions, especially GI distress and fluid retention. If GI distress is troublesome, a concomitant antacid usually provides relief.
• Apply moist heat to the affected side of the face, taking care not to burn the skin.
• Massage the patient's face with a gentle upward motion two to three times daily for 5 to 10 minutes, or have him massage his face himself. When he's ready for active exercises, teach him to exercise by grimacing in front of a mirror.
• Arrange for privacy at mealtimes.
• Offer psychological support. Give reassurance that recovery is likely within 1 to 8 weeks.

BRAIN ABSCESS

Key signs and symptoms

• Headache
• Chills
• Fever
• Confusion
• Drowsiness

Key test results

• Physical examination shows increased ICP.
• Enhanced CT scan reveals the abscess site.
• A CT-guided stereotactic biopsy may be performed to drain and culture the abscess.

Key treatments

• Penicillinase-resistant antibiotics: nafcillin (Unipen), methicillin (Staphcillin)
• Surgical aspiration or drainage of the abscess

Key interventions

• Frequently assess neurologic status, especially cognition and mentation, speech, and sensorimotor and cranial nerve function.
• Assess and record vital signs at least every hour.
• Monitor fluid intake and output carefully.
• After surgery, continue frequent neurologic assessment. Monitor vital signs and intake and output.
• Watch for signs of meningitis (nuchal rigidity, headaches, chills, sweats).
• Change a damp dressing often. Never allow bandages to remain damp.
• Position the patient on the operative side.
• Measure drainage from Jackson-Pratt or other types of drains as instructed by the surgeon.

BRAIN TUMOR

Key signs and symptoms

• Vary depending on location of tumor

Key test results

• CT scan shows location and size of tumor.
• MRI also shows location and size of tumor.

Key treatments

• Craniotomy
• Anticonvulsant: phenytoin (Dilantin)
• Glucocorticoid: dexamethasone (Decadron)
• H_2-receptor antagonists: cimetidine (Tagamet), ranitidine (Zantac), famotidine (Pepcid), nizatidine (Axid)
• Mucosal barrier fortifier: sucralfate (Carafate)

Key interventions

• Assess neurologic and respiratory status.
• Assess pain.
• Assess for increased ICP.
• Monitor for signs and symptoms of syndrome of inappropriate antidiuretic hormone (edema, weight gain, positive fluid balance, high urine specific gravity).
• Encourage the patient to express feelings about changes in body image and a fear of dying.

CATARACT

Key signs or symptoms

• Dimmed or blurred vision
• Poor night vision
• Yellow, gray, or white pupil

Key test result

• Ophthalmoscopy or slit-lamp examination confirms the diagnosis by revealing a dark area in the normally homogeneous red reflex.

Key treatment

• Extracapsular cataract extraction or intracapsular lens implant

Key interventions

• Provide a safe environment for the patient.
• Modify the environment to help patient meet self-care needs by placing items on the unaffected side.

CEREBRAL ANEURYSM

Key sign or symptom

• Headache (commonly described by the patient as the worst he's ever had)

Key test results

• Cerebral angiogram identifies the aneurysm.

(continued)

Neurosensory refresher (continued)

CEREBRAL ANEURYSM (continued)
• CT scan shows a shift of intracranial midline structures, blood in subarachnoid space.

Key treatments
• Aneurysm clipping
• Anticonvulsant: phenytoin (Dilantin)
• Calcium channel blocker: nimodipine (Nimotop) is preferred to prevent cerebral vasospasm
• Glucocorticoid: dexamethasone (Decadron)
• H_2-receptor antagonists: cimetidine (Tagamet), ranitidine (Zantac), famotidine (Pepcid)
• Stool softener: docusate sodium (Colace)

Key interventions
• Assess neurologic status.
• Administer crystalloid solutions after aneurysm clipping.
• Take vital signs every 1 to 2 hours initially, then every 4 hours when the patient becomes stable.
• Allow a rest period between nursing activities.

CEREBROVASCULAR ACCIDENT

Key signs and symptoms
• Fever
• Headache
• Mental impairment
• Seizures
• Coma
• Nuchal rigidity
• Vomiting

Key test results
• CT scan reveals intracranial bleeding, infarct (shows up 24 hours after the initial symptoms), or shift of midline structures
• Digital subtraction angiography reveals occlusion or narrowing of vessels.
• MRI shows intracranial bleeding, infarct, or shift of midline structures.

Key treatments
• Anticoagulants: heparin, warfarin (Coumadin), ticlopidine
• Anticonvulsant: phenytoin (Dilantin)
• Glucocorticoid: dexamethasone (Decadron)
• Thrombolytic therapy: tissue plasminogen activator given within the first 3 hours of an ischemic CVA, to restore circulation to the affected brain tissue and limit the extent of brain injury

Key interventions
• Take vital signs every 1 to 2 hours initially, then every 4 hours when the patient becomes stable.
• Elevate the head of the bed 30 degrees.

• Conduct a neurologic assessment every 1 to 2 hours initially, then every 4 hours when the patient becomes stable.

CONJUNCTIVITIS

Key signs and symptoms
• Excessive tearing
• Itching, burning
• Mucopurulent discharge

Key test results
• Culture and sensitivity tests identify the causative bacterial organism and indicate appropriate antibiotic therapy.

Key treatments
• Antiviral agents: vidarabine ointment (Vira-A) or oral acyclovir (Zovirax), if herpes simplex is the cause
• Corticosteroids: dexamethasone (Maxidex), fluorometholone (Fluor-Op Ophthalmic)
• Mast cell stabilizer: cromolyn (Opticrom), for allergic conjunctivitis
• Topical antibiotics according to sensitivity of infective organism (if bacterial cause)

Key interventions
• Teach proper hand-washing technique.
• Stress the risk of spreading infection to family members by sharing washcloths, towels, and pillows. Warn against rubbing the infected eye, which can spread the infection to the other eye and to other persons.
• Apply warm compresses and therapeutic ointment or drops. Don't irrigate the eye.
• Have the patient wash his hands before he uses the medication, and use clean washcloths or towels frequently.
• Teach the patient to instill eyedrops and ointments correctly — without touching the bottle tip to his eye or lashes.

CORNEAL ABRASION

Key signs and symptoms
• Burning
• Increased tearing
• Redness

Key test results
• Staining the cornea with fluorescein stain confirms the diagnosis: the injured area appears green when examined with a flashlight.

Key treatments
• Cycloplegic agent: tropicamide (Ocu-Tropic)
• Irrigation with saline solution
• Pressure patch (a tightly applied eye patch)

Neurosensory refresher (continued)

CORNEAL ABRASION (continued)

• Removal of a deeply embedded foreign body with a foreign body spud, using a topical anesthetic

Key interventions

• Assist with examination of the eye. Check visual acuity before beginning treatment.
• If foreign body is visible, carefully irrigate the eye with normal saline solution.
• Tell the patient with an eye patch to leave the patch in place for 6 to 8 hours.
• Stress the importance of instilling prescribed antibiotic eye-drops.

ENCEPHALITIS

Key signs and symptoms

• Meningeal irritation (stiff neck and back) and neuronal damage (drowsiness, coma, paralysis, seizures, ataxia, and organic psychoses)
• Sudden onset of fever
• Headache
• Vomiting

Key test results

• Blood studies identify the virus and confirm diagnosis.
• Cerebrospinal fluid (CSF) analysis identifies the virus.

Key treatments

• Endotracheal intubation and mechanical ventilation
• Nasogastric tube feedings or total parenteral nutrition
• Anticonvulsants: phenytoin (Dilantin), phenobarbital (Luminal)
• Analgesic and antipyretics: aspirin or acetaminophen (Tylenol) to relieve headache and reduce fever
• Diuretics: furosemide (Lasix) or mannitol (Osmitrol) to reduce cerebral swelling
• Corticosteroid: dexamethasone (Decadron) to reduce cerebral inflammation and edema

Key interventions

During the acute phase of the illness:

• Assess neurologic function often. Observe the patient's mental status and cognitive abilities.
• Maintain adequate fluid, but avoid fluid overload. Measure and record intake and output accurately.
• Carefully position the patient and turn him often.
• Assist with range-of-motion exercises.
• Maintain a quiet environment. Darken the room.

GLAUCOMA

Key signs and symptoms

Chronic open-angle glaucoma

• Initially asymptomatic

Acute angle-closure glaucoma

• Acute ocular pain
• Blurred vision
• Dilated pupil
• Halo vision

Key test results

• Ophthalmoscopy shows atrophy and cupping of optic nerve head.
• Tonometry shows increased intraocular pressure.

Key treatments

Chronic open-angle glaucoma

• Alpha agonist: (Alphagon)
• Beta-adrenergic antagonist: timolol (Timoptic)

Acute angle-closure glaucoma

• Cholinergic agent: pilocarpine
• Laser iridectomy or surgical iridectomy if pressure doesn't decrease with drug therapy

Key interventions

• Assess eye pain and administer medication as prescribed.
• Modify the environment.

GUILLAIN-BARRÉ SYNDROME

Key symptom

• Muscle weakness (ascending from the legs to arms)

Key test results

• A history of preceding febrile illness (usually a respiratory tract infection) and typical clinical features suggest Guillain-Barré syndrome.
• CSF protein level begins to rise, peaking in 4 to 6 weeks. The CSF white blood cell count remains normal but, in severe disease, CSF pressure may rise above normal.

Key treatments

• Anticoagulants: heparin (Liquaem), warfarin (Coumadin)
• Corticosteroid: prednisone (Deltasone)
• Endotracheal intubation or tracheotomy if the patient has difficulty clearing secretions; may require mechanical ventilation
• I.V. fluid therapy
• Nasogastric tube feedings or parenteral nutrition
• Plasmapheresis

(continued)

Neurosensory refresher (continued)

GUILLAIN-BARRÉ SYNDROME (continued)

Key interventions

• Watch for ascending sensory loss, which precedes motor loss. Also, monitor vital signs and level of consciousness.
• Assess and treat respiratory dysfunction. If respiratory muscles are weak, take serial vital capacity recordings. Use a respirometer with a mouthpiece or a facemask for bedside testing.
• Obtain arterial blood gas measurements.
• Begin respiratory support at the first sign of dyspnea (in adults, a vital capacity less than 800 ml) or a decreasing partial pressure of arterial oxygen
• If respiratory failure becomes imminent, establish an emergency airway with an endotracheal tube.
• Establish a strict turning schedule; inspect the skin (especially the sacrum, heels, and ankles) for breakdown, and reposition the patient every 2 hours.
• If aspiration can't be minimized by diet and position modification, expect to provide nasogastric feeding.
• Inspect the patient's legs regularly for signs of thrombophlebitis (localized pain, tenderness, erythema, edema, positive Homans' sign).
• Apply antiembolism stockings and give prophylactic anticoagulants, as needed.
• Encourage adequate fluid intake (2,000 ml/day), unless contraindicated.

HUNTINGTON'S DISEASE

Key signs and symptoms

• Dementia (can be mild at first but eventually disrupts the patient's personality)
• Gradual loss of musculoskeletal control, eventually leading to total dependence

Key test results

• Positron emission tomography detects the disease.
• Deoxyribonucleic acid analysis detects the disease.

Key treatments

• Antidepressant: imipramine (Tofranil) helps control choreic movements
• Antipsychotics: chlorpromazine (Thorazine) and haloperidol (Haldol) help control choreic movements
• Because Huntington's disease has no known cure, treatment is supportive, protective, and aimed at relieving symptoms.

Key interventions

• Provide physical support by attending to the patient's basic needs, such as hygiene, skin care, bowel and bladder care, and nutrition. Increase this support as mental and physical deterioration make him increasingly immobile.
• Stay alert for possible suicide attempts. Control the patient's environment to protect him from suicide or other self-inflicted injury.
• Pad the side rails of the bed but avoid restraints.

MÉNIÈRE'S DISEASE

Key signs and symptoms

• Sensorineural hearing loss
• Severe vertigo
• Tinnitus

Key test results

• Audiometric studies indicate a sensorineural hearing loss and loss of discrimination and recruitment.

Key treatments

• Restriction of sodium intake to less than 2 g/day
• Anticholinergic: Atropine may stop an attack in 20 to 30 minutes
• Antihistamine: diphenhydramine (Benadryl) may be necessary in a severe attack

Key interventions

If the patient is in the facility during an attack of Ménière's disease:
• Advise the patient against reading and exposure to glaring lights.
• Keep the side rails of the patient's bed up. Tell him not to get out of bed or walk without assistance.
• Instruct the patient to avoid sudden position changes and any tasks that vertigo makes hazardous.

Before surgery:
• If the patient is vomiting, record fluid intake and output and characteristics of vomitus. Administer antiemetics as necessary, and give small amounts of fluid frequently.

After surgery:
• Tell the patient to expect dizziness and nausea for 1 or 2 days after surgery.

MENINGITIS

Key signs and symptoms

• Chills
• Fever
• Headache
• Malaise
• Photophobia

Neurosensory refresher *(continued)*

MENINGITIS *(continued)*

- Positive Brudzinski's sign (The patient flexes hips or knees when the nurse places her hands behind his neck and bends it forward, a sign of meningeal inflammation and irritation.)
- Positive Kernig's sign (Pain or resistance when the patient's leg is flexed at the hip or knee while he's in a supine position.)
- Stiff neck and back
- Vomiting

Key test results

- A lumbar puncture shows elevated CSF pressure, cloudy or milky white CSF, high protein level, positive Gram stain and culture that usually identifies the infecting organism (unless it's a virus) and depressed CSF glucose concentration.

Key treatments

- Analgesics or antipyretics: acetaminophen (Tylenol), aspirin
- Antibiotics: penicillin G (Pfizerpen), ampicillin (Omnipen), or nafcillin (Unipen); tetracycline (Achromycin V), or chloramphenicol (Chloromycetin), if allergic to penicillin
- Anticonvulsant: phenytoin (Dilantin), phenobarbital (Luminal)
- Bed rest
- Diuretic: mannitol (Osmitrol)
- Hypothermia
- I.V. fluid administration
- Oxygen therapy, possibly with endotracheal intubation and mechanical ventilation

Key interventions

- Assess neurologic function often.
- Watch for deterioration in the patient's condition.
- Monitor fluid balance. Maintain adequate fluid intake
- Measure central venous pressure and intake and output accurately.
- Suction the patient only if necessary. Limit suctioning to 10 to 15 seconds per pass of the catheter.
- Hyperoxygenate the lungs with 100% oxygen for 1 minute before and after suctioning.
- Administer lidocaine, if prescribed, I.V. or into the endotracheal tube before suctioning.
- Position the patient carefully.
- Darken the room.
- Relieve headache with a nonnarcotic analgesic, such as aspirin or acetaminophen, as needed.

MULTIPLE SCLEROSIS

Key signs and symptoms

- Nystagmus, diplopia, blurred vision, optic neuritis
- Weakness, paresthesia, impaired sensation, paralysis

Key test results

- CT scan eliminates other diagnoses such as brain or spinal cord tumors.
- MRI eliminates other diagnoses such as brain or spinal cord tumors.

Key treatments

- Plasmapheresis (for antibody removal)
- Cholinergic: bethanechol (Urecholine)
- Glucocorticoids: prednisone (Deltasone), dexamethasone (Decadron), corticotropin (ACTH)
- Immunosuppressants: interferon beta-1b (Betaseron), cyclophosphamide (Cytoxan), methotrexate (Folex)
- Skeletal muscle relaxants: dantrolene (Dantrium), baclofen (Lioresal).

Key interventions

- Assess changes in motor coordination, paralysis, or muscular weakness and report changes.
- Encourage the patient to express feelings about changes in body image.
- Establish bowel and bladder program.
- Maintain activity, as tolerated (alternating rest and activity).

MYASTHENIA GRAVIS

Key signs and symptoms

- Dysphagia, drooling
- Muscle weakness and fatigability (Typically, muscles are strongest in the morning but weaken throughout the day, especially after exercise.)
- Profuse sweating

Key test results

- EMG shows decreased amplitude of evoked potentials.
- Neostigmine (Prostigmin) or edrophonium (Tensilon) test relieves symptoms after medication administration (which is a positive indication of the disease).

Key treatments

- Anticholinesterase: neostigmine (Prostigmin), pyridostigmine (Mestinon), ambenonium (Mytelase)
- Glucocorticoids: prednisone (Deltasone), dexamethasone (Decadron), corticotropin (ACTH)
- Immunosuppressants: azathioprine (Imuran), cyclophosphamide (Cytoxan)

Key interventions

- Assess neurologic and respiratory status.
- Assess swallow and gag reflexes.
- Watch the patient for choking while eating.

(continued)

Neurosensory refresher (continued)

OTOSCLEROSIS

Key signs and symptoms
- Progressive hearing loss
- Tinnitus

Key test result
- Audiometric testing confirms hearing loss.

Key treatments
- Stapedectomy and insertion of a prosthesis to restore partial or total hearing

Key interventions
- Develop alternative means of communication.

PARKINSON'S DISEASE

Key signs and symptoms
- "Pill-rolling" tremors, tremors at rest
- Masklike facial expression
- Shuffling gait, stiff joints, dyskinesia, "cogwheel" rigidity, stooped posture

Key test results
- EEG reveals minimal slowing of brain activity.

Key treatments
- Antidepressant: amitriptyline (Elavil)
- Antiparkinsonian agents: levodopa (Larodopa), carbidopa-levodopa (Sinemet), benztropine (Cogentin)

Key interventions
- Assess neurologic and respiratory status.
- Reinforce gait training.
- Reinforce independence in care.

RETINAL DETACHMENT

Key signs and symptoms
- Painless change in vision (floaters and flashes of light)
- With progression of detachment, painless vision loss may be described as veil, curtain or cobweb that eliminates part of visual field

Key test results
- Indirect ophthalmoscope shows retinal tear or detachment.
- Slit-lamp examination shows retinal tear or detachment.

Key treatments
- Scleral buckling to reattach the retina

Key interventions
- Postoperatively instruct the patient to lie on his back or on his unoperated side.

- Discourage straining during defecation, bending down, and hard coughing, sneezing, or vomiting.

SPINAL CORD INJURY

Key signs and symptoms
- Loss of bowel and bladder control
- Paralysis below the level of the injury
- Paresthesia below the level of the injury

Key test results
- CT scan shows spinal cord edema, vertebral fracture, and spinal cord compression.
- MRI shows spinal cord edema, vertebral fracture, and spinal cord compression.

Key treatments
- Flat position, with neck immobilized in a cervical collar
- Maintenance of vertebral alignment through Crutchfield tongs and Halo brace
- Surgery for stabilization of the upper spine, such as insertion of Harrington rods
- Antianxiety agent: lorazepam (Ativan)
- Glucocorticoid: methlyprednisolone (Solu-Medrol) given as infusion immediately following injury (improves neurologic recovery when administered within 8 hours of injury)
- H_2-receptor antagonists: cimetidine (Tagamet), ranitidine (Zantac), famotidine (Pepcid)
- Laxative: bisacodyl (Dulcolax)
- Mucosal barrier fortifier: sucralfate (Carafate)
- Muscle relaxant: dantrolene (Dantrium)

Key interventions
- Assess neurologic and respiratory status.
- Assess for spinal shock.
- Check for autonomic dysreflexia (sudden extreme rise in blood pressure).
- Provide skin care.

TRIGEMINAL NEURALGIA

Key sign or symptom
- Searing pain in the facial area

Key test results
- Observation during the examination shows the patient favoring (splinting) the affected area. To ward off a painful attack, the patient often holds his face immobile when talking. He may also leave the affected side of his face unwashed and unshaven, or protect it with a coat or shawl.

Neurosensory refresher *(continued)*

TRIGEMINAL NEURALGIA *(continued)*

Key treatments
- Anticonvulsants: carbamazepine (Tegretol) or phenytoin (Dilantin) may temporarily relieve or prevent pain
- Microsurgery for vascular decompression

Key interventions
- Observe and record the characteristics of each attack, including the patient's protective mechanisms.
- Provide adequate nutrition in small, frequent meals at room temperature.
- If the patient is receiving carbamazepine, watch for cutaneous and hematologic reactions (erythematous and pruritic rashes, urticaria, photosensitivity, exfoliative dermatitis, leukopenia, agranulocytosis, eosinophilia, aplastic anemia, thrombocytopenia) and, possibly, urine retention and transient drowsiness.

- For the first 3 months of carbamazepine therapy, complete blood count and liver function should be monitored weekly, then monthly thereafter. Warn the patient to immediately report fever, sore throat, mouth ulcers, easy bruising, or petechial or purpuric hemorrhage.
- If the patient is receiving phenytoin, watch for adverse effects, including ataxia, skin eruptions, gingival hyperplasia, and nystagmus.
- Advise the patient to place food in the unaffected side of his mouth when chewing, to brush his teeth and rinse his mouth often, and to see a dentist twice a year to detect cavities.
- After surgical decompression of the root or partial nerve dissection, check neurologic and vital signs often.

- the midbrain — mediates pupillary reflexes and eye movements; it's also the reflex center for the third and fourth cranial nerves
- the pons — helps regulate respiration; it's also the reflex center for the fifth through eighth cranial nerves and mediates chewing, tasting, saliva secretion, and equilibrium
- the medulla oblongata — contains the vomiting, vasomotor, respiratory, and cardiac centers.

Information super-highway

The **spinal cord** functions as a two-way conductor pathway between the brain stem and the peripheral nervous system. It consists of gray matter and white matter. The gray matter is made up of cell bodies and dendrites and axons. The white matter contains ascending (sensory) and descending (motor) tracts, sending signals up to the brain and motor signals out to the muscles.

Like the post office

The **peripheral nervous system** delivers messages from the spinal cord to outlying areas of the body. The main nerves of this system are grouped into:
- 31 pairs of spinal nerves, which carry mixed impulses (motor and sensory) to and from the spinal cord

- 12 pairs of cranial nerves — olfactory, optic, oculomotor, trochlear, trigeminal, abducens, facial, acoustic, glossopharyngeal, vagus, spinal accessory, and hypoglossal.

Involuntary actions

The **autonomic nervous system,** a subdivision of the peripheral nervous system, controls involuntary body functions, such as digestion, respiration, and cardiovascular function.

It's divided into two cooperating systems to maintain homeostasis: the sympathetic nervous system and the parasympathetic nervous system. The sympathetic nervous system coordinates activities that handle stress (the flight or fight response). The parasympathetic nervous system conserves and restores energy stores.

Blink and you'll miss it

The **eyes** are composed of both external and internal structures. External structures include the eyelids, conjunctiva (a thin, transparent mucous membrane that lines the lid), lacrimal apparatus (which lubricates and protects the cornea and conjunctiva by producing and absorbing tears), extraocular muscles (which hold the eyes parallel to create binocular vision), and the eyeball itself.

Memory jogger

To help you remember the cranial nerves (and their order) think of the mnemonic "On Old Olympus's Towering Tops, A Finn And German Viewed Some Hops."

Olfactory (CN I)

Optic (CN II)

Oculomotor (CN III)

Trochlear (CN IV)

Trigeminal (CN V)

Abducens (CN VI)

Facial (CN VII)

Acoustic (CN VIII)

Glossopharyngeal (CN IX)

Vagus (CN X)

Spinal accessory (CN XI)

Hypoglossal (CN XII)

An inside view

The eye also contains numerous **internal structures.** Some of the most important include:

• the iris — a thin, circular pigmented muscular structure in the eye that gives color to the eye and divides the space between the cornea and lens into anterior and posterior chambers
• the cornea — a smooth, transparent tissue that works with the sclera to give the eye its shape
• the pupil — the circular aperture in the iris that changes size as the iris adapts to amount of light entering the eye
• the lens — a biconvex, avascular, colorless, and transparent structure suspended behind the iris by the ciliary zonulae
• the vitreous body — a clear, transparent, avascular, gelatinous fluid that fills the space in the posterior portion of the eye and maintains the transparency and form of the eye
• the retina — a thin, semitransparent layer of nerve tissue that lines the eye wall
• retinal cones — visual cell segments responsible for visual acuity and color discrimination
• retinal rods — visual cell segments responsible for peripheral vision under decreased light conditions
• the optic nerve — a nerve located at the posterior portion of the eye that transmits visual impulses from the retina to the brain.

External, middle, and inner

The **ears** are composed of three sections: external, middle, and inner. The external ear includes the pinna (auricle) and external auditory canal. It's separated from the middle ear by the tympanic membrane.

The middle ear, known as the tympanum, is an air-filled cavity in the temporal bone. It contains three small bones (malleus, incus, and stapes).

The inner ear, known as the labyrinth, is the portion of the ear that consists of the cochlea, vestibule, and semicircular canals.

Keep abreast of diagnostic tests

Here are the most important tests used to diagnose neurosensory disorders, along with common nursing actions associated with each test.

Electrical graph

An **electroencephalogram** (EEG) records the electrical activity of the brain. Using electrodes, this noninvasive test gives a graphic representation of brain activity.

Nursing actions

• Determine the patient's ability to lie still.
• Reassure the patient that electrical shock won't occur.
• Explain that the patient will be subjected to stimuli, such as lights and sounds.
• Withhold medications that may interfere with the results (such as anticonvulsants, antianxiety agents, sedatives, and antidepressants) and caffeine for 24 to 48 hours before the procedure.

Brain images

A **computed tomography (CT) scan,** used to identify brain abnormalities, produces a series of tomograms translated by a computer and displayed on a monitor, which represent cross-sectional images of various layers of the brain. It can be used to identify intracranial tumors and other brain lesions. It may be performed with or without the injection of contrast dye.

Nursing actions

• Note the patient's allergies to iodine, seafood, and radiopaque dyes, if dye will be used.
• Make sure that written, informed consent has been obtained, if appropriate.
• Inform the patient about possible throat irritation and facial flushing if contrast dye is injected.

Magnetic snapshot

Magnetic resonance imaging (MRI) uses magnetic and radio waves to create a detailed visualization of the brain and its structures.

Nursing actions
• Be aware that patients with pacemakers, surgical and orthopedic clips, or shrapnel shouldn't be scanned.
• Remove jewelry and metal objects from the patient.
• Determine the patient's ability to lie still.
• Administer sedation as prescribed.

Upstairs artery exam

A **cerebral angiogram** uses a radiopaque dye, in conjunction with X-rays, to examine the cerebral arteries.

Nursing actions
Before the procedure:
• note the patient's allergies to iodine, seafood, or radiopaque dyes
• make sure that a written, informed consent has been obtained
• inform the patient about possible throat irritation and facial flushing.
After the procedure:
• monitor vital signs
• check the insertion site for bleeding and assess pulses distal to the site
• assess neurologic status
• force fluids if patient's condition allows.

Puncture reveals pressure

In a **lumbar puncture** (LP), a doctor uses a needle to collect CSF from the lumbar subarachnoid space. This allows measurement of CSF pressure as well as the injection of radiopaque dye for a myelogram.

Nursing actions
Before the procedure:
• determine the patient's ability to lie still in a flexed, lateral, recumbent position
• explain the procedure to the patient
• make sure that written, informed consent has been obtained

• be aware that the presence of increased intracranial pressure (ICP) is a contraindication for having the test.
   After the procedure:
• assess neurologic status
• keep the patient flat in bed, as directed (from 20 minutes to a few hours)
• administer analgesics as prescribed
• check the puncture site for bleeding or CSF leakage
• force fluids, if patient's condition allows.

Fluid to the lab

Cerebrospinal fluid analysis is a laboratory test of CSF obtained by lumbar puncture or ventriculostomy. It allows microscopic examination of CSF for blood, white blood cells (WBCs), immunoglobulins, bacteria, protein, glucose, and electrolytes.

Nursing actions
• Label specimens properly and send to the laboratory immediately.
• Adhere to nursing interventions that follow an LP.

Electric flex

Electromyography (EMG) uses electrodes to graphically record the electrical activity of a muscle at rest and during contraction.

Nursing actions
• Explain that the patient must flex and relax the muscles during the procedure.
• Explain that the patient will feel some discomfort but not pain.
• Administer analgesics, as prescribed, after the procedure.

See the spine

In **myelography,** an injection of radiopaque dye by LP followed by fluoroscopy allows visualization of the subarachnoid space, spinal cord, and vertebrae.

Nursing actions
Before the procedure:
• note the patient's allergies to iodine, seafood, and radiopaque dyes
• make sure that written, informed consent has been obtained

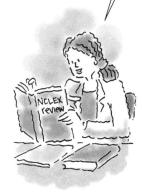

Hmmm. Contraindications count. The presence of a pacemaker rules out an MRI.

Memory jogger

To remember that increased intracranial pressure contraindicates a lumbar puncture, think:

Increased ICP — No LP.

• inform the patient about possible throat irritation and facial flushing from dye injection.

After the procedure:
• assess neurologic status
• keep the patient flat in bed, as directed
• check the puncture site for bleeding or CSF leakage
• force fluids if patient's condition allows.

Snooping on the skull
Skull X-rays give a radiographic picture of the head and neck bones.

Nursing actions
• Determine the patient's ability to lie still during the procedure.
• Explain the events that will occur during the procedure.

Marking blood flow in the brain
Positron emission tomography (PET) involves injection of a radioisotope, allowing visualization of the brain's oxygen uptake, blood flow, and glucose metabolism.

Nursing actions
• Determine the patient's ability to lie still during the procedure.
• Withhold alcohol, tobacco, and caffeine for 24 hours before the procedure.
• Withhold medications, as directed, before the procedure.
• Check the injection site for bleeding after the procedure.

Studying blood once...
A **blood chemistry test** analyzes a blood sample for potassium, sodium, calcium, phosphorus, protein, osmolality, glucose, bicarbonate, blood urea nitrogen, and creatinine.

Nursing actions
• Explain the reason for testing to the patient.
• Monitor the site for bleeding after the procedure.

...Studying blood twice...
A **hematologic study** is a laboratory test of a blood sample that analyzes for WBCs, red blood cells, erythrocyte sedimentation rate, platelets, hemoglobin, and hematocrit.

Nursing actions
• Note current drug therapy before the procedure.
• Check the venipuncture site for bleeding after the procedure.

...Studying blood three times
A **coagulation study** is a laboratory test of a blood sample which analyzes prothrombin time, international normalized ratio, and partial thromboplastin time.

Nursing actions
• Note current drug therapy before the procedure.
• Check the venipuncture site for bleeding after the procedure.

Ye olde eye chart
A **visual acuity test** measures clarity of vision using a letter chart (Snellen's) placed 20′ (6 m) from the patient. Acuity is expressed in a ratio that relates what a person with normal vision sees at 20′ to what the patient can see at 20′.

Nursing actions
• Explain the testing procedure to the patient.
• Remind the patient to bring eyeglasses or contact lenses, if presently prescribed.
• Advise the examiner if the patient is unable to read alphabet letters.
• Advise the examiner if the patient has difficulty hearing or following directions.

All lined up?
Extraocular eye muscle testing checks for parallel alignment of the eyes, muscle strength, and cranial nerve function.

Nursing actions
• Explain the testing procedure to the patient.
• Advise the examiner if the patient has difficulty hearing or following directions.

Seeing on the side
A **visual field examination** tests the degree of peripheral vision of each eye.

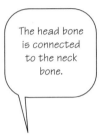

The head bone is connected to the neck bone.

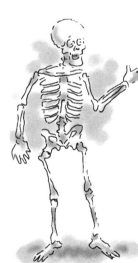

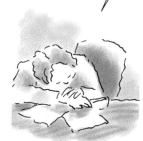

Nursing actions
- Explain the testing procedure to the patient.
- Advise the examiner if the patient has difficulty hearing or following directions.

Puff to measure pressure
A **tonometry test** measures intraocular fluid pressure using an applanation tonometer or an air-puff tonometer.

Nursing actions
- Ask the patient to remain still.
- Depending on the method of examination, advise the patient that a puff of air or the instrument may be felt touching the eye.

Tick-tock test
An **auditory acuity test** gives a general estimation of a patient's hearing. It assesses the patient's ability to hear a whispered phrase or ticking watch.

Nursing actions
- Explain the testing procedure to the patient.
- Advise the examiner if the patient has difficulty following directions.

Scope inside the ear
An **otoscopic examination** uses an otoscope to visualize the tympanic membrane.

Nursing actions
- Advise the patient to hold still during the examination.
- Explain that a gentle pull will be felt on the auricle and slight pressure will be felt in the ear.

Determining degree of deafness
Audiometry measures the patient's degree of deafness using pure-tone or speech methods.

Nursing actions
- Explain that the patient will need to wear earphones for the procedure.
- Explain that the patient will be asked to signal when a tone is heard while sitting in a soundproof room.

Polish up on patient care

Major neurosensory disorders include acute head injury, amyotrophic lateral sclerosis, Bell's palsy, brain abscess, brain tumors, cataract, cerebral aneurysm, cerebrovascular accident (CVA), conjunctivitis, corneal abrasion, encephalitis, glaucoma, Guillain-Barré syndrome, Huntington's disease, Ménière's disease, meningitis, multiple sclerosis, myasthenia gravis, otosclerosis, Parkinson's disease, retinal detachment, spinal cord injury, and trigeminal neuralgia.

Acute head injury

Acute head injury results from a trauma to the head, leading to brain injury or bleeding within the brain. Effects of injury may include edema and hypoxia. Manifestations of the injury can vary greatly from a mild cognitive effect to severe functional deficits.

A head injury is classified by brain injury type: fracture, hemorrhage, or trauma. Fractures can be depressed, comminuted, or linear. Hemorrhages are classified as epidural, subdural, intracerebral, or subarachnoid.

CAUSES
- Assault
- Automobile accident
- Blunt trauma
- Fall
- Penetrating trauma

ASSESSMENT FINDINGS
- Decreased level of consciousness (LOC)
- Disorientation to time, place, or person
- Otorrhea, rhinorrhea, frequent swallowing (if a CSF leak occurs)
- Paresthesia
- Unequal pupil size, loss of pupillary reaction (if edema is present)

DIAGNOSTIC TEST RESULTS
- CT scan shows hemorrhage, cerebral edema, or shift of midline structures.

Too much studying giving you a decreased LOC? Take a quick break — then come back ready to review some more!

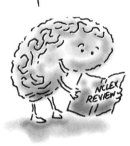

Acute head injury results from a trauma to the head, leading to brain injury or bleeding within the brain. Sounds awful.

- EEG may reveal seizure activity
- ICP monitoring shows increased ICP.
- MRI shows hemorrhage, cerebral edema, or shift of midline structures.
- Skull X-ray may show skull fracture.

NURSING DIAGNOSES

- Altered cerebral tissue perfusion
- Decreased adaptive capacity: Intracranial
- Risk for injury

TREATMENT

- Cervical collar (until neck injury is ruled out)
- Craniotomy: surgical incision into the cranium (may be necessary to evacuate a hematoma or evacuate contents to make room for swelling to prevent herniation)
- Oxygen therapy: intubation and mechanical ventilation (to provide controlled hyperventilation to decrease elevated ICP)
- Restricted oral intake for 24 to 48 hours
- Ventriculostomy: insertion of a drain into the ventricles (to drain CSF in the presence of hydrocephalus, which may occur as a result of head injury; can also be used to monitor ICP)

Drug therapy

- Analgesic: codeine phosphate
- Anesthetic: lidocaine (Xylocaine)
- Anticonvulsant: phenytoin (Dilantin)
- Barbiturate: pentobarbital (Nembutal), if unable to control ICP with diuresis
- Diuretics: mannitol (Osmitrol), furosemide (Lasix) to combat cerebral edema
- Dopamine (Intropin) to maintain cerebral perfusion pressure above 50 mm Hg (if blood pressure is low and ICP is elevated)
- Glucocorticoid: dexamethasone (Decadron) to reduce cerebral edema
- Histamine$_2$ (H$_2$)-receptor antagonists: cimetidine (Tagamet), ranitidine (Zantac), famotidine (Pepcid), nizatidine (Axid)
- Mucosal barrier fortifier: sucralfate (Carafate)
- Posterior pituitary hormone: vasopressin (Pitressin) if patient develops diabetes insipidus

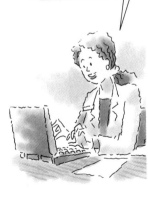

In patients with head injuries: Allow a rest period between procedures to avoid increasing ICP.

INTERVENTIONS AND RATIONALES

- Assess neurologic and respiratory status *to monitor for signs of increased ICP and respiratory distress.*
- Observe for signs of increasing ICP (including ICP greater than 20 mm Hg for more than 10 minutes) *to avoid treatment delay and prevent neurologic compromise.*
- Monitor and record vital signs and intake and output, hemodynamic variables, ICP, cerebral perfusion pressure, specific gravity, laboratory studies, and pulse oximetry *to detect early signs of compromise.*
- Assess for CSF leak as evidenced by otorrhea or rhinorrhea. *CSF leak could leave the patient at risk for infection.*
- Assess pain. *Pain may cause anxiety and increase ICP.*
- Check cough and gag reflex *to prevent aspiration.*
- Check for signs of diabetes insipidus (low urine specific gravity, high urine output) *to maintain hydration.*
- Administer I.V. fluids *to maintain hydration.*
- Administer oxygen and maintain position and patency of endotracheal tube, if present, *to maintain airway and hyperventilate the patient to lower ICP.*
- Provide suctioning; if patient is able, assist with turning, coughing, and deep breathing *to prevent pooling of secretions.*
- Maintain position, patency, and low suction of nasogastric (NG) tube *to prevent vomiting.*
- Maintain seizure precautions *to maintain patient safety.*
- Administer medications as prescribed *to decrease ICP and pain.*
- Allow a rest period between nursing activities *to avoid increase in ICP.*
- Encourage the patient to express feelings about changes in body image *to allay anxiety.*
- Provide appropriate sensory input and stimuli with frequent reorientation *to foster awareness of the environment.*
- Provide means of communication such as a communication board *to prevent anxiety.*
- Provide eye, skin, and mouth care *to prevent tissue damage.*
- Turn the patient every 2 hours or maintain in a rotating bed if condition allows *to prevent skin breakdown.*

Teaching topics
• Recognizing the signs and symptoms of decreased LOC
• Recognizing the signs of seizures
• Adhering to fluid restrictions
• Contacting the National Head Injury Foundation

Amyotrophic lateral sclerosis

Amyotrophic lateral sclerosis (ALS), commonly known as Lou Gehrig's disease, is a progressive, degenerative disorder that leads to decreased motor function in the upper and lower motor neuron systems. In ALS, myelin sheaths are destroyed and replaced with scar tissue, resulting in distorted or blocked nerve impulses. Nerve cells die and muscle fibers have atrophic changes resulting in progressive motor dysfunction. The disease affects males three times more often than females.

CAUSES
• Genetic predisposition
• Nutritional deficiency related to a disturbance in enzyme metabolism
• Slow-acting virus
• Unknown

ASSESSMENT FINDINGS
• Atrophy of tongue
• Awkwardness of fine finger movements
• Dysphagia
• Dyspnea
• Fasciculations of face
• Fatigue
• Muscle weakness of hands and feet
• Nasal quality of speech
• Spasticity

DIAGNOSTIC TEST RESULTS
• Creatinine kinase level is elevated.
• EMG shows decreased amplitude of evoked potentials.

NURSING DIAGNOSES
• Altered health maintenance
• Impaired physical mobility
• Ineffective airway clearance

TREATMENT
• Symptomatic relief

Drug therapy
• Anticholinergics: dicyclomine (Bentyl)
• Anticonvulsant: gabapentin (Neurontin)
• Antispasmodics: baclofen (Lioresal), lorazepam (Ativan)
• Investigational: thyrotropin-releasing hormone, interferon
• Neuroprotective agent: riluzole (Rilutek)

INTERVENTIONS AND RATIONALES
• Assess neurologic and respiratory status *to detect decreases in neurologic functioning.*
• Assess swallow and gag reflexes *to decrease risk of aspiration.*
• Monitor and record vital signs and intake and output *to determine baseline and detect changes from baseline assessment.*
• Administer medications as prescribed *to help patient achieve maximum potential.*
• Devise an alternate method of communication, when necessary, *to help the patient communicate and decrease the patient's anxiety and frustration.*
• Encourage the patient to verbalize his feelings and maintain his independence for as long as possible *to decrease anxiety and promote self-esteem.*
• Suction oral pharynx, as necessary, *to stimulate cough and clear airways.*
• Maintain the patient's diet *to improve nutritional status.*

Teaching topics
• Maintaining tucked chin position while eating or drinking
• Using tonsillar suction tip to clear oral pharynx
• Using prosthetic devices to assist with activities of daily living (ADLs)
• For patient's family, information about the disease, required treatment, and possible need for long-term care
• Contacting the Amyotrophic Lateral Sclerosis Association (The association may supply the patient with some of the needed equipment, such as a wheelchair and communication board.)

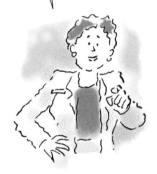

Teach the family members of a patient with ALS about a living will and options for long-term care.

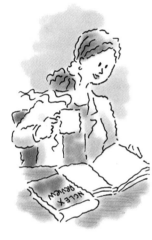

There are two facial nerves, one on each side. Bell's palsy occurs when one of those nerves becomes swollen and pinched.

Bell's palsy

This neurologic disorder affects the seventh cranial (facial) nerve and produces unilateral facial weakness or paralysis. Onset is rapid. While it affects all age-groups, it occurs most often in persons under age 60. In 80% to 90% of patients, it subsides spontaneously, with complete recovery in 1 to 8 weeks; however, recovery may be delayed in older adults. If recovery is partial, contractures may develop on the paralyzed side of the face. Bell's palsy may recur on the same or opposite side of the face.

CAUSES
• Blockage of the seventh cranial resulting from infection, hemorrhage, tumor, meningitis, or local trauma.

ASSESSMENT FINDINGS
• Eye rolls upward and tears excessively when the patient attempts to close it
• Inability to close eye completely on the affected side
• Pain around the jaw or ear
• Ringing in the ears
• Taste distortion on the affected anterior portion of the tongue
• Unilateral facial weakness

DIAGNOSTIC TEST RESULTS
• EMG helps predict the level of expected recovery by distinguishing temporary conduction defects from a pathologic interruption of nerve fibers.

NURSING DIAGNOSES
• Pain
• Sensory or perceptual alterations (gustatory)
• Body image disturbance

TREATMENT
• Electrotherapy after the 14th day of prednisone therapy to help prevent facial muscle atrophy
• Moist heat
• Facial sling

Drug therapy
• Corticosteroid: prednisone (Deltasone) to reduce facial nerve edema and improve nerve conduction and blood flow

INTERVENTIONS AND RATIONALES
• During treatment with prednisone, watch for adverse reactions, especially GI distress and fluid retention. If GI distress is troublesome, a concomitant antacid usually provides relief *to prevent further complications.*
• If the patient has diabetes, prednisone must be used with caution and necessitates frequent monitoring of serum glucose levels. *Hyperglycemia is an adverse reaction to prednisone therapy.*
• Apply moist heat to the affected side of the face, taking care not to burn the skin *to reduce pain.*
• Massage the patient's face with a gentle upward motion two to three times daily for 5 to 10 minutes, or have him massage his face himself. When he's ready for active exercises, teach him to exercise by grimacing in front of a mirror *to help maintain muscle tone.*
• Arrange for privacy at mealtimes *to reduce embarrassment.*
• Apply a facial sling *to improve lip alignment.*
• Give the patient frequent and complete mouth care, being careful to remove residual food that collects between the cheeks and gums *to prevent breakdown of oral mucosa.*
• Offer psychological support. Give reassurance that recovery is likely within 1 to 8 weeks *to allay the patient's anxiety.*

Teaching topics
• Protecting the eye by covering it with an eye patch, especially when outdoors
• Keeping warm, avoiding exposure to dust and wind, and covering face when exposure is unavoidable
• Performing facial exercises

Brain abscess

Brain abscess is a free or encapsulated collection of pus that usually occurs in the temporal lobe, cerebellum, or frontal lobes. Brain abscess is rare. Although it can occur at any age, it's most common in people ages 10 to 35 and is rare in older adults.

An untreated brain abscess is usually fatal; with treatment, the prognosis is only fair.

CAUSES
- Infection, especially otitis media, sinusitis, dental abscess, and mastoiditis
- Subdural empyema
- Physical trauma

ASSESSMENT FINDINGS
- Headache
- Chills
- Fever
- Malaise
- Confusion
- Drowsiness

Temporal lobe abscess
- Auditory-receptive dysphasia
- Central facial weakness
- Hemiparesis

Cerebellar abscess
- Dizziness
- Coarse nystagmus
- Gaze weakness on lesion side
- Tremor
- Ataxia

Frontal lobe abscess
- Expressive dysphasia
- Hemiparesis with unilateral motor seizure
- Drowsiness
- Inattention
- Mental function impairment
- Seizures

DIAGNOSTIC TEST RESULTS
- Physical examination shows increased ICP.
- Enhanced CT scan reveals the abscess site
- Arteriography highlights the abscess by a halo appearance.
- A CT-guided stereotactic biopsy may be performed to drain and culture the abscess.
- Culture and sensitivity of drainage identifies the causative organism

NURSING DIAGNOSES
- Decreased adaptive capacity: Intracranial
- Altered thought process
- Impaired physical mobility

TREATMENT
- Endotracheal (ET) intubation and mechanical ventilation
- I.V. therapy
- Surgical aspiration or drainage of the abscess

Drug therapy
- Diuretics: urea (Ureaphil), mannitol (Osmitrol)
- Corticosteroids: dexamethasone (Decadron)
- Penicillinase-resistant antibiotics: nafcillin (Unipen), methicillin (Staphcillin)
- Anticonvulsants, such as phenytoin (Dilantin) and phenobarbital (Luminal)

INTERVENTIONS AND RATIONALES
- Provide intensive care and monitoring to the patient with an acute brain abscess *to closely monitor ICP and provide necessary life-support.*
- Frequently assess neurologic status, especially cognition and mentation, speech, and sensorimotor and cranial nerve function *to detect early sign of increased ICP.* (See *Using the Glasgow Coma Scale,* page 187.)
- Assess and record vital signs at least every hour *to detect trends which may signify increasing ICP, such as increasing blood pressure and slowing heart rate.*
- Monitor fluid intake and output carefully *because fluid overload could contribute to cerebral edema.*
- If surgery is necessary, explain the procedure to the patient and answer his questions *to allay anxiety.*
- After surgery, continue frequent neurologic assessment *to detect rises in ICP and deteriorating neurologic status.* Monitor vital signs and intake and output.
- Watch for signs of meningitis (nuchal rigidity, headaches, chills, sweats) *to avoid treatment delay.*

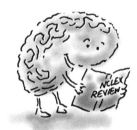

Location, location, location. Effects of a brain abscess depend upon which part of the brain is affected.

• Change a damp dressing often. Never allow bandages to remain damp. *Damp dressings are a good medium for bacterial growth.*
• Position the patient on the operative side *to promote drainage and prevent reaccumulation of the abscess.*
• Measure drainage from Jackson-Pratt or other types of drains as instructed by the surgeon *to assess effectiveness of drain and to detect signs of hemorrhage if blood should begin to accumulate in the drain.*
• If the patient remains stuporous or comatose for an extended period, give meticulous skin care *to prevent pressure ulcers*, and position him *to preserve function and prevent contractures.*
• If the patient requires isolation because of postoperative drainage, make sure he and his family understand why *to promote compliance with isolation precautions and allay anxiety.*
• Ambulate the patient as soon as possible *to prevent immobility and encourage independence.*
• Give prophylactic antibiotics as needed after a compound skull fracture or penetrating head wound *to prevent brain abscess.*

Teaching topics
• Stressing the need for treatment of otitis media, mastoiditis, dental abscess, and other infections to prevent brain abscess.

Brain tumor

A brain tumor is an abnormal mass found in the brain resulting from unregulated cell growth and division. These tumors can either infiltrate and destroy surrounding tissue or be encapsulated and displace brain tissue. The presence of the lesion causes compression of blood vessels, producing ischemia, edema, and increased ICP.

Symptoms and manifestations vary depending on the location of the tumor in the brain. The tumor can be primary (originating in the brain tissue) or secondary (metastasizing from another area of the body). Tumors are classified according to the tissue of origin, such as gliomas (composed of neuroglial cells), meningiomas (originating in the meninges), and astrocytomas (composed of astrocytes).

CAUSES
• Environmental
• Genetic

ASSESSMENT FINDINGS
A tumor in any area of the brain may lead to:
• deficits in cerebral function
• headache.
  In the frontal lobe, tumor may lead to:
• aphasia
• memory loss
• personality changes.
  In the temporal lobe, tumor may lead to:
• aphasia
• seizures.
  In the parietal lobe, tumor may lead to:
• motor seizures
• sensory impairment.
  In the occipital lobe, tumor may lead to:
• homonymous hemianopsia (defective vision or blindness affecting the right halves or the left halves of the visual field of the two eyes)
• visual hallucinations
• visual impairment.
  In the cerebellum, tumor may lead to:
• impaired coordination
• impaired equilibrium.

DIAGNOSTIC TEST RESULTS
• CT scan shows location and size of tumor.
• MRI also shows location and size of tumor.

NURSING DIAGNOSES
• Anxiety
• Risk for injury
• Sensory or perceptual alterations (kinesthetic)

TREATMENT
• Craniotomy
• High-calorie diet
• Radiation therapy

Drug therapy
• Anticonvulsant: phenytoin (Dilantin)
• Antineoplastics: vincristine (Oncovin), lomustine (CeeNu), carmustine (BiCNU)

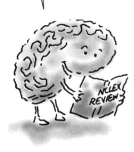

A brain tumor is an abnormal mass found in the brain resulting from unregulated cell growth and division

Using the Glasgow Coma Scale

The Glasgow Coma Scale is used to assess a patient's level of consciousness. It was designed to help predict a patient's survival and recovery after a head injury. The scale scores three observations: eye opening response, best motor response, and best verbal response. Each response receives a point value. If the patient is alert, can follow simple commands, and is completely oriented to person, place, and time, his score will total 15 points. If the patient is comatose, his score will total 7 or less. A score of 3, the lowest possible score, indicates deep coma and a poor prognosis.

OBSERVATION	RESPONSE	SCORE
Eye response	Opens spontaneously	4
	Opens to verbal command	3
	Opens to pain	2
	No response	1
Best motor response	Follows commands	6
	Localizes pain	5
	Flexion withdrawal	4
	Abnormal flexion	3
	Abnormal extension	2
	No response	1
Verbal response	Is oriented and converses	5
	Is disoriented but converses	4
	Uses inappropriate words	3
	Makes incomprehensible sounds	2
	No response	1
Total score		Ranges between 3 and 15

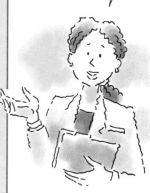

Early increases in intracranial pressure can be detected by using the Glasgow Coma Scale.

• Diuretics: mannitol (Osmitrol), furosemide (Lasix) if increased ICP
• Glucocorticoid: dexamethasone (Decadron)
• H_2-receptor antagonists: cimetidine (Tagamet), ranitidine (Zantac), famotidine (Pepcid), nizatidine (Axid)
• Mucosal barrier fortifier: sucralfate (Carafate)

INTERVENTIONS AND RATIONALES

• Assess neurologic and respiratory status *to determine baseline and deviations from baseline assessment.*
• Assess pain. *Continuous assessment correlates patient's subjective complaints and behavior with organic pathology.*

• Assess for increased ICP *to facilitate early intervention and prevent neurologic complications.*
• Monitor and record vital signs and intake and output, ICP, and laboratory studies *to determine baseline and detect early deviations from baseline assessment.*
• Monitor for signs and symptoms of syndrome of inappropriate antidiuretic hormone (edema, weight gain, positive fluid balance, high urine specific gravity) *to facilitate early intervention and prevent increased ICP through fluid restriction and I.V. infusion of normal saline solution.*
• Turn and reposition patient every 2 hours *to maintain skin integrity.*

- Maintain the patient's diet *to promote healing*.
- Encourage the patient to drink fluids *to maintain hydration*.
- Administer I.V. fluids *to maintain hydration if patient is unable to drink adequate amounts*.
- Administer oxygen *to prevent ischemia*.
- Administer enteral nutrition or total parenteral nutrition (TPN), as indicated, *to meet nutritional needs*.
- Limit environmental noise. *Auditory stimuli can contribute to increased ICP.*
- Encourage the patient to express feelings about changes in body image and a fear of dying *to decrease anxiety*.
- Monitor arterial blood gas (ABG) levels. *Hypercapnia results in vasodilation, increased cerebral blood volume, and increased ICP.*
- Maintain normothermia and control shivering. *Shivering causes isometric muscle contraction, which can increase ICP.*
- Provide rest periods. *Cerebral blood flow increases during rapid eye-movement sleep.*
- Maintain seizure precautions and administer anticonvulsants, as ordered. *Seizures increase intrathoracic pressure, decrease cerebral venous outflow, and increase cerebral blood volume, thereby increasing ICP.*

Teaching topics
- Recognizing decreased LOC
- Maintaining a safe, quiet environment
- Discussing quality of life decisions
- Arranging for hospice care, if appropriate

Cataract

A cataract occurs when the normally clear, transparent crystalline lens becomes opaque. With age, lens fibers become more densely packed, making the lens less transparent and giving the lens a yellowish hue. These changes result in vision loss.

A cataract usually develops first in one eye, but is often followed by the development of a cataract in the other eye.

CAUSES
- Aging
- Anterior uveitis

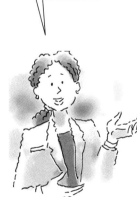

It's clear. Postoperative patient teaching is an important part of cataract care.

- Blunt or penetrating trauma
- Diabetes mellitus
- Hypoparathyroidism
- Long-term steroid treatment
- Radiation exposure
- Ultraviolet light exposure

ASSESSMENT FINDINGS
- Dimmed or blurred vision
- Disabling glare
- Distorted images
- Poor night vision
- Yellow, gray, or white pupil

DIAGNOSTIC TEST RESULTS
- Ophthalmoscopy or slit-lamp examination confirms the diagnosis by revealing a dark area in the normally homogeneous red reflex.

NURSING DIAGNOSES
- Impaired physical mobility
- Risk for injury
- Sensory or perceptual alterations (visual)

TREATMENT
- Extracapsular cataract extraction or intracapsular lens implant

INTERVENTIONS AND RATIONALES
- Provide a safe environment for the patient. *Orienting patient to surroundings reduces the risk of injury.*
- Modify the environment to help patient meet self-care needs by placing items on the unaffected side to *discourage movement or positions that would apply pressure to the operative site or cause increased intraocular pressure*.
- Provide sensory stimulation (such as large print or tapes) *to help compensate for vision loss*.

Teaching topics
- Returning for a checkup the day after surgery
- Protecting the eye from injury by wearing an eye shield
- Correctly instilling eyedrops
- Notifying the doctor immediately if patient experiences sharp eye pain
- Maintaining activity restrictions

Cerebral aneurysm

A cerebral aneurysm is an outpouching of a cerebral artery that results from weakness of the middle layer of an artery. It usually results from a congenital weakness in the structure of the artery and remains asymptomatic until it ruptures.

Cerebral aneurysms are classified by type: saccular (berry), fusiform, and giant. Saccular aneurysms, the most common, occur at the base of the brain at the juncture where the large arteries bifurcate.

CAUSES
- Atherosclerosis
- Congenital weakness
- Head trauma

ASSESSMENT FINDINGS
- Asymptomatic until aneurysm ruptures
- Decreased LOC
- Diplopia, ptosis, blurred vision
- Fever
- Headache (commonly described by the patient as the worst he's ever had)
- Hemiparesis
- Nuchal rigidity
- Seizure activity

DIAGNOSTIC TEST RESULTS
- Cerebral angiogram identifies the aneurysm.
- CT scan shows a shift of intracranial midline structures and blood in subarachnoid space.
- LP (contraindicated with increased ICP) shows increased CSF pressure, protein level, and WBCs and grossly bloody and xanthochromic CSF.
- MRI shows shift of intracranial midline structures and blood in subarachnoid space.

NURSING DIAGNOSES
- Anxiety
- Altered cerebral tissue perfusion
- Decreased adaptive capacity: Intracranial

TREATMENT
- Aneurysm and seizure precautions
- Aneurysm clipping
- Bed rest
- Head of bed elevated 30 degrees
- I.V. therapy
- Oxygen therapy (intubation and mechanical ventilation with hyperventilation, if increased ICP)

Drug therapy
- Analgesic: codeine sulfate
- Anticonvulsant: phenytoin (Dilantin)
- Antihypertensives: hydralazine (Apresoline), nitroprusside (Nitropress), labetalol (Trandate), metoprolol (Lopressor), esmolol (Brevibloc)
- Calcium channel blocker: nimodipine (Nimotop) preferred drug to prevent cerebral vasospasm
- Glucocorticoid: dexamethasone (Decadron)
- H_2-receptor antagonists: cimetidine (Tagamet), ranitidine (Zantac), famotidine (Pepcid)
- Possibly dopamine (Intropin) to maintain systolic blood pressure at 140 to 160 mm Hg
- Mucosal barrier fortifier: sucralfate (Carafate)
- Stool softener: docusate sodium (Colace)

INTERVENTIONS AND RATIONALES
- Assess neurologic status *to screen for changes in the patient's condition.*
- Keep environment and patient quiet using sedatives and pain medication *to reduce increased ICP.*
- Administer diuretics *to prevent or treat increased ICP.*
- Administer crystalloid solutions after aneurysm clipping *to induce hypervolemia and increase cerebral perfusion, thus decreasing the risk of vasospasm.*
- Administer oxygen (may require intubation and mechanical ventilation with hyperventilation). *Hypercapnia results in vasodilation, increased cerebral blood volume, and increased ICP.*
- Keep the head of the bed elevated to 30 degrees *to reduce increased ICP.*

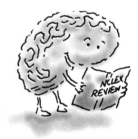

Maintain precautions for patients with cerebral aneurysm to prevent complications. Keep the lights low. No stress. No metal utensils.

• Monitor for Cushing's triad, (bradycardia, systolic hypertension, and wide pulse pressure) *which is a sign of impending hemorrhage.*

• Take vital signs every 1 to 2 hours initially, then every 4 hours when the patient becomes stable *to detect early signs of decreased cerebral perfusion pressure or increased ICP.*

• Allow a rest period between nursing activities *to reduce increased ICP.*

• Maintain seizure precautions and administer anticonvulsants, as ordered. *Seizures increase intrathoracic pressure, decrease cerebral venous outflow, and increase cerebral blood volume, thereby increasing ICP.*

• Provide skin care and turn patient every 2 hours *to prevent pressure ulcers.*

• Maintain adequate nutrition *to facilitate tissue healing, and meet metabolic needs.*

• Prevent constipation and straining at defecation *to prevent increased ICP.*

• If patient has a potentially compromised airway, use antiemetics or NG suction *to prevent nausea and vomiting, which may increase ICP.*

Teaching topics
• Recognizing decreasing LOC
• Minimizing environmental stress
• Altering ADLs to compensate for neurologic deficits
• Preventing constipation

Cerebrovascular accident

A CVA, commonly known as a stroke, results from a sudden impairment of cerebral circulation in one or more of the blood vessels supplying the brain. A CVA interrupts or diminishes oxygen supply and often causes serious damage or necrosis in brain tissues.

The sooner circulation returns to normal after CVA, the better the patient's chances for a complete recovery. However, about half of those who survive a CVA remain permanently disabled and experience a recurrence within weeks, months, or years.

CAUSES
• Cerebral arteriosclerosis

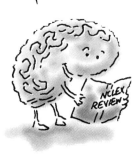

A CVA results from a sudden impairment of cerebral circulation in one or more of the blood vessels supplying the brain. Not cool.

• Embolism
• Hemorrhage
• Hypertension
• Thrombosis
• Vasospasm

ASSESSMENT FINDINGS
CVA symptoms depend on the artery affected. (See *Location, location, location.*)
  Generalized symptoms include:
• fever
• headache
• mental impairment
• seizures
• coma
• nuchal rigidity
• vomiting.

DIAGNOSTIC TEST RESULTS
• CT scan reveals intracranial bleeding, infarct (shows up 24 hours after the initial symptoms), or shift of midline structures.
• Digital subtraction angiography reveals occlusion or narrowing of vessels.
• EEG shows focal slowing in area of lesion.
• MRI shows intracranial bleeding, infarct, or shift of midline structures.

NURSING DIAGNOSES
• Altered cerebral tissue perfusion
• Risk for aspiration
• Risk for injury

TREATMENT
• Active and passive range-of-motion (ROM) and isometric exercises
• Bed rest, but out of bed when blood pressure stabilizes
• Low-sodium diet
• Physical therapy

Drug therapy
• Analgesics: codeine sulfate or codeine phosphate (if nothing- by-mouth status) to reduce headache
• Anticoagulants: heparin (Liquem), warfarin (Coumadin), ticlopidine (Ticlid)
• Anticonvulsant: phenytoin (Dilantin)
• Diuretics: mannitol (Osmitrol), furosemide (Lasix)

Location, location, location

Clinical features of cerebrovascular accident (CVA) vary with the artery affected (and, consequently, the portion of the brain the artery supplies), the severity of damage, and the extent of collateral circulation that develops to help the brain compensate for decreased blood supply.

Typical arteries affected and their associated signs and symptoms are described below.

MIDDLE CEREBRAL ARTERY
Injury to this artery causes aphasia, dysphagia, visual field cuts, and hemiparesis on the affected side (more severe in the face and arm than in the leg).

CAROTID ARTERY
If the carotid artery is affected, the patient may develop weakness, paralysis, numbness, sensory changes, and visual disturbances on the affected side; altered level of consciousness, bruits, headaches, aphasia, and ptosis.

VERTEBROBASILAR ARTERY
A CVA affecting this artery may lead to weakness on the affected side, numbness around the lips and mouth, visual field cuts, diplopia, poor coordination, dysphagia, slurred speech, dizziness, amnesia, and ataxia.

ANTERIOR CEREBRAL ARTERY
If this artery becomes affected, the patient may develop confusion, weakness, and numbness (especially in the leg) on affected side, incontinence, loss of coordination, impaired motor and sensory functions, and personality changes.

POSTERIOR CEREBRAL ARTERIES
If these arteries are affected, the patient may develop visual field cuts, sensory impairment, dyslexia, coma, and cortical blindness. Usually, paralysis is absent.

- Glucocorticoid: dexamethasone (Decadron)
- H_2-receptor antagonists: cimetidine (Tagamet), ranitidine (Zantac), famotidine (Pepcid)
- Thrombolytic therapy: tissue plasminogen activator given within the first 3 hours of an ischemic CVA to restore circulation to the affected brain tissue and limit the extent of brain injury

INTERVENTIONS AND RATIONALES
- Take vital signs every 1 to 2 hours initially, then every 4 hours when the patient becomes stable *to detect early signs of decreased cerebral perfusion pressure or increased ICP.*
- Elevate head of bed 30 degrees *to facilitate venous drainage and reduce cellular edema.*
- Maintain the patient's diet *to promote nutritional status and healing.*
- Administer I.V. fluids and monitor intake and output *to prevent volume overload or deficit.*
- Conduct a neurologic assessment every 1 to 2 hours initially, then every 4 hours when the patient becomes stable *to screen for changes in LOC and neurologic status.*

- Take patient's temperature at least every 4 hours. *Hyperthermia causes increased ICP; hypothermia causes reduced cerebral perfusion pressure.*
- Monitor hemoglobin and hematocrit and report anomalies *to prevent tissue ischemia.*
- Assess respiratory status at least every 4 hours *for signs of aspiration or respiratory depression.*
- Make sure that suction equipment is available and suction as needed *to keep airway clear.*
- Administer oxygen *to promote cerebral tissue oxygenation.*
- Assist the patient with coughing and deep breathing *to mobilize secretions.*
- Maintain position, patency, and low suction of NG tube. *Delayed gastric emptying and elevated intragastric pressure may cause regurgitation of stomach contents.*
- Administer enteral nutrition or TPN depending on the patient's condition *to facilitate tissue healing and meet metabolic needs.*

CVA care shifts focus. When the emergency has passed, care turns to rehab and recovery.

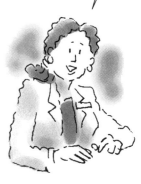

• Apply antiembolism stockings *to promote venous return and prevent thromboembolism formation.*
• Maintain seizure precautions and administer anticonvulsants, as ordered. *Seizures increase intrathoracic pressure, decrease cerebral venous outflow, and increase cerebral blood volume, thereby increasing ICP.*
• Provide passive ROM exercises *to prevent venous thrombosis and contractures.*
• Turn and position the patient every 2 hours *to prevent pressure ulcers.*
• Provide means of communication *to promote understanding and decrease anxiety.*
• Maintain routine bowel and bladder function and administer diuretics, as ordered, *to promote fluid mobilization.*
• Encourage the patient to express feelings about changes in body image and about difficulty in communicating verbally *to promote reduced anxiety and expression of feelings.*
• Maintain a quiet environment *to prevent increases in ICP.*
• Protect the patient from falls and injury and provide a safe environment *to reduce the risk of injury.*

Teaching topics
• Monitoring blood pressure
• Recognizing signs and symptoms of stroke
• Minimizing environmental stress
• Communicating effectively (for an aphasic patient)
• Using devices to assist in ADLs
• Reducing stress
• Contacting the American Heart Association and the National Stroke Association

Conjunctivitis

Conjunctivitis is characterized by inflammation of the conjunctiva, the delicate membrane that lines the eyelids and covers the exposed surface of the eyeball. It may result from infection, allergy, or chemical reactions.
 Conjunctivitis is common. Bacterial and viral conjunctivitis is highly contagious, but is also self-limiting after a couple of weeks' dura-

tion. Chronic conjunctivitis may result in degenerative changes to the eyelids.

CAUSES
The most common causative organisms are:
• bacterial: *Staphylococcus aureus, Streptococcus pneumoniae, Neisseria gonorrhoeae, N. meningitidis*
• chlamydial: *Chlamydia trachomatis* (inclusion conjunctivitis)
• viral: adenovirus types 3, 7, and 8; herpes simplex virus, type 1.

Other causes
• Allergic reactions to pollen, grass, topical medications, air pollutants, and smoke
• Fungal infections (rare)
• Occupational irritants (acids and alkalies)
• Parasitic diseases caused by *Phthirus pubis* or *Schistosoma haematobium*
• Rickettsial diseases (Rocky Mountain spotted fever)

ASSESSMENT FINDINGS
• Excessive tearing
• Hyperemia (engorgement) of the conjunctiva, sometimes accompanied by discharge and tearing
• Itching, burning
• Mucopurulent discharge

DIAGNOSTIC TEST RESULTS
• Culture and sensitivity tests identify the causative bacterial organism and indicate appropriate antibiotic therapy.

NURSING DIAGNOSES
• Risk for infection
• Sensory or perceptual alterations: Visual
• Body image disturbance

TREATMENT
• Cold compresses to relieve itching for allergic conjunctivitis
• Warm compresses to treat bacterial or viral conjunctivitis

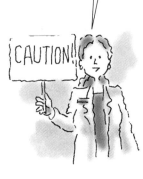

Encourage the patient with conjunctivitis to practice meticulous hygiene. The disorder can be highly contagious.

CAUTION!

Drug therapy

- Antiviral agents: vidarabine ointment (Vira-A) or oral acyclovir (Zovirax), if herpes simplex is the cause
- Corticosteroids: dexamethasone (Maxidex), fluorometholone (Fluor-Op Ophthalmic)
- Mast cell stabilizer: cromolyn (Opticrom), for allergic conjunctivitis
- Topical antibiotics according to sensitivity of infective organism (if bacterial cause)

INTERVENTIONS AND RATIONALES

- Teach proper hand-washing technique *because certain forms of conjunctivitis are highly contagious.*
- Stress the risk of spreading infection to family members by sharing washcloths, towels, and pillows. Warn against rubbing the infected eye, which can spread the infection to the other eye and to other persons. *These measures prevent the spread of infection.*
- Apply warm compresses and therapeutic ointment or drops. Don't irrigate the eye; *this will only spread infection.*
- Have the patient wash his hands before he uses the medication, and use clean washcloths or towels frequently *so he doesn't infect his other eye.*
- Teach the patient to instill eyedrops and ointments correctly—without touching the bottle tip to his eye or lashes *to prevent the spread of infection.*
- Stress the importance of safety glasses for the patient who works near chemical irritants *to prevent further episodes of conjunctivitis.*
- Notify public health authorities if cultures show *N. gonorrhoeae. Public health authorities track sexually transmitted diseases.*

Teaching topics

- Disease process and treatment options
- Proper hand washing
- Preventing the spread of infection
- Eye drop instillation

Corneal abrasion

A corneal abrasion is a scratch on the surface epithelium of the cornea, the dome-shaped

transparent structure in front of the eye. This common type of eye injury is commonly caused by a foreign body, such as a cinder or piece of dirt or by improper use of a contact lens.

CAUSES

- Improper use of contact lenses
- Trauma caused by a foreign body (such as a cinder or a piece of dust, dirt, or grit)

ASSESSMENT FINDINGS

- Burning
- Change in visual acuity (depending on the size and location of injury)
- Increased tearing
- Pain disproportionate to size of injury
- Redness
- Sensation of "something in the eye"

DIAGNOSTIC TEST RESULTS

- Staining the cornea with fluorescein stain confirms the diagnosis: the injured area appears green when examined with a flashlight.
- Slit-lamp examination discloses the depth of the abrasion.

NURSING DIAGNOSES

- Pain
- Risk for infection
- Sensory or perceptual alterations (visual)

TREATMENT

- Irrigation with saline solution
- Pressure patch (a tightly applied eye patch)
- Removal of a deeply embedded foreign body with a foreign body spud, using a topical anesthetic

Drug therapy

- Antibiotic: sulfisoxazole (Gantrisin)
- Cycloplegic agent: tropicamide (Ocu-Tropic)

INTERVENTIONS AND RATIONALES

- Assist with examination of the eye. Check visual acuity before beginning treatment *to assess visual loss from injury.*
- If foreign body is visible, carefully irrigate the eye with normal saline solution *to wash*

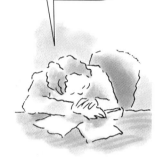

Corneal abrasions are common in people who fall asleep wearing hard contact lenses.

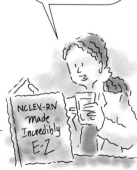

A pressure patch may be applied in corneal abrasion to prevent further corneal irritation if the patient blinks.

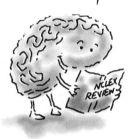

Encephalitis may produce only mild effects or it may cause permanent neurologic damage and death.

away the foreign body without damaging the eye.

• Tell the patient with an eye patch to leave the patch in place for 6 to 8 hours *to protect the eye from further corneal irritation when the patient blinks.*

• Warn the patient with an eye patch that wearing a patch alters depth perception, so advise caution in everyday activities, such as climbing stairs or stepping off a curb *to prevent injury.*

• Reassure the patient that the corneal epithelium usually heals in 24 to 48 hours *to allay anxiety.*

• Stress the importance of instilling prescribed antibiotic eyedrops *because an untreated corneal infection can lead to ulceration and permanent loss of vision.*

• Emphasize the importance of safety glasses *to protect workers' eyes from flying fragments.*

Teaching topics
• Eye drop instillation
• Proper contact use

Encephalitis

Encephalitis is a severe inflammation and swelling of the brain, usually caused by a mosquito-borne or, in some areas, a tick-borne virus. Transmission also may occur through ingestion of infected goat's milk and accidental injection or inhalation of the virus. Eastern equine encephalitis may produce permanent neurologic damage and is often fatal.

In encephalitis, intense lymphocytic infiltration of brain tissues and the leptomeninges causes cerebral edema, degeneration of the brain's ganglion cells, and diffuse nerve cell destruction.

CAUSES
• Exposure to virus

ASSESSMENT FINDINGS
• Coma (following the acute phase of illness)
• Meningeal irritation (stiff neck and back) and neuronal damage (drowsiness, coma, paralysis, seizures, ataxia, organic psychoses)

• Sensory alterations
• Sudden onset of fever
• Headache
• Vomiting

DIAGNOSTIC TEST RESULTS
• Blood studies identify the virus and confirm diagnosis
• CSF analysis identifies the virus
• Lumbar puncture discloses CSF pressure is elevated and, despite inflammation, the fluid is often clear. WBC and protein levels in CSF are slightly elevated, but the glucose level remains normal.
• EEG reveals abnormalities, such as generalized slowing of waveforms.
• CT scan may be ordered to rule out cerebral hematoma.

NURSING DIAGNOSES
• Altered thought processes
• Hyperthermia
• Impaired physical mobility

TREATMENT
• ET intubation and mechanical ventilation
• I.V. fluids
• NG tube feedings or TPN

Drug therapy
• Anticonvulsants: phenytoin (Dilantin), phenobarbital (Luminal)
• Antiviral: acyclovir (Zovirax) is effective only against herpes encephalitis and is only effective if administered before the onset of coma.
• Analgesic and antipyretics: aspirin or acetaminophen (Tylenol) to relieve headache and reduce fever.
• Diuretics: furosemide (Lasix) or mannitol (Osmitrol) to reduce cerebral swelling
• Corticosteroid: dexamethasone (Decadron) to reduce cerebral inflammation and edema
• Laxative: bisacodyl (Dulcolax)
• Sedatives: lorazepam (Ativan) for restlessness
• Stool softener: docusate (Colace)

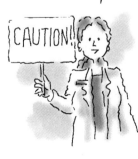

Encephalitis causes the patient to be extremely sensitive to light — keep the patient's room cool and dark.

INTERVENTIONS AND RATIONALES

During the acute phase of the illness:

• Assess neurologic function often. Observe the patient's mental status and cognitive abilities. *If the tissue within the brain becomes edematous, changes will occur in the patient's mental status and cognitive abilities.*

• Maintain adequate fluid intake *to prevent dehydration*, but avoid fluid overload, *which may increase cerebral edema.* Measure and record intake and output accurately *to assess fluid status.*

• Give acyclovir by slow I.V. infusion only. The patient must be well-hydrated and the infusion given over 1 hour *to avoid kidney damage.* Watch for adverse effects, such as nausea, diarrhea, pruritus, and rash, and adverse effects of other drugs *to prevent complications.* Check the infusion site often *to avoid infiltration and phlebitis.*

• Carefully position the patient *to prevent joint stiffness and neck pain,* and turn him often *to prevent skin breakdown.*

• Assist with ROM exercises *to maintain joint mobility.*

• Maintain adequate nutrition *to keep up with increased metabolic needs and promote healing.* It may be necessary to give the patient small, frequent meals or to supplement these meals with NG tube or parenteral feedings *to meet nutritional needs.*

• Give a stool softener or mild laxative *to prevent constipation and minimize the risk of increased ICP from straining during defecation.*

• Provide good mouth care *to prevent breakdown of oral mucous membrane.*

• Maintain a quiet environment *to promote comfort and decrease stimulation that can cause ICP to rise.* Darkening the room *may decrease photophobia and headache.*

• If the patient naps during the day and is restless at night, plan daytime activities *to minimize napping and promote sleep at night.*

• Provide emotional support and reassurance *because the patient is apt to be frightened by the illness and frequent diagnostic tests.*

• Reassure the patient and his family that behavioral changes caused by encephalitis usually disappear *to decrease anxiety.*

Teaching topics
• The disease and its effects
• Treatment and rehabilitation options

Glaucoma

In glaucoma, the patient experiences visual field loss due to damage to the optic nerve resulting from increased intraocular pressure. If left untreated, glaucoma can lead to blindness.

Glaucoma is either open-angle or angle-closure. In open-angle glaucoma, increased intraocular pressure is caused by overproduction of, or obstructed outflow of, aqueous humor (a fluid in the front of the eye). In angle-closure glaucoma, there is an obstructed outflow of aqueous humor due to anatomically narrow angles.

CAUSES
• Diabetes mellitus
• Family history of glaucoma
• Long-term steroid treatment
• Previous eye trauma or surgery
• Race (Blacks have higher incidences.)
• Uveitis

ASSESSMENT FINDINGS
Acute angle-closure glaucoma
• Acute ocular pain
• Blurred vision
• Dilated pupil
• Halo vision
• Increased intraocular pressure
• Nausea and vomiting

Chronic open-angle glaucoma
• Atrophy and cupping of optic nerve head
• Increased intraocular pressure
• Initially asymptomatic
• Narrowed field of vision
• Possible asymmetrical involvement

DIAGNOSTIC TEST RESULTS
• Gonioscopy reveals if angle is open or closed.
• Ophthalmoscopy shows atrophy and cupping of optic nerve head.
• Perimetry shows decreased field of vision

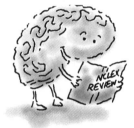

I see. Glaucoma damages the optic nerve, which sends me visual impulses for sight perception.

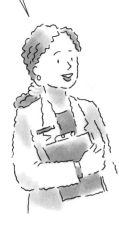

Angle-closure glaucoma is an emergency, requiring immediate treatment. If drugs don't lower intraocular pressure sufficiently, surgery follows.

• Tonometry shows increased intraocular pressure.

NURSING DIAGNOSES
• Anxiety
• Risk for injury
• Sensory or perceptual alterations (visual)

TREATMENT
Acute angle-closure glaucoma
This ocular emergency requires immediate treatment to lower intraocular pressure)
• Laser iridectomy or surgical iridectomy if pressure doesn't decrease with drug therapy

Drug therapy
Chronic open-angle glaucoma
• Alpha-adrenergic agonist: brimonidane (Alphagan)
• Beta-adrenergic antagonist: timolol (Timoptic)

Acute angle-closure glaucoma
• Cholinergic: pilocarpine

INTERVENTIONS AND RATIONALES
• Assess eye pain and administer medication as prescribed. *Medication reduces pain and may control disease process.*
• Provide a safe environment. *Orienting the patient to surroundings reduces the risk of injury.*
• Modify the environment *to meet patient's self-care needs.*
• For acute episode, limit activities that raise intraocular pressure. *Avoiding activities that increase intraocular pressure helps reduce complications.*
• Encourage the patient to express feelings about changes in body image *to aid acceptance of visual loss.*

Teaching topics
• Meticulous compliance with prescribed drug therapy to prevent an increase in intraocular pressure
• Monitoring eye for discharge, watering, blurred or cloudy vision, halos, flashes of light, and floaters

Guillain-Barré syndrome

Guillain-Barré syndrome is an acute, rapidly progressive, and potentially fatal form of polyneuritis (inflammation of several peripheral nerves at once) that causes muscle weakness and mild distal sensory loss.

Recovery is spontaneous and complete in about 95% of patients, although mild motor or reflex deficits in the feet and legs may persist. The prognosis is best when symptoms clear between 15 and 20 days after onset.

This disorder is also known as infectious polyneuritis, Landry-Guillain-Barré syndrome, and acute idiopathic polyneuritis

CAUSES AND CONTRIBUTING FACTORS
• Cell-mediated immune response with an attack on peripheral nerves in response to a virus.
• Demyelination of the peripheral nerves
• Respiratory infection

ASSESSMENT FINDINGS
• Dysphagia (difficulty swallowing) or dysarthria (poor speech caused by impaired muscular control)
• Facial diplegia (affecting like parts on both sides of the face; possibly accompanied by ophthalmoplegia [ocular paralysis]),
• Hypertonia (excessive muscle tone) and areflexia (absence of reflexes)
• Muscle weakness (ascending from the legs to arms)
• Paresthesia
• Stiffness and pain in the form of a severe "charley horse"
• Weakness of the muscles supplied by cranial nerve XI, the spinal accessory nerve; this is a less common finding; these muscles affect shoulder movement and head rotation

DIAGNOSTIC TEST RESULTS
• A history of preceding febrile illness (usually a respiratory tract infection) and typical clinical features suggest Guillain-Barré syndrome.
• CSF protein level begins to rise, peaking in 4 to 6 weeks. The CSF WBC count remains

normal, but in severe disease, CSF pressure may rise above normal.

- Blood studies reveal a complete blood count that shows leukocytosis with the presence of immature forms early in the illness, but blood study results soon return to normal.
- EMG may show repeated firing of the same motor unit, instead of widespread sectional stimulation.
- Nerve conduction velocities are slowed soon after paralysis develops. Diagnosis must rule out similar diseases, such as acute poliomyelitis.

NURSING DIAGNOSES
- Impaired physical mobility
- Ineffective breathing pattern
- Risk for injury

TREATMENT
- ET intubation or tracheotomy if the patient has difficulty clearing secretions; possible mechanical ventilation
- NG tube feedings or parenteral nutrition
- I.V. fluid therapy
- Specialty bed or support surfaces
- Plasmapheresis

Drug therapy
- Corticosteroid: prednisone (Deltasone)
- Antiarrhythmics: propranolol (Inderal), atropine
- Anticoagulants: heparin (Liquaem), warfarin (Coumadin)

INTERVENTIONS AND RATIONALES
- Watch for ascending sensory loss, which precedes motor loss. Also, monitor vital signs and LOC *to detect disease progression.*
- Assess and treat respiratory dysfunction *to prevent respiratory arrest.* If respiratory muscles are weak, take serial vital capacity recordings. Use a respirometer with a mouthpiece or a facemask for bedside testing *to ensure accurate measurement.*
- Obtain ABG measurements. *Because neuromuscular disease results in primary hypoventilation with hypoxemia and hypercapnia, watch for a partial pressure of arterial oxygen (Pao_2)*

below 70 mm Hg, which signals respiratory failure.

- Be alert for signs of a rising partial pressure of carbon dioxide (confusion, tachypnea) *to detect early signs of hypoventilation and avoid treatment delay.*
- Auscultate for breath sounds *to detect early changes in respiratory function,* and encourage coughing and deep breathing *to mobilize secretions and prevent atelectasis.*
- Begin respiratory support at the first sign of dyspnea (in adults, a vital capacity less than 800 ml) or a decreasing Pao_2 *to prevent hypoxemia.*
- If respiratory failure becomes imminent, establish an emergency airway with an ET tube *to prevent organ damage from anoxia.*
- Give meticulous skin care *to prevent skin breakdown and contractures.*
- Establish a strict turning schedule; inspect the skin (especially the sacrum, heels, and ankles) for breakdown, and reposition the patient every 2 hours. *These measures prevent skin breakdown and pressure ulcer development.*
- After each position change, stimulate circulation by carefully massaging pressure points. Also, use foam, gel, or alternating-pressure pads at points of contact *to prevent skin breakdown.*
- Perform passive ROM exercises within the patient's pain limits, perhaps using a Hubbard tank. Remember that the proximal muscle groups of the thighs, shoulders, and trunk will be the most tender and cause the most pain on passive movement and turning. *Passive ROM exercises maintain joint function.*
- When the patient's condition stabilizes, change to gentle stretching and active assistance exercises *to strengthen muscles and maintain joint function.*
- Assess the patient for signs of dysphagia (coughing, choking, "wet"-sounding voice, increased presence of rhonchi after feeding, drooling, delayed swallowing, regurgitation of food, and weakness in cranial nerves V, VII, IX, X, XI, or XII). *These measures help prevent aspiration.*

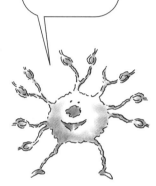

Time is on my side. The nerve damage of Guillain-Barré is usually temporary.

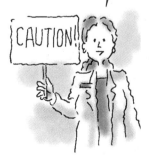

Potential complications of Guillain-Barré syndrome include mechanical ventilatory failure, aspiration pneumonia, sepsis, joint contractures, and deep vein thrombosis.

• Elevate the head of the bed, position the patient upright and leaning forward when eating, feed semisolid food, and check the mouth for food pockets *to minimize aspiration.*

• Encourage the patient to eat slowly and remain upright for 15 to 20 minutes after eating *to prevent aspiration.*

• If aspiration can't be minimized by diet and position modification, expect to provide NG feeding *to prevent aspiration and ensure that nutritional needs are met.*

• As the patient regains strength and can tolerate a vertical position, be alert for postural hypotension. Monitor blood pressure and pulse rate during tilting periods, and if necessary, apply toe-to-groin elastic bandages or an abdominal binder *to prevent postural hypotension.*

• Inspect the patient's legs regularly for signs of thrombophlebitis (localized pain, tenderness, erythema, edema, positive Homans' sign). *Thrombophlebitis is a common complication of Guillain-Barré syndrome.*

• Apply antiembolism stockings and give prophylactic anticoagulants, as needed *to prevent thrombophlebitis.*

• If the patient has facial paralysis, give eye and mouth care every 4 hours *to prevent corneal damage and breakdown of oral mucosa.*

• Protect the corneas with isotonic eyedrops and conical eye shields *to prevent corneal injury.*

• Encourage adequate fluid intake (2,000 ml/day), unless contraindicated *to prevent dehydration, constipation, and renal calculi formation.*

• Measure and record intake and output every 8 hours, and offer the bedpan every 3 to 4 hours *to monitor for urine retention.*

• Begin intermittent catheterization, as needed *to relieve urine retention.* The patient may need manual pressure on the bladder (Credé's method) before he can urinate *because the abdominal muscles are weak.*

• Offer prune juice and a high-bulk diet *to prevent and relieve constipation.* If necessary, give daily or alternate-day suppositories (glycerin or bisacodyl) or Fleet enemas *to relieve constipation.*

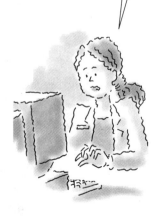

In Huntington's disease, uncontrollable body movements called chorea develop over time and are followed by mental deterioration.

• Refer the patient for physical therapy, occupational therapy, and speech therapy, as needed.

Teaching topics
• Transferring from bed to wheelchair and from wheelchair to toilet or tub and how to walk short distances with a walker or cane
• Caregiving strategies for the family, such as how to help the patient eat, compensate for facial weakness, and help avoid skin breakdown as well as the need for a regular bowel and bladder routine

Huntington's disease

Huntington's disease is a hereditary disease in which degeneration in the cerebral cortex and basal ganglia causes chronic progressive chorea (involuntary and irregular movements) and cognitive deterioration, ending in dementia.

Huntington's disease usually strikes people between ages 25 and 55 (the average age is 35). Death usually results 10 to 15 years after onset from suicide, heart failure, or pneumonia. The disorder is also called Huntington's chorea, hereditary chorea, chronic progressive chorea, and adult chorea.

CAUSES
• Genetic transmission: autosomal dominant trait. (Either sex can transmit and inherit the disease.) Each child of a parent with this disease has a 50% chance of inheriting it; however, a child who doesn't inherit it can't pass it on to his own children.

ASSESSMENT FINDINGS
• Choreic movements; rapid, often violent and purposeless; become progressively severe; may include mild fidgeting, tongue smacking, dysarthria (indistinct speech), athetoid movements (slow, sinuous, writhing movements, especially of the hands), and torticollis (twisting of the neck)
• Dementia (can be mild at first but eventually disrupts the patient's personality)
• Gradual loss of musculoskeletal control, eventually leading to total dependence

• Personality changes, such as obstinacy, carelessness, untidiness, moodiness, apathy, loss of memory, and, possibly, paranoia (in later stages of dementia)

DIAGNOSTIC TEST RESULTS
• PET detects the disease.
• Deoxyribonucleic acid analysis detects the disease.
• CT scan reveals brain atrophy.
• MRI demonstrates brain atrophy.
• Molecular genetics may detect the gene for Huntington's disease in people at risk while they're still asymptomatic.

NURSING DIAGNOSES
• Impaired physical mobility
• Altered health maintenance
• Risk for injury

TREATMENT
• Because Huntington's disease has no known cure, treatment is supportive, protective, and aimed at relieving symptoms.

Drug therapy
• Antipsychotics: chlorpromazine (Thorazine) and haloperidol (Haldol) help control choreic movements
• Antidepressant: imipramine (Tofranil) helps control choreic movements

INTERVENTIONS AND RATIONALES
• Provide physical support by attending to the patient's basic needs, such as hygiene, skin care, bowel and bladder care, and nutrition. Increase this support as mental and physical deterioration make him increasingly immobile. *These measures help prevent complications of immobility.*
• Assist in designing a behavioral plan that deals with the disruptive and aggressive behavior and impulse control problems. Reinforce positive behaviors, and maintain consistency with all caregiving. *These interventions consistently limit the patient's negative behaviors.*
• Offer emotional support to the patient and his family *to relieve anxiety and enhance coping.* Keep in mind the patient's dysarthria, and

allow him extra time to express himself, *thereby decreasing frustration.*
• Stay alert for possible suicide attempts. Control the patient's environment to protect him from suicide or other self-inflicted injury. *The patient may be unable to cope with the devastating nature of the disease.*
• Pad the side rails of the bed but avoid restraints, *which may cause the patient to injure himself with violent, uncontrolled movements.*
• If the patient has difficulty walking, provide a walker *to help him maintain his balance.*
• Refer the patient and his family to appropriate community organizations.

Teaching topics
• Disease process
• Family participation in the patient's care
• Importance of genetic counseling (Each child of a parent with this disease has a 50% chance of inheriting it.)
• Contact information for the Huntington's Disease Association

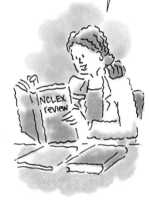

Slow down. Allow the patient with Huntington's disease extra time to express himself.

Ménière's disease

Ménière's disease is a dysfunction in the labyrinth (the part of the ear that produces balance) that produces severe vertigo, sensorineural hearing loss, and tinnitus. It usually affects adults, men slightly more often than women, between the ages of 30 and 60. After multiple attacks over several years, this disorder leads to residual tinnitus and hearing loss.

This disorder may also be called endolymphatic hydrops.

CAUSES
• Autonomic nervous system dysfunction that produces a temporary constriction of blood vessels supplying the inner ear
• Overproduction or decreased absorption of endolymph, which causes endolymphatic hydrops or endolymphatic hypertension, with consequent degeneration of the vestibular and cochlear hair cells

ASSESSMENT FINDINGS
- Sensorineural hearing loss
- Severe vertigo
- Tinnitus
- Feeling of fullness or blockage in the ear
- Severe nausea
- Vomiting
- Sweating
- Giddiness
- Nystagmus

DIAGNOSTIC TEST RESULTS
- Electronystagmography, electrocochleography, a CT scan, MRI, and X-rays of the internal meatus may be necessary for differential diagnosis.
- Audiometric studies indicate a sensorineural hearing loss and loss of discrimination and recruitment

NURSING DIAGNOSES
- Impaired physical mobility
- Risk for injury
- Sensory or perceptual alterations (auditory)

TREATMENT
- Restrict sodium intake to less than 2 g/day.
- Surgery to destroy the affected labyrinth: only if medical treatment fails; destruction of the labyrinth permanently relieves symptoms but at the expense of irreversible hearing loss.

Drug therapy
- Anticholinergic: atropine (may stop an attack in 20 to 30 minutes)
- Cardiac stimulant: epinephrine (Adrenalin)
- Diuretic to prevent excess fluid in the labyrinth (long-term management)
- Antihistamine: diphenhydramine (Benadryl) (may be necessary in a severe attack)
- Antihistamines: meclizine (Antivert), dimenhydrinate (Dramamine) (for milder attacks; may also be administered as part of prophylactic therapy)
- Sedatives: phenobarbital (Luminal), diazepam (Valium); administered as part of prophylactic therapy

INTERVENTIONS AND RATIONALES
If the patient is in the facility during an attack of Ménière's disease:
- Advise the patient against reading and exposure to glaring lights *to reduce dizziness.*
- Keep the side rails of the patient's bed up *to prevent falls.* Tell him not to get out of bed or walk without assistance *to prevent injury.*
- Instruct the patient to avoid sudden position changes and any tasks that vertigo makes hazardous *because an attack can begin quite rapidly.*

Before surgery:
- If the patient is vomiting, record fluid intake and output and characteristics of vomitus *to prevent dehydration.* Administer antiemetics as necessary, and give small amounts of fluid frequently *to prevent vomiting.*

After surgery:
- Record intake and output carefully *to monitor fluid status and direct the treatment plan.*
- Tell the patient to expect dizziness and nausea for 1 or 2 days after surgery *to relieve anxiety.*
- Give prophylactic antibiotics and antiemetics as required *to decrease the chance of infection and combat nausea.*

Teaching topics
- Disease process and treatment options
- Measures to combat dizziness, such as rising slowly from a sitting or lying position.

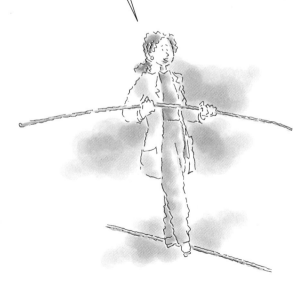

In Ménière's disease, an increase in the amount of fluid in the labyrinth increases pressure in the inner ear and leads to a disruption in the sense of balance.

Meningitis

In meningitis, the brain and the spinal cord meninges become inflamed, usually as a result of bacterial infection. Such inflammation may involve all three meningeal membranes: the dura mater, arachnoid, and pia mater.

The prognosis is good and complications are rare, especially if the disease is recognized early and the infecting organism responds to antibiotics. The prognosis is poorer for infants and elderly people. Mortality is high in untreated meningitis.

CAUSES
• Bacterial infection (may occur secondary to bacteremia [especially from pneumonia, empyema, osteomyelitis, and endocarditis], sinusitis, otitis media, encephalitis, myelitis, or brain abscess)
• Head trauma (may follow a skull fracture, a penetrating head wound, lumbar puncture, or ventricular shunting procedure)
• Virus (in aseptic viral meningitis, which is usually mild and self-limiting)
• Fungal or protozoal infection (less common)

ASSESSMENT FINDINGS
• Chills
• Coma
• Confusion
• Deep stupor
• Delirium
• Exaggerated deep tendon reflexes
• Fever
• Headache
• increased ICP
• Irritability
• Malaise
• Opisthotonos (a spasm in which the back and extremities arch backward so that the body rests on the head and heels)
• Petechial, purpuric, or ecchymotic rash on the lower part of the body (meningococcal meningitis)
• Photophobia
• Positive Brudzinski's sign, in which the patient flexes hips or knees when the nurse places her hands behind his neck and bends it forward (a sign of meningeal inflammation and irritation)
• Positive Kernig's sign (Pain or resistance when the patient's leg is flexed at the hip or knee while he's in a supine position)
• Seizures
• Stiff neck and back
• Twitching
• Visual alterations (diplopia — two images of a single object)
• Vomiting

DIAGNOSTIC TEST RESULTS
• An LP shows elevated CSF pressure, cloudy or milky white CSF, high protein level, positive Gram stain and culture that usually identifies the infecting organism (unless it's a virus) and depressed CSF glucose concentration.
• Chest X-rays may reveal pneumonitis or lung abscess, tubercular lesions, or granulomas secondary to fungal infection.
• Sinus and skull films may help identify the presence of cranial osteomyelitis, paranasal sinusitis, or skull fracture.
• WBC count reveals leukocytosis.
• CT scan can rule out cerebral hematoma, hemorrhage, or tumor.

NURSING DIAGNOSES
• Decreased adaptive capacity: Intracranial
• Hyperthermia
• Risk for injury

TREATMENT
• Bed rest
• Hypothermia
• I.V. fluid administration
• Oxygen therapy, possibly with ET intubation and mechanical ventilation

Drug therapy
• Antibiotics: penicillin G (Pfizerpen), ampicillin (Omnipen), or nafcillin (Unipen); tetracycline (Achromycin V), or chloramphenicol (Chloromycetin), if allergic to penicillin
• Digitalis glycoside: digoxin (Lanoxin)
• Diuretic: mannitol (Osmitrol)
• Anticonvulsant: phenytoin (Dilantin), phenobarbital (Luminal)

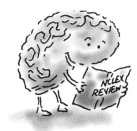

Blame it on bacteria. In meningitis, the brain and the spinal cord meninges become inflamed, usually as a result of bacterial infection.

- Analgesics or antipyretics: acetaminophen (Tylenol), aspirin
- Anesthetic: lidocaine (Xylocaine)
- Laxative: bisacodyl (Dulcolax)
- Stool softener: docusate (Colace)

INTERVENTIONS AND RATIONALES

- Assess neurologic function often *to detect early signs of increased ICP, such as plucking at the bedcovers, vomiting, seizures, a change in motor function and vital signs. Detecting early signs of increased ICP prevents treatment delay.*
- Watch for deterioration in the patient's condition, *which may signal an impending crisis.*
- Monitor fluid balance. Maintain adequate fluid intake *to avoid dehydration without causing fluid overload which may lead to cerebral edema.*
- Measure central venous pressure and intake and output accurately *to determine fluid volume status.*
- Suction the patient only if necessary. Limit suctioning to 10 to 15 seconds per pass of the catheter. *Suctioning stimulates coughing and Valsalva's maneuver; Valsalva's maneuvers increase intrathoracic pressure, decrease cerebral venous drainage, and increase cerebral blood volume, resulting in increased ICP.*
- Hyperoxygenate the lungs with 100% oxygen for 1 minute before and after suctioning. *Hypercapnia results in cerebral vasodilation, increased blood volume, and increased ICP. Preoxygenation helps avoid hypoxemia and tissue ischemia.*
- Administer lidocaine, if prescribed, I.V. or into the ET tube before suctioning. *Lidocaine suppresses the cough reflex, thereby preventing increases in ICP.*
- Watch for adverse reactions to I.V. antibiotics and other drugs *to prevent complications such as anaphylaxis.*
- Check the I.V. site often, and change the site according to facility policy *to avoid infiltration and phlebitis.*
- Position the patient carefully *to prevent joint stiffness and neck pain.*
- Turn the patient often, according to a planned positioning schedule *to prevent skin breakdown.*
- Assist with ROM exercises *to prevent contractures.*

- It may be necessary to provide small, frequent meals or supplement meals with NG tube or parenteral feedings *to maintain adequate nutrition and elimination.*
- Give the patient a mild laxative or stool softener *to prevent constipation and minimize the risk of increased ICP resulting from straining during defecation.*
- Ensure the patient's comfort *to prevent rises in ICP.*
- Provide mouth care regularly *to prevent breakdown of oral mucosa and promote patient comfort.*
- Maintain a quiet environment. *Auditory stimuli can contribute to increased ICP.*
- Darken the room *to decrease photophobia.*
- Relieve headache with a nonnarcotic analgesic, such as aspirin or acetaminophen, as needed. *Narcotics interfere with accurate neurologic assessment.*
- Provide reassurance and support. The patient may be frightened by his illness and frequent LPs. *These measures decrease anxiety; emotional upsets may increase ICP.*
- Reassure the family that the delirium and behavior changes caused by meningitis usually disappear *to allay anxiety.*
- Follow strict aseptic technique when treating patients with head wounds or skull fractures *to prevent meningitis.*

Teaching topics

- Preventing meningitis (teach patients with chronic sinusitis or other chronic infections the importance of proper medical treatment)
- Recognizing signs of meningitis
- Contagion risks; notifying anyone who came in close contact with the patient

Multiple sclerosis

Multiple sclerosis is a progressive disease that destroys myelin in the neurons of the brain and spinal cord. Degeneration of the myelin sheath results in patches of sclerotic tissue and impairs the ability of the nervous system to conduct motor nerve impulses.

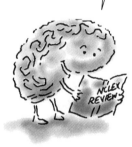

Shhh. Auditory stimuli can contribute to increased ICP. Plus, as you can see, I'm studying.

CAUSES
- Autoimmune response
- Environmental or genetic factors
- Slow-acting or latent viral infection
- Unknown

ASSESSMENT FINDINGS
- Ataxia
- Feelings of euphoria
- Heat intolerance
- Inability to sense or gauge body position
- Intention tremor
- Nystagmus, diplopia, blurred vision, optic neuritis
- Scanning speech
- Urinary incontinence or retention
- Weakness, paresthesia, impaired sensation, paralysis

DIAGNOSTIC TEST RESULTS
- CSF analysis shows increased immunoglobulin G, protein, and WBCs or it may be normal.
- CT scan eliminates other diagnoses such as brain or spinal cord tumors
- MRI eliminates other diagnoses such as brain or spinal cord tumors

NURSING DIAGNOSES
- Ineffective airway clearance
- Impaired physical mobility
- Altered nutrition: Less than body requirements

TREATMENT
- A high-calorie, high-vitamin, gluten-free, and low-fat diet
- Increased intake of fluids
- Physical therapy
- Plasmapheresis (for antibody removal)
- Speech therapy

Drug therapy
- Cholinergic: bethanechol (Urecholine)
- Glucocorticoids: prednisone (Deltasone), dexamethasone (Decadron), corticotropin (ACTH)
- Immunosuppressants: interferon beta-1b (Betaseron), cyclophosphamide (Cytoxan), methotrexate (Folex)

- Skeletal muscle relaxants: dantrolene (Dantrium), baclofen (Lioresal)

INTERVENTIONS AND RATIONALES
- Assess changes in motor coordination, paralysis, or muscular weakness *to facilitate early intervention.*
- Assess respiratory status at least every 4 hours *to detect early signs of compromise.*
- Maintain the patient's diet *to decrease risk of constipation.*
- Force fluids *to decrease risk of urinary tract infection.*
- Administer medications, as prescribed, *to improve or maintain patient's condition and functional status.*
- Encourage the patient to express feelings about changes in body image *to promote acceptance of muscular impairment.*
- Maintain active and passive exercises *to maintain ROM and prevent musculoskeletal degeneration.*
- Establish bowel and bladder program *to decrease risk of constipation and urinary retention.*
- Maintain activity, as tolerated (alternating rest and activity), *to improve muscle tone and enhance self-esteem.*
- Protect the patient from falls *to prevent injury.*
- Monitor patient's neuromuscular status and voiding pattern *to facilitate early interventions for urinary retention.*

Teaching topics
- Reducing stress
- Recognizing the signs and symptoms of exacerbation
- Avoiding exposure to people with infections
- Alternating rest and activity
- Maintaining a safe, quiet environment
- Using devices to assist with daily living
- Maintaining a sense of independence
- Avoiding temperature extremes, especially heat
- Contacting the National Multiple Sclerosis Society

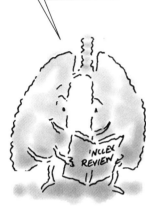

Heads up. Respiratory muscle weakness in myasthenic crisis may require an emergency airway and mechanical ventilation.

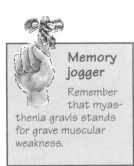

Memory jogger

Remember that myasthenia gravis stands for grave muscular weakness.

Myasthenia gravis

A neuromuscular disorder, myasthenia gravis is marked by weakness of voluntary muscles. The patient experiences sporadic, progressive weakness and abnormal fatigue of voluntary skeletal muscles.

Myasthenia gravis is characterized by a disturbance in transmission of nerve impulses at neuromuscular junctions. This transmission defect results from a deficiency in release of acetylcholine or a deficient number of acetylcholine receptor sites.

CAUSES
- Autoimmune disease
- Excessive cholinesterase
- Insufficient acetylcholine

ASSESSMENT FINDINGS
- Diplopia, ptosis, strabismus
- Dysarthria
- Dysphagia, drooling
- Impaired speech
- Masklike expression
- Muscle weakness and fatigue (Typically, muscles are strongest in the morning but weaken throughout the day, especially after exercise.)
- Profuse sweating
- Respiratory distress

DIAGNOSTIC TEST RESULTS
- EMG shows decreased amplitude of evoked potentials.
- Neostigmine (Prostigmin) or edrophonium (Tensilon) test relieves symptoms after medication administration (which is a positive indication of the disease).
- Thymus scan reveals hyperplasia or thymoma.

NURSING DIAGNOSES
- Impaired gas exchange
- Impaired physical mobility
- Impaired verbal communication

TREATMENT
- A high-calorie diet with soft foods
- Plasmapheresis (in severe exacerbations)

Drug therapy
- Anticholinesterase inhibitors: neostigmine (Prostigmin), pyridostigmine (Mestinon)
- Glucocorticoids: prednisone (Deltasone), dexamethasone (Decadron), corticotropin (ACTH)
- Immunosuppressants: azathioprine (Imuran), cyclophosphamide (Cytoxan)

INTERVENTIONS AND RATIONALES
- Assess neurologic and respiratory status. *Respiratory muscle weakness may be severe enough in myasthenic crisis to require an emergency airway and mechanical ventilation.*
- Assess swallow and gag reflexes *to prevent aspiration and determine extent of neurologic deficit.*
- Watch the patient for choking while eating *to prevent aspiration of food particles.*
- Monitor and record vital signs and intake and output *to prevent fluid overload or deficit and facilitate early intervention for deterioration of respiratory status.*
- Administer medications, as prescribed, *to relieve symptoms.*
- Maintain the patient's diet; encourage small, frequent meals *to conserve energy and meet nutritional needs.*
- Encourage the patient to express feelings about changes in body image and about difficulty in communicating verbally *to reduce patient's tendency to suppress or repress feelings about neuromuscular loss.*
- Determine the patient's activity tolerance and assist in ADLs *to conserve energy and avoid fatigue.*
- Provide rest periods *to reduce the body's oxygen demands and prevent fatigue.*
- Provide oral hygiene *to promote comfort and enhance appetite.*
- Improve environmental safety *to protect the patient from falls.*

Teaching topics
- Reducing stress
- Recognizing the signs and symptoms of respiratory distress
- Recognizing the signs and symptoms of myasthenic crisis
- Adhering to activity limitations
- Contacting the Myasthenia Gravis Foundation

Otosclerosis

Otosclerosis is marked by an overgrowth of the ear's spongy bone around the oval window and stapes footplate. This overgrowth curtails movement of the stapes in the oval window, preventing sound from being transmitted to the cochlea and resulting in conductive hearing loss.

CAUSES
• Familial tendency

ASSESSMENT FINDINGS
• Progressive hearing loss
• Tinnitus

DIAGNOSTIC TEST RESULTS
• Audiometric testing confirms hearing loss.

NURSING DIAGNOSES
• Anxiety
• Impaired verbal communication
• Sensory or perceptual alterations (auditory)

TREATMENT
• Hearing aid (air conduction aid with molded ear insert receiver)
• Stapedectomy and insertion of a prosthesis to restore partial or total hearing

Drug therapy
• Antibiotics postoperatively to prevent infection

INTERVENTIONS AND RATIONALES
• Monitor vital signs, and monitor dressing postoperatively for signs of bleeding *to detect complications.*
• Develop alternative means of communication *to decrease anxiety and communicate effectively with the patient.*

Teaching topics
• Using a hearing aid
• Avoiding loud noises and sudden pressure changes until healing is complete
• Avoiding (for at least 1 week) blowing the nose to prevent contaminated air and bacteria from entering the eustachian tube
• Protecting the ears against cold
• Avoiding activities that provoke dizziness
• Changing external ear dressings

Parkinson's disease

Parkinson's disease is a progressive, degenerative disorder of the CNS associated with dopamine deficiency. This lack of dopamine impairs the area of the brain responsible for control of voluntary movement. As a result, most symptoms relate to problems with posture and movement.

CAUSES
• Cerebral vascular disease
• Dopamine deficiency
• Drug-induced
• Imbalance of dopamine and acetylcholine in basal ganglia
• Repeated head trauma
• Unknown

ASSESSMENT FINDINGS
• "Pill-rolling" tremors, tremors at rest
• Difficulty in initiating voluntary activity
• Dysphagia, drooling
• Fatigue
• Masklike facial expression
• Shuffling gait, stiff joints, dyskinesia, "cogwheel" rigidity, stooped posture
• Small handwriting

DIAGNOSTIC TEST RESULTS
• CT scan is normal.
• EEG reveals minimal slowing of brain activity.

NURSING DIAGNOSES
• Activity intolerance
• Impaired physical mobility
• Altered nutrition: Less than body requirements

TREATMENT
• A high-residue, high-calorie, high-protein diet composed primarily of soft foods
• Physical therapy

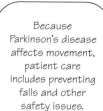

Loud noises are bad for otosclerosis patients and for NCLEX review. Find a quiet, calm place to study.

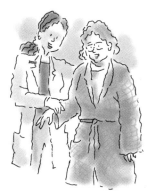

Because Parkinson's disease affects movement, patient care includes preventing falls and other safety issues.

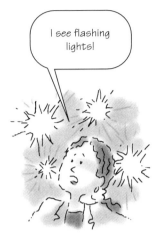

I see flashing lights!

• Stereotactic neurosurgery: thalamotomy or pallidotomy

Drug therapy
• Anticholinergics: trihexyphenidyl (Artane)
• Antidepressant: amitriptyline (Elavil)
• Antiparkinsonian agents: levodopa (Larodopa), carbidopa-levodopa (Sinemet), benztropine (Cogentin)
• Antispasmodic: procyclidine (Kemadrin)
• Antiviral agent: amantadine (Symmetrel) is used early on to reduce tremors and rigidity
• Dopamine receptor agonists: pergolide (Permax), bromocriptine (Parlodel)
• Enzyme inhibiting agent: selegiline (Eldepryl)

INTERVENTIONS AND RATIONALES
• Assess neurologic and respiratory status *to detect change in status and possible need for change in treatment.*
• Monitor and record vital signs and intake and output *to detect complications.*
• Monitor patient at mealtimes *to decrease risk of aspiration.*
• Position the patient *to prevent contractures and maintain skin integrity.*
• Administer medications, as prescribed *to improve functioning.* (Elderly patients may need smaller doses of anti-Parkinsonian drugs because of reduced tolerance. Be alert for and report orthostatic hypotension, irregular pulse, blepharospasm, and anxiety or confusion.)
• Encourage the patient to express feelings about changes in body image *to reduce anxiety and depression.*
• Promote daily ambulation *to promote independence.*
• Provide active and passive ROM exercises *to maintain mobility.*
• Maintain the patient's diet *to decrease constipation.*
• Provide skin care daily *to maintain skin integrity.*
• Provide oral hygiene *to promote self-care and improve nutritional intake.*
• Reinforce gait training *to improve mobility.*
• Reinforce independence in care *to maintain self-esteem.*

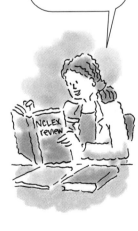

Speaking of seeing, be sure that you've got good lighting. It'll help you study longer and more comfortably.

Teaching topics
• Recognizing early signs and symptoms of respiratory distress
• Alternating rest periods with activity
• Promoting a safe environment (Shuffling gait and rigidity make patients very prone to falls, so encourage family members to remove obstacles and throw rugs.)
• Preventing choking
• Eating soft foods cut into small pieces
• Increasing intake of roughage and fluids to prevent constipation.

Retinal detachment

Retinal detachment is the separation of the retina (a thin, semitransparent layer of nerve tissue that lines the eye wall) from the choroid (the middle vascular coat of the eye between the retina and the sclera). It occurs when the retina develops a hole or tear and the vitreous seeps between the retina and choroid. If left untreated, retinal detachment can lead to vision loss.

CAUSES
• Aging
• Diabetic neovascularization
• Familial tendency
• Hemorrhage
• Inflammatory process
• Myopia
• Trauma
• Tumor

ASSESSMENT FINDINGS
• Painless change in vision (floaters and flashes of light)
• Photopsia (recurrent flashes of light)
• With progression of detachment, painless vision loss may be described as veil, curtain or cobweb that eliminates part of visual field

DIAGNOSTIC TEST RESULTS
• Indirect ophthalmoscope shows retinal tear or detachment.
• Slit-lamp examination shows retinal tear or detachment
• Ultrasound shows retinal tear or detachment in presence of cataract.

NURSING DIAGNOSES
- Anxiety
- Risk for injury
- Sensory or perceptual alterations (visual)

TREATMENT
- Complete bed rest and restriction of eye movement to prevent further detachment
- Cryopexy, if there is a hole in the peripheral retina
- Laser therapy, if there is a hole in the posterior portion of the retina
- Scleral buckling to reattach the retina

INTERVENTIONS AND RATIONALES
- Assess visual status and functional vision in unaffected eye *to determine self-care needs.*
- Postoperatively instruct the patient to lie on his back or on his unoperated side *to reduce intraocular pressure on the affected side.*
- Discourage straining during defecation, bending down, and hard coughing, sneezing, or vomiting *to avoid activities that can increase intraocular pressure.*
- Provide assistance with ADLs *to minimize frustration and strain.*
- Assist with ambulation, as needed, *to help the patient remain independent.*
- Approach patient from the unaffected side *to avoid startling the patient.*
- Orient patient to his environment *to reduce the risk of injury.*

Teaching topics
- Need for eye rest
- Keeping walkways free of clutter to prevent falls

Spinal cord injury

Spinal cord injuries usually result from traumatic force on the vertebral column, which, in turn, injures the spinal cord. Necrosis and scar tissue form in the area of the traumatized cord. Damage to the spinal cord results in sensory and motor deficits. The patient may experience partial or full loss of function of any or all extremities and bodily functions.

CAUSES
- Car accidents
- Congenital anomalies
- Diving into shallow water
- Falls
- Gunshot wounds
- Infections
- Stab wounds
- Tumors

ASSESSMENT FINDINGS
- Absence of reflexes below the level of the injury
- Flaccid muscle
- Loss of bowel and bladder control
- Neck pain
- Numbness and tingling
- Paralysis below the level of the injury
- Paresthesia below the level of the injury
- Respiratory distress

DIAGNOSTIC TEST RESULTS
- CT scan shows spinal cord edema, vertebral fracture, and spinal cord compression.
- MRI shows spinal cord edema, vertebral fracture, and spinal cord compression.
- Spinal X-rays reveal vertebral fracture.

NURSING DIAGNOSES
- Impaired physical mobility
- Posttrauma response
- Powerlessness

TREATMENT
- Flat position, with neck immobilized in a cervical collar
- Maintenance of vertebral alignment through Crutchfield tongs, Halo vest
- Specialized rotation bed
- Surgery for stabilization of the upper spine, such as insertion of Harrington rods

Drug therapy
- Antianxiety agent: lorazepam (Ativan)
- Glucocorticoid: methylprednisolone (Solu-Medrol) infusion immediately following injury (possible; improves neurologic recovery when administered within 8 hours of injury)

• H$_2$-receptor antagonists: cimetidine (Tagamet), ranitidine (Zantac), famotidine (Pepcid)
• Laxative: bisacodyl (Dulcolax)
• Mucosal barrier fortifier: sucralfate (Carafate)
• Muscle relaxant: dantrolene (Dantrium)

INTERVENTIONS AND RATIONALES

• Assess neurologic and respiratory status *to determine baseline and detect early complications.*
• Assess for spinal shock *to detect early changes in patient's condition.*
• Monitor and record vital signs and intake and output, laboratory studies, and pulse oximetry *to detect early changes in patient's condition.*
• Check for autonomic dysreflexia (sudden extreme rise in blood pressure) *to prevent life-threatening complications.*
• Administer fluids *to maintain hydration.*
• Administer oxygen as needed *to maintain oxygenation to cells.*
• Provide suctioning, if necessary, and encourage coughing and deep breathing *to maintain patent airway.*
• Administer medications, as prescribed, *to maintain or improve patient's condition.*
• Encourage the patient to express feelings about changes in body image, changes in sexual expression and function, and altered mobility *to reduce anxiety and depression.*
• Turn the patient every 2 hours using the logrolling technique (only if the patient is stabilized and not in a specialty bed) *to prevent pressure ulcers.*
• Maintain patient safety; keep tool available to open Halo vest in the case of cardiac arrest *to maintain patient safety.*
• Maintain body alignment *to maintain joint function and prevent musculoskeletal degeneration.*
• Initiate bowel and bladder retraining *to avoid stimuli that could trigger dysreflexia.*
• Provide passive ROM exercises *to maintain ROM and joint mobility.*
• Provide skin care *to avoid discomfort and loss of skin integrity because that can become a permanent impairment. Maintaining skin integrity becomes a priority after the patient is stabilized.*

• Apply antiembolism stockings *to maintain venous circulation and prevent thromboembolism.*
• Provide sexual counseling *to encourage questions and avoid misunderstandings.*

Teaching topics
• Exercising regularly to strengthen muscles
• Recognizing the signs and symptoms of autonomic dysreflexia, urinary tract infection, and upper respiratory infection
• Continuing a bowel and bladder program
• Maintaining acidic urine with cranberry juice
• Consuming adequate fluids: 3,000 ml/day
• Using assistive devices with proper body mechanics for ADLs
• Maintaining skin integrity
• Using a wheelchair and proper transfer techniques such as moving the strong part of the patient's body to the chair first
• Maintaining a sense of independence
• Contacting the National Spinal Cord Injury Association

Trigeminal neuralgia

Trigeminal neuralgia is a painful disorder of one or more branches of the fifth cranial (trigeminal) nerve that produces paroxysmal attacks of excruciating facial pain. Attacks are precipitated by stimulation of a trigger zone, a hypersensitive area of the face.

It occurs mostly in people over age 40, in women more often than men, and on the right side of the face more often than the left. Trigeminal neuralgia can subside spontaneously, with remissions lasting from several months to years. The disorder is also called tic douloureux.

CAUSES
Although the cause remains undetermined, trigeminal neuralgia may:
• reflect an afferent reflex phenomenon located centrally in the brain stem or more peripherally in the sensory root of the trigeminal nerve
• be related to compression of the nerve root by posterior fossa tumors, middle fossa tu-

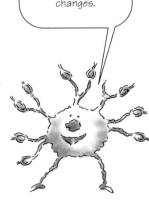

Who says I'm not sensitive? In trigeminal neuralgia, pain may be triggered by touching a sensitive area on the face or even by temperature changes.

mors, or vascular lesions (subclinical aneurysm), although such lesions usually produce simultaneous loss of sensation
• occasionally be a manifestation of multiple sclerosis or herpes zoster.

ASSESSMENT FINDINGS
• Searing pain in the facial area

Triggers
• Light touch to a sensitive area of the face (trigger zone)
• Exposure to hot or cold
• Eating, smiling, or talking
• Drinking hot or cold beverages

DIAGNOSTIC TEST RESULTS
• Observation during the examination shows the patient favoring (splinting) the affected area. To ward off a painful attack, the patient often holds his face immobile when talking. He may also leave the affected side of his face unwashed and unshaven.
• Skull X-rays, tomography, and CT scan rule out sinus or tooth infections, and tumors.

NURSING DIAGNOSES
• Pain
• Powerlessness
• Anxiety

TREATMENT
• Percutaneous radio frequency procedure, which causes partial root destruction and relieves pain
• Microsurgery for vascular decompression.
• Percutaneous electrocoagulation of nerve rootlets, under local anesthesia.

Drug therapy
• Anticonvulsants: carbamazepine (Tegretol) or phenytoin (Dilantin) may temporarily relieve or prevent pain

INTERVENTIONS AND RATIONALES
• Observe and record the characteristics of each attack, including the patient's protective mechanisms *to gain information for developing the treatment plan.*
• Provide adequate nutrition in small, frequent meals at room temperature *to ensure nutritional needs are met. Temperature extremes may cause an attack.*
• If the patient is receiving carbamazepine, watch for cutaneous and hematologic reactions (erythematous and pruritic rashes, urticaria, photosensitivity, exfoliative dermatitis, leukopenia, agranulocytosis, eosinophilia, aplastic anemia, thrombocytopenia) and, possibly, urine retention and transient drowsiness. *Identifying adverse reactions early helps to limit complications.*
• For the first 3 months of carbamazepine therapy, complete blood count and liver function should be monitored weekly, then monthly thereafter. Warn the patient to immediately report fever, sore throat, mouth ulcers, easy bruising, or petechial or purpuric hemorrhage. *Hematologic toxicity is rare but serious.*
• If the patient is receiving phenytoin, watch for adverse effects, including ataxia, skin eruptions, gingival hyperplasia, and nystagmus. *Early detection of adverse reactions limits complications with early intervention.*
• After resection of the first division of the trigeminal nerve, tell the patient to avoid rubbing his eyes and using aerosol spray. Advise him to wear glasses or goggles outdoors and to blink often *to prevent injury.*
• After surgery to sever the second or third division, tell the patient to avoid hot foods and drinks, *which could burn his mouth,* and to chew carefully *to avoid biting his mouth.*
• Advise the patient to place food in the unaffected side of his mouth when chewing, to brush his teeth often, and to see a dentist twice per year to detect cavities. *Cavities in the area of the severed nerve won't cause pain.*
• After surgical decompression of the root or partial nerve dissection, check neurologic and vital signs often *to detect early signs of postoperative complications.*
• Reinforce natural avoidance of stimulation (air, heat, cold) of trigger zones (lips, cheeks, gums) *to prevent further episodes.*

Teaching topics
• Disease process and treatment options
• Avoiding things that can trigger an attack, such as temperature extremes

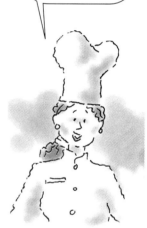

Offer the patient with trigeminal neuralgia small, frequent meals at room temperature. Temperature extremes may cause an attack.

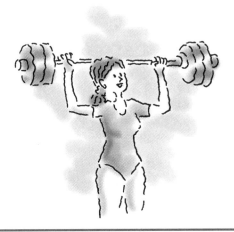

Pump up on practice questions

1. The nurse is caring for a client with a cerebral injury that impaired his speech and hearing. Most likely, the client has experienced damage to the:

A. frontal lobe.
B. parietal lobe.
C. occipital lobe.
D. temporal lobe.

Answer: D. The portion of the cerebrum that controls speech and hearing is the temporal lobe. Injury to the frontal lobe causes personality changes, difficulty speaking, and disturbances in memory, reasoning, and concentration. Injury to the parietal lobe causes sensory alterations and problems with spatial relationships. Damage to the occipital lobe causes vision disturbances.

➡ *NCLEX keys*

Nursing process step: Analysis
Client needs category: Physiological integrity
Client needs subcategory: Physiological adaptation
Taxonomic level: Comprehension

2. Stimulation of the autonomic nervous system that produces a parasympathetic response would most likely cause:

A. increased heart rate.
B. increased metabolism.
C. increased gastric motility.
D. increased systemic vascular resistance.

Answer: C. A parasympathetic response increases gastric motility but decreases heart rate, metabolism, and systemic vascular response.

➡ *NCLEX keys*

Nursing process step: Analysis
Client needs category: Health promotion and maintenance
Client needs subcategory: Prevention and early detection of disease
Taxonomic level: Comprehension

3. A client with a massive cerebral hemorrhage and loss of consciousness is scheduled for an electroencephalogram (EEG). The nurse is discussing the purpose of the test with the family. It would be most accurate for the nurse to tell family members the test will measure:

A. extent of intracranial bleeding.
B. sites of brain injury.
C. activity of the brain.
D. percent of functional brain tissue.

Answer: C. An EEG measures the electrical activity of the brain. Extent of intracranial bleeding and location of the injury site would be determined by computerized tomography or magnetic resonance imaging. Percent of functional brain tissue would be determined by a series of tests.

➡ *NCLEX keys*

Nursing process step: Implementation
Client needs category: Physiological integrity
Client needs subcategory: Physiological adaptation
Taxonomic level: Comprehension

4. The nurse is teaching a client and his family about dietary practices related to Parkinson's disease. A priority for the nurse to address is risk of:

A. fluid overload and drooling.
B. aspiration and anorexia.
C. choking and diarrhea.
D. dysphagia and constipation.

Answer: D. The eating problems associated with Parkinson's disease include dysphagia, aspiration, constipation, and risk of choking. Fluid overload, anorexia, and diarrhea aren't problems specifically related to Parkinson's disease. Drooling occurs with Parkinson's disease but doesn't take priority.

➡ NCLEX keys

Nursing process step: Implementation
Client needs category: Physiological integrity
Client needs subcategory: Reduction of risk potential
Taxonomic level: Analysis

5. In some clients with multiple sclerosis (MS), plasmapheresis diminishes symptoms. Plasmapheresis achieves this effect by removing:

A. catecholamines.
B. antibodies.
C. plasma proteins.
D. lymphocytes.

Answer: B. In plasmapheresis, antibodies are removed from the client's plasma. Antibodies attack the myelin sheath of the neuron causing the manifestations of MS. The treatment of MS with plasmapheresis isn't for the purpose of removing catecholamines, plasma proteins, or lymphocytes.

➡ NCLEX keys

Nursing process step: Evaluation
Client needs category: Physiological integrity
Client needs subcategory: Physiological adaptation
Taxonomic level: Comprehension

6. A client undergoes a surgical clipping of a cerebral aneurysm. To prevent vasospasm, postsurgical care focuses on maintaining an optimal cerebral perfusion pressure. This is best accomplished by administering:

A. diuretics such as furosemide (Lasix).
B. blood products such as cryoprecipitate.
C. the calcium channel blocker nifedipine (Procardia).
D. volume expanders such as crystalloids.

Answer: D. To prevent vasospasm following repair of a cerebral aneurysm, treatment focuses on increasing cerebral perfusion. This can be accomplished by giving volume expanders such as crystalloids. Diuretics would decrease cerebral perfusion by reducing volume. Cryoprecipitate isn't used as a volume expander. Nimodipine (Nimotop), not nifedipine (Procardia), is the calcium channel blocker indicated for use in cerebral vasospasm treatment and prevention.

➡ NCLEX keys

Nursing process step: Implementation
Client needs category: Physiological integrity
Client needs subcategory: Reduction of risk potential
Taxonomic level: Application

7. A client is diagnosed with a brain tumor. Palliative care is all that can be offered to the client. In addressing the client and family, it would be most therapeutic for the nurse to say:

A. "I'm sorry. I wish there was more we could do."
B. "Be optimistic. Others have survived equally as grave situations."
C. "I understand how this may be affecting you and I want to help."
D. "Be thankful you and your family have each other for support during this time."

Answer: C. Initially, the client and family may be in shock and disbelief. They need the nurse's understanding, support, and offer of help. The other responses communicate pity, false hope, and detachment.

➡ NCLEX keys
Nursing process step: Implementation
Client needs category: Psychosocial integrity
Client needs subcategory: Coping and adaptation
Taxonomic level: Application

8. The nurse is teaching a client with a T4 spinal cord injury and paralysis of the lower extremities how to independently transfer from bed to a wheelchair. In transferring, it is important for the client to move:
    A. the upper and lower body simultaneously into the wheelchair.
    B. his upper body to the wheelchair first.
    C. his feet to the wheelchair pedals and then his hands to the wheelchair arms.
    D. his feet to the floor and then his buttocks to the wheelchair seat.
Answer: B. The proper technique in transferring from a bed to a wheelchair when there is paralysis of the lower extremities is to move the strong part of the body to the chair first. The client should move his upper body to the wheelchair first and then move his legs from the bed to the wheelchair. Other techniques are less safe and can endanger the client.

➡ NCLEX keys
Nursing process step: Implementation
Client needs category: Physiological integrity
Client needs subcategory: Basic care and comfort
Taxonomic level: Application

9. A client who recently underwent cranial surgery develops syndrome of inappropriate antidiuretic hormone (SIADH). The nurse should anticipate that the client will:
    A. experience edema and weight gain.
    B. produce excessive amounts of urine.
    C. need vigorous fluid replacement therapy.
    D. have a low urine specific gravity.
Answer: A. SIADH is an abnormally high release of antidiuretic hormone causing water retention, which leads to edema and weight gain. Urine output is low, fluid is restricted rather than replaced, and the urine specific gravity is high.

➡ NCLEX keys
Nursing process step: Planning
Client needs category: Physiological integrity
Client needs subcategory: Reduction of risk potential
Taxonomic level: Application

10. The nurse is providing care for a client following right cataract removal surgery. In which position should the nurse place the client?
    A. Right-side lying
    B. Prone
    C. Supine
    D. Trendelenburg's
Answer: C. Positioning the client on his back or unoperative side prevents pressure on the operative eye. Operative side-lying or prone position may put external pressure on the affected eye. Trendelenburg's position may increase intraocular pressure.

➡ NCLEX keys
Nursing process step: Implementation
Client needs category: Physiological integrity
Client needs subcategory: Physiological adaptation
Taxonomic level: Application

I sense that you've completed another chapter. Keep up the good work!

Brush up on key concepts

The musculoskeletal system has two main functions: to provide support and to produce movement. In addition, the musculoskeletal system protects internal tissues and organs, produces red blood cells (RBCs) in the bone marrow, and stores mineral salts such as calcium.

At any time, you can review the major points of this chapter by consulting the *Cheat sheet* on pages 214 to 216.

Mr. Bones

The **skeleton** consists of 206 bones, which work with the muscles to support and protect internal organs.

The skeleton also stores calcium, magnesium, and phosphorus, and the bone marrow produces RBCs.

The movement machine

The **skeletal muscles**, attached to the bones by tendons, provide body movement and posture by tightening and shortening. They begin contracting when stimulated by a motor neuron, and derive energy for muscle contraction from hydrolysis of adenosine triphosphate to adenosine diphosphate and phosphate.

The skeletal muscles relax with the breakdown of acetylcholine by cholinesterase. Even then, they retain some contraction to maintain muscle tone.

Bones to bones and bones to muscles

Ligaments and **tendons** are tough bands of collagen fibers. Ligaments connect bones to bones and encircle joints to add strength and stability. Tendons connect muscles to bones.

Where bones meet

A **joint** is the articulation of two bone surfaces. Joints provide stabilization and permit locomotion. The degree of joint movement is called range of motion (ROM).

Friction reduction

The **synovium** is the membrane that lines a joint's inner surfaces. In conjunction with cartilage, the synovium reduces friction in joints through its production of synovial fluid.

Shock absorber

Cartilage is a specialized tissue that serves as a smooth surface for articulating bones. It absorbs shock to joints and serves as padding to reduce friction.

Cartilage atrophies with limited ROM or in the absence of weight-bearing bursae (small sacs of synovial fluid).

Keep abreast of diagnostic tests

Here are the most important tests used to diagnose musculoskeletal disorders, along with common nursing interventions associated with each test.

Muscle picture

Electromyography (EMG) uses electrodes to create a graphic recording of the muscle at rest and during contraction.

Nursing actions
• Explain that the patient will be asked to flex and relax muscles during the procedure.
• Instruct the patient that the procedure may cause some minor discomfort but isn't painful.

(Text continues on page 217.)

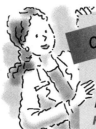

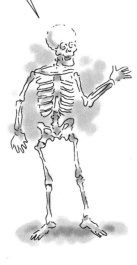

Cheat sheet

Musculoskeletal refresher

ARM AND LEG FRACTURES

Key signs and symptoms
- Loss of limb function
- Pain
- Deformity

Key test results
- Anteroposterior and lateral X-rays of the suspected fracture as well as X-rays of the joints above and below it confirm the diagnosis.

Key treatments
- Closed reduction (restoring displaced bone segments to their normal position)
- Immobilization with a splint, cast, or traction
- Open reduction during surgery to reduce and immobilize the fracture with rods, plates, and screws when closed reduction is impossible, usually followed by application of a plaster cast.
- Analgesics: morphine, acetaminophen and oxycodone (Percocet)

Key interventions
- Monitor vital signs and be especially alert for a rapid pulse, decreased blood pressure, pallor, and cool, clammy skin.
- Administer I.V. fluids as needed.
- Ease pain with analgesics as needed.
- If the fracture requires long-term immobilization with traction, reposition the patient often. Assist with active range-of-motion (ROM) exercises. Encourage deep breathing and coughing.
- Make sure that the immobilized patient receives adequate fluid intake. Watch for signs of renal calculi, such as flank pain, nausea, and vomiting.
- Provide good cast care.
- Encourage the patient to start moving around as soon as possible. Help him to walk. (Remember, the patient who has been bedridden for some time may be dizzy at first.) Demonstrate how to use crutches properly.
- After cast removal, refer the patient for physical therapy.

The musculoskeletal system has two main functions: to provide support and produce movement.

CARPAL TUNNEL SYNDROME

Key signs and symptoms
- Numbness, burning, or tingling
- Pain
- Weakness

Key test results
- A blood pressure cuff inflated above systolic pressure on the forearm for 1 to 2 minutes provokes pain and paresthesia along the distribution of the median nerve.
- Electromyography detects a median nerve motor conduction delay of more than 5 msec.

Key treatments
- Resting the hands by splinting the wrist in neutral extension for 1 to 2 weeks. (If a definite link has been established between the patient's occupation and the development of carpal tunnel syndrome, he may have to seek other work.)
- Corticosteroid injections: betamethasone (Celestone), hydrocortisone (Hydrocortone)
- Nonsteroidal anti-inflammatory drugs (NSAIDs): indomethacin (Indocin), ibuprofen (Motrin), naproxen (Naprosyn)

Key interventions
- Administer NSAIDs as needed.
- Encourage the patient to use his hands as much as possible.
- If the patient's dominant hand has been impaired, you may have to help with eating and bathing.
- After surgery, monitor vital signs and regularly check the color, sensation, and motion of the affected hand.

COMPARTMENT SYNDROME

Key signs and symptoms
- Loss of distal pulse
- Severe or increased pain in the affected area with stretching or muscle elevation that is unrelieved by narcotics
- Tense, swollen muscle

Musculoskeletal refresher *(continued)*

Key test results

• Intracompartment pressure is elevated, as indicated by a blood pressure machine.

Key treatments

• Fasciotomy
• Positioning affected extremity lower than the heart
• Removal of dressings or constrictive coverings of the area

Key interventions

• Monitor the affected extremity and perform neurovascular checks.
• Perform dressing changes postfasciotomy and reinforce dressings frequently. (A large amount of bloody drainage should be expected.)

GOUT

Key signs and symptoms

• Inflamed, painful joints

Key test results

• Blood studies show serum uric acid level above normal. The urine uric acid level is usually higher in secondary gout than in primary gout.

Key treatments

• Antigout drug: colchicine
• Uricosuric drugs: probenecid (Benemid), sulfinpyrazone (Anturane)
• Corticosteroids: betamethasone (Celestone), hydrocortisone (Hydrocortone)

Key interventions

• Encourage bed rest but use a bed cradle.
• Give pain medication, as needed, especially during acute attacks.
• Apply hot or cold packs to inflamed joints.
• Administer anti-inflammatory medication and other drugs.
• Urge the patient to drink plenty of fluids (up to 2 L/day).
• When forcing fluids, record intake and output accurately.
• Be sure to monitor serum uric acid levels regularly.
• Alkalinize urine with sodium bicarbonate or another agent, as needed.

HERNIATED NUCLEUS PULPOSUS

Key signs and symptoms

In lumbrosacral area:

• Acute pain in the lower back radiating across the buttock and down the leg
• Pain on ambulation
• Weakness, numbness, and tingling of the foot and leg

In cervical area:

• Neck pain that radiates down the arm to the hand
• Neck stiffness
• Weakness of affected upper extremities
• Weakness, numbness, and tingling of the hand

Key test results

• Myelogram shows compression of spinal cord.
• X-ray shows narrowing of disk space.

Key treatments

• Corticosteroid: cortisone (Cortone)
• NSAIDs: indomethacin (Indocin), ibuprofen (Motrin), sulindac (Clinoril), piroxicam (Feldene), flurbiprofen (Ansaid), diclofenac sodium (Voltaren), naproxen (Naprosyn), diflunisal (Dolobid)

Key interventions

• Assess neurovascular status.
• Turn the patient every 2 hours using the logrolling technique.

HIP FRACTURE

Key signs and symptoms

• Shorter appearance and outward rotation of affected leg resulting in limited or abnormal ROM
• Edema and discoloration of surrounding tissue

Key test results

• Computed tomography scan (for complicated fractures) pinpoints abnormalities.
• X-ray reveals break in continuity of bone.

Key treatments

• Abductor splint or trochanter roll between legs to prevent loss of alignment
• Surgical immobilization or joint replacement

Key interventions

• Assess neurovascular and respiratory status. Most important, check for compromised circulation, hemorrhage, and neurologic impairment in the affected extremity and pneumonia in the bedridden patient.
• Provide active and passive ROM and isometric exercises for unaffected limbs.
• Provide a trapeze.
• Maintain traction at all times.

OSTEOARTHRITIS

Key signs and symptoms

• Crepitation
• Joint stiffness
• Pain relieved by resting joints

(continued)

Musculoskeletal refresher *(continued)*

OSTEOARTHRITIS *(continued)*

Key test results

• Arthroscopy reveals bone spurs and narrowing of joint space.
• X-rays show joint deformity, narrowing of joint space, and bone spurs.

Key treatments

• Cold therapy
• Heat therapy
• NSAIDs: indomethacin (Indocin), ibuprofen (Motrin), sulindac (Clinoril), piroxicam (Feldene), flurbiprofen (Ansaid), diclofenac (Voltaren), naproxen (Naprosyn), diflunisal (Dolobid)

Key interventions

• Assess musculoskeletal status.
• Assess for increased bleeding or bruising tendency.

OSTEOMYELITIS

Key signs and symptoms

• Pain
• Tenderness
• Swelling

Key test results

• Blood cultures identify the causative organism.
• Erythrocyte sedimentation rate and C-reactive protein (CRP) are elevated. Note that CRP appears to be a better diagnostic tool.

Key treatments

• Immobilization of the affected bone by plaster cast, traction, or bed rest
• Antibiotics: large doses of I.V. antibiotics, usually a penicillinase-resistant penicillin, such as nafcillin (Unipen) and oxacillin (Bactocill), or a cephalosporin such as cefazolin (Ancef) after blood cultures are taken

Key interventions

• Use strict aseptic technique when changing dressings and irrigating wounds.
• Assess vital signs and wound appearance daily, and monitor daily for new pain.
• Check circulation and drainage: If a wet spot appears on the cast, circle it with a marking pen and note the time of appearance (on the cast). Be aware of how much drainage is expected.

Check the circled spot at least every 4 hours. Watch for any enlargement.

OSTEOPOROSIS

Key signs and symptoms

• Deformity
• Kyphosis
• Pain

Key test results

• X-rays show typical degeneration in the lower thoracic and lumbar vertebrae. The vertebral bodies may appear flattened and may look denser than normal. Loss of bone mineral becomes evident in later stages.

Key treatments

• Physical therapy of gentle exercise and activity
• Hormonal agents: conjugated estrogen (Premarin), calcitonin (Calcimar)
• Vitamin D supplements
• Antihypercalcemic: etidronate (Didronel)

Key interventions

• Check the patient's skin daily for redness, warmth, and new sites of pain. Encourage activity; help the patient walk several times daily.
• Perform passive ROM exercises or encourage the patient to perform active exercises. Make sure she regularly attends scheduled physical therapy sessions.
• Provide a balanced diet high in such nutrients as vitamin D, calcium, and protein.
• Administer analgesics and heat.

• Administer analgesics, as prescribed, after the procedure.

Direct view of a joint

Arthroscopy is a relatively simple surgical procedure, performed under local anesthesia, that allows for direct visualization of a joint.

Nursing actions

Before the procedure, you should:
• administer prophylactic antibiotics, as prescribed
• explain the procedure, skin preparation, and use of local anesthetics.
  After the procedure, you should:
• apply a pressure dressing to the injection site
• monitor neurovascular status
• apply ice to the affected joint
• limit weight bearing or joint use until allowed by the doctor
• administer analgesics, as prescribed.

Fluid removal

In **arthrocentesis**, a doctor removes synovial fluid from a joint using a needle.

Nursing actions

Before the procedure, you should:
• administer prophylactic antibiotics, as prescribed
• explain the procedure to the patient.
  After the procedure, you should:
• maintain a pressure dressing on the aspiration site
• monitor neurovascular status
• apply ice to the affected area
• limit weight bearing or joint use until allowed by the doctor
• administer analgesics, as prescribed.

Bone image

A **bone scan** is used to reveal bone abnormalities. It involves the injection of a radioisotope, which (in conjunction with a scanner) allows a visual image of bone metabolism.

Nursing actions

• Determine the patient's ability to lie still during the scan.

• Make sure that written, informed consent has been obtained before the procedure.
• Advise the patient that radioisotope will be injected I.V.
• Explain to the patient that he will be required to drink several glasses of fluid during the waiting period to enhance excretion of isotope not absorbed by bone tissue.

Vertebrae visual

A **myelogram** involves the injection of radiopaque dye into the spine during a lumbar puncture. This dye allows fluoroscopic visualization of the subarachnoid space, spinal cord, and vertebral bodies.

Nursing actions

Before the procedure, you should:
• make sure that written, informed consent has been obtained before the procedure
• note the patient's allergies to iodine, seafood, and radiopaque dyes
• inform the patient about possible throat irritation and flushing of the face from the injection.
  After the procedure, you should:
• maintain bed rest, with the patient lying flat
• inspect the insertion site for bleeding
• monitor neurologic status
• force fluids.

Solving for X

An **X-ray** provides a noninvasive radiographic examination of bones and joints.

Nursing actions

• Use caution when moving a patient with a suspected fracture.
• Explain the procedure to the patient.
• Make sure that the patient isn't pregnant (to prevent possible fetal damage from radiation exposure).

Lab exam #1

A **blood chemistry test** is a laboratory test that analyzes a blood sample for potassium, sodium, calcium, phosphorus, glucose, bicarbonate, blood urea nitrogen, creatinine, protein, albumin, osmolality, creatine kinase, serum aspartate aminotransferase, aldolase, rheumatoid factor, complement fixation, lupus

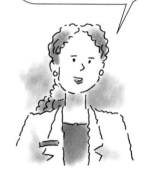

A myelogram — evaluation of the subarachnoid space — requires a lumbar puncture. Inspect the insertion site. Monitor neurologic status.

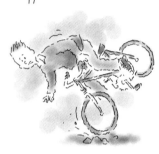

> Arm and leg fractures usually result from trauma and commonly cause substantial muscle, nerve, and other soft-tissue damage.

erythematosus cell preparation, antinuclear antibody, anti-deoxyribonucleic acid, and C-reactive protein (CRP).

Nursing actions
• Withhold food and fluid before the procedure, if appropriate.
• Monitor the venipuncture site for bleeding after the procedure.

Lab exam #2
A **hematologic study** analyzes a blood sample for white blood cells (WBCs), RBCs, platelets, prothrombin time, international normalized ratio, partial thromboplastin time, erythrocyte sedimentation rate (ESR), hemoglobin (Hb), and hematocrit (HCT).

Nursing actions
• Note current drug therapy to anticipate possible interference with test results.
• Assess the venipuncture site for bleeding after the procedure.

Polish up on patient care

Major musculoskeletal disorders include arm and leg fractures, carpal tunnel syndrome, compartment syndrome, gout, herniated nucleus pulposus, hip fracture, osteoarthritis, osteomyelitis, and osteoporosis.

Arm and leg fractures

Fractures of the arms and legs usually result from trauma and commonly cause substantial muscle, nerve, and other soft-tissue damage. The prognosis varies with the extent of disability or deformity, the amount of tissue and vascular damage, the adequacy of reduction and immobilization, and the patient's age, health, and nutritional status.

Children's bones usually heal rapidly and without deformity. Bones of adults in poor

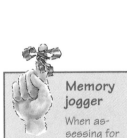

Memory jogger

When assessing for fractures, remember the "5 Ps":

Pain, Pallor, Pulse loss, Paresthesia, and Paralysis. (The last three are distal to the fracture site.)

health and with impaired circulation may never heal properly. Severe open fractures, especially of the femoral shaft, may cause substantial blood loss and life-threatening hypovolemic shock.

CAUSES
• Bone tumors
• Major trauma
• Osteoporosis

ASSESSMENT FINDINGS
• Discoloration
• Loss of limb function
• Pain
• Swelling
• Deformity
• Crepitus

DIAGNOSTIC TEST RESULTS
• Anteroposterior and lateral X-rays of the suspected fracture as well as X-rays of the joints above and below it confirm the diagnosis.

NURSING DIAGNOSES
• Pain
• Impaired physical mobility
• Anxiety

TREATMENT
Emergency care
• Splinting the limb above and below the suspected fracture
• Cold pack application
• Elevating the extremity to reduce edema and pain
• Direct pressure to control bleeding in severe fractures that cause blood loss
• Fluid replacement as soon as possible to prevent hypovolemic shock, if blood loss

After confirming diagnosis
• Closed reduction (restoring displaced bone segments to their normal position)
• Immobilization with a splint, cast, or traction
• Open reduction during surgery to reduce and immobilize the fracture using rods,

plates, and screws when closed reduction is impossible, usually followed by application of a plaster cast.
• Skin or skeletal traction (if splint or cast fails to maintain the reduction)

Open fractures
• Surgery to repair soft-tissue damage
• Thorough debridement of the wound

Drug therapy
• Analgesics: morphine, acetaminophen and oxycodone (Percocet)
• Prophylactic antibiotic: cefazolin (Ancef)
• Tetanus prophylaxis: tetanus toxoid

INTERVENTIONS AND RATIONALES
• Watch for signs of shock in the patient with a severe open fracture of a large bone such as the femur. *Open fractures can cause increased blood loss leading to hypovolemic shock.*
• Monitor vital signs and be especially alert for a rapid pulse, decreased blood pressure, pallor, and cool, clammy skin, *all of which may indicate that the patient is in shock.*
• Administer I.V. fluids as needed *to replace fluid loss.*
• Offer reassurance. *With any fracture, the patient is likely to be frightened and in pain.*
• Ease pain with analgesics as needed *to promote comfort.*
• Help the patient set realistic goals for recovery *to prevent frustration with the recovery process.*
• If the fracture requires long-term immobilization with traction, reposition the patient often *to increase comfort and prevent pressure ulcers.* Assist with active range-of-motion exercises *to prevent muscle atrophy.* Encourage deep breathing and coughing *to avoid hypostatic pneumonia.*
• Make sure that the immobilized patient receives adequate fluid intake *to prevent urinary stasis and constipation.* Watch for signs of renal calculi, such as flank pain, nausea, and vomiting *to ensure early recognition and treatment.*
• Provide good cast care *to avoid skin breakdown.*

• Encourage the patient to start moving around as soon as possible *to prevent complications of immobility.* Help him to walk. (Remember, the patient who has been bedridden for some time may be dizzy at first.) Demonstrate how to use crutches properly *to prevent injury.*
• After cast removal, refer the patient for physical therapy *to restore limb mobility.*

Teaching topics
• Cast care
• Use of assistive devices

Carpal tunnel syndrome

Carpal tunnel syndrome results from compression of the median nerve at the wrist, within the carpal tunnel. This nerve — along with blood vessels and flexor tendons — passes through to the fingers and thumb. Compression neuropathy causes sensory and motor changes in the median distribution of the hand. Carpal tunnel is the most common of the nerve entrapment syndromes.

Carpal tunnel syndrome usually occurs in women between ages 30 and 60 and poses a serious occupational health problem. Assembly-line workers and packers, typists, and persons who repeatedly use poorly designed tools are most likely to develop this disorder. Any strenuous use of the hands — sustained grasping, twisting, or flexing — aggravates this condition.

CAUSES
• Flexor tenosynovitis (often associated with rheumatic disease)
• Nerve compression
• Physical trauma
• Rheumatoid arthritis

ASSESSMENT FINDINGS
• Atrophic nails
• Numbness, burning, or tingling
• Pain
• Shiny, dry skin
• Weakness

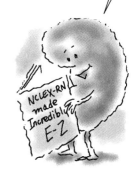

Leave no stone unturned. Immobilized patients are at risk for renal calculi.

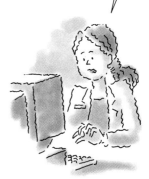

Any strenuous use of the hands, including taking the NCLEX, aggravates carpal tunnel syndrome.

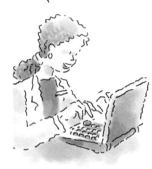

Inefficiently designed keyboards are often the culprit in cases of carpal tunnel syndrome.

DIAGNOSTIC TEST RESULTS
• Physical examination reveals decreased sensation to light touch or pinpricks in the affected fingers. Thenar muscle atrophy occurs in about half of all cases of carpal tunnel syndrome. The patient exhibits a positive Tinel's sign (tingling over the median nerve on light percussion). He also responds positively to Phalen's wrist-flexion test, in which holding the forearms vertically and allowing both hands to drop into complete flexion at the wrists for 1 minute reproduces symptoms of carpal tunnel syndrome.
• A blood pressure cuff inflated above systolic pressure on the forearm for 1 to 2 minutes provokes pain and paresthesia along the distribution of the median nerve.
• EMG detects a median nerve motor conduction delay of more than 5 msec.

NURSING DIAGNOSES
• Impaired physical mobility
• Pain
• Sensory or perceptual alterations (kinesthetic, tactile)

TREATMENT
• Resting the hands by splinting the wrist in neutral extension for 1 to 2 weeks (If a definite link has been established between the patient's occupation and the development of carpal tunnel syndrome, he may have to seek other work.)
• Correction of an underlying disorder
• Surgical decompression of the nerve by resecting the entire transverse carpal tunnel ligament or by using endoscopic surgical techniques (Neurolysis, or releasing of nerve fibers, may also be necessary.)

Drug therapy
• Nonsteroidal anti-inflammatory drugs (NSAIDs): indomethacin (Indocin), ibuprofen (Motrin), naproxen (Naprosyn)
• Corticosteroid injections: betamethasone (Celestone), hydrocortisone (Hydrocortone)

INTERVENTIONS AND RATIONALES
• Administer NSAIDs as needed *to reduce inflammation and pain.*

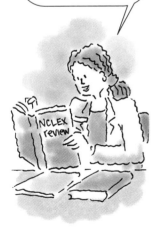

Numbers to know for compartment syndrome: Tissue damage after 30 minutes. Permanent damage after 4 hours.

NCLEX review

• Encourage the patient to use his hands as much as possible *to maintain ROM.*
• If the patient's dominant hand has been impaired, you may have to help with eating and bathing. *Mobility may be limited with carpal tunnel syndrome.*
• Regularly assess the patient's degree of physical immobility *to evaluate effectiveness of current treatment plan.*
• After surgery, monitor vital signs and regularly check the color, sensation, and motion of the affected hand *to detect signs of compromised circulation.*
• Advise the patient who's about to be discharged to occasionally exercise his hands. If the arm is in a sling, tell him to remove the sling several times each day to do exercises for his elbow and shoulder *to maintain ROM.*

Teaching topics
• Disease process and treatment options
• Applying the splint and removing it to perform gentle ROM exercises daily.
• ROM exercises
• Importance of taking NSAIDs with food or antacids to avoid stomach upset
• Reinforcing that maximum effects of drug therapy may not be seen for 2 to 4 weeks
• Contacting an occupational counselor

Compartment syndrome

Compartment syndrome occurs when the pressure within a muscle and its surrounding structures increases. If the pressure becomes greater than diastolic blood pressure, circulation can be impaired or interrupted completely. Tissue damage occurs after 30 minutes; after 4 hours, irreversible damage may occur.

If compartment syndrome is suspected, pressure within muscles is assessed by sticking a needle into a muscle. The needle is attached to an I.V. bag with tubing and a stopcock. Elevated pressure, as indicated by a blood pressure machine, indicates compartment syndrome.

CAUSES
• Application of a dressing or cast that is too tight
• Burns
• Closed fracture injury
• Crushing injuries
• Muscle swelling after exercise

ASSESSMENT FINDINGS
• Decreased movement, strength, and sensation
• Increased pain with muscle stretching
• Loss of distal pulse
• Numbness and tingling distal to the involved muscle
• Severe or increased pain in the affected area with stretching or muscle elevation that is unrelieved by narcotics
• Paralysis
• Tense, swollen muscle

DIAGNOSTIC TEST RESULTS
• Intracompartment pressure is elevated, as indicated by a blood pressure machine.

NURSING DIAGNOSES
• Impaired physical mobility
• Pain
• Risk for peripheral neurovascular dysfunction

TREATMENT
• Fasciotomy
• Positioning affected extremity lower than the heart
• Removal of dressings or constrictive coverings of the area

Drug therapy
• Narcotic analgesics

INTERVENTIONS AND RATIONALES
• Monitor vital signs *to detect early changes and prevent complications.*
• Monitor affected extremity and perform neurovascular checks *to detect signs of impaired circulation.*
• Maintain extremity in a position lower than the heart *to ensure adequate circulation in affected extremity and to reduce pressure.*
• Assess patient for pain and anxiety *as stress may lead to vasoconstriction.*

• Administer medications as ordered *to maintain or improve the patient's condition.*
• Perform dressing changes postfasciotomy and reinforce dressings frequently *to facilitate monitoring of extremity.* (A large amount of bloody drainage should be expected.)

Teaching topics
• Recognizing and reporting symptoms of compartment syndrome
• Preventing future injury

Gout

Gout is a metabolic disease marked by urate deposits in the joints, which cause painfully arthritic joints. It can strike any joint but favors those in the feet and legs. *Primary gout* usually occurs in men older than age 30 and in postmenopausal women. *Secondary gout* occurs in older people.

Gout follows an intermittent course and often leaves patients free from symptoms for years between attacks. Gout can lead to chronic disability or incapacitation and, rarely, severe hypertension and progressive renal disease. The prognosis is good with treatment.

CAUSES
• Genetic predisposition
• Increased uric acid

ASSESSMENT FINDINGS
• Hypertension
• Back pain
• Inflamed, painful joints

DIAGNOSTIC TEST RESULTS
• Arthrocentesis reveals the presence of monosodium urate monohydrate crystals or needlelike intracellular crystals of sodium urate in synovial fluid taken from an inflamed joint or a tophus.
• Blood studies show serum uric acid level above normal. The urine uric acid level is usually higher in secondary gout than in primary gout.

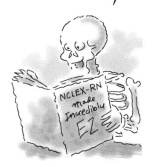

Shout about gout. Urate deposits cause painfully arthritic joints.

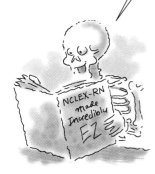

Set goals you can meet. You may be able to review this chapter in one sitting. But if that's not for you, set a shorter goal — and meet it.

• X-ray examination results are normal initially. X-rays show damage of the articular cartilage and subchondral bone in chronic gout and outward displacement of the overhanging margin from the bone contour.

NURSING DIAGNOSES
• Pain
• Impaired physical mobility
• Risk for injury

TREATMENT
• Bed rest
• Immobilization and protection of the inflamed joints
• Local application of heat and cold
• Diet changes (with the goal of weight loss)

Drug therapy
• Analgesics: acetaminophen
• Antigout drug: colchicine
• Uricosuric drugs; probenecid (Benemid), sulfinpyrazone (Anturane)
• Alkalinizing drug: sodium bicarbonate
• Corticosteroids: betamethasone (Celestone), hydrocortisone (Hydrocortone)

INTERVENTIONS AND RATIONALES
• Encourage bed rest but use a bed cradle *to keep bedcovers off extremely sensitive, inflamed joints.*
• Give pain medication, as needed, especially during acute attacks, *to promote comfort.*
• Apply hot or cold packs to inflamed joints *to promote comfort.*
• Administer anti-inflammatory medication and other drugs *to decrease inflammation and increase excretion of uric acid.*
• Be alert for GI disturbances with colchicine administration *to prevent complications.*
• Urge the patient to drink plenty of fluids (up to 2 L/day) *to prevent formation of renal calculi.*
• When forcing fluids, record intake and output accurately *to detect fluid volume excess.*
• Be sure to monitor serum uric acid levels regularly *to evaluate effectiveness of treatment plan.*
• Alkalinize urine with sodium bicarbonate or another agent, as needed, *to prevent formation of renal calculi.*

• Make sure the patient understands the importance of having serum uric acid levels checked periodically *to help ensure compliance.*
• Advise the patient receiving allopurinol, probenecid, and other drugs to report adverse effects, such as drowsiness, dizziness, nausea, vomiting, urinary frequency, and dermatitis, immediately *to prevent complications.*
• Warn the patient taking probenecid or sulfinpyrazone to avoid aspirin and other salicylates. *Their combined effect causes urate retention.*
• Inform the patient that long-term colchicine therapy is essential during the first 3 to 6 months of treatment with uricosuric drugs or allopurinol *to prevent further acute attacks.*

Teaching topics
• Avoiding alcohol, especially beer and wine
• Sparing use of purine-rich foods, such as anchovies, liver, sardines, kidneys, sweetbreads, and lentils.
• Weight loss if obese

Herniated nucleus pulposus

In herniated nucleus pulposus, the intervertebral disk ruptures, causing a protrusion of the nucleus pulposus (the soft, central portion of a spinal disk) into the spinal canal. This compresses the spinal cord or nerve roots causing pain, numbness, and loss of motor function. Commonly known as a herniated disk, herniated nucleus pulposus can be further described as lumbosacral (affecting the lumbar vertebrae L4 and L5 and the sacral vertebra S1) or cervical (affecting the cervical vertebrae C5, C6, and C7).

CAUSES
• Accidents
• Back or neck strain
• Congenital bone deformity
• Degeneration of disk
• Heavy lifting
• Trauma
• Weakness of ligaments

ASSESSMENT FINDINGS

In lumbrosacral area
- Acute pain in the lower back radiating across the buttock and down the leg
- Pain on ambulation
- Weakness, numbness, and tingling of the foot and leg

In cervical area
- Atrophy of biceps and triceps
- Neck pain that radiates down the arm to the hand
- Neck stiffness
- Straightening of normal lumbar curve with scoliosis away from the affected side
- Weakness of affected upper extremities
- Weakness, numbness, and tingling of the hand

DIAGNOSTIC TEST RESULTS

- Cerebrospinal fluid analysis shows increased protein.
- Deep tendon reflexes are depressed or absent in the upper extremities or Achilles tendon.
- EMG shows spinal nerve involvement.
- Lasègue's sign is positive.
- Myelogram shows compression of spinal cord.
- X-ray shows narrowing of disk space.

NURSING DIAGNOSES

- Impaired physical mobility
- Posttrauma response
- Pain

TREATMENT

- Bed rest with active and passive ROM and isometric exercises
- Diet that includes increased fiber and fluids
- Heating pad and moist, hot compresses
- Laminectomy
- Orthopedic devices including back brace and cervical collar
- Transcutaneous electrical nerve stimulation

Drug therapy

- Analgesic: oxycodone hydrochloride (Oxy-Contin)
- Chemonucleolysis using chymopapain (Discase)
- Corticosteroid: cortisone (Cortone)

- Muscle relaxants: diazepam (Valium), cyclobenzaprine (Flexeril)
- NSAIDs: indomethacin (Indocin), ibuprofen (Motrin), sulindac (Clinoril), piroxicam (Feldene), flurbiprofen (Ansaid), diclofenac sodium (Voltaren), naproxen (Naprosyn), diflunisal (Dolobid)
- Stool softener: docusate sodium (Colace)

INTERVENTIONS AND RATIONALES

- Assess neurovascular status *to determine baseline and detect early changes.*
- Monitor and record vital signs, intake and output, and results of laboratory studies *to detect changes in patient's condition.*
- Maintain the patient's diet; increase fluid intake *to maintain hydration.*
- Keep the patient in semi-Fowler's position with moderate hip and knee flexion *to promote comfort.*
- Administer medications, as prescribed, *to maintain or improve patient's condition.*
- Encourage the patient to express feelings about changes in body image and about fears of disability *to help patient resolve feelings.*
- Provide skin and back care *to promote comfort and prevent skin breakdown.*
- Turn the patient every 2 hours using the logrolling technique *to prevent injury.*
- Maintain bed rest and body alignment *to maintain joint function and prevent neuromuscular deformity.*
- Maintain traction, braces, and cervical collar *to prevent further injury and to promote healing.*
- Promote independence in activities of daily living (ADLs) *to maintain self-esteem.*

Teaching topics

- Exercising regularly, with special attention to exercises that strengthen and stretch the muscles
- Avoiding lifting, sleeping prone, climbing stairs, and riding in a car
- Avoiding flexion, extension, or rotation of the neck, if cervical
- Using one pillow for support while sleeping
- Using a back brace or cervical collar

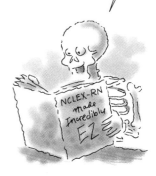

In herniated nucleus pulposus, the soft, central portion of a spinal disk protrudes into the spinal canal.

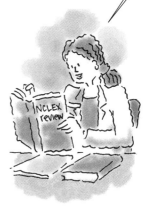

Treatment for herniated nucleus pulposus ranges from bed rest to surgery. Provide emotional support and reinforcement during the treatment and recovery period.

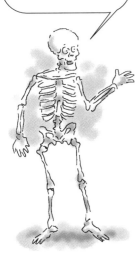

A hip fracture occurs when too much stress is placed on the bone. See what happens when you go out on a limb.

Hip fracture

A fracture occurs when too much stress is placed on the bone. As a result, the bone breaks and local tissue becomes injured causing muscle spasm, edema, hemorrhage, compressed nerves, and ecchymosis.

Sites of hip fractures include intracapsular (within the capsule of the femur), extracapsular (outside the capsule of the femur), intertrochanteric (within the trochanter), or subtrochanteric (below the trochanter).

CAUSES
• Aging
• Bone tumors
• Cushing's syndrome
• Immobility
• Malnutrition
• Multiple myeloma
• Osteomyelitis
• Osteoporosis
• Steroid therapy
• Trauma

ASSESSMENT FINDINGS
• Shorter appearance and outward rotation of affected leg resulting in limited or abnormal ROM
• Edema and discoloration of surrounding tissue
• History of a fall or other trauma to the bones
• Pain in the affected hip and leg, exacerbated by any movement

DIAGNOSTIC TEST RESULTS
• Computed tomography scan (for complicated fractures) pinpoints abnormalities.
• Hematology shows decreased Hb and HCT.
• X-ray reveals break in continuity of bone.

NURSING DIAGNOSES
• Risk for activity intolerance
• Risk for impaired skin integrity
• Altered role performance

TREATMENT
• Abductor splint or trochanter roll between legs to prevent loss of alignment

• Isometric exercises, such as tensing and relaxing the muscles of the leg
• Physical therapy to teach the patient non-weight-bearing transfers and to work with changes in weight-bearing status
• Skin traction: Buck's or Russell's
• Surgical immobilization or joint replacement

Drug therapy
• Analgesics: narcotic or nonnarcotic

INTERVENTIONS AND RATIONALES
• Assess neurovascular and respiratory status. Most important, check for compromised circulation, hemorrhage, and neurologic impairment in the affected extremity and pneumonia in the bedridden patient *to detect changes and prevent complications.*
• Monitor and record vital signs, intake and output, and results of laboratory studies *to detect early changes in patient's condition.*
• Maintain the patient's diet; increase fluid intake *to maintain hydration.*
• Keep the patient in a flat position with the foot of the bed elevated 25 degrees when in traction *to prevent further injury.*
• Keep the legs abducted *to prevent dislocation of the hip joint.*
• Administer medications, as prescribed, *to improve or maintain patient's condition.*
• Provide skin care, and logroll the patient every 2 hours *to maintain skin integrity and prevent pressure ulcers.*
• Assist with coughing, deep breathing, and incentive spirometry *to maintain patent airway.*
• Keep the hip extended *to prevent further injury and maintain circulation.*
• Promote independence in ADLs *to promote self-esteem.*
• Provide active and passive ROM and isometric exercises for unaffected limbs *to maintain joint mobility.*
• Provide a trapeze *to promote independence in self-care.*
• Maintain traction at all times *to ensure proper body alignment and promote healing.*
• Keep side rails up *to prevent injury.*
• Provide appropriate sensory stimulation with frequent reorientation *to reduce anxiety.*

- Encourage increased fiber, fluids, and activity as allowed, plus medication as needed *to prevent constipation.*
- Provide diversional activities *to promote self-esteem.*
- Apply antiembolism stockings *to promote venous circulation.*

Teaching topics
- Attending physical therapy sessions
- Avoiding putting weight on the affected limb
- Performing skin and foot care daily

Osteoarthritis

Also known as degenerative joint disease, osteoarthritis is characterized by degeneration of cartilage in weight-bearing joints, such as the spine, knees, and hips. It occurs when cartilage softens with age, narrowing the joint space. This allows bones to rub together, causing pain and limiting joint movement.

Osteoarthritis can be primary or secondary. Primary osteoarthritis, a normal part of aging, results from metabolic, genetic, chemical, and mechanical factors. Secondary osteoarthritis usually follows an identifiable cause, such as obesity and congenital deformity, and leads to degenerative changes.

CAUSES
- Aging
- Congenital abnormalities
- Joint trauma
- Obesity

ASSESSMENT FINDINGS
- Crepitation
- Enlarged, edematous joints
- Heberden's nodes
- Increased pain in damp, cold weather
- Joint stiffness
- Limited ROM
- Pain relieved by resting joints
- Smooth, taut, shiny skin

DIAGNOSTIC TEST RESULTS
- Arthroscopy reveals bone spurs and narrowing of joint space.

- Hematology shows increased ESR.
- X-rays show joint deformity, narrowing of joint space, and bone spurs.

NURSING DIAGNOSES
- Activity intolerance
- Impaired physical mobility
- Pain

TREATMENT
- Canes or walkers
- Cold therapy
- Low-calorie diet if the patient isn't at optimal weight
- Heat therapy
- Isometric exercises

Drug therapy
- Analgesic: aspirin
- NSAIDs: indomethacin (Indocin), ibuprofen (Motrin), sulindac (Clinoril), piroxicam (Feldene), flurbiprofen (Ansaid), diclofenac (Voltaren), naproxen (Naprosyn), diflunisal (Dolobid)

INTERVENTIONS AND RATIONALES
- Assess musculoskeletal status *to determine baseline and detect changes.*
- Monitor and record vital signs and intake and output *to evaluate hydration.*
- Assess pain. *Correlating patient's pain with time of day and visits may be useful in modifying tasks.*
- Determine degree of joint mobility *to determine baseline and detect changes.*
- Maintain the patient's diet *to promote nutrition and healing.*
- Keep joints extended *to prevent contractures and maintain joint mobility.*
- Administer medications, as prescribed, *to relieve pain and encourage mobility.*
- Assess for increased bleeding or bruising tendency *to facilitate early intervention for drug adverse effects.*
- Urge the patient to express feelings about changes in body image *to promote effective communication about changes.*
- Provide skin care *to promote skin integrity.*
- Provide rest periods *to conserve energy.*
- Maintain calorie count *to promote nutrition and healing.*

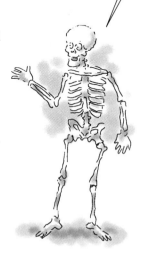

Don't get soft on me. In osteoarthritis, cartilage softens, narrowing the joint space and allowing bones to rub together.

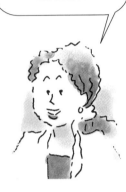

Although osteomyelitis often remains in one location, it can spread through the bone marrow and the membrane that covers the bones.

• Provide moist compresses and paraffin baths (heat therapy), as prescribed, *to promote comfort.*
• Teach proper body mechanics *to prevent injury.*
• Provide passive ROM exercises *to maintain joint mobility.*

Teaching topics

• Avoiding certain exercises (jogging, jumping, lifting)
• Identifying ways to reduce physical stress (weight loss, muscle strengthening)
• Performing complete skin and foot care daily
• Contacting the Arthritis Foundation

Osteomyelitis

Osteomyelitis is a pyogenic (pus-producing) bone infection. It may be chronic or acute and commonly results from a combination of local trauma—usually quite trivial but resulting in hematoma formation—and an acute infection originating elsewhere in the body. Although osteomyelitis commonly remains localized, it can spread through the bone to the marrow, cortex, and periosteum (the membrane that covers the bone).

Acute osteomyelitis is usually a blood-borne disease that most commonly affects rapidly growing children. Chronic osteomyelitis (rare) is characterized by multiple draining sinus tracts and metastatic lesions.

Osteomyelitis occurs more commonly in children than adults—and particularly in boys —usually as a complication of an acute, localized infection. The most common sites in children are the lower end of the femur and the upper end of the tibia, humerus, and radius. In adults, the most common sites are the pelvis and vertebrae, generally the result of contamination associated with surgery or trauma.

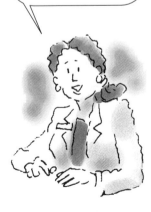

Antibiotic treatment for osteomyelitis usually includes large doses of a penicillinase-resistant penicillin and may begin even before the diagnosis is confirmed.

CAUSES

• Exposure to disease-causing organisms

ASSESSMENT FINDINGS

• Pain
• Tenderness
• Swelling

DIAGNOSTIC TEST RESULTS

• Blood cultures identify the causative organism.
• ESR and CRP are elevated. Note that CRP appears to be a better diagnostic tool.
• WBC count shows leukocytosis.

NURSING DIAGNOSES

• Impaired tissue integrity
• Impaired physical mobility
• Activity intolerance

TREATMENT

• Early surgical drainage to relieve pressure buildup and sequestrum formation (sequestrum is dead bone that has separated from sound bone)
• High-protein diet with extra vitamin C
• Immobilization of the affected bone by plaster cast, traction, or bed rest
• I.V. fluids

Drug therapy

• Antibiotics: large doses of I.V. antibiotics, usually a penicillinase-resistant penicillin, such as nafcillin (Unipen) and oxacillin (Bactocill), or a cephalosporin such as cefazolin (Ancef) after blood cultures are taken
• Analgesics: ibuprofen (Motrin), acetaminophen and oxycodone (Percocet)

INTERVENTIONS AND RATIONALES

• Use strict aseptic technique when changing dressings and irrigating wounds *to prevent infection.*
• If the patient is in skeletal traction for compound fractures, cover insertion points of pin tracks with small, dry dressings, and tell him not to touch the skin around the pins and wires *to prevent infection.*
• Administer I.V. fluids *to maintain adequate hydration as necessary.*
• Provide a diet high in protein and vitamin C *to promote healing.*

• Assess vital signs and wound appearance daily and monitor daily for new pain, *which may indicate secondary infection.*
• Support the affected limb with firm pillows. Keep the limb level with the body; don't let it sag *to prevent injury.*
• Provide good skin care. Turn the patient gently every 2 hours *to prevent skin breakdown* and watch for signs of developing pressure ulcers *to ensure early intervention and treatment.*
• Provide good cast care. Support the cast with firm pillows and "petal" the edges with pieces of adhesive tape or moleskin to smooth rough edges *to prevent skin breakdown which may lead to infection.*
• Check circulation and drainage: If a wet spot appears on the cast, circle it with a marking pen and note the time of appearance (on the cast). Be aware of how much drainage is expected. Check the circled spot at least every 4 hours. Watch for any enlargement. *These measures help detect early signs of hemorrhage.*
• Protect the patient from mishaps, such as jerky movements and falls, which may threaten bone integrity *to prevent injury.*
• Be alert for sudden pain, crepitus, or deformity. Watch for any sudden malposition of the limb *to detect fracture.*
• Provide emotional support and appropriate diversions *to reduce anxiety.*

Teaching topics
• Cleaning the wound
• Recognizing signs of infection
• Need for follow-up examinations
• Seeking prompt treatment for possible sources of recurrence—blisters, boils, styes, and impetigo

Osteoporosis

In osteoporosis, a metabolic bone disorder, the rate of bone resorption accelerates while the rate of bone formation slows down, causing a loss of bone mass. Bones affected by this disease lose calcium and phosphate salts and, thus, become porous, brittle, and abnormally vulnerable to fracture.

Osteoporosis may be primary or secondary to an underlying disease. Primary osteoporosis is often called senile or postmenopausal osteoporosis because it most commonly develops in elderly, postmenopausal women.

CAUSES
• Decreased hormonal function
• Negative calcium balance

ASSESSMENT FINDINGS
• Aged appearance
• Deformity
• Kyphosis
• Pain

DIAGNOSTIC TEST RESULTS
• Bone biopsy shows thin and porous, but otherwise normal-looking bone.
• Dual or single photon absorptiometry allows measurement of bone mass, which helps to assess the extremities, hips, and spine.
• Serum calcium, phosphorus, and alkaline phosphatase are all within normal limits, but parathyroid hormone may be elevated.
• X-rays show typical degeneration in the lower thoracic and lumbar vertebrae. The vertebral bodies may appear flattened and may look denser than normal. Loss of bone mineral becomes evident in later stages.

NURSING DIAGNOSES
• Impaired physical mobility
• Risk for injury
• Chronic pain

TREATMENT
• Physical therapy of gentle exercise and activity
• Supportive devices for weakened vertebrae
• Balanced diet high in vitamin D, calcium, and protein

Drug treatment
• Analgesics: aspirin, indomethacin (Indocin)
• Hormonal agents: conjugated estrogen (Premarin), calcitonin (Calcimar)
• Vitamin D supplements
• Antihypercalcemic drug: etidronate (Didronel)

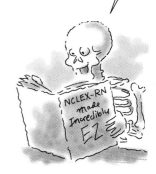

In osteoporosis, bones deteriorate faster than the body can replace them.

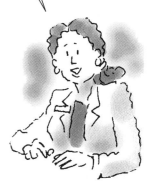

Changes in diet and activity of the patient with osteoporosis may help avoid more fractures.

INTERVENTIONS AND RATIONALES

• Focus on the patient's fragility, stressing careful positioning, ambulation, and pre-scribed exercises *to prevent injury.*

• Check the patient's skin daily for redness, warmth, and new sites of pain, *which may in-dicate new fractures.* Encourage activity; help the patient walk several times daily *to slow progress of the disease.*

• Perform passive ROM exercises or encour-age the patient to perform active exercises. Make sure she regularly attends scheduled physical therapy sessions. *These measures help slow disease progression.*

• Provide a balanced diet high in such nutri-ents as vitamin D, calcium, and protein *to sup-port skeletal metabolism.*

• Administer analgesics and heat *to relieve pain.*

• Advise the patient to sleep on a firm mat-tress *to promote comfort* and avoid excessive bed rest *to slow disease progression.*

• Make sure the patient knows how to wear her back brace *to prevent back injury.*

Teaching topics

• Using good body mechanics while lifting
• Importance of regular exercise
• Understanding the prescribed drug regi-men and reporting adverse reactions immedi-ately
• Reporting any new pain sites immediately, especially after trauma, no matter how slight
• Proper technique for self-examination of the breasts if receiving estrogen therapy
• Need for regular gynecologic examinations and reporting abnormal bleeding promptly while receiving estrogen therapy

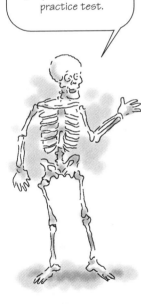

Time to give your bones a break. Take a brief stretch, then jump right in to this practice test.

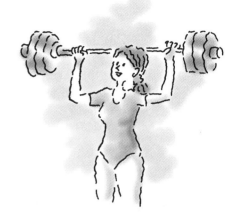

Pump up on practice questions

1. A client with a sports injury undergoes a diagnostic arthroscopy of his left knee. After the procedure, the nurse assesses the client's leg. What are the priority nursing assessment factors?

   A. Wound and skin
   B. Mobility and sensation
   C. Vascular and integumentary
   D. Circulatory and neurologic

Answer: D. Following a procedure on an ex-tremity, nursing assessment should focus on neurovascular status of the extremity. Swell-ing of the extremity can impair both neurolog-ic and circulatory function of the leg. After the neurovascular stability of the extremity has been established, the nurse can address the other concerns of skin, mobility, and pain.

➡ *NCLEX keys*
Nursing process step: Assessment
Client needs category: Physiological integrity
Client needs subcategory: Reduction of risk potential
Taxonomic level: Application

2. A client undergoes a lumbar puncture for a myelogram. Shortly after the procedure, he reports a severe headache. What should the nurse do?

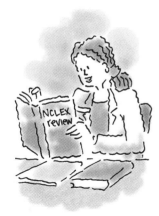

A. Increase the client's fluid intake.
B. Administer prescribed antihypertensives.
C. Offer roll lenses to the client.
D. Place cooling packs over the lumbar puncture site.

Answer: A. Headache following a lumbar puncture is usually caused by cerebrospinal fluid (CSF) leakage. Increased fluid intake will help restore CSF volume. Antihypertensives don't address the problem. Roll lenses reduce light irritation to the eyes and ice may reduce site pain, but neither intervention addresses the problem of reduced CSF volume, which caused the headache.

➡ *NCLEX keys*
Nursing process step: Implementation
Client needs category: Physiological integrity
Client needs subcategory: Reduction of risk potential
Taxonomic level: Analysis

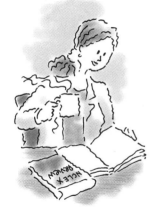

3. The nurse is assessing a client with osteoarthritis of the knees. The nurse would most likely detect crepitation during:
A. palpation.
B. percussion.
C. auscultation.
D. inspection.

Answer: A. Crepitus is a grating sensation associated with degenerative joint disease and can be felt or heard. It's best detected by palpation of the affected joint.

➡ *NCLEX keys*
Nursing process step: Assessment
Client needs category: Physiological integrity
Client needs subcategory: Physiological adaptation
Taxonomic level: Comprehension

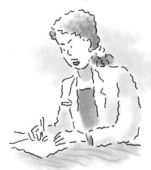

4. A client with osteoarthritis develops coagulopathy secondary to long-term nonsteroidal anti-inflammatory drug (NSAID) use. The coagulopathy is most likely the result of:
A. impaired vitamin K synthesis.
B. blocked prothrombin conversion.
C. decreased platelet adhesiveness.
D. Factor VIII destruction.

Answer: C. NSAIDs reduce platelet adhesiveness and can impair coagulation. They don't impair vitamin K synthesis, block prothrombin conversion, or destroy Factor VIII.

➡ *NCLEX keys*
Nursing process step: Analysis
Client needs category: Physiological integrity
Client needs subcategory: Physiological adaptation
Taxonomic level: Analysis

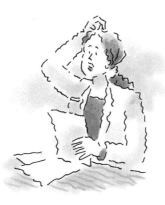

5. The nurse is teaching a client with osteoarthritis about lifestyle changes. Which lifestyle change will most likely reduce the signs and symptoms associated with osteoarthritis?

  A. Avoiding exercise
  B. Restricting caffeine
  C. Abstaining from alcohol
  D. Reducing weight

Answer: D. Osteoarthritis (degenerative joint disease) is a disorder caused by wear and tear on the joints. Excess body weight is a risk factor associated with development and progression of osteoarthritis. Weight reduction can reduce the manifestations of osteoarthritis. Certain aggravating exercises may need to be avoided but exercise can be beneficial. Caffeine isn't associated with clinical manifestations of osteoarthritis. Alcohol intake isn't prohibited.

➦ *NCLEX keys*

Nursing process step: Implementation
Client needs category: Physiological integrity
Client needs subcategory: Physiological adaptation
Taxonomic level: Comprehension

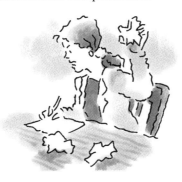

6. A client develops L5-S1 herniated nucleus pulposus, which impinges on the left nerve root. Most likely, the patient would experience pain that radiates:

  A. up the spinal column.
  B. to the lower abdomen.
  C. down the left leg.
  D. across to the right pelvis.

Answer: C. The pain associated with herniated nucleus pulposus of L5-S1 primarily affects the lower back, with radiation down one leg.

➦ *NCLEX keys*

Nursing process step: Analysis
Client needs category: Physiological integrity
Client needs subcategory: Physiological adaptation
Taxonomic level: Comprehension

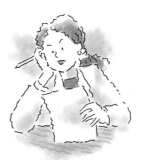

7. A nurse is walking in a local park and witnesses an elderly woman fall. The woman reports severe pain, has difficulty moving her left leg, and is unable to bear weight on the affected leg. The nurse notices her left leg appears shorter than her right. The nurse suspects a femoral fracture. The greatest risk to the client is:

  A. infection.
  B. fat embolus.
  C. neurogenic shock.
  D. hypovolemia.

Answer: D. The greatest risk to the client with a femoral fracture is hypovolemia from hemorrhage, which may be covert and can be fatal if not detected. Infection and fat emboli are potential complications less frequently seen in femoral fracture. Neurogenic shock isn't directly associated with femoral fracture.

➡ NCLEX keys
Nursing process step: Analysis
Client needs category: Physiological integrity
Client needs subcategory: Reduction of risk potential
Taxonomic level: Comprehension

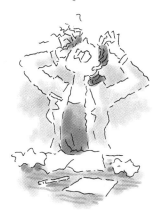

8. A client is undergoing rehabilitation following a fracture. As part of his regimen, the client performs isometric exercises. Which of the following provides the best evidence that the client understands the proper technique?
  A. Exercising of bilateral extremities simultaneously
  B. Periodic monitoring of his heart rate
  C. Forced resistance against stable objects
  D. Swinging of limbs through full range-of-motion

Answer: C. Isometric exercises involve applying pressure against a stable object, such as pressing the hands together or pushing an arm against a wall. Exercising extremities simultaneously isn't a characteristic of isometrics. Heart rate monitoring is associated with aerobic exercising. Limb swinging isn't isometric.

➡ NCLEX keys
Nursing process step: Evaluation
Client needs category: Physiological integrity
Client needs subcategory: Physiological adaptation
Taxonomic level: Application

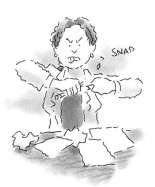

9. A client in balanced suspension traction for a fractured femur needs to be repositioned toward the head of the bed. During repositioning, the nurse should:
  A. place slight additional tension on the traction cords.
  B. release the weights and replace immediately after positioning.
  C. lift the traction and the client during repositioning.
  D. maintain the same degree of traction tension.

Answer: D. Traction is used to reduce the fracture and must be maintained at all times, including during repositioning. It isn't appropriate to increase traction tension or release or lift the traction during repositioning.

➡ NCLEX keys
Nursing process step: Implementation
Client needs category: Physiological integrity
Client needs subcategory: Physiological adaptation
Taxonomic level: Comprehension

10. A client undergoes cast placement for a fractured left radius. The nurse should suspect compartment syndrome if the client experiences pain that:
  A. intensifies with elevation of the left arm.
  B. disappears with left arm flexion.
  C. increases with the arm in a dependent position.
  D. radiates up the arm to the left scapula.

Answer: A. Pain is the most common symptom of compartment syndrome. Because the pain is the result of ischemia, elevating the limb reduces circulation, worsens the ischemia, and intensifies the pain.

➡ *NCLEX keys*

Nursing process step: Analysis
Client needs category: Physiological integrity
Client needs subcategory: Physiological adaptation
Taxonomic level: Comprehension

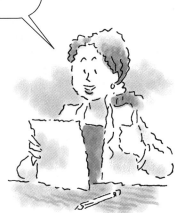

Way to go! You muscled your way through a tough chapter.

Gastrointestinal System

8

Brush up on key concepts

In this chapter, you'll review:

- components of the GI system and their function
- tests used to diagnose GI disorders
- common GI disorders.

The GI system is the body's food processing complex. The GI tract is basically a hollow, muscular tube through which food is digested. In addition, accessory organs, such as the liver and pancreas, contribute substances that are vital to digestion.

At any time, you can review the major points of this chapter by consulting the *Cheat sheet* on pages 234 to 239.

The breakdown begins
The digestive process begins in the **mouth,** where a mechanical (tongue and teeth) and chemical (saliva) combination begins to break down food.

Straight to the stomach
The **esophagus** transfers food from the oropharynx (behind the palate) to the stomach. The esophagus contains two structures, the epiglottis and the cardiac sphincter, that direct food into the stomach. The epiglottis closes to prevent food from entering the trachea, while the cardiac sphincter closes to prevent reflux of gastric contents.

Creating chyme
The **stomach** is a hollow muscular pouch that secretes pepsin, mucus, and hydrochloric acid for digestion. In the stomach, food mixes with gastric juices to become chyme, which the stomach stores before parceling it into the small intestine. The stomach also secretes the intrinsic factor necessary for absorption of vitamin B_{12}.

Digestion central
The **small intestine** consists of the duodenum, jejunum, and ileum. Nearly all digestion takes place in the small intestine, which contains digestive agents, such as bile and pancreatic secretions. The small intestine is also lined with villi, which contain capillaries and lymphatics that transport nutrients from the small intestine to the body.

Absorb, synthesize, and store
The **large intestine** consists of the ascending colon, transverse colon, descending colon, sigmoid colon, and rectum. It absorbs fluid and electrolytes, synthesizes vitamin K, and stores fecal material.

Not just bile
The **liver** is the largest organ in the body. Its many functions include:
- producing and conveying bile
- metabolizing carbohydrates, fats, and proteins
- synthesizing coagulation factors VII, IX, and X, and prothrombin
- storing copper, iron, and vitamins A, D, E, K and B_{12}
- detoxifying chemicals, excreting bilirubin, and producing and storing glycogen
- promoting erythropoiesis when bone marrow production is insufficient.

Pear-shaped storage
The **gallbladder** is a hollow, pear-shaped organ that stores bile and then delivers it through the cystic duct to the common bile duct.

Enzymes and hormones
The **pancreas** secretes three digestive enzymes: amylase, lipase, and trypsin. It also secretes the hormones insulin, glucagon, and somatostatin from the islets of Langerhans into the blood. In addition, the pancreas secretes large amounts of sodium bicarbonate, which is used to neutralize the acid in chyme.

(Text continues on page 240.)

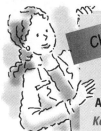

Want a 5-minute review? Check out our cheat sheet.

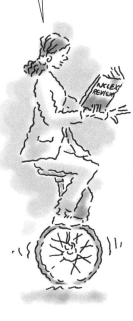

Cheat sheet

Gastrointestinal refresher

APPENDICITIS

Key signs and symptoms
- Anorexia
- Generalized abdominal pain that localizes in the right lower abdomen (McBurney's point)
- Nausea and vomiting
- Sudden cessation of pain (indicates rupture)

Key test results
- Hematology shows white blood cell count moderately elevated.

Key treatments
- Appendectomy

Key interventions
- Assess GI status and pain.
- Maintain nothing-by-mouth status until bowel sounds return postoperatively and then advance diet as tolerated.
- Monitor dressings for drainage and incision for infection postoperatively.

CHOLECYSTITIS

Key signs and symptoms
- Episodic colicky pain in epigastric area, which radiates to back and shoulder
- Indigestion or chest pain after eating fatty or fried foods
- Nausea, vomiting, and flatulence

Key test results
- Blood chemistry reveals increased alkaline phosphatase, bilirubin, direct bilirubin transaminase, amylase, lipase, aspartate aminotransferase (AST), and lactate dehydrogenase (LD) levels.
- Cholangiogram shows stones in the biliary tree.

Key treatments
- Laparoscopic cholecystectomy or open cholecystectomy
- Analgesic: meperidine (Demerol), morphine

Key interventions
- Assess abdominal status and pain.
- Provide postoperative care (monitor dressings for drainage; if open cholecystectomy, monitor and record T-tube drainage, monitor incision for signs of infection, get patient out of bed as soon as possible, encourage use of patient-controlled analgesia).
- Maintain position, patency, and low suction of nasogastric (NG) tube.

CIRRHOSIS

Key signs and symptoms
- Abdominal pain (possibly because of an enlarged liver)
- Anorexia
- Fatigue
- Nausea
- Vomiting
- Weakness

Key test results
- Liver biopsy, the definitive test for cirrhosis, detects destruction and fibrosis of hepatic tissue.
- Computed tomography scan with I.V. contrast reveals enlarged liver, identifies liver masses, and visualizes hepatic blood flow and obstruction, if present.

Key treatments
- Blood transfusions
- Gastric intubation and esophageal balloon tamponade for bleeding esophageal varices (Sengstaken-Blakemore method, esophagogastric tube method, Minnesota tube method)
- I.V. therapy using colloid volume expanders or crystalloids
- Hemostatic: vasopressin (Pitressin) for esophageal varices
- Diuretics: furosemide (Lasix), spironolactone (Aldactone) for edema (Diuretics require careful monitoring; fluid and electrolyte imbalance may precipitate hepatic encephalopathy.)
- Vitamin K: phytonadione (AquaMEPHYTON) for bleeding tendencies due to hypoprothrombinemia

Key interventions
- Assess respiratory status frequently. Position the patient to facilitate breathing.

Gastrointestinal refresher *(continued)*

CIRRHOSIS *(continued)*
- Check skin, gums, stool, and emesis regularly for bleeding.
- Observe the patient closely for signs of behavioral or personality changes—especially increased stupor, lethargy, hallucinations, and neuromuscular dysfunction.
- Wake the patient periodically.
- Monitor ammonia levels.
- Carefully evaluate before, during, and after paracentesis.

COLORECTAL CANCER
Key signs and symptoms
- Abdominal cramping
- Change in bowel habits and shape of stools
- Diarrhea and constipation
- Weight loss

Key test results
- Colonoscopy identifies and locates mass.
- Digital rectal examination reveals mass.

Key treatments
- Radiation therapy
- Surgery depending on tumor location
- Antineoplastics: doxorubicin (Adriamycin), 5-fluorouracil (Adrucil)

Key interventions
- Administer postoperative care if indicated (monitor vital signs and intake and output; make sure NG tube is kept patent; monitor dressing for drainage; assess wound for infection; assist with turning, coughing, deep breathing, and incentive spirometry; medicate for pain as necessary or guide the patient with use of patient-controlled analgesia).

CROHN'S DISEASE
Key signs and symptoms
- Abdominal cramps and spasms after meals
- Chronic diarrhea with blood
- Pain in lower right quadrant

Key test results
- Upper GI series shows classic string sign: segments of stricture separated by normal bowel.

Key treatments
- Colectomy with ileostomy in many patients with extensive disease of the large intestine and rectum
- Antibiotics: sulfasalazine (Azulfidine), metronidazole (Flagyl)
- Anticholinergics: propantheline (Pro-Banthine), dicyclomine (Bentyl)
- Antidiarrheal: diphenoxylate (Lomotil)

- Corticosteroid: prednisone (Deltasone)
- Immunosuppressants: mercaptopurine (Purinethol), azathioprine (Imuran)

Key interventions
- Assess GI status (note excessive abdominal distention) and fluid balance.
- Minimize stress and encourage verbalization of feelings.
- If surgery is necessary, provide postoperative care (monitor vital signs; monitor dressings for drainage; monitor ileostomy drainage and perform ileostomy care as needed; assess incision for signs of infection; assist with turning, coughing, and deep breathing; get the patient out of bed on the 1st postoperative day if stable).

DIVERTICULAR DISEASE
Key signs and symptoms
- Anorexia
- Change in bowel habits
- Flatulence
- Left lower quadrant pain or midabdominal pain that radiates to the back
- Nausea

Key test results
- Sigmoidoscopy shows a thickened wall in the diverticula.

Key treatments
- Colon resection (for diverticulitis refractory to medical treatment)
- Diet: bland (for diverticulosis after pain subsides) or liquid (for mild diverticulitis or diverticulosis before pain subsides)
- Temporary colostomy possible for perforation, peritonitis, obstruction, or fistula that accompanies diverticulitis
- Analgesic: meperidine (Demerol) (mild diverticulitis)
- Antibiotics: gentamicin (Garamycin), tobramycin (Nebcin), clindamycin (Cleocin) (mild diverticulitis)
- Anticholinergic: propantheline (Pro-Banthine)
- Stool softener: docusate sodium (Colace) (diverticulosis or mild diverticulitis)

Key interventions
- Assess abdominal distention and bowel sounds.
- Prepare the patient for surgery, if necessary (administer cleansing enemas, osmotic purgative, oral and parenteral antibiotics).
- Provide postoperative care (watch for signs of infection; perform meticulous wound care; watch for signs of postoperative bleeding; assist with turning, coughing, and deep breathing; teach ostomy self-care).

(continued)

Gastrointestinal refresher (continued)

ESOPHAGEAL CANCER

Key signs and symptoms
- Dysphagia
- Weight loss

Key test results
- Endoscopic examination of the esophagus, punch and brush biopsies, and an exfoliative cytologic test confirm esophageal tumors.

Key treatments
- Gastrostomy or jejunostomy to help provide adequate nutrition
- Radiation therapy
- Radical surgery to excise the tumor and resect either the esophagus alone or the stomach and the esophagus
- Antineoplastic: porfimer (Photofrin)

Key interventions
- Before surgery, answer the patient's questions and let him know what to expect after surgery (gastrostomy tubes, closed chest drainage, NG suctioning).
- After surgery, monitor vital signs and watch for unexpected changes. If surgery included an esophageal anastomosis, keep the patient flat on his back.
- Promote adequate nutrition, and assess the patient's nutritional and hydration status.
- Place the patient in Fowler's position for meals and allow plenty of time to eat.
- Provide high-calorie, high-protein, pureed food as needed.
- If the patient has a gastrostomy tube, give food slowly, using gravity to adjust the flow rate. The prescribed amount usually ranges from 200 to 500 ml. Offer him something to chew before each feeding.
- Provide emotional support for the patient and his family.

GASTRIC CANCER

Key signs and symptoms
- Anorexia
- Epigastric fullness and pain
- Nausea and vomiting
- Pain after eating that isn't relieved by antacids
- Weight loss

Key test results
- Gastric analysis shows positive cancer cells and achlorhydria.
- Gastroscopy biopsy is positive for cancer cells.

Key treatments
- Gastric surgery: gastroduodenostomy, gastrojejunostomy, partial gastric resection, total gastrectomy

- Antineoplastics: carmustine (BiCNU), 5-fluorouracil (Adrucil)
- Vitamin supplements: folic acid (Folvite), cyanocobalamin (vitamin B_{12}) for patients who have undergone total gastrectomy

Key interventions
- Assess GI status postoperatively.
- Maintain position, patency, and low suction of NG tube (without irrigating or repositioning the NG tube because it may put pressure on the suture line).

GASTRITIS

Key signs and symptoms
- Abdominal cramping
- Epigastric discomfort
- Hematemesis
- Indigestion

Key test results
- Upper GI endoscopy with biopsy confirms the diagnosis when performed within 24 hours of bleeding.

Key treatments
- I.V. fluid therapy
- NG lavage to control bleeding
- Histamine$_2$-receptor antagonists: cimetidine (Tagamet), ranitidine (Zantac), famotidine (Pepcid), nizatidine (Axid) (may block gastric secretions)

Key interventions
- If the patient is vomiting, give antiemetics and I.V. fluids.
- Monitor fluid intake and output and electrolyte levels.
- Provide a bland diet. Monitor the patient for recurrent symptoms as food is reintroduced.
- Offer smaller, more frequent meals. Eliminate foods that cause gastric upset.
- If surgery is necessary, prepare the patient preoperatively and provide appropriate postoperative care.
- Administer antacids and other prescribed medications.
- Provide emotional support to the patient.

GASTROENTERITIS

Key signs and symptoms
- Abdominal discomfort
- Diarrhea
- Nausea

Key test results
- Stool culture identifies causative bacteria, parasites, or amoebae.

Key treatments
- I.V. fluid and electrolyte replacement

Gastrointestinal refresher (continued)

GASTROENTERITIS (continued)

• Antidiarrheals: camphorated opium tincture (Paregoric), diphenoxylate with atropine (Lomotil), loperamide (Imodium)

Key interventions

• Administer medications; correlate dosages, routes, and times appropriately with the patient's meals and activities; for example, give antiemetics 30 to 60 minutes before meals.
• If the patient is unable to tolerate food, replace lost fluids and electrolytes with clear liquids and sport drinks.
• Record strict intake and output. Watch for signs of dehydration, such as dry skin and mucous membranes, fever, and sunken eyes.
• Wash your hands thoroughly after giving care.

GASTROESOPHAGEAL REFLUX

Key signs and symptoms

• Dysphagia
• Heartburn (burning sensation in the upper abdomen)

Key test results

• Barium swallow fluoroscopy indicates reflux.
• Esophagoscopy shows reflux.
• Endoscopy allows visualization and confirmation of pathologic changes in the mucosa.

Key treatments

• Positional therapy to help relieve symptoms by decreasing intra-abdominal pressure
• GI stimulant: metoclopramide (Reglan), bethanechol (Urecholine)

Key interventions

• Develop a diet for the patient that takes his food preferences into account.
• Have the patient sleep in reverse Trendelenburg's position (with the head of the bed elevated 6" to 12" [15 to 30 cm]). After surgery using a thoracic approach:
• Carefully watch and record chest tube drainage and respiratory status.
• If needed, give chest physiotherapy and oxygen.
• Place the patient with an NG tube in semi-Fowler's position.

HEPATITIS

Key signs and symptoms

During preicteric phase (usually 1 to 5 days)
• Fatigue
• Right upper quadrant pain
• Weight loss
• Clay-colored stools

During icteric phase (usually 1 to 2 weeks)
• Fatigue
• Jaundice
• Pruritus
• Weight loss

During posticteric or recovery phase (usually 2 to 12 weeks, sometimes longer in patients with hepatitis B, C, or E)
• Decreased hepatomegaly
• Decreased jaundice
• Fatigue

Key test results

• Blood chemistry shows increased alanine aminotransferase, AST, alkaline phosphatase, LD, bilirubin, and erythrocyte sedimentation rate; positive antibody to hepatitis A; positive immunoglobulin antidelta antigens (in type D); positive hepatitis B surface antigen; and positive hepatitis E antigen.

Key treatments

• Vitamins and minerals: vitamin K (AquaMEPHYTON), vitamin C (ascorbic acid), vitamin B-complex (mega-B)

Key interventions

• Assess GI status and watch for bleeding and fulminant hepatitis.
• Maintain standard precautions.

HIATAL HERNIA

Key signs and symptoms

• Dysphagia
• Regurgitation
• Sternal pain after eating

Key test results

• Barium swallow reveals protrusion of the hernia.
• Chest X-ray shows protrusion of abdominal organs into the thorax.
• Esophagoscopy shows incompetent cardiac sphincter.

Key treatments

• Bland diet with decreased intake of caffeine and spicy foods
• Anticholinergic: propantheline (Pro-Banthine)
• Histamine$_2$-receptor antagonists: cimetidine (Tagamet), ranitidine (Zantac), famotidine (Pepcid)

Key interventions

• Assess respiratory status.
• Avoid flexion at the waist in positioning the patient.

(continued)

Gastrointestinal refresher *(continued)*

INTESTINAL OBSTRUCTION

Key signs and symptoms
- Abdominal distention
- Cramping pain
- Diminished or absent bowel sounds

Key test results
- Abdominal X-ray shows increased amount of gas in bowel.
- Barium enema stops at obstruction.

Key treatments
- Bowel resection with or without anastomosis if other treatment fails
- GI decompression using NG tube, Miller-Abbott tube, or Cantor tube

Key interventions
- Assess GI status. Assess and record bowel sounds once per shift.
- Measure and record the patient's abdominal girth.
- Maintain position, patency, and low intermittent suction of NG tube and Miller-Abbott tube.
- Administer postoperative care if indicated (monitor vital signs and intake and output; make sure NG tube is kept patent; monitor dressing for drainage; assess wound for infection; assist with turning, coughing, and deep breathing; medicate for pain as necessary or guide the patient with use of postoperative patient-controlled analgesia).

IRRITABLE BOWEL SYNDROME

Key signs and symptoms
- Abdominal bloating
- Constipation, diarrhea, or both
- Lower abdominal pain
- Passage of mucus
- Pasty, pencil-like stools

Key test results
- Sigmoidoscopy may disclose spastic contractions.

Key treatments
- Elimination diet to determine if symptoms result from food intolerance (In this type of diet, certain foods, such as citrus fruits, coffee, corn, dairy products, tea, and wheat, are sequentially eliminated. Then each food is gradually reintroduced to identify which foods, if any, trigger the patient's symptoms.)
- Diet containing 15 to 20 g daily of bulky foods, such as wheat bran, oatmeal, oat bran, rye cereals, prunes, dried apricots, and figs (if the patient has constipation and abdominal pain)
- Stress management
- Antispasmodic: propantheline (Pro-Banthine)

- Antidiarrheal: diphenoxylate with atropine (Lomotil)

Key interventions
- Help the patient deal with stress, and warn against dependence on sedatives or antispasmodics.

PANCREATITIS

Key signs and symptoms
- Abdominal tenderness and distention
- Abrupt onset of pain in epigastric area that radiates to the shoulder, substernal area, back, and flank
- Aching, burning, stabbing, pressing pain
- Nausea and vomiting
- Tachycardia

Key test results
- Blood chemistry shows increased amylase, lipase, LD, glucose, AST, and lipid levels and decreased calcium and potassium levels.
- Cullen's sign is positive.
- Grey Turner's sign is positive.
- Ultrasonography reveals cysts, bile duct inflammation, and dilation.

Key treatments
- Bed rest
- I.V. fluids (vigorous replacement of fluids and electrolytes)
- Transfusion therapy with packed red blood cells
- Analgesic: meperidine (Demerol) (morphine contraindicated)
- Antidiabetic: insulin (possible infusion to stabilize blood glucose levels)
- Corticosteroid: hydrocortisone (Solu-Cortef)
- Potassium supplement: I.V. potassium chloride

Key interventions
- Assess abdominal, cardiac, and respiratory status (as the disease progresses, watch for respiratory failure, tachycardia, and worsening GI status).
- Assess fluid balance.
- Perform bedside glucose monitoring.
- Administer I.V. fluids.
- Keep the patient in bed and turn every 2 hours, or utilize a specialty rotation bed.

PEPTIC ULCER

Key signs and symptoms
- Anorexia
- Hematemesis
- Left epigastric pain 1 to 2 hours after eating
- Relief of pain after administration of antacids

PEPTIC ULCER *(continued)*

Key test results

- Barium swallow shows ulceration of gastric mucosa.
- Upper GI endoscopy shows location of ulcer.

Key treatments

- If GI hemorrhage, gastric surgery that may include gastroduodenostomy, gastrojejunostomy, partial gastric resection, and total gastrectomy
- Saline lavage by NG tube until return is clear (if bleeding is present)
- Antibiotic if *Helicobacter pylori* is present
- Histamine$_2$-receptor antagonists: cimetidine (Tagamet), ranitidine (Zantac), nizatidine (Axid), famotidine (Pepcid)
- Mucosal barrier fortifier: sucralfate (Carafate)

Key interventions

- Assess GI status.
- Assess cardiovascular status.
- Maintain position, patency, and low suction of NG tube if gastric decompression is ordered.
- Provide postoperative care if necessary (don't reposition NG tube; irrigate it gently if ordered; medicate for pain as needed and ordered; monitor dressings for drainage; assess bowel sounds; get patient out of bed as tolerated).

PERITONITIS

Key signs and symptoms

- Abdominal resonance and tympany on percussion
- Abdominal rigidity and distention
- Constant, diffuse, and intense abdominal pain
- Decreased or absent bowel sounds
- Decreased urine output
- Fever
- Rebound tenderness
- Shallow respirations
- Weak, rapid pulse

Key test results

- Abdominal X-ray shows free air in abdomen under diaphragm.

Key treatments

- Surgical intervention when the patient's condition is stabilized (Surgery is chosen to treat the cause; for example, if the patient has a perforated appendix, then an appendectomy is indicated. Drains will also be placed for drainage of infected material.)

Key interventions

- Assess abdominal and respiratory status and fluid balance.
- Monitor and record vital signs, intake and output, laboratory studies, central venous pressure, daily weight, and urine specific gravity.

- Provide routine postoperative care (monitor vital signs and intake and output, including drainage from drains; assist with turning, incentive spirometry, coughing, and deep breathing; and get the patient out of bed on the 1st postoperative day if his condition allows).

ULCERATIVE COLITIS

Key signs and symptoms

- Abdominal cramping
- Bloody, purulent, mucoid, watery stools (15 to 20 per day)
- Hyperactive bowel sounds
- Weight loss

Key test results

- Barium enema shows ulcerations.
- Sigmoidoscopy shows ulceration and hyperemia.

Key treatments

- Colectomy or pouch ileostomy
- Total parenteral nutrition (TPN) if necessary to rest the GI tract
- Antibiotic: sulfasalazine (Azulfidine)
- Anticholinergics: propantheline (Pro-Banthine), dicyclomine (Bentyl)
- Antidiarrheals: diphenoxylate (Lomotil), loperamide (Imodium)
- Antiemetic: prochlorperazine (Compazine)
- Corticosteroid: hydrocortisone (Solu-Cortef)
- Immunosuppressants: azathioprine (Imuran), cyclophosphamide (Cytoxan)

Key interventions

- Assess GI status and fluid balance.
- Monitor the number, amount, and character of stools.
- Administer I.V. fluids and TPN.
- Maintain position, patency, and low suction of NG tube.

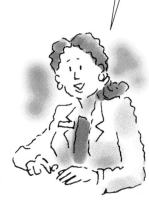

Visualize. Imagine that you're caring for a real-life patient and performing each nursing action. It will make information more meaningful and help you remember.

Keep abreast of diagnostic tests

Here are the most important tests used to diagnose GI disorders, along with common nursing interventions associated with each test.

Barium upstairs

A **barium swallow test** involves fluoroscopic examination of the pharynx and esophagus.

Nursing actions

Before the procedure, you should:
• withhold food and fluids.
  After the procedure, you should:
• force fluids unless contraindicated
• administer laxatives, as prescribed.

Barium in the middle

An **upper GI series** uses an X-ray to examine the esophagus, stomach, duodenum, and other portions of the small bowel after the patient swallows barium.

Nursing actions

Before the procedure, you should:
• withhold food and fluids
• administer I.V. fluids, cathartics, and enemas, as prescribed.
  After the procedure, you should:
• inform the patient that stool will be light-colored for several days
• administer cathartics, fluids, and enemas, as prescribed.

Barium below

A **lower GI series**, also known as a barium enema, uses an X-ray to examine the large intestine.

Nursing actions

Before the procedure, you should:
• withhold food and fluids
• administer bowel preparation (laxatives and enemas), as prescribed.
  After the procedure, you should:
• force fluids unless contraindicated

• administer enemas and laxatives, as prescribed
• monitor color and consistency of stool.

Viewing the stomach directly

Endoscopy uses an endoscope to view the esophagus and stomach.

Nursing actions

Before the procedure, you should:
• withhold food and fluids
• make sure that written, informed consent has been obtained
• obtain baseline vital signs
• administer sedatives, as prescribed.
  After the procedure, you should:
• assess gag and cough reflexes
• assess vasovagal response
• withhold food and fluids until the gag reflex returns.

Blood search

A **fecal occult blood test** analyzes stools for the presence of blood.

Nursing actions

• Document administration of aspirin, vitamin C, and anti-inflammatory drugs.

Fat search

A **fecal fat test** analyzes stool for the presence of fat.

Nursing actions

• Instruct the patient to abstain from alcohol and to maintain a high-fat diet (100 g/day) for 3 days before and during the 72-hour stool collection.
• Refrigerate the specimen.
• Document current medications.

From colon to canal

Proctosigmoidoscopy uses a lighted scope to view the sigmoid colon, rectum, and anal canal.

Nursing actions

Before the procedure, you should:
• administer bowel preparation, as prescribed

• make sure that written, informed consent has been obtained.
  After the procedure, you should:
• document iron intake
• check the patient for bleeding
• monitor the patient's vital signs.

Detailing the biliary duct

Cholangiography uses dye injection to produce a radiographic picture of the biliary duct system.

Nursing actions

Before the procedure, you should:
• encourage a low-residue, high-fat diet 1 day before the examination
• make sure that written, informed consent has been obtained
• withhold food and fluids after midnight
• note the patient's allergies to iodine, seafood, and radiopaque dyes
• inform the patient about possible throat irritation and flushing of the face.
  After the procedure, you should:
• check the injection site for bleeding
• monitor vital signs
• administer fluids to flush the dye out through the kidneys.

Liver image

A **liver scan** produces an image of blood flow in the liver using an injection of a radioisotope.

Nursing actions

Before the procedure, you should:
• determine the patient's ability to lie still during the procedure
• check the patient for possible allergies
• make sure that written, informed consent has been obtained.
  After the procedure, you should:
• assess the patient for signs of delayed allergic reaction to the radioisotope, such as itching and hives.

Acid analysis

A **gastric analysis** is performed after the patient has fasted. It measures the acidity of gastric secretions aspirated through a nasogastric (NG) tube.

Nursing actions

Before the procedure, you should:
• withhold food and fluids after midnight
• instruct the patient not to smoke for 8 to 12 hours before the test
• withhold medications that can affect gastric secretions for 24 hours before the procedure.
  After the procedure, you should:
• obtain vital signs
• note reactions to gastric acid stimulant, if used.

Organ echo

Ultrasonography uses echoes from sound waves to visualize body organs.

Nursing actions

• Assess the patient's ability to lie still during the procedure.
• Explain the procedure to the patient.

Blood study 1

Blood chemistry tests are used to analyze the patient's blood. Samples may be obtained to analyze potassium, sodium, calcium, phosphorus, glucose, bicarbonate, blood urea nitrogen, creatinine, protein, albumin, osmolality, amylase, lipase, alkaline phosphatase, ammonia, bilirubin, lactate dehydrogenase (LD), aspartate aminotransferase (AST), serum alanine aminotransferase (ALT), hepatitis-associated antigens, and carcinoembryonic antigen (CEA).

Nursing actions

• Check the venipuncture site for bleeding.

Blood study 2

A **hematologic study** analyzes a blood sample for red blood cells (RBCs), white blood cells (WBCs), platelets, prothrombin time (PT), international normalized ratio (INR), partial thromboplastin time (PTT), hemoglobin (Hb), hematocrit (HCT), fibrin split products (FSP), and erythrocyte sedimentation rate (ESR).

Nursing actions

• Note current drug therapy.
• Check venipuncture site for bleeding.

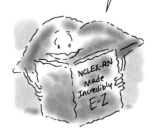

A biliary duct, also called a bile duct, is a duct by which bile passes from the liver or gallbladder to the duodenum.

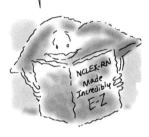

Liver biopsy involves percutaneous removal of liver tissue with a needle. Afterward, watch for signs of shock and pneumothorax.

Tissue removal

A **liver biopsy**, which is used to diagnose disorders such as cirrhosis and cancer, involves percutaneous removal of liver tissue with a needle.

Nursing actions

Before the procedure, you should:
• withhold food and fluids after midnight
• make sure that written, informed consent has been obtained
• assess baseline clotting studies and vital signs
• instruct the patient to exhale and hold his breath during insertion of the needle.
    After the procedure, you should:
• check the insertion site for bleeding
• monitor vital signs
• observe the patient for signs of shock (hypotension, tachycardia, oliguria) and pneumothorax (decreased breath sounds on the affected side, tachypnea, shortness of breath)
• position the patient on right lateral side for hemostasis.

Lighting the large intestine

Colonoscopy uses a lighted scope to directly visualize the large intestine.

Nursing actions

Before the procedure, you should:
• make sure that written, informed consent has been obtained
• provide a clear liquid diet 48 hours before the test
• administer a bowel preparation the day before the test
• explain that the patient will feel cramping and the sensation of needing to have a bowel movement
• explain the use of air to distend the bowel lumen.
    After the procedure, you should:
• monitor for gross bleeding
• withhold food and fluids for 2 hours
• check for blood in stool if polyps were removed.

Detailing ducts

Endoscopic retrograde cholangiopancreatography (ERCP) is a radiographic examination of the hepatobiliary tree and pancreatic ducts using a contrast medium and a lighted scope.

Nursing actions

Before the procedure, you should:
• make sure that written, informed consent has been obtained
• withhold food and fluids after midnight
• check for allergies to iodine or seafood.
    After the procedure, you should:
• check for respiratory depression
• check for urine retention
• assess gag reflex and withhold food until gag reflex returns.

Tracking the bile trail

Percutaneous transhepatic cholangiography is fluoroscopic examination of the biliary ducts. It involves injection of a contrast medium.

Nursing actions

Before the procedure, you should:
• inform the patient that the X-ray table will be tilted and rotated during the procedure
• make sure that written, informed consent has been obtained
• check for allergies to iodine or seafood
• check PT, INR, and PTT
• withhold food and fluids after midnight.
    After the procedure, you should:
• require the patient to rest for at least 6 hours on his side
• check for bleeding at the injection site
• monitor vital signs
• withhold food and fluids for 2 hours.

Polish up on patient care

Major GI disorders include appendicitis, cholecystitis, cirrhosis, colorectal cancer, Crohn's disease, diverticular disease, esophageal cancer, gastric cancer, gastritis, gastroenteritis, gastroesophageal reflux, hepatitis, hiatal hernia, intestinal obstruction, irritable bowel syndrome, pancreatitis, peptic ulcer, peritonitis, and ulcerative colitis.

Appendicitis

Appendicitis is an inflammation of the appendix. Although the appendix has no known function, it regularly fills with and empties itself of food. Appendicitis occurs when the appendix becomes inflamed from ulceration of the mucosa or from obstruction of the lumen.

CAUSES
- Barium ingestion
- Fecal mass
- Stricture
- Viral infection

ASSESSMENT FINDINGS
- Anorexia
- Constipation
- Generalized abdominal pain that becomes localized in the right lower abdomen (McBurney's point)
- Lies in knee-bent position
- Malaise
- Nausea and vomiting
- Sudden cessation of pain (indicates rupture)

DIAGNOSTIC TEST RESULTS
- Hematology shows WBC count moderately elevated.

NURSING DIAGNOSES
- Altered nutrition: Less than body requirements
- Pain
- Risk for infection

TREATMENT
- Appendectomy
- I.V. fluids to prevent dehydration
- Nothing by mouth

Drug therapy
- Analgesics: meperidine (Demerol), morphine (administered only when diagnosis is confirmed)

INTERVENTIONS AND RATIONALES
- Assess GI status and pain. *Sudden cessation of pain preoperatively may indicate appendix rupture.*

- Monitor and record vital signs and intake and output *to determine fluid volume.*
- Administer medications as ordered *to maintain or improve patient's condition.*
- Maintain nothing-by-mouth status until bowel sounds return postoperatively; then advance diet as tolerated *to promote healing and meet metabolic needs.*
- Assist patient with incentive spirometry, turning, coughing, and deep breathing *to mobilize secretions and promote lung expansion.*
- Monitor dressings for drainage and incision for infection postoperatively *to detect early signs of infection and prevent complications.*

Teaching topics
- Completing follow-up medical care
- Following activity restrictions
- Recognizing the signs and symptoms of infection

Cholecystitis

Cholecystitis is an acute or chronic inflammation of the gallbladder most commonly associated with cholelithiasis (presence of gallstones). It occurs when an obstruction, such as calculi or edema, prevents the gallbladder from contracting when fatty foods enter the duodenum.

CAUSES
- Cholelithiasis
- Estrogen therapy
- Infection of the gallbladder
- Obesity

ASSESSMENT FINDINGS
- Belching
- Clay-colored stools
- Dark amber urine
- Ecchymosis
- Episodic colicky pain in the epigastric area, which radiates to the back and shoulder
- Fever
- Flatulence
- Indigestion or chest pain after eating fatty or fried foods
- Jaundice
- Nausea and vomiting

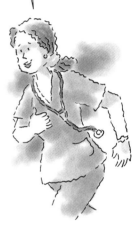

When pain suddenly stops during appendicitis, it indicates rupture. Get ready to implement emergency care.

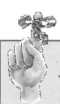

Memory jogger

Cholecystitis occurs most often in overweight women over 40 who haven't gone through menopause. To remember risk factors associated with cholecystitis, think of the 4 Fs.

Female

Fertile

Forty

Fat

- Pruritus
- Steatorrhea

DIAGNOSTIC TEST RESULTS
- Blood chemistry reveals increased alkaline phosphatase, bilirubin, direct bilirubin transaminase, amylase, lipase, AST, and LD levels.
- Cholangiogram shows stones in the biliary tree.
- Gallbladder series shows stones in the biliary tree.
- Hematology shows increased WBC count.
- Liver scan shows obstruction of the biliary tree.
- Ultrasound shows bile duct distention and calculi.

NURSING DIAGNOSES
- Fluid volume deficit
- Altered nutrition: Less than body requirements
- Risk for infection

TREATMENT
- Small, frequent meals of a low-fat, low-calorie diet high in carbohydrates, protein, and fiber with restricted intake of gas-forming foods or no foods or fluids, as directed
- Extracorporeal shock wave lithotripsy
- Incentive spirometry
- Laparoscopic cholecystectomy or open cholecystectomy

Drug therapy
- Analgesics: meperidine (Demerol), morphine
- Antibiotic: cephalothin (Keflin)
- Anticholinergics: propantheline (Pro-Banthine), dicyclomine (Bentyl)
- Antiemetic: prochlorperazine (Compazine)
- Antipruritic: diphenhydramine (Benadryl)

INTERVENTIONS AND RATIONALES
- Assess abdominal status and pain *to determine baseline and detect changes in patient's condition.*
- Monitor and record vital signs and intake and output, laboratory studies, and urine specific gravity *to assess fluid and electrolyte balance.*
- Maintain the patient's diet; withhold food and fluids *to rest the GI tract and prevent recurrence of condition.*
- Administer I.V. fluids *to provide patient with needed fluids and electrolytes.*
- Administer medications as prescribed *to treat infection, decrease pain, and promote comfort.*
- Provide postoperative care (monitor dressings for drainage; if open cholecystectomy monitor and record T-tube drainage, monitor incision for signs of infection, get patient out of bed as soon as possible, encourage use of patient-controlled analgesia) *to maintain the patient's condition and prevent postoperative complications.*
- Assist with turning, incentive spirometry, coughing, and deep breathing *to mobilize secretions and promote lung expansion.*
- Maintain position, patency, and low suction of NG tube *to prevent nausea and vomiting.*
- Keep the patient in semi-Fowler's position *to promote comfort and facilitate GI emptying.*
- Provide skin, nares, and mouth care *to promote patient comfort and prevent tissue breakdown.*
- Maintain a quiet environment *to promote rest.*

Teaching topics
- Using patient-controlled analgesia
- Completing skin care daily
- Recognizing the signs and symptoms of infection
- Limiting activity as necessary

Cirrhosis

Cirrhosis is a chronic hepatic disease characterized by diffuse destruction of hepatic cells, which are replaced by fibrous cells. Necrotic tissue yields to fibrosis. Cirrhosis alters liver structure and normal vasculature, impairs blood and lymph flow, and eventually causes hepatic insufficiency. Cirrhosis is irreversible.

In cirrhosis, drug therapy requires special caution because the cirrhotic liver can't detoxify harmful substances efficiently.

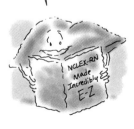

CAUSES
• Alcoholism and resulting malnutrition
• Autoimmune disease such as sarcoidosis or chronic inflammatory bowel disease
• Exposure to hepatitis (types A, B, C, and D viral hepatitis) or toxic substances

ASSESSMENT FINDINGS
• Abdominal pain (possibly because of an enlarged liver)
• Anorexia
• Constipation
• Diarrhea
• Fatigue
• Indigestion
• Muscle cramps
• Nausea
• Vomiting
• Weakness

DIAGNOSTIC TEST RESULTS
• Liver biopsy, the definitive test for cirrhosis, detects destruction and fibrosis of hepatic tissue.
• Computed tomography (CT) scan with I.V. contrast medium reveals enlarged liver, identifies liver masses, and visualizes hepatic blood flow and obstruction, if present.
• Magnetic resonance imaging can further assess hepatic nodules.
• Esophagogastroduodenoscopy reveals bleeding esophageal varices, stomach irritation or ulceration, or duodenal bleeding and irritation.
• Blood studies reveal decreased platelets and decreased levels of Hb and HCT, albumin, serum electrolytes (sodium, potassium, chloride, magnesium), and folate.
• Blood studies reveal elevated levels of globulin, ammonia, total bilirubin, alkaline phosphatase, AST, ALT, and LD and increased thymol turbidity.
• Urine studies show increased levels of bilirubin and urobilinogen.
• Stool studies reveal decreasing urobilinogen levels.

NURSING DIAGNOSES
• Altered nutrition: Less than body requirements
• Risk for injury
• Ineffective breathing pattern

TREATMENT
• Blood transfusions
• Fluid restriction (usually to 1,500 ml/day)
• Gastric intubation and esophageal balloon tamponade for bleeding esophageal varices (Sengstaken-Blakemore method, esophagogastric tube method, Minnesota tube method)
• I.V. therapy using colloid volume expanders or crystalloids
• Oxygen therapy (may require endotracheal intubation and mechanical ventilation)
• Paracentesis to reduce abdominal pressure from ascites
• Portal-systemic shunting as a last resort for patients with bleeding esophageal varices and portal hypertension
• Sclerotherapy, if the patient continues to experience repeated hemorrhagic episodes despite conservative treatment
• Sodium restriction (usually up to 500 mg/day)
• Surgical intervention: peritoneovenous shunt

Drug therapy
• Antiemetics: trimethobenzamide (Tigan), benzquinamide (Emete-Con)
• Hemostatic: vasopressin (Pitressin) for esophageal varices
• Diuretics: furosemide (Lasix), spironolactone (Aldactone) for edema (Diuretics require careful monitoring; fluid and electrolyte imbalance may precipitate hepatic encephalopathy.)
• Vitamin K: phytonadione (AquaMEPHYTON) for bleeding tendencies due to hypoprothrombinemia
• Beta-adrenergic blocker: propranolol (Inderal) to decrease pressure from varices
• Laxative: lactulose (Cephulac) to reduce serum ammonia levels

INTERVENTIONS AND RATIONALES
• Assess respiratory status frequently *because abdominal distention may interfere with lung expansion.* Position the patient *to facilitate breathing.*

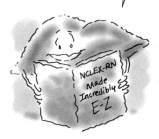

Talkin' 'bout regeneration. . . The process whereby necrotic cells are replaced by fibrous cells is called fibrotic regeneration.

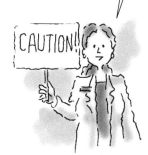

Watch ammonia levels in the patient with cirrhosis; elevated ammonia levels may lead to encephalopathy.

• Check skin, gums, stool, and emesis regularly for bleeding *to recognize early signs of bleeding and prevent hemorrhage.*
• Apply pressure to injection sites *to prevent bleeding.*
• Warn the patient against taking aspirin, straining during defecation, and blowing his nose or sneezing too vigorously *to avoid bleeding.* Suggest using an electric razor and soft toothbrush. *These measures also prevent bleeding.*
• Observe the patient closely for signs of behavioral or personality changes—especially increased stupor, lethargy, hallucinations, and neuromuscular dysfunction. *Behavioral or personality changes may indicate increased ammonia levels.*
• Wake the patient periodically *to determine his level of consciousness.*
• Watch for asterixis, *a sign of developing hepatic encephalopathy.*
• Monitor ammonia levels *to determine effectiveness of lactulose therapy.*
• Weigh the patient and measure his abdominal girth daily, inspect the ankles and sacrum for dependent edema, and accurately record intake and output *to assess fluid retention.*
• Carefully evaluate the patient before, during, and after paracentesis *because this drastic loss of fluid may induce shock.*

• Avoid using soap when bathing the patient; instead, use lubricating lotion or moisturizing agents *to prevent skin breakdown associated with edema and pruritus.*
• Handle the patient gently, and turn and reposition often *to keep skin intact.*
• Encourage rest and good nutrition *to help the patient conserve energy and decrease metabolic demands on the liver.*
• Encourage frequent, small meals *to ensure nutritional needs are met.*

Teaching topics
• Importance of avoiding infections and abstaining from alcohol
• Contacting Alcoholics Anonymous
• Avoiding activities that increase intra-abdominal pressure, such as heavy lifting, vigorous coughing, and straining during a bowel movement

Colorectal cancer

Colorectal cancer is a malignant tumor of the colon or rectum. It may be primary or metastatic. It begins when unregulated cell growth and uncontrolled cell division develop into a neoplasm. Adenocarcinomas then infiltrate and cause obstruction, ulcerations, and hemorrhage.

Battling illness

Location, location, location

Surgery for colorectal cancer depends on the location of the tumor. If the tumor is in the:
• cecum and ascending colon, surgery is a right hemicolectomy. This surgery may include resection of the terminal segment of the ileum, cecum, ascending colon, and right half of the transverse colon with corresponding mesentery.
• proximal and middle transverse colon, surgery is a right colectomy that includes the transverse colon and mesentery, or segmental resection of the transverse colon and associated midcolic vessels.
• sigmoid colon, surgery is limited to the sigmoid colon and mesentery.
• upper rectum, surgery is an anterior or low anterior resection.
• lower rectum, surgery is an abdominoperineal resection and permanent sigmoid colostomy.

CAUSES
- Aging
- Chronic constipation
- Chronic ulcerative colitis
- Diverticulosis
- Familial polyposis
- Low-fiber, high-carbohydrate diet

ASSESSMENT FINDINGS
- Abdominal cramping
- Abdominal distention
- Anorexia
- Change in bowel habits and shape of stools
- Diarrhea and constipation
- Fecal oozing
- Melena
- Pallor
- Palpable mass
- Rectal bleeding
- Vomiting
- Weakness
- Weight loss

DIAGNOSTIC TEST RESULTS
- Barium enema locates mass.
- Biopsy is positive for cancer cells.
- CEA is positive.
- Colonoscopy identifies and locates mass.
- Digital rectal examination reveals mass.
- Fecal occult blood test is positive.
- Lower GI series shows location of mass.
- Hematology shows decreased Hb and HCT.
- Sigmoidoscopy identifies and locates mass.

NURSING DIAGNOSES
- Anxiety
- Fluid volume deficit
- Pain

TREATMENT
- Radiation therapy
- Surgery depending on tumor location (see *Location, location, location*)

Drug therapy
- Antiemetics: prochlorperazine (Compazine), ondansetron (Zofran)
- Antineoplastics: doxorubicin (Adriamycin), 5-fluorouracil (Adrucil)
- Folic acid derivative: leucovorin (citrovorum factor)

- Immunomodulator: levamisole (Ergamisol)

INTERVENTIONS AND RATIONALES
- Assess GI status *to determine baseline and detect changes in patient's condition.*
- Monitor and record vital signs and intake and output, laboratory studies, and daily weight *to assess fluid and electrolyte status.*
- Monitor and record the color, consistency, amount, and frequency of stools *to detect early changes and bleeding.*
- Monitor for bleeding, infection, and electrolyte imbalance *to detect early changes and prevent complications.*
- Maintain the patient's diet *to meet metabolic needs and promote healing.*
- Keep the patient in semi-Fowler's position *to promote emptying of the GI tract.*
- Administer total parenteral nutrition *to improve nutritional status when the patient is unable to consume adequate calories through the GI tract.*
- Administer postoperative care if indicated (monitor vital signs and intake and output; make sure NG tube is kept patent; monitor dressing for drainage; assess wound for infection; assist with turning, coughing, deep breathing, and incentive spirometry; medicate for pain as necessary or guide the patient with use of patient-controlled analgesia) *to prevent complications and promote healing.*
- Encourage the patient to express feelings about changes in body image and a fear of dying, and support coping mechanisms *to increase potential for further adaptive behavior.*
- Provide skin and mouth care *to maintain tissue integrity.*
- Provide rest periods *to promote healing and conserve energy.*
- Provide postchemotherapeutic and postradiation nursing care *to promote healing and prevent complications.*
- Monitor dietary intake *to determine nutritional adequacy.*
- Administer antiemetics and antidiarrheals, as prescribed, *to prevent further fluid loss.*

Teaching topics
- Performing ostomy self-care if indicated
- Monitoring changes in bowel elimination
- Self-monitoring for infection

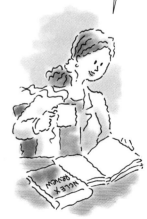

Patient-controlled analgesia allows the patient to control I.V. delivery of an analgesic, usually morphine.

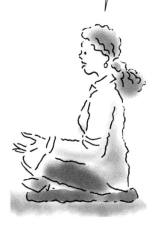

Crohn's disease is a chronic disorder. Patient care involves long-term concerns such as reducing stress.

• Alternating rest periods with activity.
• Contacting the United Ostomy Association and the American Cancer Society

Crohn's disease

Crohn's disease is a chronic inflammatory disease of the small intestine, usually affecting the terminal ileum. It also sometimes affects the large intestine, usually in the ascending colon. It's slowly progressive with exacerbations and remissions.

CAUSES
• Emotional upsets
• Fried foods
• Milk and milk products
• Unknown

ASSESSMENT FINDINGS
• Abdominal cramps and spasms after meals
• Chronic diarrhea with blood
• Fever
• Flatulence
• Nausea
• Pain in lower right quadrant
• Weight loss

DIAGNOSTIC TEST RESULTS
• Abdominal X-ray shows congested, thickened, fibrosed, narrowed intestinal wall.
• Barium enema shows lesions in terminal ileum.
• Fecal fat test shows increased fat.
• Fecal occult blood test is positive.
• Proctosigmoidoscopy shows ulceration.
• Upper GI series shows classic string sign: segments of stricture separated by normal bowel.

NURSING DIAGNOSES
• Anxiety
• Diarrhea
• Altered nutrition: Less than body requirements

TREATMENT
• Colectomy with ileostomy in many patients with extensive disease of the large intestine and rectum

• Small, frequent meals of a diet high in protein, calories, and carbohydrates and low in fat, fiber, and residue with bland foods and restricted intake of milk and gas-forming foods or no food or fluids
• Total parenteral nutrition (TPN) to rest the bowel

Drug therapy
• Analgesic: meperidine (Demerol), morphine
• Antianemics: ferrous sulfate (Feosol), ferrous gluconate (Fergon)
• Antibiotics: sulfasalazine (Azulfidine), metronidazole (Flagyl)
• Anticholinergics: propantheline (Pro-Banthine), dicyclomine (Bentyl)
• Antidiarrheal: diphenoxylate (Lomotil)
• Antiemetic: prochlorperazine (Compazine)
• Anti-inflammatory: olsalazine (Dipentum)
• Corticosteroid: prednisone (Deltasone)
• Immunosuppressants: mercaptopurine (Purinethol), azathioprine (Imuran)
• Potassium supplements: potassium chloride (K-Lor) administered with food, potassium gluconate (Kaon)

INTERVENTIONS AND RATIONALES
• Assess GI status (note excessive abdominal distention) and fluid balance *to determine baseline and detect changes in patient's condition.*
• Monitor and record vital signs and intake and output, laboratory studies, daily weight, urine specific gravity, and fecal occult blood *to detect bleeding and dehydration.*
• Monitor the number, amount, and character of stools *to detect deterioration in GI status.*
• Administer TPN *to rest the bowel and promote nutritional status.*
• Administer medications, as prescribed, *to maintain or improve patient's condition.*
• Maintain the patient's diet; withhold food and fluids as necessary *to minimize GI discomfort.*
• Minimize stress and encourage verbalization of feelings *to allay the patient's anxiety.*
• Provide skin and perianal care *to prevent skin breakdown.*
• If surgery is necessary, provide postoperative care (monitor vital signs; monitor dressings for drainage; monitor ileostomy drainage

and perform ileostomy care as needed; assess incision for signs of infection; assist with turning, coughing, and deep breathing; get the patient out of bed on the 1st postoperative day if stable) *to promote healing and prevent complications.*

Teaching topics
- Performing ileostomy self-care
- Avoiding laxatives and aspirin
- Performing perianal care daily
- Reducing stress
- Recognizing the signs and symptoms of rectal hemorrhage and intestinal obstruction

Diverticular disease

Diverticular disease has two clinical forms: diverticulosis and diverticulitis. Diverticulosis occurs when the intestinal mucosa protrudes through the muscular wall. The common sites for diverticula are in the descending and sigmoid colon, but they may develop anywhere from the proximal end of the pharynx to the anus.

Diverticulitis is an inflammation of the diverticula that may lead to infection, hemorrhage, or obstruction.

CAUSES
- Age (most common in people over age 40)
- Chronic constipation
- Congenital weakening of the intestinal wall
- Low intake of roughage and fiber
- Straining during defecation
- Stress

ASSESSMENT FINDINGS
- Anorexia
- Bloody stools
- Change in bowel habits
- Constipation and diarrhea
- Fever
- Flatulence
- Left lower quadrant pain or midabdominal pain that radiates to the back
- Nausea
- Rectal bleeding

DIAGNOSTIC TEST RESULTS
- Barium enema (contraindicated in acute diverticulitis) shows inflammation, narrow lumen of the bowel, and diverticula.
- Hematologic study shows increased WBC count and ESR.
- Sigmoidoscopy shows a thickened wall in the diverticula.

NURSING DIAGNOSES
- Constipation
- Diarrhea
- Pain

TREATMENT
- Generally no treatment for asymptomatic diverticulosis
- Colon resection (for diverticulitis refractory to medical treatment)
- Bland diet, stool softeners, and occasional doses of mineral oil for diverticulosis with pain, mild GI distress, constipation, or difficult defecation
- Diet: bland (for diverticulosis after pain subsides) or liquid (for mild diverticulitis or diverticulosis before pain subsides)
- Temporary colostomy possible for perforation, peritonitis, obstruction, or fistula that accompanies diverticulitis

Drug therapy
- Analgesic: meperidine (Demerol)
- Antibiotics: gentamicin (Garamycin), tobramycin (Nebcin), clindamycin (Cleocin) (for mild diverticulitis)
- Anticholinergic: propantheline (Pro-Banthine)
- Stool softener: docusate sodium (Colace) (for diverticulosis or mild diverticulitis)

INTERVENTIONS AND RATIONALES
- Assess abdominal distention and bowel sounds *to determine baseline and detect changes in patient's condition.*
- Monitor and record vital signs, intake and output, and laboratory studies *to assess fluid status.*
- Monitor stools for occult blood *to detect bleeding.*

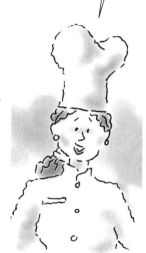

Bland or liquid? Remember that the diet for diverticular disease depends on the patient's pain status.

- Maintain the patient's diet *to improve nutritional status and promote healing.*
- Maintain position, patency, and low suction of NG tube *to prevent nausea and vomiting.*
- Keep the patient in semi-Fowler's position *to promote comfort and GI emptying.*
- Prepare the patient for surgery, if necessary (administer cleansing enemas, osmotic purgative, and oral and parenteral antibiotics), *to avoid wound contamination from bowel contents during surgery.*
- Provide postoperative care (watch for signs of infection; perform meticulous wound care; watch for signs of postoperative bleeding; assist with turning, coughing, and deep breathing; teach ostomy self-care) *to promote healing and prevent complications.*
- Administer TPN *to improve nutritional status when the patient is unable to receive nutrition through the GI tract.*
- Administer medications as prescribed *to maintain or improve the patient's condition.*

Teaching topics
- Decreasing constipation
- Following dietary recommendations and restrictions
- Avoiding corn and nuts and fruits and vegetables with seeds
- Monitoring stools for bleeding

Esophageal cancer

This form of cancer attacks the esophagus, the muscular tube that runs from the back of the throat to the stomach. Cells in the lining of the esophagus start to multiply rapidly and form a tumor that may spread to other parts of the body.

Nearly always fatal, esophageal cancer usually develops in men over age 60. This disease occurs worldwide, but incidence varies geographically. It's most common in Japan, China, the Middle East, and parts of South Africa.

CONTRIBUTING FACTORS
- Excessive use of alcohol
- Nutritional deficiency
- Smoking

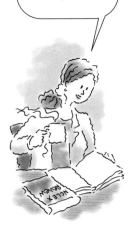

Esophageal cancer usually is advanced when diagnosed; surgery and other treatments can only relieve symptoms.

ASSESSMENT FINDINGS
- Dysphagia
- Weight loss

DIAGNOSTIC TEST RESULTS
- Endoscopic examination of the esophagus, punch and brush biopsies, and an exfoliative cytologic test confirm esophageal tumors.
- X-rays of the esophagus, with barium swallow and motility studies, reveal structural and filling defects and reduced peristalsis.

NURSING DIAGNOSES
- Altered nutrition: Less than body requirements
- Impaired swallowing
- Risk for aspiration

TREATMENT
- Endoscopic laser treatment and bipolar electrocoagulation can help restore swallowing by vaporizing cancerous tissue
- Esophageal dilation
- Gastrostomy or jejunostomy to help provide adequate nutrition
- Radiation therapy
- Radical surgery to excise the tumor and resect either the esophagus alone or the stomach and the esophagus

Drug therapy
- Antineoplastic: porfimer (Photofrin)
- Analgesics: morphine (MS Contin), fentanyl (Duragesic-25)

INTERVENTIONS AND RATIONALES
- Before surgery, answer the patient's questions and let him know what to expect after surgery (gastrostomy tubes, closed chest drainage, NG suctioning) *to allay anxiety.*
- After surgery, monitor vital signs and watch for unexpected changes *to detect early signs of complications and avoid treatment delay.* If surgery included an esophageal anastomosis, keep the patient flat on his back *to avoid tension on the suture line.*
- Promote adequate nutrition, and assess the patient's nutritional and hydration status *to determine the need for supplementary parenteral feedings.*

• Place the patient in Fowler's position for meals and allow plenty of time to eat *to avoid aspiration of food.*

• Provide high-calorie, high-protein, pureed food as needed *to meet increased metabolic demands and prevent aspiration.*

• If the patient has a gastrostomy tube, give food slowly, using gravity to adjust the flow rate *to prevent abdominal discomfort.* The prescribed amount usually ranges from 200 to 500 ml. Offer him something to chew before each feeding *to promote gastric secretions and a semblance of normal eating.*

• Instruct the family in gastrostomy tube care (checking tube patency before each feeding, providing skin care around the tube, and keeping the patient upright during and after feedings) *to avoid complications.*

• Provide emotional support for the patient and his family *to help them cope with terminal illness.*

Teaching topics
• Gastrostomy tube care
• Contacting the American Cancer Society

Gastric cancer

Gastric cancer involves a malignant stomach tumor. It may be primary or metastatic. Its precise cause is unknown, but it's often associated with gastritis, gastric atrophy, and other conditions. About one-half of gastric cancers occur in the pyloric area of the stomach.

CONTRIBUTING FACTORS
• Achlorhydria
• Chronic gastritis
• Peptic ulcer
• High intake of salted and smoked foods
• Low intake of vegetables and fruits
• Pernicious anemia

ASSESSMENT FINDINGS
• Anorexia
• Epigastric fullness and pain
• Fatigue
• Hematemesis
• Indigestion

• Malaise
• Melena
• Nausea and vomiting
• Pain after eating that isn't relieved by antacids
• Regurgitation
• Shortness of breath
• Syncope
• Weakness
• Weight loss

DIAGNOSTIC TEST RESULTS
• Blood chemistry shows increased levels of AST, LD, and amylase.
• CEA test is positive.
• Fecal occult blood test is positive.
• Gastric analysis shows positive cancer cells and achlorhydria.
• Gastroscopy biopsy is positive for cancer cells.
• Upper GI series reveals a gastric mass.
• Hematology shows decreased Hb and HCT.
• Gastric hydrochloric acid level is decreased.

NURSING DIAGNOSES
• Anxiety
• Altered GI tissue perfusion
• Risk for fluid volume deficit

TREATMENT
• Gastric surgery: gastroduodenostomy, gastrojejunostomy, partial gastric resection, total gastrectomy
• TPN
• High-calorie diet
• Radiation therapy

Drug therapy
• Analgesics: meperidine (Demerol), morphine
• Antiemetic: prochlorperazine (Compazine)
• Antineoplastics: carmustine (BiCNU), 5-fluorouracil (Adrucil)
• Vitamin supplements: folic acid (Folvite), cyanocobalamin (vitamin B_{12}) for patients who have undergone total gastrectomy

INTERVENTIONS AND RATIONALES
• Assess GI status postoperatively *to monitor the patient for dumping syndrome (weakness,*

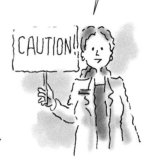

Be prepared! The patient with esophageal cancer may regurgitate food; clean his mouth carefully after each meal and keep mouthwash handy.

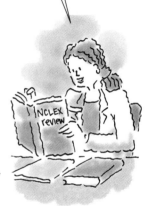

In gastric cancer, pain after eating isn't relieved by antacids and weight loss is common.

nausea, flatulence, and palpitations 30 minutes after a meal).
- Monitor and record vital signs, intake and output, laboratory studies, and daily weight *to determine baseline and early changes in condition.*
- Monitor the consistency, amount, and frequency of stools *to detect GI compromise.*
- Monitor the color of stools *to detect bleeding and prevent hemorrhage.*
- Maintain the patient's diet *to promote nutritional balance.*
- Maintain position, patency, and low suction of NG tube (without irrigating or repositioning the NG tube because it may put pressure on the suture line) *to prevent complications, nausea, and vomiting.*
- Administer TPN for 1 week or longer if gastric surgery is extensive *to meet metabolic needs and promote wound healing.*
- Administer medications, as prescribed, *to maintain or improve patient's condition.*
- Support patient coping mechanisms *to increase the potential for adaptive behavior.*
- Provide skin and mouth care *to prevent skin breakdown and damage to the oral mucosa and improve nutritional intake.*
- Provide rest periods *to conserve energy.*

Teaching topics
- Avoiding exposure to people with infections
- Alternating rest periods with activity
- Monitoring temperature
- Recognizing the signs and symptoms of wound infection
- Recognizing the signs and symptoms of ulceration
- Completing skin care daily
- Contacting the American Cancer Society

Gastritis

Gastritis is an inflammation of the gastric mucosa (the stomach lining). It may be acute or chronic.

Acute gastritis produces mucosal reddening, edema, hemorrhage, and erosion.

Chronic gastritis is common among elderly people and people with pernicious anemia. In chronic atrophic gastritis, all stomach mucosal layers are inflamed.

CAUSES
Acute gastritis
- Chronic ingestion of irritating foods, spicy foods, or alcohol
- Drugs, such as aspirin and other nonsteroidal anti-inflammatory drugs (NSAIDs) (in large doses), cytotoxic agents, caffeine, corticosteroids, antimetabolites, phenylbutazone, and indomethacin
- Ingestion of poisons, especially DDT, ammonia, mercury, carbon tetrachloride, and corrosive substances
- Endotoxins released from infecting bacteria, such as staphylococci, *Escherichia coli,* and *Salmonella.*

Chronic gastritis
- Alcohol ingestion
- Cigarette smoke
- Environmental irritants
- Peptic ulcer disease

ASSESSMENT FINDINGS
- Abdominal cramping
- Epigastric discomfort
- Hematemesis
- Indigestion

DIAGNOSTIC TEST RESULTS
- Fecal occult blood test can detect occult blood in vomitus and stools if the patient has gastric bleeding.
- Blood studies show low Hb level and HCT when significant bleeding has occurred.
- Upper GI endoscopy with biopsy confirms the diagnosis when performed within 24 hours of bleeding.
- Upper GI series may be performed to exclude serious lesions.

NURSING DIAGNOSES
- Risk for fluid volume deficit
- Altered nutrition: Less than body requirements
- Pain

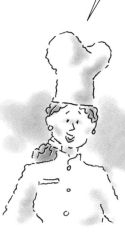

Of course we have a special diet for the patient with gastritis. Smaller, more frequent portions of bland food. Bon appetit!

TREATMENT
• Angiography with vasopressin infused in normal saline solution (when gastritis causes massive bleeding)
• Blood transfusion
• I.V. fluid therapy
• NG lavage to control bleeding
• Oxygen therapy, if necessary
• Partial or total gastrectomy (rare)
• Vagotomy and pyloroplasty (limited success when conservative treatments have failed)

Drug therapy
• Antibiotics according to sensitivity of infecting organism (if the cause is bacterial)
• Antidote according to the ingested poison (if the cause is poisoning)
• Histamine$_2$-receptor antagonists: cimetidine (Tagamet), ranitidine (Zantac), famotidine (Pepcid), nizatidine (Axid) (may block gastric secretions)

INTERVENTIONS AND RATIONALES
• If the patient is vomiting, give antiemetics and I.V. fluids *to prevent dehydration and electrolyte imbalance.*
• Monitor fluid intake and output and electrolyte levels *to detect early signs of dehydration and electrolyte loss.*
• Provide a bland diet *to prevent recurrence.* Monitor the patient for recurrent symptoms as food is reintroduced.
• Offer smaller, more frequent meals *to reduce irritating gastric secretions.* Eliminate foods that cause gastric upset *to prevent gastric irritation.*
• If surgery is necessary, prepare the patient preoperatively and provide appropriate postoperative care *to decrease preoperative anxiety and prevent intraoperative and postoperative complications.*
• Administer antacids and other prescribed medications *to promote gastric healing.*
• Urge the patient to seek immediate attention for recurring symptoms, such as hematemesis, nausea, and vomiting *to prevent complications such as GI hemorrhage.*
• Urge the patient to take prophylactic medications as prescribed *to prevent recurring symptoms.*

• Provide emotional support to the patient *to help him manage his symptoms.*

Teaching topics
• Taking antacids between meals and at bedtime and avoiding aspirin-containing compounds
• Taking steroids with milk, food, or antacids
• Contacting support groups for smoking-cessation
• Avoiding spicy foods and foods and beverages containing caffeine

Gastroenteritis

Gastroenteritis is an irritation and inflammation of the digestive tract characterized by diarrhea, nausea, vomiting, and abdominal cramping. It occurs in all age-groups and is usually self-limiting in adults.

In the United States, gastroenteritis ranks second to the common cold as a cause of lost work time and fifth as the cause of death among young children. It also can be life-threatening in elderly and debilitated persons. It's a major cause of morbidity and mortality in developing nations.

This disorder is also called intestinal flu, traveler's diarrhea, viral enteritis, and food poisoning.

CAUSES
• Amoebae, especially *Entamoeba histolytica*
• Bacteria (responsible for acute food poisoning): *Staphylococcus aureus, Salmonella, Shigella, Clostridium botulinum, Escherichia coli, Clostridium perfringens*
• Drug reactions (especially antibiotics)
• Enzyme deficiencies
• Food allergens
• Ingestion of toxins: plants or toadstools (mushrooms)
• Parasites: *Ascaris, Enterobius, Trichinella spiralis*
• Viruses (may be responsible for traveler's diarrhea): adenovirus, echovirus, or coxsackievirus

ASSESSMENT FINDINGS
• Abdominal discomfort

What's the recipe for preventing gastroenteritis? Clean utensils and cook food thoroughly. Refrigerate perishable foods. Wash hands with warm water and soap before handling foods.

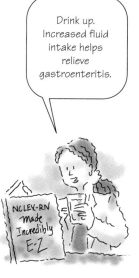

Drink up. Increased fluid intake helps relieve gastroenteritis.

- Diarrhea
- Nausea

DIAGNOSTIC TEST RESULTS
- Stool culture identifies causative bacteria, parasites, or amoebae.
- Blood culture identifies causative organism.

NURSING DIAGNOSES
- Diarrhea
- Risk for fluid volume deficit
- Pain

TREATMENT
- Increased fluid intake
- I.V. fluid and electrolyte replacement
- Nutritional support

Drug therapy
- Antibiotic therapy according to sensitivity of causative organism
- Antidiarrheals: camphorated opium tincture (Paregoric), diphenoxylate with atropine (Lomotil), loperamide (Imodium)
- Antiemetics: prochlorperazine (Compazine), trimethobenzamide (Tigan) (These medications should be avoided in patients with viral or bacterial gastroenteritis.)

INTERVENTIONS AND RATIONALES
- Administer medications; correlate dosages, routes, and times appropriately with the patient's meals and activities; for example, give antiemetics 30 to 60 minutes before meals *to prevent onset of symptoms.*
- If the patient is unable to tolerate food, replace lost fluids and electrolytes with clear liquids and sport drinks *to prevent dehydration.*
- Vary the patient's diet *to make it more enjoyable and allow some choice of foods.*
- Instruct the patient to avoid milk and milk products, *which may exacerbate the condition.*
- Record strict intake and output. Watch for signs of dehydration, such as dry skin and mucous membranes, fever, and sunken eyes *to prevent complications of dehydration.*
- Wash your hands thoroughly after giving care *to avoid spread of infection.*
- Instruct the patient to perform warm sitz baths three times per day *to relieve anal irritation.*

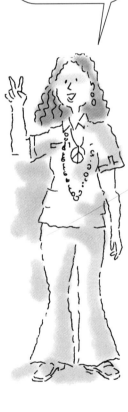

Get back. In gastroesophageal reflux, duodenal contents get back to where they don't belong — into the esophagus.

Teaching topics
- Cleaning utensils thoroughly; avoiding drinking water or eating raw fruit or vegetables when visiting a foreign country; eliminating flies and roaches in the home
- Thoroughly cooking foods, especially pork; refrigerating perishable foods, such as milk, mayonnaise, potato salad, and cream-filled pastry
- Washing hands with warm water and soap before handling food, especially after using the bathroom

Gastroesophageal reflux

Gastroesophageal reflux refers to the backflow, or reflux, of gastric and duodenal contents past the lower esophageal sphincter and into the esophagus. Reflux may or may not cause symptoms or pathologic changes. Persistent reflux may cause reflux esophagitis (inflammation of the esophageal mucosa). The prognosis varies with the underlying cause.

CAUSES AND CONTRIBUTING FACTORS
- Any action that decreases lower esophageal sphincter pressure, such as smoking cigarettes and ingesting food, alcohol, anticholinergics (atropine, belladonna, propantheline), and other drugs (morphine, diazepam, meperidine)
- Any condition or position that increases intra-abdominal pressure
- Hiatal hernia (especially in children)
- Long-term NG intubation (more than 5 days)
- Pressure within the stomach that exceeds lower esophageal sphincter pressure
- Pyloric surgery (alteration or removal of the pylorus), which allows reflux of bile or pancreatic juice

ASSESSMENT FINDINGS
- Dysphagia
- Heartburn (burning sensation in the upper abdomen)

Atypical symptoms
- Asthma

- Atypical chest pain
- Chronic cough
- Laryngitis
- Sore throat

DIAGNOSTIC TEST RESULTS
- Barium swallow fluoroscopy indicates reflux.
- Esophageal pH probe reveals reflux.
- Esophagoscopy shows reflux.
- Acid perfusion (Bernstein) test shows that reflux is the cause of symptoms.
- Endoscopy allows visualization and confirmation of pathologic changes in the mucosa.
- Biopsy allows visualization and confirmation of pathologic changes in the mucosa.

NURSING DIAGNOSES
- Risk for aspiration
- Pain
- Knowledge deficit

TREATMENT
- Oxygen therapy
- Positional therapy to help relieve symptoms by decreasing intra-abdominal pressure
- Surgery, which reduces reflux by creating an artificial closure at the gastroesophageal junction (in extreme, chronic cases)

Drug therapy
- Antacids: aluminum hydroxide (AlternaGEL) administered 1 hour and 3 hours after meals and at bedtime
- GI prokinetic: cisapride (Propulsid)
- GI stimulant: metoclopramide (Reglan), bethanechol (Urecholine)
- Histamine$_2$-receptor antagonists: cimetidine (Tagamet), ranitidine (Zantac), famotidine (Pepcid), nizatidine (Axid)

INTERVENTIONS AND RATIONALES
- Develop a diet that takes food preferences into account while helping to minimize reflux symptoms to ensure compliance.
- Have the patient sleep in reverse Trendelenburg's position (with the head of the bed elevated 6″ to 12″ [15 to 30 cm]) to reduce intra-abdominal pressure.
  After surgery using a thoracic approach:

- Carefully watch and record chest tube drainage and respiratory status to detect early signs of respiratory distress.
- If needed, give chest physiotherapy and oxygen to mobilize secretions and prevent hypoxemia.
- Place the patient with an NG tube in semi-Fowler's position to help prevent reflux.
- Offer reassurance and emotional support to help the patient cope with pain and discomfort.

Teaching topics
- Avoiding reflux through diet and lifestyle changes

Hepatitis

Hepatitis is an inflammation of liver tissue that causes inflammation of hepatic cells, hypertrophy, and proliferation of Kupffer's cells and bile stasis. Hepatitis is typically caused by one of five viruses: hepatitis A, B, C, D, or E.

CAUSES
- Hepatitis A: contaminated food, milk, water, feces (most commonly foodborne)
- Hepatitis B: parenteral (needle sticks), blood, sexual contact, secretions
- Hepatitis C: blood or serum (blood transfusion, exposure to contaminated blood), sexual contact
- Hepatitis D: similar to causes of type B virus
- Hepatitis E: fecal-oral route

ASSESSMENT FINDINGS
Assessment findings are consistent for the different types of hepatitis, but signs and symptoms progress over several stages.
During preicteric phase (usually 1 to 5 days)
- Anorexia
- Constipation and diarrhea
- Fatigue
- Fever
- Headache
- Hepatomegaly
- Malaise
- Nasal discharge
- Nausea and vomiting
- Pharyngitis

Recognizing fulminant hepatitis

A rare but severe form of hepatitis, fulminant hepatitis rapidly causes massive liver necrosis. It usually occurs in patients with hepatitis B, D, or E. Although mortality is extremely high (more than 80% of patients lapse into deep coma), patients who survive may recover completely.

ASSESSMENT
In a patient with viral hepatitis, suspect fulminant hepatitis if you assess:
• confusion
• somnolence
• ascites
• edema
• rapidly rising bilirubin level
• markedly prolonged prothrombin time.
   As the disease progresses quickly to the terminal phase, the patient may experience cerebral edema, brain stem compression, GI bleeding, sepsis, respiratory failure, cardiovascular collapse, and renal failure.

EMERGENCY ACTIONS
If you suspect fulminant hepatitis, you should:
• notify the doctor immediately
• provide supportive care, such as maintaining fluid volume, supporting ventilation through mechanical means, controlling bleeding, and correcting hypoglycemia
• restrict protein intake
• expect to administer oral lactulose or neomycin and, possibly, massive doses of glucocorticoids
• prepare the patient for a liver transplant if necessary and if the patient meets the criteria.

• Pruritus
• Right upper quadrant pain
• Splenomegaly
• Weight loss
During icteric phase (usually 1 to 2 weeks)
• Clay-colored stools
• Dark urine
• Fatigue
• Hepatomegaly
• Jaundice
• Pruritus
• Splenomegaly
• Weight loss
During posticteric or recovery phase (usually 2 to 12 weeks, sometimes longer in patients with hepatitis B, C, or E)
• Decreased hepatomegaly
• Decreased jaundice
• Fatigue
• Improved appetite

DIAGNOSTIC TEST RESULTS
• Blood chemistry shows increased ALT, AST, alkaline phosphatase, LD, bilirubin, and ESR; positive antibody to hepatitis A; positive immunoglobulin (Ig) antidelta antigens (in type D); positive hepatitis B surface antigen; and positive hepatitis E antigen.

• Hematology shows increased PT and FSP.
• Stool specimen reveals hepatitis A virus (in hepatitis A cases).
• Urine chemistry shows increased urobilinogen.

NURSING DIAGNOSES
• Fluid volume deficit
• Altered nutrition: Less than body requirements
• Pain

TREATMENT
• High-calorie, moderate-protein, high-carbohydrate, low-fat diet in small, frequent meals

Drug therapy
• Antiemetic: prochlorperazine (Compazine)
• Vitamins and minerals: vitamin K (Aqua-MEPHYTON), ascorbic acid (Vitamin C), vitamin B-complex (mega-B)

INTERVENTIONS AND RATIONALES
• Assess GI status and watch for bleeding and fulminant hepatitis *to detect early complications.* (See *Recognizing fulminant hepatitis.*)
• Maintain the patient's diet *to meet the patient's metabolic needs.*

• Monitor and record vital signs, intake and output, and laboratory studies *to detect early signs of fluid volume deficit.*
• Administer medications, as prescribed, *to maintain or improve patient's condition.*
• Maintain standard precautions. *Hand washing prevents the spread of pathogens to others.* (See *Standard precautions,* page 258.)
• Provide rest periods *to conserve patient energy and reduce metabolic demands.*
• Encourage small, frequent meals *to improve patient's nutritional status.*
• Change the patient's position every 2 hours *to reduce risk of skin breakdown.*
• Monitor for signs of bleeding *to prevent hemorrhage.*

Teaching topics
• Avoiding exposure to people with infections
• Avoiding alcohol
• Maintaining good personal hygiene
• Refraining from donating blood
• Increasing fluid intake to 3,000 ml/day (approximately 12 8-oz glasses)
• Abstaining from sexual intercourse until serum liver studies are within normal limits

Hiatal hernia

A hiatal hernia, also known as an esophageal hernia, is a protrusion of the stomach through the diaphragm into the thoracic cavity.

CAUSES
• Aging
• Congenital weakness
• Increased abdominal pressure
• Obesity
• Pregnancy
• Trauma
• Unknown

ASSESSMENT FINDINGS
• Cough
• Dysphagia
• Dyspnea
• Feeling of fullness
• Pyrosis
• Regurgitation
• Sternal pain after eating
• Tachycardia
• Vomiting

DIAGNOSTIC TEST RESULTS
• Barium swallow reveals protrusion of the hernia.
• Chest X-ray shows protrusion of abdominal organs into the thorax.
• Esophagoscopy shows incompetent cardiac sphincter.
• Gastric analysis reveals increased pH.

NURSING DIAGNOSES
• Anxiety
• Altered nutrition: Less than body requirements
• Pain

TREATMENT
• Antireflux surgical repair, if complications develop
• Bland diet with decreased intake of caffeine and spicy foods
• Weight loss, if necessary

Drug therapy
• Anticholinergic: propantheline (Pro-Banthine)
• Histamine$_2$-receptor antagonists: cimetidine (Tagamet), ranitidine (Zantac), famotidine (Pepcid)

INTERVENTIONS AND RATIONALES
• Assess respiratory status *to detect early signs of respiratory distress.*
• Monitor and record vital signs, intake and output, and daily weight *to determine baseline and detect early signs of nutritional deficit.*
• Administer oxygen *to help relieve respiratory distress.*
• Avoid flexion at the waist in positioning the patient *to promote comfort.*
• Maintain the patient's diet *to maintain and improve nutritional status.*
• Maintain position, patency, and low suction of NG tube *to prevent nausea and vomiting.*
• Keep the patient in semi-Fowler's position *to promote comfort.*
• Administer medications, as prescribed, *to improve GI function.*

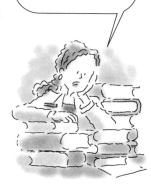

Maintaining standard precautions affects your safety and the patient's safety; it's an important topic to cover.

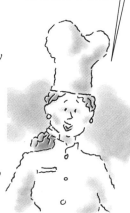

Say no to the burrito and junk the java! Remember that patients with hiatal hernia should avoid spicy foods and caffeine.

Battling illness

Standard precautions

Standard precautions apply to blood; all body fluids, secretions, and excretions except sweat, regardless of whether they contain visible blood; nonintact skin; and mucous membranes.

HAND WASHING
Wash hands after touching blood, body fluids, secretions, excretions, and contaminated items, whether or not gloves are worn. Wash hands immediately after gloves are removed, between patient contacts, and when otherwise indicated to avoid transfer of microorganisms to other patients or environments. It may be necessary to wash hands between tasks and procedures on the same patient to prevent cross contamination of different body sites.

GLOVES
Wear gloves when touching blood, body fluids, secretions, excretions, or contaminated items. Put on clean gloves just before touching mucous membranes and nonintact skin. Remove gloves promptly after use and wash hands.

MASK, EYE PROTECTION, FACE SHIELD
Wear a mask, eye protection, and a face shield to protect the mucous membranes of your eyes, nose, and mouth during procedures and patient care activities that are likely to generate splashes of blood, body fluids, secretions, or excretions.

GOWN
Wear a gown to protect skin and prevent soiling of clothing during procedures and patient care activities that are likely to generate splashes of blood, body fluids, secretions, or excretions.

Teaching topics
• Eating small, frequent meals
• Avoiding carbonated beverages and alcohol
• Remaining upright for 2 hours after eating
• Avoiding constrictive clothing
• Avoiding lifting, bending, straining, and coughing
• Sleeping with upper body elevated to reduce gastric reflux

> Complete intestinal blockage is life-threatening. It must be treated within hours.

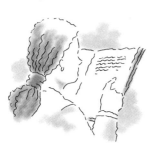

Intestinal obstruction

An intestinal obstruction occurs when the intestinal lumen becomes blocked, causing gas, fluid, and digested substances to accumulate near the obstruction and increasing peristalsis in the area of the obstruction. Water and electrolytes are then secreted into the blocked bowel, causing inflammation and inhibiting absorption.

CAUSES
• Adhesions
• Diverticulitis
• Fecal impaction
• Hernias
• Inflammation (Crohn's disease)
• Mesenteric thrombosis
• Paralytic ileus
• Tumors
• Volvulus

ASSESSMENT FINDINGS
• Abdominal distention
• Constipation
• Cramping pain
• Diminished or absent bowel sounds
• Fever

- Nausea
- Vomiting fecal material
- Weight loss

DIAGNOSTIC TEST RESULTS
- Abdominal X-ray shows increased amount of gas in bowel.
- Barium enema stops at obstruction.
- Blood chemistry shows decreased sodium and potassium levels.
- Hematologic study shows increased WBC count.

NURSING DIAGNOSES
- Altered GI tissue perfusion
- Altered nutrition: Less than body requirements
- Pain

TREATMENT
- Bowel resection with or without anastomosis if other treatment fails
- GI decompression using NG tube, Miller-Abbott tube, or Cantor tube
- Withholding food and fluids

Drug therapy
- Analgesic: meperidine (Demerol)
- Antibiotic: gentamicin (Garamycin)

INTERVENTIONS AND RATIONALES
- Assess GI status. Assess and record bowel sounds once per shift *to determine GI status.*
- Monitor and record vital signs, intake and output, and laboratory studies *to detect early signs of fluid volume deficit.*
- Withhold food and fluids *to prevent nausea and vomiting.*
- Monitor and record the frequency, color, and amount of stools *to assess and determine nutritional status.*
- Measure and record the patient's abdominal girth *to determine presence of distention.*
- Administer I.V. fluids *to maintain hydration.*
- Maintain position, patency, and low intermittent suction of NG tube and Miller-Abbott tube *to prevent nausea and vomiting and resolve the obstruction if possible.*
- Keep the patient in semi-Fowler's position *to promote comfort.*

- Administer postoperative care if indicated (monitor vital signs and intake and output; make sure NG tube is kept patent; monitor dressing for drainage; assess wound for infection; assist with turning, coughing, and deep breathing; medicate for pain as necessary or guide the patient with use of postoperative patient-controlled analgesia) *to promote healing and detect early postoperative complications.*
- Administer medications as prescribed *to maintain or improve the patient's condition.*

Teaching topics
- Avoiding constipation-causing foods
- Monitoring the frequency and color of stools
- Recognizing the signs and symptoms of diverticulitis
- Contacting the American Ostomy Association, if appropriate

Irritable bowel syndrome

Irritable bowel syndrome is marked by chronic symptoms of abdominal pain, alternating constipation and diarrhea, and abdominal distention. This disorder is extremely common; a substantial portion of patients, however, never seek medical attention.

This disorder may also be referred to as spastic colon or spastic colitis.

CAUSES AND CONTRIBUTING FACTORS
- Diverticular disease
- Irritants (caffeine, alcohol)
- Stress

ASSESSMENT FINDINGS
- Abdominal bloating
- Constipation, diarrhea, or both
- Dyspepsia
- Faintness
- Heartburn
- Lower abdominal pain
- Passage of mucus
- Pasty, pencil-like stools
- Weakness

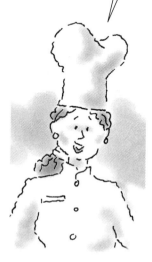

Withhold food and fluids from the patient with intestinal obstruction.

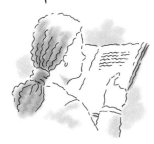

The patient with irritable bowel syndrome needs 15 to 20 g of bulk per day.

DIAGNOSTIC TEST RESULTS
- Barium enema may reveal colonic spasm and tubular appearance of the descending colon. It also rules out certain other disorders, such as diverticula, tumors, and polyps.
- Sigmoidoscopy may disclose spastic contractions.
- Stool examination for occult blood, parasites, and pathogenic bacteria is negative.

NURSING DIAGNOSES
- Constipation
- Diarrhea
- Pain

TREATMENT
- Elimination diet to determine if symptoms result from food intolerance (In this type of diet, certain foods, such as citrus fruits, coffee, corn, dairy products, tea, and wheat, are sequentially eliminated. Then each food is gradually reintroduced to identify which foods, if any, trigger the patient's symptoms.)
- Diet containing 15 to 20 g daily of bulky foods, such as wheat bran, oatmeal, oat bran, rye cereals, prunes, dried apricots, and figs (if the patient has constipation and abdominal pain)
- Increasing fluid intake to at least eight 8-oz glasses per day
- Stress management
- Heat application

Drug therapy
- Sedatives: diazepam (Valium)
- Antiflatulent: simethicone (Mylicon)
- Antispasmodic: propantheline (Pro-Banthine)
- Antidiarrheal: diphenoxylate with atropine (Lomotil)

One good reason not to get stressed out about the NCLEX. Stress contributes to development of irritable bowel syndrome.

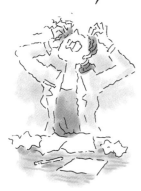

INTERVENTIONS AND RATIONALES
- Help the patient deal with stress, and warn against dependence on sedatives or antispasmodics *because stress may be the underlying cause of irritable bowel syndrome.*
- Encourage regular checkups. For patients over age 40, emphasize the need for a yearly flexible sigmoidoscopy and rectal examination. *Irritable bowel syndrome is associated*

with a higher-than-normal incidence of diverticulitis and colon cancer.

Teaching topics
- Avoiding irritating foods
- Managing stress
- Quitting smoking (smoking can increase GI motility)
- Planning diet and increasing water intake

Pancreatitis

Pancreatitis is the inflammation of the pancreas. In acute pancreatitis, pancreatic enzymes are activated in the pancreas rather than the duodenum, resulting in tissue damage and autodigestion of the pancreas.

In chronic pancreatitis, chronic inflammation results in fibrosis and calcification of the pancreas, obstruction of the ducts, and destruction of the secreting acinar cells.

CAUSES
- Alcoholism
- Bacterial or viral infection
- Biliary tract disease
- Blunt trauma to pancreas or abdomen
- Drug induced: steroids, thiazide diuretics, oral contraceptives
- Duodenal ulcer
- Hyperlipidemia
- Hyperparathyroidism

ASSESSMENT FINDINGS
- Abdominal tenderness and distention
- Abrupt onset of pain in epigastric area that radiates to the shoulder, substernal area, back, and flank
- Aching, burning, stabbing, pressing pain
- Decreased or absent bowel sounds
- Dyspnea
- Fever
- Hypotension
- Jaundice
- Nausea and vomiting
- Pain upon eating
- Knee-chest position, fetal position, or leaning forward for comfort
- Steatorrhea

- Tachycardia
- Weight loss

DIAGNOSTIC TEST RESULTS

- Arteriography reveals fibrous tissue and calcification of pancreas.
- Blood chemistry shows increased amylase, lipase, LD, glucose, AST, and lipid levels and decreased calcium and potassium levels.
- CT scan shows enlarged pancreas.
- Cullen's sign is positive.
- ERCP reveals biliary obstruction.
- Fecal fat test is positive.
- Glucose tolerance test shows decreased tolerance.
- Grey Turner's sign is positive.
- Hematology shows increased WBC count and decreased Hb and HCT.
- Ultrasonography reveals cysts, bile duct inflammation, and dilation.
- Urine chemistry shows increased amylase.

NURSING DIAGNOSES

- Fluid volume deficit
- Altered nutrition: Less than body requirements
- Pain

TREATMENT

- Bland, low-fat, high-protein diet of small, frequent meals with restricted intake of caffeine, alcohol, and gas-forming foods; as disease progresses, nothing by mouth
- Bed rest
- I.V. fluids (vigorous replacement of fluids and electrolytes)
- Dialysis
- Sequential compression device to prevent blood clot formation
- Surgical intervention to treat underlying cause, if appropriate
- Transfusion therapy with packed RBCs

Drug therapy

- Analgesic: meperidine (Demerol) (morphine contraindicated)
- Anticholinergics: propantheline (Pro-Banthine), dicyclomine (Bentyl)
- Antidiabetic: insulin (possible infusion to stabilize blood glucose levels)
- Antiemetic: prochlorperazine (Compazine)

- Calcium supplement: calcium gluconate (Kalcinate)
- Corticosteroid: hydrocortisone (Solu-Cortef)
- Digestant: pancrelipase (Pancrease)
- Histamine$_2$-receptor antagonists: cimetidine (Tagamet), ranitidine (Zantac), famotidine (Pepcid), nizatidine (Axid)
- Mucosal barrier fortifier: sucralfate (Carafate)
- Potassium supplement: I.V. potassium chloride
- Tranquilizers: lorazepam (Ativan), alprazolam (Xanax)

INTERVENTIONS AND RATIONALES

- Assess abdominal, cardiac, and respiratory status (as the disease progresses, watch for respiratory failure, tachycardia, and worsening GI status) *to determine baseline and detect early changes and signs of complications.*
- Assess fluid balance *to detect fluid volume deficit or excess.*
- Monitor and record vital signs, intake and output, laboratory studies, central venous pressure (CVP), daily weight, and urine specific gravity *to detect signs of fluid volume deficit.*
- Monitor urine and stool for color, character, and amount *to detect bleeding.*
- Maintain the patient's diet; withhold food and fluids as necessary *to rest the pancreas and prevent nausea and vomiting.*
- Perform bedside glucose monitoring *to assess for hyperglycemia.*
- Administer oxygen and maintain endotracheal tube and mechanical ventilation if necessary *to improve oxygenation* and provide suctioning as needed *to stabilize secretions.*

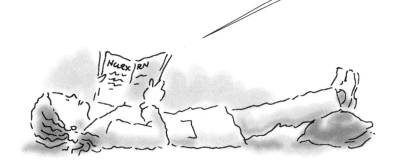

Keep the patient with pancreatitis in bed and turn him frequently to prevent pressure ulcers.

• Administer I.V. fluids *to treat or prevent hypovolemic shock and restore electrolyte balance.*
• Maintain position, patency, and low suction of NG tube *to prevent nausea and vomiting.*
• Keep the patient in semi-Fowler's position if the patient's blood pressure allows *to promote comfort and lung expansion.*
• Administer TPN. *In severe cases, reintroduction of food may be associated with pancreatic abscess. TPN is necessary to meet the patient's metabolic needs.*
• Keep the patient in bed and turn every 2 hours, or utilize a specialty rotation bed *to prevent pressure ulcers.*
• Administer medications, as prescribed, *to improve or maintain the patient's condition.*
• Provide skin, nares, and mouth care *to prevent tissue damage.*
• Provide a quiet, restful environment *to conserve energy and decrease metabolic demands.*

Teaching topics
• Monitoring blood glucose levels frequently
• Monitoring stools for steatorrhea
• Monitoring self for infection
• Recognizing the signs and symptoms of increased blood glucose levels
• Adhering to activity limitations
• Modifying risk factors

Peptic ulcer

Peptic ulcers are breaks in the continuity of esophageal, gastric, or duodenal mucosa. They may occur in any part of the GI tract that comes in contact with gastric substances, hydrochloric acid, and pepsin. The ulcers may be found in the esophagus, stomach, duodenum, or (after gastroenterostomy) jejunum.

CAUSES
• Alcohol abuse
• Drug-induced: salicylates, steroids, NSAIDs, reserpine
• Gastritis
• *Helicobacter pylori*
• Smoking
• Stress
• Zollinger-Ellison syndrome

ASSESSMENT FINDINGS
• Anorexia
• Hematemesis
• Left epigastric pain 1 to 2 hours after eating
• Melena
• Nausea and vomiting
• Relief of pain after administration of antacids
• Weight loss

DIAGNOSTIC TEST RESULTS
• Barium swallow shows ulceration of gastric mucosa.
• Fecal occult blood test is positive.
• Gastric analysis is normal.
• Hematologic study shows decreased Hb and HCT (if bleeding is present).
• Serum gastrin level is normal or increased.
• Upper GI endoscopy shows location of ulcer.

NURSING DIAGNOSES
• Anxiety
• Altered nutrition: Less than body requirements
• Pain

TREATMENT
• Endoscopic laser to control bleeding
• If GI hemorrhage, gastric surgery that may include gastroduodenostomy, gastrojejunostomy, partial gastric resection, and total gastrectomy
• Low-fiber diet with small, frequent meals
• Photocoagulation to control bleeding
• Saline lavage by NG tube until return is clear (if bleeding is present)
• Transfusion therapy with packed RBCs (if bleeding is present and Hb and HCT are low)

Drug therapy
• Antacids: magnesium and aluminum hydroxide (Maalox), aluminum hydroxide gel (AlternaGEL)
• Antibiotic if *H. pylori* is present
• Anticholinergics: propantheline (Pro-Banthine), dicyclomine (Bentyl)
• Histamine$_2$-receptor antagonists: cimetidine (Tagamet), ranitidine (Zantac), nizatidine (Axid), famotidine (Pepcid)
• Pituitary hormone: vasopressin (Pitressin) to manage bleeding

• Mucosal barrier fortifier: sucralfate (Carafate)
• Prostaglandin: misoprostol (Cytotec) to protect the stomach lining

INTERVENTIONS AND RATIONALES
• Assess GI status *to monitor for signs of bleeding.*
• Assess cardiovascular status *to detect early signs of GI hemorrhage.*
• Monitor and record vital signs, intake and output, laboratory studies, fecal occult blood, and gastric pH *to detect signs of bleeding.*
• Monitor the consistency, color, amount, and frequency of stools *to detect early signs of GI bleeding.*
• Maintain the patient's diet with small, frequent feedings *to meet metabolic needs and promote healing.*
• Maintain position, patency, and low suction of NG tube if gastric decompression is ordered *to prevent nausea and vomiting.*
• Administer medications, as prescribed, *to maintain or improve patient's condition.*
• Provide nose and mouth care *to maintain tissue integrity.*
• Provide postoperative care if necessary (don't reposition NG tube; irrigate it gently if ordered; medicate for pain as needed and ordered; monitor dressings for drainage; assess bowel sounds; get patient out of bed as tolerated) *to detect early complications and promote healing.*

Teaching topics
• Reducing stress
• Relaxation techniques
• Following dietary recommendations and restrictions such as avoiding caffeine, alcohol, and spicy and fried foods
• Following postoperative care and restrictions

Peritonitis

Peritonitis results from a localized or generalized inflammation of the peritoneal cavity. It occurs when irritants in the peritoneal area cause inflammatory edema, vascular congestion, and hypermotility of the bowel.

CAUSES
• Bacterial invasion
• Chemical invasion

ASSESSMENT FINDINGS
• Abdominal resonance and tympany on percussion
• Abdominal rigidity and distention
• Anorexia
• Constant, diffuse, and intense abdominal pain
• Decreased or absent bowel sounds
• Decreased peristalsis
• Decreased urine output
• Fever
• Malaise
• Nausea
• Rebound tenderness
• Shallow respirations
• Weak, rapid pulse

DIAGNOSTIC TEST RESULTS
• Abdominal X-ray shows free air in abdomen under diaphragm.
• Hematologic study shows increased WBC count and HCT.
• Peritoneal aspiration is positive for blood, pus, bile, bacteria, or amylase.

NURSING DIAGNOSES
• Anxiety
• Decreased cardiac output
• Fluid volume deficit

TREATMENT
• Withholding food or fluid
• Surgical intervention when the patient's condition is stabilized (Surgery is chosen to treat the cause; for example, if the patient has a perforated appendix, then an appendectomy is indicated. Drains will also be placed for drainage of infected material.)

Drug therapy
• Analgesic: meperidine (Demerol)
• Antibiotics: gentamicin (Garamycin), clindamycin (Cleocin), cephalothin (Keflin), ampicillin sodium/sulbactam sodium (Unasyn)

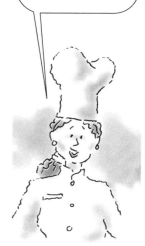

Withhold food and fluids from the patient with acute peritonitis. Provide TPN.

INTERVENTIONS AND RATIONALES

• Assess abdominal and respiratory status and fluid balance *to detect and assess signs of fluid volume deficit.*
• Monitor and record vital signs, intake and output, laboratory studies, CVP, daily weight, and urine specific gravity *to detect signs of fluid volume deficit.*
• Measure and record the patient's abdominal girth *to assess for abdominal distention.*
• Withhold food and fluids *to prevent nausea and vomiting.*
• Administer I.V. fluids *to maintain hydration and electrolyte balance.*
• Provide routine postoperative care (monitor vital signs and intake and output, including drainage from drains; assist with turning, incentive spirometry, coughing, and deep breathing; and get the patient out of bed on the 1st postoperative day if his condition allows) *to promote healing and prevent and detect early complications.*
• Maintain position, patency, and low suction of NG tube *to prevent nausea and vomiting.*
• Keep the patient in semi-Fowler's position *to promote comfort and prevent pulmonary complications.*
• Administer TPN *to meet patient's metabolic needs.*
• Administer medications, as prescribed, *to treat infection and control pain.*

Teaching topics
• Recognizing the signs and symptoms of infection
• Recognizing the signs and symptoms of GI obstruction
• Performing ostomy self-care if indicated

Ulcerative colitis

Ulcerative colitis is an inflammatory disorder of the colon. It's commonly a chronic condition and causes damage to the large intestine's mucosal and submucosal layers.

CAUSES
• Genetics
• Idiopathic cause
• Allergies
• Autoimmune disease
• Emotional stress
• Viral and bacterial infections

ASSESSMENT FINDINGS
• Dehydration
• Nausea and vomiting
• Abdominal cramping
• Abdominal distention
• Abdominal tenderness
• Anorexia
• Bloody, purulent, mucoid, watery stools (15 to 20 per day)
• Cachexia
• Debilitation
• Fever
• Hyperactive bowel sounds
• Weakness
• Weight loss

DIAGNOSTIC TEST RESULTS
• Barium enema shows ulcerations.
• Blood chemistry shows decreased potassium level and increased osmolality.
• Hematology shows decreased Hb and HCT.
• Sigmoidoscopy shows ulceration and hyperemia.
• Stool specimen is positive for blood and mucus.
• Urine chemistry displays increased urine specific gravity.

NURSING DIAGNOSES
• Diarrhea
• Fluid volume deficit
• Altered nutrition: Less than body requirements

TREATMENT
• Colectomy or pouch ileostomy
• High-protein, high-calorie, low-residue diet, with bland foods in small, frequent meals and restricted intake of milk and gas-forming foods or no food or fluids
• TPN if necessary to rest the GI tract
• Transfusion therapy with packed RBCs

Drug therapy
• Analgesic: meperidine (Demerol)
• Antianemics: ferrous sulfate (Feosol), ferrous gluconate (Fergon)

• Antibiotic: sulfasalazine (Azulfidine)
• Anticholinergics: propantheline (Pro-Banthine), dicyclomine (Bentyl)
• Antidiarrheals: diphenoxylate (Lomotil), loperamide (Imodium)
• Antiemetic: prochlorperazine (Compazine)
• Anti-inflammatory: olsalazine (Dipentum)
• Corticosteroid: hydrocortisone (Solu-Cortef)
• Immunosuppressants: azathioprine (Imuran), cyclophosphamide (Cytoxan)
• Potassium supplements: potassium chloride (K-Lor), potassium gluconate (Kaon)
• Sedative: lorazepam (Ativan)

INTERVENTIONS AND RATIONALES

• Assess GI status and fluid balance *to determine fluid volume deficit.*
• Monitor and record vital signs, intake and output, laboratory studies, daily weight, urine specific gravity, calorie count, and fecal occult blood *to determine fluid volume deficit.*
• Monitor the number, amount, and character of stools *to determine status of nutrient absorption.*
• Maintain the patient's diet; withhold food and fluids as necessary *to prevent nausea and vomiting.*
• Administer I.V. fluids and TPN *to maintain hydration and improve nutritional status.*
• Maintain position, patency, and low suction of NG tube *to prevent nausea and vomiting.*
• Keep the patient in semi-Fowler's position *to promote comfort.*
• Administer medications, as prescribed, *to maintain or improve patient's condition.*
• Provide skin, mouth, nares, and perianal care *to promote comfort and prevent skin breakdown.*

Teaching topics

• Monitoring weight
• Reducing stress and performing relaxation techniques
• Recognizing the early signs and symptoms of rectal hemorrhage and intestinal obstruction
• Contacting the United Ostomy Association and the National Foundation of Ileitis and Colitis

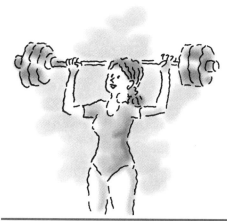

Pump up on practice questions

1. A client begins a fecal fat analysis test on a Monday. The nurse should instruct the client to begin the 3-day stool collection on:

    A. Monday.
    B. Tuesday.
    C. Wednesday.
    D. Thursday.

Answer: D. The fecal fat analysis test requires a 3-day period in which the client eats a high-fat diet. On the day after the 3-day diet, the client begins collecting his stool. In this scenario, that would be Thursday. Selecting Monday, Tuesday, or Wednesday would be erroneously teaching the client to begin the test prematurely, which may nullify the test's accuracy.

➡ *NCLEX keys*
Nursing process step: Implementation
Client needs category: Health promotion and maintenance
Client needs subcategory: Prevention and early detection of disease
Taxonomic level: Application

2. A client returns from an endoscopic procedure during which he was sedated. Before offering the client food, it's most important for the nurse to:

    A. monitor his oxygen saturation levels.
    B. assess his gag reflex.
    C. place him in the side-lying position.
    D. have him drink sips of water.

Answer: B. The sedation associated with a procedure such as endoscopy can impair the gag reflex. If a client is fed before the gag reflex returns, the client can experience airway obstruction and aspiration. Therefore, the nurse should assess the client's gag reflex before offering the client food. Monitoring hemoglobin saturation levels is important after an endoscopic procedure but its results won't support feeding the client. In this situation, the side-lying position isn't necessary. Having the client drink water isn't the proper method of assessing for a gag reflex.

➡ **NCLEX keys**
Nursing process step: Assessment
Client needs category: Physiological integrity
Client needs subcategory: Reduction of risk potential
Taxonomic level: Application

3. A client with a history of hiatal hernia reports to the nurse that he has trouble sleeping because of abdominal pain. It would be most beneficial to the client if the nurse instructed him to sleep:
    A. with his upper body elevated.
    B. in the prone position.
    C. flat or in a side-lying position.
    D. with his lower body slightly elevated.
Answer: A. Upper body elevation can reduce the gastric reflux associated with hiatal hernia. The other positions won't benefit the client.

➡ **NCLEX keys**
Nursing process step: Implementation
Client needs category: Physiological integrity
Client needs subcategory: Basic care and comfort
Taxonomic level: Analysis

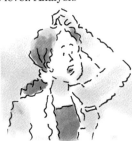

4. A client with peptic ulcer disease secondary to chronic nonsteroidal anti-inflammatory drug (NSAID) use is prescribed misoprostol (Cytotec). The nurse would be most accurate in informing the client that the drug:
    A. reduces the stomach's hydrochloric acid volume.
    B. increases the speed of gastric emptying.
    C. protects the stomach's lining.
    D. increases lower esophageal sphincter pressure.
Answer: C. Misoprostol (Cytotec) is a synthetic prostaglandin that, like prostaglandin, protects the gastric mucosa. NSAIDs decrease prostaglandin production and predispose the client to peptic ulceration. Cytotec is prescribed to clients with peptic ulcer disease who are also taking NSAIDs. Misoprostol doesn't reduce gastric acidity, improve emptying of the stomach, or increase lower esophageal sphincter pressure.

➡ **NCLEX keys**
Nursing process step: Implementation
Client needs category: Physiological integrity
Client needs subcategory: Pharmacological and parenteral therapies
Taxonomic level: Application

5. The nurse is reviewing the diagnostic data of a client suspected of having gastric cancer. What laboratory finding is the nurse most likely to find?
    A. Elevated hemoglobin and hematocrit
    B. Negative fecal occult blood test
    C. Subnormal gastric hydrochloric acid level
    D. Negative carcinoembryonic antigen (CEA) test
Answer: C. One manifestation of gastric cancer is achlorhydria, an absence of free hydrochloric acid in the stomach. In gastric cancer, a subnormal hemoglobin and hematocrit is most likely; fecal occult blood test is most likely to be positive. The CEA test would most likely be positive in gastric cancer.

➡ NCLEX keys
Nursing process step: Analysis
Client needs category: Health promotion and maintenance
Client needs subcategory: Prevention and early detection of disease
Taxonomic level: Analysis

6. A physician orders gastric decompression for a client with small bowel obstruction. The nurse should plan for the suction to be:
   A. low pressure and intermittent.
   B. low pressure and continuous.
   C. high pressure and intermittent.
   D. high pressure and continuous.
Answer: A. Gastric decompression is typically low pressure and intermittent. High pressure and continuous gastric suctioning predisposes the gastric mucosa to injury and ulceration.

➡ NCLEX keys
Nursing process step: Planning
Client needs category: Physiological integrity
Client needs subcategory: Reduction of risk potential
Taxonomic level: Application

7. A client with Crohn's disease has a serum potassium level of 3.1 mEq/dl. The client is prescribed 30 mEq of oral potassium chloride (K-lor) twice daily. The nurse should plan to give the supplement:
   A. with food or after the client eats.
   B. on an empty stomach.
   C. along with no other medications.
   D. 2 hours before or after eating.
Answer: A. Supplemental potassium can be irritating to the esophagus and stomach and is best tolerated with meals or shortly after meals. It's typically appropriate to give oral potassium at the same time other medications are being administered.

➡ NCLEX keys
Nursing process step: Planning
Client needs category: Physiological integrity
Client needs subcategory: Pharmacological and parenteral therapies
Taxonomic level: Application

8. A nurse is evaluating the effectiveness of dietary instructions in a client with diverticulitis. Regular consumption of which food would indicate that the client hasn't understood instructions?
   A. Fiber
   B. Bananas
   C. Cucumbers
   D. Milk products
Answer: C. In diverticulitis, vegetables with seeds are prohibited in the diet because the seeds can lodge in diverticula and cause flare-ups of diverticulitis. Fiber and residue are recommended in the diet. Bananas and mild products aren't contraindicated.

➡ NCLEX keys
Nursing process step: Evaluation
Client needs category: Physiological integrity
Client needs subcategory: Reduction of risk potential
Taxonomic level: Analysis

9. A client with a history of peptic ulcer disease develops a fever of 101° F (38.3° C). Which accompanying sign most strongly indicates the client has peritonitis?
   A. Leukopenia
   B. Hyperactive bowel sounds
   C. Abdominal rigidity
   D. Polyuria
Answer: C. Abdominal rigidity is a classic sign of peritonitis. The client would more likely have leukocytosis, hypoactive bowel sounds, and decreased urine output.

➡ NCLEX keys
Nursing process step: Assessment
Client needs category: Physiological integrity
Client needs subcategory: Reduction of risk potential
Taxonomic level: Analysis

10. Daily abdominal girth measurements are prescribed for a client with liver dysfunction and ascites. To increase accuracy, the nurse should use which landmark?
   A. Xiphoid process
   B. Umbilicus
   C. Iliac crest
   D. Symphysis pubis

Answer: B. The proper technique for abdominal girth measurement involves circumventing the abdomen with a tape measure using the umbilicus as a landmark. The other sites would give inaccurate measurements.

➡ *NCLEX keys*
Nursing process step: Assessment
Client needs category: Physiological integrity
Client needs subcategory: Reduction of risk potential
Taxonomic level: Application

All that talk about the GI system makes me hungry. Remember that healthy eating promotes good studying.

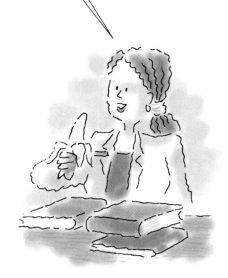

9 Endocrine System

Brush up on key concepts

The endocrine system consists of chemical transmitters called hormones and specialized cell clusters called glands.

At any time, you can review the major points of this chapter by consulting the *Cheat sheet* on pages 270 to 273.

Thermostat central

The **hypothalamus** controls temperature, respiration, and blood pressure. Its functions affect the emotional states. The hypothalamus also produces hypothalamic-stimulating hormones, which affect the inhibition and release of pituitary hormones.

Heavy on the hormones

The **pituitary gland** is composed of anterior and posterior lobes. Together these lobes produce a variety of hormones that affect the body.

The anterior lobe secretes:
- **follicle-stimulating hormone,** which stimulates graafian follicle growth and estrogen secretion in women
- **luteinizing hormone,** which induces ovulation and development of the corpus luteum in women and stimulates testosterone secretion in men
- **adrenocorticotropic hormone (ACTH),** also called corticotropin, which stimulates secretion of hormones from the adrenal cortex
- **thyroid-stimulating hormone (TSH),** which regulates the secretory activity of the thyroid gland
- **growth hormone,** which is an insulin antagonist that stimulates the growth of cells, bones, muscle, and soft tissue.

The posterior lobe secretes:

- **vasopressin** (antidiuretic hormone, also called ADH), which helps the body retain water
- **oxytocin,** which stimulates uterine contractions during labor and milk secretion in lactating women.

Growth gland

The **thyroid gland** accelerates growth and cellular reactions, including basal metabolic rate (BMR). It's controlled by the pituitary gland's secretion of TSH.

The thyroid gland produces thyrocalcitonin, triiodothyronine (T_3), and thyroxine (T_4), which are necessary for growth and development.

Coping with calcium

The **parathyroid gland** secretes parathyroid hormone (parathormone), which regulates calcium and phosphorus levels and promotes the resorption of calcium from bones.

Androgen, estrogen, and others

The **adrenal glands** are composed of the adrenal cortex and the adrenal medulla. The adrenal cortex secretes three major hormones:

- **glucocorticoids** (cortisol, cortisone, and corticosterone), which mediate the stress response, promote sodium and water retention and potassium secretion, and suppress ACTH secretion
- **mineralocorticoids** (aldosterone and deoxycorticosterone), which promote sodium and water retention and potassium secretion
- **sex hormones** (androgens, estrogens, and progesterone), which develop and maintain secondary sex characteristics and libido.

The adrenal medulla secretes two hormones:

- **norepinephrine,** which regulates generalized vasoconstriction

(Text continues on page 273.)

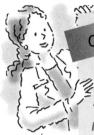

Endocrine refresher

ACROMEGALY AND GIGANTISM

Key signs and symptoms
Acromegaly
- Enlarged supraorbital ridge
- Thickened ears and nose
- Paranasal sinus enlargement
- Thickening of the tongue

Gigantism
- Excessive growth in all parts of the body

Key test results
- Plasma human growth hormone (HGH) levels measured by radioimmunoassay typically are elevated. However, because HGH secretion is pulsatile, the results of random sampling may be misleading. IGF-1 (somatomedin-C) levels offer a better screening alternative.

Key treatments
- Surgery to remove effecting tumor (transsphenoidal hypophysectomy)
- Thyroid hormone replacement therapy following surgery: levothyroxine (Synthroid)
- Corticosteroid: cortisone (Cortone)
- Inhibitor of HGH release: bromocriptine (Parlodel)
- Somatotropic hormone: octreotide (Sandostatin)

Key interventions
- Provide the patient with emotional support.
- Perform or assist with range-of-motion exercises.
- Keep in mind that this disease can also cause inexplicable mood changes. Reassure the family that these mood changes result from the disease and can be modified with treatment.
- After surgery, diligently monitor vital signs and neurologic status. Be alert for any alterations in level of consciousness, pupil equality, or visual acuity as well as vomiting, falling pulse rate, and rising blood pressure.
- Check blood glucose often.
- Measure intake and output hourly, watching for large increases.

- Encourage the patient to ambulate on the first or second day after surgery.

ADDISON'S DISEASE

Key signs and symptoms
- Hypoglycemia
- Orthostatic hypotension
- Weakness and lethargy
- Weight loss

Key test results
- Blood chemistry reveals decreased hematocrit (HCT), decreased hemoglobin (Hb), cortisol, glucose, sodium, chloride, and aldosterone levels; and increased blood urea nitrogen (BUN) and potassium level.
- Fasting blood glucose reveals hypoglycemia.
- Urine chemistry shows decreased 17-ketosteroids and hydroxycorticosteroids (17-OHCS.)

Key treatments
- In adrenal crisis, I.V. hydrocortisone given promptly along with 3 to 5 L of saline solution
- Glucocorticoids: cortisone (Cortone), hydrocortisone (Solu-Cortef)
- Mineralocorticoid: fludrocortisone (Florinef)

Key interventions
- Be prepared to administer I.V. hydrocortisone and saline solution promptly if patient is in adrenal crisis.
- Administer I.V. fluids.
- Don't allow the patient to sit up or stand quickly.

CUSHING'S SYNDROME

Key signs and symptoms
- Amenorrhea
- Hypertension
- Mood swings
- Muscle wasting
- Weight gain, especially truncal obesity, buffalo hump, and moonface

Key test results
- Blood chemistry shows increased cortisol, aldosterone, sodium, corticotropin, and glucose levels and a decreased potassium level.

> Because endocrine disorders often affect fluid balance, monitoring fluid status is a key element of patient care.

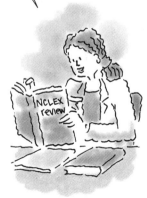

Endocrine refresher *(continued)*

CUSHING'S SYNDROME *(continued)*
• Dexamethasone suppression test shows no decrease in 17-OHCS.
• Magnetic resonance imaging shows pituitary or adrenal tumors.

Key treatments
• Hypophysectomy or bilateral adrenalectomy
• Antidiabetic agents: insulin or oral antidiabetic agents such as tolbutamide (Orinase), chlorpropamide (Diabinese), acetohexamide (Dymelor), tolazamide (Tolinase), glyburide (DiaBeta, Micronase), glipizide (Glucotrol)

Key interventions
• Perform postoperative care.
• Assess edema.
• Limit water intake.
• Weigh the patient daily.

DIABETES INSIPIDUS

Key signs and symptoms
• Polydipsia (consumption of 4 to 40 L/day)
• Polyuria (greater than 5 L/day)

Key test results
• Urine chemistry shows urine specific gravity less than 1.004, osmolality 50 to 200 mOsm/kg, decreased urine pH, and decreased sodium and potassium levels.

Key treatments
• I.V. therapy: hydration (when first diagnosed, intake and output must be matched milliliter to milliliter to prevent dehydration), electrolyte replacement
• Antidiuretic hormone replacement: vasopressin (Pitressin), lypressin (Diapid nasal spray)

Key interventions
• Assess fluid balance.
• Monitor and record vital signs, intake and output (urine output should be measured every hour when first diagnosed), urine specific gravity (check every 1 to 2 hours when first diagnosed), and laboratory studies.
• Administer I.V. fluids.

DIABETES MELLITUS

Key signs and symptoms
• Polydipsia
• Polyphagia
• Polyuria
• Weight loss

Key test results
• Fasting blood glucose level is increased (greater than or equal to 126 mg/dl).
• 2-hour postprandial blood glucose level shows hyperglycemia (greater than 200 mg/dl).

Key treatments
• Antidiabetic agents: insulins and oral agents, such as tolbutamide (Orinase), chlorpropamide (Diabinese), acetohexamide (Dymelor), tolazamide (Tolinase), glyburide (DiaBeta, Micronase), glipizide (Glucotrol)

Key interventions
• Assess acid-base and fluid balance.
• Monitor for signs of hypoglycemia (vagueness, slow cerebration, dizziness, weakness, pallor, tachycardia, diaphoresis, seizures, and coma), ketoacidosis (acetone breath, dehydration, weak or rapid pulse, Kussmaul's respirations), and hyperosmolar coma (polyuria, thirst, neurologic abnormalities, stupor).
• Be prepared to treat hypoglycemia; immediately give carbohydrates in the form of fruit juice, hard candy, or honey. If the patient is unconscious, administer glucogon or dextrose I.V.
• Be prepared to administer I.V. fluids, insulin and, usually, potassium replacement for ketoacidosis or hyperosmolar coma.
• Monitor wound healing.
• Maintain the patient's diet.
• Provide meticulous skin and foot care. Patients with diabetes are at increased risk for infection from impaired leukocyte activity.
• Foster independence.

GOITER

Key signs and symptoms
• Single or multinodular, firm, irregular enlargement of the thyroid gland
• Dizziness or syncope when the patient raises his arms above his head (Pemberton's sign)
• Dysphagia

Key test results
• Laboratory tests reveal high or normal thyroid-stimulating hormone (TSH), low serum thyroxine (T_4) concentrations, and increased iodine 131 uptake.

Key treatments
• Subtotal thyroidectomy
• Thyroid hormone replacement: levothyroxine (Synthroid)

(continued)

Endocrine refresher *(continued)*

GOITER *(continued)*
Key interventions
- Measure the patient's neck circumference. Also check for the development of hard nodules in the gland.
- Provide preoperative teaching and postoperative care if subtotal thyroidectomy is indicated.

HYPERTHYROIDISM
Key signs and symptoms
- Atrial fibrillation
- Bruit or thrill over thyroid
- Diaphoresis
- Palpitations
- Tachycardia

Key test results
- Blood chemistry shows increased tri-iodothyronine (T_3), T_4, and free thyroxine levels and decreased TSH and cholesterol levels.
- Radioactive iodine uptake (RAIU) is increased.

Key treatments
- Radiation therapy
- Thyroidectomy
- Iodine preparations: potassium iodide (SSKI), radioactive iodine

Key interventions
- Assess cardiovascular status.
- Avoid stimulants, such as drugs and foods that contain caffeine.
- Administer I.V. fluids.
- Weigh the patient daily.
- Provide postoperative nursing care.

HYPOTHYROIDISM
Key signs and symptoms
- Dry, flaky skin and thinning nails
- Fatigue
- Hypothermia
- Menstrual disorders
- Mental sluggishness
- Weight gain or anorexia

Key test results
- Blood chemistry shows decreased T_3, T_4, free thyroxine, and sodium levels, and increased TSH and cholesterol levels.
- RAIU is decreased.

Key treatments
- Thyroid hormone replacement: levothyroxine (Synthroid), liothyronine (Cytomel), thyroglobulin (Proloid)

Key interventions
- Avoid sedation; administer one-half to one-third the normal dose of sedatives or narcotics.
- Check for constipation and edema.
- Force fluids.

PANCREATIC CANCER
Key signs and symptoms
- Dull, intermittent epigastric pain (early in disease)
- Continuous pain that radiates to the right upper quadrant or dorsolumbar area, pain may be colicky, dull or vague and unrelated to activity or posture.
- Anorexia
- Rapid, profound weight loss
- Palpable mass in the subumbilical or left hypochondrial region

Key test results
- Percutaneous fine-needle aspiration biopsy of the pancreas may detect tumor cells.
- Blood studies reveal increased serum bilirubin, increased serum amylase and lipase, prolonged prothrombin time, elevated alkaline phosphatase (with biliary obstruction), and elevated aspartate aminotransferase and alanine aminotransferase (when liver cell necrosis is present).
- Fasting blood glucose may indicate hyperglycemia or hypoglycemia.

Key treatments
- Blood transfusion
- I.V. fluid therapy
- Whipple's operation or pancreatoduodenectomy (excision of the head of the pancreas along with the encircling loop of the duodenum)
- Antineoplastic combinations: fluorouracil (Adrucil), streptozocin (Zanosar), ifosfamide (Ifex), and doxorubicin (Adriamycin)
- Insulin after pancreatic resection, to provide adequate exogenous insulin supply
- Narcotic analgesics: morphine, meperidine (Demerol), and codeine, which can lead to biliary tract spasm and increase common bile duct pressure (used only when other methods fail)
- Pancreatic enzyme: pancrelipase (Pancrease)

Key interventions
Before surgery
- Give blood transfusions, vitamin K , antibiotics, and gastric lavage, as necessary.
After surgery
- Monitor fluid balance, abdominal girth, metabolic state, and weight daily. Replace nutrients I.V., orally, or by nasogastric

Endocrine refresher (continued)

PANCREATIC CANCER (continued)

tube. Impose dietary restrictions such as a low-sodium or fluid retention diet as required). Maintain a 2,500 calorie diet for the patient.

- Administer an oral pancreatic enzyme at mealtimes, if needed.
- Administer pain medication, antibiotics, and antipyretics, as necessary.
- Watch for signs of hypoglycemia or hyperglycemia; administer glucose or an antidiabetic agent as necessary. Monitor blood glucose levels.
- Apply antiembolism stockings and assist in range-of-motion exercises. If thrombosis occurs, elevate the patient's legs and give an anticoagulant or aspirin, as required.

THYROID CANCER

Key signs and symptoms
- Enlarged thyroid gland
- Painless, firm, irregular, and enlarged thyroid nodule or mass

Key test results
- Blood chemistry shows increased calcitonin, serotonin, and prostaglandin levels.
- RAIU shows a "cold," or nonfunctioning, nodule.
- Thyroid biopsy shows cytology positive for cancer cells.

Key treatments
- Radiation therapy
- Thyroidectomy (total or subtotal); total thyroidectomy and radical neck excision

Key interventions
- Assess respiratory status for signs of airway obstruction.
- Assess ability to swallow.
- Provide postoperative thyroidectomy care.

THYROIDITIS

Key signs and symptoms
- Thyroid enlargement
- Fever
- Pain
- Tenderness and reddened skin over the gland

Key test results
Precise diagnosis depends on the type of thyroiditis.
- In autoimmune thyroiditis, high titers of thyroglobulin and microsomal antibodies may be present in serum.
- In subacute granulomatous thyroiditis, tests may reveal elevated erythrocyte sedimentation rate, increased thyroid hormone levels, and decreased thyroidal RAIU.
- In chronic infective and noninfective thyroiditis, varied findings occur, depending on underlying infection or other disease.

Key treatments
- Partial thyroidectomy to relieve tracheal or esophageal compression in Riedel's thyroiditis
- Thyroid hormone replacement: levothyroxine (Synthroid) for accompanying hypothyroidism

Key interventions.
- Check vital signs and examine the patient's neck for unusual swelling, enlargement, or redness.
- If the neck is swollen, measure and record the circumference daily.

After thyroidectomy:
- Check vital signs every 15 to 30 minutes until the patient's condition stabilizes. Stay alert for signs of tetany secondary to accidental parathyroid injury during surgery. Keep 10% calcium gluconate available for I.M. use if needed.
- Assess dressings frequently for excessive bleeding.
- Watch for signs of airway obstruction, such as difficulty talking and increased swallowing; keep tracheotomy equipment handy.

- **epinephrine,** which regulates instantaneous stress reaction and increases metabolism, blood glucose levels, and cardiac output.

Endo and exo

The **pancreas** is an accessory gland of digestion. In its **exocrine function,** it secretes digestive enzymes (amylase, lipase, and trypsin). Amylase breaks down starches into smaller carbohydrate molecules. Lipase breaks down fats into fatty acids and glycerol. Trypsin breaks down proteins. Note that ex-

ocrine glands discharge secretions via a duct; the pancreas secretes enzymes into the duodenum through the pancreatic duct.

In its **endocrine function,** the pancreas secretes hormones from the Langerhans' islets (insulin, glucagon, and somatostatin). Insulin regulates fat, protein, and carbohydrate metabolism and lowers blood glucose levels by promoting glucose transport into cells. Glucagon increases blood glucose levels by promoting hepatic glyconeogenesis. Somatostatin inhibits the release of insulin, glucagon,

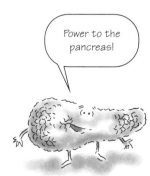

Power to the pancreas!

and somatotropin. Note that endocrine glands discharge secretions into the blood or lymph.

Keep abreast of diagnostic tests

Below are the major diagnostic tests for assessing endocrine disorders as well as common nursing actions associated with each test.

Draw blood and test, part 1

Blood chemistry tests are used to analyze blood samples for potassium, sodium, calcium, phosphorus, glucose, bicarbonate, blood urea nitrogen (BUN), creatinine, protein, albumin, osmolality, amylase, lipase, alkaline phosphatase, lactate dehydrogenase, aldosterone, cortisol, ketones, cholesterol, triglycerides, and carbon dioxide.

Nursing actions
• Check the venipuncture site for bleeding.

Draw blood and test, part 2

A **hematologic study** analyzes a blood sample for red blood cells (RBCs), white blood cells (WBCs), platelets, prothrombin time, international normalized ratio, partial thromboplastin time, hemoglobin (Hb), and hematocrit (HCT).

Nursing actions
• Note current drug therapy.
• Check the venipuncture site for bleeding.

Fast and test

The **fasting blood glucose test** measures plasma glucose levels following a 12- to 14-hour fast.

Nursing actions
• Withhold food and fluids for 12 to 14 hours before fasting sample is drawn.
• Withhold insulin until the test is completed.

Eat carbos and test

The **2-hour postprandial glucose test** uses a blood sample analysis to determine the body's insulin response to carbohydrate ingestion.

Nursing actions
• List any medications that might interfere with the test.
• Note pregnancy, trauma, or infectious disease.
• Provide the patient with a 100 g carbohydrate diet before the test and then ask him to fast for 2 hours.
• Instruct the patient to avoid smoking, caffeine, alcohol, and exercise after the meal.

Carbo absorption assessment

The **glucose tolerance test** (GTT) uses blood and urine samples to measure absorption of carbohydrates.

Nursing actions
• List any medications that might interfere with the test.
• Note pregnancy, trauma, or infectious disease.
• Provide the patient with a high-carbohydrate diet for 3 days.
• Instruct the patient to fast for 10 to 16 hours before the test.
• Advise the patient not to smoke, drink coffee or alcohol, or exercise strenuously for 8 hours before or during the test.
• Withhold any medications that may interfere with testing.
• Draw a fasting blood sample and have the patient provide a urine specimen at the same time.
• Administer the test dose of oral glucose and record the time of administration.
• Request laboratory collection of serum glucose and urine samples at 30, 60, 120, and 180 minutes.
• Refrigerate samples and assess the patient for hypoglycemia.

Months of blood glucose levels

Glycosylated Hb testing utilizes a blood sample to measure glycosylated Hb levels. This provides information about average blood glucose levels during the preceding 2 to 3 months. This test is used to evaluate the long-term effectiveness of diabetes therapy.

Nursing actions
• Explain to the patient that this test is used to evaluate diabetes therapy.
• Tell the patient that he needn't restrict food or fluids and instruct him to maintain his prescribed medication and diet regimen.

Checking for cortisol
The **adrenocorticotropic hormone (corticotropin) stimulation test** analyzes blood samples for cortisol.

Nursing actions
• List any medications that might interfere with the test.
• Know that pregnancy contraindicates this test.
• Monitor 24-hour I.V. infusion of corticotropin after baseline serum sample is drawn.

Blood analysis (with drug)
The **dexamethasone suppression test,** which involves the administration of dexamethasone, is used to analyze a blood sample for serum cortisol.

Nursing actions
• On the first day, give the patient 1 mg of dexamethasone at 11 p.m.
• On the next day, collect blood samples at 4 p.m. and 11 p.m.
• Monitor the venipuncture site; if hematoma develops, apply warm soaks.
• List any medications that might interfere with the test.

Urine analysis (24-hour collection)
The **24-hour urine test for 17-ketosteroids (17-KS) and 17-hydroxycorticosteroids (17-OHCS)** is a quantitative laboratory analysis of urine collected over 24 hours to determine hormone precursors.

Nursing actions
• Withhold all medications for 48 hours before the test.
• Instruct the patient to void and note the time (collection of urine starts with the next voiding).
• Place urine container on ice.
• Measure each voided urine collection.
• If done on an outpatient basis, instruct the patient about how to collect the 24-hour specimen.
• List any medications that might interfere with the test.

Epinephrine exam
The **urine vanillylmandelic acid test** is a quantitative analysis of urine collected over 24 hours to determine the end products of catecholamine metabolism (epinephrine and norepinephrine).

Nursing actions
• List any medications, previous tests, and medical conditions that might interfere with the test.
• Restrict foods that contain vanilla, coffee, tea, citrus fruits, bananas, nuts, and chocolate for 3 days prior to test.
• Hold any medications that might interfere with testing such as antihypertensives and aspirin.
• Instruct the patient to void and note the time (collection of urine starts with the next voiding).
• Place urine container on ice.
• Measure each voided urine.

Oxygen in, calories used
The **basal metabolic rate test** is an indirect, noninvasive measurement of BMR. The test measures oxygen consumed by the body during a given time and evaluates caloric expenditure in a 24-hour period.

Nursing actions
• List medications taken before the procedure.
• Note environmental and emotional stressors.

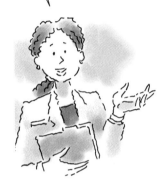

The sella turcica is located in a depression at the base of the skull and contains the pituitary gland.

Eyesight exam

Visual acuity and field testing measures the patient's central and peripheral vision.

Nursing actions

• Ask the patient to wear or bring corrective lenses for the test.

Inspecting the abdomen

Computed tomography (CT) scan allows visualization of the sella turcica and abdomen.

Nursing actions

• Note the patient's allergies to iodine, seafood, and radiopaque dyes.
• Instruct the patient to fast for 4 hours prior to the procedure.

Echo exam

Ultrasonography allows visualization of the thyroid, pelvis, and abdomen through the use of reflected sound waves.

Nursing actions

• Assess whether the patient can lie still during the procedure.

Taking thyroid tissue

A **closed percutaneous thyroid biopsy** uses the percutaneous, sterile aspiration of a small amount of thyroid tissue for histologic evaluation.

Nursing actions

Before the procedure:
• withhold food and fluids after midnight
• obtain the patient's written, informed consent.
  After the procedure:
• maintain bed rest for 24 hours
• monitor vital signs
• assess for esophageal or tracheal puncture and bleeding or respiratory distress caused by hematoma or edema.

Thyroid function test

A **thyroid uptake,** also called **radioactive iodine uptake** or **RAIU,** measures the amount of radioactive iodine taken up by the thyroid gland in 24 hours. This measurement gives doctors an indication of thyroid function.

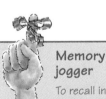

Memory jogger

To recall interventions for Sulkowitch's test, remember that hyper- comes before hypo- alphabetically. Then remember to collect a urine specimen before a meal for hypercalcemia and after for hypocalcemia.

Nursing actions

• Instruct the patient not to ingest iodine-rich foods for 24 hours before the test
• Discontinue all thyroid and cough medications 7 to 10 days before the test.

Radiograph of the 'roid'

A **thyroid scan** gives visual imaging of radioactivity distribution in the thyroid gland. Doctors use these results to assess size, shape, position, and anatomic function of the thyroid.

Nursing actions

• If iodine^{123} (^{123}I) or ^{131}I is to be used, tell the patient to fast after midnight the night before the test. Fasting isn't required if an I.V. injection of $^{99m}T_6$ pertechnetate is used.
• Hold any medications that may interfere with the procedure.
• Instruct the patient to stop consuming iodized salt, iodinated salt substitutes, and seafood one week before the procedure.
• Imaging follows oral administration (^{123}I or ^{131}I) by 24 hours, and I.V. injection ($^{99m}T_6$ pertechnetate) by 20 to 30 minutes.
• Remove dentures, jewelry, and other materials that may interfere with imaging.
• After the procedure, tell the patient he may resume medications that were suspended for testing.

Artery assessment

Arteriography gives a fluoroscopic examination of the arterial blood supply to the parathyroid, adrenal, and pancreatic glands.

Nursing actions

Before the procedure, you should:
• check for written, informed consent
• note the patient's allergies to iodine, seafood, and radiopaque dyes
• withhold food and fluids after midnight.
  After the procedure, you should:
• monitor vital signs
• check the insertion site for bleeding and assess pulses distal to the site.

Counting calcium

Sulkowitch's test analyzes urine to measure the amount of calcium being excreted.

Nursing actions

• If hypercalcemia is indicated, collect a single urine specimen *before* a meal,
• If hypocalcemia is indicated, collect a single urine specimen *after* a meal.

Polish up on patient care

Major endocrine disorders include acromegaly and gigantism, Addison's disease, Cushing's syndrome, diabetes insipidus, diabetes mellitus, goiter, hyperthyroidism, hypothyroidism, pancreatic cancer, and thyroid cancer.

Acromegaly and gigantism

Acromegaly and gigantism are marked by hormonal dysfunction and startling skeletal overgrowth. Both are chronic, progressive diseases. Both occur when the pituitary gland produces too much growth hormone, causing excessive growth.

Acromegaly occurs after epiphyseal closure, causing bone thickening and transverse growth and visceromegaly (enlargement of the viscera). In other words, acromegaly may occur any time after adolescence, when the arms and legs have stopped growing. The signs of this disorder are swelling and enlargement of the arms, legs, and face.

Gigantism begins before epiphyseal closure and causes proportional overgrowth of all body tissues. In other words, gigantism begins in childhood or adolescence when the arms and legs are still growing. That is why these patients may attain giant proportions.

CAUSES

• Oversecretion of human growth hormone (HGH)
• Tumors of the anterior pituitary gland (which lead to oversecretion of human growth hormone)

ASSESSMENT FINDINGS

Acromegaly develops slowly; gigantism develops abruptly.

Acromegaly

• Enlarged supraorbital ridge
• Thickened ears and nose
• Prognathism (projection of the jaw) becomes marked and may interfere with chewing
• Laryngeal hypertrophy
• Paranasal sinus enlargement
• Thickening of the tongue
• Oily skin
• Diaphoresis
• Severe headache
• Bitemporal hemianopia
• Loss of visual acuity
• Blindness may occur

Gigantism

• Excessive growth in all parts of the body; gigantism causes remarkable height increases, as much as six inches a year; infants and children may grow to three times the normal height for their age; adults may reach heights above 6 feet 8 inches

DIAGNOSTIC TEST RESULTS

• Plasma HGH levels measured by radioimmunoassay typically are elevated. However, because HGH secretion is pulsatile, the results of random sampling may be misleading. IGF-1 (somatomedin-C) levels offer a better screening alternative.
• Glucose normally suppresses HGH secretion; therefore, a glucose infusion that doesn't suppress the hormone level to below the accepted normal value of 2 ng/ml, when combined with characteristic clinical features, strongly suggests hyperpituitarism.
• Skull X-rays, a CT scan, arteriography, and magnetic resonance imaging (MRI) determine the presence and extent of the pituitary lesion.

NURSING DIAGNOSES

• Body image disturbance
• Pain
• Impaired physical mobility

TREATMENT

• Surgery to remove effecting tumor (transsphenoidal hypophysectomy)
• Pituitary radiation therapy

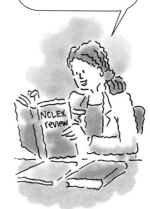

It's a question of timing. Acromegaly may occur any time after adolescence, when the arms and legs have stopped growing. Gigantism begins in childhood or adolescence when the arms and legs are still growing.

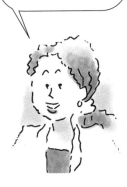

Think about therapeutic communication. The patient needs help coping with his body image as well as mood changes brought on by the disorder.

Drug therapy

- Thyroid hormone replacement therapy following surgery: levothyroxine (Synthroid)
- Corticosteroid: cortisone (Cortone)
- Inhibitor of growth hormone release: bromocriptine (Parlodel)
- Somatotropic hormone: octreotide (Sandostatin)

INTERVENTIONS AND RATIONALES

- Provide the patient with emotional support *to help him cope with his body image. Grotesque body changes characteristic of this disorder can cause severe psychological stress.*
- Examine the patient for skeletal manifestations, such as arthritis of the hands and osteoarthritis of the spine *to detect complications.*
- Administer prescribed medications *to improve the patient's condition.*
- Perform or assist with range-of-motion exercises *to promote maximum joint mobility.*
- Evaluate muscular weakness, especially in the patient with late-stage acromegaly. Check the strength of his handclasp *to monitor for disease progression.* If it's very weak, help with tasks such as cutting food.
- Keep the skin dry. Avoid using an oily lotion *because the skin is already oily.*
- Test blood glucose *to detect early signs of hyperglycemia.* Check for signs of hyperglycemia (fatigue, polyuria, polydipsia) *to avoid treatment delay.*
- Be aware that the patient's tumor may cause visual problems. If the patient has hemianopia, stand where he can see you *to reduce anxiety.*
- Keep in mind that this disease can also cause inexplicable mood changes. Reassure the family that these mood changes result from the disease and can be modified with treatment *to help the family cope with the patient's illness.*
- Before surgery, reinforce what the surgeon has told the patient, if possible, and provide a clear and honest explanation of the scheduled operation *to allay the patient's fears and anxiety.*
- If the patient is a child, explain to his parents that such surgery prevents permanent soft-tissue deformities but won't correct bone changes that have already taken place.

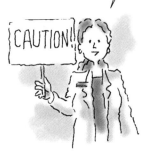

A patient with acromegaly should be periodically screened for colon polyps — incidence of polyps increases with chronic human growth hormone elevation.

Arrange for counseling, if necessary, *to help the child and parents cope with permanent defects.*

- After surgery, diligently monitor vital signs and neurologic status. Be alert for any alterations in level of consciousness, pupil equality, or visual acuity as well as vomiting, falling pulse rate, and rising blood pressure. *These changes may signal an increase in intracranial pressure due to intracranial bleeding or cerebral edema.*
- Check blood glucose often. *HGH levels usually fall rapidly after surgery, removing an insulin antagonist effect in many patients and possibly precipitating hypoglycemia.*
- Measure intake and output hourly, watching for large increases. *Transient diabetes insipidus, which sometimes occurs after surgery for hyperpituitarism, can cause such increases in urine output.*
- If the transsphenoidal approach is used, a large nasal pack is kept in place for several days. Because the patient must breathe through his mouth, give good mouth care *to prevent the breakdown of oral mucosa.*
- The surgical site is packed with a piece of tissue generally taken from a mid-thigh donor site. Watch for cerebrospinal fluid (CSF) leaks from the packed site. Look for increased external nasal drainage or drainage into the nasopharynx. CSF leaks may necessitate additional surgery to repair the leak. *These measures detect complications quickly and avoid treatment delays.*
- Encourage the patient to ambulate on the first or second day after surgery *to prevent complications of immobility.*

Teaching topics

- Receiving follow-up check-ups (there is a slight chance that the tumor that caused his condition could recur)
- Continuing hormone replacement therapy following surgery (warn against stopping the hormones suddenly)
- Wearing a medical identification bracelet at all times and bringing his hormone replacement schedule with him whenever he returns to the facility.

Addison's disease

Addison's disease, also known as adrenal hypofunction, occurs when the adrenal gland fails to secrete sufficient mineralocorticoids, glucocorticoids, and androgens.

Addisonian crisis (adrenal crisis) is a critical deficiency of mineralocorticoids and glucocorticoids. It generally occurs in patients who have chronic adrenal insufficiency and follows acute stress, sepsis, trauma, surgery, or omission of steroid therapy. It's a medical emergency that necessitates immediate, vigorous treatment.

CAUSES
• Autoimmune disease
• Histoplasmosis
• Idiopathic atrophy of adrenal glands
• Metastatic lesions from lung cancer
• Pituitary hypofunction
• Surgical removal of adrenal glands
• Trauma
• Tuberculosis

ASSESSMENT FINDINGS
• Anorexia, diarrhea, and nausea
• Bronzed skin pigmentation of nipples, scars, and buccal mucosa
• Decreased pubic and axillary hair
• Dehydration and thirst
• Depression and personality changes
• Hypoglycemia
• Orthostatic hypotension
• Weakness and lethargy
• Weight loss

DIAGNOSTIC TEST RESULTS
• Blood chemistry reveals decreased HCT; decreased Hb, cortisol, glucose, sodium, chloride, and aldosterone levels; and increased BUN and potassium levels.
• BMR is decreased.
• Electrocardiogram demonstrates prolonged PR and QT intervals.
• Fasting blood glucose reveals hypoglycemia.
• Urine chemistry shows decreased 17-KS and 17-OHCS.

NURSING DIAGNOSES
• Fluid volume deficit
• Altered nutrition: Less than body requirements
• Risk for infection

TREATMENT
• High-carbohydrate, high-protein, high-sodium, low-potassium diet in small, frequent feedings before steroid therapy; high-potassium and low-sodium diet while on steroid therapy
• In adrenal crisis, I.V. hydrocortisone administered promptly along with 3 to 5 L of normal saline solution

Drug therapy
• Antacids: magnesium and aluminum hydroxide (Maalox), aluminum hydroxide gel (Gelusil)
• Glucocorticoids: cortisone (Cortone), hydrocortisone (Solu-Cortef)
• Mineralocorticoid: fludrocortisone (Florinef)
• Vasopressor: phenylephrine (NeoSynephrine)

INTERVENTIONS AND RATIONALES
• Be prepared to administer I.V. hydrocortisone and saline solution promptly if patient is in adrenal crisis *to reverse shock and hyponatremia.*
• Assess fluid balance (and increase in fluid intake in hot weather) *to prevent addisonian crisis, which may be precipitated by salt or fluid loss in hot weather and during exercise.*
• Monitor and record vital signs, intake and output, urine specific gravity, and laboratory studies *to assess for fluid volume deficit.*
• Maintain the patient's diet *to promote nutritional balance.*
• Administer I.V. fluids *to maintain hydration and prevent addisonian crisis.*
• Weigh the patient daily *to determine nutritional status and detect fluid loss.*
• Administer medications, as prescribed, *to maintain or improve patient's condition.*
• Don't allow the patient to sit up or stand quickly *to avoid orthostatic hypotension.*
• Encourage fluid intake *to improve fluid status and prevent addisonian crisis.*

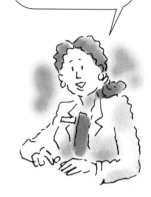

In Addison's disease, the adrenal glands don't secrete enough steroid hormones.

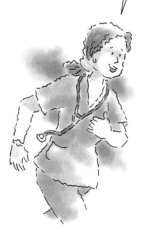

For adrenal crisis, take emergency action — I.V. hydrocortisone with 3 to 5 L of saline solution.

• Assist with activities of daily living *to conserve energy and decrease metabolic demands.*
• Maintain a quiet environment *to conserve energy and decrease metabolic demands.*

Teaching topics
• Recognizing the signs and symptoms of adrenal crisis (profound weakness, fatigue, nausea, vomiting, hypotension, dehydration and, occasionally, high fever followed by hypothermia)
• Carrying injectable dexamethasone (Decadron)
• Avoiding over-the-counter drugs
• Avoiding strenuous exercise, particularly in hot weather

Cushing's syndrome

Cushing's syndrome, also known as hypercortisolism, is the hyperactivity of the adrenal cortex. It results in excessive secretion of glucocorticoids, particularly cortisol. There is also a possible increase in mineralocorticoids and sex hormones.

CAUSES
• Adenoma or carcinoma of the adrenal cortex
• Adenoma or carcinoma of the pituitary gland
• Excessive or prolonged administration of glucocorticoids or corticotropin
• Exogenous secretion of corticotropin by malignant neoplasms in the lungs or gallbladder
• Hyperplasia of the adrenal glands
• Hypothalamic stimulation of the pituitary gland

ASSESSMENT FINDINGS
• Acne
• Amenorrhea
• Decreased libido
• Ecchymosis
• Edema
• Enlarged clitoris
• Fragile skin
• Gynecomastia
• Hirsutism

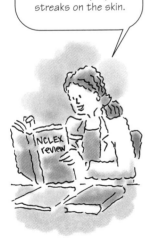

Cushing's syndrome has distinctive signs, including rapidly developing fatty tissue in the face, neck, and trunk and purple streaks on the skin.

• Hypertension
• Mood swings
• Muscle wasting
• Pain in joints
• Poor wound healing
• Purple striae on abdomen
• Recurrent infections
• Weakness and fatigue
• Weight gain, especially truncal obesity, buffalo hump, moonface

DIAGNOSTIC TEST RESULTS
• Blood chemistry shows increased cortisol, aldosterone, sodium, corticotropin and glucose levels and a decreased potassium level.
• CT scan shows pituitary or adrenal tumors.
• Dexamethasone suppression test shows no decrease in 17-OHCS.
• GTT shows hyperglycemia.
• Hematology shows increased WBC and RBC counts and decreased eosinophils.
• MRI shows pituitary or adrenal tumors.
• Ultrasonography shows pituitary or adrenal tumors.
• Urine chemistry shows increased 17-OHCS and 17-KS, decreased urine specific gravity, and glycosuria.
• X-ray shows pituitary or adrenal tumor and osteoporosis.

NURSING DIAGNOSES
• Body image disturbance
• Fluid volume deficit
• Impaired skin integrity

TREATMENT
• Hypophysectomy or bilateral adrenalectomy
• Low-sodium, low-carbohydrate, low-calorie, high-potassium, and high-protein diet
• Radiation therapy
• Potassium supplements: potassium chloride (K-Lor), potassium gluconate (Kaon)

Drug therapy
• Adrenal suppressants: metyrapone (Metopirone), aminoglutethimide (Cytadren)
• Antidiabetic agents: insulin or oral antidiabetic agents, such as tolbutamide (Orinase), chlorpropamide (Diabinese), acetohexamide

(Dymelor), tolazamide (Tolinase), glyburide (DiaBeta, Micronase), glipizide (Glucotrol)
• Diuretics: furosemide (Lasix), ethacrynic acid (Edecrin)

INTERVENTIONS AND RATIONALES
• Perform postoperative care *to prevent complications.*
• Assess fluid balance *to detect fluid deficit or overload.*
• Monitor and record vital signs, intake and output, urine specific gravity, fingersticks, urine glucose and ketones, and laboratory studies. *Changed parameters may indicate altered fluid or electrolyte status.*
• Assess edema *to detect signs of fluid volume excess.*
• Apply antiembolism stockings *to promote venous return and prevent thromboembolism formation.*
• Maintain the patient's diet *to maintain nutritional status.*
• Maintain standard precautions to *protect the patient from infection.*
• Provide meticulous skin care and reposition every 2 hours *to prevent skin breakdown.*
• Limit water intake *to prevent fluid volume excess.*
• Weigh the patient daily *to detect fluid retention.*
• Administer medications, as prescribed, *to maintain or improve patient's condition.*
• Encourage the patient to express feelings about changes in body image and sexual function *to help the patient cope effectively.*
• Provide rest periods *to prevent fatigue.*
• Provide postradiation nursing care *to prevent complications.*

Teaching topics
• Recognizing the signs and symptoms of infection and fluid retention
• Avoiding exposure to people with infections
• Self-monitoring for infection
• Carrying a medical identification card (and immediately reporting infections, which necessitate increased steroid dosage)
• Recognizing signs of inadequate steroid dosage (fatigue, weakness, and dizziness) and overdosage (severe edema, weight gain)
• Avoiding discontinuing steroid dosage

Diabetes insipidus

Diabetes insipidus stems from a deficiency of antidiuretic hormone (ADH; vasopressin) secreted by the posterior lobe of the pituitary gland. Decreased ADH reduces the ability of distal and collecting renal tubules in the kidneys to concentrate urine, resulting in excessive urination, excessive thirst, and excessive fluid intake.

CAUSES
• Brain surgery
• Head injury
• Idiopathy
• Meningitis
• Trauma to posterior lobe of pituitary gland
• Tumor of posterior lobe of pituitary gland

ASSESSMENT FINDINGS
• Dehydration
• Fatigue
• Headache
• Muscle weakness and pain
• Polydipsia (excessive thirst, consumption of 4 to 40 L/day)
• Polyuria (greater than 5 L/day)
• Tachycardia
• Weight loss

DIAGNOSTIC TEST RESULTS
• Blood chemistry shows decreased ADH by radioimmunoassay and increased potassium, sodium, and osmolality levels.
• Urine chemistry shows urine specific gravity less than 1.004, osmolality 50 to 200 mOsm/kg, decreased urine pH, and decreased sodium and potassium levels.

NURSING DIAGNOSES
• Fluid volume deficit
• Altered oral mucous membrane
• Risk for altered body temperature

TREATMENT
• I.V. therapy: hydration (when first diagnosed, intake and output must be matched milliliter to milliliter to prevent dehydration), electrolyte replacement
• Regular diet with restriction of foods that exert a diuretic effect

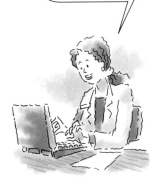

In diabetes mellitus, the body produces little or no insulin or resists the insulin it does produce.

Drug therapy
• ADH replacement: vasopressin (Pitressin), lypressin (Diapid nasal spray)
• ADH stimulant: carbamazepine (Tegretol)

INTERVENTIONS AND RATIONALES
• Assess fluid balance *to avoid dehydration.*
• Monitor and record vital signs, intake and output (urine output should be measured every hour when first diagnosed), urine specific gravity (check every 1 to 2 hours when first diagnosed), and laboratory studies *to assess for fluid volume deficit.*
• Maintain the patient's diet *to maintain nutritional balance.*
• Force fluids *to keep intake equal to output and prevent dehydration.*
• Administer I.V. fluids *to replace fluid and electrolyte loss.*
• Maintain patency of indwelling urinary catheter *to allow accurate measuring of urine output.*
• Administer medications, as prescribed, *to enable the patient to concentrate urine and prevent dehydration.*
• Weigh the patient daily *to detect fluid loss.*

Teaching topics
• Recognizing the signs and symptoms of dehydration
• Increasing fluid intake in hot weather
• Carrying medications at all times

Diabetes mellitus

Diabetes mellitus is a chronic disorder resulting from a disturbance in the production, action, and rate of utilization of insulin. There are several types of diabetes mellitus.

Type 1 (insulin-dependent diabetes mellitus) usually develops in childhood. Type 2 (non-insulin-dependent diabetes mellitus) usually develops after age 30. Gestational diabetes mellitus occurs with pregnancy. Secondary diabetes is induced by trauma, surgery, pancreatic disease, or medications and can be treated as type 1 or type 2.

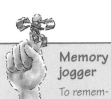

Memory jogger

To remember the classic signs of diabetes, think of the **3 P's:**

Polydipsia: excessive thirst

Polyphagia: excessive hunger

Polyuria: excessive urination.

CAUSES
• Autoimmune disease
• Blockage of insulin supply
• Cushing's syndrome
• Exposure to chemicals
• Failure of body to produce insulin
• Genetics
• Hyperpituitarism
• Hyperthyroidism
• Infection
• Medications
• Pregnancy
• Receptor defect in normally insulin-responsive cells
• Stress
• Surgery
• Trauma

ASSESSMENT FINDINGS
• Acetone breath
• Anorexia
• Atrophic muscles
• Blurred vision
• Dehydration
• Fatigue
• Flushed, warm, smooth, shiny skin
• Kussmaul's respirations
• Mottled extremities
• Multiple infections and boils
• Pain
• Paresthesia
• Peripheral and visceral neuropathies
• Polydipsia
• Polyphagia
• Polyuria
• Poor wound healing
• Retinopathy
• Sexual dysfunction
• Weakness
• Weight loss

DIAGNOSTIC TEST RESULTS
• Blood chemistry shows increased glucose, potassium, chloride, ketone, cholesterol, and triglyceride levels; decreased carbon dioxide level; and pH less than 7.4.
• Fasting blood glucose level is increased (greater than or equal to 126 mg/dl).
• Glycosylated hemoglobin assay (Hb A_{1c}) is increased.
• GTT shows hyperglycemia.

Battling illness

Treating diabetes

Effective treatment for diabetes optimizes blood glucose level and decreases complications. In type 1 diabetes, treatment includes insulin replacement, meal planning, and exercise. Current forms of insulin replacement include single-dose, mixed-dose, split-mixed-dose, and multiple-dose regimens. The multiple-dose regimen may use an insulin pump.

INSULIN ACTION
Insulin may be rapid-acting (Humalog), fast-acting (Regular), intermediate-acting (NPH and Lente), long-acting (Ultralente), or a premixed combination of fast-acting and intermediate-acting. Insulin may be derived from beef, pork, or human sources. Purified human insulin is used commonly today.

PERSONALIZED MEAL PLAN
Treatment for both types of diabetes also requires a meal plan to meet nutritional needs, to control blood glucose levels, and to help the patient reach and maintain his ideal body weight. In type 1 diabetes, the calorie allotment may be high, depending on the patient's growth stage and activity level. Weight reduction is a goal for the obese patient with type 2 diabetes.

OTHER TREATMENTS
Exercise is also useful in managing type 2 diabetes because it increases insulin sensitivity, improves glucose tolerance, and promotes weight loss. In addition, patients with type 2 diabetes may need oral antidiabetic drugs to stimulate endogenous insulin production and increase insulin sensitivity at the cellular level.

THINKING LONG-TERM
Treatment for long-term complications may include dialysis or kidney transplantation for renal failure, photocoagulation for retinopathy, and vascular surgery for large vessel disease. Pancreas transplantation is also an option.

• 2-hour postprandial blood glucose level shows hyperglycemia (greater than 200 mg/dl).
• Urine chemistry shows increased glucose and ketone levels.

NURSING DIAGNOSES
• Altered nutrition: More than body requirements
• Risk for fluid volume deficit
• Risk for impaired skin integrity

TREATMENT
• dietary restrictions
• exercise
• pancreas transplant

Drug therapy
• Antidiabetic agents: insulins and oral agents, such as tolbutamide (Orinase), chlorpropamide (Diabinese), acetohexamide (Dymelor), tolazamide (Tolinase), glyburide (DiaBeta, Micronase), glipizide (Glucotrol)
• Vitamin and mineral supplements (See *Treating diabetes.*)

INTERVENTIONS
• Assess acid-base and fluid balance *to monitor for signs of hyperglycemia.*
• Monitor for signs of hypoglycemia (vagueness, slow cerebration, dizziness, weakness, pallor, tachycardia, diaphoresis, seizures, and coma), ketoacidosis (acetone breath, dehydration, weak or rapid pulse, Kussmaul's respirations), and hyperosmolar coma (polyuria, thirst, neurologic abnormalities, stupor) *to ensure early intervention and prevent complications.*
• Be prepared to treat hypoglycemia; immediately give carbohydrates in the form of fruit juice, hard candy, or honey. If the patient is unconscious, administer glucagon or dextrose I.V. *to prevent neurologic complications*
• Be prepared to administer I.V. fluids, insulin and, usually, potassium replacement for ketoacidosis or hyperosmolar coma *to reduce the risk of potentially life-threatening complications.*
• Monitor and record vital signs, intake and output, fingersticks for blood glucose, and

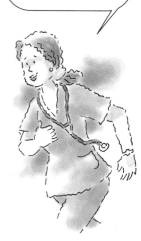

> Be prepared to treat hypoglycemia immediately. Give fruit juice, hard candy, or honey. If the patient is unconscious, administer glucagon or dextrose I.V.

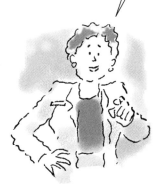

Remember, positive thinking has a lot of power. Repeat to yourself, I WILL PASS THE NCLEX EXAM!

laboratory studies *to assess fluid and electrolyte balance.*
- Monitor wound healing *to assess for infection.*
- Maintain the patient's diet *to prevent complications of diabetes, such as hyperglycemia and hypoglycemia.*
- Force fluids *to maintain patient's hydration.*
- Administer medications, as prescribed. *Diabetic control requires a dynamic balance between diet, antidiabetic agent, and exercise.*
- Encourage the patient to express feelings about diet, medication regimen, and body image changes *to facilitate coping mechanisms.*
- Encourage exercise, as tolerated, *to prevent long-term complications of diabetes.*
- Weigh the patient weekly *to determine nutritional status.*
- Provide meticulous skin and foot care. Patients with diabetes are at increased risk for infection from impaired leukocyte activity. *These health care practices minimize the risk of infection and promote early detection of health problems.*
- Maintain a warm and quiet environment *to provide rest and reduce metabolic demands.*
- Foster independence *to promote self-esteem.*
- Determine the patient's compliance to diet, exercise, and medication regimens *to help develop appropriate interventions.*

Teaching topics
- Understanding the importance of routine follow-up care
- Exercising regularly
- Quitting tobacco products
- Recognizing the signs and symptoms of hyperglycemia and hypoglycemia
- Self-monitoring for infection, skin breakdown, changes in peripheral circulation, poor wound healing, and numbness in extremities
- Adjusting diet and insulin for changes in work, exercise, trauma, infection, fever, and stress
- Administering antidiabetic agents and using the insulin pump
- Using home blood glucose monitoring technique
- Completing daily skin and foot care (avoiding foot soaks, using water-soluble lotions, and using nail files—not nail clippers)
- Carrying an emergency supply of glucose
- Avoiding over-the-counter medication and alcohol
- Adhering to the treatment regimen to prevent complications
- Contacting the American Diabetes Association

Goiter

A goiter is an enlargement of the thyroid gland. It isn't caused by inflammation or a neoplasm. This condition is commonly referred to as nontoxic or simple goiter.

Goiter is commonly classified as endemic or sporadic. With appropriate treatment, the prognosis is good for either type.

Endemic goiter usually results from inadequate dietary intake of iodine associated with such factors as iodine-depleted soil and malnutrition. Endemic goiter affects females more than males, especially during adolescence and pregnancy, when the demand on the body for thyroid hormone increases.

Sporadic goiter follows ingestion of certain drugs or foods. It doesn't affect any specific population segment more than others.

CAUSES
- Insufficient thyroid gland production
- Depletion of glandular iodine
- Ingestion of goitrogenic foods (rutabagas, cabbage, soybeans, peanuts, peaches, peas, strawberries, spinach, and radishes)
- Use of goitrogenic drugs (propylthiouracil, methimazole, iodides, and lithium)

ASSESSMENT FINDINGS
- Single or multinodular, firm, irregular enlargement of the thyroid gland
- Dizziness or syncope when the patient raises his arms above his head (Pemberton's sign)
- Dysphagia
- Respiratory distress

DIAGNOSTIC TEST RESULTS
- Test to rule out Graves' disease, Hashimoto's thyroiditis, and thyroid carcinoma.

• Laboratory tests reveal high or normal TSH, low serum T_4 concentrations, and increased iodine ^{131}I uptake.

NURSING DIAGNOSES
• Risk for suffocation
• Risk for injury
• Body image disturbance

TREATMENT
• Subtotal thyroidectomy

Drug therapy
• Thyroid hormone replacement: levothyroxine (Synthroid)
• Small doses of iodine (Lugol's or potassium iodide solution)

INTERVENTIONS AND RATIONALES
• Measure the patient's neck circumference *to check for progressive thyroid gland enlargement.* Also check for the development of hard nodules in the gland, *which may indicate carcinoma.*
• Provide preoperative teaching and postoperative care if subtotal thyroidectomy is indicated. *These measures allay the patient's anxiety and prevent postoperative complications.*

Teaching topics
• Understanding the importance of iodized salt, medications, and the symptoms of thyrotoxicosis (increased pulse rate, palpitations, diarrhea, sweating, tremors, agitation, and shortness of breath)

Hyperthyroidism

Hyperthyroidism is the increased synthesis of thyroid hormone. It can result from overactivity (Graves' disease) or a change in the thyroid gland (toxic nodular goiter).

CAUSES
• Autoimmune disease
• Genetic
• Infection
• Pituitary tumors
• Psychological or physiologic stress
• Thyroid adenomas

ASSESSMENT FINDINGS
• Anxiety and mood swings
• Atrial fibrillation
• Bruit or thrill over thyroid
• Diaphoresis
• Diarrhea
• Dyspnea
• Exophthalmos
• Fine hand tremors
• Flushed, smooth skin
• Heat intolerance
• Hyperhidrosis
• Increased hunger
• Increased systolic blood pressure
• Palpitations
• Tachycardia
• Tachypnea
• Weakness
• Weight loss

DIAGNOSTIC TEST RESULTS
• Blood chemistry shows increased T_3, T_4, and free thyroxine levels and decreased TSH and cholesterol levels.
• RAIU is increased.
• Thyroid scan shows nodules.

NURSING DIAGNOSES
• Decreased cardiac output
• Risk for altered body temperature
• Risk for injury

TREATMENT
• High-protein, high-carbohydrate, high-calorie diet; restricting stimulants, such as coffee and caffeine
• Radiation therapy
• Thyroidectomy

Drug therapy
• Adrenergic-blocking agents: propranolol (Inderal), reserpine (Serpasil), guanethidine (Ismelin)
• Antithyroid agents: methimazole (Tapazole), propylthiouracil
• Digitalis glycoside: digoxin (Lanoxin)
• Glucocorticoids: cortisone (Cortone), hydrocortisone (Solu-Cortef)
• Iodine preparations: potassium iodide (SSKI), radioactive iodine
• Sedative: oxazepam (Serax)

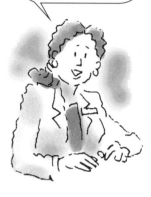

As with many endocrine disorders, therapeutic care requires helping the patient with goiter cope with a change of body image.

• Vitamins: thiamine (vitamin B_1), ascorbic acid (vitamin C)

INTERVENTIONS AND RATIONALES

• Assess cardiovascular status *to detect signs of hyperthyroidism, such as tachycardia, increased blood pressure, palpitations, and atrial arrhythmias. Presence of these signs may require a change in the treatment regimen.*
• Assess fluid balance to determine signs of fluid volume deficit.
• Monitor and record vital signs, intake and output, and laboratory studies *to detect early changes and guide treatment.*
• Maintain the patient's diet *to promote adequate nutrition.*
• Avoid stimulants, such as drugs and foods that contain caffeine, *to reduce or eliminate arrhythmias.*
• Administer I.V. fluids *to promote hydration.*
• Administer medications as prescribed *to maintain or improve patient's condition.*
• Weigh the patient daily *to provide consistent readings.*
• Provide postoperative nursing care *to promote healing and prevent complications.* (See *Caring for the thyroidectomy patient,* page 290.)
• Provide rest periods *to reduce metabolic demands.*
• Provide a quiet, cool environment *to promote comfort. Hypermetabolism causes intolerance.*
• Provide skin and eye care *to prevent complications.*
• Encourage the patient to express feelings about changes in body image *to reduce anxiety and facilitate coping mechanisms.*
• Provide postradiation nursing care *to prevent complications associated with treatment.*

Teaching topics
• Quitting tobacco products
• Recognizing the signs and symptoms of thyroid storm
• Adhering to activity limitations
• Avoiding exposure to people with infections
• Self-monitoring for infection

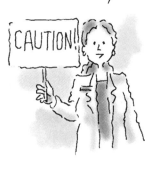

Avoid sedation. Give patients with hypothyroidism one-half to one-third the normal dose of sedatives or narcotics.

Hypothyroidism

Hypothyroidism, which affects women more often than men, occurs when the thyroid gland fails to produce sufficient thyroid hormone. This causes an overall decrease in metabolism.

CAUSES
• Hashimoto's thyroiditis
• Malfunction of pituitary gland
• Overuse of antithyroid drugs
• Thyroidectomy
• Use of radioactive iodine

ASSESSMENT FINDINGS
• Coarse hair and alopecia
• Cold intolerance
• Constipation
• Decreased diaphoresis
• Dry, flaky skin and thinning nails
• Edema
• Fatigue
• Hypersensitivity to narcotics, barbiturates, and anesthetics
• Hypothermia
• Menstrual disorders
• Mental sluggishness
• Thick tongue and swollen lips
• Weight gain and anorexia

DIAGNOSTIC TEST RESULTS
• Blood chemistry shows decreased T_3, T_4, and sodium levels and increased TSH and cholesterol levels.
• RAIU is decreased.

NURSING DIAGNOSES
• Activity intolerance
• Body image disturbance
• Decreased cardiac output

TREATMENT
• High-fiber, high-protein, low-calorie diet

Drug therapy
• Stool softener: docusate sodium (Colace)
• Thyroid hormone replacement: levothyroxine (Synthroid), liothyronine (Cytomel), thyroglobulin (Proloid)

INTERVENTIONS AND RATIONALES

• Avoid sedation: administer one-half to one-third the normal dose of sedatives or narcotics *to prevent complications. Patients taking warfarin (Coumadin) with levothyroxine may require lower doses of warfarin because levothyroxine enhances the effects of warfarin.*

• Assess fluid balance *to determine fluid volume deficit or excess.*

• Check for constipation and edema *to detect early changes.*

• Monitor and record vital signs, intake and output, and laboratory studies *to determine fluid status.*

• Maintain the patient's diet *to facilitate nutritional balance.*

• Force fluids *to maintain hydration.*

• Administer medications as prescribed *to maintain or improve patient's condition.*

• Encourage the patient to express feelings of depression *to promote coping mechanisms.*

• Encourage physical activity and mental stimulation *to enhance self-esteem.*

• Provide a warm environment *to promote comfort because the patient with hypothyroidism may be sensitive to cold.*

• Turn patient every 2 hours and provide skin care *to prevent skin breakdown.*

• Provide frequent rest periods *because patients diagnosed with hypothyroidism are often fatigued.*

Teaching topics

• Exercising regularly

• Taking thyroid medication (patient may develop myxedema coma if drug not taken)

• Recognizing the signs and symptoms of myxedema coma (progressive stupor, hypoventilation, hypoglycemia, hyponatremia, hypotension, and hypothermia)

• Self-monitoring for constipation

• Seeking additional protection and limiting exposure during cold weather

• Avoiding sedatives

• Completing skin care daily

Pancreatic cancer

Pancreatic cancer progresses rapidly and is deadly. Treatment is rarely successful because the disease has usually metastasized widely at diagnosis.

Pancreatic cancer has a swift and deadly course. Therapeutic care means helping the patient and family come to terms with the end of life.

Pancreatic tumors are almost always adenocarcinomas and most arise in the head of the pancreas. Rarer tumors are those of the body and tail of the pancreas and islet cell tumors. The two main tissue types are cylinder cell and large, fatty, granular cell.

CONTRIBUTING FACTORS

• Cigarettes

• Foods high in fat and protein

• Food additives

• Industrial chemicals, such as beta-naphthalene, benzidine, and urea.

SIGNS AND SYMPTOMS

• Dull, intermittent epigastric pain (early in disease)

• Continuous pain that radiates to the right upper quadrant or dorsolumbar area; pain may be colicky, dull or vague and unrelated to activity or posture.

• Anorexia

• Nausea

• Vomiting

• Diarrhea

• Jaundice

• Rapid, profound weight loss

• Palpable mass in the subumbilical or left hypochondrial region

DIAGNOSTIC TEST RESULTS

• Percutaneous fine-needle aspiration biopsy of the pancreas may detect tumor cells

• Laparotomy with a biopsy allows definitive diagnosis.

• Ultrasound and CT scan can identify a mass but not its histology.

• Angiography can reveal the vascular supply of a tumor.

• MRI shows tumor size and location in great detail.

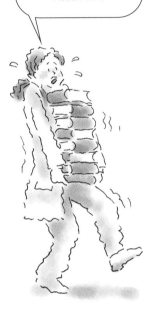

Say it 200 times:
Studying for the
NCLEX is fun.
Studying for the
NCLEX is fun.
Studying for the
NCLEX is...

• Blood studies reveal increased serum bilirubin, increased serum amylase and lipase, prolonged prothrombin time, elevated alkaline phosphatase (with biliary obstruction), aspartate aminotransferase and alanine aminotransferase are elevated (when liver cell necrosis is present).
• Fasting blood glucose may indicate hyperglycemia or hypoglycemia.
• Plasma insulin immunoassay shows measurable serum insulin in the presence of islet cell tumors.
• Stool studies may show occult blood if ulceration in the GI tract or ampulla of Vater has occurred.
• Tumor markers for pancreatic cancer, including carcinoembryonic antigen, alpha-fetoprotein, and serum immunoreactive elastase I, are elevated.

NURSING DIAGNOSES
• Pain
• Altered nutrition: Less than body requirements
• Anticipatory grieving

TREATMENT
• Blood transfusion
• I.V. fluid therapy
• Total pancreatectomy (surgical removal of the pancreas)
• Cholecystojejunostomy (surgical anastomosis of the gallbladder and the jejunum)
• Choledochoduodenostomy (surgical anastomosis of the common bile duct to the duodenum)
• Choledochojejunostomy (surgical anastomosis of the common bile duct to the jejunum)
• Whipple's operation or pancreatoduodenectomy (excision of the head of the pancreas along with the encircling loop of the duodenum)
• Gastrojejunostomy (surgical creation of an anastomosis between the stomach and the jejunum)
• Radiation therapy

Drug therapy
• Antineoplastic combinations: fluorouracil (Adrucil), streptozocin (Zanosar), ifosamide (Ifex), and doxorubicin (Adriamycin)
• Antibiotic: cefmetazole (Zefazone)–to prevent infection and relieve symptoms
• Anticholinergic: propantheline (Pro-Banthine)–to decrease GI tract spasm and motility and reduce pain and secretions
• Histamine$_2$ –receptor antagonists: cimetidine (Tagamet), ranitidine (Zantac), famotidine (Pepcid), nizatidine (Axid)
• Diuretics: furosemide (Lasix)–to mobilize extracellular fluid from ascites
• Insulin–to provide adequate exogenous insulin supply after pancreatic resection
• Narcotic analgesics: morphine, meperidine (Demerol), and codeine, which can lead to biliary tract spasm and increase common bile duct pressure (used when other methods fail)
• Pancreatic enzyme: pancrelipase (Pancrease)
• Vitamin K: phytonadione (AquaMEPHYTON)
• Stool softener: docusate (Colace)
• Laxative: bisacodyl (Dulcolax)

INTERVENTIONS AND RATIONALES
Before surgery:
• Ensure that the patient is medically stable, particularly regarding nutrition (this may take 4 to 5 days). If the patient can't tolerate oral feedings, provide total parenteral nutrition and I.V. fat emulsions *to correct deficiencies and maintain positive nitrogen balance.*
• Give blood transfusions *to combat anemia,* vitamin K *to overcome prothrombin deficiency,* antibiotics *to prevent postoperative infection,* and gastric lavage *to maintain gastric decompression,* as necessary.
• Tell the patient about expected postoperative procedures and expected side effects of radiation and chemotherapy *to allay anxiety.*
    After surgery:
• Watch for and report complications, such as fistula, pancreatitis, fluid and electrolyte imbalance, infection, hemorrhage, skin breakdown, nutritional deficiency, hepatic failure, renal insufficiency, and diabetes *to ensure early detection and treatment of complications.*

• If the patient is receiving chemotherapy, treat side effects symptomatically *to promote patient comfort and prevent complications.*

Throughout illness, provide meticulous supportive care as follows:

• Monitor fluid balance, abdominal girth, metabolic state, and weight daily *to determine fluid volume status.* Replace nutrients I.V., orally, or by NG tube *to combat weight loss.* Impose dietary restrictions such as a low-sodium or fluid retention diet as required *to combat weight gain (due to ascites).* Maintain a 2,500 calorie diet for the patient *to meet increased nutritional needs.*

• Serve small, frequent, nutritious meals by enlisting the dietitian's services *to help the patient meet increased metabolic demands.*

• Administer an oral pancreatic enzyme at mealtimes, if needed, *to aid digestion.*

• Administer laxatives, stool softeners, and cathartics as required; modify diet; and increase patient fluid intake *to prevent constipation.*

• Position the patient properly at mealtime and help him walk when he can *to increase GI motility.*

• Administer pain medication, antibiotics, and antipyretics, as necessary.

• Watch for signs of hypoglycemia or hyperglycemia; administer glucose or an antidiabetic agent as necessary *to prevent complications of hypoglycemia or hyperglycemia.* Monitor blood glucose levels *to detect early signs of hypoglycemia or hyperglycemia*

• Provide meticulous skin care *to avoid pruritus and necrosis.*

• Watch for signs of upper GI bleeding; test stools and vomitus for occult blood and keep a flow sheet of hemoglobin and hematocrit values *to prevent hemorrhage.*

• Promote gastric vasoconstriction with prescribed medication *to control active bleeding.* Replace any fluid loss *to prevent hypovolemia.*

• Ease discomfort from pyloric obstruction with an NG tube *to provide gastric decompression.*

• Apply antiembolism stockings and assist in range-of-motion exercises *to prevent thrombosis.* If thrombosis occurs, elevate the patient's legs *to promote venous return* and give an anticoagulant or aspirin as required *to decrease blood viscosity and prevent further thrombosis.*

Teaching topics
• Learning disease process and treatment options
• Contacting American Cancer Society

Thyroid cancer

Thyroid cancer is a malignant, primary tumor of the thyroid. It doesn't affect thyroid hormone secretion.

CAUSES
• Chronic overstimulation of the pituitary gland
• Chronic overstimulation of the thymus gland
• Neck radiation

ASSESSMENT FINDINGS
• Dysphagia
• Dyspnea
• Enlarged thyroid gland
• Hoarseness
• Painless, firm, irregular, and enlarged thyroid nodule or mass
• Palpable cervical lymph nodes

DIAGNOSTIC TEST RESULTS
• Blood chemistry shows increased calcitonin, serotonin, and prostaglandin levels.
• RAIU shows a "cold," or nonfunctioning, nodule.
• Thyroid biopsy shows cytology positive for cancer cells.
• Thyroid function test is normal.

NURSING DIAGNOSES
• Anxiety
• Ineffective family coping
• Pain

TREATMENT
• High-protein, high-carbohydrate, high-calorie diet with supplemental feedings
• Radiation therapy
• Thyroidectomy (total or subtotal); total thyroidectomy and radical neck excision

Drug therapy
• Antiemetics: prochlorperazine (Compazine), ondansetron (Zofran)

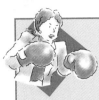

Battling illness

Caring for the thyroidectomy patient

Keep these crucial points in mind when caring for the patient who has undergone thyroidectomy.
• Keep the patient in Fowler's position to promote venous return from the head and neck and to decrease oozing into the incision.
• Watch for signs of respiratory distress (tracheal collapse, tracheal mucus accumulation, and laryngeal edema).
• Note that vocal cord paralysis can cause respiratory obstruction, with sudden stridor and restlessness.
• Keep a tracheotomy tray at the patient's bedside for 24 hours after surgery and be prepared to assist with emergency tracheotomy if necessary.

• Assess for signs of hemorrhage.
• Assess for hypocalcemia (tingling and numbness of the extremities, muscle twitching, cramps, laryngeal spasm, cramps, and positive Chvostek's and Trousseau's signs), which may occur when parathyroid glands are damaged.
• Keep calcium gluconate available for emergency I.V. administration.
• Be alert for signs of thyroid storm (tachycardia, hyperkinesis, fever, vomiting, and hypertension).

• Chemotherapy: chlorambucil (Leukeran), doxorubicin (Adriamycin), vincristine (Oncovin)
• Thyroid hormone replacements: levothyroxine (Synthroid), liothyronine (Cytomel), thyroglobulin (Proloid)

INTERVENTIONS AND RATIONALES
• Assess respiratory status for signs of airway obstruction. *A tracheotomy set should be kept at the bedside because swelling may cause airway obstruction.*
• Assess ability to swallow *to maintain a patent airway.*
• Provide postoperative thyroidectomy care *to promote healing and prevent postoperative complications.* (See *Caring for the thyroidectomy patient.*)
• Monitor and record vital signs, intake and output, and laboratory studies *to determine baseline and detect early changes that may occur with hemorrhage, airway obstruction, or hypocalcemia.*
• Administer medications as prescribed *to maintain or improve patient's condition.*
• Maintain the patient's diet *to improve nutritional status.*

• Encourage the patient to express feelings *to facilitate coping mechanisms.*
• Provide postchemotherapy and postradiation nursing care *to prevent and treat complications associated with therapy.*

Teaching topics
• Recognizing the signs and symptoms of respiratory distress, infection, myxedema coma, and difficulty swallowing
• Contacting the American Cancer Society

Thyroiditis

Thyroiditis is inflammation of the thyroid gland. It may occur in a variety of forms: autoimmune thyroiditis (long-term inflammatory disease), subacute granulomatous thyroiditis (self-limiting inflammation), Riedel's thyroiditis (rare, invasive fibrotic process), and miscellaneous thyroiditis (acute suppurative, chronic infective, and chronic noninfective).

CAUSES
• Antibodies to thyroid antigens
• Bacterial invasion
• Mumps, influenza, coxsackievirus, or adenovirus infection

ASSESSMENT FINDINGS
- Thyroid enlargement
- Fever
- Pain
- Tenderness and reddened skin over the gland

DIAGNOSTIC TEST RESULTS
Precise diagnosis depends on the type of thyroiditis:
- *autoimmune:* high titers of thyroglobulin and microsomal antibodies present in serum
- *subacute granulomatous:* elevated erythrocyte sedimentation rate, increased thyroid hormone levels, decreased thyroidal radioactive iodine uptake
- *chronic infective and noninfective:* varied findings, depending on underlying infection or other disease.

NURSING DIAGNOSES
- Risk for infection
- Pain
- Body image disturbance

TREATMENT
- Partial thyroidectomy to relieve tracheal or esophageal compression in Riedel's thyroiditis

Drug therapy
- Thyroid hormone replacement: levothyroxine (Synthroid) for accompanying hypothyroidism
- Analgesics and anti-inflammatory agents: indomethacin (Indocin) for mild subacute granulomatous thyroiditis
- Beta-adrenergic blocker: propranolol (Inderal) for transient thyrotoxicosis

INTERVENTIONS AND RATIONALES
- Before treatment, obtain a patient history *to identify underlying diseases that may cause thyroiditis, such as tuberculosis and a recent viral infection.*
- Check vital signs and examine the patient's neck for unusual swelling, enlargement, or redness *to detect disease progression and signs of airway occlusion.*

- Provide a liquid diet if the patient has difficulty swallowing, especially when due to fibrosis, *to aid swallowing and prevent aspiration.*
- If the neck is swollen, measure and record the circumference daily *to monitor progressive enlargement.*
- Check for signs of thyrotoxicosis (nervousness, tremor, weakness), which often occur in subacute thyroiditis. *Checking for early signs avoids treatment delay.*

After thyroidectomy:
- Check vital signs every 15 to 30 minutes until the patient's condition stabilizes. Stay alert for signs of tetany secondary to accidental parathyroid injury during surgery. Keep 10% calcium gluconate available for I.M. use if needed. *These measures help prevent serious postoperative complications.*
- Assess dressings frequently for excessive bleeding *to detect signs of hemorrhage.*
- Watch for signs of airway obstruction, such as difficulty talking and increased swallowing; keep tracheotomy equipment handy. *The airway may become obstructed because of postoperative edema; tracheotomy equipment should be handy to avoid treatment delay if airway becomes obstructed.*

Teaching topics
- Watching for and reporting signs of hypothyroidism (lethargy, restlessness, sensitivity to cold, forgetfulness, dry skin) — especially if he has Hashimoto's thyroiditis, which often causes hypothyroidism.
- Recognizing the need for lifelong thyroid hormone replacement therapy if permanent hypothyroidism occurs
- Recognizing the need to watch for signs of overdose, such as nervousness and palpitations

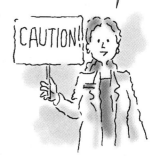

After thyroidectomy, watch for signs of airway obstruction, such as difficulty talking and increased swallowing; keep tracheotomy equipment handy.

CAUTION!

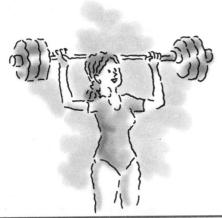

Pump up on practice questions

1. A client with a parathormone (PTH) deficiency would most likely experience abnormal serum levels of:

    A.   sodium and chloride.
    B.   potassium and glucose.
    C.   urea and uric acid.
    D.   calcium and phosphorous.

Answer: D. Because PTH regulates calcium and phosphorous metabolism, a PTH deficiency would affect calcium and phosphorous levels. PTH doesn't affect sodium, chloride, potassium, glucose, urea, and uric acid.

➡ NCLEX keys
Nursing process step: Assessment
Client needs category: Physiological integrity
Client needs subcategory: Physiological adaptation
Taxonomic level: Comprehension

2. A 28-year-old woman is scheduled for a glucose tolerance test (GTT). She asks the nurse what result indicates diabetes mellitus. The nurse should respond that the minimum parameter for indication of diabetes mellitus is a 2-hour blood glucose level greater than:

    A.   120 mg/dl.
    B.   150 mg/dl.
    C.   200 mg/dl.
    D.   250 mg/dl.

Answer: C. A GTT indicates a diagnosis of diabetes mellitus when the 2-hour blood glucose level is greater than 200 mg/dl. Confirmation occurs when at least one subsequent result is greater than 200 mg/dl.

➡ NCLEX keys
Nursing process step: Implementation
Client needs category: Health promotion and maintenance
Client needs subcategory: Prevention and early detection of disease
Taxonomic level: Comprehension

3. In interpreting a radioactive iodine uptake test, the nurse should know that:

    A.   uptake increases in hyperthyroidism and decreases in hypothyroidism.
    B.   uptake decreases in hyperthyroidism and increases in hypothyroidism.
    C.   uptake increases in both hyperthyroidism and hypothyroidism.
    D.   uptake decreases in both hyperthyroidism and hypothyroidism.

Answer: A. Iodine is necessary for the synthesis of thyroid hormones. In hyperthyroidism, more iodine is taken up by the thyroid so more thyroid hormones may be synthesized. In hypothyroidism, less iodine is taken up because fewer thyroid hormones are synthesized.

➡ NCLEX keys
Nursing process step: Assessment
Client needs category: Health promotion and maintenance
Client needs subcategory: Prevention and early detection of disease
Taxonomic level: Comprehension

4. A client is diagnosed with hyperthyroidism. The nurse should expect clinical manifestations similar to:

    A.   hypovolemic shock.
    B.   adrenergic stimulation.
    C.   benzodiazepine overdose.
    D.   Addison's disease.

Answer: B. Hyperthyroidism is a hypermetabolic state characterized by such signs as tachycardia, systolic hypertension, and anxiety—all seen in adrenergic (sympathetic) stimulation. Manifestations of hypovolemic shock, benzodiazepine overdose, and Addison's disease are more similar to a hypometabolic state.

➡ NCLEX keys
Nursing process step: Analysis
Client needs category: Physiological integrity
Client needs subcategory: Physiological adaptation
Taxonomic level: Analysis

5. A client with a history of mitral valve replacement and chronic warfarin (Coumadin) usage is diagnosed with hypothyroidism and prescribed levothyroxine. The nurse should expect the need for the warfarin:
   A. dosage to be decreased.
   B. dosage to be increased.
   C. frequency to be decreased.
   D. frequency to be increased.
Answer: A. Levothyroxine enhances the effects of warfarin; therefore, the warfarin dosage would need to be decreased.

➡ NCLEX keys
Nursing process step: Planning
Client needs category: Physiological integrity
Client needs subcategory: Pharmacological and parenteral therapies
Taxonomic level: Application

6. A client with thyroid cancer undergoes a thyroidectomy. After surgery, the client develops peripheral numbness and tingling and muscle twitching and spasms. The nurse should expect to administer:
   A. thyroid supplements.
   B. antispasmodics.
   C. barbiturates.
   D. I.V. calcium.
Answer: D. Removal of the thyroid gland can cause hyposecretion of parathormone leading to calcium deficiency. Manifestations of calcium deficiency include numbness, tingling, and muscle spasms. Treatment includes immediate administration of calcium. Thyroid supplements will be necessary following thy-

roidectomy but aren't specifically related to the identified problem. Antispasmodics don't treat the problem's cause. Barbiturates aren't indicated.

➡ NCLEX keys
Nursing process step: Implementation
Client needs category: Physiological integrity
Client needs subcategory: Pharmacological and parenteral therapies
Taxonomic level: Application

7. A client with intractable asthma develops Cushing's syndrome. Development of this complication can most likely be attributed to chronic use of:
   A. prednisone.
   B. theophylline.
   C. metaproterenol (Alupent).
   D. cromolyn (Intal).
Answer: A. Cushing's syndrome results from excessive glucocorticoids. This can occur from frequent or chronic use of corticosteroids such as prednisone. Theophylline, metaproterenol, and cromolyn don't cause Cushing's syndrome.

➡ NCLEX keys
Nursing process step: Analysis
Client needs category: Physiological integrity
Client needs subcategory: Pharmacological and parenteral therapies
Taxonomic level: Comprehension

8. During treatment of a client in adrenal crisis (addisonian crisis), it would be inappropriate for the nurse to administer I.V.:
   A. glucose.
   B. isotonic saline.
   C. vasopressors.
   D. dextrose 5% in water.
Answer: D. A client in addisonian crisis has hyponatremia. It would be inappropriate to administer a sodium-free I.V. solution such as dextrose 5% in water. Isotonic saline, glucose, and perhaps vasopressors are used in the treatment of addisonian crisis.

➡ *NCLEX keys*

Nursing process step: Implementation
Client needs category: Physiological integrity
Client needs subcategory: Pharmacological
and parenteral therapies
Taxonomic level: Application

9. A client with newly diagnosed type 1 diabetes mellitus is learning about diabetic foot care. The nurse should instruct the client to avoid:

    A.   lotions.
    B.   antiperspirants.
    C.   foot soaks.
    D.   nail files.

Answer: C. Foot soaks macerate the skin and increase the risk for breaks in the skin. Water-soluble lotions are recommended to moisturize the feet. Nail files are preferred over nail clippers or scissors. Antiperspirants may be used when foot perspiration exists.

➡ *NCLEX keys*

Nursing process step: Implementation
Client needs category: Physiological integrity
Client needs subcategory: Physiological adaptation
Taxonomic level: Knowledge

10. Which nursing diagnosis is most likely for a client with an acute episode of diabetes insipidus?

    A.   Altered nutrition
    B.   Fluid volume deficit
    C.   Impaired gas exchange
    D.   Altered tissue perfusion

Answer: B. Diabetes insipidus causes a pronounced loss of intravascular volume. The most prominent risk to the client is fluid volume deficit. Nutrition, gas exchange, and tissue perfusion are at risk because of diabetes insipidus but this risk is a result of the fluid volume deficit caused by diabetes insipidus.

➡ *NCLEX keys*

Nursing process step: Analysis
Client needs category: Physiological integrity
Client needs subcategory: Reduction of risk potential
Taxonomic level: Application

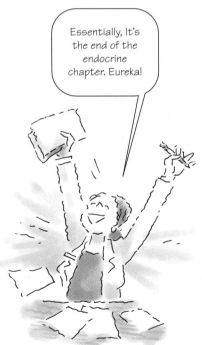

Essentially, It's the end of the endocrine chapter. Eureka!

10 Genitourinary System

Brush up on key concepts

The genitourinary system is the body's water treatment plant. This system filters waste products from the body and expels them as urine. It does this by continuously exchanging water and solutes such as hydrogen, potassium, chloride, bicarbonate, sulfate and phosphate across cell membranes.

At any time, you can review the major points of this chapter by consulting the *Cheat sheet* on pages 296 to 301.

Fluid facts

Urine is produced by a complex process centered in the kidneys. By removing water from the body in the form of urine, the kidneys also help regulate blood pressure.

Here's how urine is formed:
• Blood from the renal artery is filtered across the glomerular capillary membrane in the Bowman's capsule.
• Filtration requires adequate intravascular volume and adequate cardiac output.
• Antidiuretic hormone (ADH) and aldosterone control the reabsorption of water and electrolytes.
• Composition of formed filtrate is similar to blood plasma without proteins.
• Formed filtrate moves through the tubules of the nephron, which reabsorb and secrete electrolytes, water, glucose, amino acids, ammonia, and bicarbonate.
• What's left is excreted as urine.

Blood pressure control

Regulation of fluid volume by the **kidney** affects blood pressure. The renin-angiotensin system is activated by decreased blood pressure and can be altered by renal disease.

Urine producers

The kidneys are two bean-shaped organs that produce urine and maintain fluid and acid-base balance. To help maintain acid-base balance, the kidneys secrete hydrogen ions, reabsorb sodium and bicarbonates, acidify phosphate salts, and produce ammonia.

The kidneys have four main components:
• the cortex, which makes up the outer layer of the kidney and contains the glomeruli, the proximal tubules of the nephron, and the distal tubules of the nephron
• the medulla, which makes up the inner layer of the kidney and contains the loops of Henle and the collecting tubules
• the renal pelvis, which collects urine from the calices
• the nephron, which makes up the functional unit of the kidney. It contains Bowman's capsule and the glomerulus, as well as the renal tubule, which consists of the proximal convoluted tubule and collecting segments.

Transport tubule

The **ureter,** which transports urine from the kidney to the bladder, is a tubule that extends from the renal pelvis to the bladder floor.

Storage sac

The **bladder,** a muscular, distendable sac, can contain up to 1 liter of urine at a single time.

Tube to the outside

The **urethra,** extending from the bladder to the urinary meatus, transports urine from the bladder to the exterior of the body.

Semen secretor

The **prostate gland** surrounds the male urethra. It contains ducts that secrete the alkaline portion of seminal fluid.

(Text continues on page 301.)

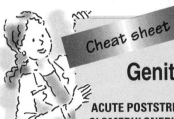

Cheat sheet

Genitourinary refresher

ACUTE POSTSTREPTOCOCCAL GLOMERULONEPHRITIS

Key signs and symptoms
- Azotemia
- Fatigue
- Oliguria

Key test results
- Blood tests show elevated serum creatinine levels.
- 24-hour urine sample shows low creatinine clearance and impaired glomerular filtration.
- Urinalysis typically reveals proteinuria and hematuria. Red blood cells, white blood cells, and mixed cell casts are common findings in urinary sediment.
- Kidney-ureter-bladder X-rays show bilateral kidney enlargement.

Key treatments
- Bed rest
- Diuretics, such as metolazone (Zaroxolyn) and furosemide (Lasix), to reduce extracellular fluid overload and an antihypertensive such as hydralazine
- Fluid restriction
- High-calorie, low-sodium, low-potassium, low-protein diet

Key interventions
- Check vital signs and electrolyte values. Monitor intake and output and daily weight. Assess renal function daily through serum creatinine and blood urea nitrogen (BUN) levels and urine creatinine clearance. Watch for signs of acute renal failure (oliguria, azotemia, and acidosis).
- Provide good nutrition, use good hygienic technique, and prevent contact with infected people.
- Bed rest is necessary during the acute phase. Encourage the patient to gradually resume normal activities as symptoms subside.

ACUTE RENAL FAILURE

Key signs and symptoms
- Urine output less than 400 ml/day for 1 to 2 weeks followed by diuresis (3 to 5 L/day) for 2 to 3 weeks
- Weight gain

Key test results
- Creatinine clearance estimates the number of functioning nephrons.
- Glomerular filtration rate (GFR) is 20 to 40 ml/minute (renal insufficiency); 10 to 20 ml/minute (renal failure); less than 10 ml/minute (end-stage renal disease).

Key treatments
- Continuous arteriovenous hemofiltration
- Low-protein, increased-carbohydrate, moderate-fat, and moderate-calorie diet with potassium, sodium, and phosphorus intake regulated according to serum levels
- Peritoneal dialysis or hemodialysis
- Beta-adrenergic blocker: dopamine (Intropin) initially to improve renal perfusion
- Diuretics: furosemide (Lasix), metolazone (Zaroxolyn)

Key interventions
- Assess fluid balance, respiratory, cardiovascular, and neurologic status.
- Monitor and record vital signs and intake and output, central venous pressure, daily weight, urine specific gravity, and laboratory studies.
- Monitor for arrhythmias.
- Maintain the patient's diet.

BENIGN PROSTATIC HYPERPLASIA

Key signs and symptoms
- Decreased force and amount of urination
- Urgency, frequency, and burning on urination

Key test results
- Cystoscopy shows enlarged prostate gland, obstructed urine flow, and urinary stasis.
- Rectal examination shows enlarged prostate gland.

> I cannot tell a lie. Sometimes I skip the chapter and just read the Cheat sheet.

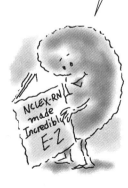

Genitourinary refresher (continued)

BENIGN PROSTATIC HYPERPLASIA (continued)

Key treatments

- Forcing fluids
- Transurethral resection of the prostate or prostatectomy

Key interventions

- Force fluids.

BLADDER CANCER

Key signs and symptoms

- Frequency of urination
- Painless hematuria
- Urgency of urination

Key test results

- Cystoscopy reveals a mass.

Key treatments

- Surgery dependent on location and progress of tumor

Key interventions

- Provide postoperative care. (Closely monitor urine output; observe for hematuria [reddish tint to gross bloodiness] or infection [cloudy, foul smelling, with sediment]; maintain continuous bladder irrigation, if indicated; assist with turning, coughing, and deep breathing.)
- Force fluids.

BREAST CANCER

Key signs and symptoms

- Cervical, supraclavicular, or axillary lymph node lump or enlargement on palpation
- Painless lump or mass in the breast or thickening of breast tissue
- Skin changes

Key test results

- Breast self-examination reveals a lump or mass in the breast or thickening of breast tissue.
- Fine-needle aspiration and excisional biopsy provide histologic cells that confirm diagnosis.
- Mammography detects a tumor.

Key treatments

- Peripheral stem cell therapy for advanced breast cancer
- Surgery; options include lumpectomy, skin-sparing mastectomy, partial mastectomy, total mastectomy, and modified radical mastectomy
- Chemotherapy: cyclophosphamide (Cytoxan), methotrexate (Folex), fluorouracil (Adrucil)
- Hormonal therapy: tamoxifen (Nolvadex), aminoglutethimide (Cytadren), diethylstilbestrol, megestrol (Megace)

Key interventions

- Assess the patient's feelings about her illness, and determine what she knows about breast cancer and her expectations.
- Provide routine postoperative care.
- Perform comfort measures.
- Administer analgesics as ordered, and monitor their effectiveness.
- Watch for treatment-related complications, such as nausea, vomiting, anorexia, leukopenia, thrombocytopenia, GI ulceration, and bleeding.

CERVICAL CANCER

Key signs and symptoms

- Preinvasive: Symptoms are absent
- Invasive: Abnormal vaginal discharge (yellowish, blood-tinged, and foul-smelling); postcoital pain and bleeding

Key test results

- Colposcopy determines the source of the abnormal cells seen on the Pap test.

Key treatments

- Preinvasive: Conization, cryosurgery
- Invasive: Radiation therapy (internal, external, or both); radical hysterectomy

Key interventions

- Encourage the patient to use relaxation techniques.
- When assisting with a biopsy, drape and prepare the patient as for a routine pelvic examination. Have a container of formaldehyde ready. Assist the doctor as needed, and provide support for the patient throughout the procedure.
- If assisting with laser therapy, drape and prepare the patient as for a routine pelvic examination. Assist the doctor as needed and provide support to the patient.
- Watch for complications related to therapy.

CHLAMYDIA

Key signs and symptoms

In women, assessment findings include:
- dyspareunia
- mucopurulent discharge
- pelvic pain.

In men, assessment findings include:
- dysuria
- erythema
- tenderness of the meatus
- urethral discharge
- urinary frequency.

(continued)

Genitourinary refresher *(continued)*

CHLAMYDIA *(continued)*

Key test results
• Antigen detection methods, including the enzyme-linked immunosorbent assay and the direct fluorescent antibody test, are the diagnostic tests of choice for identifying chlamydial infection, although tissue cell cultures are more sensitive and specific.

Key treatments
• Antibiotics: doxycycline (Vibramycin), azithromycin (Zithromax)
• For pregnant women with chlamydial infections, azithromycin (Zithromax), in a single 1-gram dose

Key interventions
• Practice standard precautions when caring for a patient with a chlamydial infection.
• Make sure that the patient fully understands the dosage requirements of any prescribed medications for this infection.
• Check newborns of infected mothers for signs of chlamydial infection.
• Obtain appropriate specimens for diagnostic testing.

CHRONIC GLOMERULONEPHRITIS

Key signs and symptoms
• Edema
• Hematuria
• Hypertension

Key test results
• Kidney biopsy identifies underlying disease and provides data needed to guide therapy.
• Blood studies reveal rising blood urea nitrogen and serum creatinine levels, which indicate advanced renal insufficiency.
• Urinalysis reveals proteinuria, hematuria, cylindruria, and red blood cell casts.

Key treatments
• Dialysis
• Kidney transplant

Key interventions
• Understand that patient care is primarily supportive, focusing on continual observation and sound patient teaching.
• Accurately monitor vital signs, intake and output, and daily weight.
• Observe for signs of fluid, electrolyte, and acid-base imbalances.
• Administer medications and provide good skin care.

CHRONIC RENAL FAILURE

Key signs and symptoms
• Azotemia
• Decreased urine output
• Heart failure
• Lethargy
• Pruritus
• Weight gain

Key test results
• Blood chemistry shows increased BUN, creatinine, phosphorus and lipid levels and decreased calcium, CO_2, and albumin levels.

Key treatments
• Limited fluids
• Low-protein, low-sodium, low-potassium, low-phosphorus, high-calorie, and high-carbohydrate diet
• Peritoneal dialysis and hemodialysis
• Antacids: aluminum hydroxide gel (AlternaGEL)
• Antiemetic: prochlorperazine (Compazine)
• Calcium supplement: calcium carbonate (Os-Cal)
• Cation exchange resin: sodium polystyrene sulfonate (Kayexalate)
• Diuretic: furosemide (Lasix)

Key interventions
• Assess renal, respiratory, and cardiovascular status and fluid balance.
• Assess dialysis access for bruit and thrill.
• Maintain standard precautions.
• Restrict fluids.

CYSTITIS

Key signs and symptoms
• Dark, odoriferous urine
• Frequency of urination
• Urgency of urination

Key test results
• Urine culture and sensitivity positively identifies organisms *(Escherichia coli, Proteus vulgaris,* and *Streptococcus faecalis).*

Key treatments
• Diet: increased intake of fluids and vitamin C

Key interventions
• Assess renal status.
• Force fluids (cranberry or orange juice) to 3 qt (3 L)/day.

Genitourinary refresher (continued)

GONORRHEA

Key signs and symptoms
- Dysuria (painful urination)
- Purulent urethral or cervical discharge
- Itching, burning, and pain

Key test results
- A culture from the site of infection (urethra, cervix, rectum, or pharynx), grown on a Thayer-Martin or Transgrow medium, usually establishes the diagnosis by isolating the organism.

Key treatments
- Antibiotics: ceftriaxone (Rocephin), doxycycline (Vibramycin), erythromycin (E-mycin)
- Prophylactic antibiotics: 1% silver nitrate or erythromycin (EryPed) eye drops to prevent infection in newborns

Key interventions
- Before treatment, establish whether the patient has any drug sensitivities, and watch closely for adverse effects during therapy.
- Practice standard precautions.
- Routinely instill two drops of 1% silver nitrate or erythromycin in the eyes of all neonates immediately after birth. Check newborn infants of infected mothers for signs of infection. Take specimens for culture from the infant's eyes, pharynx, and rectum.

HERPES SIMPLEX

Key signs and symptoms
- Blisters, which may form on any part of the mouth
- Dysuria (painful urination; occurs in genital herpes)
- Erythema
- Skin lesions

Key test results
- Confirmation requires isolation of the virus from local lesions and a histologic biopsy.

Key treatments
- Antiviral agents: idoxuridine (Herplex Liqufilm), trifluridine (Viroptic), and vidarabine (Vira-A)
- 5% acyclovir (Zovirax) ointment (possible relief to patients with genital herpes or to immunosuppressed patients with *Herpesvirus hominis* skin infections; I.V. acyclovir helps treat more severe infections)

Key interventions
- Observe standard precautions. For patients with extensive cutaneous, oral, or genital lesions, institute contact precautions.
- Administer pain medications and prescribed antiviral agents as ordered.

- Provide supportive care, as indicated, such as oral hygiene, nutritional supplementation, and antipyretics for fever.

NEUROGENIC BLADDER

Key symptom
- Altered micturition

Key test results
- Voiding cystourethrography evaluates bladder neck function, vesicoureteral reflux, and continence.

Key treatment
- Indwelling urinary catheter insertion (including teaching the patient self-catheterization techniques)

Key interventions
- Use strict aseptic technique during insertion of an indwelling urinary catheter (a temporary measure to drain the incontinent patient's bladder). Don't interrupt the closed drainage system for any reason.
- Clean the catheter insertion site with soap and water at least twice a day.
- Clamp the tubing, or empty the catheter bag before transferring the patient to a wheelchair or stretcher.
- Watch for signs of infection (fever, cloudy or foul-smelling urine).

OVARIAN CANCER

Key signs and symptoms
- Abdominal distention
- Pelvic discomfort
- Urinary frequency
- Weight loss

Key test results
- Abdominal ultrasonography, computed tomography scan, or X-ray may delineate tumor size

Key treatments
- Resection of the involved ovary
- Total abdominal hysterectomy and bilateral salpingo-oophorectomy with tumor resection, omentectomy, and appendectomy
- Antineoplastics: cisplatin (Platinol), paclitaxel (Taxol), topotecan (Hycamtin)
- Analgesics: morphine, fentanyl (Duragesic-25)

Key interventions
Before surgery
- Thoroughly explain all preoperative tests, the expected course of treatment, and surgical and postoperative procedures.

(continued)

Genitourinary refresher (continued)

OVARIAN CANCER (continued)

After surgery

• Monitor vital signs frequently.
• Monitor intake and output while maintaining good catheter care.
• Check the dressing regularly for excessive drainage or bleeding, and watch for signs of infection.
• Encourage coughing and deep breathing.
• Reposition the patient often and encourage her to walk shortly after surgery.

PROSTATE CANCER

Key signs and symptoms

• Decreased size and force of urinary stream
• Difficulty and frequency of urination
• Urine retention

Key test results

• Digital rectal examination reveals palpable firm nodule in gland or diffuse induration in posterior lobe.
• Prostatic-specific antigen is increased.

Key treatments

• Radiation implant
• Radical prostatectomy (for localized tumors without metastasis) or transurethral resection of the prostate (to relieve obstruction in metastatic disease)
• Luteinizing hormone-releasing hormone agonists: goserelin acetate and leuprolide acetate

Key interventions

• Assess renal and fluid status.
• Monitor for signs of infection.
• Assess pain and note effectiveness of analgesia.
• Maintain the patient's diet.
• Maintain patency of the urinary catheter and note drainage.

RENAL CALCULI

Key signs and symptoms

• Flank pain

Key test results

• Excretory urography reveals stones.
• KUB reveals stones.

Key treatments

• Diet: for calcium stones, acid-ash with limited intake of calcium and milk products; for oxalate stones, alkaline-ash with limited intake of foods high in oxalate (cola, tea); for uric acid stones, alkaline-ash with limited intake of foods high in purine
• Extracorporeal shock wave lithotripsy

• Surgery if other measures to remove the stone aren't effective (type of surgery dependent on location of the stone)

Key interventions

• Monitor the patient's urine for evidence of renal calculi. Strain all urine and save all solid material for analysis.
• Force fluids to 3,000 ml/day.
• If surgery was performed, check dressings regularly for bloody drainage and report excessive amounts of bloody drainage to the doctor; use sterile technique to change the dressing; maintain nephrostomy tube or indwelling urinary catheter if indicated; and monitor incision for signs of infection.

SYPHILIS

Key signs and symptoms

Primary syphilis

• Chancres on the genitalia, anus, fingers, lips, tongue, nipples, tonsils, or eyelids

Secondary syphilis

• Symmetrical mucocutaneous lesions
• Malaise
• Anorexia
• Weight loss
• Slight fever

Key test results

• Fluorescent treponemal antibody-absorption test identifies antigens of *T. pallidum* in tissue, ocular fluid, cerebrospinal fluid (CSF), tracheobronchial secretions, and exudates from lesions. This is the most sensitive test available for detecting syphilis in all stages. Once reactive, it remains so permanently.
• Venereal Disease Research Laboratory (VDRL) slide test and rapid plasma reagin test detect nonspecific antibodies. Both tests, if positive, become reactive within 1 to 2 weeks after the primary lesion appears or 4 to 5 weeks after the infection begins.

Key treatments

• Antibiotic: penicillin G benzathine (Permapen); if allergic to penicillin, then erythromycin (Erythrocin) or tetracycline (Panmycin)

Key interventions

• Check for a history of drug sensitivity before administering the first dose of penicillin.
• Urge patients to seek VDRL testing after 3, 6, 12, and 24 months. Patients treated for latent or late syphilis should receive blood tests at 6-month intervals for 2 years.

Genitourinary refresher *(continued)*

TESTICULAR CANCER

Key signs and symptoms
- Firm, painless, smooth testicular mass, varying in size and sometimes producing a sense of testicular heaviness

In advanced stages
- Ureteral obstruction
- Abdominal mass
- Weight loss
- Fatigue
- Pallor

Key test results
- Regular self-examinations and testicular palpation during a routine physical examination may detect testicular tumors.

Key treatments
- Surgery: orchiectomy (testicle removal; most surgeons remove the testicle but not the scrotum to allow for a prosthetic implant)
- High-calorie diet provided in small frequent feedings
- I.V. fluid therapy

- Antineoplastics: bleomycin (Blenoxane), carboplatin (Paraplatin), cisplatin (Platinol), dactinomycin (Cosmegen), etoposide (VePesid), ifosfamide (Ifex), plicamycin (Mithracin), vinblastine (Velban)
- Analgesics: morphine, fentanyl (Duragesic-25)
- Antiemetics: trimethobenzamide (Tigan), metoclopramide (Reglan), ondansetron (Zofran)

Key interventions
- Develop a treatment plan that addresses the patient's psychological and physical needs.

After orchiectomy
- For the first day after surgery, apply an ice pack to the scrotum and provide analgesics.
- Check for excessive bleeding, swelling, and signs of infection.
- Give antiemetics, as needed.
- Encourage small, frequent meals.
- Watch for signs of myelosuppression.

Female and male reproductive systems

The genitourinary system also encompasses the female and male reproductive systems. Here is a brief review of the female and male reproductive systems, including external and internal genitalia.

FEMALE EXTERNAL GENITALIA

The following is a brief review of the external female genitalia.

Protecting the pelvic bone

The **mons pubis** provides an adipose cushion over the anterior symphysis pubis, protects the pelvic bones, and contributes to rounded contour of the female body.

Protecting the vulval cleft

The **labia majora** are two folds that converge at the mons pubis and extend to the posterior commissure. They consist of connective tissue, elastic fibers, veins, and sebaceous glands, and they protect components of the vulval cleft.

Lubricating the vulva

The **labia minora** are within the labia majora and consist of connective tissue, sebaceous and sweat glands, nonstriated muscle fibers, nerve endings, and blood vessels. They unite to form the fourchette, the vaginal vestibule, and serve to lubricate the vulva, which adds to sexual enjoyment and fights bacteria.

Nerve center

The **clitoris** — located in the anterior portion of the vulva above the urethral opening — is made up of erectile tissue, nerves, and blood vessels and, homologous to the penis, provides sexual pleasure. The clitoris consists of:
- the glans
- the body
- two crura.

The vestibule

The **vaginal vestibule** extends from the clitoris to the posterior fourchette and consists of:
- the vaginal orifice
- the hymen — a thin, vascularized mucous membrane at the vaginal orifice

• the fossa navicularis — a depressed area between the hymen and fourchette
• Bartholin's glands — two bean-shaped glands on either side of the vagina that secrete mucus during sexual stimulation.

Episiotomy site
The **perineal body** (the area between the vagina and the anus) is the site of episiotomy during childbirth.

Urine passage
The **urethral meatus** is located ⅜ to 1″ (1 to 2.5 cm) below the clitoris.

Mucus producers
The **paraurethral glands** (Skene's glands) are located immediately inside the urethral meatus.

FEMALE INTERNAL GENITALIA
Here is a brief review of the internal female genitalia.

Copulatory and birth passage
The **vagina** is a vascularized musculomembranous tube extending from the external genitals to the uterus.

An environment for growth
Hollow and pear-shaped, the **uterus** is a muscular organ divided by a slight constriction (isthmus) into an upper portion (body or corpus) and a lower portion (cervix); the body or corpus has three layers (perimetrium, myometrium, and endometrium). The uterus receives support from broad, round, uterosacral ligaments and provides an environment for fetal growth and development.

Fertilization site
The **fallopian tubes** are about 4½″ (12 cm) long and consist of four layers (peritoneal, subserous, muscular, mucous) divided into four portions (interstitial, isthmus, ampulla, fimbria). The fallopian tubes:
• transport ovum from the ovary to the uterus
• provide a nourishing environment for zygotes
• serve as the site of fertilization.

Ovulation site
The **ovaries** are two almond-shaped glandular structures resting below and behind the fallopian tubes on either side of the uterus. They produce sex hormones (estrogen, progesterone, androgen) and serve as the site of ovulation.

Food for thought
The **breasts** consist of glandular, fibrous, and adipose tissue. Stimulated by secretions from the hypothalamus, anterior pituitary, and ovaries, they provide nourishment to the infant and transfer maternal antibodies during breast-feeding and enhance sexual pleasure.

MALE EXTERNAL GENITALIA
The following is a list of external male genitalia.

Erectile tissue
The **penis,** consisting of the body (shaft) and glans, has three layers of erectile tissue — two corpora cavernosa and one corpus spongiosum. The penis deposits spermatozoa in the female reproductive tract and provides sexual pleasure.

Protective pouch
The scrotum is a pouch-like structure composed of skin, fascial connective tissue, and smooth muscle fibers housing the testes and serving to protect spermatozoa from high body temperature.

MALE INTERNAL GENITALIA
Internal male genitalia serves to produce and transport semen and seminal fluid.

Sperm producers
The **testes** or testicles, two oval-shaped glandular organs inside the scrotum, function to produce spermatozoa and testosterone.

Sperm storage
The **epididymides** serve as the initial section of the testes' excretory duct system and store spermatozoa as they mature and become motile.

Sperm conduit

The **vas deferens** connects the epididymal lumen and the prostatic urethra, serving as a conduit for spermatozoa.

Seminal passage

The **ejaculatory ducts**—located between the seminal vesicles and the urethra—serve as passageways for semen and seminal fluid.

Excretory duct

The **urethra** extends from the bladder through the penis to the external urethral opening and serves as the excretory duct for urine and semen.

Motility aids

The **seminal vesicles** are two pouch-like structures between the bladder and the rectum that secrete a viscous fluid which aids in spermatozoa motility and metabolism.

Lubricating gland

The **prostate gland,** located just below the bladder, is considered homologous to Skene's glands in females. It produces an alkaline fluid that enhances spermatozoa motility and lubricates the urethra during sexual activity.

Peas in a pod

The **bulbourethral glands** (or Cowper's glands) are two pea-sized glands opening into the posterior portion of the urethra. They secrete a thick alkaline fluid that neutralizes acidic secretions in the female reproductive tract, thus prolonging spermatozoa survival.

Keep abreast of diagnostic tests

Below are the major diagnostic tests for assessing genitourinary disorders, as well as common nursing actions associated with each test.

Urine sample study #1

Urinalysis involves an examination of urine for color, appearance, pH, urine specific gravity, protein, glucose, ketones, red blood cells (RBCs), white blood cells (WBCs), and casts.

Nursing actions
- Wash perineal area.
- Obtain first morning urine specimen.

Urine sample study #2

A **urine culture and sensitivity test** examines a urine specimen for the presence of bacteria.

Nursing actions
- Clean perineal area and urinary meatus with bacteriostatic solution.
- Collect midstream sample in sterile container.

A day's worth of kidney function

A **24-hour urine collection** analyzes urine specimens collected over 24 hours to assess kidney function.

Nursing actions
- Instruct the patient to void and note time collection starts with the next voiding.
- Place urine container on ice.
- Measure each voided urine and place in the collection container.
- Instruct the patient to void at the end of the 24-hour period.

1st blood sample study

Blood chemistry tests are used to analyze blood samples for potassium, sodium, calcium, phosphorus, glucose, bicarbonate, BUN, creatinine, protein, albumin, osmolality, magnesium, uric acid, and carbon dioxide levels.

Nursing actions
- Withhold food and fluids before the procedure, as directed.
- Monitor venipuncture site for bleeding.

2nd blood sample study

A **hematologic study** analyzes a blood sample for WBCs, RBCs, erythrocyte sedimenta-

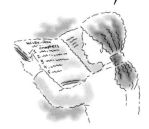

Maintain a sense of accomplishment while studying. Make a list of chapters to review this week, then cross them off one by one. That's satisfying!

tion rate, platelets, prothrombin time (PT), international normalized ratio, partial thromboplastin time (PTT), hemoglobin (Hb), and hematocrit (HCT).

Nursing actions
• Explain the purpose of the procedure.
• Check the venipuncture site for bleeding.

Picture this
A **kidney-ureter-bladder (KUB) X-ray** provides a radiographic picture of the kidneys, ureters, and bladder.

Nursing actions
• Schedule the X-ray before other examinations requiring contrast medium.
• Ensure that the patient removes metallic belts.

Scope the whole system
Excretory urography produces a fluoroscopic examination of the kidneys, ureters, and bladder.

Nursing actions
Before the procedure, you should:
• note any allergies to iodine, seafood, and radiopaque dyes
• withhold food and fluids after midnight
• administer laxatives, as prescribed
• make sure that written, informed consent has been obtained
• inform the patient that he may experience a transient burning sensation and metallic taste when the contrast is injected.
  After the procedure, you should:
• instruct the patient to drink at least 1 quart (1 liter) of fluids.

Bladder inspection
Cystoscopy uses a cytoscope to directly visualize the bladder. During the procedure the bladder is usually distended with fluid to enhance visualization.

Nursing actions
Before the procedure, you should:
• withhold food and fluids
• make sure that a written, informed consent has been obtained

• administer enemas and medications, as prescribed.
  After the procedure, you should:
• monitor vital signs and intake and output
• administer analgesics and sitz baths, as prescribed
• check the patient's urine for blood clots
• force fluids.

Examining arteries
Renal angiography provides a radiographic examination of the renal arterial supply.

Nursing actions
Before the procedure, you should:
• make sure that a written, informed consent has been obtained
• withhold food and fluids after midnight
• instruct the patient to void immediately before procedure
• administer enemas, as prescribed
• note any allergies to iodine, seafood, and radiopaque dyes.
  After the procedure, you should:
• assess vital signs and pulses below the catheter insertion site
• inspect the catheter insertion site for bleeding or hematoma formation
• force fluids.

Blood flow photo
A **renal scan** provides visual imaging of blood flow distribution to the kidneys.

Nursing actions
Before the procedure, you should:
• note any allergies
• make sure that a written, informed consent has been obtained.
  After the procedure, you should:
• assess the patient for signs of delayed allergic reaction, such as itching and hives
• wear gloves when caring for incontinent patients, and double-bag linens.

Taking kidney tissue
A **renal biopsy** is the percutaneous removal of a small amount of renal tissue for histologic evaluation.

> Remember that, after many genitourinary tests, like excretory urography, cytoscopy, and renal angiography, you need to force fluids.

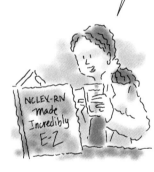

Nursing actions

Before the procedure, you should:
• assess baseline clotting studies and vital signs
• withhold food and fluids after midnight
• make sure that a written, informed consent has been obtained.

After the procedure, you should:
• monitor and record vital signs, Hb and HCT
• check biopsy site for bleeding.

Dye and shoot

A **cystourethrogram** uses a radiopaque dye and an X-ray to provide visualization of the bladder and ureters.

Nursing actions

• Note any allergies to iodine, seafood, and radiopaque dyes before the procedure.
• Make sure that a written, informed consent has been obtained.
• Advise the patient about voiding requirements during the procedure.
• Monitor voiding after the procedure.

Bladder pressure measure

Cystometrogram (CMG) graphs the pressure exerted while the bladder fills.

Nursing actions

• Advise the patient about voiding requirements during the procedure.
• Monitor voiding after the procedure.

Polish up on patient care

Major genitourinary disorders include acute poststreptococcal glomerulonephritis, acute renal failure, benign prostatic hyperplasia, bladder cancer, breast cancer, cervical cancer, chlamydia, chronic glomerulonephritis, chronic renal failure, cystitis, gonorrhea, herpes simplex, neurogenic bladder, ovarian cancer, prostate cancer, renal calculi, syphilis, and testicular cancer.

Acute poststreptococcal glomerulonephritis

Also called acute glomerulonephritis, acute poststreptococcal glomerulonephritis (APSGN) is a relatively common bilateral inflammation of the glomeruli, the kidney's blood vessels. It follows a streptococcal infection of the respiratory tract or, less often, a skin infection, such as impetigo.

CAUSES

• Trapped antigen-antibody complexes (produced as an immunologic mechanism in response to streptococci) in the glomerular capillary membranes, inducing inflammatory damage and impeding glomerular function
• Untreated pharyngitis (inflammation of the pharynx)

ASSESSMENT FINDINGS

• Azotemia
• Edema
• Fatigue
• Hematuria
• Oliguria
• Proteinuria

DIAGNOSTIC TEST RESULTS

• Blood tests show elevated serum creatinine levels.
• 24-hour urine sample shows low creatinine clearance and impaired glomerular filtration.
• Elevated antistreptolysin-O titers (in 80% of patients), elevated streptozyme and anti-Dnase B titers, and low serum complement levels verify recent streptococcal infection.
• Renal biopsy may confirm the diagnosis in a patient with APSGN or may be used to assess renal tissue status.
• Renal ultrasonography may show a normal or slightly enlarged kidney.
• Throat culture may also show group A beta-hemolytic streptococci.
• Urinalysis typically reveals proteinuria and hematuria. RBCs, WBCs, and mixed cell casts are common findings in urinary sediment.

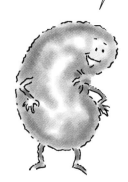

Because disorders that affect me affect fluid balance, patient care often involves monitoring and adjusting the patient's fluid status.

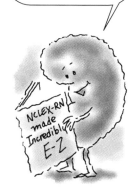

I get it. Acute poststreptococcal glomerulonephritis is a relatively common inflammation of my blood vessels.

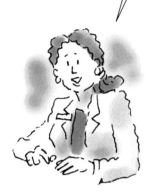

Encourage pregnant women with a history of acute poststreptococcal glomerulonephritis to have frequent medical evaluations — they're at increased risk for chronic renal failure.

• Kidney-ureter-bladder X-rays show bilateral kidney enlargement.

NURSING DIAGNOSES
• Altered urinary elimination
• Fluid volume excess
• Risk for injury

TREATMENT
• Bed rest
• Fluid restriction
• High-calorie, low-sodium, low-potassium, low-protein diet
• Dialysis (occasionally necessary)

Drug therapy
• Diuretics, such as metolazone (Zaroxolyn) and furosemide (Lasix), to reduce extracellular fluid overload and an antihypertensive such as hydralazine

INTERVENTIONS AND RATIONALES
• Check vital signs and electrolyte values. Monitor fluid intake and output and daily weight. Assess renal function daily through serum creatinine and BUN levels and urine creatinine clearance. Watch for signs of acute renal failure (oliguria, azotemia, acidosis). *These measures detect early signs of complications and guide the treatment plan.*
• Consult the dietitian *to provide a diet high in calories and low in protein, sodium, potassium, and fluids.*
• Provide good nutrition, use good hygienic technique, and prevent contact with infected people *to protect the debilitated patient against secondary infection.*
• Bed rest is necessary during the acute phase. Encourage the patient to gradually resume normal activities as symptoms subside *to prevent fatigue.*
• Provide emotional support for the patient and family. If the patient is on dialysis, explain the procedure fully. *These measures may help to ease the patient's anxiety.*

Teaching topics
• The importance of immediately reporting signs of infection such as fever and sore throat (for the patient with a history of chronic upper respiratory tract infections)
• The importance of follow-up examinations to detect chronic renal failure
• The need for regular blood pressure, urinary protein, and renal function assessments during the convalescent months to detect recurrence
• What to expect (After APSGN, gross hematuria may recur during nonspecific viral infections; abnormal urinary findings may persist for years.)
• The possibility of orthostatic hypotension when taking diuretics and the need to change position slowly
• The need for frequent medical evaluations in pregnant patients with a history of poststreptococcal glomerulonephritis (Pregnancy further stresses the kidneys, increasing the risk of chronic renal failure.)

Acute renal failure

Acute renal failure is a sudden interruption of renal function resulting from obstruction, poor circulation, or kidney disease. With treatment, this condition is usually reversible, but if untreated, it may progress to end-stage renal disease or death.

Acute renal failure is classified as prerenal (results from conditions that diminish blood flow to the kidneys), intrarenal (results from damage to the kidneys, usually from acute tubular necrosis), or postrenal (results from bilateral obstruction of urine flow).

CAUSES
• Acute glomerulonephritis
• Acute tubular necrosis
• Anaphylaxis
• Benign prostatic hyperplasia
• Blood transfusion reaction
• Burns
• Cardiopulmonary bypass
• Collagen diseases
• Congenital deformity
• Dehydration
• Diabetes mellitus

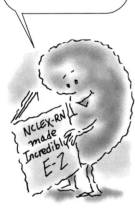

Treatment is terrific. With treatment, acute renal failure is usually reversible. Untreated, it may progress to end-stage renal disease or death.

- Heart failure, cardiogenic shock, endocarditis, malignant hypertension
- Hemorrhage
- Hypotension
- Nephrotoxins: antibiotics, X-ray dyes, pesticides, anesthetics
- Renal calculi
- Septicemia
- Trauma
- Tumor

ASSESSMENT FINDINGS
- Anorexia, nausea, and vomiting
- Circumoral numbness, tingling extremities
- Costovertebral pain
- Diarrhea or constipation
- Epistaxis
- Headache
- Irritability, restlessness
- Lethargy, drowsiness, stupor, coma
- Pallor, ecchymosis
- Stomatitis
- Thick, tenacious sputum
- Urine output less than 400 ml/day for 1 to 2 weeks followed by diuresis (3 to 5 L/day) for 2 to 3 weeks
- Weight gain

DIAGNOSTIC TEST RESULTS
- Arterial blood gas analysis (ABG) shows metabolic acidosis.
- Blood chemistry shows increased potassium, phosphorus, magnesium, BUN, creatinine, and uric acid levels and decreased calcium, carbon dioxide (CO_2), and sodium levels.
- Creatinine clearance is low.
- Excretory urography shows decreased renal perfusion and function.
- Glomerular filtration rate (GFR) is 20 to 40 ml/minute (renal insufficiency); 10 to 20 ml/minute (renal failure); less than 10 ml/minute (end-stage renal disease).
- Hematology shows decreased Hb, HCT and erythrocytes; and increased PT and PTT.
- Urine chemistry shows albuminuria, proteinuria, and increased sodium level; casts, RBCs, and WBCs; and urine specific gravity greater than 1.025, then fixed at less than 1.010.

NURSING DIAGNOSES
- Decreased cardiac output
- Fluid volume excess
- Altered renal tissue perfusion

TREATMENT
- Continuous arteriovenous hemofiltration
- Low-protein, increased-carbohydrate, moderate-fat, and moderate-calorie diet with potassium, sodium, and phosphorus intake regulated according to serum levels
- Peritoneal dialysis or hemodialysis
- Fluid intake restricted to amount needed to replace fluid loss
- Transfusion therapy with packed RBCs administered over 1 to 3 hours as tolerated

Drug therapy
- Alkalinizing agent: sodium bicarbonate
- Antacid: aluminum hydroxide gel (AlternaGEL)
- Antibiotic: cefazolin (Ancef)
- Anticonvulsant: phenytoin (Dilantin)
- Antiemetic: prochlorperazine (Compazine)
- Antipyretic: acetaminophen (Tylenol)
- Beta-adrenergic blocker: dopamine (Intropin) initially to improve renal perfusion
- Cation exchange resin: sodium polystyrene sulfonate (Kayexalate)
- Diuretics: furosemide (Lasix), metolazone (Zaroxolyn)

INTERVENTIONS AND RATIONALES
- Assess fluid balance, respiratory, cardiovascular, and neurologic status *to detect fluid overload, a complication of acute renal failure*.
- Monitor and record vital signs and intake and output, central venous pressure, daily weight, urine specific gravity, and laboratory studies *to detect early signs of fluid overload*.
- Monitor for arrhythmias *to assess for complications of fluid and electrolyte imbalance*.
- Assess for presence of dependent edema, *which may indicate fluid overload*.
- Maintain the patient's diet *to promote nutritional status*.
- Restrict fluids *to prevent fluid volume excess*.
- Administer I.V. fluids *to correct electrolyte imbalance and maintain hydration*.

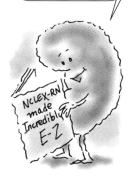

Everyone depends on me. If I fail to function, it can threaten many body systems.

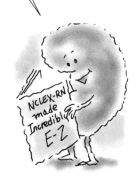

If conservative measures fail to control renal failure, hemodialysis or peritoneal dialysis may be necessary.

• Keep the patient in semi-Fowler's position *to facilitate lung expansion.*
• Administer total parenteral nutrition or enteral nutrition, if indicated, *to promote nutritional status.*
• Administer medications, as prescribed, *to maintain or improve patient's condition.*
• Encourage the patient to express feelings about changes in body image *to facilitate coping mechanisms.*
• Assist with peritoneal dialysis, if indicated; notify the doctor if return solution is cloudy, indicating infection, *to prevent complications.*
• Maintain a quiet environment *to reduce metabolic demands.*
• Assist the patient with turning, coughing, and deep breathing *to mobilize secretions and promote lung expansion.*
• Provide skin and mouth care using plain water *to promote comfort and prevent tissue breakdown.*

Teaching topics
• Avoiding over-the-counter medications
• Maintaining a quiet environment

Benign prostatic hyperplasia

In benign prostatic hyperplasia (BPH), the prostate gland enlarges enough to compress the urethra and cause urinary obstruction.

CAUSES
• Hormonal
• Unknown

ASSESSMENT FINDINGS
• Decreased force and amount of urination
• Dribbling
• Dysuria
• Hesitancy
• Nocturia
• Urgency, frequency, and burning on urination
• Urinary tract infection
• Urine retention

DIAGNOSTIC TEST RESULTS
• Blood chemistry shows increased BUN and creatinine levels.

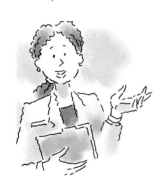

Relate assessment findings to how the disorder affects the body. BPH can compress the urethra. Decreased force and amount of urination is a key sign.

• CMG shows abnormal pressure recordings.
• Cystoscopy shows enlarged prostate gland, obstructed urine flow, and urinary stasis.
• Excretory urography shows urethral obstruction, and hydronephrosis.
• Prostate-specific antigen levels are commonly low.
• Rectal examination shows enlarged prostate gland.
• Urinary flow rate determination shows small volume, prolonged flow pattern, low peak flow.
• Urine chemistry shows bacteria, hematuria, alkaline pH, and increased urine specific gravity.

NURSING DIAGNOSES
• Sexual dysfunction
• Altered urinary elimination
• Urinary retention

TREATMENT
• Forcing fluids
• Transurethral resection of the prostate or prostatectomy

Drug therapy
• Alpha-adrenergic antagonists: prazosin (Minipress), terazosin (Hytrin)
• Alpha-adrenergic blocker: phenoxybenzamine (Dibenzyline)
• Analgesic: oxycodone hydrochloride (Tylox)
• Antianxiety: oxazepam (Serax)
• Antibiotic: trimethoprim and sulfamethoxazole (Bactrim)
• Urinary antiseptic: phenazopyridine (Pyridium)

INTERVENTIONS AND RATIONALES
• Assess fluid balance *to determine fluid deficit or overload.*
• Monitor and record vital signs and intake and output. *Accurate intake and output are essential to detect urine retention if the patient doesn't have an indwelling urinary catheter in place.*
• Monitor for urinary tract infection *to assess for complications.*
• Force fluids *to improve hydration.*
• Administer medications, as prescribed, *to maintain or improve patient's condition.*

• Encourage the patient to express feelings about changes in body image and fear of sexual dysfunction *to help pinpoint fears, establish trust, and facilitate coping.*
• Maintain position and patency of indwelling urinary catheter to straight drainage *to avoid urine reflux.*
• Maintain activity as tolerated *to promote independence.*
• Provide routine postoperative care *to prevent complications.*

Teaching topics
• Recognizing the signs and symptoms of urine retention
• Adhering to medical follow-up

Bladder cancer

Bladder cancer is a malignant tumor that invades the mucosal lining of the bladder. It may metastasize to the ureters, prostate gland, vagina, rectum, and periaortic lymph nodes.

CAUSES
• Chronic bladder irritation
• Cigarette smoking
• Drug-induced from cyclophosphamide (Cytoxan)
• Excessive intake of coffee, phenacetin, sodium, saccharin, sodium cyclamate
• Exposure to industrial chemicals
• Radiation

ASSESSMENT FINDINGS
• Anuria
• Chills
• Dysuria
• Fever
• Flank or pelvic pain
• Frequency of urination
• Painless hematuria
• Peripheral edema
• Urgency of urination

DIAGNOSTIC TEST RESULTS
• Cystoscopy reveals a mass.
• Cytologic examination is positive for malignant cells.

• Excretory urography shows mass or obstruction.
• Hematology shows decreased RBC count, Hb, and HCT.
• KUB X-ray shows mass or obstruction.
• Urine chemistry shows hematuria.

NURSING DIAGNOSES
• Incontinence
• Pain
• Altered urinary elimination

TREATMENT
• Transfusion therapy with packed RBCs
• Surgery dependent on location and progress of tumor (see *Bladder cancer treatment options,* page 310)

Drug therapy
• Analgesics: meperidine (Demerol), morphine sulfate
• Antispasmodic: phenazopyridine (Pyridium)
• Sedative: oxazepam (Serax)

INTERVENTIONS AND RATIONALES
• Assess renal status *to determine baseline and detect early changes.*
• Monitor and record vital signs and intake and output. *Accurate intake and output are essential for correct fluid replacement therapy.*
• Provide postoperative care *to promote healing and prevent complications.* (Closely monitor urine output; observe for hematuria [reddish tint to gross bloodiness] or infection [cloudy, foul smelling, with sediment]; maintain continuous bladder irrigation, if indicated; assist with turning, coughing and deep breathing.)
• Maintain the patient's diet *to improve nutrition and meet metabolic demands.*
• Force fluids *to prevent dehydration.*
• Administer I.V. fluids *to maintain hydration.*
• Administer medications, as prescribed, *to maintain or improve patient's condition.*
• Encourage the patient to express feelings about a fear of dying *to encourage adequate coping mechanisms.*
• Provide postchemotherapeutic care (watch for myelosuppression, chemical cystitis, and skin rash) and postradiation nursing care *to*

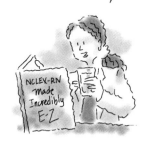

Drinking fluids is important for BPH patients — and for you. Staying hydrated will help keep your body in shape for studying.

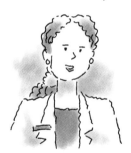

Postoperative pointer: With bladder cancer patients, be sure to monitor urine for signs of hematuria or infection.

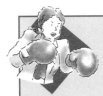

Battling illness

Bladder cancer treatment options

Treatment options for bladder cancer depend on the patient's lifestyle, other health problems, and mental outlook.

TUMOR THAT HASN'T INVADED MUSCLE
In transurethral resection, superficial bladder tumors are removed cytoscopically by transurethral resection and electrically by fulguration. The procedure is only effective if the tumor hasn't invaded muscle.
  Additional tumors may develop, and fulguration may need repeating every 3 months for years.

SUPERFICIAL TUMOR
Intravesical chemotherapy is often used to treat superficial bladder tumors (especially when tumors are in several sites). This treatment washes the bladder with drugs that fight cancer, usually thiotepa, doxorubicin, and mitomycin.

INFILTRATING TUMOR
Radical cystectomy is the choice for infiltrating bladder tumors. In this procedure, the bladder is removed and a urinary diversion is created.

REMOVAL OF A SECTION
Segmental bladder resection removes a full-thickness section of the bladder. It's only used if the tumor isn't located near the bladder neck or ureteral orifices.

---

prevent complications associated with treatment.

Teaching topics
• Contacting the American Cancer Society
• Contacting community agencies and resources for supportive services
• Skin care following radiation therapy, such as avoiding cold packs to area

Breast cancer

Breast cancer is the most common cancer in women. Although the disease may develop any time after puberty, 70% of cases occur in women over age 50. Breast cancer can also occur in men but the incidence is rare. Breast cancer is generally classified by the tissue of origin and the location of the lesion; for example:

• Adenocarcinoma, the most common form of breast cancer, arises from the epithelial tissues.
• Intraductal cancer develops within the ducts.
• Intrafiltrating cancer arises in the parenchymal tissue.
• Inflammatory cancer (rare) grows rapidly and causes the overlying skin to become edematous, inflamed, and indurated.
• Lobular cancer involves the lobes of the glandular tissue.
• Medullary or circumscribed cancer is a tumor that grows rapidly.

CAUSES
• Alcohol and tobacco use
• Antihypertensive therapy
• Being a premenopausal woman over age 40
• Benign breast disease
• Early onset menses or late menopause
• Endometrial or ovarian cancer
• Estrogen therapy

• Exact cause unknown (Scientists have discovered specific genes linked to breast cancer, which confirms that the disease can be inherited from a person's mother or father.)
• Family history of breast cancer
• First pregnancy after age 35
• High-fat diet
• Nulligravida (never pregnant)
• Obesity
• Radiation exposure

ASSESSMENT FINDINGS
• Cervical, supraclavicular, or axillary lymph node lump or enlargement on palpation
• Clear, milky, or bloody discharge
• Edema in the affected arm
• Erythema
• Nipple retraction
• Painless lump or mass in the breast or thickening of breast tissue
• Skin changes

DIAGNOSTIC TEST RESULTS
• Breast self-examination reveals a lump or mass in the breast or thickening of breast tissue.
• Chest X-rays can pinpoint chest metastases.
• Fine-needle aspiration and excisional biopsy provide histologic cells that confirm diagnosis.
• Hormonal receptor assay pinpoints whether the tumor is estrogen- or progesterone-dependent.
• Mammography detects a tumor.
• Scans of the bone, brain, liver, and other organs can detect distant metastases.
• Ultrasonography distinguishes between a fluid-filled cyst and a solid mass.

NURSING DIAGNOSES
• Body image disturbance
• Fear
• Pain

TREATMENT
• High-protein diet
• Peripheral stem cell therapy for advanced breast cancer
• Radiation therapy

• Surgery; options include lumpectomy, skin-sparing mastectomy, partial mastectomy, total mastectomy, and modified radical mastectomy
• Transfusion therapy, if needed

Drug therapy
• Analgesics: morphine
• Antiemetics: trimethobenzamide (Tigan), prochlorperazine (Compazine)
• Chemotherapy: cyclophosphamide (Cytoxan), methotrexate (Folex), fluorouracil (Adrucil)
• Hormonal therapy: tamoxifen (Nolvadex), aminoglutethimide (Cytadren), diethylstilbestrol, megestrol (Megace)

INTERVENTIONS AND RATIONALES
• Assess the patient's feelings about her illness, and determine what she knows about breast cancer and her expectations *to help identify patient needs and aid in developing a plan of care.*
• Provide routine postoperative care *to prevent postoperative complications.*
• Perform comfort measures *to promote relaxation and relieve anxiety.*
• Administer analgesics as ordered, and monitor their effectiveness *to promote patient comfort.*
• Watch for treatment-related complications, such as nausea, vomiting, anorexia, leukopenia, thrombocytopenia, GI ulceration, and bleeding, *to ensure that measures are taken to prevent further complications.*
• Monitor the patient's weight and nutritional intake *to detect evidence of malnutrition.* Encourage a high-protein diet. Dietary supplements may be necessary *to meet increased metabolic demands.*
• Assess the patient's and family's ability to cope, especially if the cancer is terminal. *Counseling may be necessary to help them cope with the fear of death and dying.*

Teaching topics
• Treatment options
• Managing adverse reactions to treatment
• Importance of immediately reporting signs of infection to the physician

- Breast self-examination
- Availability of community support services
- Contacting the American Cancer Society

Cervical cancer

The third most common cancer of the female reproductive system, cervical cancer is classified as either preinvasive or invasive. Preinvasive cancers range from minimal cervical dysplasia, in which the lower third of the epithelium contains abnormal cells, to carcinoma in situ, in which the full thickness of epithelium contains abnormally proliferating cells.

CAUSES
- Frequent intercourse at a young age (under 16)
- History of human papillomavirus or other bacterial or viral venereal infections
- Multiple pregnancies
- Multiple sex partners

ASSESSMENT FINDINGS
Preinvasive
- Symptoms are absent

Invasive
- Abnormal vaginal discharge (yellowish, blood-tinged, and foul-smelling)
- Gradually increasing flank pain
- Leakage of feces (with metastasis to the rectum with fistula development)
- Leakage of urine (with metastasis into the bladder with formation of a fistula)
- Postcoital pain and bleeding

DIAGNOSTIC TEST RESULTS
- Colposcopy determines the source of the abnormal cells seen on the Papanicolaou (Pap) test.
- Cone biopsy is performed if endocervical curettage is positive.
- Lymphangiograpy, cystography, and major organ and bone scans can detect metastasis.

NURSING DIAGNOSES
- Fear
- Impaired tissue integrity
- Pain

TREATMENT
Preinvasive
- Hysterectomy (rare)
- Laser destruction
- Total excisional biopsy

Invasive
- Pelvic exoneration (rare)
- Radiation therapy (internal, external, or both)
- Radical hysterectomy

Drug therapy
Chemotherapy is usually ineffective in treating cervical cancer. When used, it consists of hydroxyurea (Hydrea) in combination with radiation treatment.

INTERVENTIONS AND RATIONALES
- Encourage the patient to use relaxation techniques *to promote comfort during diagnostic procedures.*
- When assisting with a biopsy, drape and prepare the patient as for a routine pelvic examination. Have a container of formaldehyde ready *to preserve the specimen during transfer to the pathology laboratory.* Assist the doctor as needed and provide support for the patient throughout the procedure *to allay the patient's anxiety.*
- If assisting with laser therapy, drape and prepare the patient as for a routine pelvic examination. Assist the doctor as needed and provide support to the patient *to alleviate the patient's anxiety.*
- Watch for complications related to therapy *to ensure that measures can be instituted to prevent or alleviate complications.*
- Administer pain medication, as needed, and note effectiveness. *If pain relief isn't achieved, an alternative dose or medication may be required.*

Teaching topics
- Treatment options
- Postexcisional biopsy care (expecting discharge or spotting for about 1 week; avoiding douching, using tampons, or engaging in sexual intercourse during this time; reporting signs of infection)
- Follow-up Pap tests and pelvic examinations

Chlamydia

Chlamydia refers to a group of infections linked to one organism: *Chlamydia trachomatis*. Chlamydia infection causes urethritis in men and urethritis and cervicitis in women. Untreated, chlamydial infections can lead to such complications as acute epididymitis, salpingitis, pelvic inflammatory disease and, eventually, sterility.

Chlamydial infections are the most common sexually transmitted diseases in the United States.

CAUSES
• Exposure to *C. trachomatis* through sexual contact

ASSESSMENT FINDINGS
In women, assessment findings include:
• cervical erosion
• dyspareunia
• mucopurulent discharge
• pelvic pain.
   In men, assessment findings include:
• dysuria
• erythema
• pruritus
• tenderness of the meatus
• urethral discharge
• urinary frequency.

DIAGNOSTIC TEST RESULTS
• A swab from the site of infection (urethra, cervix, or rectum) establishes a diagnosis of urethritis, cervicitis, salpingitis, endometritis, or proctitis.
• A culture of aspirated material establishes a diagnosis of epididymitis.
• Antigen detection methods, including the enzyme-linked immunosorbent assay and the direct fluorescent antibody test, are the diagnostic tests of choice for identifying chlamydial infection, although tissue cell cultures are more sensitive and specific.

NURSING DIAGNOSES
• Altered urinary elimination
• Pain
• Knowledge deficit (disease transmission)

TREATMENT
The only treatment available for chlamydial infection is drug therapy.

Drug therapy
• Antibiotics: doxycycline (Vibramycin), azithromycin (Zithromax)
• For pregnant women with chlamydial infections, azithromycin (Zithromax), in a single 1-gram dose

INTERVENTIONS AND RATIONALES
• Practice standard precautions when caring for a patient with a chlamydial infection *to prevent the spread of infection.*
• Make sure that the patient fully understands the dosage requirements of any prescribed medications for this infection *to ensure compliance with the treatment regimen.*
• If required in your state, report all cases of chlamydial infection to the appropriate local public health authorities who will then conduct follow-up notification of the patient's sexual contacts. *These measures help ensure that an infected sexual contact will receive medical care to treat the infection.*
• Suggest that the patient and his sexual partners receive testing for human immunodeficiency virus (HIV). *Unsafe sex practices which lead to chlamydial infection also place the patient at risk for contracting HIV.*
• Check newborns of infected mothers for signs of chlamydial infection *to ensure prompt recognition and treatment of infection.* Obtain appropriate specimens for diagnostic testing *to confirm diagnosis of chlamydial infection.*

Teaching topics
• Safer sex practices
• Importance of taking all of the medication, even after symptoms subside
• Avoiding contact with eyes after touching any discharge
• Proper hand-washing technique
• Importance of follow-up medical care

Chronic glomerulonephritis

A slowly progressive disease, chronic glomerulonephritis is characterized by inflam-

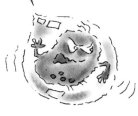

What a little microorganism can do! Chlamydia is a group of infections linked to *Chlamydia trachomatis.*

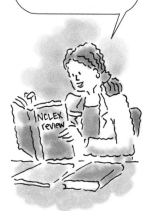

Because signs of chlamydial infection occur late in the course of illness, transmission usually occurs unknowingly.

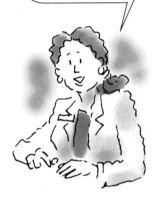

By the time chronic glomerulonephritis is diagnosed, the patient usually can't be cured and must rely on dialysis or a kidney transplant.

mation of the glomeruli (the kidney's blood vessels), which results in sclerosis, scarring and, eventually, renal failure.

By the time it produces symptoms, chronic glomerulonephritis is usually irreversible.

CAUSES
• Renal disorders
• Systemic disorders (lupus erythematosus, Goodpasture's syndrome, and diabetes mellitus)

ASSESSMENT FINDINGS
• Edema
• Hematuria
• Hypertension
• Uremic symptoms (in the late stages of the disease)

DIAGNOSTIC TEST RESULTS
• Kidney biopsy identifies underlying disease and provides data needed to guide therapy.
• Blood studies reveal rising blood urea nitrogen and serum creatinine levels, which indicate advanced renal insufficiency.
• Urinalysis reveals proteinuria, hematuria, cylindruria, and red blood cell casts.
• X-ray or ultrasonography shows smaller kidneys.

NURSING DIAGNOSES
• Altered urinary elimination
• Fluid volume excess
• Risk for injury

TREATMENT
• Dialysis
• Low-sodium, high-calorie with adequate protein diet
• Kidney transplant

Drug therapy
• Antibiotics (for symptomatic urinary tract infections)
• Antihypertensives such as metoprolol (Lopressor)
• Diuretics such as furosemide (Lasix)

INTERVENTIONS AND RATIONALES
• Understand that patient care is primarily supportive, focusing on continual observation

and sound patient teaching. *Supportive measures encourage the patient to cope with chronic disease.*
• Accurately monitor vital signs, intake and output, and daily weight *to evaluate fluid retention.*
• Observe for signs of fluid, electrolyte, and acid-base imbalances *to ensure early treatment and prevent complications.*
• Consult the dietitian *to plan low-sodium, high-calorie meals with adequate protein.*
• Administer medications and provide good skin care *to combat pruritus and edema.*
• Provide good oral hygiene *to prevent breakdown of oral mucosa.*

Teaching topics
• Continuing prescribed antihypertensives as scheduled, even if he's feeling better, and reporting any adverse effects
• Reporting signs of infection, particularly urinary tract infection, and avoiding contact with people who have infections
• Importance of follow-up examinations to assess renal function

Chronic renal failure

Chronic renal failure is the progressive, irreversible destruction of the kidneys, leading to loss of renal function. It may result from a rapidly progressing disease of sudden onset that destroys the nephrons and causes irreversible kidney damage.

CAUSES
• Congenital abnormalities
• Dehydration
• Diabetes mellitus
• Exacerbations of nephritis
• Hypertension
• Nephrotoxins
• Recurrent urinary tract infection
• Systemic lupus erythematosus
• Urinary tract obstructions

ASSESSMENT FINDINGS
• Azotemia
• Bone pain
• Brittle nails and hair

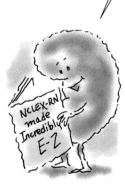

Yikes. Chronic renal failure produces major changes in all the patient's body systems.

NCLEX-RN made Incredibly E-Z

- Decreased urine output
- Ecchymosis
- Heart failure
- Lethargy
- Muscle twitching
- Paresthesia
- Pruritus
- Seizures
- Stomatitis
- Weight gain

DIAGNOSTIC TEST RESULTS

- ABG analysis shows metabolic acidosis.
- Blood chemistry shows increased BUN, creatinine, phosphorus and lipid levels and decreased calcium, CO_2, and albumin levels.
- Hematology shows decreased Hb, HCT, and platelet count.
- Urine chemistry shows proteinuria, increased WBC count, sodium level, and decreased and then fixed urine specific gravity.

NURSING DIAGNOSES

- Decreased cardiac output
- Fluid volume excess
- Altered renal tissue perfusion

TREATMENT

- Limited fluids
- Low-protein, low-sodium, low-potassium, low-phosphorus, high-calorie, and high-carbohydrate diet
- Peritoneal dialysis and hemodialysis (see *Types of dialysis,* page 316)
- Transfusion therapy with packed red blood cells and platelets

Drug therapy

- Alkalinizing agent: sodium bicarbonate
- Antacids: aluminum hydroxide gel (AlternaGEL)
- Antianemics: ferrous sulfate (Feosol), iron dextran (InFeD), epoetin alfa (recombinant human erythropoietin, Epogen)
- Antiarrhythmic: procainamide (Pronestyl)
- Antibiotic: cefazolin (Ancef)
- Antiemetic: prochlorperazine (Compazine)
- Antipyretic: acetaminophen (Tylenol)
- Beta-adrenergic blocker: dopamine (Intropin)

- Calcium supplement: calcium carbonate (Os-Cal)
- Cation exchange resin: sodium polystyrene sulfonate (Kayexalate)
- Digitalis glycoside: digoxin (Lanoxin)
- Diuretic: furosemide (Lasix)
- Stool softener: docusate sodium (Colace)
- Vitamins: pyridoxine hydrochloride (vitamin B_6), ascorbic acid (vitamin C)

INTERVENTIONS AND RATIONALES

- Assess renal, respiratory, and cardiovascular status and fluid balance. *An increase in hemodynamic status and vital signs may indicate fluid overload caused by lack of kidney function.*
- Assess dialysis access for bruit and thrill *to ensure patency and detect complications.*
- Monitor and record vital signs, intake and output, electrocardiogram values, daily weight, laboratory studies, and stools for occult blood *to assess baseline and detect early changes in patient's condition.*
- Monitor for ecchymosis and GI bleeding *because blood clotting mechanism may be affected.*
- Maintain standard precautions *to prevent spread of infection.*
- Maintain the patient's diet *to promote nutritional status.*
- Restrict fluids *to prevent fluid overload.*
- Administer medications, as prescribed, *to improve or maintain patient's condition.*
- Encourage the patient to express feelings about chronicity of illness *to encourage coping mechanisms.*
- Provide tepid baths *to promote comfort and reduce skin irritation.*
- Maintain a cool and quiet environment *to reduce metabolic demands.*
- Provide skin and mouth care using plain water *to promote comfort.*
- Avoid giving the patient I.M. injections *to prevent bleeding from injection site.*

Teaching topics

- Maintaining a quiet environment
- Completing skin and mouth care daily

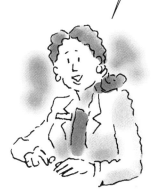

Fluid balance is achieved by restricting fluid and administering drugs that control blood pressure and reduce edema.

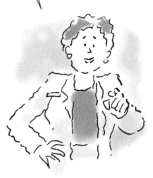

Advise the patient to take diuretics in the morning so he won't have to disrupt his sleep to void.

Battling illness

Types of dialysis

Two main types of dialysis used to treat chronic renal failure are hemodialysis and peritoneal dialysis.

REMOVING WASTE

Hemodialysis removes toxic wastes and other impurities from the blood. Blood is removed from the body through a surgically created access site, pumped through a filtration unit to remove toxins, and then returned to the body. The extracorporeal dialyzer works through osmosis, diffusion, and filtration. Hemodialysis is performed by specially trained nurses.

Nursing actions
- Monitor the venous access site for bleeding. If bleeding is excessive, maintain pressure on the site.
- Don't use the arm for blood pressure monitoring, I.V. catheter insertion, or venipuncture.
- At least four times daily, auscultate the access site for bruits and palpate for thrills.

USING THE BODY

Peritoneal dialysis removes toxins from the blood, but unlike hemodialysis, it uses the patient's peritoneal membrane as a semipermeable dialyzing membrane. Hypertonic dialyzing solution is instilled through a catheter inserted into the peritoneal cavity. Then by diffusion, excessive concentrations of electrolytes and uremic toxins in the blood move across the peritoneal membrane and into the dialysis solution. Next, by osmosis, excessive water in the blood does the same.

  After appropriate dwelling time, the dialysis solution is drained, taking toxins and wastes with it. The patient is trained to perform this procedure.

Nursing actions
- Check the patient's weight, and report any gain.
- Using aseptic technique, change the catheter dressing every 24 hours and whenever it becomes wet or soiled.
- Calculate the patient's fluid balance at the end of each dialysis session or after 8 hours in a longer session. Include oral and I.V. fluid intake as well as urine output and wound drainage. Record and report any significant imbalance, either positive or negative.

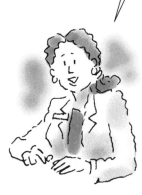

Cystitis is usually easy to cure, but reinfection and residual bacterial flare-up during treatment are possible.

Cystitis

Cystitis is the inflammation of the urinary bladder. It's usually related to a superficial infection that doesn't extend to the bladder mucosa.

CAUSES
- Diabetes mellitus
- Incorrect aseptic technique during catheterization
- Incorrect perineal care
- Kidney infection
- Obstruction of the urethra
- Pregnancy
- Radiation
- Sexual intercourse
- Stagnation of urine in the bladder

ASSESSMENT FINDINGS
- Burning or pain on urination
- Dark, odoriferous urine
- Dribbling
- Dysuria
- Flank tenderness or suprapubic pain
- Frequency of urination

- Lower abdominal discomfort
- Low-grade fever
- Nocturia
- Urge to bear down on urination
- Urgency of urination

DIAGNOSTIC TEST RESULTS
- Cystoscopy shows obstruction or deformity.
- Urine chemistry shows hematuria, pyuria, and increased protein, leukocytes, and urine specific gravity.
- Urine culture and sensitivity positively identifies organisms *(Escherichia coli, Proteus vulgaris,* or *Streptococcus faecalis).*

NURSING DIAGNOSES
- Altered urinary elimination
- Incontinence
- Pain

TREATMENT
- Diet: increased intake of fluids and vitamin C

Drug therapy
- Antibiotic: trimethoprim and sulfamethoxazole (Bactrim)
- Antipyretic: acetaminophen (Tylenol)
- Urinary antiseptic: phenazopyridine (Pyridium)

INTERVENTIONS AND RATIONALES
- Assess renal status *to determine baseline and detect changes.*
- Monitor and record vital signs, intake and output, and laboratory studies *to assess patient's status and detect early complications.*
- Maintain the patient's diet *to promote nutrition.*
- Force fluids (cranberry or orange juice) to 3 qt (3 L)/day *because dilute urine lessens the irritation to the bladder mucosa and lowering urine pH with orange juice and cranberry juice consumption helps diminish bacterial growth.*
- Administer medications, as prescribed, *to maintain or improve patient's condition.*
- Perform sitz baths and perineal care *to relieve perineal or suprapubic discomfort.*
- Encourage voiding every 2 to 3 hours. *Frequent bladder emptying decreases bladder irritation and prevents stasis of urine.*

Teaching topics
- Avoiding coffee, tea, alcohol, and cola
- Increasing intake to 3 L/day using orange juice and cranberry juice
- Voiding every 2 to 3 hours and after intercourse
- Performing perineal care correctly
- Avoiding bubble baths, vaginal deodorants, and tub baths
- Recognizing that urine may be orange while taking phenazopyridine

Gonorrhea

A common sexually transmitted disease, gonorrhea is an infection of the genitourinary tract (especially the urethra and cervix) and, occasionally, the rectum, pharynx, and eyes. Untreated gonorrhea can spread through the blood to the joints, tendons, meninges, and endocardium; in females, it can also lead to chronic pelvic inflammatory disease (PID) and sterility.

After adequate treatment, the prognosis in both males and females is excellent, although reinfection is common. Gonorrhea is especially prevalent among young people and people with multiple partners, particularly those between ages 19 and 25.

CAUSES
- Exposure to *Neisseria gonorrhoeae* through sexual contact

ASSESSMENT FINDINGS
- Dysuria
- Purulent urethral or cervical discharge
- Redness and swelling
- Itching, burning, and pain

DIAGNOSTIC TEST RESULTS
- A culture from the site of infection (urethra, cervix, rectum, or pharynx), grown on a Thayer-Martin or Transgrow medium, usually establishes the diagnosis by isolating the organism.
- A Gram stain showing gram-negative diplococci supports the diagnosis and may be sufficient to confirm gonorrhea in males.

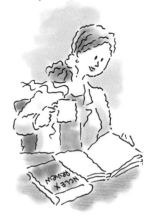

Think vitamin C for cystitis. Patients with this disorder will benefit from drinking orange or cranberry juice.

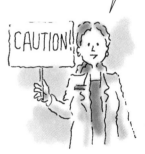

Emphasize to the patient with gonorrhea that he may be infectious even if no symptoms of the disease are present.

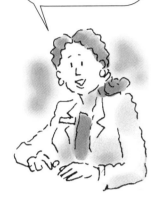

Effective treatment of all sexually transmitted diseases includes thorough patient teaching.

NURSING DIAGNOSES
- Risk for infection
- Pain
- Altered sexuality patterns

TREATMENT
- Moist heat to affected joints, if gonococcal arthritis is present

Drug therapy
- Antibiotics: ceftriaxone (Rocephin), doxycycline (Vibramycin), erythromycin (E-mycin)
- Prophylactic antibiotics: 1% silver nitrate or erythromycin (EryPed) eye drops to prevent infection in newborns

INTERVENTIONS AND RATIONALES
- Before treatment, establish whether the patient has any drug sensitivities, and watch closely for adverse effects during therapy *to prevent severe adverse reactions*.
- Warn the patient that until cultures prove negative, he's still infectious and can transmit gonococcal infection *to prevent the spread of infection to others*.
- Practice standard precautions *to prevent the spread of infection*.
- In the patient with gonococcal arthritis, apply moist heat *to ease pain in affected joints*.
- Urge the patient to inform sexual contacts of his *infection so that they can seek treatment, even if cultures are negative*. Advise them to avoid sexual intercourse until treatment is complete *to prevent the spread of infection*.
- Routinely instill two drops of 1% silver nitrate or erythromycin in the eyes of all neonates immediately after birth. Check newborn infants of infected mothers for signs of infection. Take specimens for culture from the infant's eyes, pharynx, and rectum. *These measures ensure prompt recognition and treatment of infection in the newborn*.
- Report all cases of gonorrhea in children to child abuse authorities.

Teaching topics
- Avoiding anyone even *suspected* of being infected, using condoms during intercourse, washing their genitalia with soap and water before and after intercourse, and avoiding sharing washcloths or douche equipment

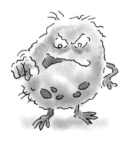

After the first infection with *Herpesvirus hominis*, the person carries the virus permanently and is vulnerable to recurrent herpes infection.

- Importance of continuing antibiotic therapy for the duration prescribed

Herpes simplex

A recurrent viral infection, herpes simplex is caused by two types of *Herpesvirus hominis* (HVH), a widespread infectious agent.

Herpes virus Type 1, which is transmitted by oral and respiratory secretions, affects the skin and mucous membranes and commonly produces cold sores and fever blisters.

Herpes virus Type 2 primarily affects the genital area and is transmitted by sexual contact. Cross-infection may result from orogenital sex.

CAUSES
- Exposure to herpes virus Type 2 through sexual contact
- Contact with herpes virus Type 1 through oral or respiratory secretions

ASSESSMENT FINDINGS
- Appetite loss
- Blisters on any part of the mouth accompanied by erythema and edema
- Conjunctivitis (herpetic keratoconjunctivitis or herpes of the eye)
- Fever
- Increased salivation
- Swelling of the lymph nodes under the jaw

Genital herpes
- Fever, swollen lymph nodes
- Fluid-filled blisters
- Painful urination

DIAGNOSTIC TEST RESULTS
- Confirmation requires isolation of the virus from local lesions and a histologic biopsy.
- Blood studies reveal a rise in antibodies and moderate leukocytosis.

NURSING DIAGNOSES
- Altered urinary elimination pattern
- Pain
- Altered oral mucous membrane

TREATMENT
Symptomatic and supportive treatment

Drug therapy
• Analgesic-antipyretic agent: acetaminophen (Tylenol) to reduce fever and relieve pain
• A drying agent such as calamine lotion (to relieve pain of genital lesions)
• Antiviral agents: idoxuridine (Herplex Liqufilm), trifluridine (Viroptic), and vidarabine (Vira-A)
• 5% acyclovir (Zovirax) ointment (possible relief to patients with genital herpes or to immunosuppressed patients with HVH skin infections; I.V. acyclovir helps treat more severe infections)

INTERVENTIONS AND RATIONALES
• Observe standard precautions. For patients with extensive cutaneous, oral, or genital lesions, institute contact precautions *to prevent the spread of infection.*
• Administer pain medications and prescribed antiviral agents as ordered *to relieve pain and treat infection.*
• Provide supportive care, as indicated, such as oral hygiene, nutritional supplementation, and antipyretics for fever. *These measures enhance the patient's well-being.*
• Abstain from direct patient care if you have herpetic whitlow (an HVH finger infection which commonly affects health care workers) *to prevent the spread of infection.*

Teaching topics
• How to care for themselves during an outbreak of HVH and how to avoid infecting others
• Importance of annual Papanicolaou test in women with genital herpes
• Avoiding kissing infants and people with eczema if a cold sore is present

Neurogenic bladder

Neurogenic bladder refers to all types of bladder dysfunction caused by an interruption of normal bladder innervation. Subsequent complications include incontinence, residual urine retention, urinary infection, stone formation, and renal failure. A neurogenic bladder may be described as spastic (resulting from an upper motor neuron lesion) or flaccid (resulting from a lower motor neuron lesion).

This disorder is also known as neuromuscular dysfunction of the lower urinary tract, neurologic bladder dysfunction, and neuropathic bladder.

CAUSES
• Acute infectious diseases such as Guillain-Barré syndrome
• Cerebral disorder (cerebrovascular accident, brain tumor [meningioma and glioma], Parkinson's disease, multiple sclerosis, dementia)
• Chronic alcoholism
• Collagen diseases such as systemic lupus erythematosus
• Disorders of peripheral innervation
• Distant effects of cancer such as primary oat cell carcinoma of the lung
• Heavy metal toxicity
• Herpes zoster
• Metabolic disturbances (hypothyroidism, porphyria, or uremia)
• Sacral agenesis
• Spinal cord disease or trauma
• Vascular diseases such as atherosclerosis

ASSESSMENT FINDINGS
• Altered micturition
• *Flaccid neurogenic bladder:* Overflow incontinence, diminished anal sphincter tone, greatly distended bladder with an accompanying feeling of bladder fullness
• Hydroureteronephrosis (distention of both the ureter and the renal pelvis and calices)
• Incontinence
• *Spastic neurogenic bladder:* involuntary or frequent scanty urination without a feeling of bladder fullness, possible spontaneous spasms of the arms and legs, increased anal sphincter tone
• Vesicoureteral reflux (passage of urine from the bladder back into a ureter)

DIAGNOSTIC TEST RESULTS
• Voiding cystourethrography evaluates bladder neck function, vesicoureteral reflux, and continence.

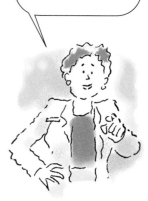

Neurogenic bladder refers to all types of bladder problems caused by disruption of normal nerve impulses to the bladder.

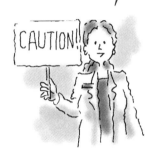

If urine output is considerable, empty the catheter bag more frequently than once every 8 hours. Bacteria can multiply in standing urine and migrate up the catheter and into the bladder.

CAUTION!

• Urodynamic studies help evaluate how urine is stored in the bladder, how well the bladder empties, and the rate of movement of urine out of the bladder during voiding.
• Retrograde urethrography reveals the presence of strictures and diverticula.

NURSING DIAGNOSES
• Altered urinary elimination
• Urge incontinence
• Urinary retention

TREATMENT
• Credé's maneuver (application of manual pressure over the lower abdomen) to evacuate the bladder)
• Valsalva's maneuver to promote complete emptying of the bladder
• Indwelling urinary catheter insertion (including teaching the patient self-catheterization techniques)
• Surgical repair if the patient has structural impairment
• Surgical insertion of an artificial urinary sphincter

Drug therapy
• Urinary tract stimulants: bethanechol (Urecholine) and phenoxybenzamine, to facilitate bladder emptying
• Antimuscarinic agents: propantheline (Pro-Banthine), flavoxate (Urispas), and dicyclomine (Antispas) to facilitate urine storage.

INTERVENTIONS AND RATIONALES
• Use strict aseptic technique during insertion of an indwelling urinary catheter (a temporary measure to drain the incontinent patient's bladder). Don't interrupt the closed drainage system for any reason *to prevent infection.*
• Obtain urine specimens with a syringe and smallbore needle inserted through the aspirating port of the catheter itself (below the junction of the balloon instillation site). Irrigate in the same manner if necessary *to prevent infection.*
• Clean the catheter insertion site with soap and water at least twice a day *to prevent infection.*

• Don't allow the catheter to become encrusted; *this is a medium for bacteria growth.*
• Use a sterile applicator to apply antibiotic ointment around the meatus after catheter care, if prescribed. Keep the drainage bag below the tubing, and don't raise the bag above the level of the bladder *to prevent urine reflux and infection.*
• Clamp the tubing or empty the catheter bag before transferring the patient to a wheelchair or stretcher *to prevent accidental urine reflux.*
• Watch for signs of infection (fever, cloudy or foul-smelling urine) *to ensure early treatment intervention and prevent complications.*
• Try to keep the patient as mobile as possible. Perform passive range-of-motion exercise if necessary. *These measures prevent complications of immobility.*
• If urinary diversion procedure is to be performed, arrange for consultation with an enterostomal therapist, and coordinate the care *to help the patient cope with his change in body image.*

Teaching topics
• Evacuation techniques as necessary (Credé's method, intermittent self-catheterization techniques)
• Preventing and identifying infection

Ovarian cancer

This cancer attacks the ovaries, the organs in women that produce the hormones estrogen and progesterone. After cancer of the lung, breast, and colon, primary ovarian cancer ranks as the most common cause of cancer deaths among American women. In women with previously treated breast cancer, metastatic ovarian cancer is more common than cancer at any other site.

The prognosis varies with the histologic type and stage of the disease but is generally poor because ovarian tumors produce few early signs and are usually advanced at diagnosis. About 40% of women with ovarian cancer survive for 5 years.

CONTRIBUTING FACTORS
- Age at menopause
- Celibacy
- Exposure to asbestos, talc, and industrial pollutants
- Familial tendency; and history of breast or uterine cancer
- High-fat diet
- Incidence is highest in women of upper socioeconomic levels between the ages of 20 and 54
- Infertility

ASSESSMENT FINDINGS
- Abdominal discomfort, dyspepsia, and other mild GI disturbances
- Abdominal distention
- Constipation
- Pelvic discomfort
- Urinary frequency
- Weight loss

DIAGNOSTIC TEST RESULTS
In ovarian cancer, diagnosis requires clinical evaluation, a complete patient history, surgical exploration, and histologic studies. Preoperative evaluation includes a complete physical examination, including pelvic examination with Pap smear (positive in only a small number of women with ovarian cancer) and the following special tests:
- Abdominal ultrasonography, computed tomography scan, or X-ray may delineate tumor size.
- Chest X-ray may reveal distant metastasis and pleural effusions.
- Barium enema (especially in patients with GI symptoms) may reveal obstruction and size of tumor.
- Lymphangiography may show lymph node involvement.
- Mammography may rule out primary breast cancer.
- Liver scan in patients with ascites may rule out liver metastasis.
- Blood tests such as ovarian carcinoma antigen, carcinoembryonic antigen, and human chorionic gonadotropin reveal presence of cancer.

Despite extensive testing, accurate diagnosis and staging are impossible without exploratory laparotomy, including lymph node evaluation and tumor resection.

NURSING DIAGNOSES
- Altered protection
- Fluid volume excess
- Altered nutrition: Less than body requirements

TREATMENT
Conservative treatment
Occasionally, in girls or young women with a unilateral encapsulated tumor who wish to maintain fertility, the following conservative approach may be appropriate:
- resection of the involved ovary
- biopsies of the omentum and the uninvolved ovary
- peritoneal washings for cytologic examination of pelvic fluid
- careful follow-up, including periodic chest X-rays to rule out lung metastasis.

Aggressive treatment
Ovarian cancer usually requires more aggressive treatment, including:
- total abdominal hysterectomy and bilateral salpingo-oophorectomy with tumor resection, omentectomy, and appendectomy
- lymph node biopsies with lymphadenectomy, tissue biopsies, and peritoneal washings.

Drug therapy
- Antineoplastics: cisplatin (Platinol), paclitaxel (Taxol), topotecan (Hycamtin)
- Analgesics: morphine, fentanyl (Duragesic-25)
- Antipyretics: aspirin, acetaminophen (Tylenol)
- Immunotherapy: bacille Calmette-Guérin vaccine

INTERVENTIONS AND RATIONALES
Before surgery:
- Thoroughly explain all preoperative tests, the expected course of treatment, and surgical and postoperative procedures *to allay anxiety.*
- In premenopausal women, explain that bilateral oophorectomy artificially induces early menopause, so they may experience hot

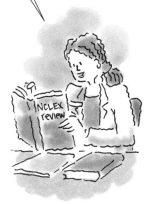

This cancer attacks the ovaries, the organs in women that produce the hormones estrogen and progesterone.

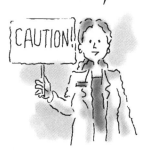

Flulike symptoms may last 12 to 24 hours after administration of immunotherapy — give aspirin or acetaminophen for fever, keep the patient well covered with blankets, and provide warm liquids to relieve chills.

flashes, headaches, palpitations, insomnia, depression, and excessive perspiration *to help the patient cope with changes in body image that occur as a result of surgery.*

After surgery:
• Monitor vital signs frequently *to detect early signs of postoperative complications, such as fluid volume deficit.*
• Monitor fluid intake and output *to detect fluid volume excess or deficit,* while maintaining good catheter care *to prevent infection.*
• Check the dressing regularly for excessive drainage or bleeding, and watch for signs of infection. *These measures detect early signs of complications and prevent treatment delay.*
• Provide abdominal support *to promote comfort,* and watch for abdominal distention, *which may indicate the presence of ascites.*
• Encourage coughing and deep breathing *to mobilize secretions and prevent postoperative pneumonia.*
• Reposition the patient often *to prevent skin breakdown,* and encourage her to walk shortly after surgery *to prevent complications of immobility.*
• Monitor and treat side effects of radiation and chemotherapy *to prevent complications.*
• Enlist the help of a social worker, chaplain, and other members of the health care team *to provide additional supportive care.*

Teaching topics
• Disease process and treatment options
• Preventing and reporting infection
• Managing adverse reactions to chemotherapy

Prostate cancer

Prostate cancer is a malignant tumor of the prostate gland, which can obstruct urine flow when encroaching on the bladder neck. It commonly metastasizes to bone, lymph nodes, brain, and lungs.

CAUSES
• Associated risk factors include family history, age, race, vasectomy, increased dietary fat
• No known etiology

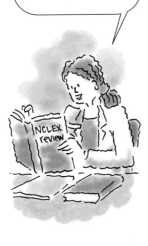

Because prostate cancer can lead to sexual dysfunction, patient care may include providing information about changes in sexual activity.

ASSESSMENT FINDINGS
• Decreased size and force of urine stream
• Difficulty and frequency of urination
• Hematuria
• Urine retention

DIAGNOSTIC TEST RESULTS
• Digital rectal examination reveals palpable firm nodule in gland or diffuse induration in posterior lobe.
• Serum acid phosphatase level is increased.
• Radioimmunoassay for acid phosphatase is increased.
• Prostatic-specific antigen is increased.
• Transurethral ultrasound studies show mass or obstruction.
• Prostate biopsy has cytology positive for cancer cells.
• Excretory urogram shows mass or obstruction.

NURSING DIAGNOSES
• Pain
• Sexual dysfunction
• Altered urinary elimination

TREATMENT
• High-protein diet with restrictions on caffeine and spicy foods
• Radiation implant
• Radical prostatectomy (for localized tumors without metastasis) or transurethral resection of the prostate (to relieve obstruction in metastatic disease)

Drug therapy
• Analgesics: oxycodone (Tylox), meperidine (Demerol), morphine
• Antiemetics: prochlorperazine (Compazine), ondansetron (Zofran)
• Antineoplastics: doxorubicin (Adriamycin), cisplatin (Platinol)
• Corticosteroid: prednisone (Deltasone)
• Immunosuppressant: cyclophosphamide (Cytoxan)
• Luteinizing hormone-releasing hormone agonists: goserelin acetate (Zoladex), leuprolide acetate (Lupron)
• Nonsteroidal anti-inflammatory drugs: indomethacin (Indocin), ibuprofen (Motrin), sulindac (Clinoril)

• Oral flutamide (Eulexin) to block circulating testosterone
• Stool softener: docusate sodium (Colace)

INTERVENTIONS AND RATIONALES
• Assess renal and fluid status *to determine baseline and detect early changes.*
• Monitor and record vital signs, fluid intake and output, and laboratory studies. *Accurate intake and output are essential for correct fluid replacement therapy.*
• Monitor for signs of infection *to assess for complications.*
• Assess pain and note effectiveness of analgesia *to promote comfort.*
• Administer medications, as prescribed, *to maintain or improve patient's condition.*
• Maintain the patient's diet *to maintain nutritional level and meet increased metabolic demands.*
• Maintain patency of the urinary catheter and note drainage *to ensure urine drainage.*
• Encourage the patient to express feelings about the changes in body image and fear of sexual dysfunction *to encourage coping and adaptation.*
• Encourage ambulation *to prevent complications of immobility.*
• Provide postoperative, postchemotherapeutic, and postradiation nursing care *to prevent complications.*

Teaching topics
• Managing changes in sexual activity
• Avoiding prolonged sitting, standing, and walking
• Avoiding the strain of exercise and lifting
• Urinating frequently
• Avoiding coffee and cola beverages
• Decreasing fluid intake during evening hours
• Performing perineal exercises
• Completing catheter care, as directed
• Self-monitoring for bloody urine, pain, burning, frequency, decreased urine output, and loss of bladder control
• Contacting the American Cancer Society
• Contacting community agencies and resources for supportive services

Renal calculi

Renal calculi, also known as kidney stones, are crystalline substances that vary in size. Under normal circumstances, calculi are dissolved and excreted in the urine. However, larger calculi can cause great pain and may become lodged in the ureter.

CAUSES
• Chemotherapy
• Dehydration
• Diet high in calcium, vitamin D, milk, protein, oxalate, alkali
• Genetics
• Gout
• Hypercalcemia
• Hyperparathyroidism
• Idiopathic origin
• Immobility
• Leukemia
• Polycythemia vera
• Urinary stasis
• Urinary tract infection
• Urinary tract obstruction

ASSESSMENT FINDINGS
• Chills and fever
• Cool, moist skin
• Costovertebral tenderness
• Diaphoresis
• Dysuria
• Flank pain
• Frequency of urination
• Nausea and vomiting
• Pallor
• Renal colic
• Syncope
• Urgency of urination

DIAGNOSTIC TEST RESULTS
• 24-hour urine collection shows increased uric acid, oxalate, calcium, phosphorus, and creatinine levels.
• Blood chemistry shows increased calcium, phosphorus, creatinine, BUN, uric acid, protein, and alkaline phosphatase levels.
• Cystoscopy visualizes stones.
• Excretory urography reveals stones.
• KUB reveals stones.

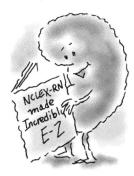

Just reading about kidney stones hurts.

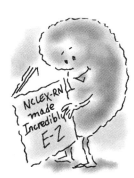

Smaller calculi may pass naturally with vigorous hydration. Larger calculi may be removed by surgery or other means. Small is better.

• Urine chemistry shows pyuria, proteinuria, hematuria, presence of WBCs, and increased urine specific gravity.

NURSING DIAGNOSES
• Pain
• Risk for infection
• Altered urinary elimination

TREATMENT
• Diet: for calcium stones, acid-ash with limited intake of calcium and milk products; for oxalate stones, alkaline-ash with limited intake of foods high in oxalate (cola, tea); for uric acid stones, alkaline-ash with limited intake of foods high in purine
• Extracorporeal shock wave lithotripsy to shatter calculi
• Increased fluid intake to 3 qt (3 L)/day
• Moist heat to flank; hot baths
• Percutaneous nephrostolithotomy
• Surgery if other measures to remove the stone aren't effective (type of surgery dependent on the location of the stone)

Drug therapy
• Acidifiers: ammonium chloride, methenamine mandelate (Mandelamine)
• Alkalinizing agents: potassium acetate, sodium bicarbonate
• Analgesic: meperidine (Demerol) or morphine sulfate
• Antibiotics: cefazolin (Ancef), cefoxitin (Mefoxin)
• Antiemetic: prochlorperazine (Compazine)
• Antigout agent: sulfinpyrazone (Anturane)

INTERVENTIONS AND RATIONALES
• Assess renal status *to determine baseline and detect complications.*
• Assess pain and effectiveness of analgesia. Assessment allows for care plan modification as needed.
• Monitor and record vital signs, intake and output, daily weight, urine specific gravity, laboratory studies, and urine pH *to assess renal status.*
• Monitor the patient's urine for evidence of renal calculi. Strain all urine and save all solid material for analysis *to facilitate spontaneous passage of calculi.*

• Force fluids to 3,000 ml/day *to moisten mucous membranes and dilute chemicals within the body.*
• Maintain the patient's diet *to promote adequate nutrition.*
• Administer medications, as prescribed, *to maintain and improve patient's condition.*
• Apply warm soaks to flank *to promote comfort.*
• If surgery was performed, check dressings regularly for bloody drainage and report excessive amounts of bloody drainage to the doctor; use sterile technique to change the dressing; maintain nephrostomy tube or indwelling urinary catheter if indicated; monitor incision for signs of infection *to promote healing and detect complications.*

Teaching topics
• Increasing fluid intake, especially during hot weather, illness, and exercise
• Voiding whenever urge is felt
• Testing urine pH
• Increasing fluids at night and voiding frequently

Syphilis

A chronic, infectious, sexually transmitted disease, syphilis begins in the mucous membranes and quickly becomes systemic, spreading to nearby lymph nodes and the bloodstream. This disease, when untreated, is characterized by progressive stages: primary, secondary, latent, and late (formerly called tertiary).

In the United States, incidence of syphilis is highest among urban populations, especially in persons between ages 15 and 39, drug users, and those infected with the human immunodeficiency virus (HIV).

CAUSES
• Exposure to the spirochete *Treponema pallidum* through sexual contact
• Transmission from an infected mother to her fetus

ASSESSMENT FINDINGS
Primary syphilis
• Chancres on the genitalia, anus, fingers, lips, tongue, nipples, tonsils, or eyelids

Secondary syphilis
• Symmetrical mucocutaneous lesions
• General lymphadenopathy
• Headache
• Malaise
• Anorexia
• Weight loss
• Nausea
• Vomiting
• Sore throat
• Slight fever

DIAGNOSTIC TEST RESULTS
• Dark-field examination identifies *T. pallidum* from a lesion. This method is most effective when moist lesions are present, as in primary, secondary, and prenatal syphilis.
• Flourescent treponemal antibody-absorption test identifies antigens of *T. pallidum* in tissue, ocular fluid, cerebrospinal fluid (CSF), tracheobronchial secretions, and exudates from lesions. This is the most sensitive test available for detecting syphilis in all stages. When reactive, it remains so permanently.
• Venereal Disease Research Laboratory (VDRL) slide test and rapid plasma reagin test detect nonspecific antibodies. Both tests, if positive, become reactive within 1 to 2 weeks after the primary lesion appears or 4 to 5 weeks after the infection begins.
• CSF examination identifies neurosyphilis when the total protein level is above 40 mg/ 100 ml, VDRL slide test is reactive, and CSF cell count exceeds five mononuclear cells/μl.

NURSING DIAGNOSES
• Altered sexuality patterns
• Impaired skin integrity
• Knowledge deficit

TREATMENT
• Antibiotic therapy is the only treatment for syphilis.

Drug therapy
• Antibiotic: penicillin G benzathine (Permapen); if allergic to penicillin, then erythromycin (Erythrocin) or tetracycline (Panmycin)

INTERVENTIONS AND RATIONALES
• Follow standard precautions when assessing the patient, collecting specimens, and treating lesions *to prevent the spread of infection.*
• Check for a history of drug sensitivity before administering the first dose of penicillin *to prevent anaphylaxis.*
• In secondary syphilis, keep lesions clean and dry. If they're draining, dispose of contaminated materials properly *to prevent the spread of infection.*
• In late syphilis, provide supportive care *to relieve the patient's symptoms during prolonged treatment.*
• In cardiovascular syphilis, check for signs of decreased cardiac output (decreased urine output, hypoxia, and decreased sensorium) and pulmonary congestion *to prevent shock and respiratory distress.*
• In neurosyphilis, regularly check level of consciousness, mood, and coherence. Watch for signs of ataxia. *These measures detect neurologic complications early and prevent treatment delay.*
• Urge patients to seek VDRL testing after 3, 6, 12, and 24 months *to detect possible relapse.* Patients treated for latent or late syphilis should receive blood tests at 6-month intervals for 2 years *to detect possible relapse.*
• Be sure to report all cases of syphilis to local public health authorities. Urge the patient to inform sexual partners of his infection *so that they can receive treatment also.*
• Refer the patient and his sexual partners for HIV testing. *High risk behaviors that caused the patient to contract syphilis also place the patient at risk for HIV.*

Teaching topics
• Safer sex practices
• Importance of completing the course of therapy even after symptoms subside
• Follow-up VDRL testing

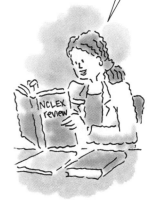

Syphilis begins in the mucous membranes and quickly becomes systemic, spreading to nearby lymph nodes and the bloodstream.

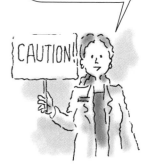

In women, syphilitic chancres may be overlooked because they often develop internally, on the cervix or vaginal wall.

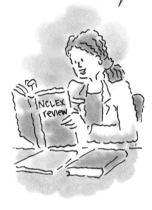

Cancer of the testicle can usually be cured easily; however, if not treated early, it can metastasize through the lymph nodes.

Testicular cancer

This type of cancer affects the testes or testicles, the two oval-shaped glandular organs inside the scrotum that produce spermatozoa and testosterone. Malignant testicular tumors primarily affect young to middle-aged men. Testicular tumors in children are rare.

Most testicular tumors originate in gonadal cells. About 40% are seminomas — uniform, undifferentiated cells resembling primitive gonadal cells. The remainder are nonseminomas — tumor cells showing various degrees of differentiation.

The prognosis varies with the cell type and disease stage. When treated with surgery and radiation, almost all patients with localized disease survive beyond 5 years.

CONTRIBUTING FACTORS
• Age (Incidence peaks between ages 20 and 40.)
• Higher incidence in men with cryptorchidism and in men whose mothers used diethylstilbestrol during pregnancy

ASSESSMENT FINDINGS
• Firm, painless, smooth testicular mass, varying in size and sometimes producing a sense of testicular heaviness

In advanced stages
• Ureteral obstruction
• Abdominal mass
• Cough
• Hemoptysis
• Shortness of breath
• Weight loss
• Fatigue
• Pallor
• Lethargy

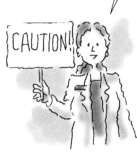

If the patient receives vinblastine, assess for neurotoxicity (peripheral paresthesia, jaw pain, and muscle cramps). If he receives cisplatin, check for ototoxicity.

DIAGNOSTIC TEST RESULTS
• Regular self-examinations and testicular palpation during a routine physical examination may detect testicular tumors.
• Transillumination can distinguish between a tumor (which doesn't transilluminate) and a hydrocele or spermatocele (which does).
• Computed tomography scan can detect metastasis.

• Scrotal ultrasonography can differentiate between a cyst and solid mass.
• Chest X-ray may show pulmonary metastasis.
• Excretory urography may reveal ureteral deviation resulting from para-aortic node involvement.
• Serum alpha-fetoprotein and beta-human chorionic gonadotropin levels — indicators of testicular tumor activity — provide a baseline for measuring response to therapy and determining the prognosis.
• Surgical excision and biopsy of the tumor and testis permits histologic verification of the tumor cell type.
• Inguinal exploration (examination of the groin) determines the extent of nodal involvement.

NURSING DIAGNOSES
• Body image disturbance
• Fear
• Sexual dysfunction

TREATMENT
• Radiation therapy
• Surgery: orchiectomy (testicle removal; most surgeons remove the testicle but not the scrotum to allow for a prosthetic implant)
• Retroperitoneal lymph node dissection (dissection of lymph nodes posterior to the peritoneum)
• Bone marrow transplantation (follows chemotherapy and radiation therapy in patients with unresponsive tumors)
• High-calorie diet provided in small frequent feedings
• I.V. fluid therapy

Drug therapy
• Diuretics: furosemide (Lasix), mannitol (Osmitrol)
• Antineoplastics: bleomycin (Blenoxane), carboplatin (Paraplatin), cisplatin (Platinol), dactinomycin (Cosmegen), etoposide (VePesid), ifosfamide (Ifex), plicamycin (Mithracin), vinblastine (Velban)
• Analgesics: morphine, fentanyl (Duragesic-25)

• Antiemetics: trimethobenzamide (Tigan), metoclopramide (Reglan), ondansetron (Zofran)
• Hormone replacement therapy (after bilateral orchiectomy)

INTERVENTIONS AND RATIONALES

• Develop a treatment plan that addresses the patient's psychological and physical needs *to enhance the patient's well-being.*

Before orchiectomy:

• Reassure the patient that sterility and impotence need not follow unilateral orchiectomy, that synthetic hormones can restore hormonal balance, and that most surgeons don't remove the scrotum. In many cases, a testicular prosthesis can correct anatomic disfigurement. *These interventions can help allay the patient's anxiety.*

After orchiectomy:

• For the first day after surgery, apply an ice pack to the scrotum *to reduce swelling* and provide analgesics *to promote comfort.*
• Check for excessive bleeding, swelling, and signs of infection *to detect early signs of complications and prevent treatment delay.*
• Provide a scrotal athletic supporter *to minimize pain during ambulation.*

During chemotherapy:

• Give antiemetics, as needed, *to treat or prevent nausea and vomiting.*
• Encourage small, frequent meals *to maintain oral intake despite anorexia.*
• Establish a mouth care regimen *to prevent breakdown of the oral mucosa* and check for stomatitis *to detect early signs and avoid treatment delay.*
• Watch for signs of myelosuppression *so precautions can be taken to avoid infection.*
• Encourage increased fluid intake and provide I.V. fluids, a potassium supplement, and diuretics *to prevent renal damage.*

Teaching topics

• Disease process and treatment options
• Preventing and reporting infection
• Managing adverse reactions to chemotherapy and radiation

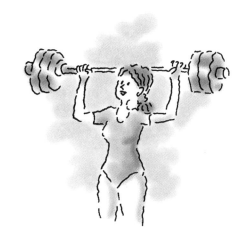

Pump up on practice questions

1. To maintain adequate glomerular filtration, it is most important for a client to have adequate:

   A.   serum albumin and stroke volume.
   B.   oncotic pressure and systemic vascular resistance.
   C.   intravascular volume and cardiac output.
   D.   hydrostatic pressure and fluid intake.

Answer: C. Adequate glomerular filtration requires adequate intravascular volume and cardiac output. The other components have some bearing on renal function but none are of the same importance.

➡ NCLEX keys

Nursing process step: Analysis
Client needs category: Physiological integrity
Client needs subcategory: Physiological adaptation
Taxonomic level: Comprehension

2. A client with fever and urinary urgency is asked to provide a urine specimen for culture and sensitivity. The nurse should instruct the client to collect the specimen from the:

    A. first stream of urine from the bladder.

    B. middle stream of urine from the bladder.

    C. final stream of urine from the bladder.

    D. full volume of urine from the bladder.

Answer: B. The midstream specimen is recommended because it is less likely to be contaminated with microorganisms from the external genitalia than other specimens. It isn't necessary to collect a full volume of urine for a urine culture and sensitivity.

➡ *NCLEX keys*

Nursing process step: Implementation
Client needs category: Physiological integrity
Client needs subcategory: Reduction of risk potential
Taxonomic level: Application

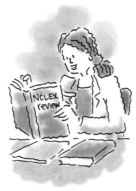

3. A client is diagnosed with cystitis. The nurse recommends the client drink cranberry juice. What assessment parameter should the nurse consider to determine if this recommendation has been effective?

    A. Urine specific gravity

    B. White cell count

    C. pH

    D. Protein

Answer: C. Because cranberry juice is an acid-ash food that lowers the urine pH, monitoring urine pH would be most useful in evaluating the effectiveness of the intervention. The other parameters won't pinpoint the effectiveness of acid-ash food.

➡ *NCLEX keys*

Nursing process step: Evaluation
Client needs category: Physiological integrity
Client needs subcategory: Physiological adaptation
Taxonomic level: Application

4. A client with dysuria is prescribed phenazopyridine (Pyridium). The nurse should teach the client to expect urine to be:

    A. greater in volume.

    B. orange in color.

    C. pungent in odor.

    D. concentrated in consistency.

Answer: B. Phenazopyridine (Pyridium) causes the urine to have an orange color. The other urine characteristics aren't caused by phenazopyridine (Pyridium).

➡ *NCLEX keys*

Nursing process step: Implementation
Client needs category: Physiological integrity
Client needs subcategory: Physiological adaptation
Taxonomic level: Application

5. A client is scheduled for extracorporeal shock wave lithotripsy (ESWL). In teaching the client about ESWL, the nurse should inform the client that the stones will be:

    A. dissolved.

    B. shattered.

    C. radiated.

    D. suctioned.

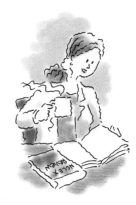

Answer: B. ESWL is a procedure in which the client's kidney stones are shattered or pulverized, not dissolved, radiated, or suctioned.

➡ *NCLEX keys*
Nursing process step: Implementation
Client needs category: Physiological integrity
Client needs subcategory: Physiological adaptation
Taxonomic level: Knowledge

6. The nurse is instructing the client about recommended daily fluid consumption. The nurse would be most helpful by telling the client to drink approximately:
    A. 4 cups per day.
    B. 8 cups per day.
    C. 12 cups per day.
    D. 16 cups per day.
Answer: C. A client with renal calculi should drink 3 L of fluid per day. This would be equivalent to 12 cups.

➡ *NCLEX keys*
Nursing process step: Implementation
Client needs category: Physiological integrity
Client needs subcategory: Reduction of risk potential
Taxonomic level: Application

7. A client with acute renal failure is being assessed to determine if the cause is prerenal, renal, or postrenal. If the cause if prerenal, which condition most likely caused it?
    A. Heart failure
    B. Glomerular nephritis
    C. Ureterolithiasis
    D. Aminoglycoside toxicity
Answer: A. By causing inadequate renal perfusion, heart failure can lead to prerenal failure. Nephritis and aminoglycoside toxicity are renal causes and ureterolithiasis is a postrenal cause.

➡ *NCLEX keys*
Nursing process step: Analysis
Client needs category: Physiological integrity
Client needs subcategory: Physiological adaptation
Taxonomic level: Comprehension

8. A client in acute renal failure becomes severely anemic and the physician prescribes two units of packed red blood cells (RBCs). The nurse should plan to administer each unit:
    A. as quickly as the client can tolerate the infusions.
    B. over 30 minutes to an hour.
    C. between 1 and 3 hours.
    D. up to 4 hours but no longer.
Answer: C. It's standard practice to infuse a unit of packed RBCs over 1 to 3 hours.

➡ *NCLEX keys*
Nursing process step: Planning
Client needs category: Physiological integrity
Client needs subcategory: Pharmacological and parenteral therapies
Taxonomic level: Application

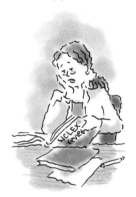

9. The nurse is teaching a client with chronic renal failure about foods to avoid. It would be most accurate for the nurse to teach the client to avoid foods high in:
    A. monosaccharides.
    B. disaccharides.
    C. iron.
    D. protein.
Answer: D. Proteins are typically restricted in clients with chronic renal failure because of their metabolites. Iron and carbohydrates aren't restricted.

➡ *NCLEX keys*
Nursing process step: Implementation
Client needs category: Physiological integrity
Client needs subcategory: Physiological adaptation
Taxonomic level: Comprehension

10. Following a diagnosis of bladder cancer, a client receives local radiation therapy and experiences a dry skin reaction. In recommending care of the skin, the nurse should instruct the client to avoid:

    A.   lubrication.
    B.   cleansers.
    C.   cold packs.
    D.   cotton garments.

Answer: C. Cold packs over the area of a dry reaction to radiation therapy are contraindicated because they reduce capillary circulation to the site and hamper healing. Lubrication, cleansers and cotton garments aren't unconditionally contraindicated.

➡ *NCLEX keys*
Nursing process step: Implementation
Client needs category: Physiological integrity
Client needs subcategory: Reduction of risk potential
Taxonomic level: Application

Ready to study the integumentary system? Meet me on the next page!

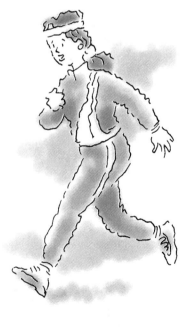

11 Integumentary System

In this chapter, you'll review:

✐ components of the integumentary system and their functions

✐ tests used to diagnose integumentary disorders

✐ common integumentary disorders.

Brush up on key concepts

The skin, hair, and nails make up the integumentary system, which serves as protection for the body's inner organs. It also helps regulate body temperature through the sweat glands.

At any time, you can review the major points of this chapter by consulting the *Cheat sheet* on pages 332 and 333.

Outer defense layer
The **skin** provides the first line of defense against microorganisms. It's composed of three layers:

✌ the **epidermis** (outer layer), which contains keratinocytes and melanocytes

✌ the **dermis** (middle layer), a collagen layer that supports the epidermis, contains nerves and blood vessels, and is the origin of hair, nails, sebaceous glands, eccrine sweat glands, and apocrine sweat glands

✌ the **hypodermis** (third layer), which is composed of loose connective tissue filled with fatty cells and provides heat, insulation, shock absorption, and a reserve of calories (also known as subcutaneous tissue).

Additional protection
Hair also provides protection and coverage for most of the body, with the exception of the palms, lips, soles of the feet, nipples, penis and labia.

Taking care of the tips
The **nails,** protecting the tips of the fingers and toes, are composed of dead cells filled with keratin.

Oil and sweat
The integumentary system also contains three types of glands:
• **sebaceous (oil) glands,** which lubricate hair and the epidermis and are stimulated by sex hormones
• **eccrine sweat glands,** which regulate body temperature through water secretion
• **apocrine sweat glands,** which are located in the axilla, nipple, anal, and pubic areas and secrete odorless fluid. (Decomposition of this fluid by bacteria causes odor.)

Keep abreast of diagnostic tests

Below are the major diagnostic tests for assessing integumentary disorders, as well as common nursing actions associated with each test.

Testing blood for this...
A **blood chemistry test** analyzes a blood sample for potassium, sodium, calcium, phosphorus, ketones, glucose, osmolality, chloride, blood urea nitrogen, and creatinine.

Nursing actions
• Withhold food and fluids before the procedure, as directed.
• Check the venipuncture site for bleeding after the procedure.

...And for that
Hematologic studies analyze a blood sample for red blood cells (RBCs), white blood cells (WBCs), erythrocyte sedimentation rate, platelets, prothrombin time, international normalized ratio, partial thromboplastin time, hemoglobin (Hb), and hematocrit (HCT).

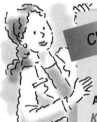

Cheat sheet

Integumentary refresher

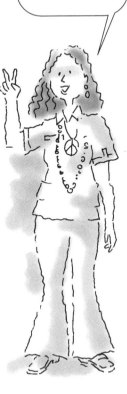

> Hair is groovy. It provides protection and coverage for most of the body.

ATOPIC DERMATITIS

Key signs and symptoms
- Erythematous lesions which eventually become scaly and lichenified
- Excessive dry skin
- Hyperpigmentation
- Skin eruptions

Key test results
- Serum immunoglobulin E levels are often elevated but this finding isn't diagnostic.

Key treatments
- Antihistamines: hydroxyzine (Atarax)
- Corticosteroid ointment, such as hydrocortisone (Dermacort)

Key interventions
- Help the patient set up an individual schedule and plan for daily skin care.
- Instruct the patient to bathe in plain water. (He may have to limit bathing, according to the severity of the lesions.) Tell him to bathe with a special nonfatty soap and tepid water (96° F [35.6° C]), to avoid using any soap when lesions are acutely inflamed, and to limit baths or showers to 5 to 7 minutes.
- For scalp involvement, advise the patient to shampoo frequently and apply corticosteroid solution to the scalp afterward.

BURNS

Key signs and symptoms
- First-degree: erythema, edema, pain, blanching
- Second-degree: pain, oozing, fluid-filled vesicles; erythema; shiny, wet subcutaneous layer after vesicles rupture
- Third-degree: eschar, edema, little or no pain
- Fourth-degree: deeply charred subcutaneous tissue muscle and bone

Key test results
- Visual examination is used to estimate extent of burn (determined by Rule of Nines and Lund and Browder chart).

Key treatments
- I.V. therapy: hydration and electrolyte replacement (I.V. administration is gauged according to the amount of fluid it takes to maintain a urine output of 30 to 50 ml/hour)
- Skin grafts
- Analgesic: morphine
- Antianxiety: lorazepam (Ativan)
- Antibiotic: gentamicin (Garamycin)
- Anti-infectives: mafenide (Sulfamylon), silver sulfadiazine (Silvadene), silver nitrate, povidone-iodine (Betadine)
- Antitetanus: tetanus toxoid
- Colloid: albumin 5% (Albuminar 5%)

Key interventions
- Assess respiratory status.
- Assess fluid status.
- Administer I.V. fluids.
- Administer oxygen.
- Administer total parenteral or enteral feedings.
- Maintain protective precautions.

HERPES ZOSTER

Key signs and symptoms
- Neuralgia
- Severe deep pain
- Unilaterally clustered skin vesicles along peripheral sensory nerves on trunk, thorax, or face

Key test results
- Skin study identifies organism.
- Visual examination shows vesicles along peripheral sensory nerves.

Key treatments
- Analgesics: acetaminophen (Tylenol), codeine
- Antianxiety agents: lorazepam (Ativan), hydroxyzine (Vistaril)
- Antipruritic: diphenhydramine (Benadryl)

Key interventions
- Assess neurologic status.
- Assess pain and note effectiveness of analgesics.
- Prevent scratching and rubbing of affected areas.

Integumentary refresher (continued)

PRESSURE ULCERS

Key signs and symptoms
• Signs determined by stage of ulceration

Key treatments
• High-protein, high-calorie diet in small frequent feedings; parenteral or enteral feedings if the patient is unable or unwilling to take adequate nutrients orally
• Topical wound care according to facility's protocol
• Wound debridement; tissue flap

Key interventions
• Assess skin integrity and watch for signs of infection.
• Check the bedridden patient for possible changes in skin color, turgor, temperature and sensation.
• Reposition the patient every 2 hours.
• Use foam mattress, bed cradle, or other device.
• Provide meticulous skin care and check bony prominences.
• Maintain patient's diet and encourage oral fluid intake.

PSORIASIS

Key signs and symptoms
• Itching
• Lesions (red and usually forming well-defined patches)
• Pustules

Key test results
• Skin biopsy is positive for the disorder.

Key treatments
• Antipsoriatic agents: calcipotriene (Dovonex), anthralin (Antraderm)
• Corticosteroid ointments: hydrocortisone (Dermacort)
• Ultraviolet light to retard cell production; may be used in conjunction with psoralen (PUVA therapy)

Key interventions
• Make sure the patient understands his prescribed therapy; provide written instructions .
• Watch for adverse reactions, especially allergic reactions to anthralin, atrophy and acne from steroids, and burning, itching, nausea, and squamous cell epitheliomas from PUVA therapy.
• Initially evaluate the patient on methotrexate weekly, then monthly for red blood cell, white blood cell, and platelet count. Liver biopsy may be performed.
• Caution the patient receiving PUVA therapy to stay out of the sun on the day of treatment, and to protect his eyes with sunglasses that screen UVA for 24 hours after treatment. Tell him to wear goggles during exposure to this light.

SKIN CANCER

Key signs and symptoms
• Change in color, size, or shape of preexisting lesion
• Irregular, circular bordered lesion with hues of tan, black, or blue (melanoma)
• Small, red, nodular lesion that begins as an erythematous macule or plaque with indistinct margins (squamous cell carcinoma)
• Waxy nodule with telangiectasis (basal cell epithelioma)

Key test results
• Skin biopsy shows cytology positive for cancer cells

Key treatments
• Chemosurgery with zinc chloride
• Cryosurgery with liquid nitrogen
• Curettage and electrodesiccation
• Antimetabolite: fluorouracil (Adrucil)

Key interventions
• Assess lesions.
• Administer medications, as prescribed.
• Provide postchemotherapy and postradiation nursing care.

Nursing actions
• Check the venipuncture site for bleeding after the procedure.

Tissue punch test

A **skin biopsy,** also known as a punch biopsy, uses a circular punch instrument to remove a small amount of skin tissue for histologic evaluation.

Nursing actions
• Make sure that a written, informed consent has been signed.
• Check the site for bleeding and infection.

Allergy exam

Skin testing uses a patch, scratch, or intradermal technique to administer an allergen to the skin's surface or into the dermis. The skin can then be analyzed for reaction.

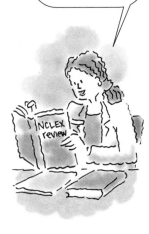

Check it out. Checking the test site for infection and bleeding is a common nursing responsibility with skin tests.

Nursing actions
• Keep the area dry.
• Record the site, date, and time of test.
• Inspect the site for erythema, papules, vesicles, edema, and induration.
• Record the date and time for follow-up site reading.

Scrape and study
A **skin scraping** involves scraping a small sample of skin, nails, or hair for evaluation under a microscope.

Nursing actions
• Check scraping site for bleeding and infection.

Under the microscope
A **skin study** is a microscopic examination of skin that includes gram stain, culture and sensitivity, cytology, and immunofluorescence.

Nursing actions
• Follow laboratory procedure guidelines.
• Note current antibiotic therapy.

UV inspection
Wood's light test uses ultraviolet (UV) light to directly examine the skin.

Nursing actions
Explain the procedure to the patient.

Polish up on patient care

Major integumentary disorders include atopic dermatitis, burns, herpes zoster, pressure ulcers, psoriasis, and skin cancer.

Atopic dermatitis

Atopic dermatitis is a chronic skin disorder characterized by superficial skin inflammation and intense itching. It may also be called atopic eczema or infantile eczema.

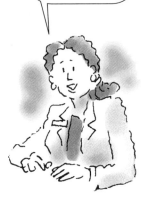

Atopic dermatitis is characterized by intense itching. Scratching the skin intensifies itching, resulting in red, weeping lesions.

Atopic dermatitis may be associated with other atopic diseases, such as bronchial asthma and allergic rhinitis. It usually develops in infants and toddlers between ages 1 month and 1 year, commonly in those with strong family histories of atopic disease. These children often acquire other atopic disorders as they grow older.

Typically, this form of dermatitis flares and subsides repeatedly before finally resolving during adolescence. However, it can persist into adulthood.

CONTRIBUTING FACTORS
• Chemical irritants
• Food allergies
• Genetic predisposition
• Immune dysfunction (possibly linked to elevated serum immunoglobulin E [IgE] levels or defective T-cell function)
• Infections (with *Staphylococcus aureus*)

ASSESSMENT FINDINGS
• Characteristic location of lesions: areas of flexion and extension such as the neck, antecubital fossa (behind the elbow), popliteal folds (posterior surface of the knee), and behind the ears
• Erythematous lesions which eventually become scaly and lichenified
• Excessive dry skin
• Hyperpigmentation
• Skin eruptions

DIAGNOSTIC TEST RESULTS
• Serum IgE levels are often elevated but this finding is not diagnostic.

NURSING DIAGNOSES
• Impaired skin integrity
• Body image disturbance
• Anxiety

TREATMENT
• Washing lesions with water and little soap
• Environmental control of offending allergens

Drug therapy
• Antihistamines: hydroxyzine (Atarax)

• Corticosteroid ointment, such as hydrocortisone (Dermacort)

INTERVENTIONS AND RATIONALES

• Warn that drowsiness is possible with the use of antihistamines to relieve daytime itching *to prevent injury.*
• If nocturnal itching interferes with sleep, suggest methods for inducing natural sleep such as drinking a glass of warm milk *to prevent overuse of sedatives.*
• Antihistamines may also be useful at bedtime *because antihistamines relieve itching and cause drowsiness.*
• Help the patient set up an individual schedule and plan for daily skin care *to help the patient cope with the chronic condition and promote compliance.*
• Instruct the patient to bathe in plain water. (He may have to limit bathing, according to the severity of the lesions.) Tell him to bathe with a special nonfatty soap and tepid water (96° F [35.6° C]), to avoid using any soap when lesions are acutely inflamed, and to limit baths or showers to 5 to 7 minutes. *These measures prevent worsening of condition.*
• For scalp involvement, advise the patient to shampoo frequently and apply corticosteroid solution to the scalp afterward *to improve skin integrity.*
• Keep fingernails short *to limit excoriation and secondary infections caused by scratching.*
• Lubricate the skin after a shower or bath *to prevent excessive dryness.*
• Apply occlusive dressings (such as plastic film) over a corticosteroid cream intermittently as necessary *to help clear lichenified skin.*
• Be careful not to show any anxiety or revulsion when touching the lesions during treatment. Help the patient accept his altered body image, and encourage him to verbalize his feelings. *Coping with disfigurement is extremely difficult, especially for children and adolescents.*

Teaching topics
• Understanding factors that exacerbate the condition (fabric, detergents, stress)
• Skin care

Burns

A burn is the destruction of skin that causes loss of intracellular fluid and electrolytes. A burn is characterized as first-, second-, third-, or fourth-degree depending on the extent (area) and degree (depth) of the burn. Most burns are a combination of degrees.
• A first-degree (superficial partial-thickness) burn involves the epidermal layer.
• A second-degree (dermal partial-thickness) burn involves the epidermal and dermal layers.
• A third-degree (full-thickness) burn involves epidermal, dermal, subcutaneous layers, and nerve endings
• A fourth-degree burn contains damage through deeply charred subcutaneous tissue to muscle and bone.

Number 9...Number 9
The rule of nines is a method used to estimate the size of a burned area. In this method, a person's skin area is divided into several sections, each representing 9 percent (or multiples of 9 percent) of the total body area. By observing the size and location of a burn and assigning the appropriate body percentage, the nurse can roughly determine what percentage of a patient's body has been burned.

Lund and Browder
The Lund and Browder chart is another method of estimating body surface area that's been burned. This method accounts for changes in body proportion that occur with age. Its greater accuracy can be used to help determine a patient's exact fluid replacement requirements after a burn injury.

CAUSES
• Chemical: acids, alkalies, vesicants
• Electrical: lightning, electrical wires
• Mechanical: friction
• Radiation: X-ray, sun, nuclear
• Thermal: flame, frostbite, scald

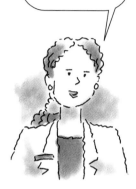

Preventing excessive dryness of the skin is critical in atopic dermatitis — use moisturizers.

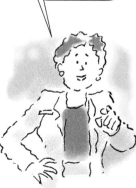

Remember your therapeutic role. Be careful not to show any anxiety or revulsion when looking at a patient with impaired skin integrity.

ASSESSMENT FINDINGS
- First-degree: erythema, edema, pain, blanching
- Second-degree: pain; oozing, fluid-filled vesicles; erythema; shiny, wet subcutaneous layer after vesicles rupture
- Third-degree: eschar, edema, little or no pain
- Fourth-degree: deeply charred subcutaneous tissue, muscle, and bone

DIAGNOSTIC TEST RESULTS
- 24-hour urine collection shows decreased creatinine clearance and negative nitrogen balance.
- Arterial blood gas shows metabolic acidosis.
- Blood chemistry test shows increased potassium level and decreased sodium, albumin, complement fixation, immunoglobulin levels.
- Hematology shows increased Hb and HCT and decreased fibrinogen and platelets and WBC count.
- Urine chemistry shows hematuria and myoglobinuria.
- Visual examination is used to estimate extent of burn (determined by Rule of Nines and Lund and Browder chart).

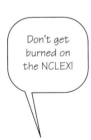

Don't get burned on the NCLEX!

NURSING DIAGNOSES
- Fluid volume deficit
- Pain
- Risk for infection

TREATMENT
- Biological dressings
- Diet high in protein, fat, calories and carbohydrates with small, frequent feedings
- Early excisional therapy
- Escharotomy (surgical excision of burned tissue)
- I.V. therapy: hydration and electrolyte replacement (I.V. administration is gauged according to the amount of fluid it takes to maintain a urine output of 30 to 50 ml/hour)
- Protective isolation to protect patient from infection
- Skin grafts
- Splints to maintain proper joint position and prevent contractures

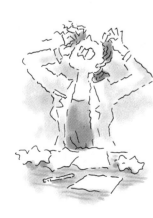

- Transfusion therapy of fresh frozen plasma, platelets, packed RBCs and plasma
- Withholding oral food and fluids until allowed

Drug therapy
- Analgesic: morphine
- Antacids: magnesium and aluminum hydroxide (Maalox), aluminum hydroxide gel (AlternaGEL)
- Antianxiety: lorazepam (Ativan)
- Antibiotic: gentamicin (Garamycin)
- Anti-infectives: mafenide (Sulfamylon), silver sulfadiazine (Silvadene), silver nitrate, povidone-iodine (Betadine)
- Antitetanus: tetanus toxoid
- Colloid: albumin 5% (Albuminar 5%)
- Diuretic: mannitol (Osmitrol)
- Histamine antagonists: cimetidine (Tagamet), ranitidine (Zantac), famotidine (Pepcid), nizatidine (Axid)
- Mucosal barrier fortifier: sucralfate (Carafate)
- Sedative: oxazepam (Serax)
- Vitamins: phytonadione (AquaMEPHYTON), cyanocobalamin (vitamin B_{12})

INTERVENTIONS AND RATIONALES
- Assess respiratory status. *Upper airway injury is common with burns to the face, neck, and chest. Edema may narrow airways.*
- Assess fluid status. *Hypovolemia is indicated by decreasing level of consciousness, urine output less than 30 ml/hour, blood pressure less than 90/60 mm Hg, heart rate greater than 100 beats/minute, dry mucous membranes, and delayed capillary refill.*
- If the patient underwent skin grafting, keep pressure off the donor side *to maintain blood flow to the site and promote wound healing.*
- Monitor for signs of infection *to determine if treatment plan must be altered.*
- Assess effectiveness of pain medication *to promote comfort.*
- Monitor and record vital signs, fluid intake and output, laboratory studies, hemodynamic variables, stool for occult blood, specific gravity, calorie count, daily weight, neurovascular checks, and pulse *to detect complications.*
- Assess bowel sounds *to determine motility of GI tract.*

- Administer I.V. fluids *to maintain hydration and replace fluid loss.*
- Administer oxygen *to meet cellular demands.*
- Provide suctioning; assist with turning, coughing, and deep breathing; perform chest physiotherapy and postural drainage *to maintain patent airway.*
- Maintain position, patency, and low suction of nasogastric tube *to prevent vomiting.*
- Administer total parenteral nutrition or enteral feedings *to meet the patient's increased metabolic demands.*
- Administer medications, as prescribed, *to maintain or improve patient's condition.*
- Encourage the patient to express feelings about disfigurement, immobility from scarring, and a fear of dying *to encourage coping mechanisms.*
- Provide treatments: range-of-motion (ROM) exercises, Hubbard tank (for immersing the patient), bed cradle, splints, and Jobst clothing *to maintain ROM and prevent complications.*
- Elevate affected extremities *to promote venous drainage and decrease edema.*
- Maintain a warm environment during acute period *because the patient is unable to regulate body temperature.*
- Maintain protective precautions *to prevent transmission of infection to the patient.*
- Provide skin and mouth care *to promote comfort.*

Teaching topics
- Following dietary recommendations and restrictions
- Avoiding restrictive clothing
- Using splints and Jobst clothing
- Contacting community agencies and resources

Herpes zoster

Herpes zoster, also known as shingles, is an acute viral infection of nerve structures caused by varicella zoster; affected areas include the spinal and cranial sensory ganglia and posterior gray matter of the spinal cord. Herpes zoster produces localized vesicular skin lesions confined to a dermatome and severe neurologic pain in peripheral areas innervated by nerves arising in the inflamed root ganglia.

CAUSES
- Cytotoxic drug-induced immunosuppression
- Debilitating disease
- Exposure to varicella zoster
- Hodgkin's disease

ASSESSMENT FINDINGS
- Anorexia
- Edematous skin
- Erythema
- Fever
- Headache
- Malaise
- Neuralgia
- Paresthesia
- Pruritus
- Severe deep pain
- Unilaterally clustered skin vesicles along peripheral sensory nerves on trunk, thorax, or face

DIAGNOSTIC TEST RESULTS
- Skin study identifies organism.
- Visual examination shows vesicles along peripheral sensory nerves.

NURSING DIAGNOSES
- Pain
- Risk for infection
- Impaired skin integrity

TREATMENT
- No specific treatment; primary goal is to relieve itching and pain

Drug therapy
- Analgesics: acetaminophen (Tylenol), codeine
- Antianxiety agents: lorazepam (Ativan), hydroxyzine (Vistaril)
- Antipruritic: diphenhydramine (Benadryl)
- Antiviral agents: acyclovir (Zovirax), famciclovir (Famvir), valacyclovir (Valtrex)
- Nerve block using lidocaine (Xylocaine)

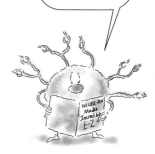

Each nerve emanates from the spine and sends signals to a skin area called a dermatome.

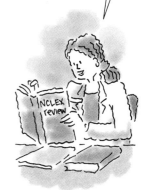

Chickenpox-like vesicles are the key sign of herpes zoster.

INTERVENTIONS AND RATIONALES

• Assess neurologic status *to determine baseline and detect changes.*
• Assess pain and note effectiveness of analgesics *to promote comfort and evaluate the need for a change in the current treatment plan.*
• Monitor and record vital signs, laboratory results, and cranial nerve function *to assess baseline and detect changes.*
• Administer medications, as directed, *to maintain or improve patient's condition.*
• Encourage the patient to express feelings about changes in physical appearance and recurrent nature of the illness *to help patient adapt to illness.*
• Prevent scratching and rubbing of affected areas *to prevent infection.*

Teaching topics

• Recognizing the signs and symptoms of hearing loss
• Avoiding wool and synthetic clothing
• Wearing lightweight, loose cotton clothing
• Keeping blisters intact

Pressure ulcers

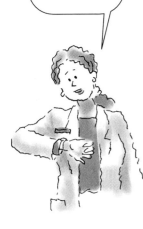

Every 2 hours: that's how often you need to reposition patients to avoid pressure ulcers.

Pressure ulcers are localized areas of cellular necrosis that occur most often in skin and subcutaneous tissue over bony prominences. These ulcers may be superficial, caused by local skin irritation with subsequent surface maceration, or deep, originating in underlying tissue. Deep lesions often go undetected until they penetrate the skin, but by then, they've usually caused subcutaneous damage.

CAUSES

• Pressure, particularly over bony prominences

ASSESSMENT FINDINGS

Signs and symptoms of pressure ulcers occur in four stages.

Stage 1

• Nonblanchable erythema of intact skin
• Skin discoloration
• Warmth and hardness

Stage 2

• Abrasion
• Blister
• Partial-thickness skin loss involving the epidermis and dermis
• Shallow crater

Stage 3

• Deep crater with or without undermining of adjacent tissue
• Full-thickness skin loss involving damage or necrosis of subcutaneous tissue that may extend down to, but not through, underlying fascia

Stage 4

• Damage to muscle, bone, tendon, or joint
• Full-thickness skin loss with extensive destruction
• Tissue necrosis

DIAGNOSTIC TEST RESULTS

• Visual inspection reveals pressure ulcer.
• Wound culture and sensitivity identify infecting organism.

NURSING DIAGNOSES

• Impaired physical mobility
• Altered nutrition: Less than body requirements
• Impaired skin integrity

TREATMENT

• High-protein, high-calorie diet in small frequent feedings; parenteral or enteral feedings if the patient is unable or unwilling to take adequate nutrients orally
• Topical wound care according to facility's protocol
• Wound debridement; tissue flap

INTERVENTIONS AND RATIONALES

• Assess skin integrity and watch for signs of infection *to detect complications.*
• Check the bedridden patient for possible changes in skin color, turgor, temperature and sensation *to prevent further skin breakdown.*
• Reposition the patient every 2 hours *to prevent pressure ulcers.*

• Use foam mattress, bed cradle, or other device *to avoid skin breakdown.*
• Provide meticulous skin care and check bony prominences *to reduce chances of pressure ulcer development.*
• Maintain patient's diet and encourage oral fluid intake *to promote wound healing.*
• Provide wound care *to promote healing.*
• Provide ROM exercises *to promote joint mobility.*

Teaching topics
• Avoiding prolonged periods of immobility
• Performing meticulous skin care
• Changing positions frequently when bedridden
• Recognizing the signs of skin breakdown
• Recognizing the signs and symptoms of infection

Psoriasis

This chronic, recurrent disease is marked by epidermal proliferation. Lesions appear as erythematous papules and plaques covered with silver scales and vary widely in severity and distribution.

Although this disorder often affects young adults, it may strike at any age, including infancy. Psoriasis is characterized by recurring partial remissions and exacerbations.

CAUSES
• Genetic predisposition

ASSESSMENT FINDINGS
• Arthritic symptoms
• Characteristic location of lesions: scalp, chest, elbows, knees, back, buttocks
• Itching
• Lesions (red and usually forming well-defined patches)
• Pain
• Patches, consisting of silver scales that flake off or thicken and cover the lesions
• Pustules

DIAGNOSTIC TEST RESULTS
• Skin biopsy is positive for the disorder.

• Blood studies reveal elevated serum uric acid level in severe cases, due to accelerated nucleic acid degradation, but indications of gout are absent.

NURSING DIAGNOSES
• Impaired skin integrity
• Risk for infection
• Body image disturbance

TREATMENT
• Tar, wet dressings, or oatmeal baths
• UV light to retard cell production; may be used in conjuction with psoralen (PUVA therapy)

Drug therapy
• Corticosteroid ointments, such as hydrocortisone (Dermacort)
• Corticosteroid: intralesional steroid injections
• Antipsoriatic agents: calcipotriene (Dovonex), anthralin (Antraderm)
• Anti-hypocalcemic agent: (Rocaltrol)
• Antineoplastic agent: methotrexate (Mexate)

INTERVENTIONS AND RATIONALES
• Make sure the patient understands his prescribed therapy; provide written instructions *to promote compliance and avoid confusion.*
• Watch for adverse reactions, especially allergic reactions to anthralin, atrophy and acne from steroids, and burning, itching, nausea, and squamous cell epitheliomas from PUVA *to prevent complications.*
• Initially evaluate the patient on methotrexate weekly, then monthly for red blood cell, white blood cell, and platelet counts *because cytotoxins may cause hepatic or bone marrow toxicity.* Liver biopsy may be done *to assess the effects of methotrexate.*
• Caution the patient receiving PUVA therapy to stay out of the sun on the day of treatment, and to protect his eyes with sunglasses that screen UVA for 24 hours after treatment. Tell him to wear goggles during exposure to this light. *These measures protect the patient from injury caused by excessive UVA exposure.*
• Be aware that psoriasis can cause psychological problems. Assure the patient that psoriasis is not contagious, and although exacer-

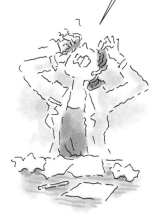

Flare-ups of psoriasis are often related to specific factors, such as stress.

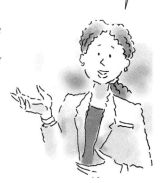

Psoriasis is marked by epidermal proliferation; the skin's outermost layer becomes overgrown.

bations and remissions occur, they're controllable with treatment. However, be sure he understands there is no cure. *Appropriate teaching helps the patient develop healthy coping strategies*
• Help the patient learn to cope with stressful situations *because stressful situations tend to exacerbate psoriasis.*

Teaching topics
• Correctly applying prescribed ointments, creams, and lotions; a steroid cream, for example, should be applied in a thin film and rubbed gently into the skin until the cream disappears
• Avoiding occlusive dressings over anthralin
• Using mineral oil, then soap and water, to remove anthralin.
• Avoiding scrubbing his skin vigorously.
• Using a soft brush to remove scales.
• Contacting the National Psoriasis Foundation

Skin cancer

Skin cancer is a malignant primary tumor of the skin. There are three types:
• Basal cell epithelioma is a tumor often caused by prolonged exposure to the sun.
• Melanoma is a neoplasm that arises from melanocytes. Melanoma spreads through the lymph and vascular systems and metastasizes to the lymph nodes, skin, liver, lungs, and central nervous system.
• Squamous cell carcinoma is a slow-growing cancer causing airway obstruction, cough, and sputum production.

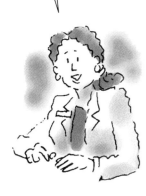

Remember: a change in color, size, or shape of a skin lesion may indicate a cancerous growth.

CAUSES
• Chemical irritants
• Friction or chronic irritation
• Heredity
• Immunosuppressive drugs
• Infrared heat or light
• Precancerous lesions: leukoplakia, nevi, senile keratoses
• Radiation
• UV rays

ASSESSMENT FINDINGS
• Change in color, size, or shape of preexisting lesion
• Irregular, circular bordered lesion with hues of tan, black, or blue (melanoma)
• Local soreness
• Oozing, bleeding, crusting lesion
• Pruritus
• Small, red, nodular lesion that begins as an erythematous macule or plaque with indistinct margins (squamous cell carcinoma)
• Waxy nodule with telangiectasis (basal cell epithelioma)

DIAGNOSTIC TEST RESULTS
• Skin biopsy shows cytology positive for cancer cells.

NURSING DIAGNOSES
• Anxiety
• Body image disturbance
• Altered oral mucous membrane

TREATMENT
• Chemosurgery with zinc chloride
• Cryosurgery with liquid nitrogen
• Curettage and electrodesiccation
• Radiation therapy

Drug therapy
• Alkylating agents: carmustine (BiCNU), dacarbazine (DTIC-Dome)
• Antiemetics: prochlorperazine (Compazine), ondansetron (Zofran)
• Antimetabolite: fluorouracil (Adrucil)
• Antineoplastics: hydroxyurea (Hydrea), vincristine sulfate (Oncovin)
• Immunotherapy for melanoma: bacille Calmette-Guérin (BCG) vaccine

INTERVENTIONS AND RATIONALES
• Monitor skin punch biopsy site *for bleeding.*
• Assess lesions. *Regular assessment prevents recurrence.*
• Monitor and record vital signs *to determine baseline and detect changes.*
• Administer medications, as prescribed, *to maintain and improve patient's condition.*
• Encourage the patient to express feelings about changes in body image and a fear of dy-

ing *to help patient accept changes in body image*.

• Provide postchemotherapy and postradiation nursing care *to promote healing*.

Teaching topics
• Avoiding contact with chemical irritants
• Using sun block and layered clothing when outdoors
• Self-monitoring for lesions and moles that don't heal or that change characteristics
• Removing moles that are subject to chronic irritation
• Contacting the Skin Cancer Foundation
• Contacting community agencies and resources

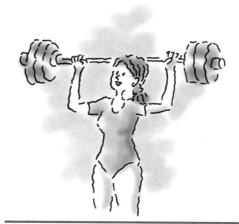

Pump up on practice questions

1. A client experiences problems in body temperature regulation associated with a skin impairment. Most likely, which gland is involved?
    A. Eccrine
    B. Sebaceous
    C. Apocrine
    D. Endocrine
Answer: A. Eccrine glands are associated with body temperature regulation; sebaceous glands lubricate the skin and hair; and apocrine glands are involved in bacteria decomposition. Endocrine glands are a group of glands that secrete hormones responsible for the regulation of body processes such as metabolism and glucose regulation.

➡ *NCLEX keys*
Nursing process step: Analysis
Client needs category: Physiological integrity
Client needs subcategory: Physiological adaptation
Taxonomic level: Comprehension

2. A client undergoes a circular skin punch to confirm a diagnosis of skin cancer. Immediately following the procedure, the nurse should observe the site for:
    A. infection.
    B. dehiscence.
    C. hemorrhage.
    D. swelling.

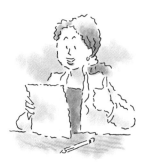

Answer: C. The nurse's main concern following a circular skin punch procedure is to monitor for bleeding. Dehiscence is more likely in larger wounds such as surgical wounds of the abdomen or thorax. Infection is a later possible consequence of a skin punch and swelling is a normal reaction associated with any event that traumatizes the skin.

➡ NCLEX keys
Nursing process step: Implementation
Client needs category: Physiological integrity
Client needs subcategory: Reduction of risk potential
Taxonomic level: Application

3. A client undergoes hypersensitivity testing with the intradermal technique. When the nurse administers the allergen, what should the angle of the needle be?
   A. 0 degrees
   B. 15 degrees
   C. 45 degrees
   D. 90 degrees
Answer: B. The proper angle for intradermal injections is 15 degrees. There are no injections requiring a 0 degree insertion. The subcutaneous angle is 45 degrees and the intramuscular is 90 degrees.

➡ NCLEX keys
Nursing process step: Implementation
Client needs category: Health promotion and maintenance
Client needs subcategory: Prevention and detection of disease
Taxonomic level: Application

4. The nurse is caring for a client admitted with severe burns. The best approach for preventing hypovolemic shock in a client with severe burns is to:
   A. administer dopamine.
   B. apply medical antishock trousers.
   C. infuse I.V. fluids.
   D. infuse fresh frozen plasma.
Answer: C. During the early postburn period, large amounts of plasma fluid extravasates into interstitial spaces. Restoring the fluid loss is necessary to prevent hypovolemic shock; this is best accomplished with crystalloid and colloid solutions. Fresh frozen plasma is expensive and carries the slight risk of disease transmission. Medical antishock trousers would be applied to treat, not prevent shock. Dopamine causes vasoconstriction and elevates blood pressure but it does not prevent hypovolemia in burn clients.

➡ NCLEX keys
Nursing process step: Implementation
Client needs category: Physiological integrity
Client needs subcategory: Physiological adaption
Taxonomic level: Application

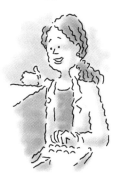

5. The Wood's light would be used during which phases of the nursing process?
   A. Assessment and implementation
   B. Planning and implementation
   C. Diagnosis and implementation
   D. Assessment and evaluation
Answer: D. The Wood's light is used to assess for certain skin conditions and to evaluate the

treatment of those conditions. It's a diagnostic tool, not a treatment device.

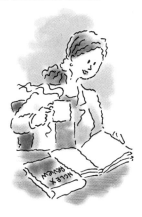

➡ NCLEX keys
Nursing process step: Assessment, Evaluation
Client needs category: Health promotion and maintenance
Client needs subcategory: Prevention and early detection of disease
Taxonomic level: Comprehension

6. The skin lesions evident in herpes zoster are similar to those seen in:
  A. impetigo.
  B. syphilis.
  C. varicella.
  D. rubella.
Answer: C. Varicella (chickenpox) characteristically has vesicles as the hallmark lesion. Impetigo has pustules. Syphilis's primary lesion is the chancre and in rubella the lesion is a maculopapular rash.

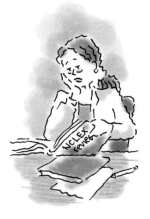

➡ NCLEX keys
Nursing process step: Assessment
Client needs category: Physiological integrity
Client needs subcategory: Physiological adaptation
Taxonomic level: Comprehension

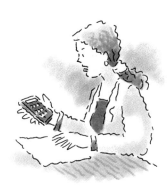

7. A client with widespread herpes zoster is placed on I.V. hydrocortisone (Solu-Cortef). The nurse should be aware that the drug can cause an elevation of which serum chemistry value?
  A. Potassium
  B. Calcium
  C. Glucose
  D. Magnesium
Answer: C. Corticosteroids are known to elevate the blood glucose level and tend to lower serum potassium and calcium levels. Their effect on magnesium isn't substantial.

➡ NCLEX keys
Nursing process step: Assessment
Client needs category: Physiological integrity
Client needs subcategory: Pharmacological and parenteral therapies
Taxonomic level: Comprehension

8. A client is admitted to a burn intensive care unit with extensive full-thickness burns. The nurse is most concerned about the client's:

    A. fluid status.
    B. risk for infection.
    C. body image
    D. level of pain.

Answer: A. In early burn care, the client's greatest need has to do with fluid resuscitation because of large-volume fluid loss through the damaged skin. Infection, body image, and pain are certainly great concerns in the nursing care of a burn client, but are less urgent than fluid management in the early phase of burn care.

➥ *NCLEX keys*
Nursing process step: Analysis
Client needs category: Physiological integrity
Client needs subcategory: Physiological adaptation
Taxonomic level: Analysis

9. Deep partial-thickness burn wounds are characterized by:

    A. erythema.
    B. blanching.
    C. eschar.
    D. fluid-filled vesicles.

Answer: D. Deep partial-thickness skin destruction (also referred to as second-degree burns) is characterized by fluid-filled vesicles. Erythema and blanching on pressure are characteristic of partial-thickness skin destruction. Eschar is a manifestation of full-thickness skin destruction.

➥ *NCLEX keys*
Nursing process step: Assessment
Client needs category: Physiological integrity
Client needs subcategory: Physiological adaptation
Taxonomic level: Knowledge

10. The nurse is caring for a client with a new donor site that was harvested to treat a burn. The nurse should position the patient to:

    A. allow ventilation of the site.
    B. make the site dependent.
    C. avoid pressure on the site.
    D. keep the site fully covered.

Answer: C. A universal concern in the care of donor sites for burn care is to keep the site away from sources of pressure. Ventilation of the site and keeping the site fully covered are practices in some institutions but aren't hallmarks of donor site care. Placing the site in a position of dependence isn't a justified aspect of donor site care.

➥ *NCLEX keys*
Nursing process step: Implementation
Client needs category: Physiological integrity
Client needs subcategory: Physiological adaptation
Taxonomic level: Application

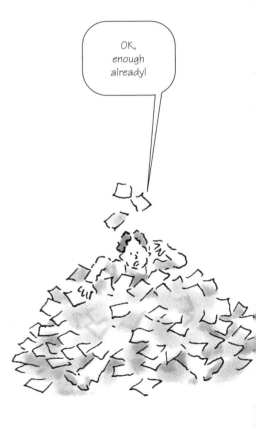

OK, enough already!

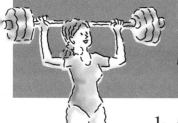

Pump up on more practice questions

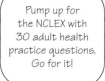

Pump up for the NCLEX with 30 adult health practice questions. Go for it!

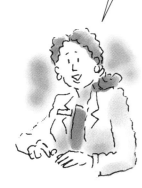

1. A client experiences abdominal pain and exhibits blood in his stools and emesis. He is scheduled to undergo several diagnostic tests. It isn't necessary for the nurse to withhold all food from the client if he's scheduled for:

A. an endoscopy.
B. a fecal occult blood test.
C. an endoscopic retrograde cholangiopancreatography.
D. a barium swallow.

Answer: B. The client may eat normally when a fecal occult blood test is scheduled; however, for endoscopic tests, an upper GI series, or a barium swallow, the client should take nothing by mouth before the test.

➡ *NCLEX keys*
Nursing process step: Planning
Client needs category: Physiological integrity
Client needs subcategory: Reduction of risk potential
Taxonomic level: Application

2. The nurse is providing patient teaching for a client with hiatal hernia. The nurse asks the client which foods he regularly consumes. What answer would indicate the need for more teaching on this topic?

A. Milk products
B. Small meals
C. Fatty foods
D. Soft drinks

Answer: D. Carbonated beverages stimulate belching and gastric reflux causing lower esophageal irritation and associated pain of hiatal hernia. Milk products, fatty foods, and small meals aren't prohibited with hiatal hernia.

➡ *NCLEX keys*
Nursing process step: Analysis
Client needs category: Physiological integrity
Client needs subcategory: Reduction of risk potential
Taxonomic level: Analysis

3. A client experiences an exacerbation of ulcerative colitis. Test results reveal elevated serum osmolality and urine specific gravity. What is the most likely explanation for these test results?

A. Renal insufficiency
B. Hypoaldosteronism
C. Diabetes insipidus
D. Fluid volume deficit

Answer: D. Ulcerative colitis causes watery diarrhea. The client will lose large volumes of fluid causing hemoconcentration and an elevated serum osmolality and urine specific gravity. Renal insufficiency, hypoaldosteronism and diabetes insipidus aren't associated with ulcerative colitis.

➡ *NCLEX keys*
Nursing process step: Analysis
Client needs category: Physiological integrity
Client needs subcategory: Reduction of risk potential
Taxonomic level: Analysis

4. A client with regional enteritis asks her nurse which food she should eat. What should the nurse recommend?

A. Celery
B. Peanut butter
C. Honey
D. Fudge

Answer: C. The dietary recommendations for regional enteritis are a diet high in protein, carbohydrates and calories and low in fat, residue, and fiber. Honey is a high calorie carbohydrate. Celery isn't recommended because it's high in residue and fiber. Peanut butter isn't recommended because it's high in fat. Fudge is typically high fat and shouldn't be recommended.

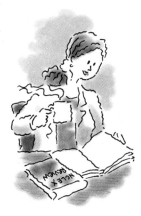

→ NCLEX keys

Nursing process step: Implementation
Client needs category: Physiological integrity
Client needs subcategory: Reduction of risk potential
Taxonomic level: Application

5. A client is diagnosed with acute diverticulitis. He is prescribed gentamicin I.V. (Garamycin). When administering gentamicin, the nurse should expect to give it:
    A.   I.V. push over 1 minute.
    B.   I.V. push over 2 minutes.
    C.   I.V. piggy back over 15 to 20 minutes.
    D.   I.V. piggy back over 30 to 60 minutes.

Answer: D. Because of the risk for nephrotoxicity, aminoglycosides such as gentamycin should be administered slowly by intermittent infusion. The recommended length of time for administration is 30 to 60 minutes. I.V. boluses or pushes should be avoided.

→ NCLEX keys

Nursing process step: Implementation
Client needs category: Physiological integrity
Client needs subcategory: Pharmacological and parenteral therapies
Taxonomic level: Application

6. A client develops hepatic cirrhosis. Laboratory tests reveal an elevated prothrombin time. Which clinical finding should the nurse expect?
    A.   Edema
    B.   Jaundice
    C.   Pruritus
    D.   Ecchymosis

Answer: D. Ecchymosis is a manifestation of a coagulation problem, which could be evidenced when prothrombin time is elevated. Edema, jaundice, and pruritus, all manifestations of hepatic cirrhosis, aren't related to abnormal prothrombin time.

→ NCLEX keys

Nursing process step: Analysis
Client needs category: Physiological integrity
Client needs subcategory: Reduction of risk potential
Taxonomic level: Comprehension

7. The nurse is seeking to meet the nutritional needs of a client with acute peritonitis. The nurse should administer:
    A.   nasal enteral feedings.
    B.   gastric enteral feedings.
    C.   oral feedings.
    D.   parenteral feedings.

Answer: D. To avoid introduction of nutritional products into the abdominal cavity through a perforation of the GI tract, the client with peritonitis is typically fed by way of the parenteral route either with total parenteral nutrition or peripheral parenteral nutrition. Feedings via a nasal cannula, gastric tube, or the oral route are avoided.

→ NCLEX keys

Nursing process step: Planning
Client needs category: Physiological integrity
Client needs subcategory: Pharmacological and parenteral therapies
Taxonomic level: Application

8. The nurse is providing discharge teaching to a client with pancreatitis. The nurse and client are discussing hyperglycemia. Which of the following symptoms is the nurse most likely to bring up in her discussion?
    A.   Thirst
    B.   Oliguria
    C.   Weight gain
    D.   Loss of appetite

Answer: A. One of the classic manifestations of hyperglycemia is polydipsia which is extreme thirst. In hyperglycemia, the expectation is polyuria rather than oliguria. Most typically weight loss is a manifestation of hyperglycemia because the cells are not being nourished due to a lack of insulin. In hyperglycemia, the client typically experiences hunger rather than a loss of appetite.

→ NCLEX keys

Nursing process step: Implementation
Client needs category: Physiological integrity
Client needs subcategory: Reduction of risk potential
Taxonomic level: Knowledge

9. Following an arteriogram for a suspected abdominal aortic aneurysm, a client reports itching skin. The nurse notes red blotches on the client's trunk. How should the nurse respond initially?

    A. Notify the physician.
    B. Administer an antihistamine.
    C. Check the vital functions.
    D. Plan to monitor finding closely.

Answer: C. An arteriogram involves administration of a radiopaque dye. Some clients are hypersensitive to the dye and exhibit related manifestations or pruritus and urticaria. More severe manifestations can occur including hypotension and dyspnea. Therefore, it's important to initially monitor vital functions. The other choices have a lesser priority.

➡ *NCLEX keys*
Nursing process step: Implementation
Client needs category: Physiological integrity
Client needs subcategory: Physiological adaptation
Taxonomic level: Application

10. A client develops recurrent urolithiasis. What mineral will most likely be restricted in the client's diet?

    A. Phosphorus
    B. Calcium
    C. Magnesium
    D. Sodium

Answer: B. Renal stones are often heavily composed of calcium; therefore, calcium-restricted diets will be prescribed in recurrent urolithiasis. The other minerals listed aren't typically restricted in the diet of the client with urolithiasis.

➡ *NCLEX keys*
Nursing process step: Implementation
Client needs category: Physiological integrity
Client needs subcategory: Reduction of risk potential
Taxonomic level: Application

11. A client diagnosed with cardiogenic shock is in the oliguric phase of acute renal failure. What laboratory test findings should the nurse anticipate?

    A. Low blood urea nitrogen (BUN), low creatinine, and high potassium
    B. High BUN, high creatinine, and low potassium
    C. High BUN, high creatinine, and high potassium
    D. Low BUN, low creatinine, and low potassium

Answer: B. During the oliguric phase of acute renal failure, the client is producing a lot of urine and losing potassium. However, the client does not excrete the metabolites that are expressed in BUN and creatinine levels. Therefore, the expected results include elevated BUN and creatinine levels and a subnormal potassium level.

➡ *NCLEX keys*
Nursing process step: Assessment
Client needs category: Physiological integrity
Client needs subcategory: Physiological adaptation
Taxonomic level: Knowledge

12. A 26-year-old client with chronic renal failure plans to receive a kidney transplant. Recently, the physician told the client he is a poor candidate for transplant because of chronic uncontrolled hypertension and diabetes mellitus. Now, the client tells the nurse, "I want to go off dialysis. I'd rather not live than be on this treatment for the rest of my life." How should the nurse respond?

    A. "We all have days when we don't feel like going on."
    B. "You're feeling upset about the news you got about the transplant."
    C. "The treatments are only three times a week. You can live with that."
    D. "Whatever decision you make, we will support you."

Answer: B. In reflecting the client's implied feelings, the nurse is promoting communication. Using platitudes such as "We all have days when we don't feel like going on" fails to address the individual client's needs. Reminding the client of the treatment frequency isn't addressing the client's need. Offering support is therapeutic but doesn't address the client's expressed need to discuss the decision to go off dialysis.

➡ *NCLEX keys*
Nursing process step: Implementation
Client needs category: Psychosocial integrity
Client needs subcategory: Coping and adaptation
Taxonomic level: Application

13. A client experiences urinary retention from benign prostatic hyperplasia and undergoes a transurethral resection of the prostate. Following the procedure, the client receives continuous bladder irrigation. The nurse notices that the drainage from the catheter has stopped. How should the nurse respond?
- A. Replace the existing catheter.
- B. Increase the infusion rate.
- C. Attempt to dislodge a clot.
- D. Notify the urologist.

Answer: C. Most likely, the apparatus is blocked by a blood clot, which the nurse may remove by either gentle aspiration of the clot from the catheter or irrigation through the out-port. It's probably unnecessary to replace the apparatus. Increasing the flow may cause bladder distention and pain. Calling the physician isn't an appropriate initial nursing response because the nurse has the autonomy to solve this problem without calling the physician first.

➡ *NCLEX keys*
Nursing process step: Implementation
Client needs category: Physiological integrity
Client needs subcategory: Physiological adaptation
Taxonomic level: Application

14. A nurse is conducting a screening clinic. A client visits the clinic to be screened for prostatic cancer. Which laboratory measure is used to screen for prostatic cancer?
- A. Creatinine kinase (CK)
- B. Aspartate aminotransferase (AST)
- C. Blood urea nitrogen (BUN)
- D. Prostate-specific antigen (PSA)

Answer: D. PSA measurement is widely used as a screening test for prostatic cancer. CK measurement is most associated with myocardial damage, the AST measurement provides information about liver damage and BUN measurement provides information about kidney function.

➡ *NCLEX keys*
Nursing process step: Assessment
Client needs category: Health promotion and maintenance
Client needs subcategory: Prevention and early detection of disease
Taxonomic level: Knowledge

15. The nurse is instructing a client regarding skin tests for hypersensitivity reactions. The nurse should teach the client to:
- A. keep skin test areas moist with a mild lotion.
- B. stay out of direct sunlight until tests are read.
- C. wash the sites daily with a mild soap.
- D. have the sites read on the correct date.

Answer: D. An important facet of evaluating skin tests is to read the skin test results at the proper time. Evaluating the skin test too late or too early will give inaccurate and unreliable results. The sites should be kept dry. There is no requirement to wash the sites with soap, and direct sunlight isn't prohibited.

➡ *NCLEX keys*
Nursing process step: Implementation
Client needs category: Health promotion and maintenance
Client needs subcategory: Prevention and early detection of disease
Taxonomic level: Application

16. A client is admitted to the hospital with an acute exacerbation of asthma. Auscultation reveals almost absent breath sounds. Thirty minutes after administering albuterol by nebulizer, the nurse auscultates diffuse inspiratory and expiratory wheezes throughout all lung fields. This finding most likely represents:
- A. increased airflow.
- B. no change in airflow
- C. decreased airflow.
- D. no correlation with airflow.

Answer: A. Changes in breath sounds provide a general indication of response to treatment.

Nearly absent breath sounds or no breath sounds indicate severe airflow obstruction. A noisy chest is a sign that air is flowing through the air passages even though they are partially obstructed.

➡ *NCLEX keys*

Nursing process step: Assessment
Client needs category: Physiological integrity
Client needs subcategory: Physiological adaptation
Taxonomic level: Application

17. A client is scheduled to perform a 24-hour urine test beginning at 8:00 a.m. on the first day and ending at 8:00 a.m. on the second day. The nurse should instruct the client to:

   A. discard the second-day 8:00 a.m. sample.
   B. discard the first and last samples.
   C. discard the first-day 8:00 a.m. sample.
   D. retain all samples collected.

Answer: C. In a 24-hour urine test, the first sample is discarded and the last sample is retained.

➡ *NCLEX keys*

Nursing process step: Implementation
Client needs category: Health promotion and maintenance
Client needs subcategory: Prevention and early detection of disease
Taxonomic level: Application

18. The nurse is planning to administer levothyroxine (Synthroid) to an adult client. Which vital signs measurements indicate that the nurse should consider withholding the dose and consulting the physician?

   A. Temperature 97.8° F (36.6° C), pulse 88 beats/minute, respirations 22 breaths/minute, blood pressure 110/70 mm Hg
   B. Temperature 98.4° F (36.9° C), pulse 54 beats/minute, respirations 16 breaths/minute, blood pressure 100/56 mm Hg
   C. Temperature 99.0° F (37.2° C), pulse 110 beats/minute, respirations 20 breaths/minute, blood pressure 136/88 mm Hg
   D. Temperature 98.8° F (37.1°C), pulse 72 beats/minute, respirations 12 breaths/minute, blood pressure 118/72 mm Hg

Answer: C. Levothyroxine can cause tachycardia, indicated here by a pulse rate of 110 beats/minute. Tachycardia is an indication of thyroid toxicity.

➡ *NCLEX keys*

Nursing process step: Planning
Client needs category: Physiological integrity
Client needs subcategory: Pharmacological and parenteral therapies
Taxonomic level: Application

19. A client is receiving treatment for Cushing's syndrome. A reduction in which laboratory measurement would provide an indication that treatment is successful?

   A. Serum potassium levels
   B. Urine sodium levels
   C. Gastric pH
   D. Serum glucose levels

Answer: D. Cushing's syndrome causes hyperglycemia, which may require exogenous insulin administration. Since Cushing's syndrome causes hypokalemia and hypernatremia, a drop in serum potassium and urine sodium levels wouldn't indicate improvement. Cushing's syndrome causes increased gastric acid secretion so a reduction in gastric pH wouldn't be a desired finding.

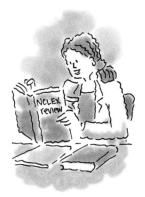

➡ *NCLEX keys*

Nursing process step: Evaluation
Client needs category: Physiological integrity
Client needs subcategory: Physiological adaptation
Taxonomic level: Analysis

20. A client scheduled for a gastroscopy has had nothing by mouth since midnight. The procedure is scheduled for 8:00 a.m. At 6:30 a.m., the nurse collects a capillary blood glucose sample that registers 40 mg/dl on the glucose monitor. The client is alert, has clear speech, and states, "I don't feel like my sugar is too low." Initially the nurse should:

A. document the finding and withhold the client's morning insulin.
B. repeat the capillary blood glucose test.
C. give the client an oral simple sugar.
D. administer dextrose 50 g I.V. immediately.

Answer: B. Because the client is asymptomatic for hypoglycemia yet the capillary blood glucose reading is significantly subnormal, an error may have occurred in obtaining the result. The nurse should repeat the test. Because the blood glucose reading is so low, responding to the reading has precedence over documenting findings. Because of the inconsistency between the 40 mg/dl reading and the absence of symptoms, rechecking the value should precede administering glucose.

➡ *NCLEX keys*
Nursing process step: Planning
Client needs category: Physiological integrity
Client needs subcategory: Physiological adaptation
Taxonomic level: Application

21. A client with systemic lupus erythematosus, who receives immunosuppressive drugs, develops a fever. The nurse should:
A. administer prescribed antipyretics.
B. place the client in isolation.
C. apply cooling measures immediately.
D. help identify the cause.

Answer: D. Immunosuppressive drugs impair the client's immunocompetence and predispose him to infection. Fever is a manifestation of infection; therefore, it is most important to discover the cause of the fever as soon as possible. Antipyretics should be withheld until cultures have been obtained. Isolation isn't indicated unless the absolute neutrophil count is less than 1,000. Cooling measures may be indicated but don't have priority over organism identification.

➡ *NCLEX keys*
Nursing process step: Planning
Client needs category: Physiological integrity
Client needs subcategory: Reduction of risk potential
Taxonomic level: Application

22. Which clinical finding distinguishes rheumatoid arthritis from osteoarthritis and gouty arthritis?
A. Crepitus with range of motion
B. Symmetry of joint involvement
C. Elevated serum uric acid levels
D. Dominance in weight-bearing joints

Answer: B. Rheumatoid arthritis is bilateral and symmetrical; by contrast, osteoarthritis and gouty arthritis are unilateral. Crepitus is most associated with osteoarthritis. Elevated serum uric acid levels are seen in gouty arthritis; weight-bearing joint dominance occurs in osteoarthritis.

➡ *NCLEX keys*
Nursing process step: Assessment
Client needs category: Physiological integrity
Client needs subcategory: Physiological adaptation
Taxonomic level: Comprehension

23. A client undergoes screening for sexually transmitted diseases. The results of an enzyme-linked immunosorbent assay (ELISA) are positive. The client asks the nurse to explain the meaning of test results. How should the nurse respond?
A. "Test results indicate that the human immunodeficiency virus is in your blood."
B. "These test results are the early evidence of acquired immunodeficiency syndrome."
C. "Test results suggest that you have contracted a viral sexually transmitted disease. The specific disease needs to be identified."
D. "Test results indicate the possibility that you have contracted the human immunodeficiency virus."

Answer: D. The ELISA is a screening test for presence of the human immunodeficiency virus. A positive result implies exposure to human immunodeficiency virus but confirmation requires a Western blot analysis.

➡ *NCLEX keys*
Nursing process step: Implementation
Client needs category: Physiological integrity
Client needs subcategory: Reduction of risk potential
Taxonomic level: Application

24. A client with aplastic anemia secondary to radiation exposure undergoes hematologic testing. What test results are most likely?
    A. Subnormal red blood cell (RBC) count, elevated WBC (white blood cell) count, subnormal platelet count.
    B. Subnormal RBC count, subnormal WBC count, subnormal platelet count.
    C. Elevated RBC count, elevated WBC count, elevated platelet count.
    D. Elevated RBC count, subnormal WBC count, elevated platelet count.
Answer: B. Aplastic anemia, also called pancytopenia, causes a reduction in erythrocytes, leukocytes and thrombocytes. Therefore, laboratory results would most likely yield low RBC count, WBC count and platelet count.

➡ *NCLEX keys*
Nursing process step: Assessment
Client needs category: Physiological integrity
Client needs subcategory: Physiological adaptation
Taxonomic level: Knowledge

25. A client with a history of severe penicillin hypersensitivity is about to undergo an arthrocentesis. The orthopedic surgeon prescribes a broad-spectrum antibiotic for prophylactic purposes. Which antibiotic is most likely to be prescribed?
    A. Ampicillin and sulbactam (Unasyn)
    B. Erythromycin (E-Mycin)
    C. Cefazolin (Zolicef)
    D. Gentamicin (Garamycin)
Answer: B. Erythromycin is a broad-spectrum antibiotic commonly used as a substitute in persons with penicillin allergy. Ampicillin is a penicillin and shouldn't be given to clients with penicillin hypersensitivity. Cefazolin is a cephalosporin. Persons allergic to penicillin can have sensitivity to cephalosporins. Gen-

tamicin is a narrow-spectrum antibiotic and not suitable for prophylaxis.

➡ *NCLEX keys*
Nursing process step: Planning
Client needs category: Physiological integrity
Client needs subcategory: Reduction in risk potential
Taxonomic level: Analysis

26. A client is scheduled for a myelogram, which requires administration of an I.V. radiopaque dye. The nurse informs the client that during the procedure he may experience:
    A. chest tightness.
    B. burning at the I.V. site.
    C. flushing of the face.
    D. increased salivation.
Answer: C. A typical response to I.V. radiopaque dye is the sensation of flushing of the face. Chest tightness is associated with a hypersensitive reaction and isn't an expected response. Neither burning at the I.V. site nor increased salivation are associated with administration of radiopaque dye.

➡ *NCLEX keys*
Nursing process step: Implementation
Client needs category: Health promotion and maintenance
Client needs subcategory: Prevention and early detection of disease
Taxonomic level: Comprehension

27. A client with herniated nucleus pulposus of the lumbar spine is scheduled for a laminotomy. The nurse is providing preoperative teaching. How should the nurse instruct the client to get out of bed following the procedure?
    A. Pulling himself up using an over-the-bed trapeze
    B. Logrolling to a side-lying position
    C. Twisting to a sitting position
    D. Avoiding use of abdominal muscles
Answer: B. Following back surgery such as a laminotomy, it is best for the client to get out of bed by initially logrolling to his side. Using an over-the-bed trapeze or twisting may put strain on the surgical site. When repositioning, the client should actually tighten abdominal muscles.

▶ NCLEX keys
Nursing process step: Implementation
Client needs category: Physiological integrity
Client needs subcategory: Reduction of risk
potential
Taxonomic level: Application

28. A client is in the first postoperative day
following a right total hip replacement. To
prevent dislocation, the nurse should avoid
positioning the client:
- A. with the right leg externally rotated.
- B. in the left lateral decubitus position.
- C. with the legs adducted.
- D. in semi-Fowler's position.

Answer: C. To prevent dislocation following a
total hip replacement, leg adduction should
be avoided. Instead, the legs should be abducted. External rotation of the affected leg is
appropriate as well as sitting at a forty-five degree angle.

▶ NCLEX keys
Nursing process step: Implementation
Client needs category: Physiological integrity
Client needs subcategory: Reduction of risk
potential
Taxonomic level: Application

29. A client with Parkinson's disease is receiving carbidopa-levodopa (Sinemet). Decrease in the frequency of what clinical manifestation of the disorder best indicates the
drug's effectiveness?
- A. Tremors
- B. Swallowing
- C. Seizures
- D. Lacrimation

Answer: A. A common sign of Parkinson's disease is tremors. Successful therapy with carbidopa-levodopa (Sinemet) should result in
diminution of tremors. Increased swallowing
and lacrimation aren't manifestations of
Parkinson's disease. Seizures aren't associated with Parkinson's disease.

▶ NCLEX keys
Nursing process step: Evaluation
Client needs category: Physiological integrity
Client needs subcategory: Pharmacological
and parenteral therapies
Taxonomic level: Application

30. The nurse is providing care for a client
experiencing a myasthenic crisis. Which body
system should the nurse monitor most care-
fully?
A. Respiratory system
B. Immune system
C. Cardiovascular system
D. Hepatic and renal system

Answer: A. The client's ability to ventilate and
oxygenate are at great risk during a myasthenic crisis. Mechanical ventilation is often
required. The immune, cardiovascular, and
hepatic and renal systems may be involved but
are not the primary body systems in jeopardy.

▶ NCLEX keys
Nursing process step: Analysis
Client needs category: Physiological integrity
Client needs subcategory: Physiological adap-
tation
Taxonomic level: Comprehension

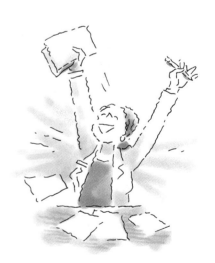

Part III Psychiatric care

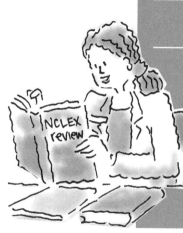

Brush up on key concepts

Effective patient care of all kinds requires consideration of both psychological and physiologic aspects of health. A patient who seeks medical help for chest pain, for example, may also need to be assessed for anxiety or depression. As a nurse, you will need a fundamental understanding of communication techniques as well as an understanding of psychiatric disorders.

The key to any relationship

Therapeutic communication is the foundation for developing a nurse-patient relationship, making it a vital topic for the NCLEX. It's the primary intervention in psychiatric nursing. Therapeutic communication requires awareness of both the patient's verbal and nonverbal messages.

To uncover and investigate the patient's inner thoughts, personal problems, and emotions, the nurse must establish trust and help the patient feel safe and respected. The therapeutic relationship helps the patient feel understood, become comfortable discussing problems, and find better ways to meet his emotional needs and develop satisfying relationships.

You got your ears on?

Listening intently to the patient enables the nurse to hear and analyze everything the patient is saying, alerting the nurse to the patient's communication patterns.

Connect the dots

Succinct **rephrasing** of key patient statements helps ensure the nurse's understanding and emphasizes important points in the patient's message. For example, the nurse might say, "You're feeling angry and you say it's because of the way your friend treated you yesterday."

Keep the door open

Using **broad openings** and **general statements** to initiate conversations encourages the patient to talk about any subject that comes to mind. These openings allow the patient to focus the conversation and demonstrate the nurse's willingness to interact. An example of this technique is: "Is there something you would like to talk about?"

Polish the rough edges

Asking the patient to **clarify** a confusing or vague message demonstrates the nurse's desire to understand what the patient is saying. It can also elicit precise information crucial to the patient's recovery. An example of clarifying is: "I'm not sure I understood what you said."

A sharper focus

In the technique called **focusing** the nurse assists the patient in redirecting attention toward something specific. It fosters the patient's self-control and helps avoid vague generalizations, thereby enabling the patient to accept responsibility for facing problems. "Let's go back to what we were just talking about," would be one example of this technique.

It's golden

Refraining from comment can have several benefits: **Silence** gives the patient time to talk, think, and gain insight into problems, and it also permits the nurse to gather more information. The nurse must use this technique judiciously, however, to avoid giving any impression of disinterest or judgment.

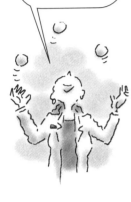

Consider all aspects of the patient's functioning: biological, psychological, and social.

Valuable assistance

When used correctly, the technique of **suggesting collaboration** gives the patient the opportunity to explore the pros and cons of a suggested approach. It must be used carefully to avoid directing the patient. An example of this technique is: "Perhaps we can meet with your parents to discuss the matter."

A two-way street

In the technique called **sharing impressions**, the nurse attempts to describe the patient's feelings and then seeks corrective feedback from the patient. This allows the patient to clarify any misperceptions and gives the nurse a better understanding of the patient's true feelings. For example, the nurse might say, "Tell me if my perception of what you're telling me agrees with yours."

Brush up on assessment

Because the nurse is commonly the health care provider who develops the closest long-term relationship with the patient the nurse is often most capable of assessing the emotional and mental health care needs of a patient, and identifying the appropriate interventions.

During the assessment stage the nurse determines a patient's psychological and physiologic status by assessing:
• the patient's history
• the patient's physical status
• laboratory and diagnostic tests.

Every therapeutic relationship calls for sensitive and attentive communication.

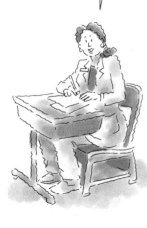

Gathering data #1: Getting history

A complete **patient history** provides information about the following:
• the patient's chief complaint or concern
• the history of the present illness
• past psychiatric illness
• personal or developmental history
• family history
• social history
• cultural considerations that may affect the patient's outcome.

Gathering data #2: Getting physical

The **physical examination** provides objective data that will help confirm or rule out assessments made during the health history interview.

In addition to the routine physical examination, the nurse should assess the patient's:
• general appearance — helps indicate the patient's emotional and mental status. The nurse should specifically note his dress and grooming.
• behavior — the nurse should note the patient's demeanor and overall attitude as well as any extraordinary behavior.
• mood — ask the patient to describe his current feelings in concrete terms and to suggest possible reasons for these feelings. Be sure to note inconsistencies between body language and mood.
• thought processes and cognitive function — the patient's orientation to time, place, or person can indicate confusion or disorientation. The presence of delusions, hallucinations, obsessions, compulsions, fantasies, and daydreams should be noted.
• coping mechanisms — a patient who is faced with a stressful situation may adopt excessive coping or defense mechanisms, which operate on an unconscious level to protect the ego. Examples include denial, regression, displacement, projection, reaction formation, and fantasy.
• potential for self-destructive behavior — a patient who has lost touch with reality may cut or mutilate body parts to focus on physical pain, which may be less overwhelming than emotional distress.

Keep abreast of diagnostic tests

Diagnosing psychiatric disorders differs from diagnosing other medical disorders. (See *The authority*.) While many medical tests involve instrumentation and physical analyses, psychological testing focuses on questioning and observing the patient.

The authority

Published by the American Psychiatric Association, the *Diagnostic and Statistical Manual of Mental Disorders (DSM)* is a standard interdisciplinary psychiatric diagnostic system designed to be used by all members of the mental health care team. The manual includes a complete description of psychiatric disorders and other conditions and describes diagnostic criteria that must be met to support each diagnosis.

The current manual is the fourth edition, commonly known as *DSM-IV*. The *DSM* is updated frequently, and new information regularly replaces old.

Performing diagnostic tests on a patient with a suspected psychiatric disorder may assist with accurate diagnosis, can reveal underlying physiologic disorders, establishes normal renal and hepatic function, and monitors for therapeutic medication levels.

Blood study #1

A **blood chemistry test** assesses a blood sample for potassium, sodium, calcium, phosphorus, glucose, bicarbonate, blood urea nitrogen, creatinine, protein, albumin, osmolality, amylase, lipase, alkaline phosphatase, ammonia, bilirubin, lactate dehydrogenase, aspartate aminotransferase, and alanine aminotransferase.

Nursing actions
- Withhold food and fluids before the procedure, as directed.
- Check the site for bleeding after the procedure.

Blood study #2

A **hematologic study** uses a blood sample to analyze red blood cells, white blood cells, prothrombin time, international normalized ratio, partial thromboplastin time, erythrocyte sedimentation rate, platelets, hemoglobin, and hematocrit.

Nursing actions
- Note current drug therapy before the procedure.
- Check the venipuncture site for bleeding after the procedure.

AIDS-related blood study #1

Enzyme-linked immunosorbent assay uses a blood sample to detect the HIV-1 antibody (acquired immunodeficiency syndrome [AIDS] can cause psychiatric complications).

Nursing actions
- Verify that informed consent has been obtained and documented.
- Provide the patient with appropriate pretest counseling.
- After the procedure, check the venipuncture site for bleeding.

AIDS-related blood study #2

A **Western blot test** uses a blood sample to detect the presence of specific viral proteins to confirm human immunodeficiency virus (HIV) infection.

Nursing actions
- Verify that informed consent has been obtained and documented.
- After the procedure, check the venipuncture site for bleeding.

Drug detection

Toxicology screening uses a urine specimen to detect unknown drugs.

Nursing actions
- Make sure that a written, informed consent has been obtained.
- Witness the procurement of the urine specimen and process according to the facility's protocol.

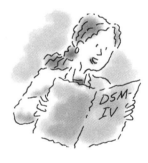

The *DSM* is updated regularly...make sure your information is up to date!

Brain meter-reading

An **electroencephalogram** records the electrical activity of the brain. Using electrodes, this noninvasive test gives a graphic representation of brain activity.

Nursing actions
• Determine the patient's ability to lie still.
• Reassure the patient that electrical shock won't occur.
• Explain that the patient will be subjected to stimuli, such as lights and sounds.
• Withhold food for 8 hours before the procedure.
• Withhold medications and caffeine for 24 to 48 hours before the procedure.

Dye job

A **computed tomography scan,** used to identify brain abnormalities, produces a finely detailed image of the brain and its structures. It may be performed with or without the injection of contrast dye.

Nursing actions
• Note the patient's allergies to iodine, seafood, and radiopaque dyes.
• Allay the patient's anxiety.
• Inform the patient about possible throat irritation and flushing of the face, if contrast dye is injected.

Mental picture

Magnetic resonance imaging uses electromagnetic energy to create a detailed visualization of the brain and its structures.

Nursing actions
• Be aware that patients with pacemakers, surgical and orthopedic clips, or shrapnel shouldn't be scanned.
• Remove jewelry and metal objects from the patient.
• Determine the patient's ability to lie still.
• Administer sedation, as prescribed.

Brain metabolism test

Positron emission tomography involves injection of a radioisotope, allowing visualization of the brain's oxygen uptake, blood flow, and glucose metabolism.

Nursing actions
• Determine the patient's ability to lie still during the procedure.
• Withhold alcohol, tobacco, and caffeine for 24 hours before the procedure.
• Withhold medications, as directed, before the procedure.
• Check the injection site for bleeding after the procedure.

Keep abreast of psychological tests

These tests evaluate the patient's mood, personality, and mental status. The following is a review of the most common psychological tests.

Pop quiz

The **Mini–Mental Status Examination** measures orientation, registration, recall, calculation, language, and motor skills.

Cognitive capacity

The **Cognitive Capacity Screening Examination** measures orientation, memory, calculation, and language.

General knowledge

The **Cognitive Assessment Scale** measures orientation, general knowledge, mental ability, and psychomotor function.

Measuring what's lost

The **Global Deterioration Scale** assesses and stages primary degenerative dementia, based on orientation, memory, and neurologic function.

Getting by

The **Functional Dementia Scale** measures orientation, affect, and the ability to perform activities of daily living.

Measuring depression

The **Beck Depression Inventory** helps diagnose depression, determine its severity, and monitor the patient's response during treatment.

What's on the menu?
The **Eating Attitudes Test** detects patterns that suggest an eating disorder.

Who are you?
The **Minnesota Multiphasic Personality Inventory** helps assess personality traits and ego function in adolescents and adults. Test results include information on coping strategies, defenses, strengths, gender identification, and self-esteem. The test pattern may strongly suggest a diagnostic category, point to a suicide risk, or indicate the potential for violence.

Alcoholism test #1
The **Michigan Alcoholism Screening Test** is a 24-item timed test in which a score of 5 or better classifies the patient as alcoholic.

Alcoholism test #2
The **CAGE Questionnaire** is a four-question tool in which two or three positive responses indicate alcoholism.

Cocaine addiction tests
The **Cocaine Addiction Severity Test** and **Cocaine Assessment Profile** are used when cocaine use is suspected.

Polish up on patient care

A variety of treatment options coexist in psychiatric and mental health care. Nurses may use one specific treatment approach or a combination of approaches to guide patient care.

One on one
Individual therapy is the establishment of a structured relationship between nurse and patient in an attempt to achieve change in the patient. The nurse works with the patient to develop an approach to resolve conflict, decrease emotional pain, and develop appropriate ways of meeting the patient's needs. This relationship with the patient consists of three overlapping phases:
• the orientation phase, in which the nurse builds a connection with the patient by establishing rapport and a sense of trust. Goals are formulated in this phase.
• the working phase, in which the patient becomes increasingly involved in self-exploration. The nurse assists the patient as he tries to develop self-understanding and encourages him to take risks in terms of changing dysfunctional behavior.
• the termination phase, in which the patient and nurse determine that closure of the relationship is appropriate. Both parties agree that the problem that initiated the relationship has been alleviated or has become manageable.

Milling around
During **milieu therapy** the nurse uses all aspects of the hospital environment in a therapeutic manner. Patients are exposed to rules, expectations, peer pressure, and social interactions. Nurses encourage communication and decision making and provide opportunities for enhancing self-esteem and learning new skills and behaviors. The goal of therapy is to enable the patient to live outside the institutional setting.

Treating disease and imbalance
Biological therapies are called for when emotional and behavioral disturbances are thought to be caused by chemical imbalances or by disease-causing organisms.
    Some examples of biological therapies are:
• psychoactive drugs
• electroconvulsive therapy
• nonconvulsive electrical stimulation
• psychosurgery.

Changing ideas
Cognitive therapy employs strategies to modify the beliefs and attitudes that influence a patient's feelings and behaviors.
    Some basic cognitive interventions include:
• teaching thought substitution
• identifying problem-solving strategies
• finding ways to modify negative self-talk
• role playing
• modeling coping strategies.

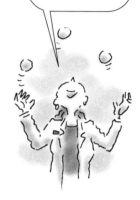

It's a balancing act! While identifying the disordered thought of a schizophrenic patient, also assess for physiologic complications.

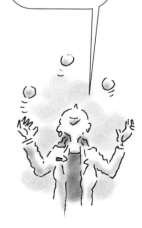

Alternatively, you may need to assess a respiratory patient for depression or suicidal thoughts.

The real world

Reality therapy focuses on assisting the patient to meet two basic emotional needs:
• loving and being loved
• feeling worthwhile and feeling that others are worthwhile.

The nurse emphasizes personal responsibility for behavior, controlling one's own life, and fulfilling basic needs.

All in the family

During **family therapy**, the entire family is considered the treatment unit. The primary goal of therapy is to improve the functioning of the family. The types of patients that can benefit most from family therapy are those involved in marital issues, intergenerational conflicts, sibling concerns, and family crises, such as death and divorce.

The gang's all here

Group therapy includes an advanced practice nurse–therapist and six to eight people who meet regularly for the purpose of increasing self-awareness, improving interpersonal relationships, and changing maladaptive behavioral problems. Like individual therapy, group therapy goes through the orientation phase, working phase, and termination phase.

Urgent care

Crisis intervention is a systemic approach of short-term therapy where the nurse works with a patient, family, or group that is experiencing an unbearable situation. The nurse initiates actions to decrease the patient's sense of personal danger and facilitate the patient's ability to control the situation.

Trance time

Hypnosis is used to induce deep relaxation by altering the patient's state of consciousness. The result of hypnotic induction is a trancelike state during which patients use memories, mental associations, and concentration to discover experiences that are connected to their current distress. Hypnosis is effective for dealing with anxiety disorders, some types of pain, repressed traumatic events, and addictive disorders.

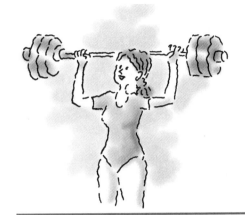

Pump up on practice questions

1. A 35-year-old client tells the nurse that he never disagrees with anyone and that he has loved everyone he's ever known. What would be the nurse's best response to this client?
    A. "How do you manage to do that?"
    B. "That's hard to believe. Most people couldn't do that."
    C. "What do you do with your feelings of dissatisfaction or anger?"
    D. "How did you come to adopt such a way of life?"

Answer: D. Inquiring about the client's way of life allows for further exploration of the message he's trying to convey. Option A has too narrow a focus and doesn't permit maximal exploration of the client's experience. Option B is incorrect because the client could misinterpret it as a challenge and become even more defensive. Option C is incorrect because the nurse shouldn't identify the client's feelings for him.

➥ **NCLEX keys**
Nursing process step: Implementation
Client needs category: Psychosocial integrity
Client needs subcategory: Coping and adaptation
Taxonomic level: Application

2. The nurse is working with a client who has just stimulated her anger by using a condescending tone of voice. Which of the following responses by the nurse would be the most therapeutic?
- A. "I feel angry when I hear that tone of voice."
- B. "You make me so angry when you talk to me that way."
- C. "Are you trying to make me angry?"
- D. "Why do you use that condescending tone of voice with me?"

Answer: A. This response allows the nurse to provide feedback without making the client responsible for the nurse's reaction. Option B is accusatory and blocks communication. Option C is a challenging remark that can lead to power struggles, lowers the client's self-esteem, and blocks opportunities for open communication. Option D is incorrect because "why" questions put the client on the defensive.

➡ *NCLEX keys*
Nursing process step: Implementation
Client needs category: Psychosocial integrity
Client needs subcategory: Coping and adaptation
Taxonomic level: Application

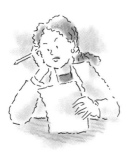

3. A client on the unit tells the nurse that his wife's nagging really gets on his nerves. He asks the nurse if she will talk with his wife about her nagging during their family session tomorrow afternoon. Which of the following would be the most therapeutic response to the client?

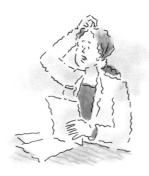

- A. "Tell me more specifically about her complaints."
- B. "Can you think why she might nag you so much?"
- C. "I'll help you think about how to bring this up yourself tomorrow."
- D. "Why do you want me to initiate this discussion in tomorrow's session rather than you?"

Answer: C. The client needs to learn how to communicate directly with his wife about her behavior. The nurse's assistance will enable him to practice a new skill and will communicate the nurse's confidence in his ability to confront this situation directly. Options A and B inappropriately direct attention away from the client and toward his wife, who isn't present. Option D implies that there might be a legitimate reason for the nurse to assume responsibility for something that rightfully belongs to the client. Instead of focusing on his problems, he will waste time convincing the nurse why she should do his work.

➡ *NCLEX keys*
Nursing process step: Implementation
Client needs category: Psychosocial integrity
Client needs subcategory: Coping and adaptation
Taxonomic level: Application

4. The nurse is caring for a client diagnosed with conversion disorder who has developed paralysis of her legs. Diagnostic tests fail to uncover a physiologic cause. During the working phase of the nurse-client relationship, the client says to her nurse, "You think I could walk if I wanted to, don't you?" Which of the following would be the nurse's best response?

- A. "Yes, if you really wanted to, you could."
- B. "Tell me why you're concerned about what I think."
- C. "Do you think you could walk if you wanted to?"
- D. "I think you are unable to walk now, whatever the cause."

Answer: D. This response answers the question honestly and nonjudgmentally and helps to preserve the client's self-esteem. Option A is an open and candid response but diminishes the client's self-esteem. Option B doesn't answer the client's question and isn't helpful. Option C would increase the client's anxiety because her inability to walk is directly related to an unconscious psychological conflict that hasn't yet been resolved.

➡ *NCLEX keys*

Nursing process step: Implementation
Client needs category: Psychosocial integrity
Client needs subcategory: Coping and adaptation
Taxonomic level: Application

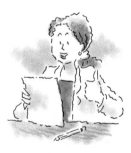

5. A 42-year-old homemaker arrives at the emergency department with uncontrollable crying and anxiety. Her husband of 17 years has recently asked her for a divorce. The patient is sitting in a chair, rocking back and forth. Which is the best response for the nurse to make?

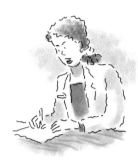

- A. "You must stop crying so that we can discuss your feelings about the divorce."
- B. "Once you find a job, you will feel much better and more secure."
- C. "I can see how upset you are. Let's sit in the office so that we can talk about how you're feeling."
- D. "Once you have a lawyer looking out for your interests, you will feel better."

Answer: C. This response validates the client's distress and provides an opportunity for her to talk about her feelings. Because clients in crisis have difficulty making decisions, the nurse must be directive as well as supportive. Option A doesn't provide the client with adequate support. Options B and D don't acknowledge the client's distress. Moreover, clients in crisis can't think beyond the immediate moment, so discussing long-range plans isn't helpful.

➡ *NCLEX keys*

Nursing process step: Implementation
Client needs category: Psychosocial integrity
Client needs subcategory: Coping and adaptation
Taxonomic level: Application

6. A 60-year-old widower is hospitalized after complaining of difficulty sleeping, extreme apprehension, shortness of breath, and a sense of impending doom. What is the best response for the nurse to make?

A. "You have nothing to worry about. You are in a safe place. Try to relax."

B. "Has anything happened recently or in the past that may have triggered these feelings?"

C. "We have given you a medication that will help to decrease these feelings of anxiety."

D. "Take some deep breaths and try to calm down."

Answer: B. This provides support, reassurance, and an opportunity to gain insight into the cause of the client's anxiety. Option A dismisses the client's feelings and offers false reassurance. Options C and D don't allow the client to discuss his feelings, which he must do to understand and resolve the cause of his anxiety.

➡ *NCLEX keys*

Nursing process step: Implementation
Client needs category: Psychosocial integrity
Client needs subcategory: Coping and adaptation
Taxonomic level: Application

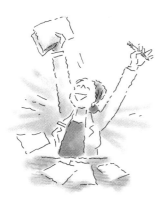

7. A 26-year-old male is admitted to an inpatient psychiatric hospital after having been picked up by the local police while walking around the neighborhood at night without shoes in the snow. He appears confused and disoriented. Which of the following is the most immediate nursing action?

A. Assess and stabilize the client's medical needs.

B. Assess and stabilize the client's psychological needs.

C. Attempt to locate the nearest family members to get an accurate history.

D. Arrange a transfer to the nearest medical facility.

Answer: A. The possibility of frostbite must be evaluated before the other interventions. Options B, C, and D don't address the client's immediate medical needs.

➡ *NCLEX keys*

Nursing process step: Implementation
Client needs category: Physiological integrity
Client needs subcategory: Reduction of risk potential
Taxonomic level: Analysis

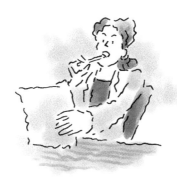

8. What occurs during the working phase of the nurse-client relationship?

A. The nurse assesses the client's needs and develops a plan of care.

B. The nurse and client together evaluate and modify the goals of the relationship.

C. The nurse and client discuss their feelings about terminating the relationship.

D. The nurse and client explore each other's expectations of the relationship.

Answer: B. The therapeutic nurse-client relationship consists of three overlapping phases, the orientation, the working, and the termination. During the working phase, the nurse and the client together evaluate and refine goals established during the orientation phase. In addition, major therapeutic work takes place, and insight is integrated into a plan of action. The orientation phase involves assessing the client, formulating a contract, exploring feelings, and establishing expectations about the relationship. During the termination phase, the nurse prepares the client for separation and explores feelings about the end of the relationship.

➡ NCLEX keys

Nursing process step: Planning
Client needs category: Psychosocial integrity
Client needs subcategory: Coping and adaptation
Taxonomic level: Knowledge

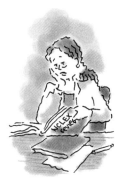

9. When preparing to conduct group therapy, the advanced practice nurse keeps in mind that the optimal number of clients in a group would be:
    A. 6 to 8.
    B. 10 to12.
    C. 3 to 5.
    D. unlimited.
Answer: A. Clinicians generally consider 6 to 8 people to be the ideal number of clients for a therapeutic group. The size allows opportunities for maximum therapeutic exchange and participation. In groups of 5 or fewer, participation commonly is inhibited by self-consciousness and insecurity. In groups larger than 8, participation and exchange among certain members may be lost.

➡ NCLEX keys

Nursing process step: Planning
Client needs category: Psychosocial integrity
Client needs subcategory: Coping and adaptation
Taxonomic level: Application

10. A therapeutic nurse-client relationship begins with the nurse's:
    A. sincere desire to help others.
    B. acceptance of others.
    C. self-awareness and understanding.
    D. sound knowledge of psychiatric nursing.
Answer: C. Although all of the options are desirable, knowledge of self is the basis for building a strong, therapeutic nurse-client relationship. Being aware of and understanding personal feelings and behavior is a prerequisite for understanding and helping clients.

➡ NCLEX keys

Nursing process step: Planning
Client needs category: Safe, effective care environment
Client needs subcategory: Management of care
Taxonomic level: Knowledge

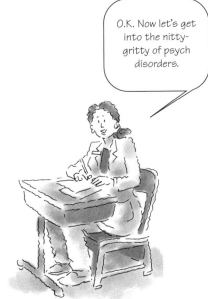

O.K. Now let's get into the nitty-gritty of psych disorders.

Brush up on key concepts

The patient with a sleep disorder commonly suffers from excessive daytime sleepiness and impaired ability to perform daily tasks safely or properly. The patient with a somato-form disorder commonly suffers physical symptoms related to an inability to handle stress. These physical symptoms have no physiologic cause but are overwhelming to the patient.

At any time, you can review the major points of each disorder by consulting the *Cheat sheet* on pages 366 and 367.

Sleep disorders

The patient with a primary sleep disorder is unable to initiate or maintain sleep. Primary sleep disorders may be categorized as dys-somnias or parasomnias.

Too much or not enough
Dyssomnias involve excessive sleep or diffi-culty initiating and maintaining sleep. Exam-ples of dyssomnias include primary insomnia, circadian rhythm sleep disorder, breathing-related sleep disorder, primary hypersomnia, and narcolepsy.

Strange things in the night
Parasomnias are physiologic or behavioral reactions *during* sleep. Examples of parasom-nias include nightmare disorder, sleep terror disorder, and sleepwalking disorder.

You are getting sleepy...
Sleep can be broken down into five distinct stages, **rapid-eye-movement** (REM) sleep and four stages of **non–rapid-eye-movement** (NREM) sleep (stages 1, 2, 3, and 4).

☝ Stage 1 NREM sleep is a transition from wakefulness to sleep and occupies about 5% of time spent asleep in healthy adults.

✌ Stage 2 NREM sleep, which is character-ized by specific EEG waveforms (sleep spin-dles and K complexes), occupies about 50% of time spent asleep.

🖐 Stages 3 and 4 NREM sleep (also known collectively as slow-wave sleep) are the deep-est levels of sleep and occupy about 10% to 20% of sleep time.

🖐 REM sleep, during which the majority of typical storylike dreams occur, occupies about 20% to 25% of total sleep.

Patterns after dark
Stages of sleep have a characteristic temporal organization. NREM stages 3 and 4 tend to occur in the first one-third to one-half of the night. REM sleep occurs in cycles throughout the night, alternating with NREM sleep about every 80 to 100 minutes. REM sleep periods increase in duration toward the morning.

Sparks in the night
Polysomnography is the monitoring of mul-tiple electrophysiologic parameters during sleep and generally includes measurement of EEG activity, electro-oculographic activity (electrographic tracings made by movement of the eye), and electromyographic activity (electrographic tracings made by skeletal muscles at rest).

Additional polysomnographic measures may include oral or nasal airflow, respiratory effort, chest and abdominal wall movement, oxyhemoglobin saturation, or exhaled carbon dioxide concentration. These measures are used to monitor respiration during sleep and

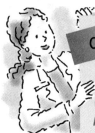

Somatoform & sleep disorders refresher

CONVERSION DISORDER

Key sign or symptom
• La belle indifference (a lack of concern about the symptoms or limitation on functioning)

Key test result
• The absence of expected diagnostic findings can confirm the disorder.

Key treatments
• Individual therapy

Key interventions
• Establish a supportive relationship that communicates acceptance of the patient but keeps the focus away from symptoms
• Review all laboratory and diagnostic study results.

DYSSOMNIAS

Key signs and symptoms
Primary insomnia
• History of light or easily disturbed sleep or difficulty falling asleep
• Insomnia
Breathing-related sleep disorder
• Abnormal breathing events during sleep including apnea, abnormally slow or shallow respirations, and hypoventilation (abnormal blood oxygen and carbon dioxide levels)
• Fatigue
• Snoring while sleeping
Primary hypersomnia
• Confusion upon awakening
• Difficulty awakening
• Poor memory
Narcolepsy
• Cataplexy (bilateral loss of muscle tone triggered by strong emotion)
• Generalized daytime sleepiness
• Hypnagogic hallucination (intense dreamlike images)
• Irresistible attacks of refreshing sleep

Key test result
• Polysomnography is diagnostic for individual sleep disorder.

Key treatment
• Hypnotics: zolpidem (Ambien)

Key interventions
For primary insomnia and circadian rhythm disturbance
• Encourage the patient to discuss concerns that may be preventing sleep.
• Schedule regular sleep and awakening times.
For breathing-related sleep disorder
• Administer continuous positive nasal airway pressure.
For primary hypersomnia and narcolepsy
• Administer medications as prescribed.
• Develop strategies to manage symptoms and integrate them into their daily routine, such as taking naps during lunch or work breaks.

HYPOCHONDRIASIS

Key signs and symptoms
• Abnormal focus on bodily functions and sensations
• Anger, frustration, depression
• Frequent visits to doctors and specialists despite assurance from health care providers that the patient is healthy
• Intensified physical symptoms around sympathetic people
• Rejection of the idea that the symptoms are stress related
• Use of symptoms to avoid difficult situations

Key treatments
• Individual therapy
• Tricyclic antidepressants: amitriptyline (Elavil), imipramine (Tofranil), doxepin (Sinequan), phenelzine (Nardil)

Key interventions
• Assess the patient's level of knowledge about how emotional issues can impact physiologic functioning.
• Encourage emotional expression.
• Respond to the patient's symptoms in a matter-of-fact way.

Falling asleep during NCLEX studying doesn't count as a sleep disorder.

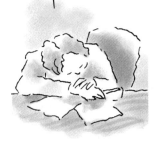

Somatoform & sleep disorders refresher *(continued)*

PAIN DISORDER

Key signs and symptoms
• Acute and chronic pain not associated with a psychological cause
• Frequent visits to multiple doctors to seek pain relief

Key test result
• Test results are inconsistent with physical findings.

Key treatments
• Individual therapy
• Tricyclic antidepressants: amitriptyline (Elavil), imipramine (Tofranil), doxepin (Sinequan)

Key interventions
• Acknowledge the patient's pain.
• Encourage the patient to recognize situations that precipitate pain.

PARASOMNIAS

Key signs and symptoms
Nightmare disorder
• Dream recall
• Mild autonomic arousal upon awakening (sweating, tachycardia, tachypnea)
Sleep terror disorder
• Autonomic signs of intense anxiety (tachycardia, tachypnea, flushing, sweating, increased muscle tone, dilated pupils)
• Inability to recall dream content
Sleepwalking disorder
• Amnesia of the episode or limited recall
• Episode may include sitting up, talking, walking, or engaging in inappropriate behavior

Key test result
• Polysomnography is diagnostic for individual sleep disorder.

Key interventions
• Lock windows and doors if sleepwalking occurs.
• Provide emotional support.

---

to detect the presence and severity of sleep apnea. Measurement of peripheral electromyographic activity may be used to detect abnormal movements during sleep.

You can do it during the daytime, too!

Most polysomnographic studies are performed during the patient's usual sleeping hours — that is, at night. However daytime polysomnographic studies are also used to quantify daytime sleepiness.

Somatoform disorders

The patient with a somatoform disorder complains of physical symptoms and typically travels from doctor to doctor in search of sympathetic and enthusiastic treatment. Physical examinations and laboratory tests, however, fail to uncover an organic basis for the patient's symptoms. Because the patient doesn't produce the symptoms intentionally or feel a sense of control over them, he's usually un-

able to accept that his illness has a psychological cause.

From mind to body

Psychosomatic is a term used to describe conditions in which a psychological state contributes to the development of a physical illness.

An expression of emotional stress

Somatization is the manifestation of physical symptoms that result from psychological distress. Anyone who feels the pain of a sore throat or the ache of flu has a somatic symptom, but it isn't considered somatization unless the physical symptoms are an expression of emotional stress.

All bottled up

Internalization refers to the condition in which a patient's anxiety, stress, and frustration are expressed through physical symptoms rather than confronted directly.

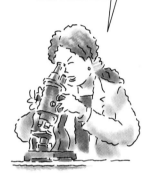

Absence means presence. The absence of expected diagnostic findings can confirm conversion disorder.

Polish up on patient care

Major somatoform disorders include conversion disorder, hypochondriasis, and pain disorder. Sleep disorders include dyssomnias (primary insomnia, circadian rhythm sleep disorder, breathing-related sleep disorder, primary hypersomnia, and narcolepsy) and parasomnias (nightmare disorder, sleep terror disorder, and sleepwalking disorder).

Conversion disorder

The patient with conversion disorder exhibits symptoms that suggest a physical disorder, but evaluation and observation can't determine a physiologic cause. The onset of symptoms is preceded by psychological trauma or conflict, and the physical symptoms are a manifestation of the conflict.

CONTRIBUTING FACTORS
• Psychological conflict
• Overwhelming stress

ASSESSMENT FINDINGS
• Aphonia (inability to produce sound)
• Blindness
• Deafness
• Dysphagia
• Impaired balance and impaired coordination
• La belle indifference (a lack of concern about the symptoms or limitation on functioning)
• Loss of touch sensation
• Lump in the throat
• Paralysis
• Seizures
• Urinary retention

DIAGNOSTIC TEST RESULTS
• Test results are inconsistent with physical findings.
• The absence of expected diagnostic findings can confirm the disorder.

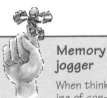

Memory jogger

When thinking of conversion disorder, think of the term *convert* which means "to change from one form or function to another." Patients with conversion disorder convert stress into physical ailments.

NURSING DIAGNOSES
• Ineffective individual coping
• Anxiety
• Self-esteem disturbance

TREATMENT
• Individual therapy

Drug therapy
• Benzodiazepines: lorazepam (Ativan), alprazolam (Xanax)

INTERVENTIONS AND RATIONALES
• Ensure and maintain a safe environment *to protect the patient.*
• Establish a supportive relationship that communicates acceptance of the patient but keeps the focus away from symptoms *to help the patient learn to recognize and express anxiety.*
• Review all laboratory and diagnostic study results *to ascertain whether any physical problems are present.*
• Encourage the patient to identify any emotional conflicts occurring before the onset of physical symptoms *to make the relationship between the conflict and the symptoms more clear.*
• Promote social interaction *to decrease the patient's level of self-involvement.*
• Identify constructive coping mechanisms *to encourage the patient to use practical coping skills and relinquish the role of being sick.*

Teaching topics
• Teach family members how to set limits on the patient's sick role behavior while continuing to provide support.
• Teach stress-reduction methods.

Dyssomnias

Dyssomnias are primary disorders of initiating or maintaining sleep or excessive sleepiness. These disorders are characterized by a disturbance in the amount, quality, or timing of sleep.

Primary insomnia is characterized by difficulty initiating or maintaining sleep that lasts for at least 1 month. Alternatively, the patient may report that sleep is not refreshing. A key symptom of primary insomnia is the patient's intense focus and anxiety about not getting sleep. Commonly, the patient reports being a "light sleeper."

In **circadian rhythm sleep disorder,** there is a mismatch between the internal sleep-wake circadian rhythm and timing and duration of sleep. The patient may report insomnia at particular times during the day and excessive sleepiness at other times. Causes can be intrinsic such as delays in the sleep phases or extrinsic as in jet lag or shift work.

Another class of sleep disorder identified by the *Diagnostic and Statistical Manual of Mental Disorders*, 4th ed., is **breathing-related sleep disorder.** Specific disorders in this class include central sleep apnea syndrome, central alveolar hypoventilation syndrome, and obstructive sleep apnea syndrome. Obstructive sleep apnea syndrome is the most commonly diagnosed breathing-related sleep disorder.

In breathing-related sleep disorder, a disturbance in breathing leads to a disruption in sleep that leads to excessive sleepiness or insomnia. Excessive sleepiness is the most common complaint of patients. Naps usually aren't refreshing and may be accompanied by a dull headache. These patients often minimize the problem by bragging that they can sleep anywhere and at any time.

In **narcolepsy,** the patient develops an overwhelming urge to sleep at any time of the day regardless of the amount of previous sleep. The patient may fall asleep two to six times a day during inappropriate times, such as while driving the car or attending class. The patient's sleepiness typically decreases after a sleep attack, only to return several hours later. The sleep attacks must occur daily over a period of 3 months to confirm the diagnosis.

In **primary hypersomnia,** the patient experiences excessive sleepiness lasting at least 1 month. The patient may take daytime naps or sleep extended periods of time at night. People with primary hypersomnia typically sleep 8 to 12 hours per night. They fall asleep easily, sleep through the night, but often have trouble awakening in the morning. Some mornings they awake confused and combat-

ive. These patients have great difficulty with morning obligations.

CONTRIBUTING FACTORS
Primary insomnia
- Illness (especially pheochromocytoma or hyperthyroidism)
- Many illegal drugs
- Older than age 65
- Stress
- Use of certain legal drugs (see *Drugs that affect sleep*, page 370)

Circadian rhythm sleep disorder
- Delayed sleep phase
- Jet lag
- Shift work

Breathing-related sleep disorder
- Instability in the respiratory control center, which causes apnea
- Obstruction or collapse of airway, which causes apnea
- Slow or shallow breathing, which causes arterial oxygen desaturation

Primary hypersomnia
- Autonomic nervous system dysfunction
- Genetic predisposition

Narcolepsy
- Genetic predisposition

ASSESSMENT FINDINGS
Primary insomnia
- Anxiety related to sleep loss
- Fatigue
- Haggard appearance
- History of light or easily disturbed sleep or difficulty falling asleep
- Insomnia
- Poor concentration
- Tension headache

Circadian rhythm sleep disorder
- Cardiovascular and GI disturbances, such as palpitations, peptic ulcer disease, and gastritis
- Fatigue

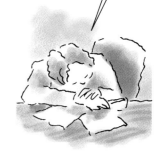

In *narcolepsy,* the patient develops an overwhelming urge to sleep at any time of the day. Zzzz.

Drugs that affect sleep

Increased total sleep time
- Barbiturates
- Benzodiazepines
- Alcohol (during the first half of the night)
- Phenothiazines

Decreased total sleep time
- Amphetamines
- Alcohol (during the second half of the night)
- Caffeine

Altered dreaming and REM sleep
- Beta-adrenergic blockers: decreased rapid-eye-movement (REM) sleep, possible nightmares

- L-Dopa: vivid dreams and nightmares
- Amphetamines: decreased REM sleep
- Tricyclic antidepressants and monoamine oxidase inhibitors: decreased REM sleep
- Barbiturates: decreased REM sleep
- Benzodiazepines: decreased REM sleep

Increased waking after sleep onset
- Steroids
- Narcotics
- Beta-adrenergic blockers

Decreased waking after sleep onset
- Benzodiazepines
- Barbiturates

- Haggard appearance
- Poor concentration

Breathing-related sleep disorder
- Abnormal breathing events during sleep including apnea, abnormally slow or shallow respirations, and hypoventilation (abnormal blood oxygen and carbon dioxide levels)
- Dull headache upon awakening
- Fatigue
- Gastroesophageal reflux
- Mild systemic hypertension with elevated diastolic blood pressure
- Snoring while sleeping

Primary hypersomnia
- Confusion upon awakening
- Difficulty awakening
- Poor memory

Narcolepsy
- Cataplexy (bilateral loss of muscle tone triggered by strong emotion)
- Frequent, intense, and vivid dreams may occur during nocturnal sleep
- Generalized daytime sleepiness
- Hypnagogic hallucination (intense dreamlike images)
- Irresistible attacks of refreshing sleep

DIAGNOSTIC TEST RESULTS
Primary insomnia
- Polysomnography shows poor sleep continuity, increased stage 1 sleep, decreased stages 3 and 4 sleep, increased muscle tension, or increased amounts of EEG alpha activity during sleep.
- Psychophysiologic testing may show high arousal (increased muscle tension or excessive physiologic reactivity to stress).

Circadian rhythm sleep disorder
- Polysomnography shows short sleep latency (length of time it takes to fall asleep), reduced sleep duration, and sleep continuity disturbances.

Breathing-related sleep disorder
- Polysomnography measures of oral and nasal airflow are abnormal and oxyhemoglobin saturation is reduced.

Primary hypersomnia
- Polysomnography demonstrates a normal to prolonged sleep duration, short sleep latency, normal to increased sleep continuity, and normal distributions of REM and NREM sleep. Some individuals may have increased amounts of slow-wave sleep.

Narcolepsy

• Polysomnography shows sleep latencies of less than 10 minutes and frequent sleep onset REM periods, frequent transient arousals, decreased sleep efficiency, increased stage 1 sleep, increased REM sleep, and increased eye movements within the REM periods. Periodic limb movements and episodes of sleep apnea are also often noted.

NURSING DIAGNOSES

• Sleep pattern disturbance
• Fatigue
• Impaired home maintenance management

TREATMENT

• Hypnosis
• Relaxation techniques
• Sleep restrictions (Patients are instructed to avoid napping and to stay in bed only when sleeping.)

Drug therapy

For primary insomnia or circadian rhythm sleep disorder:
• antidepressants: trazodone (Desyrel)
• benzodiazepines: lorazepam (Ativan), alprazolam (Xanax)
• diphenhydramine (Benadryl)
• hypnotics: zolpidem (Ambien)
   For primary hypersomnia or narcolepsy:
• stimulants: caffeine, methylphenidate (Ritalin), pemoline (Cylert), dextroamphetamine (Dexedrine)

INTERVENTIONS AND RATIONALES

• Assess the patient and document symptoms of sleep disturbance *to gain information for care plan development.*

Primary insomnia and circadian rhythm disturbance

• Encourage the patient to discuss concerns that may be preventing sleep. *Active listening helps elicit underlying causes of sleep disturbance such as stress.*
• Establish a sleep routine *to promote relaxation and sleep.*
• Schedule regular sleep and awakening times *to help ensure that progress is maintained after the patient leaves the hospital.*

• Administer medications, as prescribed, *to induce sleep and to reduce anxiety.*
• Provide warm milk at bedtime. *L-tryptophan, found in milk, is a precursor to serotonin, a neurotransmitter necessary for sleep.*
• Plan activities that require the patient to wake at a regular hour and stay out of bed during the day *to reinforce natural circadian rhythms.*

Breathing-related sleep disorder

• Administer continuous positive nasal airway pressure *to treat obstructive sleep disorders.*

Primary hypersomnia and narcolepsy

• Administer medications as prescribed *to help the patient stay awake and to maintain patient safety.*
• Develop strategies to manage symptoms and integrate them into the patient's daily routine, such as taking naps during lunch or work breaks *to help maintain patient safety and promote normal functioning.*

Teaching topics

For primary insomnia and circadian rhythm disorder
• Relaxation techniques
• Importance of limiting caffeine, alcohol, and spicy foods
• Need to avoid exercising within 3 hours before bedtime
• Ways to identify and reduce stressors
   For breathing-related sleeping disorder
• Use of home positive nasal airway pressure device
   For primary hypersomnia and narcolepsy
• Integrating nap period into daily routine

Hypochondriasis

In hypochondriasis, the patient is preoccupied by fear of a serious illness, despite medical assurance of good health. The patient with hypochondriasis interprets all physical sensations as indications of illness, impairing his ability to function normally.

I'm sick of studying for the NCLEX!

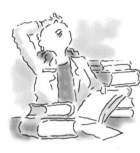

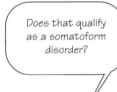

Does that qualify as a somatoform disorder?

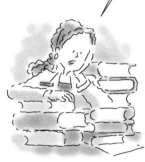

CONTRIBUTING FACTORS
- Death of someone close to the individual
- Family member with a serious illness
- Previous serious illness

ASSESSMENT FINDINGS
- Abnormal focus on bodily functions and sensations
- Anger, frustration, depression
- Frequent visits to doctors and specialists despite assurance from health care providers that the patient is healthy
- Intensified physical symptoms around sympathetic people
- Rejection of the idea that the symptoms are stress related
- Use of symptoms to avoid difficult situations
- Vague physical symptoms.

DIAGNOSTIC TEST RESULTS
- Test results are inconsistent with patient's complaint and physical findings.

NURSING DIAGNOSIS
- Knowledge deficit
- Ineffective individual coping
- Altered health maintenance

TREATMENT
- Individual therapy

Drug therapy
- Benzodiazepines: lorazepam (Ativan), alprazolam (Xanax)
- Tricyclic antidepressants: amitriptyline (Elavil), imipramine (Tofranil), doxepin (Sinequan), phenelzine (Nardil)

INTERVENTIONS AND RATIONALES
- Assess the patient's level of knowledge about how emotional issues can impact physiologic functioning *to promote understanding of the condition.*
- Encourage emotional expression *to discourage emotional repression, which can have physical consequences.*
- Respond to the patient's symptoms in a matter-of-fact way *to reduce secondary gain the patient achieves from talking about symptoms.*

Teaching topics
- Relaxation and assertiveness techniques
- Initiating conversations that focus on something other than physical maladies

Pain disorder

In pain disorder, the patient experiences pain in which psychological factors play a significant role in the onset, severity, exacerbation, or maintenance of the pain. The pain isn't intentionally produced or feigned by the patient. The pain becomes a major focus of life, and the patient is often unable to function socially or at work. The patient may have a physical ailment but shouldn't be experiencing such intense pain.

CONTRIBUTING FACTORS
- Traumatic, stressful, or humiliating experience

ASSESSMENT FINDINGS
- Acute and chronic pain not associated with a physiologic cause
- Anger, frustration, depression
- Drug-seeking behavior in an attempt to relieve pain
- Frequent visits to multiple doctors to seek pain relief
- Insomnia

DIAGNOSTIC TEST RESULTS
- Test results don't support patient complaints.
- With psychotherapy, the patient may recall a traumatic event.

NURSING DIAGNOSES
- Pain
- Ineffective individual coping
- Anxiety

TREATMENT
- Individual therapy

Drug therapy
- Anxiolytics (benzodiazepines): lorazepam (Ativan), alprazolam (Xanax)

• Tricyclic antidepressants: amitriptyline (Elavil), imipramine (Tofranil), doxepin (Sinequan)

INTERVENTIONS AND RATIONALES
• Ensure a safe, accepting environment for the patient *to promote therapeutic communication.*
• Acknowledge the patient's pain *to discourage the patient from striving to convince you that pain is real and to reinforce a therapeutic relationship.*
• Encourage the patient to recognize situations that precipitate pain *to foster an understanding of the disorder.*

Teaching topics
• Promoting social interaction
• Establishing constructive coping mechanisms
• Problem-solving techniques
• Nonpharmacologic pain management, such as guided imagery, massage, therapeutic touch, relaxation, heat, and cold

Parasomnias

Parasomnias are characterized by abnormal behavior that occurs during sleep. They include nightmare disorder, sleep terror disorder, and sleepwalking disorder.

   Nightmare disorder is characterized by the recurrence of frightening dreams that cause the patient to awaken from sleep. When the patient awakens, he is fully alert and experiences persistent anxiety or fear. Typically, the patient is able to recall details of the dream that involves physical danger.

   Sleep terror disorder is characterized by episodes of sleep terrors that cause distress or impairment of social or occupational functioning. The patient may sit up in bed screaming or crying with a frightened expression and signs of intense anxiety. During such episodes, the patient is difficult to awaken and, if he does awaken, he's generally confused or disoriented. The patient has no recollection of the dream content.

In **sleepwalking disorder,** the patient arises from bed and walks about. The patient has limited recall of the event upon awakening.

CONTRIBUTING FACTORS
• Severe psychosocial stressors
• Genetic predisposition
• Sleep deprivation
• Fever

ASSESSMENT FINDINGS
Nightmare disorder
• Anxiety
• Depression
• Dream recall
• Excessive sleepiness
• Irritability
• Mild autonomic arousal upon awakening (sweating, tachycardia, tachypnea)
• Poor concentration

Sleep terror disorder
• Autonomic signs of intense anxiety (tachycardia, tachypnea, flushing, sweating, increased muscle tone, dilated pupils)
• Inability to recall dream content
• Screaming or crying

Sleepwalking disorder
• Amnesia of the episode or limited recall
• Episode may include sitting up, talking, walking, or engaging in inappropriate behavior

DIAGNOSTIC TEST RESULTS
Nightmare disorder
• Polysomnography demonstrates abrupt awakenings from REM sleep that correspond to the individual's report of nightmares. These awakenings usually occur during the second half of the night. Heart rate and respiratory rate may increase or show increased variability before the awakening.

Sleep terror disorder
• Polysomnography reveals that sleep terrors begin during deep NREM sleep characterized by slow-frequency EEG activity.

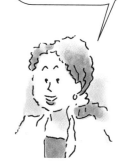

Acknowledging the patient's pain helps to discourage the patient from striving to convince you the pain is real.

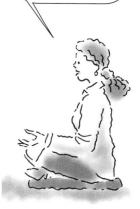

Nursing care in pain disorder may focus on pain management techniques, such as relaxation and meditation.

Sleepwalking disorder
• Polysomnography reveals episodes of sleep-walking that begin within the 1st few hours of sleep, usually during NREM stage 3 or 4 sleep.

NURSING DIAGNOSES
• Sleep pattern disturbance
• Fatigue
• Altered role performance

TREATMENT
• Hypnosis

Drug therapy
• Benzodiazepines: lorazepam (Ativan), alprazolam (Xanax)

INTERVENTIONS AND RATIONALES
• Assess the patient and document the symptoms of sleep disturbance *to aid in formulating a treatment plan.*
• Lock windows and doors if sleepwalking occurs *to maintain patient safety.*
• Provide emotional support *to allay the patient's anxiety.*
• Establish a sleep routine *to promote relaxation and sleep.*
• Schedule regular sleep and awakening times *so that the patient can learn specific planning strategies for managing sleep.*
• Administer medications as prescribed *to promote sleep.*

Teaching topics
• Safety measures for the patient with sleepwalking disorder
• Ways to identify and reduce stressors

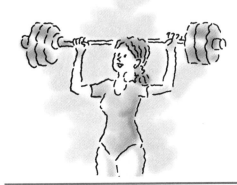

Pump up on practice questions

1. A client complains of experiencing an overwhelming urge to sleep. He states that he's been falling asleep while working at his desk. He reports that these episodes occur about five times daily. This client is most likely experiencing which sleep disorder?

   A.   Breathing-related sleep disorder
   B.   Narcolepsy
   C.   Primary hypersomnia
   D.   Circadian rhythm disorder

Answer: B. Narcolepsy is characterized by irresistible attacks of refreshing sleep that occur two to six times per day and last for 5 to 20 minutes. The client with breathing-related sleep disorder suffers interruptions in sleep that leave the client with excess sleepiness. In hypersomnia, the client suffers excess sleepiness and reports prolonged periods of nighttime sleep or daytime napping. With circadian

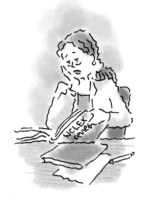

rhythm disorder, the client has periods of insomnia followed by periods of increased sleepiness.

➡ *NCLEX keys*

Nursing process step: Assessment
Client needs category: Psychosocial integrity
Client needs subcategory: Psychosocial adaptation
Taxonomic level: Application

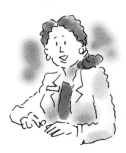

2. The nurse is caring for a client who complains of fatigue, inability to concentrate, and palpitations. The client states that she has been experiencing these symptoms for the past 6 months. Which factor in the client's history has most likely contributed to these symptoms?
   A. History of recent fever
   B. Shift work
   C. Hyperthyroidism
   D. Pheochromocytoma
Answer: B. The client is experiencing circadian rhythm sleep disorder (palpitations, GI disturbances, fatigue, haggard appearance, and poor concentration) which is typically caused by shift work, jet lag, or a delayed sleep phase. Fever is a contributing factor in parasomnias. Hyperthyroidism and pheochromocytoma are causative factors for primary insomnia.

➡ *NCLEX keys*

Nursing process step: Assessment
Client needs category: Psychosocial integrity
Client needs subcategory: Coping and adaptation
Taxonomic level: Analysis

3. A client comes to the clinic complaining of the inability to sleep over the past 2 months. He states that his inability to sleep is ruining his life because "getting sleep" is all he can think about. This client is most likely experiencing which sleep disorder?
   A. Circadian rhythm sleep disorder
   B. Breathing-related sleep disorder
   C. Primary insomnia
   D. Primary hypersomnia
Answer: C. The client with primary insomnia experiences difficulty initiating or maintaining sleep. A key symptom of primary insomnia is the client's intense focus and anxiety about not getting to sleep. The client diagnosed with circadian rhythm sleep disorder reports periods of insomnia at particular times during a 24-hour period and excessive sleepiness at other times. Excessive sleepiness is the most common complaint of clients affected by breathing-related sleep disorder. The client experiencing primary hypersomnia typically sleeps 8 to 12 hours per night. They fall asleep easily and sleep through the night, but often have trouble awakening in the morning.

➡ *NCLEX keys*

Nursing process step: Assessment
Client needs category: Psychosocial integrity
Client needs subcategory: Coping and adaptation
Taxonomic level: Analysis

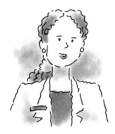

4. The nurse is preparing a teaching plan for a client diagnosed with primary insomnia. Which of the following teaching topics should be included in the plan?

A. Eating unlimited spicy foods, and limiting caffeine and alcohol
B. Exercising 1 hour before bedtime to promote sleep
C. Importance of sleeping whenever the client tires
D. Drinking warm milk before bed to induce sleep

Answer: D. Clients diagnosed with primary insomnia should be taught that drinking warm milk before bedtime can help induce sleep. They should also be taught the importance of limiting spicy foods, alcohol and caffeine; the need to avoid exercising within 3 hours before bedtime; and establishing a routine bedtime and avoid napping.

➡ *NCLEX keys*
Nursing process step: Planning
Client needs category: Psychosocial integrity
Client needs subcategory: Coping and adaptation
Taxonomic level: Application

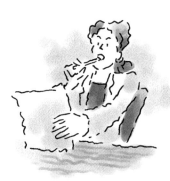

5. The nurse is caring for a client hospitalized on numerous occasions for complaints of chest pain and fainting spells, which she attributes to her deteriorating heart condition. No relatives or friends report ever actually seeing a fainting spell. After undergoing an extensive cardiac, pulmonary, gastrointestinal, and neurologic work-up, she is told that all test results are completely negative. The client remains persistent in her belief that she has a serious illness. What diagnosis is appropriate for this client?

A. Exhibitionism
B. Somatoform disorder
C. Degenerative dementia
D. Echolalia

Answer: B. Somatoform disorders are characterized by recurrent and multiple physical symptoms that have no organic or physiologic base. Exhibitionism involves public exposure of genitals. Degenerative dementia is characterized by deterioration of mental capacities. Echolalia is a repetition of words or phrases.

➡ *NCLEX keys*
Nursing process step: Assessment
Client needs category: Safe, effective care environment
Client needs subcategory: Management of care
Taxonomic level: Analysis

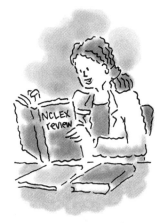

6. The nurse is caring for a client who believes he has cancer. He has visited several oncologists and undergone many tests. Thus far, no evidence of cancer has been found. The client remains convinced he is gravely ill and tells the nurse he doesn't expect to live much longer. What specific type of disorder is the client exhibiting?

A. Hypochondriasis
B. Dependency
C. Denial
D. Confabulation

Answer: A. Hypochondriasis is marked by a persistent fear or belief that one has a serious illness. Dependency involves expectations that another person should do all the work to change the client from relative illness to health. Denial is lack of awareness and is usually an unconscious defense mechanism. Confabulation is a reaction in which the client invents answers, attempting to fill in memory gaps.

➡ NCLEX keys
Nursing process step: Assessment
Client needs category: Psychosocial integrity
Client needs subcategory: Coping and adaptation
Taxonomic level: Knowledge

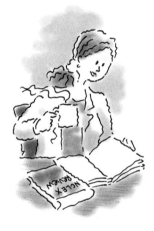

7. The nurse is caring for a client who exhibits signs of somatization. Which of the following statements is most relevant?
   A. Clients with somatization are cognitively impaired.
   B. Anxiety rarely coexists with somatization.
   C. Somatization exists when medical evidence supports the symptoms.
   D. Clients with somatization often have lengthy medical records.
Answer: D. Clients with somatization are prone to "doctor shop" and have extensive medical records as a result of their multiple procedures and tests. Clients with somatization aren't usually cognitively impaired. These clients have coexisting anxiety and depression, and no medical evidence to support a clear-cut diagnosis that is causing their symptoms.

➡ NCLEX keys
Nursing process step: Analysis
Client needs category: Psychosocial integrity
Client needs subcategory: Psychosocial adaptation
Taxonomic level: Analysis

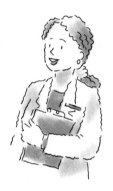

8. The nurse is caring for a client who during the admission assessment reveals symptoms of a sleep disorder. The client also admits that he has "broken down and cried for no apparent reason." Which of the following is most important for the nurse to initially consider to gain insight into the client's patterns of sleep and feelings of depression?
   A. Stressors in the client's life
   B. The client's weight
   C. Periods of apnea
   D. Sexual activity
Answer: A. Recognizing that sleep disturbances are often symptoms of stress, depression, and anxiety, the nurse is prudent to discuss these possible factors initially. If the client has a weight problem, suffers from sleep apnea, or reports sexual problems, these also can affect sleep; however, consideration of life stressors occurs first.

➡ *NCLEX keys*

Nursing process step: Analysis
Client needs category: Psychosocial integrity
Client needs subcategory: Coping and adaptation
Taxonomic level: Analysis

9. The nurse is caring for a client who displays gait disturbances, paralysis, pseudoseizures, and tremors. These symptoms may be manifestations of what psychiatric disorder?

A. Pain disorder
B. Adjustment disorder
C. Delirium
D. Conversion disorder

Answer: D. Conversion disorders are most frequently associated with psychologically mediated neurologic deficits, such as those mentioned. Pain disorders and adjustment disorders aren't generally expressed in terms of neurologic deficits. Delirium is associated with cognitive impairment.

➡ *NCLEX keys*

Nursing process step: Knowledge
Client needs category: Psychosocial integrity
Client needs subcategory: Coping and adaptation
Taxonomic level: Analysis

10. The nurse is caring for a client who complains of chronic pain. Given this complaint, why would the nurse simultaneously evaluate both general physical and psychosocial problems?

A. Depression often is characterized by pain disorders and somatic complaints.
B. Combining evaluations will save time and allow for quicker delivery of health care.
C. Most insurance plans won't cover evaluation of both as separate entities.
D. The physician doesn't have the training to evaluate for psychosocial considerations.

Answer: A. Psychosocial factors should be suspected when pain persists beyond the normal tissue healing time and physical causes have been investigated. The other choices may or may not be correct, but certainly aren't credible in all cases.

➡ *NCLEX keys*

Nursing process step: Evaluation
Client needs category: Psychosocial integrity
Client needs subcategory: Coping and adaptation
Taxonomic level: Analysis

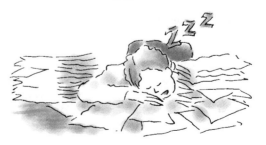

Congratulations! You've finished the chapter on sleep disorders. Now you've earned your nap.

14 Anxiety & Mood Disorders

Brush up on key concepts

Anxiety disorders are characterized by anxiety and avoidant behavior. Patients are overwhelmed by feelings of impending catastrophe, guilt, shame, and worthlessness. Patients with anxiety cling to maladaptive behaviors in an attempt to alleviate their own distress, but these behaviors only increase their symptoms.

Mood disorders are characterized by depressed or elevated moods that alter the patient's ability to cope with reality and to function normally.

At any time, you can review the major points of each disorder by consulting the *Cheat sheet* on pages 380 and 381.

Polish up on patient care

Major mood disorders include bipolar disorder and major depression. Major anxiety disorders include generalized anxiety, obsessive-compulsive disorder, panic disorder, phobias, and posttraumatic stress disorder.

Bipolar disorder

Bipolar disorder, also known as manic-depression, is a severe disturbance in affect, manifested by episodes of extreme sadness alternating with episodes of euphoria. Severity and duration of episodes vary. The exact biological basis of bipolar disorder remains unknown.

Two common patterns of bipolar disorder include:
• bipolar I, in which depressive episodes alternate with full manic episodes (hyperactive behavior, delusional thinking, grandiosity, and often hostility)
• bipolar II, characterized by recurrent depressive episodes and occasional manic episodes.

CONTRIBUTING FACTORS
• Concurrent major illness
• Environment
• Heredity
• History of psychiatric illnesses
• Seasons and circadian rhythms that affect mood
• Sleep deprivation
• Stressful events may produce limbic system dysfunction

ASSESSMENT FINDINGS
During periods of mania, look for:
• bizarre and eccentric appearance
• cognitive manifestations, such as difficulty concentrating, flight of ideas, delusions of grandeur, impaired judgment
• decreased sleep
• deteriorated physical appearance
• euphoria and hostility
• feelings of grandiosity
• impulsiveness
• increased energy, feeling of being charged up
• increased sexual interest and activity
• increased social contacts
• inflated sense of self-worth
• lack of inhibition
• rapid, jumbled speech
• recklessness.
During periods of depression, look for:
• altered sleep patterns
• amenorrhea

(Text continues on page 382.)

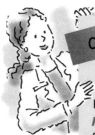

Cheat sheet

Anxiety & mood disorders refresher

BIPOLAR DISORDER

Key signs and symptoms
During periods of mania
- euphoria and hostility
- feelings of grandiosity
- inflated sense of self-worth
- increased energy, feeling of being charged up

During periods of depression
- altered sleep patterns
- anorexia and weight loss
- helplessness
- irritability
- lack of motivation
- low self-esteem
- sadness and crying

Key test results
- EEG is abnormal during the depressive episodes of bipolar I disorder and major depression.

Key treatments
- Individual therapy and family therapy
- Antimanic agents: lithium carbonate (Eskalith), lithium citrate (Cibalith-S)

Key interventions
During manic phase
- Decrease environmental stimuli by behaving consistently and supplying external controls.
- Ensure a safe environment.
- Define and explain acceptable behaviors, then set limits.
- Monitor drug levels, especially lithium.

During depressive phase
- Assess the level and intensity of the patient's depression.
- Ensure a safe environment for the patient.
- Assess the risk for suicide and formulate a safety contract with the patient, as appropriate.
- Observe the patient for medication compliance and adverse effects.
- Encourage the patient to identify current problems and stressors.

GENERALIZED ANXIETY DISORDER

Key signs and symptoms
- Easy startle reflex
- Excessive worry and anxiety
- Fatigue
- Fears of grave misfortune or death
- Motor tension
- Muscle tension

Key test results
- Laboratory tests exclude physiologic causes.

Key treatments
- Individual therapy focusing on coping skills
- Anxiolytics: alprazolam (Xanax), lorazepam (Ativan), clonazepam (Klonopin), buspirone (BuSpar)

Key interventions
- Help the patient identify and explore coping mechanisms used in the past.
- Observe for signs of mounting anxiety.

MAJOR DEPRESSION

Key signs and symptoms
- Altered sleep patterns
- Anorexia and weight loss
- Helplessness
- Irritability
- Lack of motivation
- Low self-esteem
- Sadness and crying

Key test results
- Beck depression scale indicates depression.

Key treatments
- Selective serotonin reuptake inhibitors: paroxetine (Paxil), fluoxetine (Prozac), sertraline (Zoloft)
- Tricyclic antidepressants: imipramine (Tofranil), desipramine (Norpramin), amitriptyline (Elavil)

Key interventions
- Assess the level and intensity of the patient's depression.
- Ensure a safe environment for the patient.
- Assess the risk for suicide and formulate a safety contract with the patient.

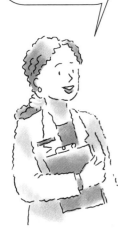

> Bipolar disorder isn't indicated by mood swings alone. It involves extreme behavior during both manic and depressive phases.

Anxiety & mood disorders refresher *(continued)*

• Observe the patient for medication compliance and adverse effects.

OBSESSIVE-COMPULSIVE DISORDER

Key signs and symptoms
• Compulsive behavior (which may include repetitive touching or counting, doing and undoing small tasks, or any other repetitive activity)
• Obsessive thoughts (which may include thoughts of contamination, repetitive worries about impending tragedy, repeating and counting images or words)

Key test results
• Positron emission tomography shows increased activity in the frontal lobe of the cerebral cortex.

Key treatments
• Behavioral therapy
• Individual therapy
• Benzodiazepines: alprazolam (Xanax), lorazepam (Ativan), clonazepam (Klonopin)

Key interventions
• Encourage the patient to express his feelings.
• Encourage the patient to identify situations that produce anxiety and precipitate obsessive-compulsive behavior.

PANIC DISORDER

Key signs and symptoms
• Diminished ability to focus, even with direction from others
• Edginess, impatience
• Loss of objectivity
• Severely impaired rational thought
• Uneasiness and tension

Key test results
• Medical tests eliminate physiologic cause.

Key treatments
• Individual therapy
• Benzodiazepines: alprazolam (Xanax), lorazepam (Ativan), clonazepam (Klonopin)

Key interventions
• During panic attacks, distract the patient from the attack.
• Approach the patient calmly and unemotionally.
• Use short, simple sentences.

PHOBIAS

Key signs and symptoms
• Panic, when confronted with the feared object
• Persistent fear of specific things, places, or situations

Key test results
• No specific tests can be used to diagnose for phobias.

Key treatments
• Benzodiazepines: alprazolam (Xanax), lorazepam (Ativan), clonazepam (Klonopin)

Key interventions
• Collaborate with the patient to identify the feared object or situation.
• Assist in desensitizing the patient.

POSTTRAUMATIC STRESS DISORDER

Key signs and symptoms
• Anxiety
• Flashbacks of the traumatic experience
• Nightmares about the traumatic experience
• Poor impulse control
• Social isolation
• Survivor guilt

Key test results
• No specific tests identify or confirm posttraumatic stress disorder.

Key treatments
• Individual therapy
• Group therapy
• Systematic desensitization
• Benzodiazepines: alprazolam (Xanax), lorazepam (Ativan), clonazepam (Klonopin)
• Tricyclic antidepressants: imipramine (Tofranil), amitriptyline (Elavil)

Key interventions
• Work with the patient to identify stressors.
• Provide for patient safety.
• Encourage the patient to explore the traumatic event and the meaning of the event.
• Assist the patient with problem solving and resolving guilt.

- anorexia and weight loss
- confusion and indecisiveness
- constipation
- decreased alertness
- delusions, hallucinations
- difficulty thinking logically
- guilt
- helplessness
- impotence and lack of interest in sex
- inability to experience pleasure
- irritability
- lack of motivation
- low self-esteem
- pessimism
- poor hygiene
- poor posture
- sadness and crying.

DIAGNOSTIC TEST RESULTS
- Abnormal dexamethasone suppression test results indicate bipolar I disorder.
- Cortisol secretion increases during manic episodes of bipolar I disorder.
- EEG is abnormal during the depressive episodes of bipolar I disorder and major depression.

NURSING DIAGNOSES
- Altered thought processes
- Bathing and hygiene self-care deficit
- Sleep pattern disturbance

TREATMENT
- Electroconvulsive therapy, if drug therapy fails
- Individual therapy and family therapy

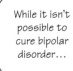

While it isn't possible to cure bipolar disorder...

...combining lithium with psychotherapy can bring manic-depressive symptoms under control.

Drug therapy
- Anticonvulsant agents: carbamazepine (Tegretol), divalproex sodium (Depakote)
- Antimanic agents: lithium carbonate (Eskalith), lithium citrate (Cibalith-S),
- Selective serotonin reuptake inhibitors (SSRIs): paroxetine (Paxil).

INTERVENTIONS AND RATIONALES
During the patient's manic phase
- Decrease environmental stimuli by behaving consistently and supplying external controls *to promote relaxation and enable sleep.*
- Ensure a safe environment *to protect the patient from himself.*
- Define and explain acceptable behaviors and then set limits *to begin a process in which the patient will eventually define and set his own limits.*
- Monitor drug levels, especially lithium, *to keep dosage within the therapeutic range.*

During the patient's depressive phase
- Assess the level and intensity of the patient's depression *because baseline information is essential for effective nursing care.*
- Ensure a safe environment for the patient *to protect the patient from self-inflicted harm.*
- Assess the risk for suicide and formulate a safety contract with the patient, as appropriate, *to ensure the patient's well-being and open lines of communication.*
- Observe the patient for medication compliance and adverse effects; *without compliance, there is little hope of progress.*
- Encourage the patient to identify current problems and stressors *so that he can begin therapeutic treatment.*
- Promote opportunities for increased involvement in activities through a structured, daily program *to help the patient feel comfortable with himself and others.*
- Select activities that ensure success and accomplishment *to increase self-esteem.*
- Help the patient to modify negative expectations and think more positively *as positive thinking will help the patient begin a healing process.*
- Spend time with the patient, even if the patient is too depressed to talk *to enhance the therapeutic relationship.*

Generalized anxiety disorder

A patient with generalized anxiety disorder worries excessively and experiences tremendous anxiety almost daily. The worry lasts for longer than 6 months, and is usually disproportionate to the situation. Both adults and children can be diagnosed with generalized anxiety disorder, though the content of the worry may differ.

CONTRIBUTING FACTORS
- Family history of anxiety
- Preexisting psychiatric problems, such as social phobia, panic disorder, and major depression

ASSESSMENT FINDINGS
- Autonomic hyperactivity
- Distractibility
- Easy startle reflex
- Excessive attention to surroundings
- Excessive worry and anxiety
- Fatigue
- Fears of grave misfortune or death
- Motor tension
- Muscle tension
- Pounding heart
- Repetitive thoughts
- Sleep disorder
- Strained expression
- Tingling of hands or feet
- Vigilance and scanning

DIAGNOSTIC TEST RESULTS
- Laboratory tests exclude physiologic causes.

NURSING DIAGNOSES
- Anxiety
- Ineffective individual coping
- Knowledge deficit

TREATMENT
- Individual therapy focusing on coping skills

Drug therapy
- Anxiolytics: alprazolam (Xanax), lorazepam (Ativan), clonazepam (Klonopin), buspirone (BuSpar)
- Beta-adrenergic blocker: propranolol (Inderal)
- Antihypertensives: clonidine (Catapres)
- Monoamine oxidase (MAO) inhibitors: phenelzine (Nardil), tranylcypromine (Parnate)
- SSRIs: paroxetine (Paxil), sertraline (Zoloft), fluoxetine (Prozac)
- Tricyclic antidepressants: imipramine (Tofranil), desipramine (Norpramin)

INTERVENTIONS AND RATIONALES
- Help the patient identify and explore coping mechanisms used in the past — *establishing a baseline for the level of current functioning will enable the nurse to build on the patient's knowledge.*
- Observe for signs of mounting anxiety *to direct measures to moderate it.*
- Negotiate a contract to work on goals *to give the patient control of his own situation.*
- Alter the environment *to reduce the anxiety or to meet the patient's needs.*
- Monitor diet and nutrition; reduce caffeine intake *to reduce anxiety.*

Teaching topics
- Recognizing signs of anxiety
- Altering diet when receiving MAO inhibitors (Caffeine can cause arrhythmias. Foods containing tyramine, such as fava beans, yeast-containing and fermented foods, and avocados, can cause a hypertensive crisis.)

Major depression

Major depression is a syndrome of persistent sad, dysphoric mood accompanied by disturbances in sleep and appetite from lethargy and an inability to experience pleasure.

Major depression can profoundly alter social functioning, but the most severe complication of major depression is the potential for suicide.

CONTRIBUTING FACTORS
- Current substance abuse

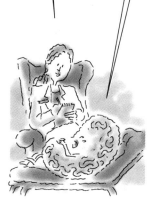

Each patient and each depression is unique.

So, finding the most effective drug and dosage is often a process of trial and error.

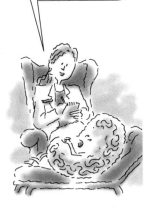

Treatment for depression usually requires collaboration with the patient to find an effective program of drug therapy and psychotherapy.

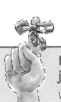
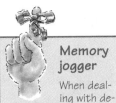

Memory jogger

When dealing with depressive patients, Think COMPARE.

Consult with staff.

Observe the suicidal patient.

Maintain personal contact.

Provide a safe environment.

Assess for clues to suicide.

Remove dangerous objects.

Encourage expression of feelings.

• Deficiencies in the receptor sites for some neurotransmitters: norepinephrine, serotonin, dopamine, and acetylcholine
• Family history of depressive disorders
• Hormonal imbalances
• Lack of social support
• Nutritional deficiencies
• Prior episode of depression
• Significant medical problems
• Stressful life events

ASSESSMENT FINDINGS
• Altered sleep patterns
• Amenorrhea
• Anorexia and weight loss
• Confusion and indecisiveness
• Constipation
• Decreased alertness
• Delusions, hallucinations
• Difficulty thinking logically
• Guilt
• Helplessness
• Impotence or lack of interest in sex
• Inability to experience pleasure
• Irritability
• Lack of motivation
• Low self-esteem
• Pessimism
• Poor hygiene
• Poor posture
• Sadness and crying

DIAGNOSTIC TEST RESULTS
• Thyroid test is abnormal in major depression.
• Beck depression inventory indicates depression.

NURSING DIAGNOSES
• Hopelessness
• Impaired social interaction
• Self-esteem disturbance

TREATMENT
• Electroconvulsive therapy (ECT)
• Individual therapy
• Family therapy
• Phototherapy

Drug therapy
• MAO inhibitors: phenelzine (Nardil)
• SSRIs: paroxetine (Paxil), fluoxetine (Prozac), sertraline (Zoloft)
• Tricyclic antidepressants: imipramine (Tofranil), desipramine (Norpramin), amitriptyline (Elavil)

INTERVENTIONS AND RATIONALES
• Assess the level and intensity of the patient's depression *because baseline information is essential for effective nursing care.*
• Ensure a safe environment for the patient *to protect the patient from self-inflicted harm.*
• Assess the risk for suicide and formulate a safety contract with the patient, as appropriate, *to ensure the patient's well-being and open lines of communication.*
• Reorient the patient undergoing ECT as needed. *Patients receiving ECT often have temporary memory loss.*
• Observe the patient for medication compliance and adverse effects; *without compliance, there is little hope of progress.*
• Encourage the patient to identify current problems and stressors *so that he can begin therapeutic treatment.*
• Promote opportunities for increased involvement in activities through a structured, daily program *to help the patient feel comfortable with himself and others.*
• Select activities that ensure success and accomplishment *to increase self-esteem.*
• Help the patient to modify negative expectations and think more positively *as positive thinking will help the patient begin a healing process.*
• Spend time with the patient, even if the patient is too depressed to talk *to enhance the therapeutic relationship.*

Teaching topics
• Learning relaxation and sleep methods
• Complying with therapy
• If taking MAO inhibitors, avoiding tyramine-containing foods such as wine, beer, cheeses, preserved fruits, meats, and vegetables

Obsessive-compulsive disorder

Obsessive-compulsive disorder is characterized by recurrent obsessions (intrusive thoughts, images, and impulses) and compulsions (repetitive behaviors in response to an obsession). The obsessions and compulsions cause intense stress and impair the patient's functioning. Some patients have simultaneous symptoms of depression.

CONTRIBUTING FACTORS
• Brain lesions
• Childhood trauma
• Lack of role models to teach coping skills
• Multiple stressors

ASSESSMENT FINDINGS
• Compulsive behavior (which may include repetitive touching or counting, doing and undoing, or any other repetitive activity)
• Obsessive thoughts (which may include thoughts of contamination, repetitive worries about impending tragedy, repeating and counting images or words)
• Social impairment

DIAGNOSTIC TEST RESULTS
• Positron emission tomography shows increased activity in the frontal lobe of the cerebral cortex.

NURSING DIAGNOSES
• Anxiety
• Ineffective individual coping
• Self-esteem disturbance

TREATMENT
• Behavioral therapy
• Individual therapy

Drug therapy
• Benzodiazepines: alprazolam (Xanax), lorazepam (Ativan), clonazepam (Klonopin)
• MAO inhibitors: phenelzine (Nardil), tranylcypromine (Parnate)
• SSRIs: paroxetine (Paxil)
• Tricyclic antidepressants: imipramine (Tofranil), desipramine (Norpramin)

INTERVENTIONS AND RATIONALES
• Encourage the patient to express his feelings *to decrease the patient's level of stress.*
• Help the patient assess how his compulsive behaviors affect his functioning. The patient needs *to realistically evaluate the consequences of his behavior.*
• Encourage the patient to identify situations that produce anxiety and precipitate obsessive-compulsive behavior *to help the patient evaluate and cope with his own condition.*
• Work with the patient to develop appropriate coping skills *to reduce anxiety.*

Teaching topics
• Understanding anxiety and obsessive-compulsive disorder

Panic disorder

While everyone experiences some level of anxiety, patients with panic disorder experience a nonspecific feeling of terror and dread, accompanied by symptoms of physiologic stress. This level of anxiety makes it difficult, if not impossible, for the patient to carry out the normal functions of everyday life.

CONTRIBUTING FACTORS
• Agoraphobia (fear of being alone or in public places)
• Asthma
• Cardiovascular disease
• Familial pattern
• GI disorders
• History of anxiety disorders
• History of depression
• Neurologic abnormalities: abnormal activity on the medial portion of the temporal lobe in the parahippocampal area, and significant asymmetrical atrophy of the temporal lobe
• Neurotransmitter involvement
• Stressful lifestyle

ASSESSMENT FINDINGS
• Abdominal discomfort or pain, nausea, heartburn, or diarrhea
• Avoidance (the patient's refusal to encounter situations that may cause anxiety)

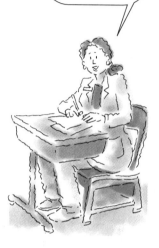

Don't worry. Feeling nervous about the NCLEX doesn't mean you've developed panic disorder.

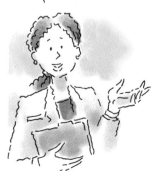

Note that depressed or anxious patients often attempt to self-medicate. Be aware of possible interactions with prescribed treatments.

• Chest pressure, lump in throat, or choking sensation
• Confusion
• Decreased ability to relate to others
• Diminished ability to focus, even with direction from others
• Edginess, impatience
• Eyelid twitching
• Fidgeting or pacing
• Flushing or pallor
• Generalized weakness, tremors
• Increased or decreased blood pressure
• Insomnia
• Loss of appetite or revulsion toward food
• Loss of objectivity
• Palpitations and tachycardia
• Physical tension
• Potential for dangerous, impulsive actions
• Rapid speech
• Rapid, shallow breathing or shortness of breath
• Severely impaired rational thought
• Startle reaction
• Sudden urge and frequent urination
• Sweating, itching
• Uneasiness and tension

DIAGNOSTIC TESTS
• Medical tests eliminate physiologic cause.
• Urine and blood tests to check for presence of psychoactive agents.

NURSING DIAGNOSES
• Anxiety
• Ineffective individual coping
• Powerlessness

TREATMENT
• Individual therapy
• Group therapy

Drug therapy
• Benzodiazepines: alprazolam (Xanax), lorazepam (Ativan), clonazepam (Klonopin)
• MAO inhibitors: phenelzine (Nardil); in patients with severe panic disorder, tranylcypromine (Parnate)
• SSRIs: paroxetine (Paxil)
• Tricyclic antidepressants: imipramine (Tofranil), desipramine (Norpramin)

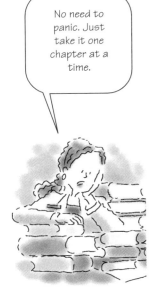

No need to panic. Just take it one chapter at a time.

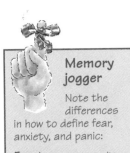

Memory jogger

Note the differences in how to define fear, anxiety, and panic:

Fear is a response to external stimuli.

Anxiety is a response to internal conflict.

Panic is an extreme level of anxiety.

INTERVENTIONS AND RATIONALES
• During panic attacks, distract the patient from the attack *to alleviate the effects of panic.*
• Discuss other methods of coping with stress *to make the patient aware of alternatives.*
• Approach the patient calmly and unemotionally *to reduce the risk of further stressing the patient.*
• Use short, simple sentences *because the patient's ability to focus and to relate to others is diminished.*
• Administer medications as needed *to ensure a therapeutic response.*

Teaching topics
• Learning decision-making and problem-solving skills
• Learning relaxation techniques

Phobias

A phobia is an intense, irrational fear of something external. It's a fear that persists, even though the patient recognizes its irrationality. Phobias are resistant to insight-oriented therapies.

CONTRIBUTING FACTORS
• Biochemical, involving neurotransmitters
• Familial patterns
• Traumatic events

ASSESSMENT FINDINGS
• Displacement (shifting of emotions from their original object) and symbolization
• Disruption in social life or work life
• Panic when confronted with the feared object
• Persistent fear of specific things, places, or situations

DIAGNOSTIC TEST RESULTS
• No specific test is used to diagnose for phobias.

NURSING DIAGNOSES
• Anxiety
• Fear
• Powerlessness

TREATMENT
- Individual therapy
- Systematic desensitization

Drug therapy
- Beta-adrenergic blocker: propranolol (Inderal) for phobia related to public speaking
- Benzodiazepines: alprazolam (Xanax), lorazepam (Ativan), clonazepam (Klonopin)
- MAO inhibitors: phenelzine (Nardil), tranylcypromine (Parnate)
- SSRIs: paroxetine (Paxil)
- Tricyclic antidepressants: imipramine (Tofranil), desipramine (Norpramin)

INTERVENTIONS AND RATIONALES
- Collaborate with the patient to identify the feared object or situation *to develop an effective treatment plan.*
- Assist in desensitizing the patient *to diminish the patient's fear.*
- Remind the patient about resources and personal strengths *to build self-esteem.*

Teaching topics
- Learning assertiveness techniques
- Learning relaxation techniques
- Participating in the desensitizing process

Posttraumatic stress disorder

Posttraumatic stress disorder (PTSD) is a group of symptoms that develop after a traumatic event. This traumatic event may involve death, injury, or threat to physical integrity. In PTSD, ordinary coping behaviors fail to relieve the anxiety. The patient may experience reactions that are acute, chronic, or delayed.

CONTRIBUTING FACTORS
- High anxiety
- Low self-esteem
- Personal experience of threatened injury or death
- Preexisting psychopathology
- Witnessing a traumatic event happen to a close friend or family member

ASSESSMENT FINDINGS
- Anger

- Anxiety
- Avoidance of people involved in the trauma
- Avoidance of places where the trauma occurred
- Chronic tension
- Detachment
- Difficulty concentrating
- Difficulty falling or staying asleep
- Emotional numbness
- Flashbacks of the traumatic experience
- Hyperalertness
- Inability to recall details of the traumatic event
- Labile affect
- Nightmares about the traumatic experience
- Poor impulse control
- Social isolation
- Survivor guilt

DIAGNOSTIC TEST RESULTS
- No specific tests identify or confirm PTSD.

NURSING DIAGNOSES
- Post-trauma syndrome
- Powerlessness
- Self-esteem disturbance

TREATMENT
- Alcohol and drug rehabilitation, when indicated
- Individual therapy
- Group therapy
- Progressive relaxation
- Systematic desensitization

Drug therapy
- Benzodiazepines: alprazolam (Xanax), lorazepam (Ativan), clonazepam (Klonopin)
- Beta-adrenergic blockers: propranolol (Inderal)
- Monoamine oxidase (MAO) inhibitors: phenelzine (Nardil), tranylcypromine (Parnate)
- Tricyclic antidepressants: imipramine (Tofranil), amitriptyline (Elavil)

INTERVENTIONS AND RATIONALES
- Work with the patient to identify stressors *to initiate effective coping.*
- Provide for patient safety *because the patient's ineffective coping, coupled with the in-*

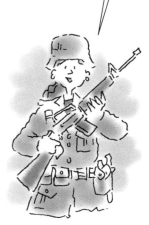

PTSD was originally called "shell shock" because participation in active combat is a common cause of this disorder.

tensity of the reaction and poor impulse control, increases the patient's risk of injury.
• Encourage the patient to explore the traumatic event and the meaning of the event *to promote effective coping.*
• Assist the patient with problem solving and resolving guilt *to help the patient understand that chance probably played a larger part in the trauma than did his personal actions, decisions, or inactions.*

Teaching topics
• Joining support groups
• Learning relaxation techniques
• Promoting social interaction

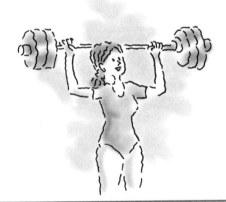

Pump up on practice questions

1. The nurse is caring for a client who is experiencing a panic attack. Which intervention would be most appropriate?
  A. Tell the client he's all right, and there is no need to panic.
  B. Speak to the client in short, simple sentences.
  C. Explain to the client that there's no need to worry because he's safe.
  D. Give the client a detailed explanation of his panic reaction.
Answer: B. The client experiencing a panic attack is unable to focus and his ability to relate to others is diminished; therefore, short, simple sentences are the most effective means of

communication. Options A, B, and C minimize the patient's anxiety.

Nursing process step: Evaluation
Client needs category: Psychosocial integrity
Client needs subcategory: Coping and adaptation
Taxonomic level: Analysis

2. The nurse is caring for a client who reports that she often feels a choking sensation in her throat, a racing heart, dizziness, and fearfulness. All of these symptoms have occurred almost daily for the past 3 months. Suspecting a psychological component to these symptoms, what would the nurse anticipate administering?
  A. Benzodiazepines
  B. Proton pump inhibitors
  C. Nitroprusside
  D. Lithium carbonate
Answer: A. Pharmacologic management would consist of either tricyclic antidepressants or benzodiazepines. Proton pump inhibitors are used for GI disorders. Nitroprusside is a potent vasodilator, used for hypertensive emergencies. Lithium carbonate is an antimanic agent.

Nursing process step: Implementation
Client needs category: Physiological integrity
Client needs subcategory: Pharmacological and parenteral therapies
Taxonomic level: Application

3. The nurse is caring for a client who complains of a choking sensation in his throat, a racing heart, dizziness, and fearfulness. Which of the following could cause these symptoms?
  A. Substance abuse
  B. Panic disorder
  C. Phobia
  D. Huntington's chorea
Answer: B. Panic disorder is diagnosed when associated symptoms occur more than four times in 1 month. Other related symptoms include rubbery legs, faintness, chest discomfort, preoccupation with health, and a feeling of going insane. Substance abuse can cause a

large spectrum of similar symptoms, but it would depend on what was ingested. Phobias are generally related to a specific phobic stimulus (heights, for instance). Huntington's chorea is a neurologic degenerative disease.

➡ **NCLEX keys**
Nursing process step: Assessment
Client needs category: Psychosocial integrity
Client needs subcategory: Coping and adaptation
Taxonomic level: Knowledge

4. A man in his mid-forties complains of severe palpitations, sweating, and intense fear when he has to speak in public. Because his job entails lecturing in auditoriums, what would the nurse suggest?
   A. Behavioral therapy and beta-adrenergic blockers
   B. Quitting his job altogether
   C. Telling jokes to reduce anxiety
   D. Monoamine oxidase (MAO) inhibitors

Answer: A. Behavioral therapy and beta-adrenergic blockers have been shown to decrease anxiety related to speaking in public. Quitting one's job is a drastic means that would only be suggested if all other therapies fail. Telling jokes wouldn't reduce anxiety in this situation for this person; in fact, this may actually increase anxiety (for example, worrying about telling the joke right). MAO inhibitors aren't indicated for such periods of episodic anxiety.

➡ **NCLEX keys**
Nursing process step: Implementation
Client needs category: Physiological integrity
Client needs subcategory: Pharmacological and parenteral therapies
Taxonomic level: Application

5. The nurse is caring for a client who complains of palpitations, sweating, and intense fear when speaking in public. What would be an appropriate diagnosis for that client?
   A. Panic attack
   B. Major depression
   C. Phobia
   D. Malingering

Answer: C. Even though a panic attack may have similar symptoms, phobias are characterized by episodic anxiety in response to a specific precipitating event. Panic attacks may not have such a specific cause. Symptoms of major depression aren't short-lived and are associated with considerable disability. Malingering occurs when an incentive for symptoms exists.

➡ **NCLEX keys**
Nursing process step: Analysis
Client needs category: Psychosocial integrity
Client needs subcategory: Coping and adaptation
Taxonomic level: Comprehension

6. The nurse is caring for a client with panic disorder and a client with a phobia. What is one major difference between those two disorders?
   A. Specific precipitants are present with panic disorders.
   B. Specific precipitants are present with phobias.
   C. The symptoms are different for each disorder.
   D. Phobias are one cause of major depressive states.

Answer: B. Phobias are characterized by episodic anxiety in response to specific precipitants, such as flying, talking in public, and insects. Both may be associated with similar, not different, symptoms. Neither phobias nor panic disorders are grouped with the depressive disorders.

➡ **NCLEX keys**
Nursing process step: Analysis
Client needs category: Psychosocial integrity
Client needs subcategory: Coping and adaptation
Taxonomic level: Comprehension

7. The nurse is caring for a client who was serving in the military during a bombing of an American embassy. Which findings would suggest posttraumatic stress disorder (PTSD)?
   A. Seizures, headache
   B. Stuttering, flashbacks, memory loss
   C. Paralysis, flashbacks, seizures
   D. Anger, depression, flashbacks

Answer: D. PTSD occurs after a person experiences trauma outside the range of normal human experiences. The disorder is characterized by nightmares, flashbacks, anxiety, and depression. The other symptoms don't apply.

➡ *NCLEX keys*

Nursing process step: Analysis
Client needs category: Psychosocial integrity
Client needs subcategory: Coping and adaptation
Taxonomic level: Knowledge

8. The nurse is caring for a client who has generalized anxiety disorder. Which statement is true about this client?
    A. The client has regular obsessions.
    B. Relaxation techniques and psychotherapy are necessary for cure.
    C. Nightmares and flashbacks are common in individuals who suffer from generalized anxiety disorder.
    D. Generalized anxiety disorder is characterized by anxiety that lasts longer than 6 months.

Answer: D. Constant patterns of anxiety that affect the client for more than 6 months and interfere with normal activities are characteristic of generalized anxiety disorder. Frequently, pharmaceutical therapy with benzodiazepines can help. Clients having regular obsessions are probably suffering from obsessive-compulsive disorder. Nightmares and flashbacks are typical symptoms of posttraumatic stress disorder.

➡ *NCLEX keys*

Nursing process step: Implementation
Client needs category: Psychosocial integrity
Client needs subcategory: Coping and adaptation
Taxonomic level: analysis

9. The nurse is caring for a client who has a mood disorder. This disorder has a very strong biological and genetic component. What disorder does this client most likely have?

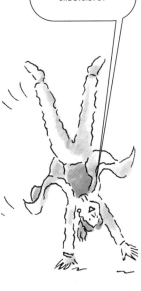

It's okay to be in a happy mood — you've finished the chapter on mood disorders!

A. Generalized anxiety disorder
B. Adjustment disorder with depressed mood
C. Posttraumatic stress disorder
D. Bipolar disorder

Answer: D. Formerly called manic-depression, bipolar disorder has a genetic link. About 10% of children who have a parent with this will develop it themselves. The other choices have no clear-cut genetic or biological link.

➡ *NCLEX keys*

Nursing process step: Analysis
Client needs category: Psychosocial integrity
Client needs subcategory: Coping and adaptation
Taxonomic level: Comprehension

10. The nurse is caring for a client who suffers from depression. Two weeks after the start of treatment, this client has gained 2 lb (0.9 kg), combs her hair, and is beginning to participate in therapy. The nurse explains that since she is showing signs of improvement, she will be able to choose her daily menu. She tells the client that she must avoid cheese, yogurt, preserved meats, and vegetables. Based on this information, the client is most likely receiving which drug therapy to treat her depression?
    A. MAO inhibitor
    B. Benzodiazepine
    C. Serotonin reuptake inhibitor
    D. Tricyclic antidepressant

Answer: A. This client is receiving an MAO inhibitor, which requires the client to avoid tyramine-rich foods, such as cheese, beer, wine, yogurt, and preserved fruits, vegetables, and meats. Benzodiazepines, serotonin reuptake inhibitors, and tricyclic antidepressants do not require dietary restrictions except avoiding alcoholic beverages.

➡ *NCLEX keys*

Nursing process step: Evaluation
Client needs category: Psychosocial integrity
Client needs subcategory: Psychosocial adaptation
Taxonomic level: Analysis

Cognitive Disorders

Brush up on key concepts

Cognitive disorders result from any condition that alters or destroys brain tissue and, in turn, impairs cerebral functioning. Symptoms of cognitive disorders include cognitive impairment, behavioral dysfunction, and personality changes. The most common cognitive disorders described in the *Diagnostic and Statistical Manual of Mental Disorders*, 4th ed., are delirium, dementia, and amnestic disorders.

At any time, you can review the major points of each disorder by consulting the *Cheat sheet* on pages 392 and 393.

Catching up on cognitive disorders

Cognitive mental disorders are characterized by the disruption of cognitive functioning. Clinically, cognitive disorders are manifested as mental deficits in patients who hadn't previously exhibited such deficits.

Cognitive disorders are difficult to identify and treat. The key to diagnosis lies in the discovery of an organic problem with the brain's tissue.

Cognitive disorders may result from:
• a primary brain disease
• the brain's response to a systemic disturbance such as a medical condition
• the brain tissue's reaction to a toxic substance as in substance abuse.

Brain disruptions

Delirium is often caused by the disruption of brain homeostasis. When the source of the disturbance is eliminated, cognitive deficits generally resolve.

Common causes of delirium include postoperative conditions or metabolic disorders, withdrawal from alcohol and drugs, and toxic substances. Toxic substances are especially difficult to deal with, as they can have residual effects. Drugs present another problem — a medication may be innocuous by itself, but deadly when taken with another medication or food. The elderly are especially susceptible to the toxic effects of medication.

Brain defects

Unlike delirium, **dementia** is caused by primary brain pathology. Consequently, reversal of cognitive defects is less likely. Dementia can easily be mistaken for delirium, so the cause needs to be thoroughly investigated.

Polish up on patient care

Major cognitive disorders include Alzheimer's-type dementia, amnesic disorder, delirium, and vascular dementia.

Alzheimer's-type dementia

A patient with Alzheimer's-type dementia suffers a global impairment of cognitive functioning, memory, and personality. The dementia occurs gradually, but with continuous decline. Damage from Alzheimer's-type dementia is irreversible. Because of the difficulty of obtaining direct pathological evidence of Alzheimer's disease, the diagnosis can be made only when the etiologies for the dementia have been eliminated.

CONTRIBUTING FACTORS
• Alterations in acetylcholine (a neurotransmitter)
• Altered immune function, with autoantibody production in the brain

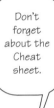

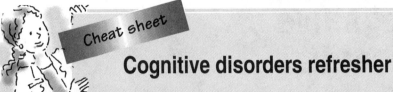

Cheat sheet

Cognitive disorders refresher

ALZHEIMER'S-TYPE DEMENTIA

Key signs and symptoms
Stage I
- Decreased concentration
- Depression
- Inability to retain new memories

Stage II
- Disorientation to person, place, and time
- Hoarding
- Inability to recognize family members
- Compulsive touching and examination of objects

Stage III
- Decreased response to stimuli
- Deterioration in motor ability

Key test results
- Cognitive assessment scale demonstrates cognitive impairment.
- Functional dementia scale shows degree of dementia.
- Magnetic resonance imaging (MRI)shows apparent structural and neuralgic changes.
- Mini–Mental Status Examination reveals disorientation and cognitive impairment.

Key treatments
- Group therapy
- Anticholinesterase agents: tacrine (Cognex), donapezil (Aricept)

Key interventions
- Remove any hazardous items or potential obstacles from the patient's environment.
- Provide verbal and nonverbal communication that is consistent and structured.
- Increase social interaction.
- Encourage the use of community resources.

AMNESTIC DISORDER

Key signs and symptoms
- Confusion, disorientation, and lack of insight
- Inability to learn and retain new information
- Tendency to remember things from very remote past better than more recent events

Key test results
- Mini–Mental Status Examination shows disorientation and lack of recall.

Key treatments
- Correction of the underlying medical cause
- Group therapy

Key interventions
- Ensure the patient's safety.
- Encourage exploration of feelings.
- Provide simple, clear medical information.

DELIRIUM

Key signs and symptoms
- Altered psychomotor activity, such as apathy, withdrawal, and agitation
- Bizarre, destructive behavior, worsening at night
- Disorganized thinking
- Distractibility
- Impaired decision making
- Inability to complete tasks
- Insomnia or daytime sleepiness
- Poor impulse control
- Rambling, bizarre, or incoherent speech

Key test results
- Laboratory results indicate delirium is a result of a physiologic condition, intoxication, substance withdrawal, toxic exposure, prescribed medicines, or a combination of these factors.

Key treatments
- Correction of underlying physiologic problem
- Cholinesterase inhibitor: physostigmine (Antilirium)
- Antipsychotic agents: risperidone (Risperdal)

Key interventions
- Determine the degree of cognitive impairment.
- Create a structured and safe environment.
- Keep room lit.

VASCULAR DEMENTIA

Key signs and symptoms
- Depression
- Difficulty following instructions

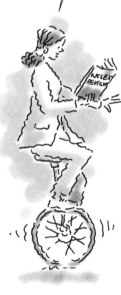

Don't forget about the Cheat sheet.

Cognitive disorders *(continued)*

VASCULAR DEMENTIA *(continued)*
- Emotional lability
- Inappropriate emotional reactions
- Memory loss
- Wandering and getting lost in familiar places

Key test results
- Cognitive assessment scale shows deterioration in cognitive ability.
- Global deterioration scale signifies degenerative dementia.
- Mini–Mental Status Examination reveals disorientation and recall difficulty.

Key treatments
- Carotid endarterectomy to remove blockages in the carotid artery
- Treatment for the underlying condition (hypertension, high cholesterol, or diabetes)
- Aspirin, to decrease platelet aggregation and prevent clots

Key interventions
- Orient the patient to his surroundings.
- Monitor the environment.
- Encourage the patient to express feelings of sadness and loss.

- Familial history, such as a first-degree relative with Alzheimer's disease or Down syndrome
- Increased brain atrophy, with wider sulci and cerebral ventricles than seen in normal aging
- Neurofibrillary tangles and beta amyloid neuritic plaques, mainly in the frontal and temporal lobes

ASSESSMENT FINDINGS
Alzheimer's-type dementia has three identifiable stages. In stage I, look for:
- agitated or apathetic mood
- attempts to cover up symptoms
- decline in personal appearance
- decline in recent memory
- decreased concentration
- depression
- disorientation regarding time
- disturbed sleep
- inability to retain new memories
- susceptibility to falls
- transitory delusions of persecution
- wandering.
  In stage II, look for:
- confabulation (unconscious filling of gaps in memory with fabricated facts and experiences)
- continuous, repetitive behaviors
- diminishing ability to understand or use language
- disorientation to person, place and time
- hoarding
- inability to recognize family members
- inability to retain new information

- incontinence of bowel and bladder
- increased appetite with no weight gain
- requiring assistance with activities of daily living
- socially unacceptable behavior
- tantrums.
  In stage III, look for:
- compulsive touching and examination of objects
- decreased response to stimuli
- deterioration in motor ability
- emaciation
- nonresponsiveness
- severe decline in cognitive functioning.

DIAGNOSTIC TEST RESULTS
- Cognitive assessment scale demonstrates cognitive impairment.
- Functional dementia scale shows degree of dementia
- Magnetic resonance imaging (MRI) shows apparent structural and neurologic changes.
- Mini–Mental Status Examination reveals disorientation and cognitive impairment.
- Spinal fluid contains increased beta amyloid.

NURSING DIAGNOSES
- Bathing, hygiene, and self-care deficit
- Impaired memory
- Caregiver role strain

TREATMENT
- Group therapy
- Hyperbaric oxygen treatment
- Palliative medical treatment

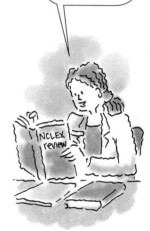

To recall symptoms, it may help to remember that Alzheimer's used to be described as "going senile."

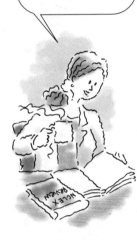

Many NCLEX questions about Alzheimer's-type dementia may focus on caregivers — who are also significantly affected by this disorder.

Because patients with Alzheimer's are confused, communication with them should be consistent, direct, and structured.

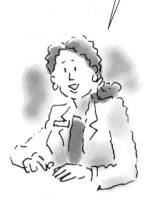

• Tissue transplantation (currently being studied)

Drug therapy

• Anticholinesterase agents: tacrine (Cognex), donapezil (Aricept)
• Antipsychotic agents: haloperidol (Haldol), risperidone (Risperdal) in low doses
• Benzodiazepines: alprazolam (Xanax)

INTERVENTIONS AND RATIONALES

• Remove any hazardous items or potential obstacles from the patient's environment *to maintain a safe environment for the patient.*
• Monitor food and fluid intake *because patient may not take in enough nutrition.*
• Provide verbal and nonverbal communication that is consistent and structured *to prevent added confusion.*
• State expectations simply and completely *to orient the patient.*
• Increase social interaction *to provide stimuli for the patient.*
• Encourage the use of community resources; make appropriate referrals as necessary *to find outside support for caregivers.*
• Promote physical activity and sensory stimulation *to alleviate symptoms of the disorder.*

Teaching topics

• Finding support and education (for caregivers)
• Learning stress-relief techniques (for caregivers)

Amnestic disorder

In amnestic disorder, the patient experiences a loss of both short-term memory and long-term memory. He is unable to recall some or many past events. The patient's abstract thinking, judgment, and personality usually remain intact. Symptoms may have a sudden or gradual onset and may be transient or long-lasting.

Amnestic disorder differs from dissociative amnesia in that it results from an identifiable physical cause, rather than psychosocial stressors.

CONTRIBUTING FACTORS

• Adverse effects of certain medications
• Brain surgery
• Cerebrovascular events
• Encephalitis
• Exposure to a toxin
• Poorly controlled type 1 diabetes
• Substance abuse
• Sustained nutritional deficiency
• Traumatic brain injury

ASSESSMENT FINDINGS

• Apathy, emotional blandness
• Confabulation in early stages
• Confusion, disorientation, and lack of insight
• Inability to learn and retain new information
• Tendency to remember things from very remote past better than more recent events

DIAGNOSTIC TEST RESULTS

• Medical tests (electrolyte levels, MRI, and computed tomography [CT] scan) confirm a physical basis.
• Mini–Mental Status Examination shows disorientation and lack of recall.
• Neuropsychological testing demonstrates memory deficits.

NURSING DIAGNOSES

• Dressing or grooming self-care deficit
• Impaired memory
• Knowledge deficit

TREATMENT

• Correction of the underlying medical cause
• Group therapy

INTERVENTIONS AND RATIONALES

• Use appropriate measures to promote the patient's safety *because the patient may be unable to maintain a safe environment.*
• Utilize environmental cues — for example, post the patient's name and schedule in his room — *to promote orientation.*
• Spend time with the patient and talk about the patient's health and self-care needs *to encourage greater self-understanding.*
• Identify realistic short-term goals *so the patient doesn't become overwhelmed.*

• Encourage exploration of feelings, *which can spark memory.*
• Provide simple, clear medical information *to help the patient understand the condition.*

Teaching topics
• Understanding the patient's underlying illness and its relationship to amnestic disorder.

Delirium

Delirium is a disturbance of consciousness accompanied by a change in cognition that can't be attributed to preexisting dementia. Delirium is characterized by an acute onset and may last from hours to a number of days. It's potentially reversible, but can be life-threatening if not treated.

CONTRIBUTING FACTORS
• Cerebral hypoxia
• Effects of medication
• Fever
• Fluid and electrolyte imbalances
• Infection (especially of the urinary tract and upper respiratory system)
• Metabolic disorders
• Multiple drug use, especially anticholinergics
• Neurotransmitter imbalance
• Pain
• Sensory overload or deprivation
• Sleep deprivation
• Stress
• Substance intoxication

ASSESSMENT FINDINGS
• Altered psychomotor activity, such as apathy, withdrawal, and agitation
• Altered respiratory depth or rhythm
• Bizarre, destructive behavior, worsening at night
• Disorganized thinking
• Disorientation (especially to time and place)
• Distractibility
• Impaired decision making
• Inability to complete tasks
• Insomnia or daytime sleepiness
• Picking at bed linen and clothes
• Poor impulse control

• Rambling, bizarre, or incoherent speech
• Tremors, generalized seizures
• Visual and auditory illusions

DIAGNOSTIC TEST RESULTS
• Laboratory results indicate delirium is a result of a physiologic condition, intoxication, substance withdrawal, toxic exposure, prescribed medicines, or a combination of these factors.

NURSING DIAGNOSES
• Risk for injury
• Impaired verbal communication
• Sensory or perceptual alterations

TREATMENT
• Correction of underlying physiologic problem
• Individual therapy

Drug therapy
• Tranquilizer: droperidol (Inapsine)
• Benzodiazepines: low-dose lorazepam (Ativan)
• Cholinesterase inhibitor: physostigmine (Antilirium)
• Antipsychotic agents: risperidone (Risperdal)

INTERVENTIONS AND RATIONALES
• Determine the degree of cognitive impairment *to understand and treat the patient.*
• Create a structured and safe environment *to prevent self-harm.*
• Institute measures to help patient relax and fall asleep *to comfort the patient.*
• Keep room lit *to allay the patient's fears and prevent visual hallucinations.*
• Monitor effects of medications *to prevent exacerbating symptoms.*

Teaching topics
• Contacting community resources
• Managing the patient's basic needs

Vascular dementia

Also called multi-infarct dementia, vascular dementia impairs the patient's cognitive func-

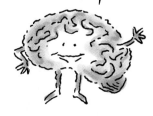

Treatment focuses on the underlying cause of delirium.

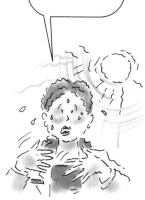

Dehydration is a common cause of delirium, especially in older patients.

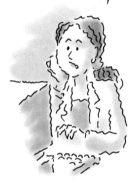

Hmmm. Slurred speech and wandering, along with stroke symptoms. That sounds like vascular dementia.

tioning, memory, and personality but doesn't affect the patient's level of consciousness. It's caused by an irreversible alteration in brain function that damages or destroys brain tissue.

CONTRIBUTING FACTORS
- Cerebral emboli or thrombosis
- Diabetes
- Heart disease
- High cholesterol level
- Hypertension (leading to stroke)
- Transient ischemic attacks

ASSESSMENT FINDINGS
- Depression
- Difficulty following instructions
- Dizziness
- Emotional lability
- Inappropriate emotional reactions
- Memory loss
- Neurologic symptoms that last only a few days
- Rapid onset of symptoms
- Slurred speech
- Wandering and getting lost in familiar places
- Weakness in an extremity

DIAGNOSTIC TEST RESULTS
- Cognitive assessment scale shows deterioration in cognitive ability.
- Global deterioration scale signifies degenerative dementia.
- Mini–Mental Status Examination reveals disorientation and recall difficulty.
- Structural and neurologic changes can be seen on MRI or CT scans.

NURSING DIAGNOSES
- Altered thought processes
- Impaired memory
- Risk for injury

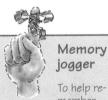

Memory jogger

To help remember the difference between delirium and dementia, think DR. DID (delirium reversible; dementia irreversible damage):

Delirium is reversible (though serious if not treated).

Dementia stems from irreversible damage.

TREATMENT
- Carotid endarterectomy to remove blockages in the carotid artery
- Low-fat diet
- Quitting smoking
- Treatment for the underlying condition (hypertension, high cholesterol, or diabetes)

Drug therapy
- Aspirin, to decrease platelet aggregation and prevent clots

INTERVENTIONS AND RATIONALES
- Orient the patient to his surroundings *to alleviate patient anxiety.*
- Monitor the environment *to prevent overstimulation.*
- Encourage the patient to express feelings of sadness and loss *to foster a healthy therapeutic environment.*

Teaching topics
- Controlling weight and diet
- Exercising to decrease cardiovascular risk factors

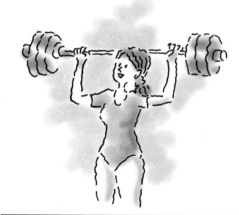

Pump up on practice questions

1. The nurse is caring for a client diagnosed with dementia and another client diagnosed with delirium. How does dementia differ from delirium?

    A. Dementia is confined to the elderly.

    B. Delirium only occurs with substance abuse.

    C. Delirium is an acute or subacute onset of confusion.

    D. They aren't different; their defining characteristics are interchangeable.

Answer: C. Delirium is characterized by an acute or subacute onset of confusion, interspersed with both alert and drowsy states. Neither disorder is age-specific. Neither disorder is restricted to individuals with histories of substance abuse. Their defining characteristics are different.

➽ *NCLEX keys*

Nursing process step: Analysis
Client needs category: Physiological integrity
Client needs subcategory: Reduction of risk potential
Taxonomic level: Comprehension

2. The nurse is caring for a 78-year-old man hospitalized with bilateral pneumonia. Shortly after admission, he became extremely belligerent, confused, hypotensive, and developed tachypnea. The nurse prepares the patient for intubation, administers anti-infectives stat, and requests that the computed tomography (CT) scan of his head be delayed. Why?

    A. His change in mental status was related to hypoxia, metabolic encephalopathy, and sepsis.

    B. Taking this client to the radiology department would jeopardize his condition.

    C. The client exhibited no signs of focal neurologic impairment.

    D. His prognosis was poor and didn't justify a CT scan.

Answer: A. Severe functional abnormalities and confusion are often caused by nonneurologic diseases, especially in the elderly. Encephalopathies such as these are reversible as the underlying cause is treated. The other choices are incorrect because poor prognosis, absence of signs of focal neurologic impairment, and an unstable condition aren't appropriate justifications for delaying a diagnostic CT scan.

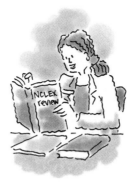

➽ *NCLEX keys*

Nursing process step: Implementation
Client needs category: Physiological integrity
Client needs subcategory: Reduction of risk potential
Taxonomic level: Analysis

3. The nurse is reading the autopsy report of a client who recently died. The report reveals senile plaques, neurofibril tangles, and atrophy. These changes are characteristic of which illness?

    A. Meningitis
    B. Delirium tremors
    C. Neurosyphilis
    D. Alzheimer's disease

Answer: D. Although some of these changes occur as part of the normal aging process, these findings are seen in Alzheimer's disease and aren't characteristic of the other three illnesses.

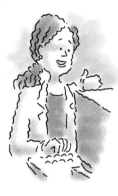

➠ *NCLEX keys*
Nursing process step: Analysis
Client needs category: Physiological integrity
Client needs subcategory: Physiological adaptation
Taxonomic level: Knowledge

4. The nurse is caring for a client diagnosed with Alzheimer's-type dementia. What of the following medications is indicated for treatment of this disorder?

    A. Donapezil
    B. Benazepril
    C. Fosinopril
    D. Lisinopril

Answer: A. Donapezil (Aricept) is an anticholinesterase drug indicated for treatment of Alzheimer's-type dementia. Benazepril, fosinopril, and lisinopril are angiotensin-converting enzyme inhibitors that are indicated for treatment of hypertension.

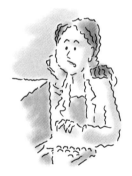

➠ *NCLEX keys*
Nursing process step: Implementation
Client needs category: Physiological integrity
Client needs subcategory: Pharmacological and parenteral therapies
Taxonomic level: Knowledge

5. The nurse is assessing a client for vascular dementia. Which of the following helps confirm the diagnosis?

    A. Drug screen for toxicology
    B. Findings upon autopsy
    C. MRI
    D. Response to electroconvulsive therapy

Answer: C. Vascular dementia is often caused by cerebrovascular disease and very small infarctions, which can be detected with MRI. Attempts to diagnosis vascular dementia wouldn't be delayed until autopsy. A positive drug screen wouldn't be helpful in diagnosing dementia caused by vascular problems. Electroconvulsive therapy is occasionally used in the treatment for selected psychiatric disorders, but isn't a diagnostic tool for dementia.

➠ *NCLEX keys*
Nursing process steps: Assessment
Client needs category: Physiological integrity
Client needs subcategory: Reduction of risk potential
Taxonomic level: Comprehension

6. The nurse is caring for a client diagnosed with delirium. Which statement is true concerning delirium?
  A. It's characterized by an acute onset and lasts about 1 month.
  B. It's characterized by a slowly evolving onset and lasts about 1 week.
  C. It's characterized by a slowly evolving onset and lasts about 1 month.
  D. It's characterized by an acute onset and lasts hours to a number of days.

Answer: D. Delirium has an acute onset and usually lasts hours to a number of days.

➡ *NCLEX keys*
Nursing process steps: Assessment
Client needs category: Physiological integrity
Client needs subcategory: Physiological adaptation
Taxonomic level: Knowledge

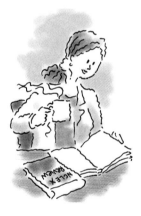

7. Which of the following can be caused by cerebral hypoxia, infection, drugs, or metabolic disorders?
  A. Dementia
  B. Anxiety disorders
  C. Delirium
  D. Amnesia

Answer: C. Delirium is often a sign of underlying medical problems, especially in older clients; it can be caused by hypoxia, infection, drugs, and metabolic disturbances. It is potentially reversible. Dementia is usually characterized by irreversible alterations in brain function. Although both amnesia and anxiety may have some association with underlying medical problems, neither is caused by such problems.

➡ *NCLEX keys*
Nursing process steps: Assessment
Client needs category: Physiological integrity
Client needs subcategory: Physiological adaptation
Taxonomic level: Comprehension

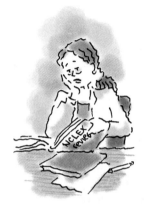

8. The nurse is caring for a client who is diagnosed with delirium. What must the nurse provide for the client?
  A. A safe environment
  B. An opportunity to release frustration
  C. Prescribed medications
  D. Medications as needed, judiciously

Answer: A. Keeping the client with delirium safe is the most important aspect of care. All other choices are logical and appropriate, but safety issues and meeting the client's basic physiologic needs are of primary importance.

➡ *NCLEX keys*
Nursing process steps: Implementation
Client needs category: Safe, effective care environment
Client needs subcategory: Safety and infection control
Taxonomic level: Application

9. The nurse is caring for a client experiencing severe psychosocial stress. This condition could trigger which disorder?

    A. Wilson's disease
    B. Huntington's disease
    C. Amnesia
    D. Multiple sclerosis

Answer: C. Amnesia is usually triggered by severe psychosocial stress, not physiologic causes. The other three choices are neurodegenerative disorders, often with physiologic causes.

➡ *NCLEX keys*

Nursing process steps: Analysis
Client needs category: Psychosocial integrity
Client needs subcategory: Coping and adaptation
Taxonomic level: Comprehension

10. A 76-year-old client is admitted to a long-term-care facility with a diagnosis of Alzheimer's-type dementia. The client has been wearing the same dirty clothes for several days and the nurse contacts the family to bring in clean clothing. Which intervention would best prevent further regression in the client's personal hygiene?

    A. Encouraging the client to perform as much self-care as possible
    B. Making the client assume responsibility for physical care
    C. Assigning a staff member to take over the client's physical care
    D. Accepting the client's desire to go without bathing

Answer: A. Clients with Alzheimer's-type dementia tend to fluctuate in their capabilities. Encouraging self-care to the extent possible will help increase the client's orientation and promote a trusting relationship with the nurse. Making the client assume responsibility for physical care is unreasonable. Assigning a staff member to take over restricts the client's independence. Accepting the client's desire to go without bathing promotes bad hygiene.

➡ *NCLEX keys*

Nursing process steps: Implementation
Client needs category: Physiological integrity
Client needs subcategory: Reduction of risk potential
Taxonomic level: Application

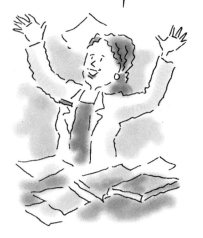

It's okay to feel a little delirious after finishing this chapter. Just remember you've taken another step toward conquering the NCLEX!

16 Personality Disorders

Brush up on key concepts

Personality traits are patterns of behavior that reflect how people perceive and relate to others and themselves. Personality disorders occur when these traits become **rigid** and **maladaptive.** According to the *Diagnostic and Statistical Manual of Mental Disorders*, 4th ed., a personality disorder is a problematic pattern occurring in two of the following four areas: cognition, affectivity, interpersonal functioning, and impulse control.

A person with a personality disorder uses maladaptive behavior to relate to others and fulfill basic emotional needs.

At any time, you can review the major points of each disorder by consulting the *Cheat sheet* on pages 402 and 403.

Polish up on patient care

Major personality disorders include antisocial personality disorder, borderline personality disorder, dependent personality disorder, and paranoid personality disorder.

Antisocial personality disorder

Antisocial personality disorder leads the patient to have a total disregard for the rights of others. Antisocial personality disorder can begin in early childhood and continue into adulthood, but the actual diagnosis requires that the patient be at least 18 years old and that the patient has displayed some symptoms of the disorder before age 15.

CONTRIBUTING FACTORS
• Childhood trauma
• Genetic predisposition
• Physical abuse
• Sexual abuse
• Social isolation
• Transient friendships
• Unstable or erratic parenting

ASSESSMENT FINDINGS
• Anxiety
• Destructive tendencies
• Excessively opinionated nature
• General disregard for the rights and feelings of others
• Impulsive actions
• Inability to maintain close personal or sexual relationships
• Inflated and arrogant self-appraisal
• Lack of remorse
• Possible concurrent psychiatric disorders
• Power-seeking behavior
• Previous violations of societal norms or rules
• Substance abuse
• Sudden or frequent changes in job, residence, or relationships
• Superficial charm, often manipulative

DIAGNOSTIC TEST RESULTS
• Minnesota Multiphasic Personality Inventory reveals antisocial personality disorder.

NURSING DIAGNOSES
• Anxiety
• Risk for violence: directed at others
• Self-esteem disturbance

TREATMENT
• Alcohol or drug rehabilitation (if appropriate)
• Behavioral therapy

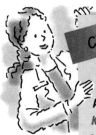

Cheat sheet

Personality disorders refresher

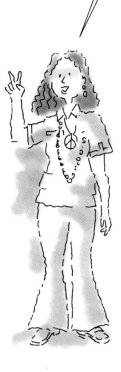

Loosen up. Personality disorders occur when traits become rigid and maladaptive.

ANTISOCIAL PERSONALITY DISORDER

Key signs and symptoms
- Destructive tendencies
- General disregard for the rights and feelings of others
- Lack of remorse
- Sudden or frequent changes in job, residence, or relationships

Key test results
- Minnesota Multiphasic Personality Inventory reveals antisocial personality disorder.

Key treatments
- Behavioral therapy
- Lithium carbonate (Eskalith) or a beta-adrenergic blocker (Inderal) for controlling aggressive outbursts

Key interventions
- Help the patient to identify manipulative behaviors.
- Establish a behavioral contract.
- Hold the patient responsible for his behavior.

BORDERLINE PERSONALITY DISORDER

Key signs and symptoms
- Destructive behavior
- Impulsive behavior
- Inability to develop a sense of self
- Inability to maintain relationships
- Moodiness
- Self-mutilation

Key test results
- Standard psychological tests reveal a high degree of dissociation.

Key treatments
- Milieu therapy
- Individual therapy
- Antimanic medications: carbamazepine (Tegretol), lithium carbonate (Eskalith)
- Anxiolytic: buspirone (BuSpar)
- Selective serotonin reuptake inhibitors (SSRIs): paroxetine (Paxil), fluoxetine (Prozac)

Key interventions
- Recognize behaviors that the patient uses to manipulate others.
- Set appropriate expectations for social interaction, and make sure these expectations are met.

DEPENDENT PERSONALITY DISORDER

Key signs and symptoms
- Clinging, demanding behavior
- Fear and anxiety about losing the people they are dependent upon
- Hypersensitivity to potential rejection and decision making
- Low self-esteem

Key test results
- Laboratory tests rule out underlying medical condition.

Key treatments
- Behavior modification through assertiveness training
- Individual therapy
- Benzodiazepines: alprazolam (Xanax), lorazepam (Ativan), clonazepam (Klonopin)
- SSRIs: paroxetine (Paxil)
- Tricyclic antidepressants: imipramine (Tofranil), desipramine (Norpramin)

Key interventions
- Support the patient in accepting increased decision making (balancing a checkbook, planning meals, paying bills).
- Help the patient to identify manipulative behaviors, focusing on specific examples.

PARANOID PERSONALITY DISORDER

Key signs and symptoms
- Feelings of being deceived
- Hostility
- Major distortions of reality
- Social isolation
- Suspiciousness, mistrusting friends and relatives

Personality disorders refresher *(continued)*

PARANOID PERSONALITY DISORDER *(continued)*

Key treatments
• Possible drug-free treatment, to reduce the chance of causing increased paranoia
• Individual therapy
• Antipsychotic agents: olanzapine (Zyprexa), risperidone (Risperdal), chlorpromazine (Thorazine), thioridazine (Mellaril), fluphenazine (Prolixin), haloperidol (Haldol).

Key interventions
• Establish a working relationship by listening and responding to the patient.
• Instruct and help the patient practice strategies that facilitate the development of social skills

• Group therapy
• Individual therapy

Drug therapy
• Lithium carbonate (Eskalith) or a beta-adrenergic blocker (Inderal) for controlling aggressive outbursts

INTERVENTIONS AND RATIONALES
• Help the patient to identify manipulative behaviors *to help the patient counteract the perception that others are extensions of the self.*
• Establish a behavioral contract *to communicate to the patient that other behavior options are available.*
• Avoid confrontations and power struggles *to maintain the opportunity for therapeutic communication.*
• Hold the patient responsible for his behavior *to promote development of a collaborative relationship with the patient.*
• Help the patient to manage anger and observe for physical and verbal signs of agitation *to maintain a healthy therapeutic environment.*

Teaching topics
• Learning appropriate behaviors
• Continuing treatments after discharge

Borderline personality disorder

Borderline personality disorder results in a pattern of instability in a person's mood, interpersonal relationships, self-esteem, self-identi-ty, behavior, and cognition. Impulsiveness is its most prominent characteristic. Borderline personality disorder appears to originate in early childhood.

CONTRIBUTING FACTORS
• Brain dysfunction in the limbic system or frontal lobe
• Decreased serotonin activity
• Early parental loss or separation
• Increased activity in alpha-2-noradrenergic receptors
• Major losses early in life
• Physical abuse
• Sexual abuse
• Substance abuse

ASSESSMENT FINDINGS
• Compulsive behavior
• Destructive behavior
• Dissociation (separating objects from their emotional significance)
• Dysfunctional lifestyle
• Emotional reactions, with few coping skills
• Extreme fear of abandonment
• High self-expectations
• Impulsive behavior
• Inability to develop a healthy sense of self
• Inability to maintain relationships
• Moodiness
• Paranoid ideation
• Self-directed anger
• Self-mutilation
• Shame
• Suicidal behavior
• View of others as either extremely good or bad

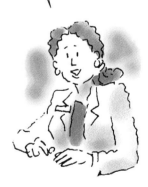

Be prepared for defensiveness. Patients suffering from a personality disorder aren't likely to recognize it in themselves.

DIAGNOSTIC TEST RESULTS
• Standard psychological tests reveal a high degree of dissociation.

NURSING DIAGNOSES
• Impaired social interaction
• Risk for violence: self-directed
• Self-esteem disturbance

TREATMENT
• Alcohol and drug rehabilitation, as indicated
• Milieu therapy
• Group therapy
• Family therapy
• Individual therapy

Drug therapy
• Antimanic medications: carbamazepine (Tegretol), lithium carbonate (Eskalith)
• Anxiolytic: buspirone (BuSpar)
• Monoamine oxidase (MAO) inhibitors: phenelzine (Nardil)
• Narcotic detoxification adjunct agent: naltrexone (ReVia)
• Selective serotonin reuptake inhibitors (SSRIs): paroxetine (Paxil), fluoxetine (Prozac)

INTERVENTIONS AND RATIONALES
• Recognize behaviors that the patient uses to manipulate others *to avoid unconsciously reinforcing these behaviors.*
• Set appropriate expectations for social interaction, and praise the patient when these expectations are met *to create a healthy therapeutic environment.*
• Respect the patient's sense of personal space *to increase trust.*

Teaching topics
• Developing problem-solving skills
• Developing therapeutic communication skills
• Implementing relaxation techniques

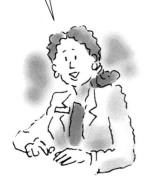

Be careful! Patients receiving drug therapy for borderline personality disorder should take medications only for targeted symptoms, and only for a short period of time.

Dependent personality disorder

The patient with dependent personality disorder experiences an extreme need to be taken care of that leads to submissive, clinging behavior and fear of separation. This pattern begins by early adulthood, when behaviors designed to elicit caring from others become predominant. These behaviors arise from the patient's perception that he's unable to function adequately without others.

CONTRIBUTING FACTORS
• Childhood traumas
• Closed family system that discourages relationships with others
• Genetic predisposition
• Physical abuse
• Sexual abuse
• Social isolation

ASSESSMENT FINDINGS
• Clinging, demanding behavior
• Exaggerated fear of losing support and approval
• Fear and anxiety about losing the people they're dependent on
• Hypersensitivity to potential rejection and decision making
• Indirect resistance to occupational and social performance
• Low self-esteem
• Tendency to be passive

DIAGNOSTIC TEST RESULTS
• Laboratory tests rule out underlying medical condition.

NURSING DIAGNOSES
• Altered family processes
• Ineffective individual coping
• Self-esteem disturbance

TREATMENT
• Behavior modification through assertiveness training
• Individual therapy
• Group therapy

Drug therapy
- Benzodiazepines: alprazolam (Xanax), lorazepam (Ativan), clonazepam (Klonopin)
- MAO inhibitors: phenelzine (Nardil)
- SSRIs: paroxetine (Paxil)
- Tricyclic antidepressants: imipramine (Tofranil), desipramine (Norpramin)

INTERVENTIONS AND RATIONALES
- Encourage activities that require decision making (balancing a checkbook, planning meals, paying bills) *to promote independence.*
- Help the patient establish and work toward goals *to foster a sense of independence.*
- Help the patient to identify manipulative behaviors, focusing on specific examples, *to decrease the perception that others are an extension of the self.*
- Limit interactions with the patient to a few consistent staff members *to increase the patient's sense of security.*

Teaching topics
- Expressing ideas and feelings assertively
- Improving social skills and promoting social interaction

Paranoid personality disorder

Paranoid personality disorder is characterized by extreme distrust of others. Paranoid people avoid relationships in which they aren't in control or have the potential of losing control.

CONTRIBUTING FACTORS
- Genetic predisposition
- Neurochemical alteration
- Parental antagonism

ASSESSMENT FINDINGS
- Bad temper, especially in children
- Delusional thinking
- Emotional reactions, including nervousness, jealousy, anger, or envy
- Feelings of being deceived
- Hostility
- Hyperactivity, especially in children
- Hypervigilance
- Irritability, especially in children
- Lack of humor

- Lack of social support systems
- Major distortions of reality
- Need to be in control
- Refusal to confide in others
- Self-righteousness
- Social isolation
- Sullen attitude
- Suspiciousness, mistrust of friends and relatives

DIAGNOSTIC TEST RESULTS
- There are no specific tests for paranoid personality disorder.

NURSING DIAGNOSES
- Anxiety
- Ineffective individual coping
- Self-esteem disturbance
- Social isolation

TREATMENT
- Possible drug-free treatment, to reduce the chance of causing increased paranoia
- Individual therapy

Drug therapy
- Antipsychotic agents: olanzapine (Zyprexa), risperidone (Risperdal), chlorpromazine (Thorazine), thioridazine (Mellaril), fluphenazine (Prolixin), haloperidol (Haldol)

INTERVENTIONS AND RATIONALES
- Establish a therapeutic relationship by listening and responding to the patient *to initiate therapeutic communication.*
- Encourage the patient to take part in social interactions *to introduce other people's perceptions and realities to the patient.*
- Help the patient to identify negative behaviors that interfere with relationships *so the patient can see how his behavior impacts others.*
- Instruct and help the patient practice strategies that facilitate the development of social skills *so the patient can gain confidence and practice interacting with others.*

Teaching topics
- Learning coping strategies
- Understanding the disorder (for family and patient)

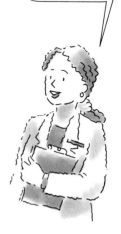

Maintain appropriate boundaries with a patient with dependent personality disorder.

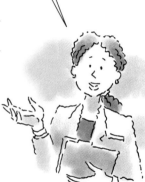

Avoid supporting the paranoid patient's delusions but don't attack the delusions directly because this will only increase anxiety.

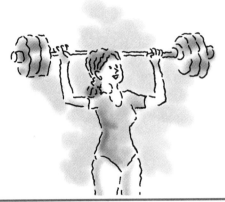

Pump up on practice questions

1. The nurse is caring for a client with a personality disorder. The client is on a general medical-surgical unit following recent surgery. The nurse deliberately interacts with this client more than she interacts with another client, who had the same surgery. Both clients are recovering equally well. Why would the nurse do this?

    A. Other caregivers often minimize contact with such clients.

    B. The nurse feels sorry for the client.

    C. One client has health insurance; the other client doesn't.

    D. The nurse suspects that the first client isn't recovering as well as reported.

Answer: A. Because clients with personality disorders are often demanding and difficult, health care providers with little psychiatric experience often try to limit their contact with them. This tends to perpetuate behavioral problems, not improve them. This nurse is acting to balance that trend. Sympathy for a client, lack of health insurance, and unfounded suspicions aren't relevant considerations.

➠ NCLEX keys
Nursing process step: Implementation
Client needs category: Safe, effective care environment
Client needs subcategory: Management of care
Taxonomic level: Application

2. The nurse is caring for a client diagnosed with paranoid personality disorder in an acute care facility. Which intervention would the nurse use to control the client's suspiciousness?

    A. Keeping messages clear and consistent, while avoiding deception

    B. Providing pharmacologic therapy

    C. Providing social interactions with others on the unit

    D. Attending to basic daily needs of the client on a consistent basis

Answer: A. Keeping messages consistent, fostering trust, and avoiding deception will help to decrease suspiciousness. Encouraging social interactions, attending to basic daily needs, and providing pharmacologic therapy are general nursing interventions that are appropriate for any psychiatric disorder.

➠ NCLEX keys
Nursing process step: Evaluation
Client needs category: Safe, effective care environment
Client needs subcategory: Management of care
Taxonomic level: Analysis

3. A client arrived on the psychiatric unit from the emergency department. His diagnosis is personality disorder, and he exhibits manipulative behavior. As the nurse reviews the unit rules with him, the client asks "Can I go to the snack shop just one time and then I will answer whatever you ask?" Which of the following is the most appropriate response?

    A. "Yes, but hurry, because I need to finish your assessment."

    B. "O.K., be back in 5 minutes."

    C. "No, you can't go."

    D. "No, you can't go. The rules here apply to everyone."

Answer: D. This response sets limits with an appropriate explanation. Options A and B give in to the manipulative behavior. Option C doesn't explain the purpose of the refusal.

▶▶ NCLEX keys

Nursing process step: Implementation
Client needs category: Psychosocial integrity
Client needs subcategory: Psychosocial adaptation
Taxonomic level: Application

4. The nurse is caring for a client who is a talented and renowned neurosurgeon. He was married several times and can't manage to keep an employee because of his constant belittling of others and preoccupation with power and control. What would be the most likely diagnosis for this physician?

    A. Personality disorder, with low self-esteem
    B. Depression, and in need of counseling
    C. Bipolar disorder with intense need for pharmacologic therapy
    D. Suffering from lingering effects of childhood abuse

Answer: A. Given as much information as presented, diagnosis of some type of personality disorder and nursing assessment of low self-esteem is appropriate. Any of the other diagnoses and treatment options are all possible concomitant problems, but further information is needed.

▶▶ NCLEX keys

Nursing process step: Assessment
Client needs category: Psychosocial integrity
Client needs subcategory: Psychosocial adaptation
Taxonomic level: Comprehension

5. The nurse is caring for a client who displays limited insight, a predilection for risky behavior, and a history of trouble with the legal system. The client moves frequently, making it difficult for him to maintain stable friendships. These characteristics are all associated with which diagnosis?

    A. Obsessive-compulsive disorder
    B. Midlife crisis
    C. Cultural awareness deprivation
    D. Antisocial personality disorder

Answer: D. The characteristics described are associated with impaired social functioning, a trait commonly attributed to clients with antisocial personality disorder. Persons with obsessive-compulsive disorder are generally less inclined to engage in risky behavior or get in trouble with the legal system. Cultural awareness deprivation and midlife crisis aren't official psychiatric diagnoses.

▶▶ NCLEX keys

Nursing process step: Analysis
Client needs category: Psychosocial integrity
Client needs subcategory: Psychosocial adaptation
Taxonomic level: Comprehension

6. The nurse is teaching a client about healthy interpersonal relationships. Which characteristic would the nurse include?

    A. Minimal self-revelation
    B. Willingness to risk self-revelation
    C. Ego-dystonic behavior
    D. Intimacy and merging of identities

Answer: B. Willingness to risk self-revelation, ego-syntonic behavior, and intimacy while maintaining separate identities are all characteristics of healthy interpersonal relationships. (Note that ego-syntonic behavior refers to thoughts, impulses, attitudes, and behavior that are felt to be acceptable and consistent with the client's personality while ego-dystonic behavior refers to thoughts, impulses, attitudes, and behavior that the client feels are distressing, repugnant, or inconsistent with the rest of his personality.)

▶▶ NCLEX keys

Nursing process step: Analysis
Client needs category: Psychosocial integrity
Client needs subcategory: Psychosocial adaptation
Taxonomic level: Analysis

7. The nurse is caring for a client with a personality disorder. What is the most significant obstacle for the nurse to overcome?

A. Clients with personality disorders generally lack the motivation to change.
B. In-house treatment is necessary, but most insurance plans don't cover such measures.
C. Appropriate pharmacologic therapy has significant, potentially lethal, adverse effects.
D. Neuroleptic medications aren't always effective in helping the client maintain control of his behavior.

Answer: A. Lack of client motivation is the most common cause of treatment failure in clients with personality disorders. The other options may contribute to treatment failure in other psychiatric disorders, but are less applicable in clients with personality disorders.

➡ NCLEX keys
Nursing process step: Evaluation
Client needs category: Psychosocial integrity
Client needs subcategory: Psychosocial adaptation
Taxonomic level: Evaluation

8. The nurse is caring for a client who has a personality disorder. Which statement is true regarding that client?
A. Personality disorders are temporary patterns of conflict within the individual.
B. Developmental growth patterns and chronologic age will halt any behavior disturbances.
C. Personality disorders are associated with high self-esteem.
D. Personality disorders are lifelong behavior patterns.

Answer: D. Personality disorders are considered to be lifelong patterns, with little relationship to age and developmental growth. Personality disorders are associated with a low self-esteem.

➡ NCLEX keys
Nursing process step: Analysis
Client needs category: Psychosocial integrity
Client needs subcategory: Psychosocial adaptation
Taxonomic level: Comprehension

9. The nurse is caring for a client who has a personality disorder. Which of the following assessment findings should the nurse expect?
A. Manipulative behavior and inflated feelings of self-worth
B. Manipulative behavior and inability to tolerate frustration
C. Suicidal ideation and starvation
D. Patterns of bulimia and starvation

Answer: B. Manipulative behavior and inability to tolerate frustration are important assessment clues. Low self-esteem — not inflated feelings of self-worth — are more likely in clients with personality disorders. The other choices are more likely to be assessed in clients with eating disorders.

➡ NCLEX keys
Nursing process step: Assessment
Client needs category: Psychosocial integrity
Client needs subcategory: Psychosocial adaptation
Taxonomic level: Comprehension

10. The nurse is caring for a client with borderline personality disorder. Which interventions should the nurse perform?
A. Setting limits on manipulative behavior
B. Allowing the client to set limits
C. Using restraints judiciously
D. Encouraging acting out behavior

Answer: A. Setting limits on manipulative behavior provides the structure that the client needs. Encouraging acting out behavior and allowing the client to set limits would be contraindicated. The need for restraints in a client with borderline personality disorder would be rare, unless coexisting disorders exist.

➡ NCLEX keys
Nursing process step: Implementation
Client needs category: Psychosocial integrity
Client needs subcategory: Psychosocial adaptation
Taxonomic level: Application

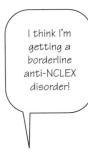

I think I'm getting a borderline anti-NCLEX disorder!

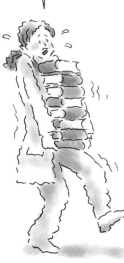

17 Schizophrenic & Delusional Disorders

Brush up on key concepts

In this chapter, you'll review:

- major characteristics of schizophrenic and delusional disorders

- common schizophrenic disorders

- treatments and interventions used in the care of schizophrenic and delusional disorders.

Schizophrenic and delusional disorders fall under the diagnostic umbrella **psychosis.** A psychotic illness is a brain disorder characterized by an impaired perception of reality, commonly coupled with mood disturbances. Psychosis can be either progressive or episodic.

Schizophrenia is characterized by disturbances (for at least 6 months) in thought content and form, perception, affect, sense of self, volition, interpersonal relationships, and psychomotor behavior.

Delusional disorders are marked by false beliefs with a plausible basis in reality. Once referred to as "paranoid disorders," delusional disorders affect less than 1% of the population.

At any time, you can review the major points of each disorder by consulting the *Cheat sheet* on pages 410 and 411.

Positive or negative

Symptoms of schizophrenia may be characterized as positive or negative. **Positive symptoms** focus on a distortion of normal functions; **negative symptoms** focus on a loss of normal functions. Examples of positive symptoms are delusions, hallucinations, disorganized speech, and grossly disorganized or catatonic behavior. Examples of negative symptoms include flat affect, alogia (poverty of speech), and avolition (lack of self-initiated behaviors).

Thought broadcasting

Delusions are mistaken beliefs based on a false or unreasonable interpretation of an experience or a perception. Commonly, delusions occur in the form of thought broadcasting, in which people believe that their personal thoughts are broadcast to the external world. Many times the patient believes that his feelings, thoughts, or actions aren't his own.

Look for a theme

Common themes characterize delusions. Delusional themes are described as **persecutory, somatic, erotomanic, jealous,** or **grandiose.** An example of a persecutory delusion is the idea that one is being followed, tricked, tormented, or made the subject of ridicule. The patient with erotomanic delusions falsely believes he shares an idealized relationship with another person, usually someone of higher status such as a celebrity. An example of a somatic delusion is a patient who believes his body is deteriorating from within. An example of jealous delusion is the patient's feeling that his or her spouse or lover is unfaithful. The patient with grandiose delusions has an exaggerated sense of self-importance.

Hearing voices

Most commonly, schizophrenics experience **auditory hallucinations.** When the patient hears voices, he perceives these voices as being separate from his own thoughts. The content of the voices is threatening and derogatory. Many times the voices tell the patient to commit an act of violence against himself or others.

All over the place

Disorganized thinking or **looseness of associations** is where speech shifts randomly from one topic to another, with only a vague connection between topics. The patient may digress to unrelated topics, make up new words (neologisms), repeat words involuntarily (perseveration) or repeat words or phrases similar in sound only (clang association).

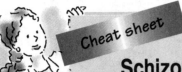

Schizophrenic & delusional disorders refresher

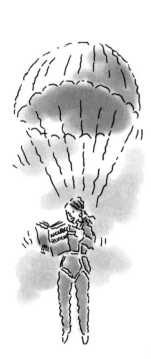

CATATONIC SCHIZOPHRENIA

Key signs and symptoms
- Bizarre postures, waxy flexibility (posture held in odd or unusual fixed positions for extended periods of time), resistance to being moved
- Displacement (switching emotions from their original object to a more acceptable substitute)
- Dissociation (separation of things from their emotional significance)
- Echolalia (repetition of another's words)
- Echopraxia (involuntary imitation of another person's movements and gestures)

Key test results
- Magnetic resonance imaging (MRI) shows possible enlargement of lateral ventricles, enlarged third ventricle and enlarged sulci.
- Patients show impaired performance on neuropsychological and cognitive tests.

Key treatments
- Milieu therapy
- Supportive psychotherapy
- Antipsychotics: fluphenazine (Prolixin), haloperidol (Haldol), olanzapine (Zyprexa), risperidone (Risperdal), thioridazine (Mellaril)

Key interventions
- Provide skin care to prevent skin breakdown.
- Monitor the patient for adverse effects of antipsychotic drugs, such as dystonic reactions and tardive dyskinesia.
- Be aware of the patient's personal space; use gestures and touch judiciously.
- Provide appropriate measures to ensure patient safety and explain to the patient why you are doing so.
- Collaborate with the patient to identify anxious behavior as well as probable causes.

DELUSIONAL DISORDER

Key signs and symptoms
- Delusions that are visual, auditory, or tactile
- Inability to trust
- Projection

Key test results
- Blood and urine tests eliminate an organic or chemical cause.
- Endocrine function tests rule out hyperadrenalism, pernicious anemia, and thyroid disorders.
- Neurologic evaluations rule out an organic cause.

Key treatments
- Milieu therapy
- Supportive psychotherapy
- Antipsychotics: chlorpromazine (Thorazine), fluphenazine (Prolixin), haloperidol (Haldol), olanzapine (Zyprexa), risperidone (Risperdal), thioridazine (Mellaril)

Key interventions
- Explore events that trigger delusions.
- Don't directly attack the delusion.
- Once the dynamics of the delusions are understood, discourage repetitious talk about delusions and refocus the conversation on the patient's underlying feelings.
- Recognize delusion as the patient's perception of the environment.

DISORGANIZED SCHIZOPHRENIA

Key signs and symptoms
- Cognitive impairment
- Fantasy
- Hallucinations
- Loose associations
- Word salads

Key test results
- Neuropsychological and cognitive tests indicate impaired performance.

Key treatments
- Milieu therapy
- Social skills training
- Supportive psychotherapy
- Antipsychotics: chlorpromazine (Thorazine), fluphenazine (Prolixin), haloperidol (Haldol), olanzapine (Zyprexa), risperidone (Risperdal), thioridazine (Mellaril)

Schizophrenic & delusional disorders refresher (continued)

DISORGANIZED SCHIZOPHRENIA *(continued)*

Key interventions
- Help the patient meet basic needs for food, comfort, and a sense of safety.
- During an acute psychotic episode, remove potentially hazardous items from the patient's environment.
- If the patient experiences hallucinations, don't attempt to reason with him or challenge his perception of hallucinations. Instead, ensure the patient's safety and provide comfort and support.
- Encourage the patient with auditory hallucinations to reveal what voices are telling him.
- First encourage the patient to participate in one-on-one interactions, and then progress to small groups.
- Provide positive reinforcement for socially acceptable behavior such as efforts to improve hygiene and table manners.
- Encourage the patient to express feelings related to experiencing hallucinations.

PARANOID SCHIZOPHRENIA

Key signs and symptoms
- Delusions and auditory hallucinations
- Dissociation
- Inability to trust

Key test results
- MRI shows possible enlargement of ventricles, and enlarged sulci. The presence of the enlarged sulci suggests cortical loss, particularly in the frontal lobe.

Key treatments
- Milieu therapy
- Supportive psychotherapy
- Antipsychotics: chlorpromazine (Thorazine), chlozapine (Clazaril), fluphenazine (Prolixin), haloperidol (Haldol), olanzapine (Zyprexa), risperidone (Risperdal), thioridazine (Mellaril).

Key interventions
- Inform the patient that you will help him control his behavior.
- Set limits on aggressive behavior and communicate your expectations to the patient.
- Maintain a low level of stimuli.

Loss of self

The patient may demonstrate a blunted, flat, or inappropriate affect manifested by poor eye contact; a distant, unresponsive facial expression; and very limited body language. The sense of self is disturbed, an experience referred to as **loss of ego boundaries.** This loss of a coherent sense of self causes the patient to experience difficulty in maintaining an ongoing sense of identity. This may make it impossible for the patient to maintain interpersonal relationships or function at work and in other life roles.

Polish up on patient care

Major psychotic disorders include catatonic schizophrenia, delusional disorder, disorganized schizophrenia, and paranoid schizophrenia.

Catatonic schizophrenia

Patients with catatonic schizophrenia show little reaction to their environments. Catatonic behavior involves remaining completely motionless or continuously repeating one motion. This behavior can last for hours at a time. Catatonic schizophrenia is the least common type of schizophrenia.

CONTRIBUTING FACTORS
- A fragile ego, which can't withstand the demands of reality
- Brain abnormalities
- Developmental abnormalities
- Genetic factors
- Hyperactivity of the neurotransmitter dopamine
- An infectious agent or autoimmune response (unproven cause)
- Social or environmental stress, interacting with the person's inherited biological makeup

ASSESSMENT FINDINGS
- Agitation at times, which may be unexpected and dangerous
- Bizarre postures, waxy flexibility (posture held in odd or unusual fixed positions for extended periods of time), resistance to being moved
- Childlike, regressed behavior
- Clang association
- Displacement (switching emotions from their original object to a more acceptable substitute)
- Dissociation (separation of things from their emotional significance)
- Echolalia (repetition of another's words)
- Echopraxia (involuntary imitation of another person's movements and gestures)
- Episodes of impulsiveness
- Fantasy
- Inability to trust
- Little reaction to environment
- Mutism
- Neologism
- Projection
- Purposeless overactivity or underactivity
- Ritualistic mannerisms
- Social isolation
- Speech resembling a word salad (string of words that are not connected in any way)

DIAGNOSTIC TEST RESULTS
- Magnetic resonance imaging (MRI) shows possible enlargement of lateral ventricles, enlarged third ventricle and enlarged sulci.
- Patients show impaired performance on neuropsychological and cognitive tests.

NURSING DIAGNOSES
- Altered thought processes
- Ineffective individual coping
- Hygiene self-care deficit

TREATMENT
- Electroconvulsive therapy
- Family therapy
- Milieu therapy
- Outpatient group therapy
- Psychoeducational programs
- Social skills training
- Stress management
- Supportive psychotherapy

Drug therapy
- Antiparkinsonian agents: benztropine (Cogentin), for adverse effects of antipsychotics
- Antipsychotics: fluphenazine (Prolixin), haloperidol (Haldol), olanzapine (Zyprexa), risperidone (Risperdal), thioridazine (Mellaril) (see Understanding antipsychotics)

INTERVENTIONS AND RATIONALES
- Provide skin care to prevent skin breakdown.
- Monitor intake and output. Body weight may decrease as a result of inadequate intake.
- Monitor the patient for adverse effects of antipsychotic drugs, such as dystonic reactions and tardive dyskinesia. Early identification of extrapyramidal effects can help diminish or eliminate the patient's anxiety about these symptoms.
- Be aware of the patient's personal space; use gestures and touch judiciously. Invading the patient's personal space can increase his anxiety.
- When discussing care, give short, simple explanations at the patient's level of understanding to increase cooperation.
- Provide appropriate measures to ensure patient safety and explain to the patient why you are doing so. Implementing and explaining safety measures can promote trust and decrease anxiety while increasing the patient's sense of security.
- Promote a trusting relationship to create a safe environment in which the patient can practice social interaction skills and prepare for social interaction.

> Here is a major difficulty in treating schizophrenia: After the patients' more troubling symptoms recede, they believe they can discontinue therapy and medication.

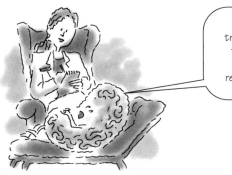

> Yet, when treatment stops, the symptoms inevitably recur in full force.

Now I get it!

Understanding antipsychotics

Antipsychotic medications act against the symptoms of schizophrenia and other psychoses and are first-line therapy for schizophrenia. These medications can't "cure" the illness, but they alleviate and eliminate symptoms. In some cases, they can shorten the course of the illness.

TRADITIONAL NEUROLEPTICS

There are a number of antipsychotic (neuroleptic) medications available. The main differences between the medications is in their potency, their therapeutic effects, and their adverse effects. Doctors consider several factors when prescribing an antipsychotic medication, including:
- the degree and type of illness
- the patient's age
- the patient's body weight
- the patient's past medical history.

TARDIVE DYSKINESIA

While maintenance treatment is helpful for many people, a drawback is the possibility of developing long-term adverse effects from long-term treatment with antipsychotics. In particular, a condition called tardive dyskinesia, characterized by involuntary movements (usually of the facial muscles), can occur. The disorder may range from mild to severe and can be irreversible.

ATYPICAL NEUROLEPTICS

In 1990, clozapine (Clozaril), an "atypical neuroleptic," was introduced in the United States. This medication is a more effective tool for treating individuals with treatment-resistant schizophrenia, and the risk of tardive dyskinesia is lower. However, because of the potential adverse effect of a serious blood disorder, agranulocytosis, patients who are on clozapine must have a blood test each week. The expense involved in this monitoring, together with the cost of the medication, has made maintenance on clozapine difficult for many persons with schizophrenia.

Since clozapine was approved in the United States, other atypical neuroleptics have been introduced. Risperidone (Risperdal) was released in 1994, olanzapine (Zyprexa) in 1996, and quetiapine (Seroquel) in 1997. While they have some adverse effects, these newer medications are generally better tolerated than either clozapine or the traditional antipsychotics such as Thorazine (chlorpromazine hydrochloride), and they don't cause agranulocytosis. Their only disadvantages are higher cost and a tendency to cause weight gain.

- Briefly explain procedures, routines, and tests *to allay the patient's anxiety.*
- Collaborate with the patient to identify anxious behavior as well as probable causes. *Involving the patient in examination of behavior can increase his sense of control.*
- Provide opportunities for the patient to learn adaptive social skills in a nonthreatening environment. *Learning new social skills can enhance the patient's adjustment after discharge.*

Teaching topics
- Accepting that feelings are valid
- Recognizing extrapyramidal effects of antipsychotic medications
- Preventing photosensitivity reactions to drugs by avoiding exposure to sunlight

Memory jogger

To remember the major needs of schizophrenic patients, think SDS.

Structure, because they tend to have too little in their lives

Diversion, to distract them from disturbing thoughts

Stress reduction, to minimize the severity of the disorder

Delusional disorder

Patients with delusional disorder hold firmly to false beliefs, despite contradictory information. The patient with delusional disorder tends to be intelligent and can have a high level of competence, but have impaired social and personal relationships. One indication of delusional disorder is an absence of hallucinations.

CONTRIBUTING FACTORS
- Brain abnormalities
- Developmental involvement
- Family history of schizophrenic, avoidant, and paranoid personality disorders
- Lower socioeconomic status
- Neurotransmitter abnormalities
- Social or environmental stress, interacting with the person's inherited biological makeup

ASSESSMENT FINDINGS
- Antagonism
- Brushes with the law
- Delusions that are visual, auditory, or tactile
- Denial
- Ideas of reference (everything in the environment takes on a personal significance)
- Inability to trust
- Irritable or depressed mood
- Marked anger and violence
- Projection
- Stalking behavior, in erotomania (belief that patient is loved by a prominent person)

DIAGNOSTIC TEST RESULTS
- Blood and urine tests eliminate an organic or chemical cause.
- Endocrine function tests rule out hyperadrenalism, pernicious anemia, and thyroid disorders.
- Neurologic evaluations rule out an organic cause.

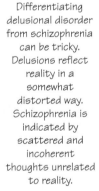

Differentiating delusional disorder from schizophrenia can be tricky. Delusions reflect reality in a somewhat distorted way. Schizophrenia is indicated by scattered and incoherent thoughts unrelated to reality.

NURSING DIAGNOSES
- Impaired social interaction
- Ineffective individual coping
- Risk for violence

TREATMENT
- Family therapy
- Group therapy
- Milieu therapy
- Psychoeducational programs
- Stress management
- Supportive psychotherapy

Drug therapy
- Antiparkinsonian agents: benztropine (Cogentin), for adverse effects of antipsychotic medications
- Antipsychotics: chlorpromazine (Thorazine), fluphenazine (Prolixin), haloperidol (Haldol), olanzapine (Zyprexa), risperidone (Risperdal), thioridazine (Mellaril)

INTERVENTIONS AND RATIONALES
- Formulate realistic, modest goals with the patient. *Including the patient when setting goals may help diminish suspicion while increasing the patient's self-esteem and sense of control.*
- Establish a therapeutic relationship *to foster trust.*
- Designate one nurse to communicate with the patient and to supervise other staff members with regard to the patient's care *to build trust and to minimize opportunities for the patient to exhibit hostility.*
- Explore events that trigger delusions. Discuss anxiety associated with triggering events. *Exploring triggers will help you understand the dynamics of the patient's delusional system.*
- Don't directly attack the delusion. *Doing so will increase the patient anxiety.* Instead, be patient in formulating a trusting relationship.
- Once the dynamics of the delusions are understood, discourage repetitious talk about delusions and refocus the conversation on the patient's underlying feelings. *As the patient identifies and explores feelings, he will decrease reliance on delusional thought.*
- Recognize delusion as the patient's perception of the environment. Avoid getting into ar-

guments with the patient regarding the content of delusions *to foster trust.*

Teaching topics
• Learning decision-making, problem-solving, and negotiating skills
• Understanding potential adverse effects of medication

Disorganized schizophrenia

Disorganized schizophrenics have a flat or inappropriate affect and incoherent thoughts. Patients with this disorder exhibit loose associations and disorganized speech and behaviors.

CONTRIBUTING FACTORS
• A fragile ego, which can't withstand the demands of external reality
• Brain abnormalities
• Developmental involvement
• Genetic factors
• Neurotransmitter abnormalities
• Social or environmental stress, interacting with the person's inherited biological makeup

ASSESSMENT FINDINGS
• Cognitive impairment
• Disorganized speech
• Displacement
• Fantasy
• Flat or inappropriate affect
• Grimacing
• Hallucinations
• Lack of coherence
• Loose associations
• Magical thinking (patient believes his thoughts can control others)
• Word salads

DIAGNOSTIC TEST RESULTS
• MRI shows possible enlargement of the ventricles and prominent cortical sulci.
• Neuropsychological and cognitive tests indicate impaired performance.

NURSING DIAGNOSES
• Altered thought processes
• Social isolation

• Sensory or perceptual alterations (auditory)

TREATMENT
• Family therapy
• Milieu therapy
• Psychoeducational programs
• Social skills training
• Stress management
• Supportive psychotherapy

Drug therapy
• Antiparkinsonian agents: benztropine (Cogentin), for adverse effects of antipsychotic medications
• Antipsychotics: chlorpromazine (Thorazine), fluphenazine (Prolixin), haloperidol (Haldol), olanzapine (Zyprexa), risperidone (Risperdal), thioridazine (Mellaril)

INTERVENTIONS AND RATIONALES
• Help the patient meet basic needs for food, comfort, and a sense of safety *to ensure the patient's well-being and build trust.*
• During an acute psychotic episode, remove potentially hazardous items from the patient's environment *to promote safety.*
• Briefly explain procedures, routines, and tests *to decrease the patient's anxiety.*
• Protect the patient from self-destructive tendencies or aggressive impulses *to ensure safety.*
• Convey sincerity and understanding when communicating *to promote a trusting relationship.*
• Formulate realistic goals with the patient. *Including the patient in formulating goals can help diminish suspicion while increasing self-esteem and sense of control.*
• If the patient experiences hallucinations, don't attempt to reason with him or challenge his perception of hallucinations. Instead, ensure the patient's safety and provide comfort and support. *Attempts to reason with the patient will increase anxiety, possibly making hallucinations worse.*
• Encourage the patient with auditory hallucinations to reveal what voices are telling him *to help prevent harm to the patient and others.*
• First, encourage the patient to participate in one-on-one interactions, and then progress to

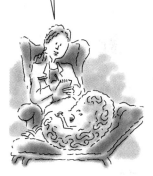

Forming a trusting relationship with the patient is a key intervention for schizophrenic patients.

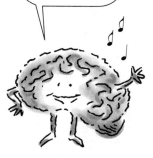

Distraction techniques, such as singing along with music, can alleviate hallucinations, helping to bring the patient back to reality.

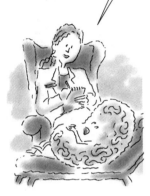

> Treatment for a patient with paranoid schizophrenia usually combines drug therapy with talk therapy.

small groups *to enable the patient to practice newly acquired social skills.*
• Provide positive reinforcement for socially acceptable behavior such as efforts to improve hygiene and table manners *to foster improved social relationships and acceptance from others.*
• Encourage the patient to express feelings related to experiencing hallucinations *to promote better understanding of the patient's experiences and to allow the patient to vent emotions, thereby reducing anxiety.*

Teaching topics
• Learning to use distraction techniques

Paranoid schizophrenia

Patients with paranoid schizophrenia have delusions unrelated to reality. Patients often display bizarre behavior, are easily angered, and are at high risk for violence. The prognosis for independent functioning is often better than for other types of schizophrenia.

CONTRIBUTING FACTORS
• A fragile ego, which cannot withstand the demands of external reality
• Brain abnormalities
• Developmental involvement
• Genetic factors
• Neurotransmitter abnormalities
• Social or environmental stress, interacting with the person's inherited biological makeup

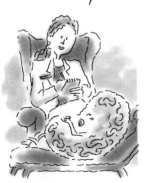

> Interventions for schizophrenia promote the patient's safety, meet physical needs, and help the patient deal with reality.

ASSESSMENT FINDINGS
• Anxiety
• Argumentativeness
• Delusions and auditory hallucinations
• Displacement
• Dissociation
• Easily angered
• Inability to trust
• Potential for violence
• Projection
• Withdrawal or aloofness

DIAGNOSTIC TEST RESULTS
• MRI shows possible enlargement of ventricles, and enlarged sulci. The presence of the enlarged sulci suggests cortical loss, particularly in the frontal lobe.
• Neuropsychological and cognitive tests indicate impaired performance.

NURSING DIAGNOSES
• Altered thought processes
• Social isolation
• Sensory or perceptual alterations (auditory)

TREATMENT
• Family therapy
• Group therapy
• Milieu therapy
• Psychoeducational programs
• Social skills training
• Stress management
• Supportive psychotherapy

Drug therapy
• Antiparkinsonian agents: benztropine (Cogentin), for adverse effects of antipsychotic drugs
• Antipsychotics: chlorpromazine (Thorazine), clozapine (Clozaril), fluphenazine (Prolixin), haloperidol (Haldol), olanzapine (Zyprexa), risperidone (Risperdal), thioridazine (Mellaril)

INTERVENTIONS AND RATIONALES
• Inform the patient that you will help him control his behavior *to promote feelings of safety.*
• Set limits on aggressive behavior and communicate your expectations to the patient *to prevent injury to the patient and others.*
• Designate one nurse to communicate with the patient and to direct other staff members who care for the patient *to foster trust and a stable environment and to minimize opportunities for the patient to exhibit hostility.*
• Maintain a low level of stimuli *to minimize the patient's anxiety, agitation, and suspiciousness.*

• Be flexible — allow the patient some control. Approach him in a calm and unhurried manner. Let the patient talk about anything he wishes, but keep the conversation light and social *to avoid entering into power struggles.*

• Don't let the patient put you on the defensive, and don't take his remarks personally. If he tells you to leave him alone, do leave but return soon. *Brief contacts with the patient may be most useful at first.*

• Don't make attempts to combat the patient's delusions with logic. Instead, respond to feelings, themes, or underlying needs — for example, "It seems you feel you've been treated unfairly." *Combatting delusions may increase feelings of persecution or hostility.*

• If the patient is taking clozapine, stress the importance of returning weekly to the facility or an outpatient setting to have his blood checked *to monitor for adverse effects and prevent toxicity.*

• Teach the patient the importance of complying with the medication regimen. Tell him to report any adverse reactions instead of discontinuing the drug *to maintain therapeutic drug levels.*

• If he takes a slow-release formulation, make sure that he understands when to return for his next dose *to promote compliance.*

Teaching topics

• Avoiding exposure to sunlight (to prevent photosensitive reactions to antipsychotics)
• Reporting any adverse affects of antipsychotic medications
• Visiting the hospital weekly to have blood chemistry monitored

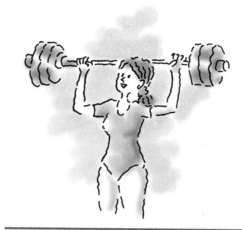

Pump up on practice questions

1. The nurse is caring for a client diagnosed with schizophrenia. Which of the following is an example of a negative symptom?

   A. Delusions
   B. Disorganized speech
   C. Flat affect
   D. Catatonic behavior

Answer: C. Negative symptoms focus on a loss of normal functions and include flat affect, alogia, and avolition. Positive symptoms focus on a distortion of normal functions and include delusions, hallucinations, disorganized speech, and grossly disorganized or catatonic behavior.

➡ *NCLEX keys*
Nursing process step: Assessment
Client needs category: Psychosocial integrity
Client needs subcategory: Psychosocial adaptation
Taxonomic level: Knowledge

2. The nurse is caring for a client who was found huddled in her apartment by the police. The client stares toward one corner of the room and seems to be responding to something not visible to others. She appears hyperalert and scared. How would the nurse assess the situation?

A. The client may be hallucinating.
B. The client is suicidal.
C. Nothing is wrong because the client isn't a threat to society.
D. The client is malingering.

Answer: A. The scenario is typical of a client who is hallucinating. Not enough information is available to suggest that she is a threat to society or to herself. Malingering refers to a medically unproven symptom that is consciously motivated.

➡ *NCLEX keys*
Nursing process step: Analysis
Client needs category: Psychosocial integrity
Client needs subcategory: Psychosocial adaptation
Taxonomic level: Analysis

3. The nurse is caring for a client whom she suspects is paranoid. How would the nurse confirm this assessment?
A. Indirect questioning
B. Direct questioning
C. Lead-in sentences
D. Open-ended sentences

Answer: B. Direct questions (such as "Do you hear voices?" or "Do you feel safe right now?") are the most appropriate technique for eliciting verifiable responses from a psychotic client. The other options may not elicit helpful responses.

➡ *NCLEX keys*
Nursing process step: Implementation
Client needs category: Psychosocial integrity
Client needs subcategory: Psychosocial adaptation
Taxonomic level: Application

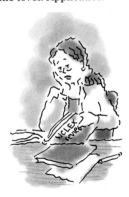

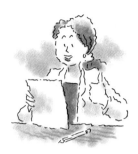

4. The nurse is caring for a client who is experiencing auditory hallucinations. What would be most crucial for the nurse to assess?
A. Possible hearing impairment
B. Family history of psychosis
C. Content of the hallucinations
D. Possible sella turcica tumors

Answer: C. To prevent the client from harming himself or others, the nurse should encourage the client to reveal the content of auditory hallucinations. Family history, although important because of a possible genetic component, isn't an immediate concern. Olfactory hallucinations, not auditory hallucinations, are associated with sella turcica tumors. Assessing for hearing impairment would be inappropriate.

➡ *NCLEX keys*
Nursing process step: Analysis
Client needs category: Safe, effective care environment
Client needs subcategory: Management of care
Taxonomic level: Application

5. The nurse is caring for a client who is experiencing an acute confusional state. What are the two most common causes of such a condition?
A. Advanced age and alcohol intake
B. Sensory deprivation and physical challenges
C. Acute schizophrenia and bipolar illness
D. Cardiac arrhythmias and cerebrovascular accidents

Answer: C. Acute schizophrenia and bipolar illness are the two most frequently cited causes of acute confusional states. Advanced age, alcohol intake, and sensory deprivation can cause confusion, but these are more likely to be chronic or subacute causes. Cardiac and cerebral causes are less likely to occur in a psychiatric setting.

➡ *NCLEX keys*
Nursing process step: Analysis
Client needs category: Psychosocial integrity
Client needs subcategory: Psychosocial adaptation
Taxonomic level: Knowledge

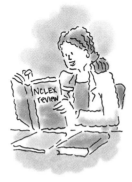

6. The nurse is preparing to care for a client diagnosed with catatonic schizophrenia. In anticipation of this client's arrival, what should the nurse do?
   A. Notify security.
   B. Prepare a magnesium sulfate drip.
   C. Place a specialty mattress overlay on the bed.
   D. Communicate the client's nothing-by-mouth status to the dietary department.

Answer: C. The nurse should first focus on meeting the client's immediate physical needs and preventing complications related to the catatonic state. The need for intervention from security personnel is unlikely. A magnesium sulfate drip isn't indicated. Nutritional status should be addressed after the client is fully assessed and admitted.

➡ *NCLEX keys*
Nursing process step: Planning
Client needs category: Physiological integrity
Client needs subcategory: Basic care and comfort
Taxonomic level: Application

7. The nurse is caring for a client with disorganized schizophrenia. The client is responding well to therapy but has had limited social contact with others. Which of the following interventions is most appropriate?
   A. Discourage the client from interacting with others because if his efforts fail it will be too traumatic for him.
   B. Encourage the client to attend a party thrown for the residents of the facility.
   C. Encourage the client to participate in one-on-one interactions.
   D. Encourage the client to place a personal advertisement in the local newspaper, but not to reveal his mental disability.

Answer: C. First, encourage the client to participate in one-on-one interactions, then progress to small groups to enable the client to practice newly acquired social skills.

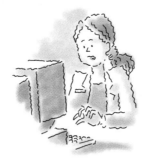

➡ *NCLEX keys*
Nursing process step: Implementation
Client needs category: Psychosocial integrity
Client needs subcategory: Coping and adaptation
Taxonomic level: Application

8. What is the least common type of schizophrenia?

    A. Undifferentiated
    B. Paranoid
    C. Residual
    D. Catatonic

Answer: D. Catatonic schizophrenia is the least common type.

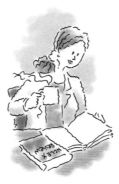

➡ *NCLEX keys*
Nursing process step: Assessment
Client needs category: Psychosocial integrity
Client needs subcategory: Psychosocial adaptation
Taxonomic level: Knowledge

9. For which type of schizophrenia should the nurse expect to provide the most physical care?

    A. Disorganized type
    B. Catatonic type
    C. Paranoid type
    D. Undifferentiated type

Answer: B. In catatonic schizophrenia, the client exhibits little reaction to environment, although periods of excitement may surface at times. Bizarre postures and the inability to feed, wash, and dress oneself are also evident in the catatonic type. Activities of daily living may be affected in varying degrees with the other types, but to a lesser extent.

➡ *NCLEX keys*
Nursing process step: Assessment
Client needs category: Psychosocial integrity
Client needs subcategory: Psychosocial adaptation
Taxonomic level: Knowledge

10. The nurse is caring for a client who has schizophrenia. What is the first-line treatment for this client?

    A. Group therapy
    B. Thyroid replacement therapy in selected individuals
    C. Milieu therapy
    D. Antipsychotics

Answer: D. Antipsychotics are used as the first-line treatment for such disorders. Although thyroid disorders can be a cause of psychotic-like symptoms, they aren't a cause of schizophrenia. Milieu therapy may be helpful but isn't first-line treatment. Group therapy wouldn't be a first-line treatment.

➡ *NCLEX keys*
Nursing process step: Implementation
Client needs category: Physiological integrity
Client needs subcategory: Pharmacological and parenteral therapies
Taxonomic level: Application

If you can't get enough of psych disorders, you're in luck. We've got more coming up in the very next chapter.

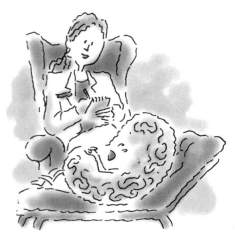

Substance-Related Disorders

Brush up on key concepts

The relationship between mental illness and substance use and abuse is complex. Alcohol and psychoactive drugs alter a person's perceptions, feelings, and behavior. People may use substances for just that reason. Many people who suffer from emotional disorders or mental illness turn to drugs and alcohol to self-medicate, as a way of tolerating feelings. Yet, this method of self-treating seldom works in the long run and frequently makes matters worse.

Nursing care for a substance abuser begins with a thorough assessment to determine which substance is being abused. During the acute phase, care focuses on maintaining the patient's vital functions and safety. Rehabilitation involves helping the patient to realize his substance abuse problem and find alternative methods of dealing with stress. The nurse helps the patient to achieve recovery and stay drug-free.

At any time, you can review the major points of each disorder by consulting the *Cheat sheet* on page 422.

Social use?

Substance intoxication is the development of a reversible substance-specific syndrome due to the ingestion of or exposure to a substance. The clinically significant maladaptive behavior or psychological changes vary from substance to substance.

It's a problem

The essential feature of **substance abuse** is a maladaptive pattern of substance use coupled with recurrent and significant adverse consequences.

The monkey ON the back

Substance dependence is characterized by physical, behavioral, and cognitive changes resulting from persistent substance use. Persistent drug use results in tolerance and withdrawal.

Just can't get enough

Tolerance is defined as an increased need for a substance or a need for an increased amount of the substance to achieve an effect.

The monkey OFF the back

Withdrawal occurs when the tissue and blood levels of the substance decrease in a person who has engaged in prolonged, heavy use of the substance.

When uncomfortable withdrawal symptoms persist, the person usually takes the drug to relieve the symptoms. Withdrawal symptoms vary from substance to substance.

Classes of controlled substances

Each class of controlled substance has a different affect on the body and thus produces different reactions. Common classes of controlled substances include:
• cannabis
• depressants
• designer drugs
• hallucinogens
• inhalants
• opiates
• phencyclidine
• stimulants.

CANNABIS

Tetrahydrocannabinol, the active ingredient in hashish and marijuana, produces a type of euphoria, increased appetite, sensory alter-

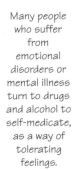

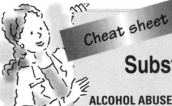

Substance-related disorders refresher

ALCOHOL ABUSE DISORDER

Key signs and symptoms
- Blackouts
- Liver damage
- Pathologic intoxication

Key test results
- CAGE questionnaire indicates alcoholism.
- Michigan Alcoholism Screening test indicates alcoholism.

Key treatments
- Alcoholics Anonymous
- Individual therapy
- Rehabilitation
- Benzodiazepines: chlordiazepoxide (Librium), diazepam (Valium), or lorazepam (Ativan)
- Disulfiram (Antabuse) to prevent relapse into alcohol abuse (The patient must be alcohol-free for 12 hours before administering this drug.)
- Naltrexone (Trexan) to prevent relapse into alcohol abuse
- Selective serotonin reuptake inhibitors: bupropion (Wellbutrin), fluoxetine (Prozac), paroxetine (Paxil)

Key interventions
- Assess the patient's use of denial as a coping mechanism.
- Set limits on denial and rationalization.
- Have the patient formulate goals for maintenance of a drug-free lifestyle.

COCAINE-USE DISORDER

Key signs and symptoms
- Elevated energy and mood
- Grandiose thinking
- Impaired judgment

Key test results
- Drug screening is positive for cocaine.

Key treatments
- Detoxification
- Rehabilitation (inpatient or outpatient)
- Narcotics Anonymous
- Individual therapy

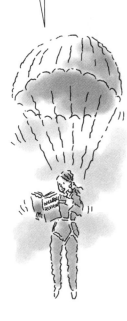

> Many people who suffer from emotional disorders or mental illness turn to drugs and alcohol to self-medicate, as a way of tolerating feelings.

- Anxiolytics: lorazepam (Ativan), Alprazolam (Xanax)
- Dopamine agent: bromocriptine (Parlodel)
- Selective serotonin reuptake inhibitors: fluoxetine (Prozac), paroxetine (Paxil)

Key interventions
- Establish a trusting relationship with the patient.
- Provide the patient with well-balanced meals.
- Set limits on the patient's attempts to rationalize behavior.

SUBSTANCE ABUSE DISORDER

Key signs and symptoms
- Blaming others for problems
- Development of biological or psychological need for a substance
- Dysfunctional anger
- Feelings of grandiosity
- Impulsiveness
- Use of denial and rationalization to explain consequences of behavior

Key test results
- Positive blood and urine drug screenings confirm the diagnosis.

Key treatments
- Individual therapy
- Clonidine (Catapres) for opiate withdrawal symptoms
- Methadone maintenance for opiate addiction detoxification

Key interventions
- Ensure a safe, quiet environment free of stimuli to provide a therapeutic setting and to alleviate withdrawal symptoms.
- Monitor for withdrawal symptoms, such as tremors, seizures, and anxiety.
- Help the patient understand the ultimate consequences of substance abuse.
- Encourage the patient to vent fear and anger.

ations, tachycardia, lack of coordination, and impaired judgment and memory.

DEPRESSANTS
These substances slow down central nervous system (CNS) functioning, causing slurred speech, impaired judgment, and mood swings. Common depressants include:
• alcohol
• barbiturates
• benzodiazepines.

DESIGNER DRUGS
These substances are similar to other classes of drugs, but slight chemical changes make them legal (and often more dangerous). The following substances are the most common:
• china white (synthetic type of heroin)
• ecstasy.

HALLUCINOGENS
These substances produce euphoria, sympathetic and parasympathetic stimulation, and hallucinations, dissociative states, and bizarre, maniclike behavior:
• lysergic acid diethylamide (LSD)
• mushrooms (psilocybin)
• mescaline (from peyote cactus).

INHALANTS
Use of these substances is called "huffing." These aren't drugs, but some people have found that they can "catch a buzz" from inhaling the fumes. The following products are commonly used:
• glue
• cleaning solutions
• nail polish remover
• aerosols
• petroleum products
• paint thinners.

OPIATES AND RELATED ANALGESICS
These substances dull the senses, resulting in sedation and a dream-like state, and can cause respiratory depression and cardiac arrest:
• heroin
• morphine
• codeine
• opium
• methadone
• meperidine.

PHENCYCLIDINE
Phencyclidine (PCP), also known as angel dust, heightens CNS function, distorts perception, and has powerful analgesic effects.

STIMULANTS
These substances stimulate the CNS:
• amphetamines
• cocaine (including crack cocaine)
• caffeine
• nicotine.

Polish up on patient care

Almost any controlled substance can potentially become addictive. Though specific circumstances may vary, causes and treatments remain similar for each substance.

Alcohol abuse disorder

Though alcohol abuse is considered a substance abuse disorder, assessment findings and treatment differ somewhat from that for other substances. Alcohol is a sedative but creates a feeling of euphoria. Sedation increases with the amount ingested.

CAUSES
• Familial tendency
• Gender (males have increased likelihood of addiction)
• History of abuse, depression, or anxiety
• Influence of nationality and ethnicity
• Personality disorders
• Religious or family taboos regarding alcohol consumption

ASSESSMENT FINDINGS
• Adrenocortical insufficiency
• Alcoholic cardiomyopathy
• Alcoholic cirrhosis
• Alcoholic hepatitis
• Alcoholic paranoia
• Blackouts
• Erection problems
• Esophageal varices

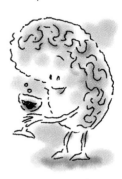

Note that alcohol is a depressant.

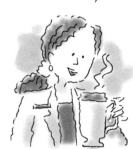

Caffeine and nicotine are classified as stimulants because of the effect they have on the body.

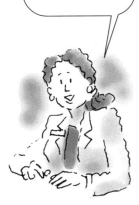

Because alcohol use is widely accepted, therapeutic communication may involve dealing with a patient's rationalizations.

- Gastritis or gastric ulcers
- Hallucinations
- Korsakoff's psychosis
- Liver damage
- Muscular myopathy
- Pancreatitis
- Pathologic intoxication
- Peripheral neuropathy
- Wernicke's encephalopathy.

DIAGNOSTIC TEST RESULTS
- Positive blood and urine drug screenings confirm the diagnosis.
- CAGE questionnaire indicates alcoholism. (See *The CAGE questionnaire*.)
- Michigan Alcoholism Screening test indicates alcoholism.

NURSING DIAGNOSES
- Ineffective denial
- Ineffective individual coping
- Risk for injury

TREATMENT
- Alcoholics Anonymous
- Individual therapy
- Rehabilitation

Drug therapy
- Antidepressants: bupropion (Wellbutrin)
- Benzodiazepines: chlordiazepoxide (Librium), diazepam (Valium), or lorazepam (Ativan)
- Disulfiram (Antabuse) to prevent relapse into alcohol abuse (The patient must be alcohol-free for 12 hours before administering this drug.)
- Naltrexone (Trexan) to prevent relapse into alcohol abuse
- Selective serotonin reuptake inhibitors: fluoxetine (Prozac), paroxetine (Paxil)

INTERVENTIONS AND RATIONALES
- Assess the patient's use of denial as a coping mechanism *to begin a therapeutic relationship.*
- Encourage the verbalization of anger, fear, inadequacy, grief, and guilt *to promote healthy coping behaviors.*

- Set limits on denial and rationalization *to help the patient gain control and perspective.*
- Have the patient formulate goals for maintenance of a drug-free lifestyle *to help avoid relapses.*

Teaching topics
- Understanding substance abuse and relapse prevention
- Maintaining good nutrition

Cocaine-use disorder

Cocaine-use disorder results from the potent euphoric effects of the drug. Individuals exposed to cocaine develop dependence after a very short period of time. Maladaptive behavior follows, resulting in social dysfunction.

CONTRIBUTING FACTORS
- Genetic predisposition
- History of abuse, depression, or anxiety
- Personality disorder

ASSESSMENT FINDINGS
- Assault or violent behavior
- Elevated energy and mood
- Grandiose thinking
- Impaired judgment
- Impaired social functioning

DIAGNOSTIC TEST RESULTS
- Drug screening is positive for cocaine.

NURSING DIAGNOSES
- Altered health maintenance
- Altered nutrition: Less than body requirements
- Risk for violence

TREATMENT
- Detoxification
- Rehabilitation (inpatient or outpatient)
- Narcotics Anonymous
- Individual therapy

The CAGE questionnaire

This questionnaire is a brief, unscored examination meant to provide a standard for assessing alcohol addiction. Any two positive responses to these four yes or no questions strongly suggest alcohol dependence.

1. Have you ever felt you should **C**ut down on your drinking?
2. Have people **A**nnoyed you by criticizing your drinking?
3. Have you ever felt bad or **G**uilty about your drinking?
4. Have you ever had an **E**ye-opener first thing in the morning because of a hangover, or just to get the day started?

Drug therapy

• Anxiolytics: lorazepam (Ativan), alprazolam (Xanax)
• Dopamine agent: bromocriptine (Parlodel)
• Selective serotonin reuptake inhibitors: fluoxetine (Prozac), paroxetine (Paxil)

INTERVENTIONS AND RATIONALES

• Establish a trusting relationship with the patient *to alleviate any anxiety or paranoia.*
• Provide the patient with well-balanced meals *to compensate for nutritional deficits.*
• Provide a safe environment. *The patient may pose a risk to self or others.*
• Set limits on the patient's attempts to rationalize behavior *to reduce inappropriate behavior.*

Teaching topics

• Contacting Narcotics Anonymous
• Coping strategies
• Managing stress

Substance abuse disorder

Substance abuse disorder includes all patterns of abuse excluding alcohol and cocaine. Abuse disorders have a great deal in common, though symptoms vary depending upon the abused substance.

CONTRIBUTING FACTORS

• Familial tendency

• Gender (Females have increased likelihood of abusing prescription drugs; males have generally increased likelihood of addiction.)
• History of abuse, depression, or anxiety
• Influence of nationality and ethnicity
• Personality disorders

ASSESSMENT FINDINGS

• Attempts to avoid anxiety and other emotions
• Attempts to avoid conscious feelings of guilt and anger
• Attempts to meet needs by influencing others
• Blaming others for problems
• Development of biological or psychological need for a substance
• Dysfunctional anger
• Feelings of grandiosity
• Impulsiveness
• Manipulation and deceit
• Need for immediate gratification
• Pattern of negative interactions
• Possible malnutrition
• Symptoms of withdrawal
• Use of denial and rationalization to explain consequences of behavior

DIAGNOSTIC TEST RESULTS

• Positive blood and urine drug screenings confirm the diagnosis.

NURSING DIAGNOSES

• Altered health maintenance
• Altered nutrition: Less than body requirements
• Risk for violence

During a psychiatric evaluation, always rule out drug or alcohol use; they produce symptoms that mimic those of mental illness.

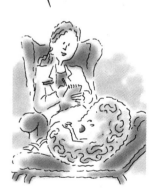

TREATMENT
- Behavior modification
- Employee assistance programs
- Family counseling
- Group therapy
- Halfway houses
- Individual therapy
- Informal social support
- Self-help groups

Drug therapy
- Clonidine (Catapres) for opiate withdrawal symptoms
- Methadone maintenance for opiate addiction detoxification

INTERVENTIONS AND RATIONALES
- Ensure a safe, quiet environment free of stimuli *to provide a therapeutic setting and to alleviate withdrawal symptoms.*
- Monitor for withdrawal symptoms, such as delirium tremors, seizures, or anxiety *to provide the most comfortable environment possible.*
- Assess the patient for polysubstance abuse *to plan appropriate interventions.*
- Help the patient understand the ultimate consequences of substance abuse *to assist recovery.*
- Provide measures to induce sleep *to help the patient manage the discomfort of withdrawal.*
- Encourage the patient to vent fear and anger *so that he can begin the healing process.*

Teaching topics
- Contacting addiction support agencies
- Learning healthy coping mechanisms

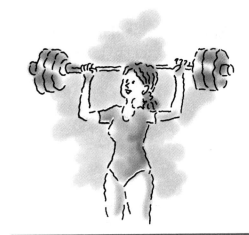

Pump up on practice questions

1. The nurse is talking to a client about amphetamines, cocaine, and caffeine. How would the nurse classify these substances?
- A. Opiates
- B. Analgesics
- C. Stimulants
- D. Depressants

Answer: C. Amphetamines, cocaine, and caffeine are stimulants. Stimulation is not a chief effect of drugs in the other three categories.

➡ **NCLEX keys**
Nursing process step: Assessment
Client needs category: Physiological integrity
Client needs subcategory: Reduction of risk potential
Taxonomic level: Knowledge

2. The nurse is caring for a client who has a history of alcohol abuse. Why would the client act as if he didn't have a problem?
- A. The client has never taken the CAGE questionnaire.
- B. Denial is a defense mechanism commonly used by alcoholics.
- C. Thought processes are distorted.
- D. Alcohol is inexpensive.

Answer: B. Denial is a defense mechanism commonly used by alcoholics. The CAGE questionaire is a direct method of discovering whether the client is a substance abuser, but the client is likely to deny the problem regardless of whether he's familiar with this assessment tool. Distorted thought processes and the cost of alcohol are less likely to influence the client's use of denial.

➨ *NCLEX keys*
Nursing process step: Evaluation
Client needs category: Psychosocial integrity
Client needs subcategory: Coping and adaptation
Taxonomic level: Analysis

3. The nurse is caring for a client who exhibits pinpoint pupils as well as decreased blood pressure, pulse, respirations, and temperature. These symptoms may be a sign of which disorder?
   A. Opiate intoxication
   B. Amphetamine intoxication
   C. Cannabis intoxication
   D. Alcohol intoxication
Answer: A. Opiates, such as morphine or heroin, cause these changes. Amphetamines dilate pupils. Cannabis intoxication causes tachycardia, dry mouth, and increased appetite. Alcohol intoxication causes unsteady gait, incoordination, nystagmus, and flushed face.

➨ *NCLEX keys*
Nursing process step: Assessment
Client needs category: Physiological integrity
Client needs subcategory: Physiological adaptation
Taxonomic level: Application

4. The nurse is caring for a client in a substance abuse clinic. The client tells the nurse he needs an increased amount of heroin to produce the same effect that he experienced a number of weeks ago. How would the nurse describe this condition?
   A. Tolerance
   B. Dependence
   C. Withdrawal delirium
   D. Compulsion
Answer: A. Tolerance occurs when an increased amount of a substance is required to produce the same effect. Dependence is a physiologic dependence on a substance.

Withdrawal delirium occurs when cessation of a substance produces physiologic symptoms. Compulsion refers to an unwanted repetitive act.

➨ *NCLEX keys*
Nursing process step: Analysis
Client needs category: Physiological integrity
Client needs subcategory: Physiological adaptation
Taxonomic level: Application

5. The nurse is interviewing a client who's currently under the influence of a controlled substance and shows signs of becoming agitated. What should the nurse do?
   A. Use confrontation.
   B. Express disgust with the client's behavior.
   C. Be aware of hospital security.
   D. Communicate a scolding attitude to intimidate the client.
Answer: C. The nurse, for her own protection, should be aware of hospital security and other assisting personnel. The other options may cause a relatively docile client to become belligerent.

➨ *NCLEX keys*
Nursing process step: Planning
Client needs category: Safe, effective care environment
Client needs subcategory: Management of care
Taxonomic level: Application

6. Which common substances is the client most likely to inhale to become intoxicated?
   A. Glue, cleaning solutions, insecticides
   B. Glue, nail polish remover, aerosols
   C. Paint thinners, insecticides, spray paint
   D. Cleaning solutions, insecticides, spray paint
Answer: B. Glue, nail polish remover, aerosols, paint thinners, and cleaning solutions are inhalants used for a "high." Insecticide inhalation would likely cause illness, and inhaling a spray paint would color the person's face, an obvious detriment.

➡ *NCLEX keys*

Nursing process step: Analysis
Client needs category: Psychosocial integrity
Client needs subcategory: Psychosocial adaptation
Taxonomic level: Comprehension

7. The nurse is caring for a client with a history of substance abuse. Depending on the substance abused, what might treatment include?

A. Antabuse or methadone
B. Morphine
C. Demerol
D. Lithium

Answer: A. Antabuse assists in recovery from alcoholism; methadone maintenance is used for opiate abusers. Morphine and Demerol are controlled substances and aren't used in substance abuse treatment. Lithium is used to treat bipolar disorder.

➡ *NCLEX keys*

Nursing process step: Planning
Client needs category: Physiological integrity
Client needs subcategory: Pharmacological and parenteral therapies
Taxonomic level: Application

8. The nurse is using the CAGE questionaire as a screening tool for alcohol problems. What do these initials represent?

A. Cut down, Annoyed, Guilty, Eyeopener
B. Consumed, Angry, Gastritis, Esophageal varices
C. Cancer, Alcoholic liver, Gastric ulcer, Erosive gastritis
D. Cunning, Anger, Guilt, Excess

Answer: A. CAGE stands for "Have you felt the need to Cut down on your drinking? Have you ever been Annoyed by criticism of your drinking? Have you felt Guilty about your drinking? Have you felt the need for an Eyeopener in the morning?"

➡ *NCLEX keys*

Nursing process step: Assessment
Client needs category: Psychosocial integrity
Client needs subcategory: Coping and adaptation
Taxonomic level: Analysis

9. The nurse is administering disulfiram (Antabuse) to a client with a history of alcohol abuse. Before receiving therapy, which of the following is required of the client?

A. Be committed to attending AA meetings weekly
B. Admit to himself and another person that he's an alcoholic
C. Remain alcohol-free for 6 hours
D. Remain alcohol-free for 12 hours

Answer: D. The client must be alcohol-free for 12 hours before initiating disulfiram therapy. Attending AA and acknowledging alcoholism aren't necessary before therapy.

➡ *NCLEX keys*

Nursing process step: Implementation
Client needs category: Physiological integrity
Client needs subcategory: Pharmacological and parenteral therapies
Taxonomic level: Application

10. A client with a history of alcoholism returns to the hospital 3 hours later than the time specified on his day pass. His breath smells of alcohol and his gait is unsteady. What should the nurse say?

A. "Why are you 3 hours late?"
B. "How much did you drink tonight? Drinking is against the rules."
C. "I'm disappointed that you weren't responsible with your day pass."
D. "Please go to bed now. We'll talk in the morning."

Answer: D. The patient can best discuss his behavior when he's no longer under the influence of alcohol. Option A encourages the patient to invent excuses. Option B is judgmental and discourages open communication, and option C is also judgmental.

➡ *NCLEX keys*

Nursing process step: Implementation
Client needs category: Psychosocial integrity
Client needs subcategory: Psychosocial adaptation
Taxonomic level: Analysis

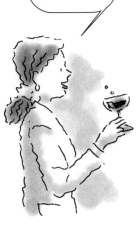

You finished another chapter. Reward yourself — but remember, moderation in all things.

19 Dissociative Disorders

Brush up on key concepts

In this chapter, you'll review:

- basic facts about dissociative disorders
- tests used to diagnose dissociative disorders
- common dissociative disorders.

A patient with a **dissociative disorder** experiences a disruption in the usual relationship between memory, identity, consciousness, and perceptions. This disturbance may occur suddenly or appear gradually. Typically, dissociation is a mechanism used to protect the self and gain relief from overwhelming anxiety.

At any time, you can review major points of each disorder by consulting the *Cheat sheet* on page 430.

Polish up on patient care

Common dissociative disorders include depersonalization disorder, dissociative amnesia, and dissociative identity disorder.

Depersonalization disorder

In depersonalization disorder, the patient experiences a loss of identity. The patient may feel like a detached observer, passively watching his mental or physical activity as if in a dream. The onset of depersonalization is sudden and the progression of the disorder is chronic, characterized by remissions and exacerbations.

CONTRIBUTING FACTORS
- History of physical and emotional abuse
- History of substance abuse
- Neurophysiologic predisposition
- Obsessive-compulsive disorder
- Sensory deprivation
- Severe stress, such as military combat, violent crime, or other traumatic events

ASSESSMENT FINDINGS
- Anxiety symptoms
- Depressive symptoms
- Disturbance in sense of time
- Fear of going insane
- Impaired occupational functioning
- Impaired social functioning
- Low self-esteem
- Persistent or recurring feelings of detachment from mind and body

DIAGNOSTIC TEST RESULTS
- Standard dissociative disorder tests demonstrate a high degree of dissociation. These tests include the:
  - diagnostic drawing series
  - dissociative experience scale
  - dissociative interview schedule
  - structured clinical interview for dissociative disorders.

NURSING DIAGNOSES
- Impaired memory
- Posttrauma response
- Sensory or perceptual alterations

TREATMENT
- Individual psychotherapy

Drug therapy
- Benzodiazepines: alprazolam (Xanax), lorazepam (Ativan), clonazepam (Klonopin)

INTERVENTIONS AND RATIONALES
- Establish a trusting relationship by conveying acceptance and respect *to provide a safe environment for the patient to express distressing feelings.*
- Encourage the patient to recognize that depersonalization is a defense mechanism used to deal with anxiety and trauma *because the*

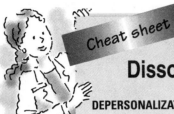

Cheat sheet

Dissociative disorders refresher

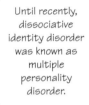

> Until recently, dissociative identity disorder was known as multiple personality disorder.

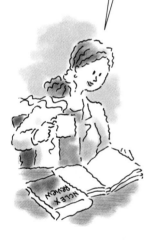

DEPERSONALIZATION DISORDER

Key signs and symptoms
- Fear of going insane
- Impaired occupational functioning
- Impaired social functioning
- Persistent or recurring feelings of detachment from mind and body

Key test results
- Standard dissociative disorder tests demonstrate a degree of dissociation. These tests include:
  – dissociative experience scale
  – dissociative interview schedule.

Key interventions
- Encourage the patient to recognize that depersonalization is a defense mechanism used to deal with anxiety and trauma.
- Assist the patient in establishing supportive relationships.

DISSOCIATIVE AMNESIA

Key signs and symptoms
- Low self-esteem
- Altered identity
- No conscious recollection of a traumatic event, yet colors, sounds, sites, or odors of the event may trigger distress or depression
- Sudden onset of amnesia and inability to recall personal information

Key test results
- Standard dissociative disorder tests demonstrate a degree of dissociation. These tests include:
  – diagnostic drawing series
  – dissociative experience scale
  – dissociative interview schedule
  – structured clinical interview for dissociative disorders.

Key treatments
- Individual therapy
- Benzodiazepines: alprazolam (Xanax), lorazepam (Ativan)

- Selective serotonin reuptake inhibitors (SSRIs): paroxetine (Paxil)

Key interventions
- Encourage the patient to verbalize feelings of distress.
- Encourage the patient to recognize that memory loss is a defense mechanism used to deal with anxiety and trauma.

DISSOCIATIVE IDENTITY DISORDER

Key signs and symptoms
- Guilt and shame
- Lack of recall (beyond ordinary forgetfulness)
- Presence of two or more distinct identities or personality states

Key test results
- Standard dissociative disorder tests demonstrate a degree of dissociation. These tests include:
  – diagnostic drawing series
  – dissociative experience scale
  – dissociative interview schedule
  – structured clinical interview for dissociative disorders.
- Electroencephalogram (EEG) readings may vary markedly among the different identities.

Key treatments
- Long-term reconstructive psychotherapy
- Benzodiazepines: alprazolam (Xanax), lorazepam (Ativan), clonazepam (Klonopin)
- SSRIs: paroxetine (Paxil)
- Tricyclic antidepressants: imipramine (Tofranil), desipramine (Norpramin)

Key interventions
- Assist the patient in identifying each personality.
- Encourage the patient to identify emotions that occur under duress.

patient needs to first recognize how depersonalization works.
• Assist the patient in establishing supportive relationships *because social interaction reduces the tendency toward depersonalization.*

Teaching topics
• Effective stress management

Dissociative amnesia

In dissociative amnesia, acute memory loss is triggered by severe psychological stress. The patient may repress disturbing memories or dissociate from anxiety-laden experiences. The patient may not recall important life events in an attempt to avoid traumatic memories. Recovery from dissociative amnesia is usually complete, and recurrences are rare.

CONTRIBUTING FACTORS
• Emotional abuse
• Low self-esteem
• Past traumatic event
• Physical abuse
• Sexual abuse

ASSESSMENT FINDINGS
• Altered identity
• Clinically significant distress or impairment in social functioning
• Depression
• Emotional numbness
• Low self-esteem
• No conscious recollection of a traumatic event, yet colors, sounds, sites, or odors of the event may trigger distress or depression
• Self-mutilation, suicidal or aggressive urges
• Sudden onset of amnesia and inability to recall personal information

NURSING DIAGNOSES
• Anxiety
• Impaired memory
• Social isolation

DIAGNOSTIC TEST RESULTS
• Standard dissociative disorder tests demonstrate a degree of dissociation. These tests include:

– diagnostic drawing series
– dissociative experience scale
– dissociative interview schedule
– structured clinical interview for dissociative disorders.

TREATMENT
• Hypnosis
• Individual therapy

Drug therapy
• Benzodiazepines: alprazolam (Xanax), lorazepam (Ativan)
• Selective serotonin reuptake inhibitors (SSRIs): paroxetine (Paxil)
• Tricyclic antidepressants: imipramine (Tofranil), desipramine (Norpramin)

INTERVENTIONS AND RATIONALES
• Encourage the patient to verbalize feelings of distress *to help the patient deal with anxiety before it escalates.*
• Encourage the patient to recognize that memory loss is a defense mechanism used to deal with anxiety and trauma *to help the patient understand his condition.*

Teaching topics
• Promoting positive coping skills
• Utilizing relaxation techniques

Dissociative identity disorder

In dissociative identity disorder, formerly known as multiple personality disorder, the patient has at least two unique identities. Each identity can have unique behavior pat-

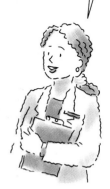

Remember, when working with patients who have dissociative disorders, keep the focus on the <u>patient</u>, not on the <u>symptoms</u>.

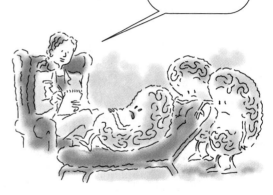

Establishing a support system is a key intervention for depersonalization disorder.

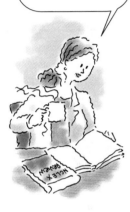

Many patients suffering from dissociative identity disorder have experienced severe childhood abuse and incest.

terns and unique memories, though usually one primary identity is associated with the patient's name. The patient may also have traumatic memories that intrude into his awareness. This disorder tends to be chronic and recurrent.

CONTRIBUTING FACTORS
- Emotional, physical, or sexual abuse
- Genetic predisposition
- Lack of nurturing experiences to assist recovery from abuse
- Low self-esteem
- Traumatic experience before the age of 15

ASSESSMENT FINDINGS
- Eating disorders
- Guilt and shame
- Hallucinations (auditory and visual)
- Lack of recall (beyond ordinary forgetfulness)
- Low self-esteem
- Posttraumatic symptoms (flashbacks, startle responses, nightmares)
- Presence of two or more distinct identities or personality states
- Recurrent depression
- Sexual dysfunction and difficulty forming intimate relationships
- Sleep disorders
- Somatic pain syndromes
- Substance abuse
- Suicidal tendencies

DIAGNOSTIC TEST RESULTS
- Standard dissociative disorder tests demonstrate a degree of dissociation. These tests include:
– diagnostic drawing series
– dissociative experience scale
– dissociative interview schedule
– structured clinical interview for dissociative disorders.
- Electroencephalogram (EEG) readings may vary markedly among the different identities.

NURSING DIAGNOSES
- Impaired verbal communication
- Personal identity disturbance
- Self-esteem disturbance

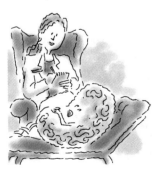

Help psychiatric patients recognize strengths as well as weaknesses to bolster confidence as they begin to cope with trauma.

TREATMENT
- Hypnosis, for the purpose of revisiting the trauma
- Implementation of suicide precautions, if necessary
- Long-term reconstructive psychotherapy
- Medications, sparingly
- Treatment for eating disorders, sleeping disorders, and sexual dysfunction

Drug therapy
- Benzodiazepines: alprazolam (Xanax), lorazepam (Ativan), clonazepam (Klonopin)
- Monoamine oxidase inhibitors: phenelzine (Nardil), tranylcypromine (Parnate)
- SSRIs: paroxetine (Paxil)
- Tricyclic antidepressants: imipramine (Tofranil), desipramine (Norpramin)

INTERVENTIONS AND RATIONALES
- Establish a trusting relationship. *Because of a history of abuse, the patient will have trouble developing a trusting relationship.*
- Assist the patient in identifying each personality *to work toward integration.*
- Encourage the patient to identify emotions that occur under duress *to demonstrate that extreme emotions are a normal result of stress.*

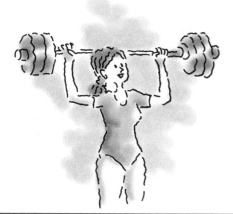

Pump up on practice questions

1. The nurse is caring for several clients diagnosed with dissociative disorders. Which of the following clients has the best chance of a complete recovery and is least likely to experience a recurrence of symptoms?

    A. A client with depersonalization disorder

    B. A client with dissociative amnesia

    C. A client with dissociative personality disorder

    D. A client with multiple personality disorder

Answer: B. A client diagnosed with dissociative amnesia experiences complete recovery, and recurrences are rare. A client diagnosed with depersonalization disorder often experiences remissions and exacerbations. Dissociative identity disorder tends to be chronic and recurrent despite extensive treatment. Multiple personality disorder is the former name for dissociative personality disorder.

➧ *NCLEX keys*

Nursing process step: Assessment
Client needs category: Psychosocial integrity
Client needs subcategory: Psychosocial adaptation
Taxonomic level: Knowledge

2. The nurse is caring for a client diagnosed with dissociative amnesia. The client recently experienced a divorce. How should the nurse help the client deal with traumatic memories?

    A. Discourage the client from verbalizing feelings because they will be too traumatic.

    B. Force the client to confront her memories about the divorce in a direct, confrontational manner.

    C. Tell the client that everything will be alright.

    D. Encourage the client to verbalize feelings of distress.

Answer: D. Encouraging the client to verbalize feelings of distress helps her deal with her anxieties before they escalate. Forcing the client to confront her memories will increase her anxiety. Telling the client that everything will be alright offers false reassurance. Discouraging the client from verbalizing her feelings may cause anxiety to escalate.

➧ *NCLEX keys*

Nursing process step: Implementation
Client needs category: Psychosocial integrity
Client needs subcategory: Coping and adaptation
Taxonomic level: Application

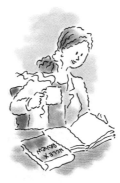

3. The nurse is caring for a client who frequently complains of vague, inconsistent symptoms. Which nursing intervention would be the most appropriate?

A. Screen the client for recent life changes and symptoms of depression, while focusing on physical symptoms.
B. Attempt to minimize physical symptoms, while screening the client for psychological disorders.
C. Exhaust all diagnostic options in ruling out disease before focusing on psychological issues.
D. Refer the client to a psychiatrist.

Answer: A. It's important not to minimize physical symptoms so that the nurse can demonstrate empathy and establish rapport. The nurse should simultaneously investigate recent life changes and the risk of depression. Although tests and imaging studies may be done in certain cases, review of previous medical records and a physical examination should first be performed to determine the likelihood of physical findings. Referral may be indicated, but not enough information is available.

➡ NCLEX keys
Nursing process step: Evaluation
Client needs category: Psychosocial integrity
Client needs subcategory: Psychosocial adaptation
Taxonomic level: Analysis

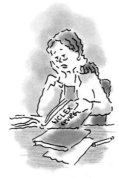

4. The nurse is caring for a client who reports feeling "estranged and separated from himself." How would the nurse describe such symptoms?

A. Intoxication
B. Antimotivational syndrome
C. Existentialism
D. Depersonalization

Answer: D. Depersonalization is characterized by feelings of separateness from oneself. Intoxication is described as feelings of calm, omnipotence, or euphoria. When a relative lack of motivation occurs within an individual, antimotivational syndrome is present. Existentialism is the philosophy that a person finds meaning in life through experiences.

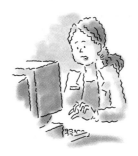

➡ NCLEX keys
Nursing process step: Analysis
Client needs category: Psychosocial integrity
Client needs subcategory: Psychosocial adaptation
Taxonomic level: Comprehension

5. The nurse is caring for a client named Susan who has been diagnosed with dissociative identity disorder. Usually, the client arrives to therapy sessions dressed in a tasteful business suit. One day, the client comes to the clinic dressed in a gold lamé mini-dress and insists that her name is Ruby. How should the nurse respond?

A. Ask the client why she's wearing that ridiculous outfit.
B. Refuse to call the client anything but Susan.
C. Ignore the client's behavior.
D. Help the client explore the characteristics of this newly emerged personality.

Answer: D. The nurse should help the client explore the characteristics of this newly emerged personality in order to work toward integration. Option A would further decrease the client's self-esteem. Not calling the client by the name she requests would jeopardize the trusting nurse-client relationship. Ignoring the behavior doesn't help the client work toward integration.

➡ NCLEX keys
Nursing process step: Implementation
Client needs category: Psychosocial integrity
Client needs subcategory: Psychosocial adaptation
Taxonomic level: Application

6. The nurse is caring for a client who has a dissociative identity disorder. Which statement would be true about this client?
A. The client's sense of selfhood, which sustains an integrated personality structure, is diminished.
B. The client's sense of selfhood continuously sustains an integrated personality structure.
C. The physician has requested that the client dissociate from his usual medical caregivers and be referred to a psychiatrist.
D. The client is experiencing a gender identity crisis.

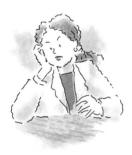

Answer: A. Identity is described as a person's sense of selfhood that sustains an integrated personality structure. In a client with a dissociative identity disorder, this sense is altered. The other choices aren't logical. Gender identity isn't necessarily an issue with this type of disorder.

7. The nurse is caring for a client who seems to lack spontaneity, have difficulty distinguishing himself from others, and have difficulty distinguishing between internal and external stimuli. The client describes a vague feeling of estrangement. Which statement would describe this client?
A. He is depressed and should be placed on antidepressants.
B. He may have a depersonalization disorder.
C. He may benefit from electroconvulsive therapy.
D. He should be placed on suicide precautions.

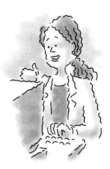

Answer: B. The client has characteristics of a depersonalization disorder. He may indeed suffer from depression also, but antidepressants aren't indicated given the available information. Electroconvulsive therapy wouldn't be appropriate. At this point, the client's behavior doesn't seem suicidal; therefore, such precautions aren't needed.

➡ NCLEX keys
Nursing process step: Assessment
Client needs category: Psychosocial integrity
Client needs subcategory: Psychosocial adaptation
Taxonomic level: Analysis

8. The nurse is caring for a client who has a depersonalization disorder. Which clear and explicit outcomes should the nurse work toward?

A. Emphasizing strengths, rather than the pathologic condition
B. Focusing on past accomplishments, rather than the current condition
C. Increasing confidence and active participation in planning and implementation of treatment
D. Eliciting empathetic responses from the client

Answer: C. These outcomes are measurable. The active involvement expected of this client will allow for concise documentation of this. The other options are vague and inappropriate.

➡ *NCLEX keys*

Nursing process step: Planning
Client needs category: Psychosocial integrity
Client needs subcategory: Psychosocial adaptation
Taxonomic level: Application

9. The nurse is caring for a client who has a dissociative disorder. What should the nurse do to assist the client in goal achievement?

A. Provide opportunities for the client to experience success.
B. Praise the client frequently, whether warranted or not.
C. Evaluate components of the client's self-concept.
D. Discuss with the client three categories of behavior commonly associated with an altered self-concept.

Answer: A. Providing opportunities for the client to experience success would assist him in achieving goals. Praise, if offered in unwarranted situations, will inevitably cause the client to question the caregiver's sincerity. The other two choices are merely academic exercises and won't assist the client in achieving goals.

➡ *NCLEX keys*

Nursing process step: Planning
Client needs category: Psychosocial integrity
Client needs subcategory: Psychosocial adaptation
Taxonomic level: Application

10. The nurse is caring for a client who has a dissociative disorder and is experiencing amnesia. What could have triggered the amnesia?

A. Severe psychosocial stress
B. Short-acting sedation
C. Conscious sedation
D. Syndrome of inappropriate antidiuretic hormone (SIADH)

Answer: A. Amnesia in the client with a dissociative disorder can be triggered by severe psychosocial stress. Certain pharmacologic agents given for sedation actually do have an amnesic affect, but this doesn't qualify as a dissociative disorder. SIADH isn't associated with amnesia.

➡ *NCLEX keys*

Nursing process step: Analysis
Client needs category: Psychosocial integrity
Client needs subcategory: Psychosocial adaptation
Taxonomic level: Evaluation

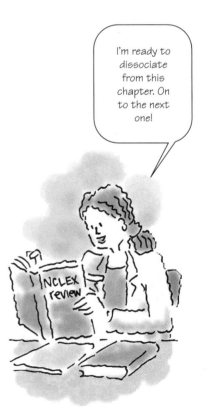

I'm ready to dissociate from this chapter. On to the next one!

Brush up on key concepts

Sexual disorders described in the *Diagnostic and Statistical Manual of Mental Disorders,* 4th ed., (*DSM-IV*) include **gender identity disorder, paraphilias,** and **sexual dysfunctions.** Gender identity disorder is characterized by an intense and ongoing cross-gender identification. Paraphilias are characterized by an intense, recurring sexual urge centered on inanimate objects or on human suffering and humiliation. Sexual dysfunctions are characterized by a deficiency or loss of desire for sexual activity or by a disturbance in the sexual response cycle.

At any time, you can review the major points of each disorder by consulting the *Cheat sheet* on page 438.

Polish up on patient care

This section discusses care for patients with gender identity disorders, paraphilias, and sexual dysfunctions.

Gender identity disorder

Patients with a gender identity disorder want to become or be like the opposite sex and are extremely uncomfortable with their assigned gender roles. This disorder can occur in childhood, adolescence, or adulthood.

CONTRIBUTING FACTORS
• Concurrent paraphilias, especially transvestic fetishism
• Feelings of sexual inadequacy
• Generalized anxiety disorder
• Personality disorders

ASSESSMENT FINDINGS
• Anxiety
• Attempts to mask or remove sex organs
• Cross-dressing
• Depression
• Disturbance in body image
• Dreams of cross-gender identification
• Fear of abandonment by family and friends
• Finding one's own genitals "disgusting"
• Ineffective coping strategies
• Peer ostracism
• Persistent distress about sexual orientation
• Preoccupation with appearance
• Self-hatred
• Self-medication such as hormonal therapy
• Strong attraction to stereotypical activities of the opposite sex
• Suicide attempts

DIAGNOSTIC TEST RESULTS
• Karyotyping for sex chromosomes (not usually indicated) may reveal abnormality.
• Psychological testing may reveal cross-gender identification or behavior patterns.
• Sex hormones assay (not usually indicated) may reveal abnormality.

NURSING DIAGNOSES
• Body image disturbance
• Chronic low self-esteem
• Personal identity disturbance

TREATMENT
• Group and individual psychotherapy
• Hormonal therapy
• Sex-change surgery

INTERVENTIONS AND RATIONALES
• Be careful to demonstrate a nonjudgmental attitude at all times. Under no circumstances

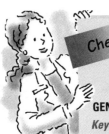

Cheat sheet

Sexual disorders refresher

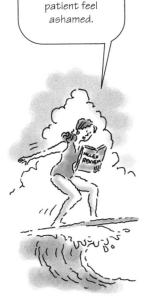

Be careful to demonstrate a nonjudgmental attitude at all times. Don't say anything that would make the patient feel ashamed.

GENDER IDENTITY DISORDER

Key signs and symptoms
- Dreams of cross-gender identification
- Finding one's own genitals "disgusting"
- Persistent distress about sexual orientation
- Preoccupation with appearance
- Self-hatred

Key test results
- Psychological testing may reveal cross-gender identification or behavior patterns.

Key treatments
- Group and individual psychotherapy
- Hormonal therapy
- Sex-change surgery

Key interventions
- Be careful to demonstrate a nonjudgmental attitude at all times. Don't say anything that would make the patient feel ashamed.
- Help the patient to identify the positive aspects of self.

PARAPHILIAS

Key signs and symptoms
- Development of a hobby or change in occupation that makes the paraphilia more accessible
- Recurrent paraphilic fantasies
- Social isolation
- Troubled social or sexual relationships

Key treatments
- Individual therapy

Key interventions
- Be careful to demonstrate a nonjudgmental attitude at all times. Don't say anything that would make the patient feel ashamed.
- If the patient is a threat to others, institute safety precautions per facility protocol.
- Initiate a discussion about how emotional needs for self-esteem, respect, love, and intimacy influence sexual expression.

- Encourage the patient to identify feelings, such as pleasure, reduced anxiety, increased control, and shame, associated with sexual behavior and fantasies.

SEXUAL DYSFUNCTIONS

Key signs and symptoms
- Anxiety
- Decreased sexual desire (sexual desire disorder)
- Delayed or absent orgasm (orgasmic disorder)
- Depression
- Inability to maintain an erection (sexual arousal disorder)
- Pain with sexual intercourse (sexual pain disorder)
- Premature ejaculation (orgasmic disorder)

Key test results
- Diagnostic tests are used to determine medical cause for dysfunction.

Key treatments
- Individual therapy
- Hormone replacement
- Sildenafil citrate (Viagra) for impotence

Key interventions
- Encourage the patient to discuss feelings and perceptions about his sexual dysfunction.
- Teach the patient and his partner alternative ways of expressing affection.
- Encourage the patient to seek evaluation and therapy from a qualified professional.

say anything that would make the patient feel ashamed. *It's the patient's needs and feelings, not your opinions, that matter.*
• Provide emotional support and empathy as the patient discusses fears and concerns *to help the patient deal with anxiety.*
• Help the patient to identify the positive aspects of self *to alleviate feelings of shame and distress.*
• Encourage the patient to participate in support groups *so the patient can gain empathy from others and find a safe environment to discuss concerns.*

Teaching topics
• Available treatment options and follow-up care

Paraphilias

A paraphilia is defined as a recurrent, intense sexual urge or fantasy, generally involving nonhuman subjects, children, nonconsenting partners, or the degradation, suffering, and humiliation of the patient or partners. The patient may report that the fantasy is always present but there are periods of time when the frequency of the fantasy and intensity of the urge vary. The disorder tends to be chronic and lifelong, but in adults, both the fantasy and behavior often diminish with advancing age. Inappropriate sexual behavior may increase in response to psychological stressors, in relation to other mental disorders, or when opportunity to engage in the paraphilia becomes more available.

Common paraphilias include:
• exhibitionism (exposing genitals and occasionally masturbating in public)
• fetishism (use of an object to become sexually aroused)
• frotteurism (rubbing one's genital on another nonconsenting person to become aroused)
• pedophilia (sexual activity with a child)
• sexual masochism (being humiliated or feeling pain to become aroused)
• sexual sadism (causing physical or emotional pain to another to become aroused)
• transvestic fetishism (cross-dressing)
• voyeurism (when arousal comes from watching others who are nude or engaging in sex).

CONTRIBUTING FACTORS
• Childhood incest
• Concurrent mental disorders
• Emotional trauma
• Gender (more likely in males)
• Personality disorders
• Central nervous system tumors
• Closed head injury
• Neuroendocrine disorders
• Psychosocial stressors
• Lack of knowledge about sex
• Sexual trauma

ASSESSMENT FINDINGS
• Anxiety
• Depression
• Development of a hobby or change in occupation that makes the paraphilia more accessible
• Disturbance in body image
• Guilt or shame
• Ineffective coping
• Multiple paraphilias at the same time
• Purchase of books, films, or magazines related to the paraphilia
• Recurrent paraphilic fantasies
• Sexual dysfunction
• Social isolation
• Troubled social or sexual relationships

DIAGNOSTIC TEST RESULTS
• Penile plethysmography testing may measure sexual arousal in response to visual imagery; however, the results of this procedure can be unreliable.

NURSING DIAGNOSES
• Altered sexuality patterns
• Chronic low self-esteem
• Risk for violence: Directed at others

TREATMENT
• Behavior therapy
• Cognitive therapy
• Individual therapy

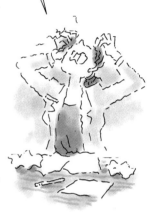

Inappropriate sexual behavior may increase in response to stress.

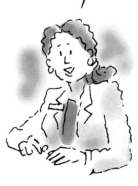

Institute safety precautions if the patient with paraphilias is a threat to others.

INTERVENTIONS AND RATIONALES

• Be careful to demonstrate a nonjudgmental attitude at all times. Under no circumstances say anything that would make the patient feel ashamed. *It's the patient's needs and feelings, not your opinions, that matter.*

• If the patient is a threat to others, institute safety precautions per facility protocol *to protect the patient and others.*

• Initiate a discussion about how emotional needs for self-esteem, respect, love, and intimacy influence sexual expression *to help the patient understand the disorder.*

• Encourage the patient to identify feelings, such as pleasure, reduced anxiety, increased control, or shame associated with sexual behavior and fantasies *to provide insight for developing appropriate interventions.*

• Help the patient distinguish between practices that are distressing because they don't conform to social norms or personal values and those that may place him or others in serious emotional, medical, or legal jeopardy *to reinforce the need to stop behaviors that could harm the patient or others.*

Teaching topic

• Contacting Sexaholics Anonymous

Sexual dysfunctions

Sexual dysfunctions are characterized by a disturbance during one or more phases of the sexual response cycle. The most common dysfunctions are:

• orgasmic disorders. The *DSM-IV* lists female orgasmic disorder, male orgasmic disorder, and premature ejaculation. Male and female orgasmic disorders are characterized by a persistent or recurrent delay in or absence of orgasm following a normal sexual excitement phase. Premature ejaculation is marked by persistent and recurrent onset of orgasm and ejaculation with minimal sexual stimulation.

• sexual arousal disorders. These include female sexual arousal disorder and male erectile disorder. With female sexual arousal disorder, the patient has a persistent or recurrent inability to attain or maintain adequate lubrication, swelling, and response of sexual excitement until the completion of sexual activity. In male erectile disorder, the patient has a persistent or recurrent inability to attain or maintain an adequate erection until completion of sexual activity.

• sexual desire disorders. This category includes hypoactive sexual desire disorder and sexual aversion disorder. The key feature of hypoactive sexual desire disorder is a deficiency or absence of sexual fantasies and the desire for sexual activity. The patient usually doesn't initiate sexual activity and may only engage in it reluctantly when it's initiated by the partner. With sexual aversion disorder, the patient has an aversion to and active avoidance of genital sexual contact with a sexual partner.

• sexual dysfunction due to a medical condition. Sexual dysfunction may occur as a result of a physiologic problem.

• sexual pain disorders. This category includes dyspareunia and vaginismus. The essential feature of dyspareunia is genital pain associated with sexual intercourse. Most commonly experienced during intercourse, dyspareunia may also occur before or after intercourse. The disorder can occur in both males and females. Vaginismus is recurrent or persistent involuntary contraction of the perineal muscles surrounding the outer third of the vagina when vaginal penetration is attempted. In some patients, even the anticipation of vaginal insertion may result in muscle spasm. The contractions may be mild to severe.

• substance-induced sexual dysfunction. This term is used to describe sexual dysfunction resulting from direct physiologic effects of a substance such as from drug abuse, medication use, or toxin exposure.

CONTRIBUTING FACTORS

• Anger or hostility
• Depression
• Drugs or alcohol
• Endocrine disorders
• Genital surgery
• Genital trauma
• Infections
• Lifestyle disruptions
• Medications

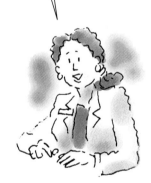

Sexual dysfunction often accompanies other medical situations, such as surgery, pregnancy, or pharmacologic treatment.

- Paraphilias
- Pregnancy
- Religious or cultural taboos that reinforce guilt feelings about sex
- Stress

ASSESSMENT FINDINGS
- Anxiety
- Decreased sexual desire (sexual desire disorder)
- Delayed or absent orgasm (orgasmic disorder)
- Depression
- Disturbance in body image
- Frustration and feelings of being unattractive
- Inability to maintain an erection (sexual arousal disorder)
- Ineffective coping
- Pain with sexual intercourse (sexual pain disorder)
- Poor self-concept
- Premature ejaculation (orgasmic disorder)
- Social isolation

DIAGNOSTIC TEST RESULTS
- Diagnostic tests are used to determine medical cause of dysfunction.

NURSING DIAGNOSES
- Impaired social interaction
- Self-esteem disturbance
- Sexual dysfunction

TREATMENT
- Changing medications to decrease symptoms (as appropriate)
- Individual therapy
- Marital or couples therapy
- Penile implant or vacuum pump, for erectile dysfunction
- Sex therapy
- Treatment of underlying medical condition
- Vaginal dilators
- Vascular surgery for erectile dysfunction

Drug therapy
- Hormone replacement
- Sildenafil citrate (Viagra) for impotence
- Alprostadil (Caverject) intracavernously to induce erection

INTERVENTIONS AND RATIONALES
- Establish a therapeutic relationship with the patient *to provide a safe and comfortable atmosphere for discussing sexual concerns.*
- Encourage the patient to discuss feelings and perceptions about his sexual dysfunction *to help validate his perceptions and reduce emotional distress.*
- Teach the patient and his partner alternative ways of expressing sexual intimacy and affection. *Alternative expressions of intimacy may raise the patient's self-esteem.*
- Encourage the patient to seek evaluation and therapy from a qualified professional *to enable the patient to obtain proper diagnosis and treatment.*

Teaching topics
- Understanding sexual response
- Using alternative sexual positions to promote comfort
- Performing relaxation exercises
- Performing Kegel exercises to improve urethral and vaginal tone
- Contacting self-help groups

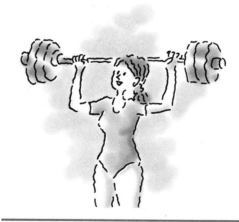

Pump up on practice questions

1. The nurse is caring for a client who is experiencing hypoactive sexual desire. How would the nurse classify this condition?

A. Sexual arousal disorder
B. Sexual pain disorder
C. Sexual desire disorder
D. Orgasmic disorder

Answer: C. Sexual desire disorders include both sexual aversion and hypoactive sexual desire disorder. Sexual arousal disorders include male erectile and female arousal disorders. Examples of sexual pain disorders include dyspareunia and vaginismus. Orgasmic disorders affect both males and females, and include premature ejaculation.

➡ NCLEX keys

Nursing process step: Assessment
Client needs category: Psychosocial integrity
Client needs subcategory: Psychosocial adaptation
Taxonomic level: Application

2. The nurse is caring for a client who was accused of voyeurism by his neighbors. Which term most appropriately describes such behavior?
A. Paraphilia
B. Depersonalization disorder
C. Dissociative fugue
D. Gender identity disorder

Answer: A. Paraphilia is a general diagnosis that encompasses such disorders as exhibitionism, fetishism, pedophilia, and voyeurism. Depersonalization disorder is characterized by a feeling of detachment or estrangement from one's self. Dissociative fugue is characterized by sudden, unexpected travel away from home, accompanied by an inability to recall one's past. Gender identity disorder is a separate diagnostic category and isn't related to the paraphilias.

➡ NCLEX keys

Nursing process step: Assessment
Client needs category: Psychosocial integrity
Client needs subcategory: Psychosocial adaptation
Taxonomic level: Application

3. The nurse is caring for a female client who is about to begin thrombolytic therapy, to treat acute MI. When the physician questions the client about her last menstrual period, she becomes embarrassed and asks him to leave the room. She then tells the nurse that she underwent a sex change operation. What would be the nurse's most appropriate response?
A. "I understand your reluctance to tell the physician, but it may have an impact on your treatment."
B. "Based on client confidentiality, I won't tell the physician if you wish."
C. "Your sex change and your hormones have nothing to do with your heart attack."
D. "Tell me about your sexual preference. Are you attracted to men or women?"

Answer: A. During the history and physical examination of any female client being screened for thrombolytic therapy, the physician must know about the last menstrual period before the myocardial infarction (MI). Although not an absolute contraindication to thrombolytics, the possibility of pregnancy or menstruation must be documented. According to the ethics of client confidentiality, information may be shared in a professional manner with those who require it for the client's care. Hormones are an important factor in the pathogenesis of MI. Estrogen is cardioprotective, while replacement hormones after a sex change operation can impact on how prone a person is to MI. The client's sexual preference is of no consequence in this situation.

➡ NCLEX keys

Nursing process step: Implementation
Client needs category: Physiological integrity
Client needs subcategory: Reduction of risk potential
Taxonomic level: Application

4. A 42-year-old research analyst arrives at her physician's office crying. Her husband of 17 years has asked her for a divorce. She admits that recently she has avoided having sexual intercourse with him. Which response by the nurse would be most appropriate when talking with this client?

A. "Please stop crying so that we can discuss your feelings about the divorce."
B. "Once you have intercourse with him, you'll be able to get your relationship back on track."
C. "I can see how upset you are. Let's sit in the office so that we can talk about how you're feeling."
D. "Find a good lawyer who'll look out for your interests, then you'll feel better."

Answer: C. This response validates the client's distress and provides her the opportunity to talk about her feelings. Because clients in crisis have difficulty making decisions, the nurse must be directive as well as supportive. Option A doesn't provide the client with adequate support. Options B and D don't acknowledge the client's distress. Moreover, clients in crisis can't think beyond the immediate moment, so discussing long-range plans isn't helpful.

➡️ *NCLEX keys*
Nursing process step: Implementation
Client needs category: Psychosocial integrity
Client needs subcategory: Psychosocial adaptation
Taxonomic level: Application

5. A client describes being under a lot of stress recently because of overwhelming demands from work and home. She has lost interest in sexual intercourse, which is placing a strain on her marriage. Based on this information, which type of sexual dysfunction does the client suffer from?
A. Hypoactive sexual desire disorder
B. Sexual aversion disorder
C. Sexual pain disorder
D. Paraphilia

Answer: A. Hypoactive sexual desire disorder is characterized by deficiency or absence of desire for sexual activity. Sexual aversion disorder is defined as the active avoidance of genital sexual contact. The client with sexual pain disorder experiences genital pain that is associated with sexual intercourse. Paraphilia is characterized by recurrent, intense sexual urges or fantasies generally involving nonhuman subjects, children, nonconsenting partners, or the degradation, suffering, and humiliation of the client or partners.

➡️ *NCLEX keys*
Nursing process step: Assessment
Client needs category: Psychosocial integrity
Client needs subcategory: Psychosocial adaptation
Taxonomic level: Knowledge

6. The nurse is caring for a client with type 1 diabetes mellitus who is experiencing erectile disorder related to his medical condition. Which statement is true about this sexual dysfunction?
A. It's unrelated to psychosocial problems.
B. It's not considered a sexual disorder.
C. It's not likely to cause infertility.
D. It can impact the client's psychosocial well-being.

Answer: D. Any general medical condition that impairs sexual function has the ability to impact the client's psychosocial well-being, as well as the ability to conceive. Regardless of the cause, sexual dysfunction is considered to be a disorder.

➡️ *NCLEX keys*
Nursing process step: Analysis
Client needs category: Psychosocial integrity
Client needs subcategory: Psychosocial adaptation
Taxonomic level: Comprehension

7. A client is diagnosed with erectile disorder. Which drug may be beneficial in treating a client with this disorder?
A. Methyldopa (Aldomet)
B. Alprostadil (Caverject)
C. Benazepril (Lotensin)
D. Clonidine (Catapres)

Answer: B. Alprostadil is indicated for erectile disorder. It can be administered intracavernously prior to sexual intercourse. Methyldopa, benazepril, and clonidine are antihypertensive agents that can cause erectile disorder.

➡ *NCLEX keys*
Nursing process step: Assessment
Client needs category: Psychosocial integrity
Client needs subcategory: Psychosocial adaptation
Taxonomic level: Analysis

8. The nurse is caring for a male client awaiting a sex-change operation. When interacting with this client, it's important that the nurse should:
- A. discourage the client from undergoing the procedure.
- B. demonstrate a nonjudgmental attitude.
- C. discuss with the client the option of undergoing hypnosis as an alternative to the sex-change procedure.
- D. Tell the client that his life will be less complicated and more peaceful once sex-change surgery is complete.

Answer: B. When caring for a client with gender identity disorder, the nurse should demonstrate a nonjudgmental attitude toward the client. It's the client's needs and feelings that matter most, not the nurse's opinions. The nurse shouldn't discourage the client's decision to go ahead with the procedure. Hypnosis isn't a treatment for gender identity disorder and it isn't appropriate for the nurse to suggest hypnosis to the client. Telling the client his life will be less complicated and more peaceful after sex-change surgery offers false reassurance.

Wow. We just did "sex and the NCLEX."

➡ *NCLEX keys*
Nursing process step: Implementation
Client needs category: Psychosocial integrity
Client needs subcategory: Psychosocial adaptation
Taxonomic level: Analysis

9. Which of the following are examples of paraphilias?
- A. Sexual masochism, transvestic fetishism, voyeurism
- B. Transvestic fetishism, voyeurism, orgasmic disorders
- C. Pedophilia, exhibitionism, orgasmic disorders
- D. Dyspareunia, vaginismus, sexual sadism

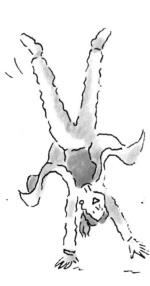

Answer: A. All the choices presented are examples of paraphilias, except dyspareunia, vaginismus, and orgasmic disorders.

➡ *NCLEX keys*
Nursing process step: Assessment
Client needs category: Psychosocial integrity
Client needs subcategory: Coping and adaptation
Taxonomic level: Comprehension

10. A 14-year old male who prefers to dress in female clothing is brought to the psychiatric crisis room by his mother. The client's mother states, "He is always dressing in female clothing. There must be something wrong with him." Which of the following responses from the nurse is most appropriate?
- A. "Your son will be evaluated shortly."
- B. "I will explain to your son that his behavior isn't appropriate."
- C. "I see you're upset. Would you like to talk?"
- D. "You're being judgmental. There is nothing wrong with a boy wearing female clothing."

Answer: C. Acknowledging the mother's feelings and offering her an opportunity to verbalize her concerns provides a forum for open communication. The nurse shouldn't offer an opinion regarding whether the client's behavior is acceptable. Telling the boy's mother that he will be evaluated shortly doesn't address the mother's concerns. Telling the client that his behavior is inappropriate isn't therapeutic.

➡ *NCLEX keys*
Nursing process step: Assessment
Client needs category: Psychosocial integrity
Client needs subcategory: Psychosocial adaptation
Taxonomic level: Application

Brush up on key concepts

Eating disorders are characterized by severe disturbances in eating behaviors. The two most common disorders, anorexia nervosa and bulimia nervosa, put the patient at risk for severe cardiovascular and GI complications and can ultimately result in death.

Patients with these disorders exhibit severe disturbances in body image and self-perception. Their behavior may include self-starvation, bingeing, and purging. The causes of eating disorders aren't fully understood.

At any time, you can review the major points of each disorder by consulting the *Cheat sheet* on page 446.

Polish up on patient care

Here is a review of anorexia nervosa and bulimia nervosa, the two most common eating disorders.

Anorexia nervosa

In anorexia nervosa, the patient deliberately starves herself or engages in binge eating and purging. A patient with anorexia nervosa wants to become as thin as possible and refuses to maintain an appropriate weight. A key clinical finding is a refusal to sustain weight at or above minimum requirements for age and height. If left untreated, anorexia nervosa can cause the patient's death.

CONTRIBUTING FACTORS
• Age (most prominent in adolescents)
• Distorted body image
• Gender (primarily affects females)
• Genetic predisposition
• Low self-esteem
• Neurochemical changes
• Poor family relations
• Poor self-esteem
• Preoccupation with weight and dieting
• Sexual abuse

ASSESSMENT FINDINGS
• Amenorrhea, fatigue, loss of libido, infertility
• Body image disturbance
• Cognitive distortions, such as overgeneralization, dichotomous thinking, or ideas of reference
• Compulsive behavior
• Decreased blood volume, evidenced by lowered blood pressure, and postural hypertension
• Dependency on others for self-worth
• Electrolyte imbalance, evidenced by muscle weakness, seizures, or arrhythmias
• Emaciated appearance
• GI complications, such as constipation or laxative dependence
• Guilt associated with eating
• Impaired decision making
• Need to achieve and please others
• Obsessive rituals concerning food
• Overly compliant attitude
• Perfectionist attitude
• Refusal to eat

DIAGNOSTIC TEST RESULTS
• Eating attitude test suggests eating disorder.
• Electrocardiogram (ECG) reveals nonspecific ST interval, prolonged PR interval, and T-wave changes.
• Laboratory tests show elevated blood urea nitrogen and electrolyte imbalances.

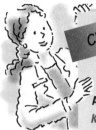

Eating disorders refresher

ANOREXIA NERVOSA

Key signs and symptoms

- Decreased blood volume, evidenced by lowered blood pressure, and postural hypertension
- Electrolyte imbalance, evidenced by muscle weakness, seizures, or arrhythmias
- Emaciated appearance
- Need to achieve and please others
- Obsessive rituals concerning food
- Refusal to eat

Key test results

- Eating attitude test suggests eating disorder.
- Electrocardiogram (ECG) reveals nonspecific ST interval, prolonged PR interval, and T-wave changes.
- Laboratory tests show elevated blood urea nitrogen level and electrolyte imbalances.
- Female patients exhibit low estrogen levels.
- Male patients exhibit low serum testosterone levels.

Key treatments

- Individual therapy
- Nutritional counseling
- Antianxiety agents: lorazepam (Ativan), alprazolam (Xanax)
- Antidepressants: amitriptyline (Elavil), imipramine (Tofranil)
- Selective serotonin reuptake inhibitors (SSRIs): paroxetine (Paxil), fluoxetine (Prozac)

Key interventions

- Contract for amount to be eaten.
- Provide one-on-one support before, during, and after meals.
- Prevent the patient from using the bathroom for 2 hours after eating.

These patients are commonly high achievers who manipulate their own body weight as a way to deal with feelings of helplessness.

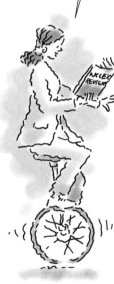

- Help patient identify coping mechanisms for dealing with anxiety.
- Weigh patient once or twice a week at same time of day using the same scale.
- Help patient understand the anorectic cycle.

BULIMIA NERVOSA

Key signs and symptoms

- Alternating episodes of binge eating and purging
- Constant preoccupation with food
- Disruptions in interpersonal relationships
- Extreme need for acceptance and approval
- Irregular menses
- Russell sign (bruised knuckles due to induced vomiting)
- Sporadic, excessive exercise

Key test results

- Beck Depression Inventory may reveal depression.
- Eating Attitudes test suggests eating disorder.
- Metabolic acidosis may occur from diarrhea caused by enemas and excessive laxative use.
- Metabolic alkalosis may occur from frequent vomiting.

Key interventions

- Explain the purpose of a nutritional contract.
- Avoid power struggles around food.
- Prevent the patient from using the bathroom for 2 hours after eating.
- Provide one-on-one support before, during, and after meals.
- Weigh patient once or twice a week at same time of day using the same scale.
- Help patient identify cause of the disorder.
- Point out cognitive distortions.

- Female patients exhibit low estrogen levels.
- Leukopenia and mild anemia are apparent.
- Male patients exhibit low serum testosterone levels.
- Thyroid study findings are low.

NURSING DIAGNOSES

- Altered nutrition: Less than body requirements
- Body image disturbance
- Self-esteem disturbance

TREATMENT
- Behavioral modification
- Group therapy
- Individual therapy
- Nutritional counseling

Drug therapy
- Antianxiety agents: lorazepam (Ativan), alprazolam (Xanax)
- Antidepressants: amitriptyline (Elavil), imipramine (Tofranil)
- Selective serotonin reuptake inhibitors (SSRIs): paroxetine (Paxil), fluoxetine (Prozac)

INTERVENTIONS AND RATIONALES
- Obtain a complete physical assessment *to identify complications of anorexia nervosa.*
- Contract for amount to be eaten *to avoid argument and conflict between staff and patient.*
- Provide one-on-one support before, during, and after meals *to foster a strong nurse-patient relationship and to ensure that the patient is eating.*
- Prevent the patient from using the bathroom for 2 hours after eating *to break the purging cycle.*
- Encourage verbal expression of feelings *to foster open communications about body image.*
- Help patient identify coping mechanisms for dealing with anxiety *to promote health-coping techniques.*
- Weigh patient once or twice a week at same time of day using the same scale *to accurately monitor weight gains.*
- Help understand the anorectic cycle *to prevent future anorectic behavior.*
- Discuss the patient's perception of her appearance. Help her understand how arbitrary social standards for beauty have affected her self-perception. Point out that she doesn't have to accept society's equation of thinness with beauty. Explain that she has a right to think of herself as beautiful regardless of how she compares with others *to build self-esteem.*
- Discuss the patient's progress with her *to increase awareness of achievements and promote continued effort.*

Teaching topics
- Need for gradual weight gain

- Nutritional support measures
- Treatment options
- Support services and community resources

Bulimia nervosa

Bulimia is characterized by episodic bingeing on food, followed by purging in the form of vomiting. The patient's weight may remain normal or close to normal. The severity of the disorder depends on the frequency of the binge and purge cycle as well as physical complications. The patient often views food as a source of comfort.

CONTRIBUTING FACTORS
- History of sexual abuse
- Low self-esteem
- Neurochemical changes
- Poor family relations

ASSESSMENT FINDINGS
- Alternating episodes of binge eating and purging
- Anxiety
- Avoidance of conflict
- Cognitive distortions, such as with anorexia nervosa
- Constant preoccupation with food
- Disruptions in interpersonal relationships
- Dissatisfaction with body image
- Extreme need for acceptance and approval
- Feelings of helplessness
- Focus on changing a specific body part
- Frequent lies and excuses to explain behavior
- Guilt and self-disgust
- Irregular menses
- Perfectionist attitude
- Parotid and salivary gland swelling
- Pharyngitis
- Physiologic problems as in anorexia nervosa (amenorrhea, fatigue, loss of libido, infertility, electrolyte imbalance, GI complications)
- Possible use of amphetamines or other drugs to control hunger
- Problems caused by frequent vomiting
- Repression of anger and frustration

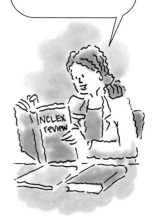

The largest obstacle to treating anorexia is that patients don't want to be treated. Yet quick intervention is essential. Anorexia nervosa can be fatal!

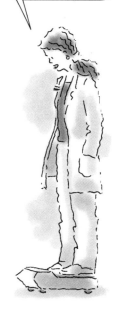

Weigh the patient once or twice each week, but not more, because weighing too often reinforces the focus on weight.

• Russell sign (bruised knuckles due to induced vomiting)
• Sporadic, excessive exercise

DIAGNOSTIC TEST RESULTS
• Beck Depression Inventory may reveal depression.
• Eating Attitudes test suggests eating disorder.
• Metabolic acidosis may occur from diarrhea caused by enemas and excessive laxative use.
• Metabolic alkalosis (the most common metabolic complication) may occur from frequent vomiting.

NURSING DIAGNOSES
• Altered nutrition: Less than body requirements
• Anxiety
• Powerlessness

TREATMENT
• Cognitive therapy (to identify triggers for bingeing and purging)
• Family therapy

Drug therapy
• SSRIs: paroxetine (Paxil), fluoxetine (Prozac); note that drug therapy is most effective when combined with cognitive therapy.

INTERVENTIONS AND RATIONALES
• Perform a complete physical assessment *to identify complications associated with bulimia nervosa.*
• Explain the purpose of a nutritional contract *to encourage a dietary change without initiating argument or struggle.*
• Avoid power struggles around food *to keep the focus on establishing and maintaining a positive self-image and self-esteem.*
• Prevent the patient from using the bathroom for 2 hours after eating *to help the patient avoid purging behavior.*
• Provide one-on-one support before, during, and after meals *to monitor and assist the patient with eating.*

• Encourage the patient to express her feelings *to facilitate conversation and promote understanding.*
• Weigh patient once or twice a week at same time of day using the same scale *to monitor weight.*
• Help patient identify cause of the disorder *to help her gain understanding and work toward wellness.*
• Point out cognitive distortions *to help identify sources of the problem.*
• Discuss the patient's perception of her appearance. Help her understand how arbitrary social standards for beauty have affected her self-perception. Point out that she doesn't have to accept society's equation of thinness with beauty. Explain that she has a right to think of herself as beautiful regardless of how she compares with others *to build self-esteem.*
• Discuss the patient's progress with her *to increase awareness of achievements and promote continued effort.*

Teaching topics
• Need to gain weight gradually
• Treatment options
• Support services and community resources

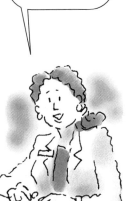

Tell the patient that she has a right to think of herself as beautiful regardless of how she compares with others.

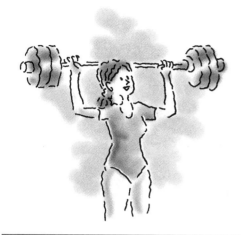

Pump up on practice questions

1. The nurse is caring for a client who is deliberately starving herself to become as thin as possible. What is the appropriate diagnosis for this client?

   A. Anorexia nervosa
   B. Eating disorder
   C. Bulimia nervosa
   D. Genu valgum

Answer: A. The scenario describes anorexia nervosa. Eating disorder encompasses both anorexia nervosa and bulimia nervosa. Bulimia nervosa is episodic bingeing and purging. Genu valgum is the medical term for "knock knees."

➥ *NCLEX keys*
Nursing process step: Assessment
Client needs category: Psychosocial integrity
Client needs subcategory: Psychosocial adaptation
Taxonomic level: Comprehension

2. The nurse is monitoring a client diagnosed with anorexia nervosa. In addition to monitoring the client's eating, the nurse should do which of the following after meals?

   A. Encourage the client to go for a walk to get some exercise.
   B. Prevent the client from using the bathroom for 2 hours after eating.
   C. Tell the client to lie down for 2 hours after eating.
   D. Instruct the client to get plenty of exercise.

Answer: B. After observing the client while she eats, the nurse should prevent the client from using the bathroom for at least 2 hours to break the purging cycle. Exercise should be restricted until the client has shown adequate weight gain, and then it should be encouraged in moderation. It isn't necessary for the client to lie down for 2 hours after eating.

➥ *NCLEX keys*
Nursing process step: Implementation
Client needs category: Physiological integrity
Client needs subcategory: Reduction of risk potential
Taxonomic level: Application

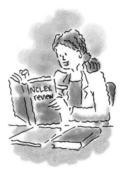

3. The nurse is caring for a client who has been binge eating. Which of the following descriptions of the client's behavior is most appropriate?

   A. The client has been slowly consuming a large amount of food over 3 hours.
   B. The client has been rapidly consuming a large amount of food.
   C. The client became extremely hungry and then consumed a large amount of food.
   D. The client is extremely thin, but still highly concerned about her weight?

Answer: B. Binge eating is the rapid consumption of a large amount of food over a given period of time. Hunger doesn't directly affect binge eating associated with mental health disorders. Bulimic people aren't necessarily thin; in fact, they're usually of normal body size and, in many cases, slightly overweight prior to onset of the disorder.

▶▶ *NCLEX keys*
Nursing process step: Assessment
Client needs category: Physiological integrity
Client needs subcategory: Physiological adaptation
Taxonomic level: Comprehension

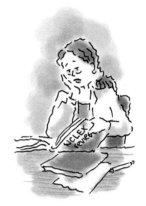

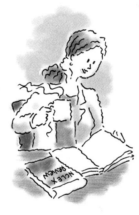

4. The nurse is caring for a bulimic client. What physical findings would the nurse expect?
   A. Parotid and salivary gland swelling, pharyngitis
   B. Facial ecchymoses, bruised knuckles, and excessive torso fat stores
   C. Depression, parotid gland swelling
   D. Depression, bruised knuckles
Answer: A. All findings listed, except excessive torso fat, are characteristic of bulimic clients. Depression; however, is a psychosocial, not a physical finding.

▶▶ *NCLEX keys*
Nursing process step: Assessment
Client needs category: Physiological integrity
Client needs subcategory: Physiological adaptation
Taxonomic level: Comprehension

5. The nurse is caring for a client diagnosed with bulimia and notices the Russell sign. What did the nurse notice?
   A. Dental enamel erosions
   B. Facial ecchymoses
   C. Pharyngitis
   D. Bruised knuckles
Answer: D. Bulimic clients often have bruised knuckles, due to self-induced vomiting. This symptom is called the Russell sign.

▶▶ *NCLEX keys*
Nursing process step: Assessment
Client needs category: Physiological integrity
Client needs subcategory: Physiological adaptation
Taxonomic level: Comprehension

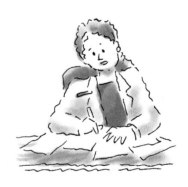

6. The nurse is caring for a client who has bulimia. What would be the most common metabolic complication for this client?

A Metabolic alkalosis
B. Respiratory alkalosis
C. Respiratory acidosis
D. Metabolic acidosis

Answer: A. With repeated emesis, the client loses stomach acids, thus becoming alkalotic. Respiratory pH disturbances aren't directly related to bulimia.

➡ NCLEX keys

Nursing process step: Assessment
Client needs category: Physiological integrity
Client needs subcategory: Physiological adaptation
Taxonomic level: Comprehension

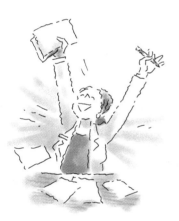

7. The nurse is caring for a client who has bulimia. Which treatment option is most effective?

A. Antidepressants
B. Cognitive-behavioral therapy
C. Antidepressants and cognitive-behavioral therapy
D. Total parenteral nutrition and antidepressants

Answer: C. The combined approach of antidepressants and cognitive-behavioral therapy has been effective, even when clients don't present with depression. Total parenteral nutrition isn't indicated.

➡ NCLEX keys

Nursing process step: Implementation
Client needs category: Physiological integrity
Client needs subcategory: Pharmacological and parenteral therapies
Taxonomic level: Application

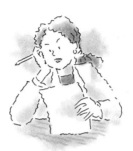

8. The nurse is caring for several clients who have eating disorders. Based on appearance, how would the nurse distinguish bulimic clients from anorectic clients?

A. By their teeth
B. By body size and weight
C. By looking for Mallory-Weiss tears
D. The clients are indistinguishable upon physical examination.

Answer: B. Behaviors of the anorectic client and the bulimic client are commonly similar, especially because both implement rituals to lose weight; however, the bulimic client tends to eat much more, due to the binge episodes, and therefore can be near-normal weight. Not all persons with the purge disorder have loss of enamel on teeth, especially if the disorder has developed recently. Mallory Weiss tears are small tears in the esophageal mucosa caused by forceful vomiting, but they aren't always present in bulimic clients.

➡ NCLEX keys

Nursing process step: Implementation
Client needs category: Physiological integrity
Client needs subcategory: Physiological adaptation
Taxonomic level: Application

9. The nurse is caring for a bulimic client and an anorectic client. What cognitive characteristics would be similar for both of these clients?

    A. Perfectionism, preoccupation with food

    B. Relaxed personality, but preoccupied with food

    C. No similarities

    D. Preoccupation with exercise

Answer: A. Cognitive distortions are similar in both disorders. Rarely do people with eating disorders have relaxed personalities. The anorectic client is more likely than the bulimic client to over-exercise for weight control.

➧ *NCLEX keys*

Nursing process step: Assessment
Client needs category: Psychosocial integrity
Client needs subcategory: Coping and adaptation
Taxonomic level: Comprehension

10. The nurse is caring for a client who has an eating disorder. Which nursing interventions would be appropriate for this client?

    A. Weigh the client once or twice a week, and contract for amount of food to be eaten.

    B Weigh the client daily, and allow the client to use the bathroom one-half hour after eating.

    C. Provide one-on-one support before meals.

    D. Contract amount of food to be eaten, and weigh client twice daily.

Answer: A. Weighing the client more often than once or twice per week reinforces the the client's excessive emphasis on weight. The client shouldn't be allowed to use the bathroom any sooner than 2 hours after eating. One-on-one support for the client must be undertaken before, during, and after meals — not just before meals.

➧ *NCLEX keys*

Nursing process step: Implementation
Client needs category: Psychosocial integrity
Client needs subcategory: Psychosocial adaptation
Taxonomic level: Application

It's been a long, strange trip through the mind, but you've finished the section on psych disorders! Congratulations!

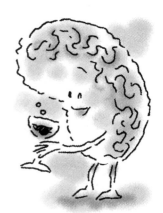

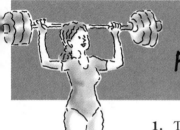
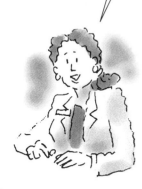

> Pump up for the
> NCLEX with 30
> psych practice
> questions.
> Go for it!

1. The nurse is caring for a client who's sarcastic and critical and often expresses feelings that are the opposite of what he's actually feeling. This client is exhibiting which type of behavior?

    A. Passive
    B. Aggressive
    C. Passive-aggressive
    D. Assertive

Answer: C. The person who is passive-aggressive is often sarcastic and critical and expresses feelings that are the opposite of what he actually feels. He defends his rights through resistance. The goal is to dominate through retaliation. Passive behavior is characterized by denying one's own rights to please others. Aggressive behavior is characterized by trying to violate the rights of others, controlling through humiliation. Assertive behavior is characterized by honest, direct assertion of one's rights through effective communication.

➡ *NCLEX keys*
Nursing process step: Assessment
Client needs category: Psychosocial integrity
Client needs subcategory: Coping and adaptation
Taxonomic level: Application

2. The nurse is teaching a client about the antidepressant drug fluoxetine (Prozac). Which of the following statements is true of this drug?

    A. The therapeutic effect may not be seen for 3 to 4 weeks.
    B. Fluoxetine doesn't cause orthostatic hypotension.
    C. Fluoxetine should be stopped immediately if adverse reactions occur.
    D. The client should avoid exposure to the sun because of photosensitivity reactions.

Answer: A. Effects of fluoxetine may not be seen for 3 to 4 weeks after the initiation of therapy. Clients taking fluoxetine should be warned to move from a sitting to a standing position very slowly because of the risk of orthostatic hypotension. Fluoxetine shouldn't be stopped abruptly by the client unless advised by the physician. Fluoxetine doesn't cause photosensitivity.

➡ *NCLEX keys*
Nursing process step: Implementation
Client needs category: Physiological integrity
Client needs subcategory: Pharmacological and parenteral therapies
Taxonomic level: Knowledge

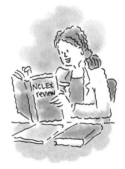

3. The nurse is teaching a client receiving a monoamine oxidase (MAO) inhibitor about his drug therapy. The client demonstrates understanding by expressing the need to avoid tyramine-containing foods and that even moderate amounts of tyramine must be avoided to prevent hypertensive crisis. The nurse asks the patient to list specific tyramine-containing foods. The client would be correct in naming which of the following foods?

    A. Swiss cheese
    B. Cream cheese
    C. Milk
    D. Ice cream

Answer: A. Fermented, aged, or smoked foods tend to be high in tyramine and should be avoided. Cream cheese, milk, and ice cream are unfermented milk products that may be taken with MAO inhibitors without incident.

➡ **NCLEX keys**
Nursing process step: Evaluation
Client needs category: Physiological integrity
Client needs subcategory: Pharmacological and parenteral therapies
Taxonomic level: Application

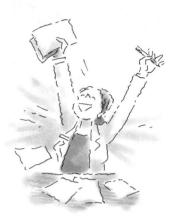

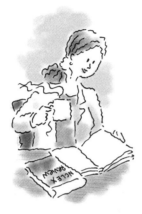

4. When caring for a client who is receiving lithium, the nurse should monitor the client for which adverse effect?
    A. Hypertension
    B. Fine hand tremors
    C. Weight loss
    D. Fluid retention
Answer: B. Fine hand tremors are an adverse effect of lithium therapy that may require a dosage adjustment. Other adverse effects include hypotension, weight gain, polyuria, and dehydration. Hypertension, weight loss, and fluid retention aren't adverse effects associated with lithium therapy.

➡ **NCLEX keys**
Nursing process step: Assessment
Client needs category: Physiological integrity
Client needs subcategory: Pharmacological and parenteral therapies
Taxonomic level: Knowledge

5. The client on antipsychotic drugs begins to exhibit bizarre facial and tongue movements. Based on these findings, the client is most likely exhibiting signs and symptoms of which disorder?
    A. Akinesia
    B. Pseudoparkinsonism
    C. Tardive dyskinesia
    D. Oculogyric crisis
Answer: C. Clients who are on long-term antipsychotic therapy are at risk for tardive dyskinesia, which causes bizarre facial and tongue movements. Symptoms are potentially irreversible. Pseudoparkinsonism may also occur in clients on antipsychotic drugs; signs and symptoms include drooling and a shuffling gait. Akinesia causes symptoms much like pseudoparkinsonism. Both are extrapyramidal adverse effects. Oculogyric crisis is uncontrolled rolling back of the eyes, which sometimes occurs in epidemic encephalitis or postencephalitic parkinsonism.

➡ **NCLEX keys**
Nursing process step: Assessment
Client needs category: Physiological integrity
Client needs subcategory: Pharmacological and parenteral therapies
Taxonomic level: Application

6. Electroconvulsive (ECT) therapy is most effective in treating which disorder?
    A. Schizophrenia
    B. Major depression
    C. Dissociative disorder
    D. Seizure disorder

Answer: B. ECT therapy is most effective in clients with major depression, especially those with associated psychosis. Treatment is initiated only after drug therapy has been unsuccessful. ECT is sometimes effective in inducing remission in clients with schizophrenia. ECT isn't effective in treating dissociative disorder or seizure disorder. Brief seizure activity occurs during ECT.

➡ *NCLEX keys*

Nursing process step: Implementation
Client needs category: Psychosocial integrity
Client needs subcategory: Psychosocial adaptation
Taxonomic level: Knowledge

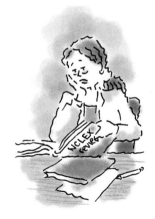

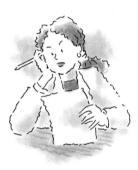

7. When preparing the client and his family for electroconvulsive therapy (ECT), the nurse should alert them about which adverse affect?

   A. Permanent memory loss
   B. Temporary memory loss
   C. Brain damage
   D. Increased intracranial pressure

Answer: B. Temporary memory loss and confusion commonly occur in clients who have undergone ECT. These effects may last for weeks or months. Permanent memory loss, brain damage, and increased intracranial pressure aren't adverse effects of ECT.

➡ *NCLEX keys*

Nursing process step: Planning
Client needs category: Physiological integrity
Client needs subcategory: Reduction of risk potential
Taxonomic level: Comprehension

8. Which nursing diagnosis would be most appropriate for the client who has undergone the full course of electroconvulsive therapy (ECT)?

   A. Knowledge deficit related to memory loss
   B. Noncompliance related to knowledge deficit
   C. Altered thought processes related to adverse effects of ECT
   D. Fear related to the unknown

Answer: C. Because memory loss is a common adverse effect of ECT, *altered thought processes* is the most appropriate nursing diagnosis for this client. Every attempt should be made to educate the client's family so they can adequately care for the client at home. Fear related to the unknown would be an appropriate diagnosis for the client before ECT. Noncompliance isn't an appropriate diagnosis for a client who has undergone a full course of therapy.

➡ *NCLEX keys*

Nursing process step: Analysis
Client needs category: Psychosocial integrity
Client needs subcategory: Coping and adaptation
Taxonomic level: Analysis

9. Which nursing intervention is most appropriate when planning care for the client with anorexia nervosa?

A. Have the client weigh herself at the same time every day.
B. Have the client record her food intake after she has eaten.
C. Remain with the client during mealtime and observe her for 1 hour after eating.
D. Recommend that the client not eat snacks so that she will be able to eat at mealtime.

Answer: C. Clients with eating disorders require supervision during and after meals to ensure that the client eats and doesn't try to vomit after eating. The client may record her weight, but the nurse must be present to weigh the client to ensure that the weight is recorded accurately. The nurse should leave snacks for the client so food is always available.

➡️ *NCLEX keys*
Nursing process step: Implementation
Client needs category: Physiological integrity
Client needs subcategory: Reduction of risk potential
Taxonomic level: Application

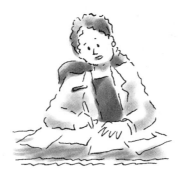

10. The nurse is assessing an elderly client for dementia. Which of the following is a primary symptom of dementia?
A. Psychosis
B. Memory loss
C. Neurosis
D. Loss of impulse control

Answer: B. Memory loss is the primary symptom of dementia. Short-term memory (retaining new information) loss is more prominent but long-term memory (recollection of events that occurred in the past) may also be

affected. Psychosis, neurosis, and loss of impulse control aren't symptoms of dementia.

➡️ *NCLEX keys*
Nursing process step: Assessment
Client needs category: Psychosocial integrity
Client needs subcategory: Psychosocial adaptation
Taxonomic level: Comprehension

11. Which intervention by the nurse takes top priority when caring for the client with dementia?
A. Providing foods that are easy for the client to eat
B. Providing the opportunity for rest and sleep
C. Keeping the incontinent client clean and dry
D. Creating a safe environment

Answer: D. Client safety takes top priority when caring for the client with dementia. Providing foods that are easy to eat, providing rest and sleep, and keeping the incontinent client clean and dry are all important when caring for the client with dementia, but client safety takes top priority.

➡️ *NCLEX keys*
Nursing process step: Implementation
Client needs category: Psychosocial integrity
Client needs subcategory: Psychosocial adaptation
Taxonomic level: Application

12. The nurse is caring for a client with alcohol dependence. When talking to the client about his treatment options, the nurse states that the only effective treatment for alcohol dependence is which of the following?
A. Attending Alcoholics Anonymous
B. Psychotherapy
C. Limiting alcohol consumption to one drink each day
D. Total abstinence

Answer: D. Total abstinence is the only effective treatment for alcohol dependence. Psychotherapy and Alcoholics Anonymous are effective ways to help the client maintain total abstinence.

➡ NCLEX keys
Nursing process step: Implementation
Client needs category: Psychosocial integrity
Client needs subcategory: Psychosocial adaptation
Taxonomic level: Comprehension

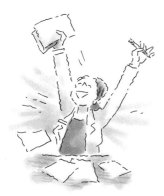

13. An alcohol dependent client is admitted for evaluation of depression. Because the client has no access to alcohol, the nurse should observe for which early signs and symptoms of alcohol withdrawal?

   A. Hypotension and agitation
   B. Seizures and nausea
   C. Anxiety, nausea, insomnia
   D. Violent behavior and tachycardia

Answer: C. Initial signs and symptoms of alcohol withdrawal include anxiety, nausea, tachycardia, fever, anxiety, agitation, and insomnia. As symptoms progress, the client may experience hallucinations, increased blood pressure, excessive sweating, and seizures. If untreated, this syndrome can cause serious medical complications, such as pneumonia, fluid and electrolyte imbalance, and dehydration. Hypotension and violent behavior aren't early signs and symptoms of alcohol withdrawal.

➡ NCLEX keys
Nursing process step: Assessment
Client needs category: Physiological integrity
Client needs subcategory: Reduction of risk potential
Taxonomic level: Knowledge

14. The nurse is providing an educational session for colleagues in the emergency department about the effects of cocaine. Which of the following is a true statement about cocaine?

   A. Cocaine is sometimes prescribed for weight control.
   B. Cocaine can only be inhaled or injected.
   C. Effects of cocaine last for 1 to 8 hours.
   D. Cocaine is occasionally used as a local anesthetic.

Answer: D. Cocaine is occasionally used as an anesthetic before nasal surgery. It isn't prescribed for weight control. Individuals who abuse cocaine may inject it I.V., inhale it, or smoke it. Cocaine's duration of action is 15 minutes to 2 hours.

➡ NCLEX keys
Nursing process step: Implementation
Client needs category: Physiological integrity
Client needs subcategory: Pharmacological and parenteral therapies
Taxonomic level: Knowledge

15. A client with a history of alcohol abuse successfully completes a few days of abstinence. The client may benefit from which drug that interferes with the metabolism of the alcohol?

   A. Chlordiazepoxide
   B. Diazepam
   C. Disulfiram
   D. Sertraline

Answer: C. Disulfiram (Antabuse) interferes with alcohol metabolism causing the client to experience a throbbing headache, tachycardia, tachypnea, and sweating within 5 to 15 minutes of alcohol consumption. Nausea and vomiting may follow within an hour. Chlordiazepoxide (Librium) and diazepam (Valium) are drugs sometimes used to ease the client through the withdrawal process. Sertraline (Zoloft) is indicated for the treatment of depression.

➡ NCLEX keys
Nursing process step: Implementation
Client needs category: Physiological integrity
Client needs subcategory: Pharmacological and parenteral therapies
Taxonomic level: Knowledge

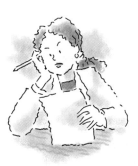

16. The nurse is caring for a client with Wernicke's encephalopathy. When developing a teaching plan for the client and his family the nurse should stress the importance of including which vitamin in his diet?
    A. Niacin
    B. Riboflavin
    C. Ascorbic acid
    D. Thiamin
Answer: D. Wernicke's encephalopathy is a neurologic disorder seen in clients with chronic alcohol abuse that results from thiamin deficiency. The client should be encouraged to eat a diet rich in thiamin. Niacin, riboflavin, and ascorbic acid deficiencies aren't implicated in Wernicke's encephalopathy.

➡ NCLEX keys
Nursing process step: Planning
Client needs category: Physiological integrity
Client needs subcategory: Reduction of risk potential
Taxonomic level: Analysis

17. A client with alcohol dependence has completed a rehabilitation program and now attends Alcoholics Anonymous (AA) meetings three times per week. Which statement by the client best reflects an understanding of Alcoholics Anonymous?

    A "I have to attend these meetings until I can control my drinking."
    B. "The organization will see that I get therapy if I begin to drink again."
    C. "AA will help me remain sober."
    D. "AA will help me find shelter and a job."
Answer: C. AA is a self-help organization that helps attendees maintain sobriety through mutual support. Total abstinence is the only effective treatment for alcohol abuse. Social drinking isn't possible for the alcoholic. AA doesn't provide counseling, shelter, or jobs.

➡ NCLEX keys
Nursing process step: Evaluation
Client needs category: Psychosocial integrity
Client needs subcategory: Coping and adaptation
Taxonomic level: Analysis

18. The nurse is interviewing a client admitted to the facility with a diagnosis of schizophrenia. The client states, "I run apple, train, grass, window." This response by the client is known as:
    A. Echopraxia
    B. A word salad
    C. Flight of ideas
    D. Neologisms
Answer: B. A word salad is an illogical word grouping. Echopraxia is an involuntary repetition of movements. Flight of ideas is a rapid succession of unrelated ideas. Neologisms are bizarre words that have meaning only to the client.

➡ NCLEX keys
Nursing process step: Assessment
Client needs category: Psychosocial integrity
Client needs subcategory: Psychosocial adaptation
Taxonomic level: Knowledge

19. The nurse is caring for a client who exhibits magical thinking. Which of the following best describes magical thinking?

A. Strong positive and negative feelings that cause conflict
B. Returning to earlier developmental stage
C. Meaningless repetition of words
D. The belief that thoughts or wishes can control other people or events

Answer: D. When a client exhibits magical thinking, he believes that his thoughts or wishes can control others or events. For example, the client may believe that through wishing he can make a plane fall from the sky. Ambivalence is the co-existence of positive and negative thoughts. Returning to an earlier stage of development is termed regression. A meaningless repetition of words is called echolalia.

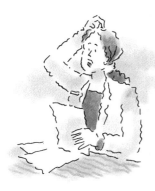

➡ *NCLEX keys*
Nursing process step: Assessment
Client needs category: Psychosocial integrity
Client needs subcategory: Psychosocial adaptation
Taxonomic level: Comprehension

20. The client tells the nurse that he can't eat because his food has been poisoned. This statement is an indication of which of the following?
A. Paranoia
B. Delusion of persecution
C. Hallucination
D. Illusion

Answer: A. Paranoia is described as extreme suspiciousness of others and their intentions. Delusions of persecution are feelings that others intend harm or persecution. A hallucina-

tion is a false sensory perception associated with real external stimuli. Illusions are misperceptions of real external stimuli.

➡ *NCLEX keys*
Nursing process step: Assessment
Client needs category: Psychosocial integrity
Client needs subcategory: Psychosocial adaptation
Taxonomic level: Application

21. A client tells the nurse that a voice keeps telling him to crawl on his hands and knees like a dog. Which response by the nurse is the most appropriate for this client?
A. "They are just imaginary voices and they will go away."
B. "If it makes you feel better, do what the voices tell you."
C. "I don't hear them, but I understand that you do."
D. "Even though I don't hear the voices, I understand that you do."

Answer: D. By telling the client that she doesn't hear the voices, the nurse lets the client know that the voices aren't real to her. The nurse follows with a validation of the client's statement that opens a line of communication and encourages the client to talk about his hallucinations. By using the words "they" and "them" in describing the voices, the nurse is reinforcing the client's perception that they actually exist.

➡ *NCLEX keys*
Nursing process step: Implementation
Client needs category: Psychosocial integrity
Client needs subcategory: Psychosocial adaptation
Taxonomic level: Analysis

22. The nurse is developing a teaching plan for the client receiving clozapine. The nurse should include the importance of which aspect of follow-up care?
A. A monthly EEG
B. A cardiology consult
C. An echocardiogram
D. Routine complete blood count with differential

Answer: D. Clozapine can cause a potentially fatal blood dyscrasia characterized by decreased white blood cells and severe neutropenia. Although this adverse effect is rare, it's potentially fatal if not detected early. Clozapine can also cause drowsiness, sedation, excessive salivation, tachycardia, dizziness, and seizures. A monthly EEG, cardiology consult, and echocardiogram aren't a necessary part of follow-up care for the client taking clozapine.

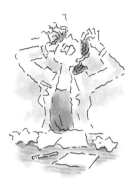

➦ *NCLEX keys*
Nursing process step: Planning
Client needs category: Physiological integrity
Client needs subcategory: Pharmacological and parenteral therapies
Taxonomic level: Application

23. A client is admitted to the hospital in the manic phase of bipolar disorder. When placing a diet order for the client, which foods would be most appropriate?
    A. A bowl of soup, crackers, and a dish of peaches
    B. A cheese sandwich, carrot sticks, fresh grapes, and cookies
    C. Roast chicken, mashed potatoes, and peas
    D. A tuna sandwich, an apple, and a dish of ice cream
Answer: B. The client may have a difficult time sitting long enough to eat his meal; therefore, finger foods that can be eaten easily are most appropriate. The other foods require the client to sit and eat, a task the client will be unable to achieve at this time.

➦ *NCLEX keys*
Nursing process step: Implementation
Client needs category: Physiological integrity
Client needs subcategory: Basic care and comfort
Taxonomic level: Application

24. A client with a history of panic attacks seeks to increase social interaction. Each time the client tries to go to the day room, she begins to perspire and becomes short of breath. Which action by the nurse will help ease the client's feelings of panic?
    A. Have other clients volunteer to accompany the client.
    B. Tell the client she has to overcome her fear.
    C. Allow the client to stay in her room.
    D. Walk with the client and stay with her while she's in the day room.
Answer: D. The client may find security in the presence of a trusted person. Her fears are very real and she'll need the emotional support of caring professionals to overcome them. Telling the client she has to overcome her fears minimizes her feelings. Allowing the client to stay in her room doesn't help the client overcome her feelings of panic.

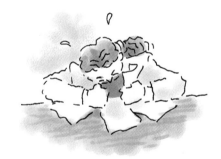

➦ *NCLEX keys*
Nursing process step: Implementation
Client needs category: Psychosocial integrity
Client needs subcategory: Psychosocial adaptation
Taxonomic level: Application

25. During the night, a 50-year-old Vietnam veteran with posttraumatic stress syndrome wakens shaking and tells you that someone is trying to smother him. What is the appropriate response for the nurse in this situation?

- A. "It was a bad dream. You are safe. I'll stay here with you until you go back to sleep."
- B. "We can talk about it tomorrow. Try to see if you can get back to sleep."
- C. "It was only a dream. There's nothing to be frightened about."
- D. " I'll call the physician and see whether I can get you medication to help you go back to sleep."

Answer: A. The important intervention is to assist the client to feel safe. Staying with him until he is able to sleep again or listening to him if he wants to talk is the most appropriate action for the nurse to take in this situation. Talking about it in the morning won't comfort the client when he's most upset. Stating that it was only a dream trivializes his experience. Calling the physician for a sleeping aide doesn't help the client cope with stress.

➡ *NCLEX keys*
Nursing process step: Implementation
Client needs category: Psychosocial integrity
Client needs subcategory: Psychosocial adaptation
Taxonomic level: Application

26. A 45-year-old female has constant complaints of dizziness and weakness. The client has been referred to specialists for evaluation. All tests have been negative. The physician has concluded that the client has a somatic disorder. How should the nurse deal with this client?

- A. Review the test results with the client so she understands there is nothing physically wrong with her.
- B. Tell the client that if she develops more outside interests she won't focus on her physical symptoms so much.
- C. Accept the fact that the physical complaint is real to the client.
- D. Ignore the client's complaints.

Answer: C. To deny the client's physical complaint is nontherapeutic and prevents the development of a trusting, therapeutic relationship. The nurse should accept the client's problem despite the fact that it isn't organic.

➡ *NCLEX keys*
Nursing process step: Implementation
Client needs category: Psychosocial integrity
Client needs subcategory: Psychosocial adaptation
Taxonomic level: Application

27. The nurse is caring for a client recently diagnosed with borderline personality disorder. Which characteristic is most notable in the client with borderline personality?

- A. Changes actions quickly and has an intense affect
- B. Does a poor job on things that he doesn't like to do
- C. Avoids responsibilities by saying that he forgot
- D. Resents useful suggestions

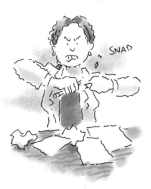

Answer: A. The changes in a borderline personality can occur within a matter of minutes, hours, or days. Commonly they exhibit an intense affective tone such as anger. The other responses are characteristics of the passive-aggressive personality disorder.

➡ *NCLEX keys*
Nursing process step: Assessment
Client needs category: Psychosocial integrity
Client needs subcategory: Psychosocial adaptation
Taxonomic level: Knowledge

28. The nurse is performing an admission interview with a client who exhibits signs of narcissistic personality disorder. Which behavior pattern is most characteristic of narcissistic personality disorder?
- A. The client has no close friends.
- B. The client is reticent in social situations.
- C. The client has a grandiose sense of self-importance.
- D. The client avoids work or school activities.

Answer: C. The client with a narcissistic personality disorder exhibits a pervasive pattern of grandiosity, lack of empathy, and hypersensitivity to the evaluation of others. The other three characteristics are behavior patterns of the avoidant personality.

➡ *NCLEX keys*
Nursing process step: Assessment
Client needs category: Psychosocial integrity
Client needs subcategory: Psychosocial adaptation
Taxonomic level: Knowledge

29. A client with borderline personality disorder has been asked to spend 1 hour in his room. The client asks the nurse for permission to go to another client's room to borrow a book. What behavior pattern is this client demonstrating?
- A. Manipulation
- B. Rationalizing
- C. Impulsivity
- D. Distancing

Answer: A. Manipulation is a technique used by the person with borderline personality to achieve whatever result he wants. Rationalizing is the substitution of acceptable reasons for the actual reasons motivating behavior. Impulsivity is poor impulse control. Distancing is becoming angry and hostile to keep another at a distance.

➡ *NCLEX keys*
Nursing process step: Assessment
Client needs category: Psychosocial integrity
Client needs subcategory: Psychosocial adaptation
Taxonomic level: Knowledge

30. A male client approaches the nurse and says "Hey cutie, can you take me outside for a smoke?" The nurse is aware that the patient isn't supposed to go out to smoke for another 15 minutes. Which response by the nurse is most therapeutic?
- A. "Sure, I'm not busy right now."
- B. "You can ask the technician. I'm busy right now."
- C. "You'll be able to smoke in 15 minutes. Calling me cutie is disrespectful."
- D. "You know the rules. It isn't time yet for you to go out to smoke."

Answer: C. The client's behavior indicates that he has difficulty adhering to limits and respecting boundaries. The nurse must place limits on the client's manipulative behavior. Taking the client outside for a smoke is inappropriate because the nurse is allowing the client to manipulate her. Referring the client to the technician is incorrect because the nurse isn't addressing the client's manipulative behavior. Option D is an abrupt response that may cause the client to act defensively.

➡ *NCLEX keys*
Nursing process step: Implementation
Client needs category: Psychosocial integrity
Client needs subcategory: Coping and adaptation
Taxonomic level: Application

Part IV Maternal-neonatal care

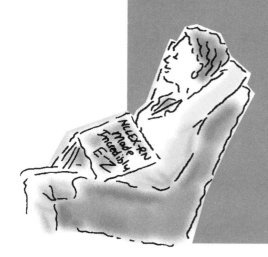

22 Antepartum Care

Brush up on key concepts

In this chapter, you'll review:

✐ basics of antepartum care

✐ antepartum tests and procedures

✐ common antepartum disorders and complications.

Antepartum care refers to care of a mother before childbirth. Knowledge of the physiologic changes that accompany pregnancy and of fetal development is essential to understanding patient care during the antepartum period.

At any time, you can review the major points of this chapter by consulting the *Cheat sheet* on pages 466 to 468.

Normal antepartum period

Nursing care during the normal antepartum period includes taking a thorough maternal history, performing a complete physical examination, and educating the patient about antepartum health.

SIGNS AND SYMPTOMS OF PREGNANCY
The patient may experience presumptive, probable, or positive signs of pregnancy.

Could be
Presumptive signs of pregnancy include:
• amenorrhea or slight, painless spotting of unknown cause in early gestation
• breast enlargement and tenderness
• fatigue
• increased skin pigmentation
• nausea and vomiting
• quickening (first recognizable movement of fetus)
• thinning and softening of fingernails
• urinary frequency and urgency.

Probably is
Probable signs of pregnancy include:

• ballottement (passive fetal movement in response to tapping of the lower portion of the uterus or cervix)
• Braxton Hicks contractions (painless uterine contractions that occur throughout pregnancy)
• Chadwick's sign (color of the vaginal walls changes from normal light pink to deep violet)
• Goodell's sign (softening of the cervix)
• Hegar's sign (softening of the lower uterine segment) may be present at 6 to 8 weeks gestation
• positive pregnancy test results
• uterine enlargement.

Definitely is
Positive signs of pregnancy include:
• detection of fetal heartbeat (by 17 to 20 weeks of gestation)
• detection of fetal movements (after 16 weeks of gestation)
• ultrasonography findings (as early as 6 weeks of gestation).

PHYSIOLOGIC ADAPTATIONS
Here is a review of how body systems adapt to pregnancy.

My ever changin' heart
Cardiovascular system changes include:
• cardiac hypertrophy from increased blood volume and cardiac output
• displacement of the heart upward and to the left from pressure on the diaphragm
• progressive increase in blood volume, peaking in the third trimester at 30% to 50% of levels before pregnancy
• resting pulse rate fluctuations, with increases ranging from 0 to 15 beats/minute at term
• pulmonic systolic and apical systolic murmurs resulting from decreased blood viscosity and increased blood flow

(Text continues on page 469.)

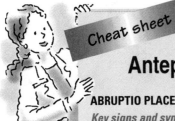

Cheat sheet

Antepartum care refresher

ABRUPTIO PLACENTAE

Key signs and symptoms
- Acute abdominal pain
- Hemorrhage, either concealed or apparent, with dark red vaginal bleeding
- Rigid abdomen

Key test results
- Ultrasonography locates the placenta, and a clot or hematoma may be apparent.

Key treatments
- Transfusion: packed red blood cells (RBCs), platelets, and fresh frozen plasma, if necessary
- Cesarean delivery

Key interventions
- Avoid pelvic or vaginal examinations and enemas.
- Administer fresh whole blood, packed RBCs, platelets, or plasma.
- Position the patient in a left lateral recumbent position.

ACQUIRED IMMUNODEFICIENCY SYNDROME

Key signs and symptoms
- Diarrhea
- Fatigue
- Kaposi's sarcoma
- Mild flu-like symptoms
- Opportunistic infections, such as toxoplasmosis, oral and vaginal candidiasis, herpes simplex, *Pneumocystis carinii*, *Candida* esophagitis
- Weight loss

Key test results
- CD4+ T-cell level is less than 200 cells/μl
- Enzyme-linked immunosorbent assay test shows positive HIV antibody titer.
- Western blot test is positive.

Key treatments
- If patient is newly diagnosed, zidovudine (Retrovir) treatment initiated between weeks 14 and 34 of gestation

Key interventions
- Assess whether the patient will be able to care for her infant after delivery.

ADOLESCENT PREGNANCY

Key signs and symptoms
- Denial of pregnancy, which may delay the patient from seeking medical attention early in pregnancy

Key treatments
- Formulation of diet with caloric intake that supports the growing adolescent and her developing fetus

Key interventions
- Monitor the patient's weight gain.
- Monitor urine protein and glucose levels.
- Assess fundal height.
- Assess fetal heart sounds.
- Advise the patient of her options, including terminating the pregnancy, continuing the pregnancy and giving up the infant for adoption, and continuing the pregnancy and keeping the infant.

DIABETES MELLITUS

Key signs and symptoms
- Glycosuria
- Ketonuria
- Polyuria

Key test results
- One-hour glucose tolerance test reveals glucose level greater than 140 mg/dl.

Key treatments
- 1,800- to 2,200-calorie diet divided into three meals and three snacks; diet should also include low fat and cholesterol, and high fiber
- Administration of insulin

Key interventions
- Encourage adherence to dietary regulations.
- Encourage the patient to exercise moderately.
- Prepare the patient for antepartum fetal surveillance testing, including oxytocin challenge testing, nipple stimulation stress testing, amniotic fluid index, biophysical profile, and nonstress test.

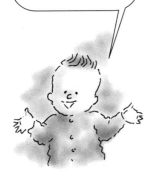

Don't forget, pregnancy itself is NOT a disorder. Often, effective nursing care will involve listening to, and reassuring healthy mothers.

Antepartum care refresher *(continued)*

ECTOPIC PREGNANCY

Key signs and symptoms

• Irregular vaginal bleeding and dull abdominal pain on the affected side early in pregnancy
• Positive Cullen's sign (bluish discoloration around the umbilicus)
• Rupture of tubes, causing sudden and severe abdominal pain, syncope, and referred shoulder pain as the abdomen fills with blood

Key test result

• Human chorionic gonadotroprin (HCG) titers are abnormally low.

Key treatment

• Laparotomy to ligate the bleeding vessels and remove or repair damaged fallopian tube
• If the tube hasn't ruptured, methotrexate (Folex) followed by leucovorin (Wellcovorin) to stop the trophoblastic cells from growing (therapy continues until negative HCG levels are achieved)

Key intervention

• Monitor for signs of rupturing ectopic pregnancy, such as severe abdominal pain, orthostatic hypotension, tachycardia, and dizziness.
• Administer I.V. fluid replacement.
• Administer blood products.

HEART DISEASE

Key sign and symptom

• Crackles at the base of the lungs
• Diastolic murmur at the heart's apex
• Dyspnea
• Fatigue
• Tachycardia

Key test results

• Echocardiography, electrocardiography, and chest X-ray may reveal cardiac abnormalities, arrhythmias, impaired cardiac function, increased workload on the heart, and cardiovascular decompensation.

Key treatments

For class III and class IV disease

• Anticoagulants, such as heparin (Liquaemin)
• Antiarrhythmics, such as digoxin (Lanoxin), quinidine (Quinora), procainamide (Pronestyl), and beta-blockers
• Thiazide diuretics and furosemide to control heart failure if activity restriction and reduced sodium intake don't prevent it

Key interventions

• Assess cardiovascular and respiratory status.
• Administer oxygen by nasal cannula or face mask during labor.
• Position the patient on her left side with her head and shoulders elevated during labor.

HYDATIDIFORM MOLE

Key signs and symptoms

• Intermittent or continuous bright red or brownish vaginal bleeding by the 12th week of gestation
• Absence of fetal heart tones

Key test results

• HCG levels are much higher than normal.
• Ultrasound fails to reveal a fetal skeleton.

Key treatments

• Therapeutic abortion (suction and curettage) if a spontaneous abortion doesn't occur
• Weekly monitoring of HCG levels until they remain normal for 3 consecutive weeks
• Periodic follow-up for 1 to 2 years because of increased risk of neoplasm

Key interventions

• Monitor vaginal bleeding.
• Send contents of uterine evacuation to the laboratory for analysis.

HYPEREMESIS GRAVIDARUM

Key signs and symptoms

• Continuous, severe nausea and vomiting
• Dehydration
• Oliguria

Key test results

• Arterial blood gas analysis reveals alkalosis.
• Hemoglobin level and hematocrit are elevated.
• Serum potassium level reveals hypokalemia.

Key treatments

• Restoration of fluid and electrolyte balance

Key interventions

• Provide small, frequent meals.
• Maintain I.V. fluid replacement and total parenteral nutrition.

(continued)

Antepartum care refresher *(continued)*

MULTIFETAL PREGNANCY

Key signs and symptoms
- More than one set of fetal heart sounds
- Uterine size greater than expected for dates

Key test results
- Alpha-fetoprotein levels are elevated.
- Ultrasonography is positive for multifetal pregnancy.

Key treatments
- Bed rest if early dilation occurs or at 24 to 28 weeks' gestation
- Biweekly nonstress test to document fetal growth, beginning with the 28th week of gestation
- Increased intake of calories, iron, folate, and vitamins
- Ultrasound examinations monthly to document fetal growth

Key interventions
- Monitor fetal heart sounds.
- Monitor maternal vital signs, including weight.
- Monitor cardiovascular and pulmonary status.

PLACENTA PREVIA

Key signs and symptoms
- Painless, bright red vaginal bleeding, especially during the third trimester

Key test results
- Early ultrasound evaluation reveals the placenta implanted in the lower uterine segment.

Key treatments
- Depends on gestational age, when first episode occurs, and amount of bleeding
- If gestational age less than 34 weeks, hospitalizing the patient and restricting her to bed rest to avoid preterm labor
- Surgical intervention by cesarean birth depending on the placental placement and maternal and fetal stability

Key interventions
- Don't perform rectal or vaginal examinations unless equipment is available for vaginal and cesarean delivery.

PREGNANCY-INDUCED HYPERTENSION

Key signs and symptoms
Gestational hypertension
- Blood pressure 140/90 mm Hg or systolic pressure elevated 30 mm Hg above prepregnancy level
- No proteinuria.
Mild eclampsia
- Blood pressure of 140/90 mm Hg, systolic pressure elevated more than 30 mm Hg above prepregnancy level, or diastolic pressure elevated 15 mm Hg above prepregnancy level

- Proteinuria of 1+ to 2+
- Weight gain more than 2 lb (0.9 kg) per week in the second trimester and 1 lb (0.45 kg) per week in the third trimester
Severe preeclampsia
- Blood pressure of 160/110 mm Hg (noted on two readings taken 6 hours apart while on bed rest)
- Proteinuria of 3+ to 4+
- Oliguria (500 ml or less in 24 hours)
- Frontal headaches, blurred vision, hyperreflexia, nausea, vomiting, irritability, cerebral disturbances, and epigastric pain
- Presence of HELLP syndrome (hemolysis, elevated liver enzymes, and low platelet count)

Key test results
- Blood chemistry reveals increased blood urea nitrogen, creatinine, and uric acid levels and elevated liver function studies

Key treatments
- Bed rest in a lateral position
- Delivery: in mild preeclampsia, once the fetus is mature and safe induction is possible; in severe preeclampsia, regardless of gestational age
- High-protein diet with restriction of excessively salty foods
- Restriction of I.V. fluid administration during labor
- In severe preeclampsia: antihypertensives such as hydralazine (Apresoline) or diazoxide (Hyperstat); betamethasone (Celestone) administered to accelerate fetal lung maturation
- Magnesium sulfate to reduce the amount of acetylcholine produced by motor nerves, thereby preventing seizures

Key interventions
For all patients
- Assess the patient for edema and proteinuria.
- Maintain seizure precautions.
- Encourage bed rest in a left lateral recumbent position.
For severe preeclampsia
- Assess maternal blood pressure every 4 hours or more frequently if unstable.
- Monitor serum magnesium levels.
- Be prepared to obtain a blood sample for typing and cross-matching.
- Be prepared to administer I.V. magnesium sulfate.
- Monitor serum blood levels while the patient is receiving I.V. magnesium sulfate.
- Be prepared to administer calcium gluconate (antidote to magnesium sulfate) at first sign of magnesium sulfate toxicity (elevated serum levels, decreased deep tendon reflexes, muscle flaccidity, central nervous system depression, and decreased respiratory rate and renal function).

• increased femoral venous pressure caused by impaired circulation from the lower extremities (resulting from the pressure of the enlarged uterus on the pelvic veins and inferior vena cava)
• decreased cerebrospinal fluid space from enlargement of the vessels surrounding the spinal cord's dura mater
• increased fibrinogen levels (up to 50% at term) from hormonal influences
• increased levels of blood coagulation factors VII, IX, and X, leading to a hypercoagulable state
• increase of about 33% in total red blood cell (RBC) volume, despite hemodilution and decreasing erythrocyte count
• hematocrit (HCT) decrease of about 7%
• increase of 12% to 15% in total hemoglobin level; this is less than the overall plasma volume increase, thus reducing hemoglobin concentration and leading to physiologic anemia of pregnancy
• leukocyte production equal to or slightly greater than blood volume increase (average leukocyte count is 10,000 to 11,000/µl; this peaks at 25,000/µl during labor, possibly through an estrogen-related mechanism).

Cravings and more

GI system changes include:
• gum swelling from increased estrogen levels; gums may be spongy and hyperemic
• lateral and posterior displacement of the intestines
• superior and lateral displacement of the stomach
• delayed intestinal motility and gastric and gallbladder emptying time from smooth-muscle relaxation caused by high placental progesterone levels
• nausea and vomiting (usually subside after the first trimester)
• hemorrhoids late in pregnancy from venous pressure
• constipation from increased progesterone levels, resulting in increased water absorption from the colon
• displacement of the appendix from McBurney's point (making diagnosis of appendicitis difficult).

Hormonal changes

Endocrine system changes include:
• increased basal metabolic rate (up 25% at term) caused by demands of the fetus and uterus and by increased oxygen consumption
• increased iodine metabolism from slight hyperplasia of the thyroid caused by estrogen levels
• slight hyperparathyroidism from increased requirement for calcium and vitamin D
• elevated plasma parathyroid hormone levels, peaking between 15 and 35 weeks of gestation
• slightly enlarged pituitary gland
• increased production of prolactin by the pituitary gland late in pregnancy
• increased estrogen levels and hypertrophy of the adrenal cortex
• increased cortisol levels to regulate protein and carbohydrate metabolism
• possibly decreased maternal blood glucose levels
• decreased insulin production early in pregnancy
• increased production of estrogen, progesterone, and human chorionic somatomammotropin by the placenta and increased levels of maternal cortisol, which reduce the mother's ability to use insulin, thus ensuring an adequate glucose supply for the fetus and placenta.

Altered breathing

Respiratory system changes include:
• increased vascularization of the respiratory tract caused by estrogen levels
• shortening of the lungs caused by the enlarging uterus
• upward displacement of the diaphragm by the uterus
• increased tidal volume, causing slight hyperventilation
• increased chest circumference (by about 2⅜" [6 cm])
• altered breathing, with abdominal breathing replacing thoracic breathing as pregnancy progresses
• slight increase (2 breaths/minute) in respiratory rate
• lowered threshold for carbon dioxide due to increased levels of progesterone.

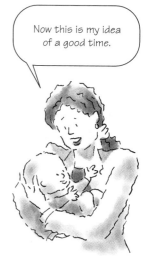

Now this is my idea of a good time.

Now I get it!

What causes weight gain in pregnancy?

- Fetus (7.5 lb [3.4 kg])
- Placenta and membranes (1.5 lb [0.7 kg])
- Amniotic fluid (2 lb [0.9 kg])
- Uterus (2.5 lb [1.1 kg])
- Breasts (3 lb [1.4 kg])
- Blood volume (2 to 4 lb [0.9 to 1.8 kg])
- Extravascular fluid and fat reserves (4 to 9 lb [1.8 to 4.1 kg])

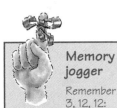

Memory jogger

Remember 3, 12, 12:

Maternal weight gain is commonly estimated at 3, 12, and 12 pounds for the first, second, and third trimesters.

Everything increases

Metabolic system changes include:
- increased water retention caused by higher levels of steroidal sex hormones, decreased serum protein levels, and increased intracapillary pressure and permeability
- increased levels of serum lipids, lipoproteins, and cholesterol
- increased iron requirements caused by fetal demands
- increased carbohydrate needs
- increased protein retention from hyperplasia and hypertrophy of maternal tissues
- weight gain of 25 to 30 lb (11.3 to 13.6 kg). (See *What causes weight gain in pregnancy?*)

Is it getting hot in here?

Integumentary system changes include:
- hyperactive sweat and sebaceous glands
- changing pigmentation from the increase of melanocyte-stimulating hormone caused by increased estrogen and progesterone levels (darkened line from symphysis pubis to umbilicus known as linea nigra)
- nipples, areola, cervix, vagina, and vulva darken
- nose, cheeks, and forehead show pigmentary changes known as facial chloasma.

Increase, decrease

Changes to the genitourinary system include:
- dilated ureters and renal pelvis caused by progesterone and pressure from the enlarging uterus

- increased glomerular filtration rate (GFR) and renal plasma flow (RPF) early in pregnancy; elevated GFR until delivery, but a near-normal RPF level by term
- increased clearance of urea and creatinine from increased renal function
- decreased blood urea and nonprotein nitrogen values from increased renal function
- glucosuria from increased glomerular filtration without an increase in tubular reabsorptive capacity
- decreased bladder tone
- increased sodium retention from hormonal influences
- increases in dimensions of uterus from about 2½″ to 12½″ (6.5 to 32 cm) in length; 1½″ to 9½″ (4 to 24 cm) in width; 8⅝″ to 10″ (22 to 25 cm) in depth; 2 to 42 oz (57 to 1,191 g) in weight; ⅛ to 170 oz (3.5 to 5,028 ml) in volume
- hypertrophied uterine muscle cells (5 to 10 times normal size)
- increased vascularity, edema, hypertrophy, and hyperplasia of the cervical glands
- increased vaginal secretions with a pH of 3.5 to 6
- discontinued ovulation and maturation of new follicles
- thickening of vaginal mucosa, loosening of vaginal connective tissue, and hypertrophy of small muscle cells. (See *Estimating delivery dates and gestational age*.)

Estimating delivery dates and gestational age

• Nägele's rule determines the estimated date of delivery by subtracting 3 months from the first day of the last menstrual period and adding 7 days, for example, October 5 - 3 months = July 5 + 7 days = July 12.
• Quickening is described as light fluttering and usually is felt between 16 and 22 weeks of gestation.
• Fetal heart sounds can be detected at 12 weeks of gestation with a Doppler ultrasound and can be auscultated with a fetoscope at 16 to 20 weeks.
• Fetal crown-to-rump measurements, determined by ultrasonography, can be used to assess the fetus's age until the head can be defined.
• Biparietal diameter is the widest transverse diameter of the fetal head. Measurements can be made by about 12 to 13 weeks' gestation.
• McDonald's rule uses fundal height to determine the duration of pregnancy in either lunar months or weeks. To use this rule, place a tape measure at the symphysis pubis and measure up and over the fundus. Fundal height in centimeters $\times$ ⅔ = duration of pregnancy in lunar months; fundal height in centimeters $\times$ ⅞ = duration of pregnancy in weeks.

Not just pickles and milkshakes

Nutritional needs also change during pregnancy. For example:
• Calorie requirements during pregnancy exceed prepregnancy needs by 300 calories/day (from 2,100 to 2,400 kcal/day).
• Protein requirements during pregnancy exceed prepregnancy needs by 30 g/day (from 46 to 76 g/day).
• Intake of all vitamins should increase, and a prenatal vitamin is usually recommended.
• Folic acid intake is particularly important to help prevent fetal anomalies, such as neural tube defect. Intake should be increased from 400 to 800 mg/day. Dietary sources of folic acid include green, leafy vegetables; eggs; milk; and whole-grain breads.
• Intake of all minerals, especially iron, should be increased. (See *Battling discomforts of pregnancy*, page 472.)

Fetal development and structures

Structures unique to the fetus include fetal membranes, the umbilical cord, the placenta, and amniotic fluid.

His and hers cells

Intrauterine development begins with **gametogenesis,** the production of specialized sex cells, called gametes.
• The male gamete (spermatozoon) is produced in the seminiferous tubules of the testes during spermatogenesis.
• The female gamete (ovum) is produced in the graafian follicle of the ovary during oogenesis.
• As gametes mature, the number of chromosomes they contain is halved (through meiosis) from 46 to 23.

The moment of truth

Conception, or fertilization, occurs with the fusion of a spermatozoon and an ovum (oocyte) in the ampulla of the fallopian tube.
• The fertilized egg is called a **zygote.**
• The diploid number of chromosomes (a pair of each chromosome; 44 autosomes and 2 sex chromosomes) is restored when the zygote is formed.
• A male zygote is formed if the ovum is fertilized by a spermatozoon carrying a Y chromosome.
• A female zygote is formed if the ovum is fertilized by a spermatozoon carrying an X chromosome.

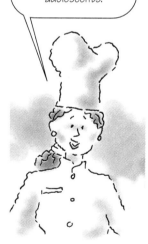

Attending to the patient's increased nutritional needs can help prevent complications. Nutritional care is especially important for pregnant adolescents.

Now I get it!

Battling discomforts of pregnancy

Education plays an important role in helping the patient deal with discomforts.

FIRST-TRIMESTER DISCOMFORTS

Nausea and vomiting
Symptoms may occur at any time during pregnancy but are most prevalent during the first trimester. Teach the patient to avoid greasy, highly seasoned foods; to eat small, frequent meals; and to eat dry toast or crackers before arising in the morning.

Nasal stuffiness, discharge, or obstruction
Advise the patient to use a cool vaporizer.

Breast enlargement and tenderness
Tell the patient to wear a well-fitting bra.

Urinary frequency and urgency
Instruct the patient to decrease fluid intake in the evening to prevent nocturia; to avoid caffeine-containing fluids; and to respond to the urge to void immediately to prevent bladder distention and urinary stasis. Also teach the patient how to perform Kegel exercises, and tell her to promptly report signs of urinary tract infections.

Increased leukorrhea
Advise the patient to bathe daily and wear absorbent cotton underwear.

SECOND- AND THIRD-TRIMESTER DISCOMFORTS

Heartburn
Encourage the patient to eat small, frequent meals; avoid fatty or fried foods; remain upright for at least 1 hour after eating; and use antacids that don't contain sodium bicarbonate.

Constipation
Encourage the patient to exercise daily, increase fluid and dietary fiber intake, and maintain regular elimination patterns.

Hemorrhoids
Tell the patient to avoid constipation, prolonged standing, and constrictive clothing, and advise her to use topical ointments, warm soaks, and anesthetic ointments to relieve symptoms.

Backache
Instruct the patient how to use proper body mechanics and maintain good posture. Also tell her to avoid wearing high heels.

Leg cramps
Instruct the patient to alter calcium and phosphorous intake, frequently rest with legs elevated, wear warm clothing and, during a leg cramp, pull the toes up toward the leg while pressing down on the knee.

Shortness of breath
Encourage the patient to maintain proper posture, especially when standing, and to use semi-Fowler's position when sleeping.

Ankle edema
Advise the patient to wear loose-fitting garments, elevate the legs during rest periods, and ensure dorsiflexion of the feet if standing or sitting for prolonged periods.

May I suggest you eat small, frequent meals and avoid fatty or fried foods.

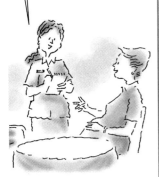

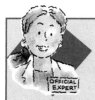

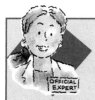

Advice from the experts

Gestational age development

By the 4th week of gestation, a normal fetus begins to show noticeable signs of growth in all areas assessed. Failure to feel fetal movement after the 20th week of gestation must be investigated by the health care provider.

A place to stay

Implantation occurs when the cellular wall of the blastocyst (trophoblast) implants itself in the endometrium of the anterior or posterior fundal region, about 7 to 9 days after fertilization.
• Primary villi appear within weeks after implantation.
• After implantation, the endometrium is called the decidua.

The beginning of the placenta

During **placentation,** chorionic villi invade the decidua and become the fetal portion of the future placenta. By the 4th week of gestation, a normal fetus begins to show noticeable signs of growth. (See *Gestational age development.*)

Fetal linings

Two fetal membranes are unique to the fetus:
• The **chorion** is the fetal membrane closest to the uterine wall; it gives rise to the placenta.
• The **amnion** is the thin, tough, inner fetal membrane that lines the amniotic sac.

Construction under way

Embryonic germ layers generate these fetal tissues:
• The **ectoderm** generates the epidermis, nervous system, pituitary gland, salivary glands, optic lens, lining of the lower portion of the anal canal, hair, and tooth enamel.
• The **endoderm** generates the epithelial lining of the larynx, trachea, bladder, urethra, prostate gland, auditory canal, liver, pancreas, and alimentary canal.

• The **mesoderm** generates the connective and sclerous tissues; the blood and vascular system; the musculature; teeth (except enamel); mesothelial lining of the pericardial, pleural, and peritoneal cavities; and kidneys and ureters.

The lifeline

The **umbilical cord** serves as the lifeline from the embryo to the placenta. At term, it measures from 20″ to 22″ (51 to 56 cm) in length and about 0.8″ (2 cm) in diameter. The umbilical cord contains two arteries, one vein, and Wharton's jelly (which prevents kinking of the cord in utero). Blood flows through the cord at about 400 ml/minute.

Red on the outside, gray on the inside

The **placenta,** weighing about 1 to 1.3 lb (454 to 590 g) and measuring from 6″ to 10″ (15 to 25 cm) in diameter, contains 15 to 20 subdivisions called cotyledons and is 1″ to 1¼″ (2.5 to 3.2 cm) thick at term. Rough in texture, the placenta appears red on the maternal surface and shiny and gray on the fetal surface. The placenta:
• functions as a transport mechanism between the mother and the fetus
• has a life span and function that depends on oxygen consumption and maternal circulation; circulation to the fetus and placenta improves when the mother lies on her left side
• receives maternal oxygen by way of diffusion
• produces hormones, including human chorionic gonadotropin, human placental lactogen, gonadotropin-releasing hormone, thy-

If this is the patient's first pregnancy, she is referred to as a primigravida; otherwise, she is referred to as a multigravida.

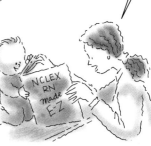

rotropin-releasing factor, corticotropin, estrogen, and progesterone
• supplies the fetus with carbohydrates, water, fats, protein, minerals, and inorganic salts
• carries end products of fetal metabolism to the maternal circulation for excretion
• transfers passive immunity by way of maternal antibodies.

Fetal protection

The **amniotic fluid** prevents heat loss, preserves constant fetal body temperatures, cushions the fetus, and facilitates fetal growth and development. Amniotic fluid is replaced every 3 hours.

At term, the uterus contains 800 to 1,200 ml of amniotic fluid, which is clear and yellowish and has a specific gravity of 1.007 to 1.025 and a pH of 7.0 to 7.25. Maternal serum provides amniotic fluid in early gestation, with increasing amounts derived from fetal urine late in gestation. Amniotic fluid contains:
• albumin
• bilirubin
• creatinine
• enzymes
• fat
• lanugo
• lecithin
• leukocytes
• sphingomyelin
• urea.

Blood movers

Fetal circulation structures include the:
• umbilical vein, which carries oxygenated blood to the fetus from the placenta
• umbilical arteries, which carry deoxygenated blood from the fetus to the placenta
• foramen ovale, which serves as the septal opening between the atria of the fetal heart
• ductus arteriosus, which connects the pulmonary artery to the aorta, allowing blood to shunt around the fetal lungs
• ductus venosus, which carries oxygenated blood from the umbilical vein to the inferior vena cava, bypassing the liver.

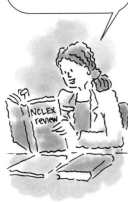

After amniocentesis, monitor the patient for hemorrhage, infection, premature labor, and amnionitis.

Keep abreast of diagnostic tests

Here's a brief review of tests performed as part of antepartum care.

The routine

These routine laboratory tests can confirm pregnancy and reveal maternal complications:
• **blood type, Rh, and abnormal antibodies** to identify the fetus at risk for erythroblastosis fetalis or hyperbilirubinemia
• **immunologic tests** such as rubella antibodies to detect the presence of rubella, rapid plasma reagin to detect untreated syphilis, and hepatitis B surface antigen to detect hepatitis B.
• **urine tests** to measure human chorionic gonadotropin (HCG) to confirm pregnancy.
• **hematologic studies** use blood samples to analyze and measure RBCs, white blood cells (WBCs), erythrocyte sedimentation rate (ESR), prothrombin time (PT), partial thromboplastin time (PTT), platelets, hemoglobin (Hb), and HCT.
• **genital cultures** such as a gonorrhea smear and chlamydia test to detect sexually transmitted disease.
• **triple screen** between 15 and 20 weeks' gestation to identify fetus at increased risk for Down syndrome and neural tube defect.
• **alpha-fetoprotein** uses a blood sample to measure alpha-fetoprotein levels. High maternal serum levels may suggest fetal neural tube defects, such as spina bifida and anencephaly.

Check your fluid?

Amniocentesis is usually performed after the14th week of gestation, when amniotic fluid is sufficient and the uterus has moved into the abdominal cavity. This procedure involves transabdominal insertion of a spinal needle into the uterus to aspirate amniotic fluid. This procedure helps determine:
• gestational age by way of a lecithin-sphingomyelin ratio

• fetal lung maturity by analyzing lecithin/sphingomyelin ratio, two key components of surfactant.
• creatinine levels.

Amniocentesis is used to diagnose genetic disorders, such as chromosomal aberrations, sex-linked disorders, inborn errors of metabolism, and neural tube defect. It may also be used to diagnose and evaluate isoimmune disease, including Rh sensitization and ABO blood type incompatibility.

Nursing actions
Before the procedure:
• Use ultrasonography to locate the fetus, placenta, and amniotic fluid.
  After the procedure:
• Monitor the fetal heart rate and uterine activity with an external fetal monitor for at least 30 minutes.
• Monitor for maternal hemorrhage, infection, premature labor, fetal hemorrhage, and amnionitis.
• Rh-negative mothers must receive Rh_0 (D) immune globulin (RhI [G]; Rh_0GAM) to prevent fetal isoimmunization.

Tissue sample
Chorionic villi sampling can be performed as early as the 8th week of gestation. It involves removal and analysis of a small tissue specimen from the fetal portion of the placenta. This test helps determine the genetic makeup of the fetus, providing earlier diagnosis and allowing earlier and safer abortion if the fetus carries the risk of spontaneous abortion, infection, hematoma, fetal limb defects, and intrauterine death.

Nursing actions
After the procedure:
• An Rh-negative mother must receive Rh_0(D) immune globulin (RhIG) to prevent sensitization.
• Monitor the fetal heart rate and uterine activity with an external fetal monitor for at least 30 minutes.

Sound picture
Ultrasonography, a noninvasive and painless procedure, uses ultrasonic waves reflected by

tissues of different densities to visualize deep structures of the body. Reflected signals are then amplified and processed to produce a visual display, providing immediate results without harm to fetus or mother. Ultrasound can detect fetal death, malformation, malpresentation, placental abnormalities, multiple gestation, and hydramnios or oligohydramnios.

Nursing actions
• Instruct the patient to drink a glass of water every 15 minutes beginning 1½ hours before the procedure.
• Instruct the patient not to void until immediately after the procedure.

Stress-free
The **nonstress test** (NST) is used to detect fetal heart accelerations in response to fetal movement. This noninvasive test provides simple, inexpensive, immediate results without contraindications or complications. It may be indicated for a patient at risk for uteroplacental insufficiency or for altered fetal movements.

The NST can be given between 32 and 34 weeks of gestation. A nonreactive test result indicates the possibility of fetal hypoxia, fetal sleep cycle, or the effects of drugs. The results may be inconclusive if the patient is extremely obese.

Nursing actions
• Before the procedure, explain the process to the patient.

Contraction action
The **oxytocin challenge test** (OCT) evaluates fetal ability to withstand an oxytocin-induced contraction. This test, given after a nonreactive NST result, requires I.V. administration of oxytocin in increasing doses every 15 to 20 minutes until three high-quality uterine contractions are obtained within 10 minutes.

The OCT is performed on a patient at risk for uteroplacental insufficiency or fetal compromise from diabetes, heart disease, hypertension, or renal disease or on a patient with a history of stillbirth. The OCT isn't indicated

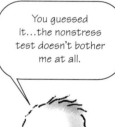

You guessed it...the nonstress test doesn't bother me at all.

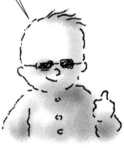

for those with previous classic cesarean section or third-trimester bleeding or for those at high risk for preterm labor.

Nursing actions
• Before performing the OCT, administer an NST.
• During and after the OCT, monitor fetal heart rate and maternal contractions.

Breast test
The **nipple stimulation stress test** induces contractions by activating sensory receptors in the areola, triggering the release of oxytocin by the posterior pituitary gland. The receptors are activated by rolling the nipple manually or by applying a warm washcloth. This test has the same reactive pattern as the reactive NST result.

Nursing actions
• Monitor fetal heart rate and uterine contractions on external fetal monitor during and after the procedure.

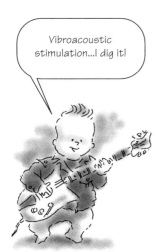

Vibroacoustic stimulation...I dig it!

Good vibrations
The **vibroacoustic stimulation** test uses vibration and sound to induce fetal reactivity during an NST. Vibration is produced by an artificial larynx or a fetal acoustic stimulator (over the fetus's head for 1 to 5 seconds). This test is noninvasive, quick, and convenient.

Nursing actions
• Monitor fetal heart rate during and after the procedure.

Five profiles in one
The **biophysical profile** assesses four to six parameters — fetal breathing movements, body movements, muscle tone, amniotic fluid volume, heart rate reactivity and placental grade — using real-time ultrasound. This test is noninvasive and quick and can detect central nervous system depression.

Nursing actions
• Perform an NST to obtain information for the profile.

• Perform a sonogram to obtain information for the profile.

How does the flow go?
Fetal blood flow studies use umbilical or uterine Doppler velocimetry to evaluate vascular resistance, especially in patients with hypertension, diabetes, isoimmunization, and lupus. These studies are useful when congenital anomalies or cardiac arrhythmias are suspected.

Nursing actions
• Before the procedure, obtain a baseline fetal heart rate.
• During the procedure, continue to monitor the patient and the fetus for signs of problems such as changes in vital signs or fetal heart rate or continuation of uterine contractions.

Risky business
Percutaneous umbilical blood sampling (PUBS) is an invasive procedure that involves inserting a spinal needle into the umbilical cord to obtain fetal blood samples or to transfuse the fetus in utero.

Usually performed during the second or third trimester, PUBS is indicated when the fetus is at risk for congenital and chromosomal abnormalities, congenital infection, or anemia. It carries a 1% to 2% risk of fetal loss.

Nursing actions
• Rh-negative mothers must receive $Rh_o D$ immune globulin after PUBS to prevent sensitization.
• Monitor the fetus by performing the NST before and after the PUBS to assess for uterine contractions.
• Monitor fetal and maternal status throughout the procedure.

Catch up on complications

Common antepartum complications and accompanying conditions include abruptio placentae, acquired immunodeficiency syn-

Grading abruptio placentae

Separation of the placenta from the uterine wall is classified as minimal, moderate, or extreme. Hemorrhaging may or may not be apparent, even with complete separation.

GRADE	CRITERIA
0	Maternal and fetal signs don't indicate difficulty. Premature separation isn't apparent until the placenta is examined after delivery.
1	Minimal separation causes vaginal bleeding and alterations in maternal vital signs, but hemorrhagic shock and fetal distress don't appear.
2	Moderate separation produces signs of fetal distress. The uterus is tense and painful when palpated.
3	Extreme separation occurs, possibly causing maternal shock and fetal death without immediate intervention.

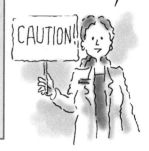

Prevent placental disruption. Avoid vaginal examinations for patients with abruptio placentae.

drome, adolescent pregnancy, diabetes mellitus, ectopic pregnancy, heart disease, hydatidiform mole, hyperemesis gravidarum, multifetal pregnancy, placenta previa, and pregnancy-induced hypertension.

Abruptio placentae

Abruptio placentae refers to premature separation of the placenta from the uterine wall after 20 to 24 weeks of gestation. It may occur as late as the first or second stage of labor. Placental separation is measured by degree (from grades 0 to 3) to determine the fetal and maternal outcome. (See *Grading abruptio placentae.*)

Perinatal mortality depends on the degree of placental separation and fetal level of maturity. Most serious complications stem from hypoxia, prematurity, and anemia. The maternal mortality rate is about 6% and depends on the severity of the bleeding, the presence of coagulation defects, hypofibrinogenemia, and the time lapse between placental separation and delivery.

CAUSES
- Abdominal trauma
- Cocaine use
- Decreased blood flow to the placenta

- Hydramnios
- Multifetal pregnancy
- Other risk factors (low serum folic acid levels, vascular or renal disease, pregnancy-induced hypertension)

ASSESSMENT FINDINGS
- Acute abdominal pain
- Frequent, low-amplitude contractions (noted with external fetal monitor)
- Hemorrhage, either concealed or apparent, with dark red vaginal bleeding
- Rigid abdomen
- Shock
- Uteroplacental insufficiency

DIAGNOSTIC TEST RESULTS
- Ultrasonography locates the placenta and a clot or hematoma may be apparent.
- Hematology may show disseminated intravascular coagulation (DIC) — increased PTT and PT, elevated level of fibrinogen degradation products, decreased fibrinogen level, or decreased platelet count.

NURSING DIAGNOSES
- Anxiety
- Fluid volume deficit
- Altered tissue perfusion (cardiopulmonary)

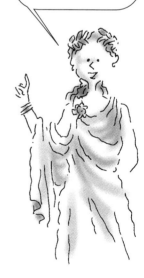

Friends, Romans, countrymen. Emergency cesarean delivery is indicated in cases of moderate to severe placental separation.

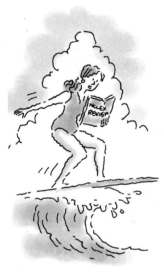

Put it together. Determination and knowledge. That's what you need to pass the NCLEX.

Treatment
• Transfusion: packed RBCs, platelets, and fresh frozen plasma, if necessary
• Cesarean delivery

INTERVENTIONS AND RATIONALES
• Monitor maternal vital signs, fetal heart rate, uterine contractions, and vaginal bleeding *to assess maternal and fetal well-being.*
• Assess fluid and electrolyte balance *to assess kidney function.*
• Avoid pelvic or vaginal examinations and enemas *to prevent further placental disruption.*
• Administer fresh whole blood, packed RBCs, platelets, or plasma *to replace blood volume.*
• Provide oxygen by mask *to minimize fetal hypoxia.*
• Evaluate maternal laboratory values *to assess for DIC.*
• Position the patient in a left lateral recumbent position *to help relieve pressure on the vena cava from an enlarged uterus, which could further compromise fetal circulation.*
• Provide emotional support *to allay patient anxiety.*

Acquired immunodeficiency syndrome

A female patient may be first identified as positive for human immunodeficiency virus (HIV) antibodies during pregnancy or when the newborn's HIV status is identified. Because of the effects of pregnancy on immunosuppression, the progression from HIV infection to full-blown acquired immunodeficiency syndrome (AIDS) may be expedited during pregnancy.

CAUSES
• Exposure to HIV through blood transfusions, contaminated needles, and handling of blood
• Exposure to semen or vaginal secretions containing HIV

ASSESSMENT FINDINGS
• Diarrhea
• Fatigue
• HIV-associated dementia
• Kaposi's sarcoma
• Mild flu-like symptoms
• Opportunistic infections, such as toxoplasmosis, oral and vaginal candidiasis, herpes simplex, *Pneumocystis carinii, Candida* esophagitis
• Weight loss

DIAGNOSTIC TEST RESULTS
• Blood chemistry shows increased transaminase, alkaline phosphatase, and gamma globulin levels; and decreased albumin level.
• CD4+ T-cell level is less than 200 cells/μl.
• Enzyme-linked immunosorbent assay shows positive HIV antibody titer.
• Hematology shows decreased WBC, RBC, and platelet counts.
• Western blot test is positive.

NURSING DIAGNOSES
• Altered protection
• Anxiety
• Ineffective individual coping

TREATMENT
• Care during pregnancy and delivery same as that for any other patient with HIV
• If patient is newly diagnosed, zidovudine (Retrovir) treatment is initiated between weeks 14 and 34 of gestation
• Fetus monitored closely; serial ultrasounds performed to identify intrauterine growth restrictions; NST performed weekly after 32 weeks

INTERVENTIONS AND RATIONALES
• Provide routine care for patients with AIDS. (See "Acquired immunodeficiency syndrome," page 127.)
• Assess for pyrexia (fever), chest tightness, and shortness of breath *to evaluate for possible recurrent acute pneumonia or pulmonary tuberculosis, which may indicate AIDS.*
• Provide emotional support to the patient and her family *to allay the patient's fears.*

• Assess whether the patient will be able to care for her infant after delivery *to evaluate the need for additional support services.*

Teaching topics
• Treatment options
• Preventing the spread of infection
• Increased risk of transmission to the fetus caused by repeated exposure to HIV through unsafe sex practices or I.V. drug use
• Information requested by the patient to help her decide whether or not to terminate the pregnancy

Adolescent pregnancy

A teenage mother is at risk for such complications as pregnancy-induced hypertension, cephalopelvic disproportion, anemia, and nutritional deficiencies. Teenagers also have a high incidence of sexually transmitted diseases (STDs), posing a concern for both the mother and the neonate.

Infants born to teenage mothers are at risk for such complications as prematurity and low birth weight.

CONTRIBUTING FACTORS
• Desire to gain love, adulthood, and independence through pregnancy
• Fear of reporting sexual activity to parents
• High level of adolescent sexual activity
• Lack of appropriate role models
• Limited access to contraceptives
• Low level of education correlated with incorrect use of contraceptives
• Naiveté about ability to become pregnant
• Sporadic use of contraception

ASSESSMENT FINDINGS
• Amenorrhea
• Denial of pregnancy, which may delay the patient from seeking medical attention early in pregnancy

DIAGNOSTIC TEST RESULTS
• Pregnancy test is positive.
• Ultrasound confirms presence of fetus.

NURSING DIAGNOSES
• Knowledge deficit
• Altered nutrition: Less than body requirements
• Altered family processes

TREATMENT
• Formulation of diet with caloric intake sufficient to support the growing adolescent and her developing fetus

Drug therapy
• Antibiotics for STDs, if necessary

INTERVENTIONS AND RATIONALES
• Monitor the patient's weight gain *to assess for nutritional deficiencies.*
• Monitor urine protein *to detect possible pregnancy-induced hypertension* and glucose levels *to detect possible gestational diabetes.*
• Assess fundal height *to detect how pregnancy is progressing.*
• Assess fetal heart sounds *to monitor fetal well-being.*
• Assess the patient's knowledge of her pregnancy *to determine need for further teaching.*
• Assess the patient's family and available support *to determine need for referrals.*
• Provide nutritional support and encouragement *to promote well-being of mother and fetus.*
• Stress the importance of attending scheduled prenatal appointments *to promote well-being of mother and fetus.*
• Advise the patient of her options, including terminating the pregnancy, continuing the pregnancy and giving up the infant for adoption, and continuing the pregnancy and keeping the infant *to promote informed decision making.*
• Allow the patient to express her feelings about her pregnancy and herself *to promote mental and emotional well-being.*

Teaching topics
• Encouraging attendance at prenatal and birthing classes and infant care classes

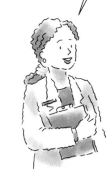

Be aware! Pregnant adolescents are at risk for insufficient or delayed medical care.

Diabetes mellitus

In gestational diabetes mellitus, the patient's pancreas, stressed by the normal adaptations to pregnancy, can't meet the increased demands for insulin.

A patient may have preexisting diabetes or may develop gestational diabetes while she's pregnant. Gestational diabetes is associated with an increased risk of congenital anomalies, hydramnios, macrosomia, pregnancy-induced hypertension, spontaneous abortion, and fetal death. Additionally, the infant of a diabetic is at risk for developing sacral agenesis, a congenital anomaly characterized by incomplete formation of the vertebral column.

The patient with gestational diabetes has an increased risk of developing diabetes mellitus.

RISK FACTORS
- Chronic hypertension
- Family history of diabetes
- Gestational diabetes in previous pregnancies
- Maternal age older than 25

ASSESSMENT FINDINGS
- Glycosuria
- Ketonuria
- Polyuria
- Possible monilial infection (vaginal yeast infection)

DIAGNOSTIC TEST RESULTS
- One-hour glucose tolerance test reveals glucose level greater than 140 mg/dl.
- Three-hour glucose tolerance test reveals fasting serum glucose level of 105 mg/dl or greater.
- Three-hour glucose tolerance test reveals one-hour serum glucose level of 190 mg/dl or greater.
- Three-hour glucose tolerance test reveals 2-hour serum glucose level of 165 mg/dl or greater.
- Three-hour glucose tolerance test reveals 3-hour serum glucose level of 145 mg/dl or greater.

NURSING DIAGNOSES
- Altered nutrition: more than body requirements
- Risk for fluid volume deficit
- Ineffective individual coping

TREATMENT
- 1,800- to 2,200-calorie diet, divided into three meals and three snacks that should also include low fat and cholesterol and high fiber
- Administration of insulin
- Oral antidiabetic agents contraindicated because of adverse effects on the fetus

INTERVENTIONS AND RATIONALES
- Monitor fetal heart rate *to assess fetal well-being.*
- Encourage adherence to dietary regulations *to maintain euglycemia.*
- Encourage the patient to exercise moderately *to reduce blood glucose levels and decrease the need for insulin.*
- Prepare the patient for antepartum fetal surveillance testing, including oxytocin challenge testing, nipple stimulation stress testing, amniotic fluid index, biophysical profile, and nonstress test *to assess fetal well-being.*
- Encourage the patient to verbalize her feelings *to allay her fears.*
- Provide emotional support *to reduce anxiety.*

Teaching topics
- Performing serum glucose monitoring and insulin regulation and administration
- Performing fetal "kick counts" to assess fetal well-being during the third trimester
- Learning about normal pregnancy care and concerns

Ectopic pregnancy

Ectopic pregnancy refers to implantation of the fertilized ovum outside the uterine cavity. Most commonly, ectopic pregnancy occurs in a fallopian tube; other sites include the cervix, ovary, and abdominal cavity. It's the second most frequent cause of vaginal bleeding early in pregnancy.

CAUSES
- Hormonal factors
- Malformed fallopian tubes
- Ovulation induction drugs
- Progestin-only oral contraceptives
- Tubal atony
- Tubal damage from pelvic inflammatory disease
- Tubal damage from previous pelvic or tubal surgery
- Tubal spasms
- Use of intrauterine devices

ASSESSMENT FINDINGS
- Falling blood pressure
- Irregular vaginal bleeding and dull abdominal pain on the affected side early in pregnancy
- Nausea and vomiting
- Positive Cullen's sign (bluish discoloration around the umbilicus)
- Rapid, thready pulse
- Rupture of tubes, causing sudden and severe abdominal pain, syncope, and referred shoulder pain as the abdomen fills with blood
- Shock with profuse hemorrhage

DIAGNOSTIC TEST RESULTS
- HCG titers are abnormally low.
- Ultrasound is positive for ruptured tube and collective pelvic fluid.
- Vaginal examination reveals a palpable tender mass in Douglas's cul-de-sac.

NURSING DIAGNOSES
- Fluid volume deficit
- Risk for infection
- Pain

TREATMENT
- Laparotomy to ligate the bleeding vessels and remove or repair damaged fallopian tube
- Transfusion therapy: packed RBCs (if bleeding is uncontrolled)

Drug therapy
- If the tube hasn't ruptured, methotrexate (Folex) followed by leucovorin (Wellcovorin) to stop the trophoblastic cells from growing (therapy continues until negative HCG levels are achieved)

INTERVENTIONS AND RATIONALES
- Monitor vital signs and intake and output *to assess for intense blood loss and shock.*
- Monitor for severe abdominal pain, orthostatic hypotension, tachycardia, and dizziness, *which may indicate rupturing ectopic pregnancy.*
- Monitor WBC and erythrocyte sedimentation rate *for signs of infection.*
- Administer I.V. fluid replacement *to accommodate for blood loss.*
- Administer blood products *to replace volume loss.*
- Administer Rh_oD immune globulin *to combat isoimmunization in the patient who is Rh-negative.*
- Provide routine postoperative care *if surgical intervention is necessary.*
- Provide emotional support *for parents grieving over the loss of the pregnancy.*

Teaching topics
- Adverse effects of methotrexate therapy, such as nausea, mouth ulceration, abdominal discomfort, and altered liver enzyme levels
- Importance of follow-up medical care

Heart disease

Heart disease occurs in about 1% of pregnant patients. Pregnancy may reveal an underlying heart condition that was previously asymptomatic or it may aggravate a known heart condition. A patient with heart disease is at greatest risk when blood volume peaks between the 28th and 32nd week of gestation.

Successful delivery of a healthy baby depends on the type and extent of the disease. Decreased placental perfusion may lead to intrauterine growth retardation, fetal distress, and prematurity.

Pregnant patients with heart disease are graded at a level of I to IV. (See *Heart disease and pregnancy,* page 482.)

CAUSES
- Regurgitation, which permits blood to leak through an incompletely closed valve, thereby increasing workload on heart chambers on either side of affected valve

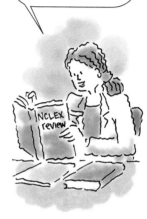

Hmmm. Irregular vaginal bleeding and dull abdominal pain may be early signs of ectopic pregnancy.

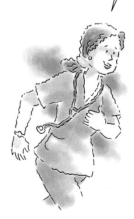

Severe abdominal pain, orthostatic hypotension, tachycardia, and dizziness may indicate a rupturing ectopic pregnancy.

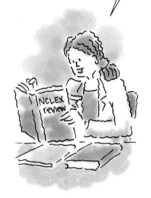

During labor, position the patient with heart disease on her left side with her head and shoulders elevated.

Heart disease and pregnancy

A patient with heart disease may or may not experience a difficult pregnancy; success depends on the type and extent of the disease, as shown below. A patient with class I or II heart disease usually completes a successful pregnancy and delivery without major complications. One with class III heart disease must maintain strict bed rest to complete the pregnancy. One with class IV heart disease is a poor candidate for pregnancy.

CLASS I
Physical activity is unrestricted. Ordinary activity causes no discomfort, cardiac insufficiency, or anginal pain.

CLASS II
There is a slight limitation on physical activity. Ordinary activity causes excessive fatigue, palpitations, dyspnea, or anginal pain.

CLASS III
There is moderate to marked limitation on activity. With less than ordinary activity, the patient experiences excessive fatigue, palpitations, dyspnea, or anginal pain.

CLASS IV
The patient can't engage in any physical activity without discomfort. Cardiac insufficiency or anginal pain occurs even at rest.

• Valvular stenosis, which decreases blood flow through a valve, increasing workload on heart chambers located before the stenotic valve

ASSESSMENT FINDINGS
• Cough
• Crackles at the base of the lungs
• Diastolic murmur at the heart's apex
• Dyspnea
• Fatigue
• Hemoptysis
• Tachycardia

DIAGNOSTIC TEST RESULTS
• Echocardiography, electrocardiography, and chest X-ray may reveal cardiac abnormalities, arrhythmias, impaired cardiac function, increased workload on the heart, and cardiovascular decompensation.

NURSING DIAGNOSES
• Activity intolerance
• Fluid volume excess
• Increased cardiac output

TREATMENT

Class I and Class II
• Sodium restriction

• Antibiotics, such as ampicillin and gentamicin, to prevent bacterial endocarditis

Class III and Class IV
• Anticoagulants, such as heparin (Liquaemin)
• Antiarrhythmics, such as digoxin (Lanoxin), quinidine (Quinora), procainamide (Pronestyl), and beta-adrenergic blockers
• Antibiotics, such as ampicillin and gentamicin, to prevent bacterial endocarditis
• Thiazide diuretics and furosemide to control heart failure if activity restriction and reduced sodium intake don't prevent it

INTERVENTIONS AND RATIONALES
• Monitor maternal and fetal vital signs *to assess for maternal and fetal well-being.*
• Assess cardiovascular and respiratory status *to assess for signs of maternal cardiac decompensation (tachycardia, tachypnea, moist crackles, exhaustion).*
• Monitor PTT, activated thromboplastin time, and platelet count *to achieve adequate anticoagulation.*
• Administer anticoagulants, antiarrhythmics, antibiotics, and diuretics, as prescribed *to achieve therapeutic regimens.*
• Encourage the patient to monitor her intake *to avoid excessive weight gain.*

• Encourage the patient to limit her physical activity according to her ability and symptoms *to ensure adequate rest.*
• Monitor I.V. fluid intake and output *to maintain proper fluid levels.*
• Administer oxygen by nasal cannula or face mask during labor *to maintain fetal oxygenation.*
• Position the patient on her left side with her head and shoulders elevated during labor *to prevent supine hypotension syndrome.*
• Continue to monitor the patient during the postpartum period *to assess for signs of cardiac decompensation, even if distress is absent during pregnancy and labor.*

Teaching topics
• Achieving a healthy diet
• Avoiding infection

Hydatidiform mole

Also known as gestational trophoblastic disease, hydatidiform mole is a developmental anomaly of the placenta that converts the chorionic villi into a mass of clear vesicles (hydatid vesicles). There are two types:
• *complete mole,* in which there is neither an embryo nor an amniotic sac
• *partial mole,* in which there is an embryo (usually with multiple abnormalities) and an amniotic sac.

CAUSES
• Possibly poor maternal nutrition or a defective ovum

ASSESSMENT FINDINGS
• Disproportionate enlargement of the uterus
• Excessive nausea and vomiting
• Intermittent or continuous bright red or brownish vaginal bleeding by the 12th week of gestation
• Absence of fetal heart tones
• Passage of clear fluid-filled vesicles along with vaginal bleeding
• Symptoms of pregnancy-induced hypertension before the 20th week of gestation

DIAGNOSTIC TEST RESULTS
• HCG levels are extremely high for early pregnancy.
• Ultrasonography fails to reveal a fetal skeleton.

NURSING DIAGNOSES
• Fluid volume deficit
• Anticipatory grieving
• Pain

TREATMENT
• Therapeutic abortion (suction and curettage) if a spontaneous abortion doesn't occur
• Pelvic examinations and chest X-rays at regular intervals
• Weekly monitoring of HCG levels until they remain normal for 3 consecutive weeks.
• Periodic follow-up for 1 to 2 years because of increased risk of neoplasm

Drug therapy
• Methotrexate prophylactically (the drug of choice for choriocarcinoma)

INTERVENTIONS AND RATIONALES
• Monitor and record vital signs and intake and output *to assess for changes that may indicate complications.*
• Provide emotional support for the grieving couple. *This demonstrates concern and understanding for the patient and family.*
• Monitor vaginal bleeding *to assess for hemorrhage.*
• Send contents of uterine evacuation to the laboratory for analysis *to assess for the presence of hydatid vesicles.*
• Advise the patient to avoid pregnancy until HCG levels are normal (may take up to 2 years) *to avoid future complications.*

Teaching topics
• Dealing with an unsure obstetric and medical future
• Managing birth control to avoid pregnancy

Hyperemesis gravidarum

Hyperemesis gravidarum is persistent, uncontrolled vomiting that begins in the 1st weeks

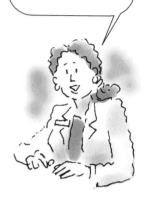

Hydatidiform mole is a chorionic tumor. The chorion is the fetal membrane closest to the uterine wall; it gives rise to the placenta.

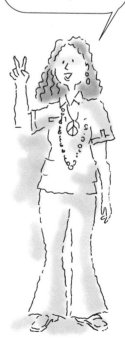

Loosen up. Don't tense up as you study...Keep it loose to tap into your full mental power.

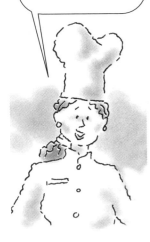

Patients with multifetal pregnancies have nutritional needs exceeding those of other pregnant patients. Try some calories, iron, folate, and vitamins.

of pregnancy and may continue throughout pregnancy. Unlike "morning sickness," hyperemesis can have serious complications, including severe weight loss, dehydration, and electrolyte imbalance.

CAUSES
- Gonadotropin production
- Psychological factors
- Trophoblastic activity

ASSESSMENT FINDINGS
- Continuous, severe nausea and vomiting
- Dehydration
- Dry skin and mucous membranes
- Electrolyte imbalance
- Jaundice
- Metabolic acidosis
- Nonelastic skin turgor
- Oliguria

DIAGNOSTIC TEST RESULTS
- Arterial blood gas analysis reveals alkalosis.
- Hb level and HCT are elevated.
- Serum potassium level reveals hypokalemia.
- Urine ketone levels are elevated.
- Urine specific gravity is increased.

NURSING DIAGNOSES
- Altered nutrition: less than body requirements
- Fluid volume deficit
- Pain

TREATMENT
- Total parenteral nutrition (TPN)
- Restoration of fluid and electrolyte balance

Drug therapy
- Antiemetics, as necessary, for vomiting

INTERVENTIONS AND RATIONALES
- Monitor vital signs and fluid intake and output *to assess for fluid volume deficit.*
- Obtain blood samples and urine specimens *for laboratory tests, including Hb level, HCT, urinalysis, and electrolyte levels.*
- Provide small, frequent meals *to maintain adequate nutrition.*

- Maintain I.V. fluid replacement and TPN *to reduce fluid deficits and pH imbalances.*
- Provide emotional support *to help the patient cope with her condition.*

Teaching topics
- Using salt on foods to replace sodium lost by vomiting

Multifetal pregnancy

A multifetal pregnancy, also known as multiple gestation, occurs when two or more embryos or fetuses exist simultaneously. Multifetal pregnancies are formed as follows:
- Single-ovum (monozygotic, identical) twins usually have one chorion, one placenta, two amnions, and two umbilical cords and are of the same sex.
- Double-ova (dizygotic, nonidentical) twins have two chorions, two placentas, two amnions, and two umbilical cords and may be of the same or different sex.
- Multifetal pregnancies of three or more fetuses may be single-ovum conceptions, multiple-ova conceptions, or a combination of both.

CAUSES
- In vitro fertilization
- Gamete intrafallopian tube transfer
- Ovulation stimulation with such drugs as clomiphene (Clomid)

ASSESSMENT FINDINGS
- More than one set of fetal heart sounds
- Uterine size greater than expected for dates

DIAGNOSTIC TEST RESULTS
- Alpha-fetoprotein levels are elevated.
- Ultrasonography is positive for multifetal pregnancy.

NURSING DIAGNOSES
- Anxiety
- Knowledge deficit
- Risk for injury

TREATMENT
- Activity as tolerated with increased rest periods

• Bed rest if early dilation occurs or at 24 to 28 weeks' gestation to improve uterine blood flow and, possibly, increase birth weight of the fetus
• Biweekly NST to document fetal growth, beginning with the 28th week of gestation
• Increased intake of calories, iron, folate, and vitamins
• Prenatal visits every 2 weeks, increasing to weekly between 24 and 28 weeks' gestation; cervical examinations performed at each visit to check for premature dilation
• Ultrasound examinations monthly to document fetal growth

INTERVENTIONS AND RATIONALES
• Monitor fetal heart sounds *to evaluate fetal well-being.*
• Monitor maternal vital signs including weight *to assess maternal well-being.*
• Monitor cardiovascular and pulmonary status *to assess for signs of pregnancy-induced hypertension.*
• Measure fundal height *to assess for possible hydramnios, which could result in preterm labor.*
• Ensure adequate nutrition and increased intake of folate, calories, vitamins, and iron *to ensure adequate weight gain.*
• Encourage the patient to take frequent rest periods, especially during the third trimester, or to maintain bed rest, if indicated, *to prevent fatigue.*
• Provide emotional support and encouragement *to reduce anxiety.*
• Advise the patient to return for ultrasound examination and NST as scheduled *to assess for fetal well-being.*

Teaching topics
• Notifying health care provider immediately if signs of premature labor occur
• Refraining from coitus during the third trimester

Placenta previa

In placenta previa, the placenta is implanted in the lower uterine segment (low implanta-tion). The placenta can occlude the cervix partially or totally.

RISK FACTORS
• Maternal age older than 35
• Multiple pregnancies
• Placental villi torn from the uterine wall as the lower uterine segment contracts and dilates in the third trimester
• Uterine fibroid tumors
• Uterine scars from surgery
• Uterine sinuses exposed at the placental site and bleeding

ASSESSMENT FINDINGS
• Painless, bright red vaginal bleeding, especially during the third trimester (possibly increasing with each successive incident)

DIAGNOSTIC TEST RESULTS
• Early ultrasound evaluation reveals the placenta implanted in the lower uterine segment.

NURSING DIAGNOSES
• Fear
• Fluid volume deficit
• Risk for injury

TREATMENT
• Depends on gestational age, when first episode occurs, and amount of bleeding
• If gestational age less than 34 weeks, hospitalizing the patient and restricting her to bed rest to avoid preterm labor
• Administering supplemental iron if anemia is present
• Restricting maternal activities (for example, no lifting heavy objects, long-distance travel, or sexual intercourse)
• Transfusion of packed RBCs if Hb level and HCT are low.
• Treatment of choice: surgical intervention (by cesarean birth) but depends on the placental placement and maternal and fetal stability.

INTERVENTIONS AND RATIONALES
• Monitor maternal vital signs, including uterine activity *to assess for maternal well-being.*
• Monitor for vaginal bleeding *to estimate blood loss.*

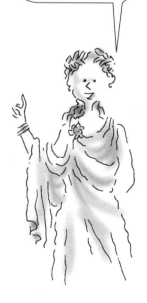

Friends, Romans, countrymen. Placenta previa may be treated by cesarian birth, depending on placental placement and maternal and fetal stability.

• Monitor fetal heart rate, using electronic fetal monitoring, *to assess for complications.*
• Don't perform rectal or vaginal examinations unless equipment is available for vaginal and cesarean delivery *to avoid stimulating uterine activity.*
• Obtain blood samples for HCT, Hb level, PT and PTT, fibrinogen level, platelet count, and typing and crossmatching *to assess for complications.*
• Provide routine postoperative care if cesarean delivery is performed *to ensure the patient's well-being.*
• Monitor for postpartum hemorrhage *because patients with placenta previa are more prone to hemorrhage.*
• Provide emotional support *to reduce anxiety.*
• Provide I.V. fluids as ordered *to reduce fluid loss.*
• Be prepared to administer betamethasone *to increase fetal lung maturity if preterm labor can't be halted.*

Teaching topics
• Activity limitations
• Reporting increased bleeding immediately
• Possible need for preterm delivery

Pregnancy-induced hypertension

Pregnancy-induced hypertension (PIH) is characterized by hypertension, proteinuria, and edema. The patient is at risk for cerebral hemorrhage, circulatory collapse, heart failure, hepatic rupture, or renal failure. If delivery occurs before term, fetal prognosis is poor because of hypoxia, acidosis, and immaturity.

If uncontrolled, PIH may progress to seizures (eclampsia). The maternal mortality from eclampsia is 10% to 15%, usually resulting from intracranial hemorrhage and heart failure.

RISK FACTORS
• Adolescent mother
• Antiphospholipid antibodies
• Diabetes mellitus
• Familial tendency

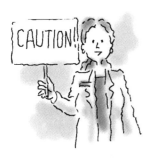

The patient with pregnancy-induced hypertension is at risk for cerebral hemorrhage, circulatory collapse, heart failure, hepatic rupture, or renal failure.

• Hydatidiform mole
• Hydramnios
• Hydrops fetalis
• Hypertension
• Malnutrition
• Maternal age older than 35
• Multifetal pregnancy
• Obesity
• Renal disease

ASSESSMENT FINDINGS
PIH usually appears between the 20th and 24th weeks of gestation and disappears within 42 days after delivery. It's classified as gestational hypertension, mild eclampsia, severe preeclampsia, or eclampsia, depending on the degree of hypertension and other symptoms.

Gestational hypertension
• Blood pressure 140/90 mm Hg or systolic pressure elevated 30 mm Hg above prepregnancy level
• No proteinuria

Mild eclampsia
• Blood pressure of 140/90 mm Hg, systolic pressure elevated more than 30 mm Hg above prepregnancy level, or diastolic pressure elevated 15 mm Hg above prepregnancy level
• Proteinuria of 1+ to 2+
• Weight gain more than 2 lb (0.9 kg) per week in the second trimester and 1 lb (0.45 kg) per week in the third trimester
• Mild edema in upper extremities or face

Severe preeclampsia
• Blood pressure of 160/110 mm Hg (noted on two readings taken 6 hours apart while on bed rest)
• Proteinuria of 3+ to 4+
• Oliguria (500 ml or less in 24 hours)
• Pulmonary edema with shortness of breath
• Peripheral edema, severe facial edema
• Frontal headaches, blurred vision, hyperreflexia, nausea, vomiting, irritability, cerebral disturbances, and epigastric pain
• Presence of HELLP syndrome (hemolysis, elevated liver enzymes, and low platelet count)

Eclampsia
- Blood pressure higher than 160/100 mm Hg
- Tonic-clonic seizure

DIAGNOSTIC TEST RESULTS
- Blood chemistry reveals increased blood urea nitrogen, creatinine, and uric acid levels and elevated liver function studies.
- Hematology reveals thrombocytopenia (HELLP syndrome).

NURSING DIAGNOSES
- Activity intolerance
- Fluid volume excess
- Risk for injury

TREATMENT
- Bed rest in a lateral position.
- Delivery: in mild preeclampsia, once the fetus is mature and safe induction is possible; in severe preeclampsia, regardless of gestational age
- High-protein diet with restriction of excessively salty foods
- Restriction of I.V. fluid administration during labor

Drug therapy
- In severe preeclampsia: antihypertensives, such as hydralazine (Apresoline) and diazoxide (Hyperstat); Betamethasone (Celestone) to accelerate fetal lung maturation
- Magnesium sulfate to reduce the amount of acetylcholine produced by motor nerves, thereby preventing seizures

INTERVENTIONS AND RATIONALES
For all patients
- Assess the patient for edema and proteinuria, *which may indicate impending eclampsia.*
- Monitor daily weight *to identify sodium and water retention.*
- Maintain a high-protein diet with moderate sodium restriction *as a measure against PIH.*
- Maintain seizure precautions *to ensure patient safety.*
- Encourage bed rest in a left lateral recumbent position *to improve uterine and renal profusion.*

- Monitor fetal heart rate continuously during labor *to assess fetal well-being.*

For severe preeclampsia
- Assess maternal blood pressure every 4 hours or more frequently if unstable *to assess for abnormalities.*
- Monitor fetal heart rate *to assess for decreased variability after magnesium sulfate administration.*
- Monitor serum magnesium levels *to assess for toxicity.*
- If necessary, prepare the patient for amniocentesis *to assess fetal maturity.*
- Administer I.V. fluids, as prescribed. *I.V. fluids are restricted to 60 to 150 ml/hour in the preeclamptic patient in labor.*
- Obtain blood samples *for complete blood count, platelet count, and liver function studies and to determine serum levels of blood urea nitrogen, creatinine, and fibrin degradation products.* Be aware that patients are at risk for developing DIC.
- Be prepared to obtain a blood sample for typing and crossmatching *because the patient is at risk for developing placenta previa.*
- Obtain urine specimens to determine urine protein levels and specific gravity and perform 24-hour urine collection for protein and creatinine, as ordered, *to evaluate renal function.*
- Be prepared to administer I.V. magnesium sulfate *to evaluate for toxicity evidenced by deep tendon reflexes.*
- Monitor serum blood levels while the patient is receiving I.V. magnesium sulfate *to assess for magnesium sulfate toxicity.*
- Monitor urine output *to assess for complications.*
- Be prepared to administer calcium gluconate (*antidote to magnesium sulfate*) at first sign of magnesium sulfate toxicity (elevated serum levels, decreased deep tendon reflexes, muscle flaccidity, central nervous system depression, and decreased respiratory rate and renal function).
- Promote relaxation *to reduce fatigue.*
- Encourage the patient to verbalize her feelings *to allay anxiety.*

Memory jogger

Some women who develop preeclampsia also develop HELLP syndrome, so be alert if you notice the following signs.

Hemolysis

ELevated liver enzyme levels

Low **P**latelet count

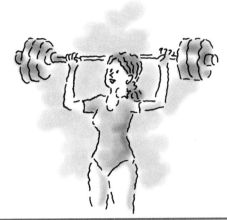

Pump up on practice questions

1. The caloric increase in nutritional requirements during pregnancy for a patient of normal weight is:
    A.   300 kcal.
    B.   400 kcal.
    C.   500 kcal.
    D.   1,000 kcal.
Answer: A. The recommended daily allowance in kilocalories during pregnancy is 300 kcal greater than the recommended daily allowance before pregnancy. The suggested daily allowance in kilocalories during lactation is 500 kcal more than the suggested daily allowance before pregnancy. An additional 1,000 kcal leads to excess weight gain. The amount recommended for underweight women may be more than 300 kcal.

➡ NCLEX keys
Nursing process step: Planning
Client needs category: Health promotion and maintenance
Client needs subcategory: Growth and development through the life span
Taxonomic Level: Knowledge

2. During prenatal screening of a diabetic client, the nurse should keep in mind that the client is at increased risk for:
    A.   Rh incompatibility.
    B.   placenta previa.
    C.   hyperemesis.
    D.   stillbirth.
Answer: D. Diabetic clients are at increased risk for intrauterine fetal death after 36 weeks' gestation. This factor must be weighed against the risks of delivery before 37 weeks and prematurity. The risk of Rh incompatibility, placenta previa, or hyperemesis isn't increased in the diabetic client.

➡ NCLEX keys
Nursing process step: Analysis
Client needs category: Physiological integrity
Client needs subcategory: Reduction of risk potential
Taxonomic level: Knowledge

3. When caring for the preeclamptic client during labor, the nurse should:
    A.   give a fluid bolus before the second stage.
    B.   give extra fluids throughout labor.
    C.   restrict the amount of fluid administered.
    D.   refrain from administering fluids during labor.
Answer: C. The volume of fluids administered to the preeclamptic client should be restricted. Clients usually receive between 60 and 150 ml/hour.

➡ NCLEX keys
Nursing process step: Implementation
Client needs category: Physiological integrity
Client needs subcategory: Physiological adaptation
Taxonomic level: Application

4. When caring for a preeclamptic client during labor, fetal monitoring should be performed:
    A.   before each contraction throughout labor.
    B.   between contractions throughout labor.
    C.   during each contraction throughout labor.
    D.   continuously throughout labor.

Answer: D. During labor, the fetus should be monitored continuously for signs of distress. Intermittent fetal monitoring isn't recommended for the preeclamptic client.

➡ NCLEX keys
Nursing process step: Planning
Client needs category: Health promotion and maintenance
Client needs subcategory: Growth and development through the life span
Taxonomic level: Knowledge

5. A pregnant client who is positive for human immunodeficiency virus asks the nurse about drug therapy. The nurse should tell the client to expect to:
A. start taking zidovudine between the 14th and 34th weeks.
B. delay taking zidovudine until after the fetus is born.
C. delay taking zidovudine until the third trimester.
D. delay starting zidovudine therapy in the newborn until age 6 months.

Answer: A. Zidovudine treatment should be initiated between weeks 14 and 34 of gestation. By taking zidovudine throughout pregnancy and labor, the risk of transmission to the fetus is significantly decreased. Zidovudine therapy in the newborn should be started immediately.

➡ NCLEX keys
Nursing process step: Planning
Client needs category: Physiological integrity
Client needs subcategory: Pharmacological and parenteral therapies
Taxonomic level: Knowledge

6. Which of the following medications promote fetal lung maturity in cases of preterm labor?
A. Terbutaline
B. Betamethasone
C. Co-trimoxazole
D. Clarithromycin

Answer: B. When the client experiences preterm labor and the probability of a continued pregnancy is in doubt, concern is raised regarding the fetus's respiratory potential.

Therefore the use of betamethasone, which stimulates the development of surfactant in the lung, is employed. Terbutaline is a beta-adrenergic agonist used to treat preterm labor. Co-trimoxazole is a sulfonamide often used to treat urinary tract infections, while clarithromycin is an antibiotic used to treat upper respiratory tract infections.

➡ NCLEX keys
Nursing process step: Planning
Client needs category: Physiological integrity
Client needs subcategory: Reduction of risk potential
Taxonomic level: Application

7. The client, a multigravida in her 38th week of gestation, has come to the emergency department complaining of chest pain. She tells the nurse that she has recently inhaled crack cocaine. The nurse's top priority is to assess the patient for:
A. abruptio placentae.
B. placenta accreta.
C. malnutrition.
D. hypotension.

Answer: A. The use of crack cocaine during pregnancy is associated with abruptio placentae, along with hypertension, cerebrovascular accident, tachycardia, hemorrhage, low birth weight, and preterm neonates. Crack cocaine isn't associated with placenta accreta (unusually deep attachment of the placenta to the uterine myometrium) or hypotension. Although malnutrition may exist, it isn't life-threatening at this point.

➡ NCLEX keys
Nursing process step: Assessment
Client needs category: Physiological integrity
Client needs subcategory: Reduction of risk potential
Taxonomic level: Analysis

8. The client, a multigravida in her 39th week of gestation, is diagnosed with PIH and HELLP syndrome. The nurse's top priority is to assess the client's:

A. white blood cell (WBC) count.
B. blood glucose levels.
C. plasma levels.
D. platelet count.

Answer: D. Women diagnosed with the HELLP syndrome have hemolysis of the red blood cells, elevated liver enzyme levels, and low platelet counts. This syndrome can lead to disseminated intravascular coagulation or hemorrhage. Monitoring the client's WBC count, blood glucose levels, and plasma levels isn't a priority for clients diagnosed with HELLP syndrome.

➡ NCLEX keys

Nursing process step: Assessment
Client needs category: Physiological integrity
Client needs subcategory: Reduction of risk potential
Taxonomic level: Analysis

9. Which of the following signs should the nurse expect to find during physical assessment of a primigravida in her 8th week of gestation?
    A. Ballottement
    B. Quickening
    C. Palpation of the fetal outline
    D. Hegar's sign

Answer: D. Hegar's sign (softening of the uterine isthmus) may be present at 6 to 8 weeks' gestation. Palpation of the fetal outline, quickening, and ballottement aren't detectable at 8 weeks' gestation.

➡ NCLEX keys

Nursing process step: Assessment
Client needs category: Health promotion and maintenance
Client needs subcategory: Growth and development through the life span
Taxonomic level: Knowledge

10. During her first clinic visit, the client reports that her last menstrual period (LMP) began on September 12. Based on Nägele's rule, what is the client's estimated date of delivery (EDD)?
    A. June 1
    B. June 19
    C. July 10
    D. July 29

Answer: B. The EDD is June 19. It equals the LMP (September 12) minus 3 months (June 12) and plus 7 days (June 19).

➡ NCLEX keys

Nursing process step: Assessment
Client needs category: Health promotion and maintenance
Client needs subcategory: Growth and development through the life span
Taxonomic level: Knowledge

Whew! Reviewing this chapter felt a bit like undergoing pregnancy. I need a rest.

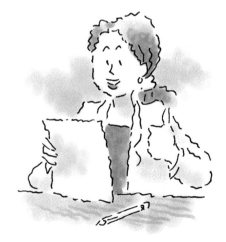

23 Intrapartum Care

Brush up on key concepts

In this chapter, you'll review:

- components and stages of labor
- how to perform maternal and fetal evaluations
- common complications of labor and delivery, such as preterm labor and prolapsed umbilical cord
- patient care for such situations as preterm labor and cesarean birth.

Intrapartum care refers to care of the patient during labor. In this section, you'll find a brief review of the signs and symptoms that indicate the onset of labor, the patient's physiologic and psychosocial responses to labor, basic obstetric procedures, and methods of monitoring the patient and fetus.

At any time, you can review the major points of this chapter by consulting the *Cheat sheet* on page 492.

Components of labor

The three important components of labor are the passage, the passenger, and the power. These components must work together for labor to progress normally.

Long and winding road

Passage refers to the maternal pelvis and soft tissues, the passageway through which the fetus exits the body. This area is affected by the shape of the inlet, structure of pelvis, and pelvic diameters.

Coach or first class?

Passenger refers to the fetus and its ability to move through the passage. This ability is affected by such fetal features as:
- the fetal skull
- the lie (relationship of the long axis [spine] of the fetus to the long axis of the mother)
- presentation (portion of the fetus that enters the pelvic passageway first)
- position (relationship of the presenting part of the fetus to the front, back, and sides of the maternal pelvis).

The fetal head can flex or extend 45 degrees and rotate 180 degrees, allowing its smallest diameters to move down the birth canal and pass through the maternal pelvis. Pressure exerted by the maternal pelvis and birth canal during labor and delivery causes the sutures of the skull to allow the cranial bones to shift, resulting in molding of the fetal head.

What kind of engine?

Power refers to uterine contractions, which cause complete cervical effacement and dilation.

Along for the ride

Other factors that affect labor are:
- accomplishment of the tasks of pregnancy
- coping mechanisms
- mother's ability to bear down (voluntary use of abdominal muscles to push during the second stage of labor)
- past experiences
- placental positioning
- preparation for childbirth
- psychological readiness
- support systems.

Let's get this show on the road

Preliminary signs that indicate the onset of labor include:
- lightening, or fetal descent into the pelvis, which usually occurs 2 to 3 weeks before term in a primiparous patient and later or during labor in a multiparous patient
- Braxton Hicks contractions, which can occur irregularly and intermittently throughout pregnancy and may become uncomfortable and produce false labor
- cervical changes, including softening, effacement, and slight dilation several days before the initiation of labor
- bloody show as the mucous plug is expelled from the cervix

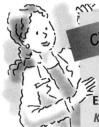

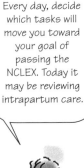

Cheat sheet

Intrapartum care refresher

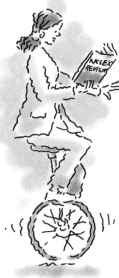

> Every day, decide which tasks will move you toward your goal of passing the NCLEX. Today it may be reviewing intrapartum care.

EMERGENCY BIRTH

Key signs and symptoms

For prolapsed umbilical cord
- Cord visible at the vaginal opening
- Variable decelerations or bradycardia noted on fetal monitor strip

For uterine rupture
- Abdominal pain and tenderness especially at the peak of a contraction or the feeling that "something ripped"
- Excessive external bleeding
- Late decelerations, reduced fetal heart rate (FHR) variability, tachycardia and bradycardia, cessation of FHR
- Palpation of the fetus outside the uterus

For amniotic fluid embolism
- Chest pain
- Coughing with pink, frothy sputum
- Increasing restlessness and anxiety
- Sudden dyspnea
- Tachypnea

Key test results

For prolapsed umbilical cord
- Ultrasonography confirms that the cord is prolapsed.

For uterine rupture
- Ultrasonography may reveal the absence of the amniotic cavity within the uterus.

For amniotic fluid embolism
- Arterial blood gas analysis reveals hypoxemia.

Key treatments

- Administration of oxygen by nasal cannula or mask (endotracheal intubation and mechanical ventilation may be necessary in the case of amniotic fluid embolism)
- Emergency cesarean delivery

Key interventions

- Monitor maternal vital signs, pulse oximetry, intake and output, and FHR.
- Administer maternal oxygen by cannula or mask at 8 to 10 L/minute.
- Initiate and maintain I.V. fluid replacement.

- Obtain blood samples to determine hematocrit, hemoglobin level, prothrombin and partial thromboplastin times, fibrinogen level, and platelet count and to type and crossmatch blood.
- Administer blood products, as necessary.

PRETERM LABOR

Key signs and symptoms

- Feeling of pelvic pressure or abdominal tightening
- Increased vaginal discharge
- Intestinal cramping
- Uterine contractions that result in cervical dilation and effacement

Key test results

- Electronic fetal monitoring confirms uterine contractions.
- Vaginal examination confirms cervical effacement and dilation.

Key treatments

- Betamethasone (Celestone) administered I.M. at regular intervals over 48 hours to increase fetal lung maturity in a fetus expected to be delivered preterm
- Tocolytic agents, such as terbutaline (Brethine) and ritodrine (Yutopar) to inhibit uterine contractions

Key interventions

- Monitor maternal vital signs, contractions, and FHR every 15 minutes during tocolytic therapy (otherwise, provide continuous fetal monitoring).
- Monitor for maternal adverse reactions to terbutaline or ritodrine.
- Monitor for magnesium sulfate toxicity and make sure calcium gluconate is available.
- Assess the neonate for possible adverse affects of indomethacin such as premature closure of the ductus arteriosus.

• rupture of membranes, occurring before the onset of labor in about 12% of patients and within 24 hours for about 80% of patients
• a sudden burst of energy before the onset of labor, commonly demonstrated by housecleaning activities and called the nesting instinct. (See *True or False?*)

Evaluating the mother during labor

Here is a review of methods and techniques used to monitor the progress of labor and the mother's condition.

Starting to open
Observe **dilation.** The external os opening should increase from 0 to 10 cm.

The thick and thin of it
Observe **effacement,** cervical thinning and shortening, which is measured from 0% (thick) to 100% (paper thin).

What's the situation?
Using abdominal palpation (Leopold's maneuvers), determine **fetal position and presentation.** The process consists of four maneuvers.

Palpate the fundus to identify the occupying fetal part: the fetus's head is firm and rounded and moves freely; the breech is softer and less regular and moves with the trunk.

Palpate the abdomen to locate the fetus's back; the back should feel firm, smooth, and convex, whereas the front is soft, irregular, and concave.

Determine the level of descent of the head by grasping the lower portion of the abdomen above the symphysis pubis to identify the fetal part presenting over the inlet; an unengaged head can be rocked from side to side.

Determine head flexion by moving fingers down both sides of the uterus to assess the descent of the presenting part into the pelvis; greater resistance is met as the fingers move downward on the cephalic prominence (brow) side.

What's the relationship?
Check the **station,** the relationship of the presenting part to the pelvic ischial spines.
• The presenting part is even with the ischial spines at 0 station.
• The presenting part is above the ischial spines at −3, −2, or −1.
• The presenting part is below the ischial spines at +1, +2, or +3.

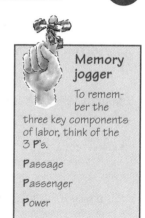

Memory jogger

To remember the three key components of labor, think of the 3 P's.

Passage

Passenger

Power

True or false?

Use the chart below to help distinguish between true and false labor.

TRUE LABOR	FALSE LABOR
Regular contractions	Irregular, brief contractions
Back discomfort that spreads to the abdomen	Discomfort that is localized in the abdomen
Progressive cervical effacement and dilation	No cervical change
Gradually shortened intervals between contractions	No change or irregular change in intervals between contractions
Increased intensity of contractions with ambulation	Contractions may be relieved with ambulation
Contractions that increase in duration and intensity	Usually no change in duration and intensity of contractions

Maternal responses to labor

During labor, the mother undergoes physiologic changes.

CARDIOVASCULAR SYSTEM
• Increased intrathoracic pressure during pushing in the second stage
• Increased peripheral resistance during contractions, which elevates blood pressure and decreases pulse rate
• Increased cardiac output

FLUID AND ELECTROLYTE BALANCE
• Increased water loss from diaphoresis and hyperventilation
• Increased evaporative water volume from increased respiratory rate

RESPIRATORY SYSTEM
• Increased oxygen consumption
• Increased respiratory rate

HEMATOPOIETIC SYSTEM
• Increased plasma fibrinogen level and leukocyte count
• Decreased blood coagulation time and blood glucose levels

GI SYSTEM
• Decreased gastric motility and absorption
• Prolonged gastric emptying time

RENAL SYSTEM
• Forward and upward displacement of the bladder base at engagement
• Possibly proteinuria from muscle breakdown
• Possibly impaired blood and lymph drainage from the bladder base, resulting from edema caused by the presenting fetal part
• Decreased bladder sensation if epidural anesthetic has been administered

Thirsty?
Monitor the patient for signs of **dehydration,** such as poor skin turgor, decreased urine output, and dry mucous membranes.

I need a little rest
Use an external pressure transducer to monitor the patient for **tetanic contractions,** sustained prolonged contractions with little rest between.

Measuring contractions
Phases of **uterine contractions** include increment (buildup and longest phase), acme (peak of the contraction), and decrement (letting-down phase). Contractions are measured by duration, frequency, and intensity. Here's how to measure each:
• **Duration** is measured from the beginning of the increment to the end of the decrement and averages 30 seconds early in labor and 60 seconds later in labor.
• **Frequency** is measured from the beginning of one contraction to the beginning of the next and averages 5 to 30 minutes apart early in labor and 2 to 3 minutes apart later in labor.

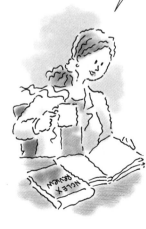

Key terms related to contractions: increment, acme, decrement, duration, frequency, and intensity.

• **Intensity** is assessed during the acme phase and can be measured with an intrauterine catheter or by palpation (normal resting pressure when using an intrauterine catheter is 5 to 15 mm Hg; pressure increases to 30 to 50 mm Hg during the acme).

All around adaptations
Labor also prompts a series of responses throughout the mother's body, including changes in the cardiovascular, respiratory, and GI systems. (See *Maternal responses to labor*.)

Evaluating the fetus during labor

Evaluation of uterine contractions and fetal heart rate (FHR) during labor involves both external and internal monitoring.

Heart check
FHR can be monitored either intermittently with a handheld device or continuously with a large fetal monitor. (See *Fetal heart rate patterns*.)

Pressure check

Contraction frequency and intensity is monitored externally with a **tocotransducer.** This pressure-sensitive device records uterine motion during contractions.

Electrode application

Internal electronic fetal monitoring can evaluate fetal status during labor more accurately than external methods. A spiral electrode attached to the presenting fetal part provides the baseline FHR and allows evaluation of FHR variability.

Intrauterine pressure check

To determine the true intensity of contractions, a **pressure-sensitive catheter** is inserted into the uterine cavity alongside the fetus.

Stages of labor

The labor process is divided into four stages, ranging from the onset of true labor, through delivery of the fetus and placenta, to the first hour after delivery.

Fetal heart rate patterns

Here is a quick review of fetal heart rate (FHR) patterns.

DECELERATIONS OF FHR
Decelerations of FHR can be a reassuring sign but may also indicate complications.

Slow going early on
Early decelerations are caused by head compression in the fetus. They are smooth, uniformly shaped waveforms that inversely mirror the corresponding contractions. Early decelerations:
- normally range from 120 to 160 beats/minute
- are a reassuring pattern not associated with fetal difficulties
- provide patient reassurance.

Slow going later on
Later decelerations are caused by uteroplacental insufficiency. They are smooth, uniformly shaped waveforms that inversely mirror the contractions but are late in onset and may remain after the contraction is over. Later decelerations:
- are usually within the normal range with a high baseline but may drop to below 100 beats/minute when severe
- are considered an ominous sign if they are persistent and uncorrected; the pattern is associated with decreased Apgar scores, fetal hypoxia, and acidosis
- may require emergency cesarean birth if persistent.

Slow going, here and there
Variable decelerations of FHR are due to umbilical cord compression. They vary in onset, occurrence, and waveform. Characteristics of variable decelerations are:
- a heart rate that may (in severe cases) decelerate below 70 beats/minute for more than 30 seconds with a slow return to baseline

- an occurrence in about 50% of labors
- usually transient and correctable
- not associated with low Apgar scores.

ACCELERATIONS OF FHR
Accelerations of FHR are normally caused by fetal movements but can also occur with contractions. Accelerations of FHR:
- can be uniformly or variably shaped
- are usually above 150 beats/minute.

VARIABILITY OF FHR
Normal cardiac irregularity is caused by continuous interplay of the parasympathetic and sympathetic nervous systems. This normal variability can be long term (rhythmic fluctuations and waves occurring three to five times/minute) or short term (beat-to-beat changes between 6 and 10 beats/minute).

Beware of increase
Increased variability can be caused by early, mild hypoxia and fetal stimulation. This is the earliest sign of mild fetal hypoxia that accompanies fetal vein compression. Carefully evaluate the FHR tracing for signs of fetal distress.

Beware of decrease
Decreased variability can be caused by hypoxia, acidosis, central nervous system depressants, or medications and may require fetal blood sampling or internal monitoring. Decreased variability is:
- benign when associated with analgesics
- ominous if caused by hypoxia or associated with late decelerations.

FIRST STAGE

The first stage is measured from the onset of true labor to complete dilation of the cervix. This period lasts from 6 to 18 hours in a primiparous patient and from 2 to 10 hours in a multiparous patient. There are three phases of stage one.

This is getting exciting

During the **latent phase,** the cervix is dilated 0 to 3 cm, contractions are irregular, and the patient may experience anticipation, excitement, or apprehension.

This is getting serious

During the **active phase,** the cervix is dilated 4 to 7 cm. Contractions are about 5 to 8 minutes apart and last 45 to 60 seconds with moderate to strong intensity. During this phase, the patient becomes serious and concerned about the progress of labor; she may ask for pain medication or use breathing techniques. If membranes have not ruptured spontaneously, amniotomy may be performed.

Whole lotta shakin' going on

During the **transitional phase,** the cervix is dilated 8 to 10 cm. Contractions are about 1 to 2 minutes apart and last 60 to 90 seconds with strong intensity. During this phase, the patient may lose control, thrash in bed, groan, or cry out.

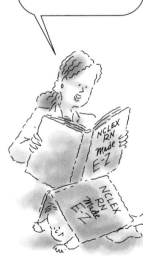

Remember that the patient shouldn't try to push until the cervix is completely dilated.

Nursing care during labor and delivery

Nursing actions include interventions that correspond to all stages of labor as well as those that apply only to certain stages.

CARE DURING ALL STAGES OF LABOR

- Monitor and record vital signs, I.V. fluid intake, and urine output.
- Provide emotional support to the patient and her coach.
- Assess the need for pain medication, and evaluate the effectiveness of pain-relief measures.
- Maintain aseptic technique and standard precautions.
- Maintain the patient's comfort by offering mouth care, ice chips, and a change of bed linen.
- Explain the purpose of all nursing actions and medical equipment.

CARE DURING FIRST AND SECOND STAGES

- Inform the patient of labor progress, such as dilation, station, effacement, and fetal well-being.
- Monitor the frequency, duration, and intensity of contractions.
- Monitor fetal heart rate (FHR) during and between contractions, noting rate, accelerations, decelerations, and variability.

- Observe for rupture of membranes, noting the time, color, odor, amount, and consistency of amniotic fluid.
- Observe for prolapsed cord and check FHR immediately after rupture of membranes.
- Assess for signs of hypotensive supine syndrome; if blood pressure falls, position the patient on the left side, increase the I.V. flow rate, and administer oxygen through a face mask at 6 to 10 L/minute.
- During the second stage, observe the perineum for show and bulging.

CARE DURING FIRST, SECOND, AND THIRD STAGES

- Assist with breathing techniques.
- Encourage rest between contractions.

CARE DURING THE FOURTH STAGE

- Assess lochia and the location and consistency of the fundus.
- Encourage bonding.
- Initiate breast-feeding.

SECOND STAGE

The second stage of labor extends from complete dilation to delivery. This stage lasts an average of 40 minutes (20 contractions) for the primiparous patient and 20 minutes (10 contractions) for the multiparous patient. It may last longer if the patient has had epidural anesthesia.

The patient may become exhausted and dehydrated as she moves from coping with contractions to actively pushing. During this stage, the fetus is moved along the birth canal by the mechanisms of labor listed below.

A brief engagement

The fetus's head is considered to be **engaged** when the biparietal diameter passes the pelvic inlet.

Going down

The movement of the presenting part through the pelvis is called **descent.**

Flex that chin

During **flexion,** the head flexes so that the chin moves closer to the chest.

Head rotation I

Internal rotation is the rotation of the head in order to pass through the ischial spines.

Stretch

Extension is when the head extends as it passes under the symphysis pubis.

Head rotation II

External rotation involves the external rotation of the head as the shoulders rotate to the anteroposterior position in the pelvis.

THIRD STAGE

The third stage of labor extends from delivery of the neonate to expulsion of the placenta and lasts from 5 to 30 minutes.

Pain, then placenta

During this period, the patient typically focuses on the neonate's condition. The patient may experience discomfort from uterine contractions before expelling the placenta.

FOURTH STAGE

The fourth stage of labor is the 1st hour after delivery, when the primary activity is the promotion of maternal-neonatal bonding.

For a review of nursing actions during the delivery process, see *Nursing care during labor and delivery.*

Pain relief during labor and delivery

Pain relief is an important element of patient care during labor and delivery. Pain relief during labor includes nonpharmacologic methods, analgesics, and general and regional anesthetics.

Just rub it

Effleurage, a light abdominal stroking with the fingertips in a circular motion, is effective for mild to moderate discomfort.

Hey, look over here

Distraction can divert attention from mild discomfort early in labor.

Breathing, breathing, breathing

Three patterns of controlled chest breathing, called **Lamaze breathing,** are used primarily during the active and transitional phases of labor.

Ancient pain relief

The stimulation of key trigger points with needles (**acupuncture**) or finger pressure (**acupressure**) can reduce pain and enhance energy flow.

Pain relief but not without risk

Opioids such as meperidine (Demerol) can be used to relieve pain. If medication is given within 2 hours of delivery, it can cause neonatal respiratory depression, hypotonia, and lethargy.

Knockout drops

General anesthetics can be administered I.V. or through inhalation, resulting in unconsciousness. General anesthetics should be

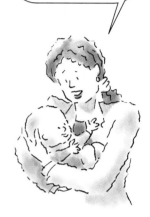

Helping to promote maternal-neonatal bonding is a key nursing responsibility in the 1st hour after delivery.

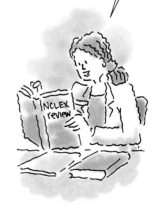

Pain relief during labor includes nonpharmacologic methods, analgesics, and general and regional anesthetics.

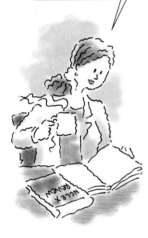

Hypotension after an epidural is uncommon but may occur if the patient doesn't receive enough fluids beforehand.

used only if regional anesthetics are contraindicated or in a rapidly developing emergency.

I.V. anesthetics, which are usually reserved for patients with massive blood loss, include:
• thiopental (Pentothal)
• ketamine (Ketalar).
   Inhalation anesthetics include:
• nitrous oxide
• isoflurane (Forane)
• halothane (Fluothane).

Less pain but still awake

Lumbar epidural anesthesia requires an injection of medication into the epidural space in the lumbar region, leaving the patient awake and cooperative. An epidural provides analgesia for the first and second stages of labor and anesthesia for delivery without adverse fetal effects. Hypotension is uncommon, but its incidence increases if the patient doesn't receive a proper fluid load before the procedure. Epidural anesthesia may decrease the woman's urge to push.

Urgent cases

Spinal anesthesia involves an injection of medication into the cerebrospinal fluid in the spinal canal. Because of its rapid onset, spinal anesthesia is useful for urgent cesarean deliveries.

Delivery relief

Local infiltration involves an injection of anesthesia into the perineal nerves. It offers no relief from discomfort during labor but relieves pain during delivery.

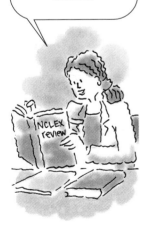

Here are two numbers to remember: a fetal blood pH of 7.25 or higher is normal. A blood pH lower than 7.2 indicates severe acidosis.

Pain blocker I

A **pudendal block** involves blockage of the pudendal nerve. This procedure is used only for delivery.

Pain blocker II

A **paracervical block** involves the blockage of nerves in the peridural space at the sacral hiatus, which provides analgesia for the first and second stages of labor and anesthesia for delivery. This procedure increases the risk of forceps delivery.

Keep abreast of diagnostic tests

The key diagnostic test in the intrapartum period is fetal blood sampling.

Blood acid-base balance

Fetal blood sampling is a method of monitoring fetal blood pH when indefinite or suspicious FHR patterns occur. The blood sample is usually taken from the scalp but may also be taken from the presenting part if the fetus is in a breech presentation. Fetal blood sampling requires that:
• membranes be ruptured
• the cervix be dilated 2 to 3 cm
• the presenting part must be no higher than –2 station.

A pH of 7.25 and higher is normal, 7.20 to 7.24 is preacidotic, and lower than 7.2 constitutes severe acidosis.

Nursing actions

• After the procedure, observe the FHR and observe the patient for vaginal bleeding, which may indicate fetal scalp bleeding.

Catch up on complications

Some common intrapartum complications are dystocia, premature rupture of membranes, amniotic fluid embolism, prolapsed umbilical cord, inverted uterus, early postpartum hemorrhage, and fetal distress.

Harder than it should be

Dystocia, or difficult labor, can be caused by a contracted pelvis or obstructive tumors in the mother or by malpresentation or malformation of the fetus. Functional causes include hypertonic or hypotonic uterine patterns.

Assessment findings

• Arrested descent
• Hypertonic contractions

- Hypotonic contractions
- Prolonged active phase
- Prolonged deceleration phase
- Protracted latent phase
- Uncoordinated contractions

Care measures
- Administration of I.V. fluids
- Support and encouragement
- Placing the patient in a side-lying position.
- Urging the patient to void every 2 hours

It's a little early for this
In **premature rupture of membranes,** rupture occurs 1 or more hours before the onset of labor. Chorioamnionitis may occur if the time between rupture of membranes and onset of labor is longer than 24 hours.

Assessment findings
- Fetal tachycardia
- Foul-smelling amniotic fluid
- Maternal fever
- Uterine tenderness

Care measures
- Assessment for signs of infection or fetal distress
- Induction of labor or cesarean delivery if labor doesn't start within 24 hours of membrane rupture
- Possible administration of antibiotics

That seemed awfully quick
Precipitate labor lasts 3 hours or less. It's usually caused by lack of maternal tissue resistance to the passage of the fetus.

Assessment findings
- Cervical dilation greater than 5 cm/hr in a nulliparous woman; more than 10 cm/hr in a multiparous woman

Care measures
- Monitoring of fetal heart rate and variability
- Possible administration of tocolytic drugs to reduce force and frequency of contractions

Dangerous fluid escape
In **amniotic fluid embolism,** amniotic fluid escapes into the maternal circulation because of a defect in the membranes after rupture or partial abruptio placentae. During labor (or in the postpartum period), solid particles such as skin cells enter the maternal circulation and reach the lungs as small emboli, forcing a massive pulmonary embolism.

Assessment findings
- Chest pain
- Coughing with pink, frothy sputum
- Cyanosis
- Hemorrhage
- Increasing restlessness and anxiety
- Shock disproportionate to blood loss
- Sudden dyspnea
- Tachypnea

Care measures
- Administration of blood replacement, platelets, or fibrinogen to correct coagulation defects, as necessary
- Administration of oxygen, blood, and heparin
- Cardiopulmonary resuscitation, if necessary
- Fluid replacement, as ordered
- Immediate delivery of infant
- Insertion of a central venous pressure line
- Mechanical ventilation, if necessary
- Monitoring cardiovascular status

Cord first
A **prolapsed umbilical cord** occurs when the umbilical cord descends into the vagina before the presenting part.

Assessment findings
- Cord palpable during vaginal examination
- Cord visible at the vaginal opening
- Variable decelerations or bradycardia noted on fetal monitor strip

Care measures
- Placing the patient in Trendelenburg's position (position the woman's hips higher than her head in a knee-to-chest position) to relieve pressure on the umbilical cord and restore blood flow to the fetus
- Applying warm saline-moistened towels to the protruding cord to prevent drying and retard cooling of the cord

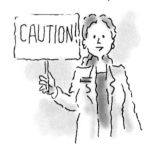

If the membrane ruptures 1 or more hours before labor begins, it may indicate infection or other fetal distress.

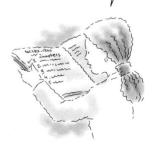

In amniotic fluid embolism, amniotic fluid escapes into the maternal circulation. It's an emergency situation that may require cardiopulmonary resuscitation.

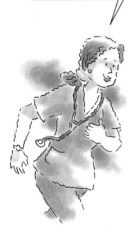

Umbilical cord prolapse, when the umbilical cord descends into the vagina before the presenting fetal part, is an emergency that requires prompt action to save the fetus.

• Maintaining the patient with her hips elevated with pillows and in side-lying position
• Immediately delivering the fetus. With a sterile gloved hand, push the presenting fetal part upward until delivery is accomplished; do not attempt to replace any part of the protruding cord back into the vagina. This could reduce blood flow further and, possibly, traumatize the cord.

Inside out
An **inverted uterus** can occur during delivery of the placenta. The inversion can be partial or total.

Assessment findings
• Hemorrhage
• Inability to palpate the fundus
• Severe uterine pain
• Uterine mass within the vaginal canal

Care measures
• Administration of fluids, blood, and oxygen
• Manually replacing the uterus immediately
• Monitoring vital signs
• Possible emergency hysterectomy

Postdelivery blood loss
Early postpartum hemorrhage indicates blood loss of 500 ml or more during the 1st hour after delivery.

Assessment findings
• Uterine atony

Care measures
• Administration of oxytocin I.V.
• Assessing for bladder distention
• Examination of possible bleeding sites in vagina
• Massaging the uterus
• Monitoring amount and color of vaginal bleeding
• Monitoring postdelivery uterine contractions
• Monitoring vital signs every 15 minutes until stable

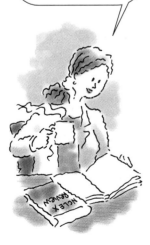

Here's a number to know: 500 ml or more of blood loss within 1 hour of delivery indicates postpartum hemorrhage.

Stressful and potentially lethal
Fetal distress refers to a fetal compromise that results in a stressful and potentially lethal condition.

Care measures
• Administering oxygen by face mask according to facility protocol or the doctor's order (typically 6 to 8 L/minute)
• Discontinuing oxytocin infusion
• Monitoring FHR, fetal activity, and fetal heart variability
• Notifying the doctor immediately
• Positioning the patient on her left side
• Possible placement of an internal fetal monitor
• Fetal scalp blood sampling to determine blood pH
• Amnioinfusion, if the fetus exhibits variable deceleration not relieved by oxygen, positioning, or discontinuation of oxytocin infusion (See *Understanding amnioinfusion*.)

Degrees of tear
Laceration refers to tears in the perineum, vagina, or cervix from the stretching of tissues during delivery. Lacerations are classified as first, second, third, or fourth degree.

First-degree laceration involves the vaginal mucosa and the skin of the perineum and fourchette.

Second-degree laceration involves the vagina, perineal skin, fascia, levator ani muscle, and perineal body.

Third-degree laceration involves the entire perineum and the external anal sphincter.

Fourth-degree laceration involves the entire perineum, rectal sphincter, and portions of the rectal mucosa.

Assessment findings
• Increased vaginal bleeding after delivery of placenta

Now I get it

Understanding amnioinfusion

Amnioinfusion is the replacement of amniotic fluid volume through intrauterine infusion of a saline solution, using a pressure catheter. This procedure is indicated for the treatment of repetitive variable decelerations not alleviated by maternal position change and oxygen administration.

Amnioinfusion relieves umbilical cord compression in such conditions as:
- oligohydramnios associated with postmaturity
- intrauterine growth retardation
- premature rupture of membranes.

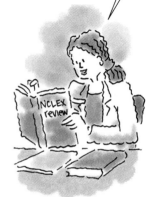

Hmmm. Lacerations can be first-, second-, third-, or fourth- degree.

Care measures
- Preparing for insertion of an underlying urinary catheter
- Providing maternal support and explaining the procedure
- Refraining from taking rectal temperature or administering suppositories or enemas to a patient with a third- or fourth-degree laceration

Blood trouble
Disseminated intravascular coagulation (DIC) refers to increased production of prothrombin, platelets, and other coagulation factors, leading to widespread thrombus formation, depletion of clotting factors, and hemorrhage.

Assessment findings
- Decreased fibrinogen level and platelet count
- Prolonged prothrombin time
- Partial thromboplastin time
- Thrombocytopenia

Care measures
- Administration of blood and fibrinogen transfusions
- Treatment of underlying condition
- Administration of heparin
- Immediate delivery of fetus

Something ripped
A **uterine rupture** occurs when the uterus undergoes more strain than it can bear. It can be caused by prolonged labor, faulty presentation, multiple gestation, obstructed labor, and trauma.

Assessment findings
- Abdominal pain and tenderness, especially at the peak of a contraction, or the feeling that "something ripped"
- Cessation of uterine contractions
- Chest pain or pain on inspiration
- Excessive external bleeding
- Hypovolemic shock caused by hemorrhage
- Late decelerations, reduced FHR variability, tachycardia and bradycardia, cessation of FHR
- Palpation of the fetus outside the uterus
- Pathological retraction ring (indentation apparent across abdomen and over the uterus)

Care measures
- Administration of a tocolytic drug to reduce the intensity of the contractions
- Blood replacement, as necessary

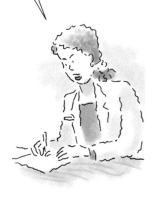

Note the most common complications indicating emergency birth: prolapsed umbilical cord, uterine rupture, and amniotic fluid embolism.

Emergency birth and preterm labor

Emergency birth and preterm labor are two examples of conditions requiring nursing care that may occur during the intrapartum period.

Emergency birth

Emergency delivery of the fetus may become necessary when the well-being of the mother or fetus is in jeopardy. Causes may include a prolapsed umbilical cord, uterine rupture, or amniotic fluid embolism.

CAUSES

Contributing factors vary for each emergency birth situation.

Prolapsed umbilical cord
• Fetus at high fetal station
• Hydramnios (excess of amniotic fluid)
• Multifetal pregnancy
• Small fetus or breech presentation
• Transverse lie

Uterine rupture
• Blunt abdominal trauma
• High parity with thin uterine wall
• Intense uterine contractions (natural or oxytocin-induced), especially with fetopelvic disproportion
• Previous uterine surgery

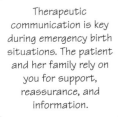

Therapeutic communication is key during emergency birth situations. The patient and her family rely on you for support, reassurance, and information.

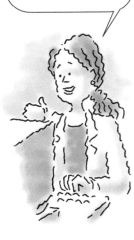

Amniotic fluid embolism
• Fetal particulate matter (skin, hair, vernix, cells, meconium) in the fluid that obstructs the maternal pulmonary vessels

ASSESSMENT FINDINGS
Assessment findings vary for each emergency birth situation.

Prolapsed umbilical cord
• Cord palpable during vaginal examination
• Cord visible at the vaginal opening
• Variable decelerations or bradycardia noted on fetal monitor strip

Uterine rupture
• Abdominal pain and tenderness especially at the peak of a contraction or the feeling that "something ripped"
• Cessation of uterine contractions
• Chest pain or pain on inspiration
• Excessive external bleeding
• Hypovolemic shock caused by hemorrhage
• Late decelerations, reduced FHR variability, tachycardia and bradycardia, cessation of FHR
• Palpation of the fetus outside the uterus

Amniotic fluid embolism
• Chest pain
• Coughing with pink, frothy sputum
• Cyanosis
• Hemorrhage
• Increasing restlessness and anxiety
• Shock disproportionate to blood loss
• Sudden dyspnea
• Tachypnea

DIAGNOSTIC TEST RESULTS

Prolapsed umbilical cord
• Ultrasonography confirms that the cord is prolapsed.

Uterine rupture
• Urinalysis can detect gross hematuria.
• Ultrasonography may reveal the absence of the amniotic cavity within the uterus.

Amniotic fluid embolism
• Arterial blood gas analysis reveals hypoxemia.
• Hematology reveals thrombocytopenia, decreased fibrinogen level and platelet count, prolonged prothrombin time, and a partial thromboplastin time consistent with DIC.

NURSING DIAGNOSES
• Ineffective individual coping
• Pain
• Risk of infection

TREATMENT
• Administration of I.V. fluid
• Administration of oxygen by nasal cannula or mask (endotracheal intubation and me-

Cesarean delivery

Cesarean delivery is the planned or emergency removal of the neonate from the uterus through an abdominal incision. The surgical incision may be midline and vertical (classic), allowing easy access to the fetus, and is usually the approach of choice in emergency situations. A low-segment, transverse, or Pfannenstiel's (bikini) incision is usually chosen in a planned cesarean birth.

NURSING ACTIONS

During a cesarean birth, you should:
• provide emotional support and reassurance to the patient and family, including reassurance about the well-being of the fetus
• assess fetal heart rate, maternal vital signs, and intake and output
• monitor uterine contractions and labor progress, when appropriate
• obtain blood samples for hematocrit, hemoglobin level, prothrombin and partial thromboplastin times, fibrinogen level, platelet count, and typing and crossmatching
• initiate and maintain I.V. fluid replacement, as necessary
• prepare the patient for surgery, including shaving of the abdomen and perineal area as necessary
• insert an indwelling urinary catheter, as ordered
• provide preoperative teaching as necessary
• administer preoperative sedation as ordered
• provide immediate postoperative care after surgery.

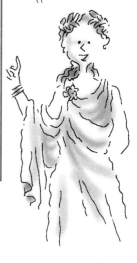

Friends, Romans, countrymen. Cesarean delivery is the most common method of treating emergency birth situations.

chanical ventilation may be necessary in the case of amniotic fluid embolism)
• Emergency cesarean delivery (See *Cesarean delivery.*)
• Emergency hysterectomy (with uterine rupture)
• Possible transfusion of packed red blood cells, fresh frozen plasma, or platelets

INTERVENTIONS AND RATIONALES
• Monitor maternal vital signs, pulse oximetry, intake and output, and FHR *to assess for complications.*
• Administer maternal oxygen by cannula or mask at 8 to 10 L/minute *to maintain uteroplacental oxygenation.*
• Initiate and maintain I.V. fluid replacement *to replace volume loss.*
• Provide emotional support and reassurance to the patient *to allay fears and reduce anxiety.*
• Obtain blood samples to determine hematocrit, hemoglobin level, prothrombin and partial thromboplastin times, fibrinogen level, and platelet count and type and crossmatch blood *to establish baseline values.*

• Administer blood products as necessary *to replace volume loss.*
• Prepare the patient and her family for the possibility of cesarean delivery *to reduce anxiety.*

Teaching topics
• Information about procedures
• Preoperative instruction
• Breathing techniques

Preterm labor

Preterm labor, also known as premature labor, occurs before the end of the 37th week of gestation. Preterm labor can place both the patient and the fetus at high risk.

CAUSES AND RISK FACTORS
Causes and risk factors of preterm labor can be maternal or fetal.

Maternal causes
• Abdominal surgery or trauma
• Cardiovascular and renal disease

• Dehydration
• Diabetes mellitus
• Incompetent cervix
• Infection
• Placental abnormalities
• Pregnancy-induced hypertension
• Premature rupture of membranes

Fetal causes
• Hydramnios
• Infection
• Multifetal pregnancy

ASSESSMENT FINDINGS
• Feeling of pelvic pressure or abdominal tightening
• Increased vaginal discharge
• Intestinal cramping
• Menstrual-like cramps
• Persistent, low, dull backache
• Uterine contractions that result in cervical dilation and effacement
• Vaginal spotting

DIAGNOSTIC TEST RESULTS
• Electronic fetal monitoring confirms uterine contractions.
• Vaginal examination confirms cervical effacement and dilation.

NURSING DIAGNOSES
• Anxiety
• Knowledge deficit
• Risk for injury

TREATMENT
• Suppression of preterm labor (if fetal membranes are intact, there is no evidence of bleeding, the well-being of the fetus and mother isn't in jeopardy, cervical effacement is no more than 50%, and cervical dilation is less than 4 cm)

Drug therapy
• Betamethasone (Celestone) administered I.M. at regular intervals over 48 hours to increase fetal lung maturity in a fetus expected to be delivered preterm
• Nifedipine (Procardia), a calcium channel blocker, to decrease the production of calcium, a substance associated with the initiation

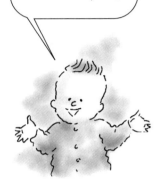

What can I say...some times I show up late, some times I show up early!

of labor; adverse maternal effects include dizziness, nausea, bradycardia, and flushing.
• Indomethacin (Indocin) to decrease the production of prostaglandins and lipid compounds associated with the initiation of labor; adverse maternal effects include nausea, vomiting, and dyspepsia; premature closure of the fetus's ductus arteriosus can occur if indomethacin is given before 32 weeks' gestation.
• Magnesium sulfate to prevent a reflux of calcium into the myometrial cells, thereby maintaining a relaxed uterus
• Tocolytic agents, such as terbutaline sulfate (Brethine) and ritodrine (Yutopar), to inhibit uterine contractions

INTERVENTIONS AND RATIONALES
• Monitor maternal vital signs, contractions, and FHR every 15 minutes during tocolytic therapy (otherwise, provide continuous fetal monitoring) *to assess maternal and fetal well-being.*
• Assess the mother's respiratory status *to assess for pulmonary edema, an adverse effect associated with tocolytic therapy).*
• Monitor for maternal adverse reactions to terbutaline or ritodrine *to detect possible tachycardia, diarrhea, nervousness, tremors, nausea, vomiting, headache, hyperglycemia, hypoglycemia, hypokalemia, or pulmonary edema.*
• Notify the doctor if the maternal pulse rate exceeds 120 beats/minute or the FHR exceeds 180 beats/minute *to expedite medical evaluation of maternal and fetal status.*
• Provide emotional support to the mother *to ease anxiety and establish a therapeutic relationship.*
• Monitor laboratory results *to detect abnormalities and initiate early intervention.*
• Place the patient in the lateral position *to increase placental perfusion.*
• Be prepared to administer propranolol (Inderal) *to counteract an adverse reaction or an overdose of terbutaline or ritodrine.*
• Monitor for magnesium sulfate toxicity, *which causes central nervous system depression in the mother and fetus,* and make sure calcium gluconate is available *to reverse these effects.*

• Assess the neonate for possible adverse effects (premature closure of the ductus arteriosus) *if indomethacin was administered before 32 weeks' gestation.*
• Administer nifedipine (Procardia), and monitor for adverse maternal effects, such as dizziness, nausea, bradycardia, and flushing, *which may compromise maternal and fetal well-being.*

Teaching topics
• Instructions for ongoing tocolytic therapy, if appropriate

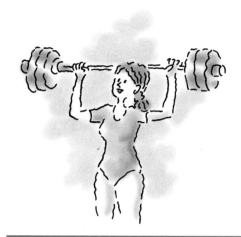

Pump up on practice questions

1. A client in the 28th week of gestation comes to the emergency department because she thinks that she's in labor. To confirm a diagnosis of preterm labor, the nurse would expect physical examination to reveal:
    A. irregular uterine contractions with no cervical dilation.
    B. painful contractions with no cervical dilation.
    C. regular uterine contractions with cervical dilation.
    D. regular uterine contractions with no cervical dilation.
Answer: C. Regular uterine contractions (every 10 minutes or more) along with cervical dilation before 36 weeks' gestation or rupture of fluids indicates preterm labor. Uterine contractions without cervical change don't indicate preterm labor.

➡ *NCLEX keys*
Nursing process step: Analysis
Client needs category: Health promotion and maintenance
Client needs subcategory: Prevention and early detection of disease
Taxonomic level: Knowledge

2. A client in the active phase of labor has a reactive fetal monitor strip and has been encouraged to walk. When she returns to bed for a monitor check, she complains of an urge to push. When performing a vaginal examination, the nurse accidentally ruptures the amniotic membranes, and as she withdraws her hand, the umbilical cord comes out. What should the nurse do next?

    A. Put the client in a knee-to-chest position.
    B. Call the physician or midwife.
    C. Push down on the uterine fundus.
    D. Set up for a fetal blood sampling to assess for fetal acidosis.

Answer: A. The knee-to-chest position gets the weight off the baby and umbilical cord, which would prevent blood flow. Calling the physician or midwife and setting up for blood sampling are important, but they have a lower priority than getting the baby off the cord. Pushing down on the fundus would increase the danger by further compromising blood flow.

➡ *NCLEX keys*
Nursing process step: Implementation
Client needs category: Physiological integrity
Client needs subcategory: Reduction of risk potential
Taxonomic level: Analysis

3. A client is attempting to deliver vaginally despite the fact that her previous delivery was by cesarean section. Her contractions are 2 to 3 minutes apart, lasting from 75 to 100 seconds. Suddenly, the client complains of intense abdominal pain and the fetal monitor stops picking up contractions. The nurse recognizes that which of the following has occurred?

    A. Abruptio placentae
    B. Prolapsed cord
    C. Partial placenta previa
    D. Complete uterine rupture

Answer: D. In complete uterine rupture, the client would feel a sharp pain in the lower abdomen and contractions would cease. Fetal heart rate would also cease within a few minutes. Uterine irritability would continue to be indicated by the fetal heart monitor tracing with abruptio placentae. With a prolapsed cord, contractions would continue and there would be no pain from the prolapse itself. There would be vaginal bleeding with a partial placenta previa, but no pain outside of the expected pain of contractions.

➡ *NCLEX keys*
Nursing process step: Assessment
Client needs category: Physiological integrity
Client needs subcategory: Physiological adaptation
Taxonomic level: Application

4. A client with gravida 3 para 2 (three pregnancies and two children) at 40 weeks' gestation is admitted with spontaneous contractions. The physician performs an amniotomy to augment her labor. The priority nursing action is to:

    A. explain the rationale for the amniotomy to the client.
    B. assess fetal heart tones after the amniotomy.
    C. ambulate the client to strengthen the contraction pattern.
    D. position the client in a lithotomy position to administer perineal care.

Answer: B. The nurse should assess fetal heart tones. After an amniotomy is performed, the umbilical cord may be washed down below the presenting part and cause umbilical cord compression, which would be indicated by variable deceleration on the fetal heart tracing. An explanation of the rationale for amniotomy would be given before the procedure. After assessing the fetal response to the amniotomy, perineal care is provided. The nurse would ambulate the client only if the presenting part were engaged.

➡ *NCLEX keys*
Nursing process step: Implementation
Client needs category: Physiological integrity
Client needs subcategory: Reduction of risk potential
Taxonomic level: Knowledge

5. The nurse can consider the fetus's head to be engaged when:
 A. the presenting part moves through the pelvis.
 B. the fetal head rotates to pass through the ischial spines.
 C. the fetal head extends as it passes under the symphysis pubis.
 D. the biparietal diameter passes the pelvic inlet.

Answer: D. The fetus's head is considered engaged when the biparietal diameter passes the pelvic inlet. The presenting part moving through the pelvis is called descent. The head flexing so that the chin moves closer to the chest is called flexion. Rotation of the head to pass through the ischial spines is called internal rotation. Extension of the head as it passes under the symphysis pubis is called extension.

➡ **NCLEX keys**
Nursing process step: Assessment
Client needs category: Health promotion and maintenance
Client needs subcategory: Prevention and early detection of disease
Taxonomic level: Analysis

6. A client is experiencing true labor when her contraction pattern shows:
 A. occasional irregular contractions.
 B. irregular contractions that increase in intensity.
 C. regular contractions that remain the same.
 D. regular contractions that increase in frequency and duration.

Answer: D. Regular contractions that increase in frequency and duration as well as intensity indicate true labor. The other choices don't describe the contraction pattern of true labor.

➡ **NCLEX keys**
Nursing process step: Assessment
Client needs category: Safe, effective care management
Client needs subcategory: Safety and infection control
Taxonomic level: Knowledge

7. A client is admitted to the hospital with contractions that are about 1 to 2 minutes apart and last for 60 seconds. Vaginal examination reveals that her cervix is dilated 8 cm. The client is in which stage of labor?
 A. The latent phase
 B. The active phase
 C. The third stage
 D. The transitional phase

Answer: D. The client is in the transitional phase of labor. This phase of labor is characterized by cervical dilation of 8 to 10 cm and contractions that are about 1 to 2 minutes apart and last for 60 to 90 seconds with strong intensity. In the latent phase, the cervix is dilated 0 to 3 cm and contractions are irregular. During the active phase, the cervix is dilated 4 to 7 cm, and contractions are about 5 to 8 minutes apart and last 45 to 60 seconds with moderate to strong intensity. The third stage of labor extends from delivery of the neonate to expulsion of the placenta and lasts from 5 to 30 minutes.

➡ **NCLEX keys**
Nursing process step: Assessment
Client needs category: Health promotion and maintenance
Client needs subcategory: Growth and development through the life span
Taxonomic level: Knowledge

8. A client in the second stage of labor experiences rupture of the membranes. The most appropriate intervention by the nurse is to:
 A. assess the client's vital signs immediately.
 B. observe for prolapsed cord and monitor fetal heart rate (FHR).
 C. administer oxygen through a face mask at 6 to 10 L/minute.
 D. position the client on her left side.

Answer: B. The nurse should immediately check for prolapsed cord and monitor FHR. When the membranes rupture, the cord may become compressed between the fetus and maternal cervix or pelvis, thus compromising fetoplacental perfusion. It isn't necessary to position the client on her left side, monitor maternal vital signs, or administer oxygen when the client's membranes rupture.

➡ *NCLEX keys*

Nursing process step: Implementation
Client needs category: Health promotion and maintenance
Client needs subcategory: Growth and development through the life span
Taxonomic level: Application

9. A client in labor is being monitored by an internal electronic device to evaluate fetal status. The nurse measures the duration of her contractions by:

    A. measuring from the beginning of the increment to the end of the decrement.

    B. measuring from the beginning of one contraction to the beginning of the next.

    C. measuring from the beginning of the decrement to the end of the increment.

    D. using an intrauterine catheter that measures increases in contraction pressures.

Answer: A. The duration of a contraction is measured from the beginning of the increment to the end of the decrement. Measuring from the beginning of one contraction to the beginning of the next reveals frequency. Measuring during the acme phase of a contraction reveals intensity (measured with an intrauterine catheter or by palpation).

➡ *NCLEX keys*

Nursing process step: Assessment
Client needs category: Health promotion and maintenance
Client needs subcategory: Growth and development through the life span
Taxonomic level: Comprehension

10. A client is receiving magnesium sulfate to help suppress preterm labor. The nurse should watch for which sign of magnesium toxicity?

    A. Headache

    B. Loss of deep tendon reflexes

    C. Palpitations

    D. Dyspepsia

Answer: B. Magnesium toxicity causes signs of central nervous system depression, such as loss of deep tendon reflexes, paralysis, respiratory depression, drowsiness, lethargy, blurred vision, slurred speech, and confusion. Headache may be an adverse effect of calcium channel blockers, which are sometimes used to treat preterm labor. Palpitations are an adverse effect of terbutaline and ritodrine, which are also used to treat preterm labor. Dyspepsia may occur as an adverse effect of indomethacin, a prostaglandin synthetase inhibitor, used to suppress preterm labor.

➡ *NCLEX keys*

Nursing process step: Assessment
Client needs category: Physiological integrity
Client needs subcategory: Pharmacological and parenteral therapies
Taxonomic level: Application

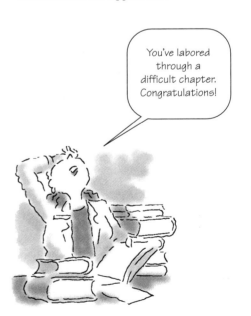

You've labored through a difficult chapter. Congratulations!

24 Postpartum Care

Brush up on key concepts

The mother undergoes both physiologic and psychological changes after delivery. Understanding these changes is essential to providing safe, effective patient care.

At any time, you can review the major points of this chapter by consulting the *Cheat sheet* on page 510.

Physiologic changes after delivery

Here is a brief review of body system changes that occur immediately after delivery.

Circulation gyration
In the **vascular system,** blood volume decreases and hematocrit increases after vaginal delivery. Excessive activation of blood-clotting factors also occurs. Blood volume returns to prenatal levels within 3 weeks.

Reproductive regeneration
In the **reproductive system,** uterine involution occurs rapidly immediately after delivery. Progesterone production ceases until the patient's first ovulation. Endometrial regeneration begins after 6 weeks. The cervical opening is permanently altered from a circle to a jagged slit.

No more pickles and milkshakes!
Gastrointestinal system changes include:
- increased hunger after labor and delivery
- delayed bowel movement from decreased intestinal muscle tone and perineal discomfort

- increased thirst from fluids lost during labor and delivery.

Increasing capacity
Genitourinary system changes include:
- increased urine output during the first 24 hours after delivery due to increased glomerular filtration rate and a drop in progesterone levels
- increased bladder capacity
- proteinuria caused by the catalytic process of involution (in 50% of women)
- decreased bladder-filling sensation caused by swollen and bruised tissues
- return of dilated ureters and renal pelvis to prepregnancy size after 6 weeks.

Hormone readjustment
In the **endocrine system,** thyroid function and the production of anterior pituitary gonadotropic hormones is increased. Simultaneously, the production of other hormones, including estrogen, aldosterone, progesterone, human chorionic gonadotropin, corticoids, and ketosteroids, decreases.

Psychological changes after pregnancy

More than 50% of women experience transient mood alterations immediately after pregnancy. This mood change is called **postpartum depression,** or the "baby blues," and signs and symptoms include sadness, crying, fatigue, and low self-esteem. Possible causes include hormonal changes, genetic predisposition, and adjustment to an altered role and self-concept.

Teach the patient that mood swings and bouts of depression are normal postpartum responses; they typically occur during the

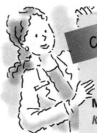

Cheat sheet

Postpartum care refresher

MASTITIS

Key signs and symptoms

- Chills
- Localized area of redness and inflammation
- Temperature of 101.1° F (38.4° C) or higher

Key test results

- Culture of purulent discharge may test positive for *Staphylococcus aureus*.

Key treatments

- incision and drainage if abscess occurs
- moist heat application
- pumping breasts to preserve breast-feeding ability
- Analgesics: acetaminophen (Tylenol), ibuprofen (Advil)
- Antibiotics: cephalexin (Keftab), cefaclor (Ceclor), clindamycin (Cleocin)

Key interventions

- Administer antibiotic therapy.
- Apply moist heat.

POSTPARTUM HEMORRHAGE

Key signs and symptoms

- Blood loss greater than 500 ml within the first 24 hours after delivery
- Signs of shock (tachycardia, hypotension, oliguria)
- Uterine atony

Key test results

- Hematology studies show decreased hemoglobin and hematocrit levels, low fibrinogen level, and decreased partial thromboplastin time.

Key treatments

- Bimanual compression of the uterus and dilatation and curettage to remove clots
- I.V. replacement of fluids and blood
- Parenteral administration of methylergonovine
- Rapid I.V. infusion of dilute oxytocin

Key interventions

- Massage the fundus and express clots from the uterus.
- Perform a pad count.

- Monitor the fundus for location.
- Administer I.V. infusion of dilute oxytocin.

PSYCHOLOGICAL MALADAPTATION

Key signs and symptoms

- Inability to stop crying
- Increased anxiety about self and infant's health
- Overall feeling of sadness
- Unwillingness to be left alone

Key treatments

- Counseling for the patient and family at risk
- Psychotherapy for the patient
- Antidepressants: imipramine (Tofranil), nortriptyline (Pamelor)

Key interventions

- Obtain a health history during the antepartum period to assess risk for postpartum depression.
- Assess the patient's support systems.
- Assess maternal-infant bonding.
- Provide emotional support and encouragement.

PUERPERAL INFECTION

Key signs and symptoms

- Abdominal pain and tenderness
- Purulent, foul-smelling lochia
- Tachycardia

Key test results

- A complete blood count may show an elevated white blood cell count in the upper ranges of normal (more than 30,000/µl) for the postpartum period.
- Cultures of the blood or the endocervical and uterine cavities may reveal the causative organism.

Key treatments

- Broad-spectrum I.V. antibiotic therapy unless a causative organism is identified

Key interventions

- Monitor vital signs every 4 hours.
- Place the patient in Fowler's position.
- Initiate and maintain I.V. fluid administration as ordered.
- Administer antibiotics as prescribed.

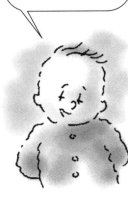

Expecting mothers spend 9 months imagining what I MIGHT be like...it takes them a little while to get used to the real me!

first 3 weeks after delivery and subside within 1 to 10 days.

Maternal behavior after delivery is divided into three phases:
• taking-in phase
• taking-hold phase
• letting-go phase.

What have I got myself into?

During the **taking-in phase** (1 to 2 days after delivery), the mother is passive and dependent, directing energy toward herself instead of toward her infant. She may relive her labor and delivery experience to integrate the process into her life and may have difficulty making decisions.

Getting to know you

During the **taking-hold phase** (about 2 to 7 days after delivery), the mother has more energy and begins to act independently and initiate self-care activities. Although she may express a lack of confidence in her abilities, she accepts responsibility for her neonate and becomes receptive to infant care and patient teaching about self-care activities.

Assuming the role

During the **letting-go phase** (about 7 days after delivery), the mother begins to readjust to family members, assuming the mother role and the responsibility that comes with it. She relinquishes the infant she has imagined during her pregnancy, and accepts her real infant as an entity separate from herself.

Keep abreast of postpartum assessment

The period immediately after labor and delivery is crucial to good postpartum nursing care. An understanding of normal and abnormal assessment findings is essential.

Monitor, monitor, monitor

The patient's respiratory rate should return to normal after delivery. Other findings are listed below.
• The patient's temperature may be elevated to 100.4° F (38° C) from dehydration and the exertion of labor.
• Blood pressure is usually normal within 24 hours of delivery.
• Bradycardia of 50 to 70 beats/minute is common during the first 6 to 10 days after delivery because of reductions in cardiac strain, stroke volume, and the vascular bed.

Nursing actions

• Monitor vital signs every 15 minutes for the first 1 to 2 hours, then every 4 hours for the first 24 hours, and then during every shift.

Fundal features

Check the tone and location of the **fundus** (the uppermost portion of the uterus) every 15 minutes for the first 1 to 2 hours after delivery and then during every shift. The involuting uterus should be at the midline. The fundus is usually:
• midway between the umbilicus and symphysis 1 to 2 hours after delivery
• 1 cm above or at the level of the umbilicus 12 hours after delivery
• 3 cm below the umbilicus by the 3rd day after delivery
• firm to the touch.

The fundus will continue to descend about 1 cm/day until it's not palpable above the symphysis (about 9 days after delivery). The uterus shrinks to its prepregnancy size 5 to 6 weeks after delivery.

A firm uterus helps control postpartum hemorrhage by clamping down on uterine blood vessels. The doctor may prescribe oxytocin (Pitocin), ergonovine maleate (Ergotrate), or methylergonovine (Methergine) to maintain uterine firmness.

Nursing actions

• Massage a boggy (soft) fundus gently; if the fundus doesn't respond, use a firmer touch.
• Be aware that the uterus may relax if overstimulated by massage or medications.

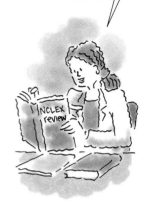

Studying for a big test can also cause mood swings — sometimes you may feel confident, other times anxious. Remind yourself that it's a normal reaction.

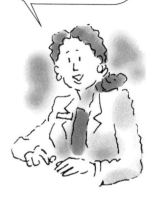

Don't worry! Patients often exhibit a slightly elevated temperature — up to 100.4° F — just after delivery.

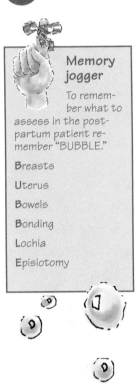

Don't forget to communicate with my mother...she may have questions or may just need a little reassurance.

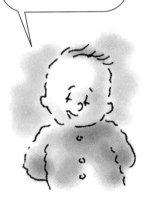

• Suspect a distended bladder if the uterus isn't firm at the midline. A distended bladder can impede the downward descent of the uterus by pushing it upward and, possibly, to the side.
• Assess maternal-infant bonding by observing how the mother responds to her newborn.
• Assess for excessive vaginal bleeding.

Discharge diagnosis
Lochia is the discharge from the sloughing of the uterine decidua.
• **Lochia rubra** is the vaginal discharge that occurs for the first 2 to 3 days after delivery; it has a fleshy odor and is bloody with small clots.
• **Lochia serosa** refers to the vaginal discharge that occurs during days 3 through 9; it is pinkish or brown with a serosanguineous consistency and fleshy odor.
• **Lochia alba** is a yellow to white discharge that usually begins about 10 days after delivery; it may last from 2 to 6 weeks.
    Some lochia characteristics may indicate the need for further intervention, for example:
• Foul-smelling lochia may indicate an infection.
• Continuous seepage of bright red blood may indicate a cervical or vaginal laceration.
• Lochia that saturates a sanitary pad within 45 minutes usually indicates an abnormally heavy flow.
• Lochia may diminish after a cesarean delivery.
• Numerous large clots should be evaluated further; they may interfere with involution.
• Lochia may be scant but should never be absent; absence may indicate postpartum infection.

Nursing action
Assess the lochia during every shift, and note its color, amount, odor, and consistency.

Breast check
Assess the size and shape of the patient's **breasts** every shift, noting reddened areas, tenderness, and engorgement. Check the nipples for cracking, fissures, and soreness.

Nursing actions
• Advise the patient to wear a support bra to maintain shape and enhance comfort.
• Tell the patient that she can relieve discomfort from engorged breasts by wearing a support bra, applying ice packs, and taking prescribed medications.
• If the patient is breast-feeding, advise her that she can relieve breast engorgement by eating frequent meals, applying warm compresses, and expressing milk manually.

Elimination examination
Assess the patient's **elimination** patterns. The patient should void within the first 6 to 8 hours after delivery. Assess for a distended bladder, which can interfere with elimination, within the first few hours after delivery.

Nursing actions
• The patient may use pain medication before urination. Pour warm water over the perineum to eliminate the fear of pain.
• The patient who can't void may require catheterization.
• Encourage the patient to have a bowel movement within 1 to 2 days after delivery to avoid constipation.
• The patient with hemorrhoids may require ice packs or analgesic preparations.
• Encourage the patient to increase her fluid and roughage intake.
• Alleviate maternal anxieties regarding pain from or damage to the episiotomy site.
• The patient may require laxatives, stool softeners, suppositories, or enemas.
• A patient with a fourth-degree laceration should never have a rectal temperature reading, nor should she be administered an enema.

Evaluating episiotomy
The site of **episiotomy** (surgical incision into the perineum and vagina) should be assessed every shift to evaluate healing, noting erythema, intactness of stitches, edema, and any odor or drainage. Twenty-four hours after delivery, the edges of an episiotomy are usually sealed.

Nursing actions

• Administer medications to relieve discomfort from the episiotomy, uterine contractions, incisional pain, or engorged breasts, as prescribed. Medications may include analgesics, stool softeners and laxatives, or oxytocic agents.

Teaching topics

Teach the patient with an episiotomy to:
• change perineal pads frequently, removing from front to back
• report lochia with a foul odor, heavy flow, or clots
• shower daily to relieve discomfort of normal postpartum diaphoresis
• follow instructions on sexual activity and contraception
• perform Kegel exercises to help strengthen the pubococcygeal muscles
• request assistance getting out of bed the first several times after delivery to minimize dizziness and fainting from medications, blood loss, and decreased fluid intake
• sit with legs elevated for 30 minutes if lochia increases or lochia rubra returns, either of which may indicate excessive activity; if excessive vaginal discharge persists, notify the doctor
• increase protein and caloric intake to restore body tissues (if breast-feeding, increase daily caloric intake by 200 kcal over the pregnancy requirement of 2,400 kcal)
• relieve perineal discomfort from an episiotomy by using ice packs (for the first 8 to 12 hours to minimize edema); spray peri bottles; sitz baths; anesthetic sprays, creams, and pads; and prescribed pain medications.

Catch up on complications

Common postpartum complications include mastitis, postpartum hemorrhage, puerperal infection, and psychological maladaptation.

Mastitis

Mastitis is an infection of the lactating breast. It most often occurs during the 2nd and 3rd weeks after birth but can potentially occur at any time.

CAUSES

• *Staphylococcus aureus* (the most common causative pathogen)

Risk factors

• Altered immune response
• Constriction from a bra that is too tight (may interfere with complete emptying of the breast)
• Engorgement and stasis of milk (usually precede mastitis)
• Injury to nipple; causative organism may enter through an injured area of the nipple, such as a crack or blister

ASSESSMENT FINDINGS

• Aching muscles
• Chills
• Fatigue
• Headache
• Localized area of redness and inflammation
• Malaise
• Purulent drainage
• Temperature of 101.1° F (38.4° C) or higher

DIAGNOSTIC TEST RESULTS

• Culture of the purulent discharge may test positive for the *S. aureus* bacteria.

NURSING DIAGNOSES

• Ineffective individual coping
• Pain
• Situational low self-esteem

TREATMENT

• Incision and drainage if abscess occurs
• Moist heat application
• Pumping breasts to preserve breast-feeding ability

Drug therapy

• Analgesics: acetaminophen (Tylenol), ibuprofen (Advil)

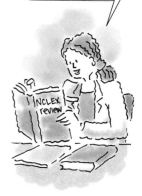

During assessment, position the patient with a mediolateral episiotomy on her side to provide better visibility and less discomfort.

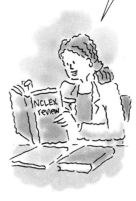

Position the patient with a midline episiotomy on her side or back.

• Antibiotics: cephalexin (Keftab), cefaclor (Ceclor), clindamycin (Cleocin)

INTERVENTIONS AND RATIONALES
• Monitor vital signs *to assess for complications.*
• Administer antibiotic therapy *to treat infection.*
• Apply moist heat *to increase circulation and reduce inflammation and edema.*

Teaching topics
• Positioning the infant during breast-feeding to avoid trauma to the nipples and milk stasis
• Avoiding bras that are too tight and may restrict the flow of milk
• Breast-feeding every 2 to 3 hours and completely emptying the breasts
• Changing nipple shields as soon as they become wet to prevent infection
• Using a breast pump and discarding milk if breast abscess has developed

Postpartum hemorrhage

Postpartum hemorrhage is maternal blood loss from the uterus greater than 500 ml within a 24-hour period. It can occur immediately after delivery (within the first 24 hours) or later (during the remaining days of the 6-week puerperium).

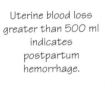

Uterine blood loss greater than 500 ml indicates postpartum hemorrhage.

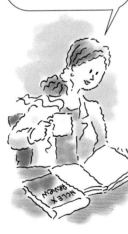

CAUSES
• Administration of magnesium sulfate
• Cesarean birth
• Clotting disorders
• Disseminated intravascular coagulation
• General anesthesia
• Low implantation of placenta or placenta previa
• Multiparity
• Overdistention of uterus (multifetal pregnancy, hydramnios, large infant)
• Perineal laceration
• Precipitate labor or delivery
• Previous postpartum hemorrhage
• Previous uterine surgery
• Prolonged labor
• Retained placental fragments

• Soft, boggy uterus, indicating relaxed uterine tone
• Use of tocolytic drugs

ASSESSMENT FINDINGS
• Blood loss greater than 500 ml within the first 24 hours after delivery
• Perineal lacerations
• Retained placental fragments
• Signs of shock (tachycardia, hypotension, oliguria)
• Uterine atony

DIAGNOSTIC TEST RESULTS
• Hematology studies show decreased hemoglobin and hematocrit levels, a low fibrinogen level, and decreased partial thromboplastin time.

NURSING DIAGNOSES
• Altered tissue perfusion
• Fluid volume deficit
• Risk for infection

TREATMENT
• Bimanual compression of the uterus and dilatation and curettage to remove clots
• I.V. replacement of fluids and blood
• Abdominal hysterectomy if other interventions fail to control blood loss

Drug therapy
• Parenteral administration of methylergonovine (Methergine)
• Rapid I.V. infusion of dilute oxytocin

INTERVENTIONS AND RATIONALES
• Monitor vital signs *to assess for complications.*
• Massage the fundus, and express clots from the uterus *to increase uterine contraction and tone.*
• Perform a pad count *to assess the amount of vaginal bleeding.*
• Monitor lochia, including amount, color, and odor *to assess for infection.*
• Monitor the fundus for location *to assess for uterine displacement.*
• Administer I.V. infusion of dilute oxytocin as ordered *to increase uterine contraction and tone.*

• Administer methylergonovine as ordered *to increase uterine contraction and tone.*
• Administer blood products and I.V. fluids as prescribed *to replace volume loss.*
• Provide emotional support *to help alleviate any fears and anxiety.*

Teaching topics
• Information about surgical procedures, if appropriate
• Reporting changes in vaginal bleeding

Psychological maladaptation

Psychological maladaptation is depression of a significant depth and duration after childbirth. Many postpartum patients experience some level of mood swings; psychological maladaptation refers to depression that lasts longer than 2 days, indicating a serious problem.

CAUSES AND RISK FACTORS
• History of depression
• Hormonal shifts as estrogen and progesterone levels decline
• Lack of support from family and friends
• Lack of self-esteem
• Stress in the home or work
• Troubled childhood

ASSESSMENT FINDINGS
• Extreme fatigue
• Inability to make decisions
• Inability to stop crying
• Increased anxiety about self and infant's health
• Overall feeling of sadness
• Postpartum psychosis (hallucinations, delusions, potential for suicide or homicide)
• Psychosomatic symptoms (nausea, vomiting, diarrhea)
• Unwillingness to be left alone

NURSING DIAGNOSES
• Fatigue
• Ineffective individual coping
• Social isolation

TREATMENT
• Counseling for the patient and family at risk
• Group therapy
• Psychotherapy

Drug therapy
• Antidepressants: imipramine (Tofranil), nortriptyline (Pamelor)

INTERVENTIONS AND RATIONALES
• Obtain a health history during the antepartum period *to assess whether the patient is at risk for postpartum depression.*
• Assess the patient's support systems *to assess the need for additional help.*
• Assess maternal-infant bonding *to assess for signs of depression.*
• Provide emotional support and encouragement *to reduce anxiety.*
• Notify a skilled professional *if you observe psychotic symptoms in the patient.*

Teaching topics
• Understanding that continued depression may require psychiatric counseling

Puerperal infection

Puerperal infection occurs after childbirth in 2% to 5% of all women who have vaginal deliveries and in 15% to 20% of those who have cesarean deliveries. Puerperal infection is one of the leading causes of maternal death.

CAUSES AND RISK FACTORS
• Catheterization
• Cesarean delivery
• Colonization of lower genital tract with pathogenic organisms, such as group B streptococcus, *Chlamydia trachomatis, S. aureus, Escherichia coli,* and *Gardnerella vaginalis*
• Excessive number of vaginal examinations
• History of previous infection
• Low socioeconomic status
• Medical conditions such as diabetes mellitus
• Poor general health
• Poor nutrition
• Prolonged labor
• Prolonged rupture of membranes

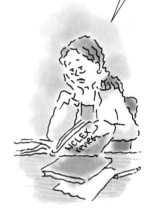

Although many patients experience some depression after childbirth, depression that lasts longer than 2 days should trigger your assessment alarm.

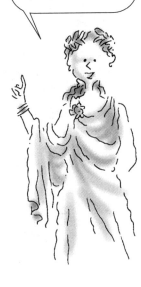

Friends, Romans, countrymen. Women who have undergone cesarean delivery are at higher risk for puerperal infection.

- Retained placental fragments
- Trauma

ASSESSMENT FINDINGS
- Abdominal pain and tenderness
- Anorexia
- Chills
- Fever
- Lethargy
- Malaise
- Purulent, foul-smelling lochia
- Subinvolution
- Tachycardia
- Uterine cramping

DIAGNOSTIC TEST RESULTS
- A catheterized urine specimen may reveal the causative organism.
- A complete blood count may show an elevated white blood cell count in the upper ranges of normal (more than 30,000/µl) for the postpartum period.
- Cultures of the blood or of the endocervical and uterine cavities may reveal the causative organism.

NURSING DIAGNOSES
- Pain
- Risk for infection
- Social isolation

TREATMENT
- Administration of I.V. fluids (if hydration is needed)

Drug therapy
- Broad-spectrum I.V. antibiotic therapy, unless a causative organism is identified

INTERVENTIONS AND RATIONALES
- Monitor vital signs every 4 hours *to assess for complications.*
- Place the patient in Fowler's position *to facilitate drainage of lochia.*
- Administer pain medication as ordered *to relieve pain and discomfort.*
- Provide emotional support and reassurance *to ease anxiety.*
- Initiate and maintain I.V. fluid administration as ordered *to replace volume loss.*
- Administer antibiotics as prescribed *to fight infection.*

Teaching topics
- Recognizing signs and symptoms of a worsening condition, such as nausea, vomiting, absent bowel sounds, abdominal distention, and severe abdominal pain

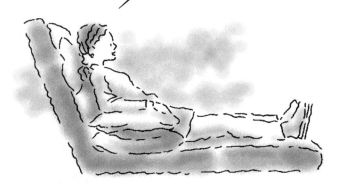

Placing the patient in Fowler's position will help with the drainage of lochia.

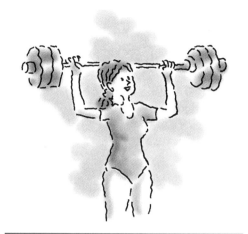

Pump up on practice questions

1. When assessing a postpartum client for uterine bleeding, the nurse finds the fundus to be boggy. After fundal massage by the nurse, the physician prescribes 0.2 mg of methylergonovine (Methergine) by mouth. What should the nurse tell the client?

   A. "Methergine is commonly used to help the uterus contract so that the bleeding will decrease. You may experience more cramping as your uterus becomes firmer."

   B. "You will probably take this medication until you are discharged from the hospital. Every patient usually needs to take this medication."

   C. "If your blood pressure is low, you won't be able to take this medication; I will establish a new I.V. line so I can start Pitocin again."

   D. "Most people don't experience additional pain or cramping from taking this medication."

Answer: A. Methylergonovine, an ergot alkaloid, is commonly given to stimulate sustained uterine contraction. It allows the uterus to remain contracted and firm, thus decreasing postpartum bleeding. Abdominal cramping, which may become painful, is a common adverse effect. Methergine is discontinued when the lochia flow has decreased or the client complains of severe cramping. Clients may need only a few doses of Methergine to keep the uterus contracted. Taking Methergine is contraindicated in clients with hypertension.

➡ *NCLEX keys*
Nursing process step: Implementation
Client needs category: Physiological integrity
Client needs subcategory: Pharmacological and parenteral therapies
Taxonomic level: Application

2. The nurse is providing care for a postpartum client. Which of the following conditions would place this client at greater risk for a postpartum hemorrhage?

   A. Hypertension
   B. Uterine infection
   C. Placenta previa
   D. Severe pain

Answer: C. The client with placenta previa is at greatest risk for postpartum hemorrhage. In placenta previa, the lower uterine segment doesn't contract as well as the fundal part of the uterus; therefore, more bleeding occurs. Hypertension, severe pain, and uterine infection don't place the client at increased risk for postpartum hemorrhage.

➡ *NCLEX keys*
Nursing process step: Planning
Client needs category: Health promotion and maintenance
Client needs subcategory: Growth and development through the life span
Taxonomic level: Comprehension

3. A client has delivered twins. What is the most important intervention for the nurse to perform?

   A. Assess fundal tone and lochia flow.
   B. Apply a cold pack to the perineal area.
   C. Administer analgesics as ordered.
   D. Encourage voiding by offering the bedpan.

Answer: A. Women who experience a twin delivery are at a higher risk for postpartum hemorrhage due to overdistention of the uterus, which causes uterine atony. Assessing fundal tone and lochia flow helps to determine risks for hemorrhage. Applying cold packs to the perineum, administering analgesics as ordered, and offering the bedpan are all significant nursing interventions; however, detecting and preventing postpartum hemorrhage is most important.

➡ NCLEX keys

Nursing process step: Implementation
Client needs category: Health promotion and maintenance
Client needs subcategory: Growth and development through the life span
Taxonomic level: Comprehension

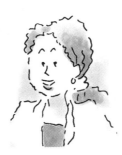

4. Which of the following is a normal physiological response in the early postpartum period?
   A. Urinary urgency and dysuria
   B. Rapid diuresis
   C. Decrease in blood pressure
   D. Increased motility of the GI system

Answer: B. In the early postpartum period there is an increase in the glomerular filtration rate and a drop in progesterone levels, which result in rapid diuresis. There should be no urinary urgency, although a woman may be anxious about voiding. There is minimal change in blood pressure following childbirth and a residual decrease in gastrointestinal motility.

➡ NCLEX keys

Nursing process step: Assessment
Client needs category: Physiological integrity
Client needs subcategory: Physiological adaptation
Taxonomic level: Knowledge

5. During the 3rd postpartum day, which of the following would the nurse be most likely to find in the client?
   A. She's interested in learning more about newborn care.
   B. She talks a lot about her birth experience.
   C. She sleeps whenever the baby isn't present.
   D. She requests help in choosing a name for the baby.

Answer: A. The 3rd to 10th days of postpartum care are the "taking-hold" phase, in which the new mother strives for independence and is eager for her baby. Options B, C, and D describe the phase in which the mother relives her birth experience.

➡ NCLEX keys

Nursing process step: Evaluation
Client needs category: Health promotion and maintenance
Client needs subcategory: Growth and development through the life span
Taxonomic level: Analysis

6. Which of the following circumstances is most likely to cause uterine atony, leading to postpartum hemorrhage?
   A. Hypertension
   B. Cervical and vaginal tears
   C. Urine retention
   D. Endometritis

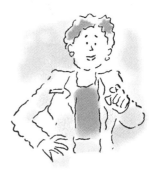

Answer: C. Urine retention is most likely to cause uterine atony and subsequent postpartum hemorrhage. Urine retention causes a distended bladder to displace the uterus above the umbilicus and to the side, which prevents the uterus from contracting. The uterus needs to remain contracted if bleeding is to stay within normal limits. Cervical and vaginal tears can cause postpartum hemorrhage, but in the postpartum period, a full bladder is the most common cause of uterine bleeding. Endometritis, an infection of the inner lining of the endometrium, and maternal hypertension don't cause postpartum hemorrhage.

➡ *NCLEX keys*
Nursing process step: Implementation
Client needs category: Health promotion and maintenance
Client needs subcategory: Growth and development through the life span
Taxonomic level: Knowledge

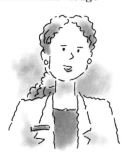

7. When assessing a client's episiotomy, the nurse should be especially careful to observe:
  A. location.
  B. discharge and odor.
  C. edema and approximation.
  D. subinvolution.
Answer: C. An episiotomy should be assessed for edema and approximation of incision. An edematous perineum causes more tension of the suture line and increases pain. Although the sutures may be difficult to visualize, the suture line should be intact. Episiotomy location is important, but not as important as the presence of edema. Discharge and odor refer to an assessment of lochia. Subinvolution refers to the complete return of the uterus to its prepregnancy size and shape.

➡ *NCLEX keys*
Nursing process step: Assessment
Client needs category: Physiological integrity
Client needs subcategory: Reduction of risk potential
Taxonomic level: Comprehension

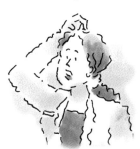

8. In performing a routine fundal assessment, the nurse finds that the client's fundus is boggy. The nurse should first:
  A. call the physician.
  B. massage the fundus.
  C. assess lochia flow.
  D. obtain an order for methylergonovine.
Answer: B. The nurse should begin to massage the uterus so that it will be stimulated to contract. Assessing lochia flow can be done while the uterus is being massaged. The nurse shouldn't leave the client to call the physician. If the fundus remains boggy and the uterus continues to bleed, the nurse should use the call button to ask another nurse to call the physician. Methylergonovine may be prescribed, if needed.

➡ *NCLEX keys*
Nursing process step: Implementation
Client needs category: Physiological integrity
Client needs subcategory: Reduction of risk potential
Taxonomic level: Application

9. Which type of lochia should the nurse expect to find in a client who is 2 days postpartum?

    A. Foul-smelling
    B. Serosa
    C. Alba
    D. Rubra

Answer: D. Lochia rubra lasts about 4 days followed by lochia serosa, which extends through the 7th day, and then lochia alba, which occurs during the 2nd and 3rd postpartum weeks. Foul-smelling lochia is a sign of infection.

➡ *NCLEX keys*
Nursing process step: Assessment
Client needs category: Health promotion and maintenance
Client needs subcategory: Growth and development through the life span
Taxonomic level: Knowledge

10. A client treated with magnesium sulfate during labor is now on the postpartum unit. The nurse should be aware that the client is at risk for which of the following complications of magnesium sulfate therapy?

    A. Hypotension
    B. Uterine infection
    C. Postpartum hemorrhage
    D. Postpartum depression

Answer: C. Because magnesium sulfate produces a smooth-muscle depressive effect, the uterus should be assessed for uterine atony. The uterus may be unable to maintain a firm tone, thus increasing the risk of postpartum hemorrhage. Uterine infection and postpartum depression aren't associated with magnesium sulfate therapy. Magnesium sulfate does decrease blood pressure, but it's considered more of an anticonvulsant drug than an antihypertensive drug.

➡ *NCLEX keys*
Nursing process step: Evaluation
Client needs category: Physiological integrity
Client needs subcategory: Pharmacological and parenteral therapies
Taxonomic level: Comprehension

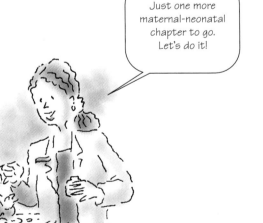

Just one more maternal-neonatal chapter to go. Let's do it!

Brush up on key concepts

A neonate experiences many changes as he adapts to life outside the uterus. Knowledge of these changes and of the normal physiologic characteristics of the neonate provides the basis for normal neonatal care.

At any time, you can review the major points of this chapter by consulting the *Cheat sheet* on pages 522 and 523.

Adaptations to extrauterine life

Here is a review of how the neonate's body systems change.

Heart seals
The **cardiovascular system** changes from the very first breath, which expands the neonate's lungs and decreases pulmonary vascular resistance. Clamping the umbilical cord increases systemic vascular resistance and left atrial pressure, which functionally closes the foramen ovale (fibrosis may take from several weeks to a year).

Every breath you take
The **respiratory system** also begins to change with the first breath. The neonate's breathing is a reflex triggered in response to noise, light, and temperature and pressure changes. Air immediately replaces the fluid that filled the lungs before birth.

A delicate balance
Renal system function doesn't fully mature until after the 1st year of life; as a result, the neonate has a minimal range of chemical bal-

ance and safety. The neonate's limited ability to excrete drugs, coupled with excessive neonatal fluid loss, can rapidly lead to acidosis and fluid imbalances.

Digestive difficulties
The **GI system** is also not fully developed because normal bacteria aren't present in the neonate's GI tract. The lower intestine contains meconium at birth; the first meconium (sterile, greenish black, and viscous) usually passes within 24 hours. Some aspects of GI development include:
• audible bowel sounds 1 hour after birth
• uncoordinated peristaltic activity in the esophagus for the first few days of life
• a limited ability to digest fats because amylase and lipase are absent at birth
• frequent regurgitation because of an immature cardiac sphincter.

Heat miser
Changes in neonatal **thermogenesis** depend on environment. In an optimal environment, the neonate can produce sufficient heat, but rapid heat loss may occur in a suboptimal thermal environment.

Disease control
The neonatal **immune system** depends largely on three immunoglobulins: immunoglobulin G (IgG), IgM, and IgA. IgG (detected in the fetus at the 3rd month of gestation) is a placentally transferred immunoglobulin, providing antibodies to bacterial and viral agents. The infant synthesizes its own IgG during the first 3 months of life, thus compensating for concurrent catabolism of maternal antibodies. By the 20th week of gestation, the fetus synthesizes IgM, which is undetectable at birth because it doesn't cross the placenta.

High levels of IgM in the neonate indicate a nonspecific infection. Secretory IgA (which

Because the neonate's renal system hasn't fully matured yet, the neonate can easily develop acidosis and fluid imbalances.

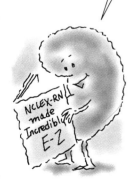

NCLEX-RN made Incredibly E-Z

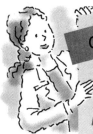

Cheat sheet

Neonatal care refresher

FETAL ALCOHOL SYNDROME

Key sign or symptom
- Central nervous system dysfunction (decreased I.Q., developmental delays, neurologic abnormalities)
- Prenatal and postnatal growth retardation

Key test results
- Chest X-ray may reveal congenital heart defect.

Key interventions
- Provide a stimulus-free environment for the neonate; darken the room if necessary.
- Provide gavage feedings as necessary.

HUMAN IMMUNODEFICIENCY VIRUS (HIV)

Key sign or symptom
- Asymptomatic at birth

Key test results
- Test interpretation is problematic because most neonates with an HIV-positive mother test positive at birth. Uninfected neonates lose this maternal antibody at 8 to 15 months, and infected neonates remain seropositive. Therefore, testing should be repeated at age 15 months.

Key treatments
- Antimicrobial therapy to treat opportunistic infections
- Prophylactic trimethoprim-sulfamethoxazole (Bactrim) for babies 4 weeks of age or older
- Zidovudine (Ritrovir) administration based on the neonate's lymphocyte count

Key interventions
- Assess cardiovascular and respiratory status.
- Protect the neonate from further exposure to maternal body fluids.
- Maintain standard precautions.
- Keep the umbilical stump meticulously clean.

HYPOTHERMIA

Key signs and symptoms
- Kicking and crying (a mechanism used to increase the metabolic rate to produce body heat)
- Core body temperature lower than 97.7° F (36.5° C)

Key test results
- Arterial blood gas analysis shows hypoxemia.
- Blood glucose level reveals hypoglycemia.

Key treatment
- Radiant warmer

Key interventions
- Dry the newborn immediately.
- Allow the mother to hold the neonate.
- Monitor vital signs every 15 to 30 minutes.
- Provide a knitted cap for the newborn.
- Place the neonate in a radiant warmer.

NEONATAL DRUG DEPENDENCY

Key signs and symptoms
- High-pitched cry
- Irritability
- Jitteriness
- Poor sleeping pattern
- Tremors

Key treatment
- Gavage feedings, if necessary
- Paregoric and phenobarbital (Barbita) to treat withdrawal symptoms; methadone shouldn't be given to neonates because of its addictive nature

Key interventions
- Monitor cardiovascular status.
- Use tight swaddling for comfort.
- Place the neonate in a dark, quiet environment.
- Encourage use of a pacifier (in cases of heroin withdrawal).
- Be prepared to administer gavage (in cases of methadone withdrawal).
- Maintain fluid and electrolyte balance.

NEONATAL INFECTIONS

Key signs and symptoms
- Feeding pattern changes, such as poor sucking or decreased intake
- Sternal retractions
- Subtle, nonspecific behavioral changes, such as lethargy or hypotonia
- Temperature instability

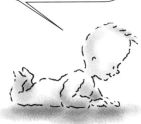

Time for a change. I experience many changes as I adapt to life outside the uterus.

Neonatal care refresher (continued)

NEONATAL INFECTIONS (continued)

Key test results
• Blood and urine cultures are positive for causative organism, most commonly gram-positive beta-hemolytic streptococci and the gram-negative *Escherichia coli, Aerobacter, Proteus,* and *Klebsiella.*
• Complete blood count shows an increased white blood cell count.

Key treatments
• I.V. therapy to provide adequate hydration
• Antibiotic therapy: broad-spectrum until causative organism is identified and then specific antibiotic

Key interventions
• Assess cardiovascular and respiratory status.
• Administer broad-spectrum antibiotics before culture results are received and specific antibiotic therapy after results are received.

NEONATAL JAUNDICE

Key signs and symptoms
• Jaundice
• Lethargy

Key test result
• Bilirubin levels exceed 12 mg/dl in premature or term neonates.

Key treatments
• Increased fluid intake
• Phototherapy

Key interventions
• Assess neurologic status.
• Monitor serum bilirubin levels.
• Initiate and maintain phototherapy (provide eye protection while under phototherapy lights and remove eye shields promptly when removed from the phototherapy lights).

RESPIRATORY DISTRESS SYNDROME

Key signs and symptoms
• Expiratory grunting
• Fine crackles and diminished breath sounds
• Seesaw respirations
• Sternal and substernal retractions
• Tachypnea (more than 60 breaths/minute)

Key test results
• Arterial blood gas analysis reveals respiratory acidosis.
• Chest X-rays reveal bilateral diffuse reticulogranular density.

Key treatments
• Endotracheal intubation and mechanical ventilation
• Nutrition supplements (total parenteral nutrition [TPN] or enteral feedings, if possible)
• Surfactant replacement by way of endotracheal tube
• Temperature regulation with a radiant warmer

Key interventions
• Assess cardiovascular, respiratory, and neurologic status.
• Monitor continuous electrocardiography and vital signs.
• Initiate and maintain ventilatory support status.
• Administer medications, including endotracheal surfactant, as prescribed.
• Provide adequate nutrition through enteral feedings, if possible, or TPN.

TRACHEOESOPHAGEAL FISTULA

Key signs and symptoms
• Difficulty feeding, such as choking or aspiration; cyanosis during feeding
• Signs of respiratory distress

Key test result
• Abdominal X-ray shows the fistula and a gas-free abdomen.

Key treatments
• Emergency surgical intervention to prevent pneumonia, dehydration, and fluid and electrolyte imbalances
• Maintenance of patent airway

Key interventions
• Monitor cardiovascular, respiratory, and GI status.
• Place the neonate in high Fowler's position.
• Keep a laryngoscope and endotracheal tube at bedside.
• Provide the neonate with a pacifier.
• Provide gastrostomy tube feedings postoperatively.

---

limits bacterial growth in the GI tract) is found in colostrum and breast milk.

Blood volume

In the neonatal **hematopoietic system,** blood volume accounts for 80 to 85 ml/kg of body weight. The neonate experiences prolonged coagulation time because of decreased levels of vitamin K.

Nervous energy

The full-term neonate's **neurologic system** should produce equal strength and symmetry in responses and reflexes. Diminished or ab-

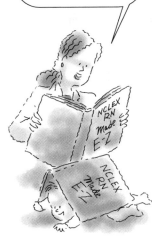

Physiologic jaundice is a mild jaundice of the neonate that lasts for the first few days after birth.

sent reflexes may indicate a serious neurologic problem, and asymmetrical responses may indicate trauma during birth, including nerve damage, paralysis, or fracture. Some neonatal reflexes gradually weaken and disappear during the early months.

Liver concerns
Jaundice is a major concern in the neonatal **hepatic system** because of increased serum levels of unconjugated bilirubin from increased red blood cell (RBC) lysis, altered bilirubin conjugation, or increased bilirubin reabsorption from the GI tract. Physiologic jaundice appears after the first 24 hours of extrauterine life; pathologic jaundice is evident at birth or within the first 24 hours of extrauterine life; and breast milk jaundice appears after the 1st week of extrauterine life when physiologic jaundice is declining.

Keep abreast of neonatal assessment

Neonatal assessment includes initial and ongoing assessment as well as a thorough physical examination.

Do this right away
Initial neonatal assessment involves draining secretions, assessing abnormalities, and keeping accurate records.

Nursing actions
• Ensure a proper airway by suctioning, and administer oxygen as needed.
• Dry the neonate under the warmer while keeping the head lower than the trunk (to promote drainage of secretions).
• Apply a cord clamp and monitor the neonate for abnormal bleeding from the cord; check the number of cord vessels.
• Observe the neonate for voiding and meconium; document the first void and stools.
• Assess the neonate for gross abnormalities and clinical manifestations of suspected abnormalities.

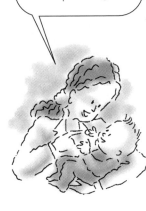

Administering erythromycin ointment and vitamin K to neonates is an important nursing responsibility.

• Continue to assess the neonate by using the Apgar score criteria even after the 5-minute score is received. (See *Apgar scoring*.)
• Obtain clear footprints and fingerprints (the neonate's footprints are kept on a record that includes the mother's fingerprints).
• Apply identification bands with matching numbers to the mother (one band) and neonate (two bands) before they leave the delivery room.
• Promote bonding between the mother and neonate.

Keep doing this
Ongoing neonatal physical assessments include observing and recording vital signs and administering prescribed medications.

Nursing actions
• Assess the neonate's vital signs.
• Take the first temperature by the axillary route (rectal route isn't recommended because of possible rectal mucosa damage).
• Take the apical pulse for 60 seconds (normal rate is 120 to 160 beats/minute).
• Count respirations with a stethoscope for 60 seconds (normal rate is 30 to 60 breaths/minute).
• Measure and record blood pressure (normal reading ranges from 60/40 mm Hg to 90/45 mm Hg).
• Measure and record the neonate's vital statistics.
• Complete a gestational age assessment.
• Administer prescribed medications such as vitamin K (AquaMEPHYTON), which is a prophylactic against transient deficiency of coagulation factors II, VII, IX, and X.
• Administer erythromycin ointment (Ilotycin), the drug of choice for neonatal eye prophylaxis, to prevent damage and blindness from conjunctivitis caused by *Neisseria gonorrhoeae* and *Chlamydia;* treatment is required by law.
• Administer first hepatitis B vaccine within 12 hours after birth.
• Perform laboratory tests.
• Monitor glucose levels and hematocrit (test results aid in assessing for hypoglycemia and anemia).

Apgar scoring

The Apgar scoring system provides a way to evaluate the neonate's cardiopulmonary and neurologic status. The assessment is performed at 1 and 5 minutes after birth and repeated every 5 minutes until the infant stabilizes. A score of 8 to 10 indicates that the neonate is in no apparent distress; a score below 8 indicates that resuscitative measures may be needed.

SIGN	0	1	2
Heart rate	Absent	Less than 100 beats/minute	Greater than 100 beats/minute
Respiratory effort	Absent	Slow, irregular	Good crying
Muscle tone	Flaccid	Some flexion of extremities	Active motion
Reflex irritability	None	Grimace	Vigorous cry
Color	Pale, blue	Body pink, blue extremities	Completely pink

Neonatal physical examination

The neonate should receive a thorough visual and physical examination of each body part. The following is a brief review of normal and abnormal neonatal physiology.

Heads up

The neonate's head is about one-fourth of body size. The term **molding** refers to asymmetry of the cranial sutures due to difficulties during labor and delivery. Cranial abnormalities include:
• cephalhematoma, a collection of blood between a skull bone and the periosteum that doesn't cross suture lines
• caput succedaneum, localized swelling over the presenting part that can cross suture lines.

Closing time

The neonatal skull has two **fontanels**: a diamond-shaped anterior fontanel and a triangular-shaped posterior fontanel. The anterior fontanel is located at the juncture of the frontal and parietal bones, measures 1⅛″ to 1⅝″ (3 to 4 cm) long and ¾″ to 1⅛″ (2 to 3 cm) wide, and closes in about 18 months. The posterior fontanel is located at the juncture of the occipital and parietal bones, measures about

¾″ across, and closes in 8 to 12 weeks. The fontanels:
• should feel soft to the touch
• shouldn't be depressed — a depressed fontanel indicates dehydration
• shouldn't bulge — bulging fontanels require immediate attention, as they may indicate increased intracranial pressure.

Where'd ya get those peepers?

• The neonate's eyes are usually blue or gray because of scleral thinness. Permanent eye color is established within 3 to 12 months.
• Lacrimal glands are immature at birth, resulting in tearless crying for up to 2 months.
• The neonate may demonstrate transient strabismus.
• Doll's eye reflex (when the head is rotated laterally, the eyes deviate in the opposite direction) may persist for about 10 days.
• Subconjunctival hemorrhages may appear from vascular tension changes during birth.

Nasal phase

Because infants are obligatory nose breathers for the first few months of life, nasal passages must be kept clear to ensure adequate respiration. Neonates instinctively sneeze to remove obstruction.

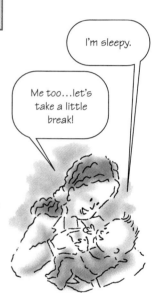

I'm sleepy.

Me too…let's take a little break!

Dry mouth

The neonate's mouth usually has scant saliva and pink lips. Epstein's pearls may be found on the gums or hard palate, and precocious teeth may also be apparent.

Do you hear what I hear?

The neonate's ears are characterized by incurving of the pinna and cartilage deposition. The top of the ear should be above or parallel to an imaginary line from the inner to the outer canthus of the eye. Low-set ears are associated with several syndromes, including chromosomal abnormalities.

Flexi-neck

The neonate's neck is typically short and weak with deep folds of skin.

Flexi-chest

The neonatal chest is characterized by a cylindrical thorax and flexible ribs. Breast engorgement from maternal hormones may be apparent, and supernumerary nipples may be located below and medially to the true nipples.

Nice abs

The neonatal abdomen is usually cylindrical with some protrusion. A scaphoid appearance indicates diaphragmatic hernia. The umbilical cord is white and gelatinous with two arteries and one vein and begins to dry within 1 to 2 hours after delivery.

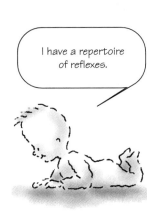

I have a repertoire of reflexes.

Boys and girls

Characteristics of a male neonate's genitalia include rugae on the scrotum and testes descended into the scrotum. The urinary meatus is located in one of three places:
• at the penile tip (normal)
• on the dorsal surface (epispadias)
• on the ventral surface (hypospadias).
   In the female neonate, the labia majora cover the labia minora and clitoris, vaginal discharge from maternal hormones appears, and the hymenal tag is present.

Extreme measures

All neonates are bowlegged and have flat feet. Some neonates may have abnormal extremities. They may be polydactyl (more than five digits on an extremity) or syndactyl (two or more digits fused together).

Soldier straight

The neonatal spine should be straight and flat, and the anus should be patent without any fissure. Dimpling at the base of the spine is commonly associated with spina bifida.

Baby-smooth skin

The skin of a neonate can indicate many conditions — some quite normal and others requiring more serious attention. Assessment findings include:
• acrocyanosis (cyanosis of the hands and feet resulting from adjustments to extrauterine circulation) for the first 24 hours after birth
• milia (clogged sebaceous glands) on the nose or chin
• lanugo (fine, downy hair) appearing after 20 weeks of gestation on the entire body except the palms and soles
• vernix caseosa (a white, cheesy protective coating composed of desquamated epithelial cells and sebum)
• erythema toxicum neonatorum (a transient, maculopapular rash)
• telangiectasia (flat, reddened vascular areas) appearing on the neck, upper eyelid, or upper lip
• port-wine stain (nevus flammeus), a capillary angioma located below the dermis and commonly found on the face
• strawberry hemangioma (nevus vasculosus), a capillary angioma located in the dermal and subdermal skin layers indicated by a rough, raised, sharply demarcated birthmark.

Reflections on reflexes

Normal neonates display a number of reflexes, which include:
• sucking: sucking motion begins when a nipple is placed in the neonate's mouth
• Moro's: when lifted above the crib and suddenly lowered, the arms and legs symmetrically extend and then abduct while the fingers spread to form a "C"

• rooting: when the cheek is stroked, the neonate turns his head in the direction of the stroke
• tonic neck (fencing position): when the neonate's head is turned while the neonate is lying supine, the extremities on the same side straighten while those on the opposite side flex
• Babinski's: when the sole on the side of the small toe is stroked, the neonate's toes fan upward
• grasping: when a finger is placed in each of the neonate's hands, the neonate's fingers grasp tightly enough to be pulled to a sitting position
• stepping: when held upright with the feet touching a flat surface, the neonate exhibits dancing or stepping movements
• startle: a loud noise such as a hand clap elicits neonatal arm abduction and elbow flexion; the neonate's hands stay clenched
• trunk incurvature: when a finger is run laterally down the neonate's spine, the trunk flexes and the pelvis swings toward the stimulated side.

Catch up on complications

Common neonatal complications and disorders include fetal alcohol syndrome, human immunodeficiency virus, hypothermia, drug dependency, infections, jaundice, respiratory distress syndrome, and tracheoesophageal fistula.

Fetal alcohol syndrome

Fetal alcohol syndrome (FAS) results from a mother's chronic or periodic intake of alcohol during pregnancy. The degree of alcohol consumption necessary to cause the syndrome varies. Because alcohol crosses the placenta in the same concentration as is present in the maternal bloodstream, alcohol consumption (particularly binge drinking) is especially dangerous during critical periods of organogene-

sis. The fetal liver isn't mature enough to detoxify alcohol.

CAUSES
• Risk of teratogenic effects increases proportionally with daily alcohol intake; FAS has been detected in neonates of even moderate drinkers (1 to 2 oz of alcohol daily)

ASSESSMENT FINDINGS
• Central nervous system dysfunction (decreased I.Q., developmental delays, neurologic abnormalities)
• Facial anomalies (microcephaly, microophthalmia, maxillary hypoplasia, short palpebral fissures)
• Prenatal and postnatal growth retardation
• Sleep disturbances (either always awake or always asleep, depending on the mother's alcohol level close to birth)
• Weak sucking reflex

DIAGNOSTIC TEST RESULTS
• Chest X-ray may reveal congenital heart defect.

NURSING DIAGNOSES
• Altered nutrition: Less than body requirements
• Altered growth and development
• Risk for altered parenting

TREATMENT
• Swaddling

Drug therapy
• I.V. phenobarbital (to control hyperactivity and irritability)

INTERVENTIONS AND RATIONALES
• Refer mother to alcohol treatment center *for ongoing support and rehabilitation.*
• Provide a stimulus-free environment for the neonate; darken the room if necessary *to minimize stimuli.*
• Provide gavage feedings as necessary *to provide adequate nutrition for the infant.*

Teaching topics
• Avoiding alcohol during pregnancy

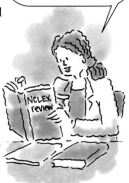

Binge drinking is even more detrimental than moderate daily consumption.

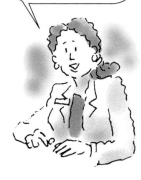

Prevention point: Administering zidovudine to HIV-positive pregnant women significantly reduces the risk of HIV transmission to the neonate.

Human immunodeficiency virus

A mother can transmit the human immunodeficiency virus (HIV) to her infant transplacentally at various gestational ages, perinatally through maternal blood and bodily fluids, and postnatally through breast milk. Administration of zidovudine to HIV-positive pregnant women significantly reduces the risk of transmission to the neonate.

CAUSES
• Transmission of the virus to the fetus or neonate from an HIV-positive mother

ASSESSMENT FINDINGS
• Asymptomatic (at birth)
• Opportunistic infections (may appear by 3 to 6 months of age)

DIAGNOSTIC TEST RESULTS
• Test interpretation is problematic because most neonates with an HIV-positive mother test positive at birth. Uninfected neonates lose this maternal antibody at 8 to 15 months, and infected neonates remain seropositive. Therefore, testing should be repeated at age 15 months.
• HIV-DNA polymerase chain reaction or viral cultures for HIV should be performed at birth and again at 1 to 2 months of age.

NURSING DIAGNOSES
• Altered nutrition: Less than body requirements
• Altered protection
• Risk for infection

TREATMENT
• Intravenous fluid administration
• Nutritional supplements to prevent weight loss

Drug therapy
• Antimicrobial therapy to treat opportunistic infections
• Pentamidine (NebuPent) beginning at 6 months of age

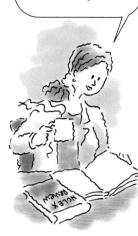

Because HIV-positive neonates are prone to opportunistic infections, keep the umbilical stump meticulously clean.

• Prophylactic trimethoprim-sulfamethoxazole (Bactrim) for babies 4 weeks of age or older
• Routine immunizations with killed viruses with the exception of oral polio and varicella vaccines
• Zidovudine (Retrovir) administration based on the neonate's lymphocyte count

INTERVENTIONS AND RATIONALES
• Assess the neonate's cardiovascular and respiratory status *to assess for complications.*
• Monitor vital signs and fluid intake and output *to assess for dehydration.*
• Monitor fluid and electrolyte status *to guide fluid and electrolyte replacement therapy.*
• Maintain standard precautions *to prevent the spread of infection..*
• Keep the umbilical stump meticulously clean *to prevent opportunistic infection.*
• Assist with blood sample and urine specimen collection *to prevent the spread of infection.*
• Administer medications, as indicated *to treat infection and improve immune function.*
• Provide emotional support to the family *to allay anxiety.*

Teaching topics
• Providing the child with all necessary immunizations

Hypothermia

A neonate's temperature is about 99° F (37.2° C) at birth. Inside the womb, the fetus was confined in an environment where the temperature was constant. At birth, this temperature can fall rapidly.

CAUSES
• Cold temperature in delivery environment
• Heat loss due to evaporation, conduction, or convection
• Immature temperature-regulating system
• Inability to conserve heat due to little subcutaneous fat

ASSESSMENT FINDINGS
• Kicking and crying (a mechanism to increase the metabolic rate to produce body heat)
• Core body temperature lower than 97.7° F (36.5° C)

DIAGNOSTIC TEST RESULTS
• Arterial blood gas analysis shows hypoxemia.
• Blood glucose level reveals hypoglycemia.

NURSING DIAGNOSES
• Hypothermia
• Ineffective thermoregulation
• Risk for altered parent/infant attachment

TREATMENT
• Radiant warmer

INTERVENTIONS AND RATIONALES
• Dry the neonate immediately *to prevent heat loss.*
• Allow the mother to hold the neonate *to provide warmth.*
• Monitor vital signs every 15 to 30 minutes *to assess temperature fluctuations and complications.*
• Provide a knitted cap for the neonate *to prevent heat loss through the head.*
• Place the neonate in a radiant warmer *to maintain thermoregulation.*

Teaching topics
• Infant-parent bonding (See *Teaching neonatal care to parents,* page 530.)

Neonatal drug dependency

Infants born to drug-addicted mothers are at risk for preterm birth, aspiration pneumonia, meconium-stained fluid, and meconium aspiration. Drug-dependent infants may also experience withdrawal from substances such as heroin and cocaine.

CAUSES
• Drug addiction in the mother

ASSESSMENT FINDINGS
• Diarrhea
• Frequent sneezing and yawning
• High-pitched cry
• Hyperactive reflexes
• Increased tendon reflexes
• Irritability
• Jitteriness
• Poor feeding habits
• Poor sleeping pattern
• Tremors
• Vigorous sucking on hands
• Withdrawal symptoms (depend on the length of maternal addiction, the drug ingested, and the time of last ingestion before delivery; usually appear within 24 hours of delivery)

DIAGNOSTIC TEST RESULTS
• Drug screen reveals agent abused by mother

NURSING DIAGNOSES
• Altered nutrition: Less than body requirements
• Risk for fluid volume deficit
• Risk for injury

TREATMENT
• Gavage feedings, if necessary
• I.V. therapy to maintain hydration

Drug therapy
• Paregoric and phenobarbital (Barbita) to treat withdrawal symptoms; methadone shouldn't be given to neonates because of its addictive nature

INTERVENTIONS AND RATIONALES
• Monitor cardiovascular status *to detect cardiovascular compromise.*
• Monitor vital signs and fluid intake and output *to assess for complications.*
• Encourage the mother to hold the infant *to promote maternal-infant bonding.*
• Use tight swaddling *for comfort.*
• Place the neonate in a dark, quiet room *to provide a stimulus-free environment.*
• Encourage the use of a pacifier *to meet sucking needs* (in cases of heroin withdrawal).

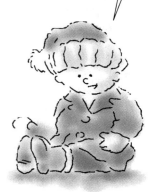

In the womb, the temperature was constant. At birth, my temperature may fall rapidly.

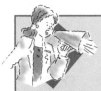

Listen up!

Teaching neonatal care to parents

Here are some topics to include when teaching parents about caring for their newborn.

CORD CARE
With every diaper change, wipe the umbilical cord with alcohol, especially around the base. Report any odor, discharge, or signs of skin irritation around the cord. Fold the diaper below the cord until the cord falls off after 7 to 10 days.

CUT CARE
Gently clean the circumcised penis with water, and apply fresh petroleum gauze with each diaper change. Loosen the petroleum gauze stuck to the penis by pouring warm water over the area. Don't remove yellow discharge that covers the glans after circumcision; this is part of normal healing. Report any foul-smelling, purulent discharge promptly. Apply diapers loosely until the circumcision heals after about 5 days.

UNCUT CARE
Don't retract the foreskin when washing the uncircumcised penis because the foreskin is adhered to the glans.

POTTY PATTERNS
Become familiar with the infant's voiding and elimination patterns.
• The infant's first stools are called meconium; they are odorless, dark green, and thick.
• Transitional stools occur about 2 to 3 days after ingestion of milk; they are greenish brown and thinner than meconium.
• The stools change to pasty yellow and pungent (bottle-fed infant) or loose yellow and sweet-smelling (breast-fed infant) by the 4th day.
• Change diapers before and after every feeding; expose the infant's buttocks to the air and light several times a day for about 20 minutes to treat diaper rash; apply ointment to minimize contact with urine and feces.

BATH TIME
Give the infant sponge baths until the cord falls off; then wash the infant in a tub containing 3" to 4" (7.6 to 10 cm) of warm water.

MEALTIME, PART ONE
Initiate breast-feeding as soon as possible after delivery and then feed the infant on demand.
• Position the infant's mouth slightly differently at each feeding to reduce irritation at one site.
• Burp the infant before switching to the other breast.
• Insert the little finger into a corner of the baby's mouth to separate the baby from the nipple.
• Experiment with various breast-feeding positions.
• Perform thorough breast care to promote cleanliness and comfort.
• Follow a diet that ensures adequate nutrition for the mother and infant (drink at least four 8-oz glasses of fluid daily, increase caloric intake by 200 kcal over the pregnancy requirement of 2,400 kcal, avoid foods that cause irritability, gas, or diarrhea).
• Consult the doctor before taking any medication.
• Know that ingested substances (caffeine, alcohol, and medications) can pass into breast milk.

MEALTIME, PART TWO
Follow the pediatrician's instructions for preparing and feeding with formula.
• Feed the infant in an upright position, and keep the nipple full of formula to minimize air swallowing.
• Burp the infant after each ounce of formula or more frequently if the infant spits up.

• Be prepared to administer gavage feeding *because of the neonate's poor sucking reflex* (in cases of methadone withdrawal).
• Maintain fluid and electrolyte balance *to replace fluid loss.*
• Monitor bilirubin levels and assess for jaundice (in cases of methadone withdrawal) *to assess for liver damage.*

Teaching topics
• Avoiding breast-feeding

Neonatal infections

A neonate may contract an infection before, during, or after delivery. Maternal IgM doesn't cross the placenta and IgA requires time to reach optimum levels after birth, limiting the neonate's immune response. Dysmaturity caused by intrauterine growth retardation, preterm birth, or postterm birth can further compromise the neonate's immune system and predispose him to infection.

Sepsis is one of the most significant causes of neonatal morbidity and mortality. Toxoplasmosis, syphilis, rubella, cytomegalovirus, and herpes are common perinatal infections known to affect infants.

CAUSES
- Chorioamnionitis
- Low birth weight or premature birth
- Maternal substance abuse
- Maternal urinary tract infections
- Meconium aspiration
- Nosocomial infection
- Premature labor
- Prolonged maternal rupture of membranes

ASSESSMENT FINDINGS
- Abdominal distention
- Apnea
- Feeding pattern changes, such as poor sucking or decreased intake
- Hyperbilirubinemia
- Pallor
- Petechiae
- Poor weight gain
- Sternal retractions
- Subtle, nonspecific behavioral changes, such as lethargy or hypotonia
- Temperature instability
- Vomiting
- Diarrhea

DIAGNOSTIC TEST RESULTS
- Blood and urine cultures are positive for causative organism, most commonly gram-positive beta-hemolytic streptococci and the gram-negative *Escherichia coli, Aerobacter, Proteus,* and *Klebsiella.*
- Blood chemistry shows increased direct bilirubin levels.
- Complete blood count shows an increased white blood cell count.
- Lumbar puncture is positive for causative organisms.

NURSING DIAGNOSES
- Altered nutrition: Less than body requirements
- Hypothermia
- Risk for fluid volume deficit

TREATMENT
- Gastric aspiration
- I.V. therapy to provide adequate hydration

Drug therapy
- Antibiotic therapy: broad-spectrum until causative organism is identified and then specific antibiotic

INTERVENTIONS AND RATIONALES
- Assess cardiovascular and respiratory status *to assess for complications.*
- Monitor vital signs and transcutaneous blood oxygen tension *to assess for complications.*
- Monitor fluid and electrolyte status *to assess the need for fluid replacement.*
- Initiate and maintain respiratory support as needed *to maintain respiratory filtration.*
- Administer broad-spectrum antibiotics before culture results are received and specific antibiotic therapy after results are received *to treat infection.*
- Provide the family with reassurance and support *to reduce anxiety.*
- Provide the neonate with physiologic supportive care *to maintain a neutral thermal environment.*
- Initiate and maintain I.V. therapy as ordered *to replace fluid loss.*
- Obtain blood samples and urine specimens *to assess antibiotic therapy efficacy.*

Teaching topics
- Importance of continuing drug therapy for the duration prescribed
- Preventing infection

Neonatal jaundice

Also called hyperbilirubinemia, neonatal jaundice is characterized by a bilirubin level that:
- exceeds 6 mg/dl within the first 24 hours after delivery

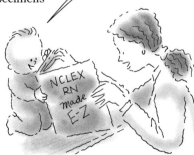

Studying sure gets hard…how did we get ourselves into this, anyway?

What do you mean we? I'm not taking the NCLEX…I'm a BABY!

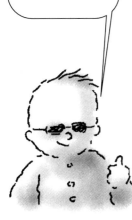

Phototherapy is the treatment of choice for neonatal jaundice.

• remains elevated beyond 7 days (in a full-term neonate)
• remains elevated for 10 days (in a premature neonate).

The neonate's bilirubin levels rise as bilirubin production exceeds the liver's capacity to metabolize it. Unbound, unconjugated bilirubin can easily cross the blood-brain barrier, leading to kernicterus (an encephalopathy).

CAUSES
• Absence of intestinal flora needed for bilirubin passage in the bowel
• Enclosed hemorrhage
• Erythroblastosis fetalis (hemolytic disease of the neonate)
• Hypoglycemia
• Hypothermia
• Impaired hepatic functioning
• Neonatal asphyxia (respiratory failure in the neonate)
• Polycythemia
• Prematurity
• Reduced bowel motility and delayed meconium passage
• Sepsis

ASSESSMENT FINDINGS
• Decreased reflexes
• High-pitched crying
• Jaundice
• Lethargy
• Opisthotonos
• Seizures

DIAGNOSTIC TEST RESULTS
• Bilirubin levels exceed 12 mg/dl in premature or term neonates.
• Conjugated (direct) bilirubin levels exceed 2 mg/dl.
• Bilirubin level rises by more than 5 mg/day.

NURSING DIAGNOSES
• Altered parenting
• Fluid volume deficit
• Risk for injury

TREATMENT
• Exchange transfusion to remove maternal antibodies and sensitized RBCs if phototherapy fails.

• Increased fluid intake
• Phototherapy (preferred treatment)
• Treatment for anemia if jaundice is caused by hemolytic disease

INTERVENTIONS AND RATIONALES
• Assess neurologic status *to assess for signs of encephalopathy, which indicates the potential for permanent damage.*
• Maintain a neutral thermal environment *to prevent hypothermia.*
• Monitor serum bilirubin levels *to assess for reduction of bilirubin.*
• Initiate and maintain phototherapy (provide eye protection while the neonate is under phototherapy lights and remove eye shields promptly when he is removed from the phototherapy lights) *to prevent complications.*
• Allow time for maternal infant bonding and interaction during phototherapy *to promote bonding.*
• Keep the neonate's anal area clean and dry. *Frequent, greenish stools result from bilirubin excretion and can lead to skin irritations.*
• Provide the parents with support, reassurance, and encouragement *to reduce anxiety.*

Teaching topics
• Encouraging frequent feedings to maintain adequate caloric intake and hydration and to facilitate excretion of wastes.

Respiratory distress syndrome

Respiratory distress syndrome occurs most often in preterm infants, infants of diabetic mothers, and infants delivered by cesarean section. In respiratory distress syndrome, a hyaline-like membrane lines the terminal bronchioles, alveolar ducts, and alveoli, preventing exchange of oxygen and carbon dioxide.

CAUSES
• Inability to maintain alveolar stability
• Low level or absence of surfactant

ASSESSMENT FINDINGS
- Cyanosis
- Expiratory grunting
- Fine crackles and diminished breath sounds
- Hypothermia
- Nasal flaring
- Respiratory acidosis
- Seesaw respirations
- Sternal and substernal retractions
- Tachypnea (more than 60 breaths/minute)

DIAGNOSTIC TEST RESULTS
- Arterial blood gas analysis reveals respiratory acidosis.
- Chest X-rays reveal bilateral diffuse reticulogranular density.

NURSING DIAGNOSES
- Altered nutrition: Less than body requirements
- Altered tissue perfusion
- Impaired gas exchange

TREATMENT
- Acid-base balance maintenance
- Endotracheal intubation and mechanical ventilation
- Nutrition supplements (total parenteral nutrition [TPN] or enteral feedings, if possible)
- Surfactant replacement by way of endotracheal tube
- Temperature regulation with a radiant warmer

Drug therapy
- Indomethacin (Indocin) to promote closure of ductus arteriosus (a fetal blood vessel connecting the left pulmonary artery to the descending aorta)

INTERVENTIONS AND RATIONALES
- Assess cardiovascular, respiratory, and neurologic status *to assess for respiratory distress.*
- Monitor continuous electrocardiography (ECG) and vital signs *to observe for changes.*
- Initiate and maintain ventilatory support status *to maintain air supply.*

- Administer medications, including endotracheal surfactant, as prescribed *to improve respiratory function.*
- Assess hydration status *to assess fluid loss.*
- Initiate and maintain I.V. therapy *to maintain fluid levels.*
- Provide adequate nutrition through enteral feedings, if possible, or TPN *to provide adequate nutrition.*
- Maintain thermoregulation *to reduce cold stress.*
- Obtain blood samples as necessary *to assess for complications.*

Teaching topics
- Promoting maternal-infant bonding

Tracheoesophageal fistula

Tracheoesophageal fistula is a congenital anomaly in which the esophagus and trachea don't separate normally. Most commonly, the esophagus ends in a blind pouch, with the trachea communicating by a fistula with the lower esophagus and stomach.

CAUSES
- Abnormal development of the trachea and esophagus during the embryonic period

ASSESSMENT FINDINGS
- Difficulty feeding, such as choking or aspiration; cyanosis during feeding
- Difficulty passing a nasogastric tube
- Excessive mucous secretions
- Maternal polyhydramnios (because fetus can't swallow amniotic fluid)
- Signs of respiratory distress (tachypnea, cyanosis, sternal and substernal retractions)

DIAGNOSTIC TEST RESULTS
- Abdominal X-ray shows the fistula and a gas-free abdomen.
- Bronchoscopy shows a blind pouch.

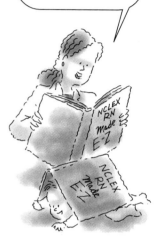

Because infants with respiratory distress syndrome can deteriorate rapidly, monitor ECG and vital signs.

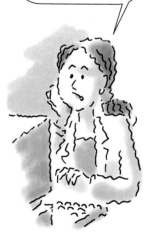

Neonate exhibits difficulty feeding and respiratory distress? That might mean tracheoesophageal fistula.

NURSING DIAGNOSES
• Altered nutrition: Less than body requirements
• Impaired gas exchange
• Risk for aspiration

TREATMENT
• Emergency surgical intervention to prevent pneumonia, dehydration, and fluid and electrolyte imbalances
• Gastrostomy tube placement
• Maintenance of patent airway

Drug therapy
• Antibiotics (as prophylaxis for aspiration pneumonia)

INTERVENTIONS AND RATIONALES
• Monitor cardiovascular, respiratory, and GI status *to assess for complications.*
• Monitor vital signs, fluid intake and output, and transcutaneous blood oxygen tension *to assess fluid replacement needs.*
• Place the neonate in high-Fowler's position *to prevent aspiration of gastric contents.*
• Keep a laryngoscope and endotracheal tube at bedside *in case extreme edema causes obstruction.*
• Provide frequent shallow suctioning for very short periods *to maintain airway patency.*
• Provide the neonate with a pacifier *to meet sucking needs.*
• Provide gastrostomy tube feedings postoperatively *to maintain nutrition.*
• Maintain I.V. fluid therapy *to replace fluid volume.*

Teaching topics
• Promoting maternal-infant bonding

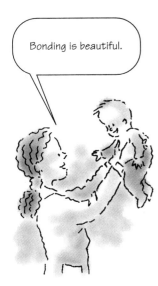

Bonding is beautiful.

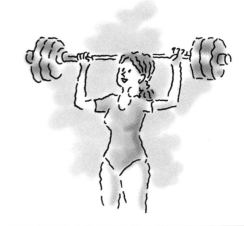

Pump up on practice questions

1. A baby weighing 1,503 g (3 lb, 5 oz) is born at 32 weeks' gestation. During an assessment 12 hours after birth, the nurse notices these signs and symptoms: hyperactivity, persistent shrill cry, frequent yawning and sneezing, and jitteriness. These symptoms indicate which of the following?
    A. Sepsis
    B. Hepatitis
    C. Drug dependence
    D. Hypoglycemia
Answer: C. These classic symptoms of drug dependency usually appear within the first 24 hours after birth. Sepsis is indicated by temperature instability and tachycardia. Hepatitis will manifest itself as jaundice. Hypothermia, muscle twitching, diaphoresis, and respiratory distress may be signs of hypoglycemia.

➡ **NCLEX keys**
Nursing process step: Implementation
Client needs category: Physiological integrity
Client needs subcategory: Physiological adaptation
Taxonomic level: Analysis

2. Which of the following is a preferred treatment for neonatal jaundice?
   A. Exchange transfusion
   B. Phototherapy
   C. Observing and monitoring bilirubin levels
   D. Stool softener

Answer: B. The preferred treatment of choice for neonatal jaundice is phototherapy. Exchange transfusion is performed when the bilirubin levels rapidly rise despite the use of phototherapy or hydration. Neonates with high bilirubin levels shouldn't be just observed; intervention is necessary. Stool softeners aren't a part of medical management for neonatal jaundice.

➡ *NCLEX keys*
Nursing process step: Implementation
Client needs category: Physiological integrity
Client needs subcategory: Physiological adaptation
Taxonomic level: Knowledge

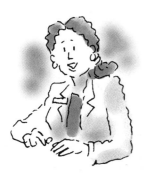

3. The nurse is assessing a 4-hour-old neonate. Which of the following would be a cause of concern?
   A. Anterior fontanel is ¾" (2 cm) wide, head is molded, and sutures are overriding.
   B. Hands and feet are cyanotic, abdomen is rounded, and the infant hasn't voided or passed meconium.
   C. Color is dusky, axillary temperature is 97° F (36.1° C), and the baby is spitting up excessive mucus.

   D. Irregular abdominal respirations and intermittent tremors in the extremities.

Answer: C. Skin color is expected to be pink-tinged or ruddy, saliva should be scant, and the normal axillary temperature ranges from 97.7° to 98.6° F (36.5° to 37° C). Overriding sutures and molding, when present, may persist for a few days. Acrocyanosis may be present for 2 to 6 hours. The neonate would be expected to pass meconium and void within 24 hours. Neonatal tremors are common in a full-term neonate; however, they must be evaluated to differentiate them from seizures.

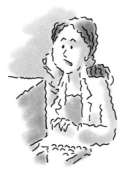

➡ *NCLEX keys*
Nursing process step: Assessment
Client needs category: Health promotion and maintenance
Client needs subcategory: Growth and development through the life span
Taxonomic level: Application

4. Which of the following neonates is at greatest risk for developing respiratory distress syndrome?
   A. A neonate with a history of intrauterine growth retardation
   B. A neonate born at less than 35 weeks' gestation
   C. A neonate whose mother experienced prolonged rupture of membranes
   D. A neonate born at 38 weeks' gestation

Answer: B. Respiratory distress syndrome is predominantly seen in premature infants; the more premature the infant, the more severe the disease. Intrauterine growth retardation and prolonged rupture of membranes are unlikely to be associated with development of respiratory distress syndrome. A 38-week gestation neonate usually has mature lungs and isn't at risk for respiratory distress syndrome.

➡ *NCLEX keys*
Nursing process step: Assessment
Client needs category: Physiological integrity
Client needs subcategory: Reduction of risk potential
Taxonomic level: Knowledge

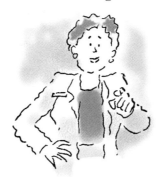

5. Which of the following infections can be acquired by the neonate during labor and delivery?
   A. Group B streptococci
   B. Rubella
   C. Hepatitis
   D. Syphilis
Answer: A. Group B streptococci may contaminate the maternal genital tract during labor and delivery. Rubella is acquired in utero. Hepatitis is a postnatal infection. Syphilis is also acquired in utero.

➡ *NCLEX keys*
Nursing process step: Analysis
Client needs category: Health promotion and maintenance
Client needs subcategory: Prevention and early detection of disease
Taxonomic level: Knowledge

6. The nurse assesses a neonate's respiratory rate at 46 breaths/minute 6 hours after birth. Respirations are shallow, with periods of apnea lasting up to 5 seconds. Which action should the nurse take next?
   A. Attach an apnea monitor.
   B. Continue routine monitoring.
   C. Follow respiratory arrest protocol.
   D. Call the pediatrician immediately to report findings.
Answer: B. The normal respiratory rate is 30 to 60 breaths/minute. Attaching the apnea monitor, following respiratory arrest protocol, and notifying the pediatrician of findings aren't necessary, as the listed findings are normal respiratory patterns in neonates.

➡ *NCLEX keys*
Nursing process step: Implementation
Client needs category: Health promotion and maintenance
Client needs subcategory: Growth and development through the life span
Taxonomic level: Application

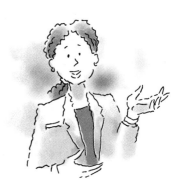

7. Which of the following statements is true?
   A. Binge drinking is less detrimental to the fetus than low-level chronic drinking.
   B. The mother's blood alcohol level is greater than that of the fetus.
   C. The fetus can stay drunk for many days.
   D. Fetal blood alcohol levels drop off quickly.
Answer: C. The fetal liver isn't mature enough to detoxify the alcohol. Binge drinking is more detrimental to the fetus than chronic

low-level drinking for this reason as well. Alcohol goes directly from mother to the fetus at the same level of concentration. High fetal blood alcohol levels stay that way for a long time.

➡ NCLEX keys

Nursing process step: Evaluation
Client needs category: Physiological integrity
Client needs subcategory: Reduction of risk potential
Taxonomic level: Analysis

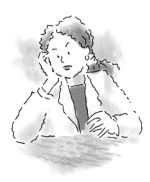

8. The only way to prevent fetal alcohol syndrome (FAS) is for a pregnant woman to:
   A. only drink on social occasions.
   B. stop drinking once she becomes pregnant.
   C. decrease alcohol intake while attempting to become pregnant.
   D. abstain from drinking before becoming pregnant and during the entire pregnancy.

Answer: D. The only prevention is to abstain from alcohol before and during pregnancy. Decreasing alcohol intake may not prevent intrauterine growth retardation. Social drinking can have adverse effects on an unborn child. Because the fetus can be damaged before the mother realizes that she's pregnant, stopping drinking once the pregnancy becomes known may not prevent FAS.

➡ NCLEX keys

Nursing process step: Analysis
Client needs category: Health promotion and maintenance

Client needs subcategory: Prevention and early detection of disease
Taxonomic level: Analysis

9. A baby girl delivered at 38-weeks' gestation weighs 2,325 grams (5 lb, 2 oz) and is having difficulty maintaining body temperature. Which nursing intervention would best prevent cold stress?
   A. Immediately after birth, dry the neonate and place her under a radiant heater for 2 hours.
   B. Administer oxygen for the first 30 minutes after birth.
   C. Decrease integumentary stimulation after birth.
   D. Maintain the environmental temperature at a constant level.

Answer: A. Drying the neonate and placing her in a radiant warmer helps prevent loss of body heat. Administering oxygen and decreasing integumentary circulation would have no effect in preventing cold stress. Maintaining environmental temperature wouldn't prevent loss of heat via conduction, evaporation, or convection.

➡ NCLEX keys

Nursing process step: Implementation
Client needs category: Physiological integrity
Client needs subcategory: Physiological adaptation
Taxonomic level: Application

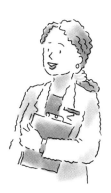

10. The nurse is caring for a drug-dependent neonate. Which intervention should the nurse perform?

    A.   Limit sensory stimulation of the neonate.

    B.   Cluster activities.

    C.   Wrap the neonate loosely in blankets.

    D.   Increase environmental stimuli.

Answer: A. Limiting sensory stimulation allows for extensive rest periods. The nurse may want to modulate sensory input as tolerated by the neonate. The neonate needs to be swaddled tightly in a flexed position. Increasing environmental stimuli may exacerbate irritability and restlessness.

➡ *NCLEX keys*

Nursing process step: Planning
Client needs category: Physiological integrity
Client needs subcategory: Physiological adaptation
Taxonomic level: Application

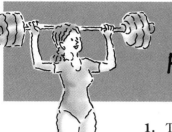

Pump up on more practice questions

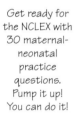

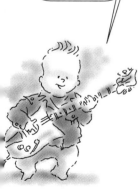

1. The nurse is assessing an infant with tracheoesophageal fistula. Which finding would the nurse expect to encounter?

    A. Increase in saliva
    B. Gastric tube easily passed
    C. Feeding without difficulty
    D. Normal chest X-ray

Answer: A. The infant's inability to swallow saliva leads to an increase in saliva. The other options aren't likely findings in tracheoesophageal fistula. The infant is unable to pass a gastric tube. During feedings, the infant is at risk for choking and cyanosis. Pulmonary infiltrates, lobar collapse, and atelectasis frequently appear on the chest X-ray.

➡ **NCLEX keys**
Nursing process step: Assessment
Client needs category: Physiological integrity
Client needs subcategory: Physiological adaptation
Taxonomic level: Knowledge

2. A client is scheduled for amniocentesis. When preparing her for the procedure, the nurse should:

    A. ask her to void.
    B. instruct her to drink 1 L (1 qt) of fluid.
    C. prepare her for I.V. anesthesia.
    D. place her on her left side.

Answer: A. To prepare a client for amniocentesis, the nurse should ask the client to empty her bladder to reduce the risk of bladder perforation. The nurse may instruct the client to drink 1 L of fluid to fill the bladder before transabdominal ultrasound (unless ultrasound is done before amniocentesis to locate the placenta). I.V. anesthesia isn't given for amniocentesis. The client should be supine during the procedure; afterward, she should be placed on her left side to avoid supine hypotension, promote venous return, and ensure adequate cardiac output.

➡ **NCLEX keys**
Nursing process step: Implementation
Client needs category: Safe, effective care environment
Client needs subcategory: Safety and infection control
Taxonomic level: Knowledge

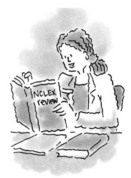

3. Six hours after birth, a neonate is transferred to the nursery. The nurse is planning interventions to prevent hypothermia. What is a common source of radiant heat loss?

    A. Low room humidity
    B. Cold weight scale
    C. Cool incubator walls
    D. Cool room temperature

Answer: C. Common sources of radiant heat loss include cool incubator walls and windows. Low room humidity promotes evaporative heat loss. When the skin directly contacts a cooler object, such as a cold weight scale, conductive heat loss may occur. A cool room temperature may lead to convective heat loss.

➡ **NCLEX keys**
Nursing process step: Planning
Client needs category: Health promotion and maintenance
Client needs subcategory: Growth and development through the lifespan
Taxonomic level: Knowledge

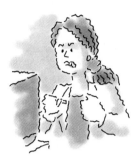

4. A client is in the 25th week of pregnancy. Which procedure is used to detect fetal anomalies?
   A. Amniocentesis
   B. Chorionic villi sampling
   C. Fetoscopy
   D. Ultrasound

Answer: D. Ultrasound is used between 18 and 40 weeks' gestation to identify normal fetal growth and detect fetal anomalies and other problems. Amniocentesis is done during the third trimester to determine fetal lung maturity. Chorionic villi sampling is performed at 8 to 12 weeks' gestation to detect genetic disease. Fetoscopy is done at about 18 weeks' gestation to observe the fetus directly and obtain a skin specimen or blood sample.

➡ *NCLEX keys*
Nursing process step: Implementation
Client needs category: Health promotion and maintenance
Client needs subcategory: Prevention and early detection of disease
Taxonomic level: Knowledge

5. Which nursing intervention has priority when feeding an infant with a cleft lip or palate?
   A. Directing the flow of milk in the center of mouth
   B. Providing frequent, small feedings
   C. Avoiding breast-feeding
   D. Infrequent burping

Answer: B. Frequent, small feedings help to prevent fatigue and frustration in the infant. The flow of milk should be directed to side of the mouth. Breast-feeding may be possible. These infants need frequent burping because of the large amount of air swallowed while feeding.

➡ *NCLEX keys*
Nursing process step: Implementation
Client needs category: Physiological integrity
Client needs subcategory: Physiological adaptation
Taxonomic level: Analysis

6. During a physical examination, a client in her 32nd week of pregnancy becomes pale, dizzy, and light-headed while supine. Which intervention takes priority?
   A. Turning the client onto her left side
   B. Asking the client to breathe deeply
   C. Listening to fetal heart tones
   D. Measuring the client's blood pressure

Answer: A. As the uterus enlarges, pressure on the inferior vena cava increases, compromising venous return and causing blood pressure to drop. This may lead to syncope and other symptoms when the client is supine. Turning the client onto her left side relieves pressure on the vena cava, restoring normal venous return and blood pressure. Deep breathing wouldn't relieve this client's symptoms. Listening to fetal heart tones and measuring the client's blood pressure don't provide relevant information.

➡ *NCLEX keys*
Nursing process step: Implementation
Client needs category: Safe, effective care environment
Client needs subcategory: Safety and infection control
Taxonomic level: Comprehension

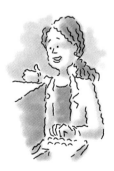

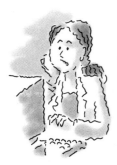

7. A client has meconium-stained amniotic fluid. The fetal monitoring strip shows fetal bradycardia. Fetal blood sampling indicates a pH of 7.12. Based on these findings, which nursing intervention is called for?

    A. Administer oxygen, as prescribed.
    B. Prepare for cesarean delivery.
    C. Reposition the client.
    D. Start I.V. oxytocin infusion, as prescribed.

Answer: B. Fetal blood pH of 7.19 or lower signals severe fetal acidosis; meconium-stained amniotic fluid and bradycardia are additional signs of fetal distress that warrant cesarean delivery. Oxygen administration and client repositioning may improve uteroplacental perfusion but are only temporary measures. Oxytocin administration increases contractions, exacerbating fetal stress.

➡ *NCLEX keys*
Nursing process step: Implementation
Client needs category: Physiological integrity
Client needs subcategory: Reduction of risk potential
Taxonomic level: Comprehension

8. Which of the following phases of uterine contractions is described as the letting-down phase?

    A. Increment
    B. Decrement
    C. Acme
    D. Variability

Answer: B. Decrement is the letting-down phase of uterine contractions. Increment refers to the building-up phase, and acme is the peak of the contraction. Variability refers to the normal variation in the heart rate, caused by continuous interplay of the parasympathetic and sympathetic nervous systems.

➡ *NCLEX keys*
Nursing process step: Assessment
Client needs category: Health promotion and maintenance
Client needs subcategory: Growth and development through the life span
Taxonomic level: Knowledge

9. Which diagnostic procedure will best determine whether a client in labor has spontaneous rupture of amniotic membranes?

    A. Complete blood count
    B. Fern test
    C. Urinalysis
    D. Vaginal examination

Answer: B. A fern test indicates spontaneous rupture of amniotic membranes. The name of this test refers to the microscopic fernlike pattern produced by sodium chloride crystallization in dried amniotic fluid, which indicates the presence of ruptured amniotic membranes. A complete blood count might indicate infection (if white blood cells are increased), but it won't indicate whether the amniotic sac had ruptured. Urinalysis doesn't test for the presence of amniotic fluid. A vaginal examination may determine whether the membranes have ruptured but isn't conclusive.

➡ *NCLEX keys*
Nursing process step: Assessment
Client needs category: Safe, effective care environment
Client needs subcategory: Safety and infection control
Taxonomic level: Analysis

10. A client is admitted to the hospital in preterm labor. To halt her uterine contractions, the nurse expects to administer:

    A. magnesium sulfate.
    B. dinoprostone.
    C. ergonovine maleate.
    D. terbutaline.

Answer: D. Terbutaline, a beta$_2$-receptor agonist, is used to inhibit preterm uterine contractions. Magnesium sulfate is used to treat pregnancy-induced hypertension. Dinoprostone is used to induce fetal expulsion and promote cervical dilation and softening. Ergonovine maleate is used to stop uterine blood flow, for example, in hemorrhage.

➡ *NCLEX keys*
Nursing process step: Planning
Client needs category: Physiological integrity
Client needs subcategory: Pharmacological and parenteral therapies
Taxonomic level: Comprehension

11. The nurse reviews the history of a postpartum client. Which factor most strongly indicates that this client is at risk for experiencing afterpains?
    A. The client delivered at 39 weeks' gestation.
    B. The client smokes cigarettes.
    B. The client has decided to bottle-feed her neonate.
    D. The client is a gravida 6, para 5.
Answer: D. In a multiparous client, decreased uterine muscle tone leads to alternating relaxation and contraction during uterine involution; this, in turn, causes afterpains. A gestation of 39 weeks and a history of cigarette smoking don't contribute directly to afterpains. A bottle-feeding client may experience afterpains from lack of oxytocin release, which stimulates the uterus to contract and thus enhances involution. The mere decision to bottle-feed doesn't cause afterpains.

➡ *NCLEX keys*
Nursing process step: Planning
Client needs category: Health promotion and maintenance
Client needs subcategory: Growth and development through the life span
Taxonomic level: Evaluation

12. The nurse is providing care for a client who has undergone an amniotomy. A strip obtained from an external fetal monitor shows large variable decelerations in the fetal heart rate (FHR). These findings signify:

    A an infection.
    B. umbilical cord prolapse.
    C. start of the second stage of labor.
    D. need for labor induction.
Answer: B. After an amniotomy, a significant change in the FHR may indicate umbilical cord prolapse; an external fetal monitor may show large variable decelerations during cord compression. The other options aren't associated with FHR changes. An infection causes a temperature elevation. The second stage of labor starts with complete cervical dilation. Labor induction is indicated if the client's labor fails to progress.

➡ *NCLEX keys*
Nursing process step: Assessment
Client needs category: Health promotion and maintenance
Client needs subcategory: Growth and development through the life span
Taxonomic level: Evaluation

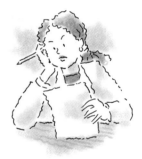

13. A fetal monitor strip shows a fetal heart rate (FHR) deceleration, which occurs about 30 seconds after each contraction begins; the FHR returns to baseline after the contraction is over. This type of deceleration is probably caused by:
    A. fetal head compression.
    B. umbilical cord compression.
    C. uteroplacental insufficiency.
    D. cardiac anomalies.
Answer: C. The fetal monitoring strip is showing late decelerations caused by uteroplacental insufficiency — inadequate fetal oxygenation resulting from decreased blood flow during uterine contractions. Uteroplacental insufficiency may result from maternal hy-

potension, tetanic contractions, postmaturity, abruptio placentae, or pregnancy-induced hypertension. Fetal head compression typically causes early decelerations, which begin and end at about the same time as the contractions. Umbilical cord compression results in variable decelerations, which are unpredictable in time of onset, duration, and appearance. Cardiac anomalies don't cause decelerations.

➡ NCLEX keys

Nursing process step: Assessment
Client needs category: Health promotion and maintenance
Client needs subcategory: Growth and development through the life span
Taxonomic level: Knowledge

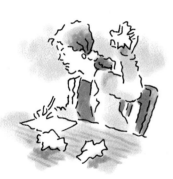

14. The nurse is reviewing laboratory results for a postpartum client. What happens to the level of human chorionic gonadotropin (HCG) during the postpartum period?

A. The circulating HCG level remains high for 2 to 4 weeks.
B. The serum HCG level diminishes over 6 weeks.
C. Circulating HCG disappears within 24 hours.
D The serum HCG level remains high until the client's next pregnancy.

Answer: C. Circulating HCG disappears within 8 to 24 hours after delivery in both lactating and nonlactating clients.

➡ NCLEX keys

Nursing process step: Assessment
Client needs category: Health promotion and maintenance
Client needs subcategory: Growth and development through the life span
Taxonomic level: Knowledge

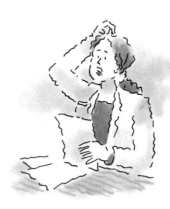

15. A client has been in labor for 6 hours, and her contractions are occurring every 2 minutes and lasting 80 seconds. She is diaphoretic, restless, and irritable and tells the nurse that she "can't take it anymore." Which stage or phase of labor is the client in?

A. Transitional phase
B. Latent phase
C. Second stage
D. Third stage

Answer: A. During the transitional phase, cervical dilation is between 8 and 10 cm and contractions occur every 1 to 2 minutes, last 60 to 90 seconds, and are strongly intense. Also during this phase, the client may feel overwhelmed and unable to continue with labor, become irritable and restless, groan or cry out, and experience diaphoresis and, possibly, nausea and vomiting. In the latent phase of the first stage, contractions are mild to moderate and irregular. The second stage of labor begins with full cervical dilation and ends with the delivery of the neonate. The third stage begins immediately after delivery.

➠ NCLEX keys
Nursing process step: Assessment
Client needs category: Health promotion and maintenance
Client needs subcategory: Growth and development through the life span
Taxonomic level: Knowledge

16. The nurse is assessing a client who is resting comfortably 4 hours after delivery. Which of the following findings is considered normal?
   A.   A thready pulse
   B.   An irregular pulse
   C.   Tachycardia
   D.   Bradycardia

Answer: D. During the client's first postpartum rest or sleep, which usually occurs 2 to 4 hours after delivery, the heart rate typically decreases, possibly slowing to 50 beats/ minute (bradycardia). This probably results from supine positioning and such normal physiologic phenomena as the postpartum rise in stroke volume and a reduction in vascular bed size. An irregular pulse is never normal. Tachycardia may indicate excessive blood loss, especially if accompanied by a thready pulse and other signs, such as pallor, an increased respiratory rate, and diaphoresis.

➠ NCLEX keys
Nursing process step: Assessment
Client needs category: Health promotion and maintenance
Client needs subcategory: Growth and development through the life span
Taxonomic level: Knowledge

17. The nurse should advise the pregnant client to use which body position to enhance cardiac output and renal function?
   A   Right lateral
   B.   Left lateral
   C.   Supine
   D.   Semi-Fowler's

Answer: B. The left lateral position shifts the enlarged uterus away from the vena cava and aorta, enhancing cardiac output, kidney perfusion, and kidney function. The right lateral and semi-Fowler's positions don't alleviate pressure of the enlarged uterus on the vena

cava. The supine position reduces sodium and water excretion because the enlarged uterus compresses the vena cava and aorta; this decreases cardiac output, leading to decreased renal blood flow, which in turn impairs kidney function.

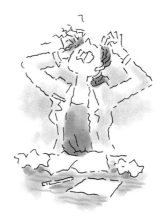

➠ NCLEX keys
Nursing process step: Implementation
Client needs category: Health promotion and maintenance
Client needs subcategory: Growth and development through the life span
Taxonomic level: Knowledge

18. The nurse is preparing a postpartum client for discharge. The nurse should instruct her to report:
   A.   scant lochia alba 2 to 3 weeks after delivery.
   B.   a temperature of 99.7° F (37.6° C) for 24 hours or more.
   C.   breast tenderness that is relieved by analgesics.
   D.   a red, warm, painful area in the breast.

Answer: D. Postpartum warning signs include a red, warm, painful area in either breast; heavy vaginal bleeding or passage of clots or tissue fragments; and a temperature of 100.2° F (37.9° C) or higher for 24 hours or longer. Scant lochia alba 2 to 3 weeks after delivery, a temperature of 99.7° F for 24 hours or longer, and breast tenderness that is relieved by analgesics are normal postpartum findings.

NCLEX keys

Nursing process step: Implementation
Client needs category: Health promotion and maintenance
Client needs subcategory: Growth and development through the life span
Taxonomic level: Knowledge

19. Just after delivery, axillary measurement reveals the neonate's temperature to be 94.1° F (34.5° C). What should the nurse do?

  A. Rewarm the neonate gradually.
  B. Rewarm the neonate rapidly.
  C. Observe the neonate at least hourly.
  D. Notify the physician when the neonate's temperature is normal.

Answer: A. A neonate with a temperature of 94.1° F is experiencing cold stress. To correct cold stress while avoiding hyperthermia and its complications, the nurse should rewarm the neonate gradually, observing closely and checking vital signs every 15 to 30 minutes. Rapid rewarming may cause hypothermia. Hourly observation is not frequent enough because cold stress increases oxygen, calorie, and fat expenditure, putting the neonate at risk for anabolic metabolism and, possibly, metabolic acidosis. A neonate with cold stress requires intervention; the nurse should notify the physician of the problem as soon as it's identified.

NCLEX keys

Nursing process step: Implementation
Client needs category: Safe, effective care environment
Client needs subcategory: Safety and infection control
Taxonomic level: Comprehension

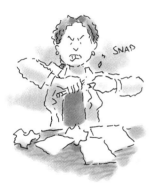

20. When does the postpartum client begin to accept the neonate as a separate individual?

  A. Letting-go phase
  B. Taking-hold phase
  C. Dependent phase
  D. Taking-in phase

Answer: A. Rubin identified three phases during which a woman adapts to the maternal role. During the taking-in (dependent) phase, which usually lasts 1 to 2 days after delivery, the client usually is exhausted and dependent on others, focusing on her own needs. During the taking-hold (dependent-independent) phase, which may last from 3 days to 8 weeks, the client vacillates between seeking nurturing and acceptance for herself and seeking to resume an independent role. During the letting-go (independent) phase, the client begins to accept the neonate as an individual who is separate from herself.

NCLEX keys

Nursing process step: Assessment
Client needs category: Psychosocial integrity
Client needs subcategory: Psychological adaptation
Taxonomic level: Knowledge

21. A neonate is born at 32 weeks' gestation to a mother who has admitted to using heroin. Which neonatal assessment takes priority?

  A. Auscultation of breath sounds for signs of pulmonary problems
  B. Careful observation of respiratory effort because of the neonate's prematurity
  C. Evaluation for signs of drug withdrawal
  D. Observation for jaundice

Answer: C. After delivery, a neonate born to a substance abuser may exhibit signs of drug withdrawal, such as irritability, poor feeding, and continual crying. Auscultating breath sounds, observing respiratory effort, and observing for jaundice are appropriate assessments for *any* neonate, not just the neonate of a substance abuser.

➠ NCLEX keys
Nursing process step: Assessment
Client needs category: Health promotion and maintenance
Client needs subcategory: Growth and development through the life span
Taxonomic level: Comprehension

22. The nurse is developing a teaching plan for a client who is about to be discharged after delivering a hydatidiform molar pregnancy. Which expected outcome takes highest priority?

 A. Client states that she may attempt another pregnancy after 3 months of follow-up care.
 B. Client schedules her first follow-up Papanicolaou test and gynecologic examination for 6 months after discharge.
 C. Client states that she won't attempt another pregnancy until her human chorionic gonadotropin (HCG) level rises.
 D. Client uses a reliable contraceptive method until her follow-up care is complete in 1 year and her HCG level is negative.

Answer: D. After a hydatidiform molar pregnancy, the client should receive follow-up care, including regular HCG testing, for 1 year because of the risk of developing chorionic carcinoma. After removal of a hydatidiform mole, the HCG level gradually falls to a negative reading unless chorionic carcinoma is developing, in which case the HCG level rises. A Papanicolaou test isn't an effective indicator of a hydatidiform molar pregnancy. A follow-up examination would be scheduled within weeks of the client's discharge. The client must not become pregnant during follow-up care because pregnancy causes the HCG level to rise, making it indistinguishable from this early sign of chorionic carcinoma.

➠ NCLEX keys
Nursing process step: Planning
Client needs category: Health promotion and maintenance
Client needs subcategory: Growth and development through the life span
Taxonomic level: Knowledge

23. A client expresses concern that her 3-hour-old neonate is difficult to awaken. The nurse explains that this behavior indicates:

 A a physiologic abnormality.
 B. probable hypoglycemia.
 C. normal progression into the sleep cycle.
 D. normal progression into a period of neonatal reactivity.

Answer: C. Three hours after birth, the neonate typically is difficult to awaken. This finding suggests normal progression into the sleep cycle. During this period, the neonate shows minimal response to external stimuli. Hypoglycemia is characterized by irregular respirations, apnea, and tremors. Periods of neonatal reactivity are characterized by alertness and attentiveness.

➠ NCLEX keys
Nursing process step: Assessment
Client needs category: Health promotion and maintenance
Client needs subcategory: Growth and development through the life span
Taxonomic level: Knowledge

24. The nurse assesses a postpartum client for signs and symptoms of cardiac decompensation. During the postpartum period, which condition may lead to cardiac decompensation?

 A. Decreased renal function
 B. Increased pain
 C. Increased cardiac output
 D. Decreased hepatic blood flow

Answer: C. Cardiac output increases immediately after delivery, as blood that had been diverted to the uterus reenters the central circulation. A client who can't tolerate these postpartum changes may experience cardiac decompensation and heart failure. After delivery, renal function increases as urine production and bladder filling increase. Pain seldom worsens after delivery, although some uterine cramps, breast tenderness, and perineal discomfort may occur. Although hepatic blood flow typically falls to prepregnancy levels after delivery, this doesn't affect cardiac function.

➡ NCLEX keys

Nursing process step: Assessment
Client needs category: Physiological integrity
Client needs subcategory: Physiological adaptation
Taxonomic level: Knowledge

25. A client expresses concern that her 2-day-old breast-feeding neonate isn't getting enough to eat. The nurse should teach the client that breast-feeding is effective if:
    A. the neonate voids once or twice every 24 hours.
    B. the neonate breast-feeds four times in 24 hours.
    C. the neonate loses 10% to 15% of birth weight within the first 2 days after birth.
    D. the neonate latches onto the areola and swallows audibly.

Answer: D. Breast-feeding is effective if the infant latches onto the mother's areola properly and if swallowing is audible. A breast-feeding neonate should void at least six to eight times per day and should breast-feed every 2 to 3 hours. Over the first few days after birth, an acceptable weight loss is 5% to 10% of the birth weight.

➡ NCLEX keys

Nursing process step: Implementation
Client needs category: Health promotion and maintenance
Client needs subcategory: Growth and development through the life span
Taxonomic level: Comprehension

26. A client who used heroin during her pregnancy delivers a neonate. When assessing the neonate, the nurse expects to find:
    A. lethargy 2 days after birth.
    B. irritability and poor sucking.
    C. a flattened nose, small eyes, and thin lips.
    D. congenital defects, such as limb anomalies.

Answer: B. Neonates of heroin-addicted mothers are physically dependent on the drug and experience withdrawal when the drug is no longer supplied. Signs of heroin withdrawal include irritability, poor sucking, and restlessness. Lethargy isn't associated with neonatal heroin addiction. A flattened nose, small eyes, and thin lips are seen in infants with fetal alcohol syndrome. Heroin use during pregnancy hasn't been linked to specific congenital anomalies.

➡ NCLEX keys

Nursing process step: Assessment
Client needs category: Health promotion and maintenance
Client needs subcategory: Growth and development through the life span
Taxonomic level: Evaluation

27. When assessing a neonate 1 hour after delivery, the nurse measures an axillary temperature of 95.8° F (35.4° C), an apical pulse of 110 beats/minute, and a respiratory rate of 64 breaths/minute. Which nursing diagnosis takes highest priority?
    A. Hypothermia related to heat loss
    B. Altered parenting related to the addition of a new family member
    C. Risk for fluid volume deficit related to insensible fluid losses
    D. Risk for infection related to transition to the extrauterine environment

Answer: A. The neonate's temperature should range from 96° to 97.7° F (35.6° to 36.5° C) and the respiratory rate should be less than 60 breaths/minute. (The respiratory rate increases as hypothermia develops.) Because this neonate's temperature is below normal and because cold stress can lead to respiratory distress and hypoglycemia, hypothermia related to heat loss takes highest priority. The other options may be appropriate but don't take precedence over hypothermia, a potentially life-threatening condition.

➡ NCLEX keys

Nursing process step: Planning
Client needs category: Health promotion and maintenance
Client needs subcategory: Growth and development through the life span
Taxonomic level: Knowledge

28. During a nonstress test (NST), the nurse notes three fetal heart rate (FHR) increases of 20 beats/minute, each lasting 20 seconds. These increases occur only with fetal movement. What does this finding suggest?

    A. The client should undergo an oxytocin challenge test.

    B. The test is inconclusive and must be repeated.

    C. The fetus is nonreactive and hypoxic.

    D. The fetus isn't in distress at this time.

Answer: D. In an NST, reactive (favorable) results include two to three FHR increases of 15 beats/minute or more, each lasting 15 seconds or more and occurring with fetal movement. An oxytocin challenge test isn't performed to stimulate uterine contractions. Instead, a nipple stimulation contraction test may be ordered. A nonreactive NST result occurs when the FHR doesn't rise 15 beats/minute or more over the specified time; a nonreactive result may indicate fetal hypoxia.

➡ NCLEX keys

Nursing process step: Assessment
Client needs category: Health promotion and maintenance
Client needs subcategory: Growth and development through the life span
Taxonomic Level: Comprehension

29. The nurse places a neonate with hyperbilirubinemia under a phototherapy lamp. The goal of phototherapy is:

    A. to prevent hypothermia.

    B. to promote respiratory stability.

    C. to decrease the serum conjugated bilirubin level.

    D. to decrease the serum unconjugated bilirubin level.

Answer: D. The goal of phototherapy is to reduce the serum unconjugated bilirubin level because a high level may lead to bilirubin encephalopathy (kernicterus). Phototherapy doesn't prevent hypothermia or promote respiratory stability. It has no effect on conjugated bilirubin, a water-soluble substance excreted easily in urine and stools.

➡ NCLEX keys

Nursing process step: Planning
Client needs category: Health promotion and maintenance
Client needs subcategory: Growth and development through the life span
Taxonomic level: Knowledge

30. The nurse assesses a 1-day-old neonate. Which nursing assessment indicates that the neonate's oxygen needs aren't being adequately met?

    A. Respiratory rate of 54 breaths/minute

    B. Abdominal breathing

    C. Nasal flaring

    D. Acrocyanosis

Answer: C. Signs of respiratory distress include a respiratory rate above 60 breaths/minute, labored respirations, grunting, nasal flaring, generalized cyanosis, and retractions. Abdominal breathing is a normal finding in neonates. Acrocyanosis (a bluish tinge to the hands and feet) is normal on the 1st day after birth.

➡ NCLEX keys

Nursing process step: Evaluation
Client needs category: Health promotion and maintenance
Client needs subcategory: Growth and development through the life span
Taxonomic level: Knowledge

You did it!

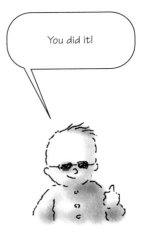

Part V Care of the child

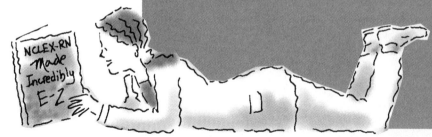

Growth & Development

Brush up on key concepts

Growth and development are fundamental concepts in pediatric nursing. Each developmental stage presents unique patient care challenges in such areas as nutrition, language, safety education, medication administration, and pain management.

You can review the major points of this chapter by consulting the *Cheat sheet* on page 552.

An infant's developmental milestones

A child is considered an infant from the time he's born until age 1. During this time, development is marked by five major periods:
• the neonatal period
• 1 to 4 months
• 5 to 6 months
• 7 to 9 months
• 10 to 12 months.

NEONATAL PERIOD
The neonatal period covers the time from birth to 28 days old.

Reflexes reign
During this period, these findings are noted:
• Head and chest circumferences are approximately equal.
• Behavior is under reflex control.
• Extremities are flexed.
• Vision is poor (the neonate fixates momentarily on light).
• Hearing and touch are well developed.
When prone, the neonate can lift the head slightly off the bed.

Rapid pulse and respiration
• Normal pulse rate ranges from 110 to 160 beats/minute.
• Normal respiratory rate is 32 to 60 breaths/minute.
• Respirations are irregular and from the abdomen.
• The neonate is an obligate nose breather.

Blood pressure and temperature
• Normal blood pressure is 82/46 mm Hg.
• Temperature regulation is poor.

1 TO 4 MONTHS
At age 3 months, the most primitive reflexes begin to disappear, except for the protective and postural reflexes (blink, parachute, cough, swallow, and gag reflexes), which remain for life. The infant reaches out voluntarily but is uncoordinated.

Heads up
During this period, the posterior fontanel closes. In addition, the infant:
• begins to hold up the head
• begins to put hand to mouth
• develops binocular vision
• cries to express needs
• smiles (The instinctual smile appears at 2 months and the social smile at 3 months.)
• laughs in response to the environment (at 4 months).

5 TO 6 MONTHS
At 5 to 6 months, birth weight doubles. In addition, the infant:
• rolls over from stomach to back
• cries when the parent leaves
• attempts to crawl when prone
• voluntarily grasps and releases objects.

7 TO 9 MONTHS
At 7 to 9 months, the infant can self-feed crackers and a bottle. When physically and

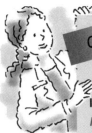

Cheat sheet

Growth & development refresher

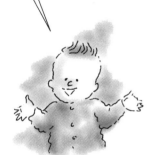

Ha, ha. That's a good one. At 4 months, I laugh in response to the environment.

INFANT (BIRTH TO AGE 1)

Neonatal period
• All behavior is under reflex control; extremities are flexed.
• Normal pulse rate ranges from 110 to 160 beats/minute.
• Normal respiratory rate is 32 to 60 breaths/ minute. Respirations are irregular and from the abdomen; the neonate is an obligate nose breather.
• Normal blood pressure is 82/46 mm Hg.
• Temperature regulation is poor.

1 to 4 months
• The posterior fontanel closes.
• The infant begins to hold up the head.
• The infant cries to express needs.

5 to 6 months
• The infant rolls over from stomach to back.
• The infant cries when the parent leaves.

7 to 9 months
• The infant sits alone with assistance.
• The infant creeps on hands and knees with belly off floor.
• The infant verbalizes all vowels and most consonants but speaks no intelligible words.
• Fear of strangers appears to peak during the 8th month.

10 to 12 months
• The infant holds on furniture while walking (cruising) at age 10 months, walks with support at age 11 months, and stands alone and takes first steps at age 12 months.
• The infant says "mama" and "dada" and responds to own name at age 10 months; can say about five words, but understands many more.

TODDLER (AGES 1 TO 3)
• Normal pulse rate is 100 beats/minute.
• Normal respiratory rate is 26 breaths/minute.
• Normal blood pressure is 99/64 mm Hg.
• Separation anxiety arises.
• The child is toilet-trained; day dryness is achieved by ages 18 months to 3 years and night dryness by ages 2 to 5.

PRESCHOOL CHILD (AGES 3 TO 5)
• Normal pulse rate ranges from 90 to 100 beats/minute.
• Normal respiratory rate is 25 breaths/minute.
• Normal blood pressure ranges from 85/60 to 90/70 mm Hg.
• The child may express fear of animal noises, new experiences, and the dark.

SCHOOL-AGE CHILD (AGES 5 TO 12)
• Normal pulse rate ranges from 75 to 115 beats/minute.
• Normal blood pressure ranges from 106/69 to 117/76 mm Hg.
• Normal respiratory rate ranges from 20 to 25 breaths/minute.
• The child plays with peers, develops a first true friendship, and develops a sense of belonging, cooperation, and compromise.
• The child learns to read and spell.
• Accidents are a major cause of death and disability during this period.

ADOLESCENT (AGES 12 TO 18)
• The adolescent experiences puberty-related changes in body structure and psychosocial adjustment.
• Peers influence behavior and values.
• Vital signs approach adult values.

emotionally ready, the infant can be weaned. The infant understands the word "no." Efforts to enforce discipline are appropriate at this time. Fear of strangers appears to peak during the 8th month. Attempts to assess breath and heart sounds should be made while the mother holds the infant.

Sit, creep, and prespeak
In addition, the infant:
• sits alone with assistance

Advice from the experts

Infants and nutrition

Here is a rundown of primary nutrition guidelines for a child's 1st year of life.
• Begin with formula or breast milk; give no more than 30 oz (887 ml) of formula each day.
• Iron supplements may be necessary after 4 months.
• No solid foods should be given for the first 6 months.
• Provide rice cereal as the first solid food, followed by any other cereal except wheat.
• Yellow and green vegetables may be given at 8 to 9 months.
• Provide noncitrus fruits at 6½ to 8 months, followed by citrus fruits late in the 1st year.
• Give junior foods or soft table foods after 9 months.

Goo goo. Ga ga. (Translation: I verbalize all vowels and most consonants but don't articulate intelligible words.)

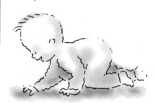

• creeps on hands and knees with belly off floor
• verbalizes all vowels and most consonants but doesn't articulate intelligible words.

10 TO 12 MONTHS
At 10 to 12 months, birth weight triples, and birth length increases about 50%. The anterior fontanel normally closes between ages 9 and 18 months. In addition, the infant:
• may walk while holding onto furniture (cruising) at age 10 months
• walks with support at age 11 months, and stands alone and takes first steps at age 12 months
• says "mama" and "dada" and responds to own name at age 10 months
• can say about five words, but understands many more
• is ready to be weaned from the bottle and breast. (See *Infants and nutrition*.)

Toddler developmental milestones

The toddler period includes ages 1 to 3. This is a slow growth period with a weight gain of 4 to 9 lb (2 to 4 kg) over 2 years.

Vital measurements
• Normal pulse rate is 100 beats/minute.

• Normal respiratory rate is 26 breaths/minute.
• Normal blood pressure is 99/64 mm Hg.

Me, myself, and I
The toddler exhibits the following behavioral and psychological characteristics:
• egocentricity
• frequent temper tantrums, especially when confronted with the conflict of achieving autonomy and relinquishing dependence on others
• follows the parent wherever he or she goes
• experiences separation anxiety
• lacks the concept of sharing
• prefers solitary play and has little interaction with others; this progresses to parallel play (toddler plays alongside but not with another child).

Look, Ma
The toddler:
• plants his feet wide apart and walks by age 15 months
• climbs stairs at 21 months, runs and jumps by age 2, and rides a tricycle by age 3
• uses at least 400 words as well as two- to three-word phrases and comprehends many more (by age 2)
• uses about 11,000 words (by age 3)
• undergoes toilet training; day dryness should be achieved by ages 18 months to 3 years and night dryness by ages 2 to 5.

I mellow with age. At ages 1 to 3, my heart rate is 100 beats/minute. By ages 3 to 5, it may slow to 90 beats/minute.

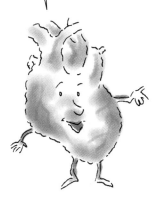

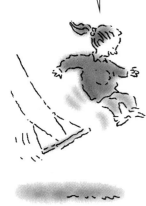

> Look out. Accidents are the major cause of school-age disability.

Preschool developmental milestones

The preschool period encompasses ages 3 to 5. Slow growth continues during this period. Birth length doubles by age 4.

Vital measurements
• Normal pulse rate ranges from 90 to 100 beats/minute.
• Normal respiratory rate is 25 breaths/ minute.
• Normal blood pressure ranges from 85/60 to 90/70 mm Hg.

Facing fear
The child may begin to express fear. Anticipate the child's fear of animal noises, new experiences, and the dark. Provide adhesive bandages for cuts because the child may fear losing blood. Using dolls for role-playing may reduce the preschool child's anxiety.

Playtime progress
The child:
• exhibits parallel play, associative play, group play in activities with few or no rules, and independent play accompanied by sharing or talking
• develops a body image
• may count but not understand what numbers mean
• may recognize some letters of the alphabet
• dresses without help but may be unable to tie shoes
• speaks in grammatically correct, complete sentences
• gets along without parents for short periods.

> As the child moves into adolescence, nutritional needs increase significantly — remember, most eating disorders emerge during adolescence.

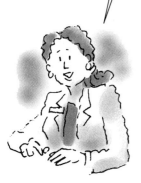

School-age developmental milestones

The school-age years last from ages 5 to 12.

Beat, blood, breath
• Normal pulse rate ranges from 75 to 115 beats/minute.
• Normal blood pressure ranges from 106/69 to 117/76 mm Hg.
• Normal respiratory rate ranges from 20 to 25 breaths/minute.

Watch out
• Accidents are a major cause of death and disability during this period.
• Height increases about 2″ (5 cm) a year, and weight doubles between ages 6 and 12.
• The first primary tooth is displaced by a permanent tooth at age 6, and permanent teeth erupt by age 12 except for final molars.
• Vision matures by age 6.

Look, Ma!
The child:
• engages in cooperative play
• plays with peers, develops a first true friendship, and develops a sense of belonging, cooperation, and compromise
• develops concepts of time and place, cause and effect, reversibility, conversation, and numbers
• learns to read and spell
• engages in fantasy play and daydreaming.

Adolescent developmental milestones

Ages 12 to 18 encompass the adolescent period. Adolescence is a period of rapid growth characterized by puberty-related changes in body structure and psychosocial adjustment.

What's happening to me?
During adolescence, these changes are noted:
• Vital signs approach adult levels.
• Peers influence behavior and values.
• Nutritional needs increase significantly.

Ch..ch..changes
Other milestones in adolescent development include:
• increased ability to engage in abstract thinking and to analyze, synthesize, and use logic
• increased attraction to the opposite sex (or same sex)
• breast development in females (the first sign of puberty; begins at about age 9 with the bud stage)
• the onset of menses in females (between ages 8 and 16; possibly irregular initially)
• testicular enlargement in males (the first sign of puberty).

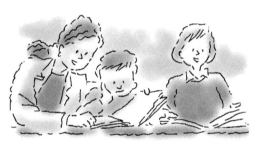

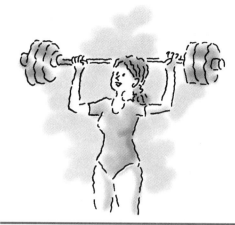

Pump up on practice questions

1. A parent brings a 19-month-old toddler to the clinic for a well checkup. When palpating the toddler's fontanels, the nurse would expect to find:
    A. closed anterior fontanel and open posterior fontanel.
    B. open anterior fontanel and closed posterior fontanel.
    C. closed anterior and posterior fontanels.
    D. open anterior and posterior fontanels.
Answer: C. By age 18 months, the anterior and posterior fontanels should be closed. The diamond-shaped anterior fontanel normally closes between ages 9 and 18 months. The triangular posterior fontanel normally closes between ages 2 and 3 months.

➡ *NCLEX keys*
Nursing process step: Assessment
Client needs category: Health promotion and maintenance
Client needs subcategory: Growth and development through the life span
Taxonomic level: Knowledge

2. The nurse is instructing a mother about the nutritional needs of her full-term, breast-feeding infant, age 2 months. Which of the following responses shows that the mother understands the infant's dietary needs?

- A. "We won't start any new foods now."
- B. "We'll start the baby on skim milk."
- C. "We'll introduce cereal into the diet now."
- D. "We should add new fruits to the diet one at a time."

Answer: A. Because breast milk provides all the nutrients that a full-term infant needs for the first 6 months, the parents shouldn't introduce new foods into the infant's diet at this point. They shouldn't provide skim milk because it doesn't have sufficient fat for infant growth. The parents also shouldn't provide solid foods, such as cereal and fruit, before age 6 months because the infant's GI tract doesn't tolerate them well.

➡ NCLEX keys
Nursing process step: Evaluation
Client needs category: Health promotion and maintenance
Client needs subcategory: Growth and development through the life span
Taxonomic level: Application

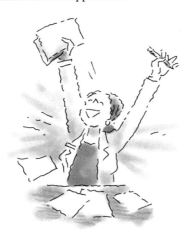

3. The nurse is assessing the sexual development of a preteenage girl. What is the first sign of sexual maturation in females?

- A. Onset of menstruation
- B. Breast development
- C. Appearance of pubic hair
- D. Appearance of axillary hair

Answer: B. The first sign of sexual maturation in females is the development of breast buds (elevation of the nipples and areolae). Then sexual development progresses, causing the appearance of pubic hair and axillary hair and the onset of menstruation.

➡ NCLEX keys
Nursing process step: Assessment
Client needs category: Health promotion and maintenance
Client needs subcategory: Growth and development through the life span
Taxonomic level: Knowledge

4. A preschooler is admitted to the hospital the day before scheduled surgery. This is the child's first hospitalization. Which of the following actions will best help reduce the child's anxiety about the upcoming surgery?

- A. Begin preoperative teaching immediately.
- B. Describe preoperative and postoperative procedures in detail.
- C. Give the child dolls and medical equipment to play out the experience.
- D. Explain that the child will be put to sleep during surgery and won't feel anything.

Answer: C. By playing with medical equipment and acting out the experience with dolls, the preschooler can begin to reduce anxiety. The nurse should schedule teaching shortly before surgery because preschoolers have little concept of time and because a delay between teaching and surgery may increase anxiety by giving the child time to worry. Detailed explanations are inappropriate for this developmental stage and may promote anxiety. The nurse should avoid such phrases as "put to sleep" because they might have a negative meaning to the child.

➡ NCLEX keys
Nursing process step: Implementation
Client needs category: Psychosocial integrity
Client needs subcategory: Coping and adaptation
Taxonomic level: Application

5. Before a well checkup in the pediatrician's office, an 8-month-old infant is sitting contentedly on the mother's lap, chewing a toy. When preparing to examine this infant, which of the following steps should the nurse do first?

    A. Obtain body weight.
    B. Auscultate heart and breath sounds.
    C. Check pupillary response.
    D. Measure the head circumference.

Answer: B. Heart and lung auscultation shouldn't distress the infant, so it should be done early in the assessment. Placing a tape measure on the infant's head, shining a light in the eyes, or undressing the infant before weighing may cause distress, making the rest of the examination more difficult.

➡ *NCLEX keys*

Nursing process step: Planning
Client needs category: Health promotion and maintenance
Client needs subcategory: Growth and development through the life span
Taxonomic level: Comprehension

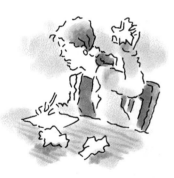

6. The nurse is teaching a mother who plans to discontinue breast-feeding after 5 months. The nurse should advise her to include which of the following foods in her infant's diet?

    A. Iron-rich formula and baby food
    B. Whole milk and baby food
    C. Skim milk and baby food
    D. Iron-rich formula only

Answer: D. The American Academy of Pediatrics recommends that infants at age 5 months should receive iron-rich formula and that they shouldn't receive solid food — even baby food — until age 6 months. The Academy doesn't recommend whole milk until age 12 months or skim milk until after age 2 years.

➡ *NCLEX keys*

Nursing process step: Implementation
Client needs category: Health promotion and maintenance
Client needs subcategory: Growth and development through the life span
Taxonomic level: Knowledge

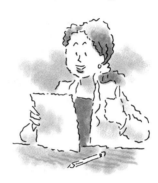

7. A mother tells the nurse that her 22-month-old child says "no" to everything. When scolded, the toddler becomes angry and starts crying loudly, but then immediately wants to be held. What is the best interpretation of this behavior?

    A. The toddler isn't effectively coping with stress.
    B. The toddler's need for affection isn't being met.
    C. This is normal behavior for a 2-year-old child.
    D. This behavior suggests the need for counseling.

Answer: C. Because toddlers are confronted with the conflict of achieving autonomy, yet relinquishing the much-enjoyed dependence on the affection of others, their negativism is a necessary assertion of self-control. Therefore, this behavior is a normal part of the child's growth and development. Nothing about the behavior indicates that the child is under stress, isn't receiving sufficient affection, or requires counseling.

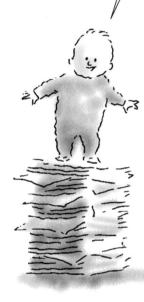

Reviewing this chapter was good preparation for the pediatric chapters ahead. Good luck, and remember to focus on patient care.

➡ NCLEX keys

Nursing process step: Evaluation
Client needs category: Health promotion and maintenance
Client needs subcategory: Growth and development through the life span
Taxonomic level: Comprehension

8. Which of the following observations signals the onset of puberty in male adolescents?
A. Appearance of pubic hair
B. Appearance of axillary hair
C. Testicular enlargement
D. Nocturnal emissions

Answer: C. Testicular enlargement signifies the onset of puberty in the male adolescent. Then sexual development progresses, causing the appearance of pubic hair and axillary hair and the onset of nocturnal emissions.

➡ NCLEX keys

Nursing process step: Assessment
Client needs category: Health promotion and maintenance
Client needs subcategory: Growth and development through the life span
Taxonomic level: Knowledge

9. The nurse is teaching the parents of a school-age child. Which of the following teaching topics should take priority?
A. Accident prevention
B. Keeping a night light on to allay fears
C. Normalcy of fears about body integrity
D. Encouraging the child to dress without help

Answer: A. Accidents are the major cause of death and disability during the school-age years. Therefore accident prevention should take priority when teaching parents of school-age children. Preschool children are afraid of the dark, have fears concerning body integrity, and should be encouraged to dress without help (with the exception of tying shoes), but none of these should take priority over accident prevention.

➡ NCLEX keys

Nursing process step: Planning
Client needs category: Health promotion and maintenance
Client needs subcategory: Growth and development through the life span
Taxonomic level: Knowledge

10. A mother brings her infant to the pediatrician's office for his 2-week-old checkup. The nurse is evaluating whether the mother has understood patient teaching points discussed during a previous visit. Which of the following indicates that further teaching is needed?
A. "I don't understand why my baby doesn't look at me."
B. "I know I should keep my baby's nasal passages clear."
C. "I should limit my baby's exposure during bath time."
D. "I should cover my baby's head when he's wet or cold."

Answer: A. Further teaching is indicated if the mother states that she doesn't understand why her 2-week-old infant doesn't look at her. The infant at this period of development has poor vision, is only able to fixate on light momentarily, and can't distinguish objects. The 2-week-old infant should have his nasal passages kept clear because he's an obligate nose breather; he should have limited exposure at bath time; and he should have his head covered when he's wet or cold.

➡ NCLEX keys

Nursing process step: Evaluation
Client needs category: Health promotion and maintenance
Client needs subcategory: Growth and development through the life span
Taxonomic level: Analysis

Brush up on key concepts

The cardiovascular system consists of the heart and central and peripheral blood vessels. A child's cardiovascular system closely resembles that of an adult. The system's main functions are to pump and circulate blood throughout the body.

At any time, you can review the major points of this chapter by consulting the *Cheat sheet* on page 560.

Communication breakdown

A child may have congenital heart defects that impair the movement of blood between the heart's chambers. For example, some congenital heart defects cause a **left-to-right shunt,** in which increased pressure on the left side of the heart forces blood back to the right side. This can lead to tissue hypertrophy on the right side and increased blood flow to the lungs.

Not closed

The blood vessels surrounding the heart may also suffer congenital defects. Soon after birth, the ductus arteriosus (located between the aorta and the pulmonary artery) normally closes. If it doesn't, the infant may experience **patent ductus arteriosus,** in which blood shunts from the aorta to the pulmonary artery. If a large patent ductus arteriosus remains uncorrected, pressure within the pulmonary arteries may increase dramatically and cause blood to flow from the right side of the heart to the left, eventually leading to heart failure.

Keep abreast of diagnostic tests

The most important tests used to diagnose cardiovascular disorders include cardiac catheterization and echocardiography.

Cardiac cath

In **cardiac catheterization,** a catheter is inserted into an artery or vein (in the arm or leg) and advanced to the heart. This procedure is used to:
• evaluate ventricular function
• measure heart pressures
• measure the blood's oxygen saturation level.

Nursing actions

Before the procedure, you should:
• describe the sensations the child will experience
• weigh the child
• check the child's color, pulse rate, blood pressure, and temperature of extremities
• check the child's activity level
• prepare the child by using doll play and hospital play. Show where the catheter is inserted. Make a security object (for example, a teddy bear or toy) available.

After the procedure, you should:
• keep the affected extremity immobile after catheterization to prevent hemorrhage
• keep the catheter site clean and dry and monitor for hematoma formation
• compare postcatheterization assessment data to precatheterization baseline data, comparing all four extremities
• ensure adequate intake (I.V. and oral) to compensate for blood loss during the procedure, nothing-by-mouth status, and diuretic action of some dyes used.

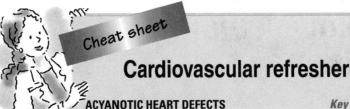

Cheat sheet

Cardiovascular refresher

ACYANOTIC HEART DEFECTS

Key signs and symptoms
- Congested cough
- Diaphoresis
- Fatigue
- Machinelike heart murmur (in patent ductus arteriosus)
- Mild cyanosis (if the condition leads to right-sided heart failure)
- Respiratory distress
- Tachycardia
- Tachypnea

Key test result
- Chest X-ray results and cardiac catheterization confirm type of acyanotic heart defect.

Key treatments
- Digoxin (Lanoxin)
- Diuretic such as furosemide (Lasix)
- Surgical repair

Key interventions
- Monitor vital signs, pulse oximetry, and intake and output.
- Assess cardiovascular and respiratory status.
- Take apical pulse for 1 minute before giving digoxin. (Bradycardia is considered to be a pulse below 100 beats/minute in infants.)
- Monitor fluid status.

CYANOTIC HEART DEFECTS

Key signs and symptoms
- Clubbing
- Crouching position assumed frequently
- Cyanosis
- History of inadequate feeding
- Irritability
- Tachycardia
- Tachypnea

Key test results
- Arterial blood gas analysis shows diminished arterial oxygen saturation.
- Complete blood count shows polycythemia.

Key treatments
- For transposition of the great vessels or arteries: corrective surgery to redirect blood flow
- For tetralogy of Fallot: complete repair or palliative treatment
- For hypoplastic left-heart syndrome: surgery to restructure the heart or heart transplantation

Key interventions
- Assess cardiovascular and respiratory status.
- Monitor vital signs, pulse oximetry, and intake and output.
- Administer prophylactic antibiotics.

RHEUMATIC FEVER

Key signs and symptoms

Major rheumatic fever
- Carditis
- Chorea
- Erythema marginatum (temporary, disk-shaped, nonpruritic, reddened macules that fade in the center, leaving raised margins)
- Polyarthritis
- Subcutaneous nodules

Key test results
- Erythrocyte sedimentation rate is increased.
- Electrocardiogram shows prolonged PR interval.

Key treatments
- Bed rest until the sedimentation rate normalizes
- Penicillin to prevent additional damage from future attacks

Key intervention
- Monitor vital signs and intake and output.

Heart mapping

Echocardiography is a noninvasive test used to evaluate the size, shape, and motion of cardiac structures by recording the echoes of ultrasonic waves of those structures.

Nursing action

• Explain to the child and parents that the child may have to lie on his left side, inhale and exhale slowly, or hold his breath during the test.

Polish up on patient care

Major cardiovascular disorders in pediatric patients include acyanotic heart defects, cyanotic heart defects, and rheumatic fever. (See *From high to low,* page 562.)

Acyanotic heart defects

In an acyanotic defect, blood is usually shunted from the left (oxygenated) side to the right (unoxygenated) side of the heart. Acyanotic defects include:

• **aortic stenosis** — a narrowing or fusion of the aortic valves, interfering with left ventricular outflow
• **atrial septal defect** — a defect stemming from a patent foramen ovale or the failure of a septum to develop completely between the atria
• **coarctation of the aorta** — a narrowing of the aortic arch, usually distal to the ductus arteriosus beyond the left subclavian artery
• **patent ductus arteriosus** — a defect resulting from the failure of the ductus to close, causing shunting of blood to the pulmonary artery
• **pulmonary artery stenosis** — a narrowing or fusing of valve leaflets at the entrance of the pulmonary artery, interfering with right ventricular outflow
• **ventricular septal defect** — a defect occurring when the ventricular septum fails to

complete its formation between the ventricles, resulting in a left-to-right shunt.

CAUSES

• Defects between structures that inhibit blood flow to the system or alter pulmonary resistance
• Defects in the septa that lead to left-to-right shunt

ASSESSMENT FINDINGS

• Congested cough
• Diaphoresis
• Fatigue
• Frequent respiratory infections
• Hepatomegaly
• Machinelike heart murmur (in patent ductus arteriosus)
• Mild cyanosis (if the condition leads to right-sided heart failure)
• Poor growth and development due to increased energy expenditure for breathing
• Respiratory distress
• Tachycardia
• Tachypnea

DIAGNOSTIC TEST RESULTS

Chest X-ray results and cardiac catheterization confirm type of acyanotic heart defect.
• In **aortic stenosis,** chest X-ray shows left ventricular hypertrophy and prominent pulmonary vasculature. Cardiac catheterization helps determine the degree of shunting and extent of pulmonary vascular disease.
• In **atrial septal defect,** chest X-ray shows enlarged right atrium and ventricle and prominent pulmonary vasculature. Cardiac catheterization shows right atrial blood that is more oxygenated than superior vena cava blood. It also helps determine the degree of shunting and extent of pulmonary vascular disease.
• In **coarctation of the aorta,** chest X-ray shows left ventricular hypertrophy, wide ascending and descending aorta, and prominent collateral circulation. Cardiac catheterization shows affected collateral circulation and pressures in the right and left ventricles.
• In **patent ductus arteriosus,** chest X-ray shows prominent pulmonary vasculature and enlargement of the left ventricle and aorta.

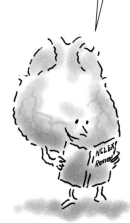

Well, I'll be. Mild cyanosis can occur in an acyanotic heart defect.

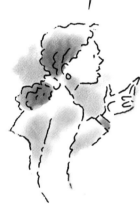

Chest X-ray and cardiac catheterization distinguish the various acyanotic heart defects.

From high to low

When cardiac anomalies involve communication — movement of blood through a common opening — between chambers, blood flows from areas of high pressure to areas of low pressure. For example, a left-to-right shunt may result when increased pressure on the left side of the heart causes increased blood flow to the right.

DEFECTS THAT DON'T INVOLVE CHAMBERS
In defects that don't involve the cardiac chambers, blood can also flow from high-pressure to low-pressure areas. In patent ductus arteriosus, for instance, the ductus arteriosus (located between the aorta and pulmonary artery) remains open after birth. This causes blood to shunt from the aorta to the pulmonary artery.

Cardiac catheterization helps determine the extent of pulmonary vascular disease and shows an oxygen content higher in the pulmonary artery than in the right ventricle.
- In **pulmonary artery stenosis,** chest X-ray shows right ventricular hypertrophy. Cardiac catheterization provides evidence of the degree of shunting.
- In **ventricular septal defect,** chest X-ray may be normal for small defects or show cardiomegaly with a large left atrium and ventricle. In a large defect, chest X-ray may show prominent pulmonary vasculature. Cardiac catheterization helps determine the size and exact location of ventricular septal defect and the degree of shunting.

NURSING DIAGNOSES
- Anxiety
- Decreased cardiac output
- Impaired gas exchange

TREATMENT
- **Aortic stenosis:** surgery (valvulotomy or commissurotomy)
- **Atrial septal defect:** surgery to patch the hole (mild defects may close spontaneously)
- **Coarctation of the aorta:** inoperable if coarctation is proximal to the ductus arteriosus; closed heart resection if coarctation is distal to the ductus arteriosus
- **Patent ductus arteriosus:** ligation of the patent ductus arteriosus in closed-heart operation
- **Pulmonary artery stenosis:** open-heart surgery to separate the pulmonary valve leaflets

- **Ventricular septal defect:** pulmonary artery banding to prevent heart failure and permanent correction with a patch later when heart is larger (spontaneous closure of the ventricular septal defect may occur in some children by age 3)

Drug therapy
- Digoxin (Lanoxin)
- Diuretic such as furosemide (Lasix)
- Indomethacin (Indocin) to achieve pharmacologic closure (in patent ductus arteriosus)
- Prophylactic antibiotics to prevent endocarditis

INTERVENTIONS AND RATIONALES
- Explain the heart defect and answer any questions *to prepare the child for cardiac catheterization.*
- Monitor vital signs, pulse oximetry, and intake and output *to assess renal function and detect change.*
- Assess cardiovascular and respiratory status *to detect early signs of decompensation.*
- Take apical pulse for 1 minute before giving digoxin and hold the drug if the heart rate is below 100 beats/minute (bradycardia in infants is a heart rate below 100 beats/minute) *to prevent toxicity.*
- Monitor fluid status, enforcing fluid restrictions as appropriate *to prevent fluid overload.*
- Weigh the child daily *to determine fluid overload or deficit.*
- Organize physical care and anticipate the child's needs *to reduce the child's oxygen demands.*

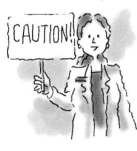

Remember to take an apical pulse for 1 minute before giving digoxin. You're checking for bradycardia, which in infants is a rate below 100 beats/minute.

CAUTION!

• Give the child high-calorie, easy-to-chew, and easy-to-digest foods *to maintain adequate nutrition and decrease oxygen demands.*
• Maintain normal body temperature *to prevent cold stress.*
• Raise the head of the bed or place the infant in an infant car seat *to ease breathing.*

Teaching topics
• Preparing the child and parents for the sights and sounds of the intensive care unit

Cyanotic heart defects

Cyanotic heart defects result in unoxygenated blood or a mixture of oxygenated and unoxygenated blood being shunted through the cardiovascular system. This shunting can lead to left-sided heart failure, decreased oxygen supply to the body, and the development of collateral circulation. Cyanotic heart defects include:
• **transposition of the great vessels or arteries** — a defect in which the aorta arises from the right ventricle and the pulmonary artery arises from the left ventricle
• **tetralogy of Fallot** — a defect consisting of pulmonary artery stenosis, ventricular septal defect, hypertrophy of the right ventricle, and an overriding aorta
• **hypoplastic left-heart syndrome** — a defect consisting of aortic valve atresia, mitral atresia or stenosis, diminutive or absent left ventricle, and severe hypoplasia of the ascending aorta and aortic arch.

CAUSES
• Any condition that increases pulmonary vascular resistance
• Structural defects

ASSESSMENT FINDINGS
• Clubbing
• Crouching position assumed frequently
• Cyanosis
• History of inadequate feeding
• Increasing cyanosis as the foramen ovale or ductus arteriosus closes (in transposition of the great vessels), leading to loss of con-

sciousness, also known as a tet spell (in tetralogy of Fallot)
• Increasing dyspnea, cyanosis, and tachypnea during the first few days after birth; without treatment, heart failure after closure of the ductus (in hypoplastic left-heart syndrome).
• Irritability
• Tachycardia
• Tachypnea

DIAGNOSTIC TEST RESULTS
• Arterial blood gas analysis shows diminished arterial oxygen saturation.
• Cardiac catheterization results confirm the diagnosis through visualization of defects and measurement of oxygen saturation level.
• Complete blood count shows polycythemia. (Hypoxia stimulates the body to increase red blood cell production.)

NURSING DIAGNOSES
• Impaired gas exchange
• Anxiety
• Decreased cardiac output

TREATMENT
For transposition of the great vessels or arteries, several therapies are possible, including:
• corrective surgery to redirect blood flow by switching the position of the major blood vessels; performed around age 1
• palliative surgery to provide communication between the chambers.
    For tetralogy of Fallot, the doctor can use:
• complete repair or palliative treatment during the 1st year to increase blood flow to the lungs by bypassing pulmonic stenosis (Blalock-Taussig anastomosis of the right pulmonary artery to the right subclavian artery)
• oxygen therapy
• repair of ventricular septal defect and stenosis (may be done in stages).
    For hypoplastic left-heart syndrome, the doctor may perform:
• heart transplant
• Norwood procedure, a two-stage procedure that involves restructuring the heart (without surgery, death occurs in early infancy).

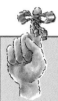

Memory jogger

When a child has a cyanotic heart defect, check for the 4 C's:

Cyanosis, especially increasing with crying

Crabbiness or irritability

Clubbing of digits

Crouching, or squatting, which increases systemic venous return, shunts blood from the extremities to the head and trunk, and decreases cyanosis.

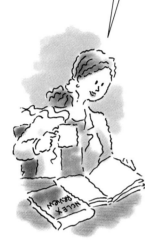

Infants with cyanotic defects have less energy for sucking; use a preemie nipple.

Drug therapy

• Morphine during tet spell
• Prophylactic propranolol (Inderal)
• Prostaglandin E to keep the ductus arteriosus patent

INTERVENTIONS AND RATIONALES

• Assess cardiovascular and respiratory status *to detect early signs of compromise.*
• Monitor vital signs and pulse oximetry to *detect hypoxia*
• Monitor intake and output *to assess renal status.*
• Provide oxygen when necessary *to compensate for impaired oxygen exchange.*
• Anticipate needs and prevent distress *to decrease oxygen demands on the child.*
• Use a preemie nipple *to decrease the energy needed for sucking.*
• Provide adequate hydration *to prevent sequelae of polycythemia.*
• Administer prophylactic antibiotics *to prevent endocarditis.*
• Provide thorough skin care *to prevent skin breakdown.*
• Prepare the child for cardiac catheterization *to decrease anxiety.*

Teaching topics

• Preparing the child and parents for the sights and sounds of the intensive care unit
• Explaining the difference between palliative and corrective procedures

Rheumatic fever

Rheumatic fever is an inflammatory disease of childhood. It first occurs 1 to 3 weeks after a group A beta-hemolytic streptococcal infection and may recur. Rheumatic fever results in antigen-antibody complexes that ultimately destroy heart tissue.

Rheumatic heart disease refers to the cardiac effects of rheumatic fever and includes pancarditis (inflammation of the heart muscle, heart lining, and sac around the heart) during the early acute phase and chronic heart valve disease later.

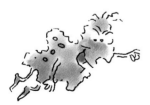

In rheumatic fever, antibodies manufactured to combat streptococci react and produce lesions at specific tissue sites, especially in the heart and joints.

CAUSES

• Production of antibodies against group A beta-hemolytic *Streptococcus*
• Untreated group A beta-hemolytic *Streptococcus* infection (1% to 5% of children infected with *Streptococcus* develop rheumatic fever.)

ASSESSMENT FINDINGS

The Jones criteria for assessing major rheumatic fever include:
• carditis
• chorea
• erythema marginatum (temporary, disk-shaped, nonpruritic, reddened macules that fade in the center, leaving raised margins)
• polyarthritis
• subcutaneous nodules.
   The Jones criteria for assessing minor rheumatic fever include:
• arthralgia
• evidence of a *Streptococcus* infection
• fever
• history of rheumatic fever.

DIAGNOSTIC TEST RESULTS

• Antistreptolysin-O titer is elevated.
• Erythrocyte sedimentation rate is increased.
• Electrocardiogram shows prolonged PR interval.

NURSING DIAGNOSES

• Decreased cardiac output
• Impaired gas exchange
• Altered nutrition: Less than body requirements

TREATMENT

• Bed rest until the sedimentation rate returns to normal.

Drug therapy

• Aspirin for arthritis pain
• Penicillin to prevent additional damage from future attacks (taken until age 20 or for 5 years after the attack, whichever is longer).

INTERVENTIONS AND RATIONALES

• Monitor vital signs and intake and output *to detect fluid volume overload or deficit.*

• Institute safety measures for chorea; maintain a calm environment, reduce stimulation, avoid the use of forks or glass, and assist in walking *to prevent injury.*
• Provide appropriate passive stimulation *to maintain growth and development.*
• Provide emotional support for long-term convalescence *to help relieve anxiety.*
• Use sterile technique in dressing changes and standard precautions *to prevent reinfection.*

Teaching topics
• Understanding the need to inform health care providers of existing medical conditions

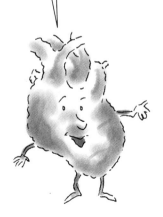

Effective treatment eliminates strep infection, relieves symptoms, and prevents recurrence, reducing the chance I'll suffer permanent damage. Thanks.

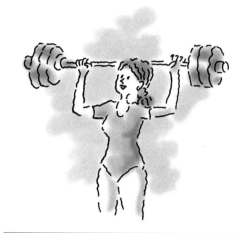

Pump up on practice questions

1. A pediatric client returns to his room after a cardiac catheterization. Which of the following nursing interventions is most appropriate?

   A. Maintain the client on bed rest with no further activity restrictions.
   B. Maintain the client on bed rest with the affected extremity immobilized.
   C. Allow the client to get out of bed to go to the bathroom, if necessary.
   D. Allow the client to sit in a chair with the affected extremity immobilized.

Answer: B. The pediatric client should be maintained on bed rest with the affected extremity immobilized after cardiac catheterization to prevent hemorrhage. Allowing the client to move the affected extremity while on bed rest, allowing the client bathroom privileges, or allowing the client to sit in a chair with the affected extremity immobilized places the client at risk for hemorrhage.

➡️ *NCLEX keys*
Nursing process step: Implementation
Client needs category: Physiological integrity
Client needs subcategory: Reduction of risk potential
Taxonomic level: Knowledge

2. A pediatric client is scheduled for echocardiography. The nurse is providing teaching to the client's mother. Which of the following statements about echocardiography indicates the need for further teaching?

    A. "I'm glad my child won't have an I.V. catheter inserted for this procedure."

    B. "I'm glad my child won't need to have dye injected into him before the procedure."

    C. "How am I ever going to explain to my son that he can't have anything to eat before the test?"

    D. "I know my child may need to lie on his left side and breathe in and out slowly during the procedure."

Answer: C. Echocardiography is a noninvasive procedure used to evaluate the size, shape, and motion of various cardiac structures. Therefore, it isn't necessary for the client to have an I.V. catheter inserted, dye injected, or have nothing by mouth, as would be the case with a cardiac catheterization. The child may need to lie on his left side and inhale and exhale slowly during the procedure.

➡ *NCLEX keys*
Nursing process step: Evaluation
Client needs category: Physiological integrity
Client needs subcategory: Reduction of risk potential
Taxonomic level: Analysis

3. An infant with a ventricular septal defect is receiving digoxin (Lanoxin). Which of the following interventions by the nurse is most appropriate before digoxin administration?

    A. Take the infant's blood pressure.

    B. Check the infant's respiratory rate for 1 minute.

    C. Check the infant's radial pulse for 1 minute.

    D. Check the infant's apical pulse for 1 minute.

Answer: D. Before administering digoxin, the nurse should check the infant's apical pulse for 1 minute. Checking the radial pulse may be inaccurate. Checking the blood pressure and respiratory rate isn't necessary before digoxin administration because the medication doesn't affect these parameters.

➡ *NCLEX keys*
Nursing process step: Implementation
Client needs category: Physiological integrity
Client needs subcategory: Pharmacological and parenteral therapies
Taxonomic level: Knowledge

4. The nurse checks an infant's apical pulse before digoxin administration and finds that the pulse rate is 90 beats/minute. Which of the following actions is most appropriate for the nurse?

    A. Withhold the digoxin, and notify the physician.

    B. Administer the digoxin, and notify the physician.

    C. Administer the digoxin, and document the infant's pulse rate.

    D. Withhold the digoxin, and document the infant's pulse rate.

Answer: A. The nurse should withhold the digoxin and notify the physician because an apical pulse below 100 beats/minute in an infant is considered bradycardic. The nurse should also document her findings and interventions in the medical record. Administering the drug to the infant already bradycardic could further decrease his heart rate and compromise his status. Withholding the drug and not notifying the physician could compromise the existing treatment plan.

➡ *NCLEX keys*
Nursing process step: Implementation
Client needs category: Physiological integrity
Client needs subcategory: Pharmacological and parenteral therapies
Taxonomic level: Application

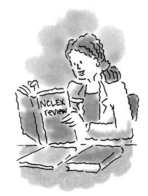

5. A pediatric client has been diagnosed with rheumatic fever. Which of the following statements by the mother indicates an effective understanding of rheumatic fever?

    A. "I should avoid giving my child aspirin for the arthritic pain."

    B. "It's very upsetting that my child must take penicillin until he's 20 years old."

    C. "I need to wear a gown, gloves, and mask to stay in my child's room."

    D. "I don't know how I'll be able to keep my child away from his sister when he gets home."

Answer: B. Rheumatic fever is an acquired autoimmune-complex disorder that occurs 1 to 3 weeks after an infection of group A beta-hemolytic *streptococci,* in many cases as a result of strep throat that hasn't been treated with antibiotics. To prevent additional heart damage from future attacks, the child must take penicillin or another antibiotic until the age of 20 or for 5 years after the attack, whichever is longer. Rheumatic fever isn't contagious, so isolation precautions aren't necessary.

➡ *NCLEX keys*
Nursing process step: Evaluation
Client needs category: Physiological integrity
Client needs subcategory: Reduction of risk potential
Taxonomic level: Analysis

6. The nurse is caring for a pediatric client with a cyanotic heart defect. Which of the following signs would the nurse expect to observe?

    A. Cyanosis, hypertension, clubbing, and lethargy

    B. Cyanosis, hypotension, crouching, and lethargy

    C. Cyanosis, crabbiness, clubbing, and crouching

    D. Cyanosis, confusion, clonus, and crouching

Answer: C. The pediatric client with a cyanotic heart defect has cyanosis along with crabiness (irritability), clubbing of the digits, and crouching or squatting. The client with cyanotic heart defect doesn't typically have hypertension, lethargy, confusion, or clonus.

➡ *NCLEX keys*
Nursing process step: Assessment
Client needs category: Physiological integrity
Client needs subcategory: Physiological adaptation
Taxonomic level: Comprehension

7. The nurse is caring for an infant with tetralogy of Fallot. Which of the following drugs should the nurse anticipate administering during a tet spell?

    A. Propranolol (Inderal)

    B. Morphine

    C. Meperidine (Demerol)

    D. Furosemide (Lasix)

Answer: B. The nurse should anticipate administering morphine during a tet spell to decrease the associated infundibular spasm. Propranolol may be administered as a preventive measure in an infant with tetralogy of Fallot but isn't administered during a tet spell. Furosemide and meperidine aren't appropriate agents for an infant experiencing a tet spell.

➡ *NCLEX keys*
Nursing process step: Planning
Client needs category: Physiological integrity
Client needs subcategory: Pharmacological and parenteral therapies
Taxonomic level: Knowledge

8. An infant is diagnosed with patent ductus arteriosus. Which of the following drugs may be administered in hopes of achieving pharmacologic closure of the defect?

    A. Digoxin (Lanoxin)

    B. Prednisone

    C. Furosemide (Lasix)

    D. Indomethacin (Indocin)

Answer: D. Indomethacin is administered to an infant with patent ductus arteriosus in hopes of closing the defect. Digoxin and furosemide may be used to treat the symptoms associated with patent ductus arteriosus but they don't achieve closure. Prednisone isn't used to treat the condition.

➡ *NCLEX keys*
Nursing process step: Planning
Client needs category: Physiological integrity
Client needs subcategory: Pharmacological and parenteral therapies
Taxonomic level: Comprehension

9. An infant, age 2 months, has a tentative diagnosis of congenital heart defect. During physical assessment, the nurse notes that the infant has a pulse rate of 168 beats/minute and respiratory rate of 72 breaths/minute. In which of the following positions should the nurse place the infant?
   A. Upright in an infant seat
   B. Lying on the back
   C. Lying on the abdomen
   D. Sitting in high Fowler's position

Answer: A. Because these signs suggest development of respiratory distress, the nurse should position the infant with the head elevated at a 45-degree angle to promote maximum chest expansion. This can be accomplished by placing the infant in an infant seat. Placing an infant flat on the back or abdomen or in high Fowler's position could increase respiratory distress by preventing maximum chest expansion.

➡ *NCLEX keys*
Nursing process step: Implementation
Client needs category: Physiological integrity
Client needs subcategory: Physiological adaptation
Taxonomic level: Application

10. An infant client with a congenital cyanotic heart defect has a complete blood count drawn, revealing an elevated red blood cell (RBC) count. Which of the following conditions do these findings indicate?
   A. Anemia
   B. Dehydration
   C. Jaundice
   D. Hypoxia compensation

Answer: D. A congenital cyanotic heart defect alters blood flow through the heart and lungs, which produces hypoxia. To compensate for this, the body increases the oxygen-carrying capacity by increasing RBC production, which causes the hemoglobin level and hematocrit to increase. The hemoglobin level and hematocrit are typically decreased in anemia. Altered electrolyte levels and other laboratory values provide better evidence of dehydration. An elevated hemoglobin level and hematocrit aren't associated with jaundice.

➡ *NCLEX keys*
Nursing process step: Evaluation
Client needs category: Physiological integrity
Client needs subcategory: Physiological adaptation
Taxonomic level: Analysis

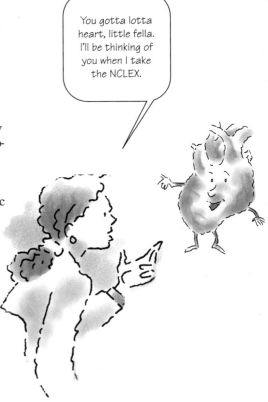

You gotta lotta heart, little fella. I'll be thinking of you when I take the NCLEX.

28 Respiratory System

Brush up on key concepts

The primary function of the respiratory system is to distribute air to the alveoli in the lungs, where gas exchange takes place. Gas exchange includes:
• the addition of oxygen (O_2) to pulmonary capillary blood
• the removal of carbon dioxide (CO_2) from pulmonary capillary blood.

At any time, you can review the major points of this chapter by consulting the *Cheat sheet* on page 570 and 571.

Upper and lower
The parts of the respiratory system include the **upper airway** and the **lower airway.** The upper airway includes:
• nasopharynx
• oropharynx
• larynx.

The lower airway includes:
• trachea
• bronchi
• bronchioles
• alveoli.

Take a deep breath
Breathing delivers inspired gas to the lower respiratory tract and alveoli. Contraction and relaxation of the respiratory muscles move air into and out of the lungs. Here are some important aspects of the breathing process.
• **Ventilation** begins with the contraction of the inspiratory muscles: The diaphragm (the major muscle of respiration) descends while the external intercostal muscles move the rib cage upward and outward.
• Air then enters the lungs in response to the pressure gradient between the atmosphere and the lungs.

• The lungs adhere to the chest wall and diaphragm because of the vacuum created by negative pleural pressure.
• As the thorax expands, the lungs also expand, causing a decrease in pressure in the lungs.
• The accessory muscles of inspiration, which include the scalene and sternocleidomastoid muscles, raise the clavicles, upper ribs, and sternum.
• To reach the capillary lumen, O_2 diffuses across the alveolocapillary membrane into the blood.
• Normal expiration is passive; the inspiratory muscles cease to contract, and the elastic recoil of the lungs causes the lungs to contract.
• These actions increase the pressure in the lungs above atmospheric pressure, moving air from the lungs to the atmosphere.

Little one's lungs
A **child's respiratory tract** differs anatomically from an adult's in ways that predispose the child to many respiratory problems. A child's respiratory tract differs from an adult's in the following ways:
• Lungs aren't fully developed at birth.
• Alveoli continue to grow and increase in size through age 8.
• A child's respiratory tract has a narrower lumen than an adult's until age 5; the narrow airway makes the young child prone to airway obstruction and respiratory distress from inflammation, mucus secretion, or a foreign body.
• Elastic connective tissue becomes more abundant with age in the peripheral part of the lung.
• A child's respiratory rate decreases as body size increases.

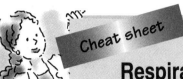

Respiratory refresher

ASTHMA

Key signs and symptoms
- Diaphoresis
- Dyspnea
- Prolonged expiration with an expiratory wheeze; in severe distress, may hear an inspiratory wheeze
- Unequal or decreased breath sounds
- Use of accessory muscles

Key test result
- Oxygen saturation via pulse oximetry may show decreased O_2 saturation.
- Arterial blood gas measurement may show increased partial pressure of arterial carbon dioxide from respiratory acidosis.

Key treatments
- Bronchodilator: albuterol (Proventil)
- Chromone derivative: cromolyn (Intal)

Key interventions
- Assess respiratory and cardiovascular status.
- Monitor vital signs.

During an acute attack
- Allow the child to sit upright to ease breathing; provide moist oxygen, if necessary.
- Monitor for alterations in vital signs (especially cardiac stimulation and hypotension).

BRONCHIOLITIS

Key signs and symptoms
- Sternal retractions
- Tachypnea

Key test result
- Bronchial mucus culture shows respiratory syncytial virus.

Key treatments
- Humidified oxygen
- I.V. fluids

Key interventions
- Monitor vital signs and pulse oximetry.
- Assess respiratory and cardiovascular status.
- Administer humidified oxygen therapy.

BRONCHOPULMONARY DYSPLASIA

Key signs and symptoms
- Atelectasis
- Crackles, rhonchi, wheezes
- Dyspnea
- Sternal retractions

Key test result
- Chest X-ray reveals pulmonary changes (bronchiolar metaplasia and interstitial fibrosis).

Key treatments
- Chest physiotherapy
- Continued ventilatory support and oxygen

Key interventions
- Assess respiratory and cardiovascular status.
- Monitor vital signs, pulse oximetry, and intake and output.

CROUP

Key signs and symptoms
- A barking, brassy cough or hoarseness
- Inspiratory stridor with varying degrees of respiratory distress

Key test results
- Laryngoscopy may reveal inflammation and obstruction in epiglottis and laryngeal areas.
- Neck X-ray shows areas of upper airway narrowing and edema in subglottic folds.

Key treatments
- Cool humidification during sleep with a cool mist tent or room humidifier
- Inhaled racemic epinephrine and corticosteroids such as methylprednisolone sodium succinate
- Tracheostomy, oxygen administration

Key interventions
- Monitor vital signs and pulse oximetry.
- Administer oxygen therapy and maintain the child in a cool mist tent, if needed.

Respiratory refresher (continued)

CYSTIC FIBROSIS

Key signs and symptoms
- History of a chronic, productive cough and recurrent respiratory infections, often due to *Pseudomonas* infections
- Parents' report of a salty taste on the child's skin

Key test result
- Sweat test using pilocarpine iontophoresis is positive.

Key treatment
- Oral pancreatic enzyme replacement

Key interventions
- Assess respiratory and cardiovascular status.
- Administer pancreatic enzymes with meals and snacks.
- Encourage breathing exercises and perform chest physiotherapy two to four times a day.

EPIGLOTTITIS

Key signs and symptoms
- Difficult and painful swallowing
- Increased drooling
- Restlessness
- Stridor

Key test result
- Lateral neck X-ray shows enlarged epiglottis.

Key treatments
- Emergency endotracheal intubation or a tracheotomy
- Oxygen therapy or cool mist tent
- 10-day course of parenteral antibiotics

Key interventions
- Monitor vital signs and pulse oximetry.
- Assess respiratory and cardiovascular status.
- Defer inspecting the throat until the arrival of emergency personnel and supplies.

SUDDEN INFANT DEATH SYNDROME (S.I.D.S.)

Key sign and symptom
- Death takes place during sleep without noise or struggle

Key test result
- Autopsy is the only way to diagnose SIDS.

Key treatment
- Resuscitation of the infant

Key interventions
- Let parents touch, hold, and rock infant.
- Reinforce the fact that the death wasn't the parents' fault.

Keep abreast of diagnostic tests

Here are the most important tests used to diagnose respiratory disorders, along with common nursing interventions associated with each test.

Check the gas

Arterial blood gas (ABG) analysis is used to assess gas exchange.
- Decreased partial pressure of arterial oxygen (Pao_2) may indicate hypoventilation, ventilation-perfusion mismatch, or shunting of blood away from gas exchange sites.
- Increased partial pressure of arterial carbon dioxide ($Paco_2$) reflects hypoventilation or marked ventilation-perfusion mismatch.
- Decreased $Paco_2$ reflects increased alveolar ventilation.

- Changes in pH may reflect metabolic or respiratory dysfunction.

Nursing actions
- Explain the procedure to the parents and child.
- Check arterial circulation before making the arterial puncture.
- After the sample is obtained, apply firm pressure to the arterial site.
- Keep the sample on ice and transport it immediately to the laboratory.
- Assess the puncture site for bleeding or hematoma formation.

Oxygen observation

Pulse oximetry is a painless alternative to ABG analysis for measuring O_2 saturation only. This test may be less effective in jaundiced children or those with dark skin.

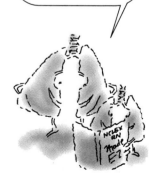

It says here that a decreased Pao_2 and an increased $Paco_2$ may indicate hypoventilation or ventilation-perfusion mismatch.

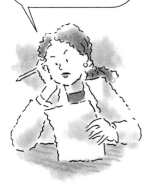

Hmmm. ABG analysis helps to assess gas exchange: pH, $Paco_2$, and Pao_2. Pulse oximetry is used to measure oxygen saturation only.

Nursing actions
• Place the oximeter on a site with adequate circulation such as the finger, toe, or nose.
• Periodically rotate sites to prevent skin breakdown and pressure ulcers.
• Ensure that pulse readings in the site used for oximetry correlate with the child's heart rate before performing oximetry.

Lung function
Pulmonary function tests are used to measure lung volume, flow rates, and compliance. Pulmonary function test results may not be accurate because the young child has trouble following directions.

Nursing actions
• Explain the procedure to the child and his parents.
• Instruct the child and his parents that he should have only a light meal before the test.
• If appropriate, tell the child that he shouldn't smoke for 4 to 6 hours before the tests.
• Tell the parents to withhold bronchodilators and intermittent positive-pressure breathing therapy.
• Just before the test tell the child to void and loosen tight clothing.

Chest check
Chest X-rays show conditions such as atelectasis, pleural effusion, infiltrates, pneumothorax, lesions, mediastinal shifts, and pulmonary edema.

Asthma typically causes prolonged expiration with an expiratory wheeze. However, during severe distress, you may hear an inspiratory wheeze.

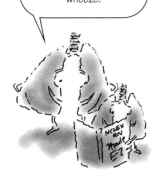

Nursing actions
• Ensure adequate protection by covering the child's gonads and thyroid gland with a lead apron.

Polish up on patient care

Major respiratory disorders in pediatric patients include asthma, bronchiolitis, bronchopulmonary dysplasia, croup, cystic fibrosis, epiglottitis, and sudden infant death syndrome.

For information about special respiratory treatments for pediatric patients, see *Respiratory assistance for children.*

Asthma

Asthma is a reversible, diffuse, obstructive pulmonary disease that produces the following effects:
• inflammation of the mucous membranes
• smooth muscle bronchospasm
• increased mucus secretion leading to airway obstruction and air trapping.

CAUSES
• Hyperresponsiveness of the lower airway (may be idiopathic or intrinsic, or caused by a hyperresponsive reaction to an allergen, exercise, or environmental change)

ASSESSMENT FINDINGS
• Alteration in chest contour from chronic air trapping
• Altered cerebral function
• Diaphoresis
• Dyspnea
• Exercise intolerance
• Fatigue and apprehension
• Prolonged expiration with an expiratory wheeze; in severe distress, may hear an inspiratory wheeze
• Unequal or decreased breath sounds
• Use of accessory muscles

DIAGNOSTIC TEST RESULTS
• Oxygen saturation via pulse oximetry may show decreased O_2 saturation.
• ABG measurement may show increased $Paco_2$ from respiratory acidosis.
• Skin test identifies the source of the allergy.
• Sputum analysis rules out respiratory infection.

NURSING DIAGNOSES
• Anxiety
• Impaired gas exchange
• Ineffective airway clearance

Respiratory assistance for children

The oxygen tent, the cool mist tent, the nasal cannula, and chest physiotherapy are specialized treatments used in pediatric respiratory disorders. Here are the nursing actions associated with each treatment.

OXYGEN TENT
• Keep the plastic sides down and tucked in; because oxygen is heavier than air, oxygen loss is greater at the bottom of the tent.
• Keep the plastic away from the child's face.
• Prevent the use of toys that produce sparks or friction.
• Frequently assess oxygen concentration.
• To return the child to a tent, put the tent sides down, turn on the oxygen, wait until the oxygen is at the prescribed concentration, and then place the child in the tent.

COOL MIST TENT (CROUP TENT)
• Explain that the cool mist thins mucus, facilitating expectoration.
• Provide the same care as with an oxygen tent.
• Expect the child to be fearful if the mist obscures vision.
• Encourage the use of transitional objects in the tent, except for stuffed toys, which may become damp and promote bacterial growth.
• Keep the child dry by changing bed linens and pajamas frequently.

• Maintain a steady body temperature.
• Teach the parents about cool mist vaporizers for home use; tell them to clean the vaporizers frequently to prevent germs from being sprayed into the air.

NASAL CANNULA
• Remove nasal secretions from the end of tubing frequently.
• Administer saline nose drops or nasal spray to moisten passages.
• Change tubing every 8 hours to prevent infection or necrosis.

CHEST PHYSIOTHERAPY
• Perform at least 30 minutes before meals.
• Use a cupped hand over a covered rib cage for 2 to 5 minutes on the five major positions (upper anterior lobes, upper posterior lobes, lower posterior lobes, and right and left sides) for a maximum of 30 minutes; for infants, preformed rubber percussors are available.
• Avoid these measures during acute bronchoconstriction (for example, asthma) or airway edema (for example, croup) to prevent mucus plugs from loosening and causing airway obstruction.
• Administer aerosol-nebulized medications immediately before percussion and postural drainage.

TREATMENT
• Chest physiotherapy (once edema has abated)
• Hyposensitization through the use of allergy shots, if appropriate
• Parenteral fluids to thin mucus secretions.
• Oxygen therapy, as tolerated

Drug therapy
• Bronchodilator: albuterol (Proventil)
• Chromone derivative: cromolyn (Intal) to prevent the release of mast cell products after an antigen-antibody union has taken place
• Inhaled corticosteroids to decrease edema of the mucous membranes (for chronic asthma, daily doses to control chronic inflammation)

INTERVENTIONS AND RATIONALES
• Assess respiratory and cardiovascular status. *Tachycardia, tachypnea, and quiet breath sounds signal worsening respiratory status.*
• Monitor vital signs *to detect changes and prevent complications.*
• Assess the nature of the child's cough (hacking, unproductive progressing to productive), especially at night in the absence of infection. *Early detection and treatment lessens respiratory distress.*

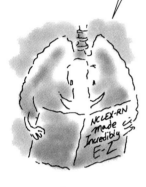

During an acute attack, allow the child to sit upright to ease breathing. Also provide moist oxygen, if necessary.

• Modify the environment to avoid an allergic reaction; remove the offending allergen. *Allergens can trigger an asthma attack.*
• Rinse the child's mouth after he inhales medication *to promote comfort and prevent irritation to the oral mucosa.*
• For exercise-induced asthma, give prophylactic treatments of cromolyn or beta-adrenergic blockers 10 to 15 minutes before the child exercises. *Premedication before exercise may prevent an asthma attack.*
• Forbid smoking in the child's environment. *Secondhand smoke can trigger an asthma attack.*

During an acute attack
• Allow the child to sit upright *to ease breathing;* provide moist oxygen, if necessary. *This position promotes chest expansion; moist oxygen promotes mobilization of secretions.*
• Monitor for alterations in vital signs (especially cardiac stimulation and hypotension) *to detect signs of impending respiratory arrest and cardiac decompensation.*
• Monitor urine for glucose if the child is receiving corticosteroids *to detect early signs of hyperglycemia.*
• Administer inhaled medications via a metered-dose inhaler and monitor peak flow rates. *Peak flow rates indicate the degree of lung impairment.*
• Maintain a calm environment; provide emotional support and reassurance *to decrease anxiety and decrease oxygen demands.*
• Monitor effectiveness of drug therapy. *Failure to respond to drugs during an acute attack can result in status asthmaticus.*

Teaching topics
• Breathing exercises to increase ventilatory capacity
• Proper use of inhalers
• Avoiding allergens

Bronchiolitis

Bronchiolitis is a lower respiratory infection that is spread by respiratory secretions, rather than droplets. It typically affects infants younger than age 6 months in the winter and spring. Mortality in this age-group is 1% to 6%.

CAUSES
• Respiratory syncytial virus

ASSESSMENT FINDINGS
• Possible air trapping and atelectasis
• Sternal retractions
• Tachypnea
• Thick mucus

DIAGNOSTIC TEST RESULT
• Bronchial mucus culture shows respiratory syncytial virus.

NURSING DIAGNOSES
• Impaired gas exchange
• Ineffective airway clearance
• Ineffective breathing pattern

TREATMENT
• Cool mist tent
• Humidified oxygen
• I.V. fluids

Drug therapy
• Bronchodilator: albuterol (Proventil)
• Respiratory syncytial virus immune globulin, administered I.V.

INTERVENTIONS AND RATIONALES
• Monitor vital signs and pulse oximetry *to determine oxygenation needs and to detect deterioration or improvement in the child's condition.*
• Assess respiratory and cardiovascular status. *Tachycardia may result from hypoxia or effects of bronchodilator use.*
• Use gloves, gowns, and aseptic hand washing as secretion precautions *to prevent spread of infection.*
• Administer chest physiotherapy after edema has abated. *Chest physiotherapy helps loosen mucus that may be blocking small airways.*
• Administer humidified oxygen therapy *to liquefy secretions and reduce bronchial edema.*
• Administer and maintain I.V. therapy *to promote hydration and replace electrolytes.*

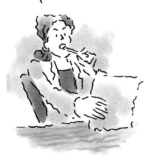

Key findings in bronchiolitis: sternal retractions and tachypnea.

Teaching topics
- Review of medications, dosages, and adverse reactions
- Providing adequate nutrition and hydration
- Importance of humidified environment
- Avoiding people with cold symptoms

Bronchopulmonary dysplasia

Bronchopulmonary dysplasia is a chronic lung disease that begins in infancy. It occurs in newborns who require ventilatory support with high positive airway pressure and oxygen in the first 2 weeks of life. Infants at risk may be born prematurely or may have a respiratory disorder.

In this disorder, an acute insult to the neonate's lungs, such as respiratory distress syndrome, pneumonia, or meconium aspiration, requires positive-pressure ventilation and a high concentration of oxygen over time. These therapies result in tissue and cellular injury to the immature lung.

CONTRIBUTING FACTORS
- Damage to the bronchiolar epithelium (from hyperoxia and positive pressure)
- Difficulty clearing mucus from the lungs
- Illness such as respiratory distress syndrome, pneumonia, or meconium aspiration
- Oxygen toxicity from administration of high concentration of oxygen and long-term assisted ventilation
- Possibly genetic factors
- Prematurity

ASSESSMENT FINDINGS
- Atelectasis
- Crackles, rhonchi, wheezes
- Delayed development
- Dyspnea
- Hypoxia without ventilator assistance
- Fatigue, delayed muscle growth
- Pallor, circumoral cyanosis
- Prolonged capillary filling time
- Respiratory distress
- Right-sided heart failure
- Sternal retractions
- Weight loss or difficulty feeding

DIAGNOSTIC TEST RESULTS
- ABG analysis reveals hypoxemia.
- Chest X-ray reveals pulmonary changes (bronchiolar metaplasia and interstitial fibrosis).

NURSING DIAGNOSES
- Altered growth and development
- Altered nutrition: Less than body requirements
- Impaired gas exchange

TREATMENT
- Chest physiotherapy
- Continued ventilatory support and oxygen
- Enteral or total parenteral nutrition
- Supportive measures to enhance respiratory function

Drug therapy
- Bronchodilators such as albuterol (Proventil) to counter increased airway resistance
- Dexamethasone (Decadron) therapy to reduce inflammation
- Diuretics such as furosemide (Lasix)

INTERVENTIONS AND RATIONALES
- Assess respiratory and cardiovascular status. *Monitoring is essential because children with bronchopulmonary dysplasia are susceptible to lower respiratory tract infections, hypertension, and respiratory failure.*
- Monitor vital signs, pulse oximetry, and intake and output *to assess and maintain adequate hydration, which is necessary to liquefy secretions and to detect early signs of respiratory compromise.*
- Provide adequate time for rest *to decrease oxygen demands.*
- Provide chest physiotherapy *to mobilize secretions that interfere with oxygenation.*
- Administer medications, as ordered, *to improve pulmonary function and improve oxygenation.*
- Provide a quiet environment. *Unnecessary noise or activity may increase the child's anxiety and cause respiratory distress.*

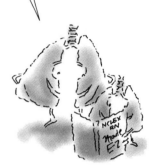

Oxygen may cause injury to the immature lung.

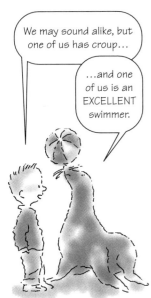

We may sound alike, but one of us has croup...

...and one of us is an EXCELLENT swimmer.

Teaching topics
• Visiting and becoming involved in the child's care, especially if child requires lengthy hospitalization

Croup

Croup is a group of related upper airway respiratory conditions that commonly affect toddlers. It includes acute spasmodic laryngitis, acute obstructive laryngitis, and acute laryngotracheobronchitis.

CAUSES
• Virus-induced edema around the larynx

ASSESSMENT FINDINGS
• Barking, brassy cough or hoarseness, sometimes described as a "seal bark" cough
• Condition usually begins at night and during cold weather and frequently recurs
• Crackles and decreased breath sounds (indicate condition has progressed to bronchi)
• Increased dyspnea and lower accessory muscle use
• Inspiratory stridor with varying degrees of respiratory distress
• Onset may be sudden or gradual

DIAGNOSTIC TEST RESULTS
• If bacterial infection is the cause, throat cultures may identify the organisms and their sensitivity to antibiotics as well as rule out diphtheria.
• Laryngoscopy may reveal inflammation and obstruction in epiglottal and laryngeal areas.
• Neck X-ray shows areas of upper airway narrowing and edema in subglottic folds and rules out the possibility of foreign body obstruction as well as masses and cysts.

NURSING DIAGNOSES
• Anxiety
• Ineffective breathing pattern
• Risk for fluid volume deficit

TREATMENT
• Clear liquid diet to keep mucus thin
• Cool humidification during sleep with a cool mist tent or room humidifier

• Rest from activity
• Tracheostomy, oxygen administration

Drug therapy
• Antipyretics, such as acetaminophen (Tylenol)
• Inhaled racemic epinephrine (Asthma-Nefrin) and corticosteroids such as methylprednisolone sodium succinate (Solu-Medrol) to alleviate respiratory distress

INTERVENTIONS AND RATIONALES
• Assess respiratory and cardiovascular status *to detect any indications that obstruction is worsening.*
• Monitor vital signs and pulse oximetry *to detect early signs of respiratory compromise.*
• Administer oxygen therapy and maintain the child in a cool mist tent, if needed. *Cool mist helps liquefy secretions.*
• Administer medications, as ordered, and note effectiveness *to maintain or improve child's condition.*
• Provide emotional support for the parents *to decrease anxiety.*
• Provide age-appropriate activities for the child confined to the mist tent *to ease anxiety.*
• Monitor for rebound obstruction when administering racemic epinephrine; *the drug's effects are short term and may result in rebound obstruction.*

Teaching topics
• Keeping the child calm to ease respiratory effort and conserve energy
• Methods of decreasing laryngeal spasm, such as taking the child into the bathroom, turning on the shower, and letting the room fill with steam
• Using a vaporizer near the child's bed

Cystic fibrosis

Cystic fibrosis is a generalized dysfunction of the exocrine glands that affects multiple organ systems. This disorder is characterized by:
• airway obstruction caused by the increased and constant production of mucus

• little or no release of pancreatic enzymes (lipase, amylase, and trypsin).

Transmitted as an autosomal recessive trait, cystic fibrosis is the one of the most common inherited diseases in children and one of the most common causes of childhood death. The disease occurs equally in both sexes. With improvements in treatment over the past decade, the average life expectancy has risen dramatically. The clinical effects may become apparent soon after birth or take years to develop.

CAUSES
• Genetic inheritance (Research suggests that there may be as many as 300 genes that code for cystic fibrosis.)

ASSESSMENT FINDINGS
• Bulky, greasy, foul-smelling stools that contain undigested food
• Distended abdomen and thin arms and legs from steatorrhea
• Failure to thrive from malabsorption
• History of a chronic, productive cough and recurrent respiratory infections, often due to *Pseudomonas* infections
• Meconium ileus in the newborn from a lack of pancreatic enzymes
• Parents' report of a salty taste on the child's skin
• Sweat that contains two to five times the normal levels of sodium and chloride
• Voracious appetite from undigested food lost in stools

DIAGNOSTIC TEST RESULTS
• Chest X-ray indicates early signs of obstructive lung disease.
• Sweat test using pilocarpine iontophoresis is positive.
• Stool specimen analysis indicates the absence of trypsin.

NURSING DIAGNOSES
• Altered nutrition: Less than body requirements
• Impaired gas exchange
• Risk for infection

TREATMENT
• Chest physiotherapy
• Multivitamins twice a day, especially fat-soluble vitamins
• High-protein formula, such as Probana, if needed

Drug therapy
• Mucolytic (dornase alfa [Pulmozyme]), bronchodilator, or antibiotic nebulizer inhalation treatment before chest physiotherapy
• I.V. antibiotics for a *Pseudomonas* infection when infection interferes with daily functioning
• Oral pancreatic enzyme replacement with pancrelipase (Pancrease)

INTERVENTIONS AND RATIONALES
• Assess respiratory and cardiovascular status *for early detection of hypoxia*.
• Monitor vital signs and intake and output *to detect dehydration, which may worsen respiratory status*.
• Monitor pulse oximetry *to detect early signs of hypoxia*.
• Administer pancreatic enzymes with meals and snacks *to aid digestion and absorption of nutrients*.
• Provide high-calorie, high-protein foods with added salt *to replace sodium loss and promote normal growth*.
• Encourage breathing exercises and perform chest physiotherapy two to four times a day *to mobilize secretions, to maintain lung capacity, and to increase oxygenation*.
• Encourage physical activity *to promote normal development*.

Teaching topics
• Avoiding cough suppressants and antihistamines because the child must be able to cough and expectorate
• Genetic counseling for the family
• Promoting as normal a life for the child as possible

Epiglottitis

Epiglottitis, a potentially life-threatening infection, causes inflammation and edema of the

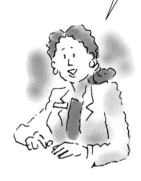

Exocrine glands, such as sweat glands and salivary glands, discharge their secretions through a duct opening on an internal or external surface of the body.

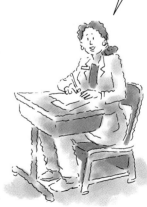

Parents may report a salty taste on the child's skin. In cystic fibrosis, the child's sweat contains two to five times the normal levels of sodium and chloride.

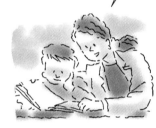

Key assessment findings for epiglottitis: difficulty swallowing, increased drooling, restlessness, and stridor.

epiglottis, a lidlike cartilaginous structure overhanging the entrance to the larynx and serving to prevent food from entering the larynx and trachea while swallowing. Epiglottitis is most common among preschoolers.

CAUSES
• Bacterial *Haemophilus influenzae* (most common causative organism)
• Pneumococci and group A beta-hemolytic streptococci

ASSESSMENT FINDINGS
• Cough
• Difficult and painful swallowing
• Extending the neck in a sniffing position
• Fever
• Increased drooling
• Irritability
• Lower rib retractions
• Pallor
• Rapid pulse rate
• Rapid respirations
• Refusal to drink
• Restlessness
• Sore throat
• Stridor
• Use of accessory muscles

DIAGNOSTIC TEST RESULTS
• Lateral neck X-ray shows an enlarged epiglottis.
• Throat examination reveals a large, edematous, bright red epiglottis.

NURSING DIAGNOSES
• Anxiety
• Ineffective airway clearance
• Ineffective breathing pattern

TREATMENT
• Emergency endotracheal intubation or a tracheotomy
• Oxygen therapy or cool mist tent
• I.V. fluid to prevent dehydration

Drug therapy
• Parenteral antibiotics according to causative organism: 10-day course

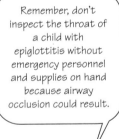

Remember, don't inspect the throat of a child with epiglottitis without emergency personnel and supplies on hand because airway occlusion could result.

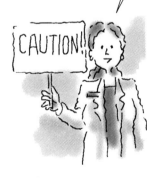

CAUTION!

INTERVENTIONS AND RATIONALES
• Monitor vital signs and pulse oximetry *to detect any changes in oxygenation.*
• Assess respiratory and cardiovascular status *to determine the severity of the child's condition and prevent respiratory failure or arrest.*
• Defer inspecting the throat until the arrival of emergency personnel and supplies *to avoid a spasm of the epiglottis that may lead to airway occlusion.*
• Reduce the number of examining personnel *to decrease the child's anxiety.*
• Allow the child to sit on a parent's lap; *sitting on a parent's lap makes breathing easier and decreases the child's anxiety.*
• Have equipment ready for a tracheotomy or intubation. *Emergency intubation and tracheostomy equipment should be on hand in case complete obstruction occurs.*
• Maintain oxygen therapy if necessary. *Humidified oxygen prevents secretions from thickening.*
• Administer medications as ordered *to treat infection and improve respiratory function.*
• Provide emotional support for the child and family *to decrease anxiety.*

Teaching topics
• Understanding signs and symptoms of this disorder and recognizing those that need immediate medical attention

Sudden infant death syndrome

Sudden infant death syndrome (SIDS) is the sudden death of an infant in which a postmortem examination fails to confirm the cause of death. The peak age is 3 months; 90% of cases occur before age 6 months, especially during the winter and early spring months.

Children who are diagnosed with SIDS are typically described as healthy with no previous medical problems. They are usually found dead sometime after being put down to sleep.

CAUSES
• May result from an abnormality in the control of ventilation, causing prolonged apneic periods with profound hypoxia and cardiac arrhythmias
• Undetected abnormalities, such as an immature respiratory system and respiratory dysfunction

ASSESSMENT FINDINGS
• History of low birth weight
• History of siblings with SIDS
• Death takes place during sleep without noise or struggle

DIAGNOSTIC TEST RESULTS
• Autopsy is the only way to diagnose SIDS. Autopsy findings indicate pulmonary edema, intrathoracic petechiae, and other minor changes suggesting chronic hypoxia.

NURSING DIAGNOSES
• Altered cardiopulmonary tissue perfusion
• Anticipatory grieving
• Inability to sustain spontaneous ventilation

TREATMENT
• If parents bring the infant to the emergency department, the doctor decides whether to try to resuscitate.
• If successfully resuscitated, the child is temporarily placed on mechanical ventilation. After he's extubated, the child is tested for infantile apnea and the parents are given a home apnea monitor.

Drug therapy
• If resuscitation is attempted, drugs are administered according to Pediatric Advanced Life Support protocols; drug therapy may include epinephrine, atropine and, after ABG analysis, sodium bicarbonate if appropriate.

INTERVENTIONS AND RATIONALES
• Because most infants can't be resuscitated, focus your interventions on providing emotional support for the family. Keep in mind grief may be coupled with guilt. Also, the parents may express anger at emergency department personnel, each other, or anyone involved with the child's care. Stay calm and let them express their feelings. *Parents need to express feelings to prevent dysfunctional grieving.*
• Let the parents touch, hold, and rock the infant if desired, and allow them to say goodbye to the infant *to facilitate the grieving process.*
• Provide literature on SIDS and support groups; suggest psychological support for the surviving children *to help prevent maladaptive emotional responses to loss, to promote a realistic perspective on the tragedy, and to promote coping.*
• Reinforce the fact that the death wasn't the parents' fault *to help alleviate guilt.*

Teaching topics
• Preparing the family for how the infant will look and feel if members touch and hold him
• Contacting a minister, priest, or rabbi; relatives; friends; and local support groups for grieving parents

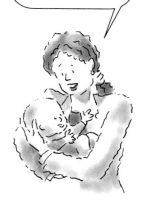

Research indicates a decreased incidence of SIDS in infants maintained in a supine position.

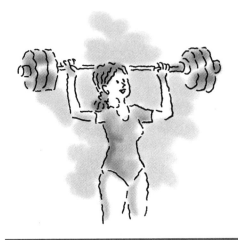

Pump up on practice questions

1. A parent brings her child to the pediatrician's office because of difficulty breathing and a "barking" cough. These signs are associated with which of the following conditions?

A. Cystic fibrosis
B. Asthma
C. Epiglottitis
D. Croup

Answer: D. A "seal bark" cough and difficulty breathing would indicate croup. Cystic fibrosis produces a chronic productive cough and recurrent respiratory infections. Asthma may cause prolonged expiration with an expiratory wheeze on auscultation, dyspnea, and accessory muscle use. Epiglottitis results in increased drooling, difficulty swallowing, tachypnea, and stridor.

➼ *NCLEX keys*
Nursing process step: Assessment
Client needs category: Physiological integrity
Client needs subcategory: Physiological adaptation
Taxonomic level: Knowledge

2. A woman with a child who awakes at night with a "barking" cough asks the nurse for advice. The nurse should instruct the mother to:

A. take the child in the bathroom, turn on the shower, and let the room fill with steam.
B. bring the child to the emergency department immediately.
C. notify the pediatrician immediately.
D. call emergency medical services to transport the child to the hospital for emergency tracheotomy.

Answer: A. The nurse should instruct the mother to take her child into the bathroom, close the door, turn on the shower's hot-water spigot full-force, and sit with the child as the room fills with steam; this should decrease laryngeal spasm. Epiglottitis is a potentially life-threatening infection that causes inflammation and edema of the epiglottis. If a child demonstrates symptoms associated with epiglottitis, not croup (increased drooling, stridor, tachypnea), the mother should notify the pediatrician immediately and call the emergency medical services to transport the child to the hospital; emergency tracheotomy may be necessary. Taking the child to the hospital by herself could jeopardize the child's condition if that condition deteriorates en route.

➼ *NCLEX keys*
Nursing process step: Implementation
Client needs category: Physiological integrity
Client needs subcategory: Reduction of risk potential
Taxonomic level: Application

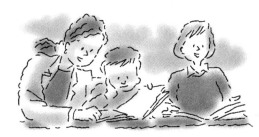

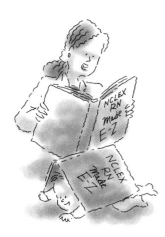

3. A child with croup is placed in a cool mist tent. Which statement should the nurse include when teaching the mother about this type of therapy?

    A. "You won't be able to touch your child while he's in the cool mist tent."

    B. "The cool mist is necessary because it will thin the child's mucus, making it easier to expectorate."

    C. "You can bring in your child's favorite stuffed animal to comfort him while he's in the cool mist tent."

    D. "You can bring in any of your child's favorite toys so he can play while he's in the cool mist tent."

Answer: B. The mother should be taught the purpose of the cool mist tent, which is to thin mucus and facilitate expectoration. The mother is able to touch her child while he's in the cool mist tent. She should be encouraged to bring in toys for the child to play with but to avoid stuffed toys, which may become damp and promote bacterial growth, and toys that produce sparks or friction.

➤ *NCLEX keys*
Nursing process step: Planning
Client needs category: Physiological integrity
Client needs subcategory: Reduction of risk potential
Taxonomic level: Application

4. The physician orders chest physiotherapy for a pediatric client. The nurse shouldn't perform chest physiotherapy when the client is experiencing:

    A. a productive cough.

    B. retained secretions.

    C. acute bronchoconstriction.

    D. hypoxia.

Answer: C. The nurse shouldn't administer chest physiotherapy during episodes of acute bronchoconstriction or airway edema (loosening mucus plugs could cause airway obstruction). Chest physiotherapy aids the elimination of secretions and reexpansion of lung tissue. Successful treatment with chest physiotherapy produces improved breath sounds, improved oxygenation, and increased sputum production and airflow. Therefore, it should be performed when a productive cough, retained secretions, or hypoxia is present.

➤ *NCLEX keys*
Nursing process step: Implementation
Client needs category: Physiological integrity
Client needs subcategory: Reduction of risk potential
Taxonomic level: Application

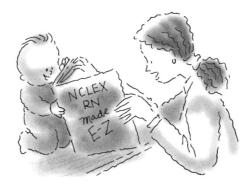

5. When preparing to teach the parents of an infant about preventing sudden infant death syndrome (SIDS), the nurse should include:

    A. positioning the infant on his stomach when sleeping.
    B. positioning the infant in an infant seat to sleep.
    C. positioning the infant on his back to sleep.
    D. positioning the infant in a side-lying position to sleep.

Answer: C. The parents should be instructed to position the infant on his back to sleep to decrease the risk of SIDS. Infants may be positioned in an infant seat during periods of respiratory distress to encourage lung expansion but it shouldn't be encouraged as a routine position for sleep. Research demonstrates an increased incidence of SIDS in infants positioned on their stomachs to sleep. The side-lying position should also be avoided because those infants can reposition themselves into a prone (stomach-lying) position.

➡ NCLEX keys

Nursing process step: Planning
Client needs category: Health promotion and maintenance
Client needs subcategory: Growth and development through the life span
Taxonomic level: Comprehension

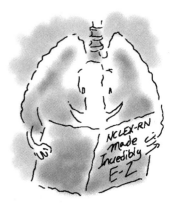

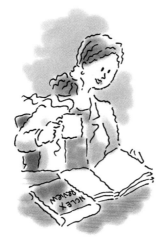

6. Which of the following test results is a key finding in the child with cystic fibrosis?

    A. Chest X-ray that reveals interstitial fibrosis
    B. Neck X-ray showing areas of upper airway narrowing
    C. Lateral neck X-ray revealing an enlarged epiglottis
    D. Positive pilocarpine iontophoresis sweat test

Answer: D. A child with cystic fibrosis has a positive pilocarpine iontophoresis sweat test. The child sweats normally, but this sweat contains two to five times the normal levels of sodium and chloride. Chest X-ray findings that reveal bronchiolar metaplasia and interstitial fibrosis are associated with bronchopulmonary dysplasia. A neck X-ray that reveals upper airway narrowing and edema in the subglottic folds indicates croup. A lateral neck X-ray that reveals an enlarged epiglottis indicates epiglottitis.

➡ NCLEX keys

Nursing process step: Assessment
Client needs category: Physiological integrity
Client needs subcategory: Reduction of risk potential
Taxonomic level: Knowledge

7. When communicating with the grieving family after a death from sudden infant death syndrome (SIDS), the nurse should:
   A. instruct the parents to place other infants on their backs to sleep.
   B. stress that the death isn't the parents' fault.
   C. stress that an autopsy must be done to confirm diagnosis.
   D. stress that the parents are still young and can have more children.

Answer: B. It's most important for the nurse to stress that death from SIDS is not predictable or preventable and that it isn't the parents' fault. Although it's important to inform the parents that an autopsy is necessary, that's secondary. Instructing the parents to place other infants on their backs to sleep implies that the parents did something wrong to cause the infant's death. Stressing that the parents are still young and can have other children minimizes their grief.

➥ *NCLEX keys*
Nursing process step: Implementation
Client needs category: Psychosocial integrity
Client needs subcategory: Coping and adaptation
Taxonomic level: Application

8. Which of the following client histories is most consistent with the diagnosis of sudden infant death syndrome (SIDS)?
   A. The child was physically abused in the past.
   B. The infant had a history of many medical problems.
   C. The infant was healthy and was found shortly after being put down to sleep.
   D. The infant was described as lethargic, irritable, and feeding poorly before being put down to sleep.

Answer: C. Children who are diagnosed with SIDS are typically described as healthy with no previous medical problems. They are usually found dead sometime after being put down to sleep. Depending on how long the infant has been dead, the infant may have a mottled complexion with extreme cyanosis of the lips, fingertips, or pooling of blood in the legs and feet that may be mistaken for bruising.

➥ *NCLEX keys*
Nursing process step: Assessment
Client needs category: Physiological integrity
Client needs subcategory: Physiological adaptation
Taxonomic level: Knowledge

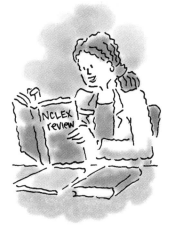

9. The nurse is teaching the parents of a child with cystic fibrosis. The nurse should teach the parents to avoid:
   A. encouraging their child to be physical active.
   B. administering pancreatic enzymes with meals and snacks.
   C. administering cough suppressants.
   D. encouraging their child to live as normal a life as possible.

Answer: C. The parents of a child with cystic fibrosis should be taught to avoid administering cough suppressants and antihistamines to their child. Administration of these drugs interferes with the child's ability to cough and expectorate. The parents should encourage the child to be physically active and lead as normal a life as possible. Pancreatic enzymes should be administered with meals and snacks.

NCLEX keys

Nursing process step: Implementation
Client needs category: Physiological integrity
Client needs subcategory: Reduction of risk potential
Taxonomic level: Knowledge

10. Which is the most appropriate nursing diagnosis for the child with epiglottitis?
   A. Anxiety related to separation from parent
   B. Decreased cardiac output related to bradycardia
   C. Ineffective airway clearance related to laryngospasm
   D. Impaired gas exchange related to noncompliant lungs

Answer: C. Epiglottitis is a life-threatening emergency that results from laryngospasm and edema. Therefore, ineffective airway clearance is the most appropriate diagnosis for this child. Anxiety related to separation shouldn't apply because the child doesn't need to be separated from the parent. The child will most likely be tachycardiac, not bradycardiac, unless respiratory failure ensues. The child has impaired gas exchange from impeded airflow, not from a noncompliant lung.

NCLEX keys

Nursing process step: Analysis
Client needs category: Physiological integrity
Client needs subcategory: Physiological adaptation
Taxonomic level: Analysis

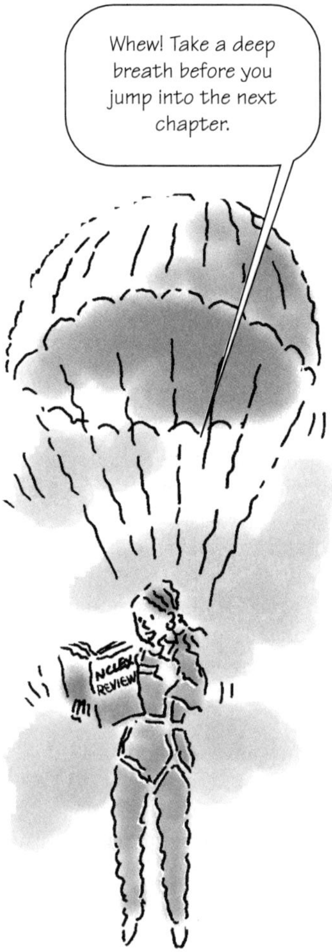

29 Hematologic & Immune Systems

Brush up on key concepts

The hematologic and immune system consists of blood and blood-forming tissues, as well as structures such as the lymph nodes, thymus, spleen, and tonsils. Reviewing the functions of this system and the development of a child's immune response will lay the groundwork for effective patient care.

At any time, you can review the major points of this chapter by consulting the *Cheat sheet* on pages 586 and 587.

What blood does

The functions of blood include:
• regulating body temperature by transferring heat from deep within the body to small vessels near the skin
• providing cell nutrition by carrying nutrients from the GI tract to the tissues and removing waste products by transporting them to the lungs, kidneys, liver, and skin for excretion
• defending against foreign antigens by transporting leukocytes and antibodies to the sites of infection, injury, and inflammation
• transporting hormones from endocrine glands to various parts of the body
• maintaining acid-base balance
• carrying oxygen to tissues and removing carbon dioxide.

Each little component does its part

Blood is composed of several components. These include:
• **erythrocytes** (red blood cells [RBCs]), which carry oxygen to the tissues and remove carbon dioxide
• **leukocytes** (white blood cells [WBCs]), which include lymphocytes, monocytes, and granulocytes; these participate in the immune response
• **thrombocytes** (platelets), which contribute to clotting
• **plasma** (the fluid part of blood), which carries antibodies and nutrients to tissues and carries wastes away.

It's common

Communicable diseases and **infections** are commonly seen during the time a child's immune system develops. Over time, a child receives protection from communicable diseases either naturally or artificially.

It's natural

• **Natural (innate) immunity** is present at birth. Examples of natural immunity include barriers against disease, such as skin and mucous membranes, and bacteriocidal substances of body fluids, such as intestinal flora and gastric acidity.
• In **naturally acquired active immunity,** the immune system makes antibodies after exposure to disease. It requires contact with the disease.
• In **naturally acquired passive immunity,** no active immune process is involved. The antibodies are passively received through placental transfer by immunoglobulin G (the smallest immunoglobulin) and breast-feeding (colostrum).

It's artificial

Artificially acquired immunity can be active or passive. In **artificially acquired active immunity,** medically engineered substances are ingested or injected to stimulate the immune response against a specific disease. Immunizations are an example of this kind of immunity.

In **artificially acquired passive immunity,** antibodies are injected without stimulating the immune response. Examples include

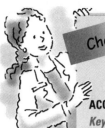

Hematologic & immune refresher

ACQUIRED IMMUNODEFICIENCY SYNDROME

Key signs and symptoms

- Failure to thrive
- Mononucleosis-like prodromal symptoms
- Night sweats
- Recurring diarrhea
- Weight loss

Key test results

- CD4+ T-cell count measures the severity of immunosuppression.
- Enzyme-linked immunosorbent assay and Western blot are positive for human immunodeficiency virus (HIV) antibody.
- Viral culture or p24 antigen test reveals presence of HIV in children under age 18 months.

Key treatments

- Antibiotic therapy according to sensitivity of infecting organisms
- Antiviral agents such as zidovudine
- Monthly gamma globulin administration

Key interventions

- Monitor vital signs, intake and output, and growth and development.
- Assess respiratory and neurologic status.
- Maintain standard precautions.

HEMOPHILIA

Key signs and symptoms

- Multiple bruises without petechiae
- Prolonged bleeding after circumcision, immunizations, or minor injuries

Key test result

- Prolonged partial thromboplastin time (PTT)

Key treatment

- Cryoprecipitate (frozen factor VIII) administration, to maintain an acceptable serum level of the clotting factor; usually done by the family at home
- Fresh frozen plasma

Key interventions

- Monitor vital signs and intake and output.
- When bleeding occurs:
- elevate the affected extremity above the heart
- immobilize the site to prevent clots from dislodging
- decrease anxiety to lower the child's heart rate.

IRON DEFICIENCY ANEMIA

Key signs and symptoms

- Fatigue, listlessness
- Increased susceptibility to infection
- Pallor
- Tachycardia
- Numbness and tingling of the extremities
- Vasomotor disturbances

Key test results

- Hemoglobin, hematocrit, and serum ferritin levels are low.
- Serum iron levels are low, with high binding capacity.

Key treatments

- Oral preparation of iron or a combination of iron and ascorbic acid (which enhances iron absorption)

Key interventions

- Administer iron before meals with citrus juice (iron is best absorbed in an acidic environment).
- Give liquid iron through a straw to prevent staining the child's skin and teeth; for infants, administer by oral syringe toward the back of the mouth.
- Don't give iron with milk products, as they interfere with absorption.

LEUKEMIA

Key signs and symptoms

- History of infections
- Low-grade fever
- Lymphadenopathy
- Pallor
- Petechiae and ecchymosis
- Poor wound healing and oral lesions

Key test results

- Blast cells appear in the peripheral blood.
- Blast cells may be as high as 95% in the bone marrow.

Hematologic and immune refresher (continued)

• Initial white blood cell (WBC) count may be 10,000/μl at time of diagnosis in a child with acute lymphocytic leukemia between the ages of 3 and 7.

Key treatments

• Bone marrow transplantation
• Radiation therapy
• Chemotherapy

Key interventions

• Provide pain relief.
• Monitor vital signs and intake and output.
• Inspect the skin frequently.
• Provide nursing measures to ease adverse effects of radiation and chemotherapy.

REYE'S SYNDROME

Key signs and symptoms

• Stage 5: seizures, loss of deep tendon reflexes, flaccidity, respiratory arrest (Death is usually a result of cerebral edema or cardiac arrest.)

Key test results

• Blood test results show elevated serum ammonia levels; serum fatty acid and lactate levels are also elevated.
• Coagulation studies reveal prolonged prothrombin time and PTT.
• Liver biopsy shows fatty droplets distributed through cells.
• Liver function studies show aspartate aminotransferase and alanine aminotransferase as elevated to twice normal levels.

Key treatments

• Endotracheal intubation and mechanical ventilation
• Exchange transfusion
• Induced hypothermia

Key interventions

• Monitor vital signs and pulse oximetry.

• Assess cardiac, respiratory, and neurologic status.
• Monitor fluid intake and output.
• Monitor blood glucose levels.
• Maintain seizure precautions.
• Keep head of bed at 30-degree angle.
• Closely monitor cardiovascular status with a pulmonary artery catheter or central venous pressure line.
• Maintain oxygen therapy, which may include intubation and mechanical ventilation.
• Administer blood products as necessary.
• Administer medications, as ordered, and monitor for adverse effects.
• Maintain hypothermia blanket as needed and monitor temperature every 15 to 30 minutes while in use.
• Check for loss of reflexes and signs of flaccidity.

SICKLE CELL ANEMIA

Key signs and symptoms

• In infants, colic and splenomegaly
• In toddlers and preschoolers, hypovolemia, shock, and pain at site of crisis
• In school-age children and adolescents, enuresis, extreme pain at site of crisis, and priapism

Key test results

• A level of more than 50% hemoglobin S indicates sickle cell disease; a lower level of hemoglobin S indicates sickle cell trait.

Key treatments

• Hydration with I.V. fluid administration
• Transfusion therapy as necessary
• Treatment for acidosis
• Analgesics (meperidine) for pain

Key interventions

• Monitor vital signs and intake and output.
• Administer pain medications and note effectiveness.

---

tetanus antitoxin, hepatitis B immune globulin, and varicella zoster immune globulin.

Keep abreast of diagnostic tests

Here are the most important tests used to diagnose hematologic and immunologic disorders, along with common nursing interventions associated with each test.

Not my type?

Blood typing is used to determine the antigens present in a patient's RBCs. A reaction with standardized sera indicates the presence of specific antigens.

Nursing actions

• Explain the procedure to the child and family.

- Handle the sample gently to prevent hemolysis.
- Apply pressure to the venipuncture site to prevent hematoma or bleeding.

Tuning into the immune system

Laboratory studies, such as **CD4+ T-cell count** and **enzyme-linked immunosorbent assay (ELISA)**, are used to assess immunosuppression.

Nursing actions

- Explain the procedure to the child and family.
- Handle the sample gently to prevent hemolysis.
- Apply pressure to the venipuncture site to prevent hematoma or bleeding.

Clot measure

A **coagulation study** tests a blood sample to analyze platelet function, platelet count, prothrombin time (PT), international normalized ratio, partial thromboplastin time (PTT), coagulation time, and bleeding time.

Nursing actions

- Note the child's current drug therapy before procedure.
- Check the venipuncture site for bleeding after the procedure.

A look at the liver

Liver function studies measure levels of hepatic enzymes such as aspartate aminotransferase (AST) and alanine aminotransferase (ALT).

Nursing actions

- Before the test, prepare the child for venipuncture.
- After the test, check the venipuncture site for bleeding.

Polish up on patient care

Major hematologic and immune disorders in pediatric patients include acquired immunodeficiency syndrome, hemophilia, iron deficiency anemia, leukemia, Reye's syndrome, and sickle cell anemia.

Acquired immunodeficiency syndrome

In acquired immunodeficiency syndrome (AIDS), the human immunodeficiency virus (HIV) attacks helper T cells. AIDS may be spread through sexual contact, percutaneous or mucous membrane exposure to needles or other sharp instruments contaminated with blood or bloody body fluid (for example, in I.V. drug abuse), or mother to infant transmission before or around the time of birth. Most children in the United States with AIDS either have parents at high risk for the disorder or received the virus through blood products.

HIV has a much shorter incubation period in children than adults. In adults, the incubation period may last 10 years or more. By contrast, children who receive the virus by placental transmission are usually HIV-positive by age 6 months and develop clinical signs by age 3.

Because of passive antibody transmission, all infants born to HIV-infected mothers test positive for antibodies to the HIV virus up to about age 18 months. Confirmation of diagnosis during this time requires detection of the HIV antigen.

CAUSES

- Contaminated blood products
- Infected parent

ASSESSMENT FINDINGS

- Failure to thrive
- Lymphadenopathy
- Mononucleosis-like prodromal symptoms
- Neurologic impairment, such as loss of motor milestones and behavioral changes
- Night sweats
- Recurrent opportunistic infections
- Recurring diarrhea
- Weight loss

DIAGNOSTIC TEST RESULTS
• CD4+ T-cell count measures the severity of immunosuppression.
• Culture and sensitivity tests reveal infection with opportunistic organisms.
• ELISA and Western blot are positive for HIV antibody.
• Viral culture or p24 antigen test reveals presence of HIV in children under age 18 months.

NURSING DIAGNOSES
• Altered protection
• Altered nutrition: Less than body requirements
• Fluid volume deficit

TREATMENT
• Blood administration, if necessary
• Follow-up laboratory studies
• High-calorie diet provided in small frequent meals
• I.V. fluids to maintain hydration
• Nutrition supplements, if necessary
• Parenteral nutrition, if necessary

Drug therapy
• Antibiotic therapy according to sensitivity of infecting opportunistic organism
• Antiviral agents such as zidovudine (Retrovir)
• Monthly gamma globulin administration
• Prophylactic antibiotic therapy with co-trimoxazole (Bactrim) to prevent *Pneumocystis carinii* pneumonia
• Routine immunizations (Varicella vaccine, however, isn't recommended for HIV-infected children.)

INTERVENTIONS AND RATIONALES
• Monitor vital signs, intake, and output *to detect tachycardia, dyspnea, hypertension, or decreased urine output, which may indicate fluid volume deficit or electrolyte imbalance.*
• Monitor developmental progress at regular intervals *to detect changes in level of functioning and, as appropriate, adapt activity program.*
• Provide appropriate play activities *to promote development.*

• Encourage fluid intake *to prevent dehydration.*
• Assess respiratory and neurologic status *to detect early signs of compromise.*
• Maintain standard precautions *to prevent the spread of infection.*
• Administer medications, as ordered, *to help boost immune response and prevent opportunistic infections.*
• Provide psychosocial support. *An AIDS diagnosis is devastating for child and family.*
• Assess the child's support system and provide referrals. *The child may have no one to care for him.*

Teaching topics
• Controlling infection in the home using sanitary measures
• Avoiding consumption of raw or undercooked meats
• Avoiding swimming in a lake or river
• Avoiding contact with young farm animals
• Understanding risk factors from pets (especially cats)
• Recognizing signs and symptoms of infection and getting immediate treatment
• Practicing safe sex, if appropriate

Hemophilia

Hemophilia results from a deficiency in one of the coagulation factors. Hemophilia affects 1 in 5,000 males.

The types of hemophilia are:
• hemophilia A (also called factor VIII deficiency or classic hemophilia), the most common type (75% of all cases)
• hemophilia B (also called factor IX deficiency or Christmas disease)
• hemophilia C (factor XI deficiency).

Hemophilia is an X-linked recessive disorder. The inheritance pattern is described below:
• If the father has the disorder and the mother doesn't, all daughters will be carriers, but sons won't have the disease.
• If the mother is a carrier and the father doesn't have hemophilia, each son has a 50% chance of getting hemophilia and each daughter has a 50% chance of being a carrier.

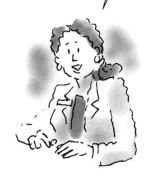

As with adults, children with AIDS exhibit nonspecific signs and symptoms.

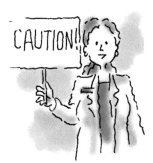

Children with HIV or AIDS and their families must maintain strict personal hygiene.

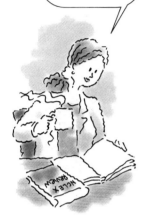

A classic sign of hemophilia: prolonged bleeding after minor injuries.

CAUSES
• Genetic inheritance

ASSESSMENT FINDINGS
• Bleeding into the throat, mouth, and thorax
• Hemarthrosis
• Multiple bruises without petechiae
• Peripheral neuropathies from bleeding near peripheral nerves
• Prolonged bleeding after circumcision, immunizations, or minor injuries

DIAGNOSTIC TEST RESULTS
• Prolonged PTT.

NURSING DIAGNOSES
• Altered protection
• Risk for fluid volume deficit
• Risk for injury

TREATMENT
• Avoiding aspirin, sutures, and cauterization, which may aggravate bleeding
• Blood transfusion if necessary
• Cryoprecipitate administration, to maintain an acceptable serum level of the clotting factor; usually done by the family at home
• Frequently assessing HIV status (Child is at increased risk for acquiring HIV through blood product transfusions.)
• Administration of fresh frozen plasma to restore deficient coagulation factors
• Promoting vasoconstriction during bleeding episodes by applying ice, pressure, and hemostatic agents

Drug therapy
• Desmopressin acetate (DDAVP) to promote release of factor VIII in individuals with mild or moderate hemophilia A

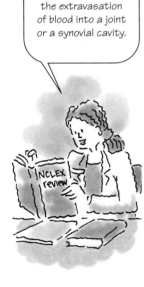

Hemarthrosis is the extravasation of blood into a joint or a synovial cavity.

INTERVENTIONS AND RATIONALES
• Monitor vital signs and intake and output *to assess renal status and monitor for fluid overload or dehydration.*
• Assess cardiovascular status and check for signs of bleeding; *fever, tachycardia, or hypotension may indicate hypovolemia.*
• Measure the joint's circumference and compare it to that of an unaffected joint *to assess*

for bleeding into the joint, which may lead to hypovolemia.
• Note swelling, pain, or limited joint mobility. *Changes may indicate progressive decline in function.*
• Assess for joint degeneration from repeated hemarthroses *to detect extent of damage.*
• Pad toys and other objects in the child's environment *to promote child safety and prevent bleeding.*
• Recommend protective headgear, soft foam Toothettes (instead of bristle toothbrushes), and stool softeners as appropriate *to prevent bleeding.*
• Discourage abnormal weight gain, *which increases the load on joints.*

When bleeding occurs
• Elevate the affected extremity above the heart *to decrease circulation to affected area and promote venous return.*
• Immobilize the site *to prevent clots from dislodging.*
• Decrease anxiety *to lower the child's heart rate.*

To treat hemarthrosis
• Immobilize the affected extremity; elevate it in a slightly flexed position *to prevent further injury.*
• Decrease pain and anxiety *to lower the child's heart rate and minimize blood loss.*
• Avoid excessive handling or weight bearing for 48 hours *to prevent bleeding and to rest the site.*
• Begin mild range-of-motion exercises after 48 hours *to facilitate absorption and prevent contractures.*

Teaching topics
• Genetic counseling for parents
• Avoiding contact sports

Iron deficiency anemia

The most common nutritional anemia during childhood, iron deficiency anemia is characterized by poor RBC production. Insufficient body stores of iron lead to:
• depleted RBC mass

- decreased hemoglobin concentration (hypochromia)
- decreased oxygen-carrying capacity of the blood.

   Most commonly, iron deficiency anemia occurs when the child experiences rapid physical growth, low iron intake, inadequate iron absorption, or loss of blood.

CAUSES
- Blood loss secondary to drug-induced GI bleeding (from anticoagulants, aspirin, steroids) or due to heavy menses, hemorrhage from trauma, GI ulcers, or cancer
- Inadequate dietary intake of iron (less than 1 to 2 mg/day), which may occur following prolonged unsupplemented breast-feeding or bottle-feeding of infants, or during periods of stress such as rapid growth in children and adolescents
- Iron malabsorption, as in chronic diarrhea, partial or total gastrectomy, and malabsorption syndromes, such as celiac disease and pernicious anemia
- Intravascular hemolysis-induced hemoglobinuria or paroxysmal nocturnal hemoglobinuria
- Mechanical erythrocyte trauma caused by a prosthetic heart valve or vena cava filters

ASSESSMENT FINDINGS
Anemia progresses gradually, and many children are initially asymptomatic, except for symptoms of an underlying condition. Children with advanced anemia display the following symptoms:
- dyspnea on exertion
- fatigue
- headache
- inability to concentrate
- irritability
- listlessness
- pallor
- susceptibility to infection
- tachycardia.

   In cases of chronic iron deficiency anemia, children display the following symptoms:
- cracks in corners of the mouth
- dysphagia
- neuralgic pain
- numbness and tingling of the extremities
- smooth tongue

- spoon-shaped, brittle nails
- vasomotor disturbances.

DIAGNOSTIC TEST RESULTS
- Bone marrow studies reveal depleted or absent iron stores and normoblastic hyperplasia.
- Hemoglobin, hematocrit, and serum ferritin levels are low.
- Mean corpuscular hemoglobin is decreased in severe anemia.
- RBC count is low, with microcytic and hypochromic cells. (In early stages, RBC count may be normal, except in infants and children.)
- Serum iron levels are low, with high binding capacity.

NURSING DIAGNOSES
- Altered nutrition: Less than body requirements
- Fatigue
- Impaired gas exchange

TREATMENT
- Increased iron intake (for children and adolescents) by adding foods rich in iron to diet, or (for infants) adding iron supplements

Drug therapy
- Oral preparation of iron or a combination of iron and ascorbic acid (which enhances iron absorption)
- Cyanocobalamin (vitamin B_{12}) if intrinsic factor is lacking
- Iron dextran (InFeD) if additional therapy is needed

INTERVENTIONS AND RATIONALES
- Carefully assess a child's drug history. *Certain drugs, such as pancreatic enzymes and vitamin E, may interfere with iron metabolism and absorption and other drugs, such as aspirin and steroids, may cause GI bleeding.*
- Provide passive stimulation; allow frequent rest; give small, frequent feedings; and elevate the head of the bed *to decrease oxygen demands.*
- Implement proper hand washing *to decrease risk of infection.*
- Provide foods high in iron (liver, dark leafy vegetables, and whole grains) *to replenish iron stores.*

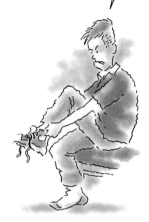

Anemia can follow periods of stress, such as rapid growth.

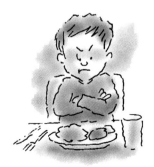

Please. Just try some of the liver.

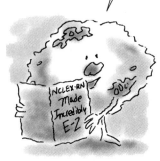

Blast it. In leukemia, I can't get the nutrition I need!

• Administer iron before meals with citrus juice. *Iron is best absorbed in an acidic environment.*

• Give liquid iron through a straw *to prevent staining the child's skin and teeth.* For infants, administer by oral syringe toward the back of the mouth.

• Don't give iron with milk products. *Milk products may interfere with absorption of iron.*

• Be supportive of the family and keep them informed of the child's status *to decrease anxiety.*

Teaching topics

• Keeping iron supplements safely stored out of the child's reach at home

• Brushing teeth after iron administration

• Reporting reactions to iron supplementation, such as nausea, vomiting, diarrhea, constipation, fever, or severe stomach pain, which may require a dosage adjustment

Leukemia

Leukemia is the abnormal, uncontrolled proliferation of WBCs. In leukemia, WBCs are produced so rapidly that immature cells (blast cells) are released into the circulation. These blast cells are nonfunctional, can't fight infection, and are formed continuously without respect to the body's needs. This proliferation robs healthy cells of sufficient nutrition.

In children, the most common type of leukemia is acute lymphocytic leukemia (ALL). This type of leukemia is marked by extreme proliferation of immature lymphocytes (blast cells). In adolescents, acute myelogenous leukemia (AML) is more common and is believed to result from a malignant transformation of a single stem cell.

CAUSES AND CONTRIBUTING FACTORS

• Chemical exposure and viruses
• Chromosomal disorders
• Down syndrome
• Ionizing radiation

ASSESSMENT FINDINGS

Clinical findings for leukemia may appear with surprising abruptness in children with few, if any warning signs. The following are common leukemia assessment findings:

• blood in urine, stool, or emesis
• bone and joint pain
• decrease in all blood cells, when bone marrow undergoes atrophy (leads to anemia, bleeding disorders, and immunosuppression)
• history of infections
• lassitude
• low-grade fever
• lymphadenopathy
• pallor
• pathologic fractures (when bone marrow undergoes hypertrophy)
• petechiae and ecchymosis
• poor wound healing and oral lesions.

DIAGNOSTIC TEST RESULTS

• Blast cells appear in the peripheral blood (where they normally don't appear).

• Blast cells may be as high as 95% in the bone marrow (they are normally less than 5%) as measured by marrow aspiration in the posterior iliac crest (the sternum can't be used in children).

• Initial WBC count may be less than 10,000/µl at the time of diagnosis in a child with ALL between ages 3 and 7. (This child has the best prognosis.)

• Lumbar puncture indicates if leukemic cells have crossed the blood-brain barrier.

NURSING DIAGNOSES

• Altered protection
• Pain
• Risk for infection

Marrow may be transfused from a twin or another HLA-identical donor.

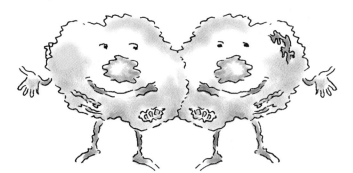

TREATMENT
- Bone marrow transplantation (Marrow from a twin or another donor with identical human leukocyte antigen [HLA], usually a sibling, is transfused to repopulate the recipient's bone marrow with normal cells.)
- High-protein, high-calorie, bland diet
- I.V. fluids, as necessary
- Oxygen therapy if needed
- Radiation therapy
- Transfusion therapy as needed

Drug therapy
- Analgesics
- Antiemetics: hydroxyzine (Atarax) and ondansetron (Zofran)
- Chemotherapy with agents such as ara-C (Cytosar-U); intrathecal chemotherapy usually with methotrexate (Folex)
- Corticosteroids: prednisone (Deltasone)

INTERVENTIONS AND RATIONALES
- Monitor vital signs and intake and output *to determine fluid volume deficit and renal status.*
- Give special attention to mouth care *to prevent infection and bleeding.*
- Inspect the skin frequently *to assess for skin breakdown.*
- Give increased fluids *to flush chemotherapeutic drugs through the kidneys.*
- Provide a high-protein, high-calorie, bland diet with no raw fruits or vegetables. *Eliminating raw fruits and vegetables helps prevent infection. A diet meeting the child's caloric requirements helps ensure that the child's maintenance and growth needs are met.*
- Provide pain relief as ordered and document effectiveness and adverse effects. *Analgesics depress the central nervous system (CNS), thereby reducing pain.*
- Monitor the CNS *to assess for changes such as confusion that may result from cerebral damage.*
- Provide nursing measures to ease the adverse reactions of radiation and chemotherapy *to promote comfort and encourage adequate nutritional intake.*

Teaching topics
- Avoiding infection
- Adjusting to changes in body image
- Contacting support groups
- Recognizing signs and symptoms of infection and the need to seek immediate medical attention

Reye's syndrome

Reye's syndrome is an acute illness that causes fatty infiltration of the liver, kidneys, brain, and myocardium. It can lead to hyperammonemia, encephalopathy, and increased intracranial pressure (ICP).

CAUSES
- Acute viral infection, such as upper respiratory tract, type B influenza, or varicella (Reye's syndrome almost always follows within 1 to 3 days of infection.)
- Concurrent aspirin use (high incidence)

ASSESSMENT FINDINGS
Reye's syndrome develops in five stages. The severity of signs and symptoms varies with degree of encephalopathy and cerebral edema.
- Stage 1: vomiting, lethargy, hepatic dysfunction
- Stage 2: hyperventilation, delirium, hyperactive reflexes, hepatic dysfunction
- Stage 3: coma, hyperventilation, decorticate rigidity, hepatic dysfunction
- Stage 4: deepening coma, decerebrate rigidity, large fixed pupils, minimal hepatic dysfunction
- Stage 5: seizures, loss of deep tendon reflexes, flaccidity, respiratory arrest. Death is usually a result of cerebral edema or cardiac arrest.

DIAGNOSTIC TEST RESULTS
- Blood test results show elevated serum ammonia levels; serum fatty acid and lactate levels are also increased.
- Cerebrospinal fluid (CSF) analysis shows WBC less than 10/µl; with coma, there's increased CSF pressure.
- Coagulation studies reveal prolonged PT and PTT.
- Liver biopsy shows fatty droplets uniformly distributed throughout cells.

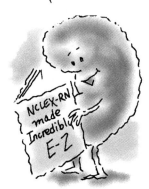

Increased fluids help to flush chemotherapeutic drugs through the kidneys.

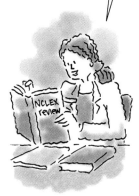

Acute infection plus aspirin use equals risk of Reye's syndrome.

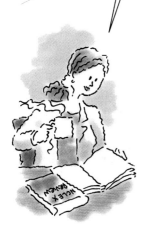

To prevent Reye's syndrome, use nonsalicylate analgesics and antipyretics.

• Liver function studies show AST and ALT are elevated to twice normal levels.

NURSING DIAGNOSES
• Decreased adaptive capacity: intracranial
• Ineffective thermoregulation
• Risk for fluid volume deficit

TREATMENT
• Decompressive craniotomy
• Endotracheal intubation and mechanical ventilation to control partial pressure of arterial carbon dioxide levels
• Enteral or parenteral nutrition as needed
• Exchange transfusion
• Induced hypothermia
• Transfusion of fresh frozen plasma

Drug therapy
• Osmotic diuretics: mannitol (Osmitrol)
• Vitamins: Phytonadione (AquaMEPHYTON)

INTERVENTIONS AND RATIONALES
• Monitor ICP with a subarachnoid screw or other invasive device *to closely assess for increased ICP.*
• Monitor vital signs and pulse oximetry *to determine oxygenation status.*
• Assess cardiac, respiratory, and neurologic status *to evaluate the effectiveness of interventions and monitor for complications such as seizures.*
• Monitor fluid intake and output *to prevent fluid overload.*
• Monitor blood glucose levels *to detect hyperglycemia or hypoglycemia and prevent complications.*
• Maintain seizure precautions *to prevent injury.*
• Keep head of bed at 30-degree angle *to decrease ICP and promote venous return.*
• Assess pulmonary artery catheter pressures *to assess cardiopulmonary status.*
• Maintain oxygen therapy, which may include intubation and mechanical ventilation, *to promote oxygenation and maintain thermoregulation.*
• Administer blood products as necessary *to increase oxygen-carrying capacity of blood and prevent hypovolemia.*

• Administer medications, as ordered, and monitor for adverse effects *to detect complications.*
• Maintain hypothermia blanket as needed and monitor temperature every 15 to 30 minutes while in use *to prevent injury and maintain thermoregulation.*
• Check for loss of reflexes and signs of flaccidity *to determine degree of neurologic involvement.*
• Provide good skin and mouth care and range-of-motion exercises *to prevent alteration in skin integrity and to promote joint motility.*
• Provide postoperative craniotomy care if necessary *to promote wound healing and prevent complications.*
• Be supportive of the family and keep them informed of the child's status *to decrease anxiety.*

Teaching topics
• Avoiding aspirin products
• Explaining all procedures and nursing care measures to family
• Referring family to support groups as indicated

Sickle cell anemia

In sickle cell anemia, a defect in the hemoglobin molecule changes the oxygen-carrying capacity and shape of RBCs. The altered hemoglobin molecule is referred to as hemoglobin S. In this disorder, RBCs acquire a sickle shape.

The child may experience periodic, painful attacks called sickle cell crises. A sickle cell crisis may be triggered or intensified by:
• dehydration
• deoxygenation
• acidosis.

CAUSES
• Genetic inheritance (sickle cell anemia is an autosomal recessive trait; the child inherits the gene that produces hemoglobin S from two healthy parents who carry the defective gene)

ASSESSMENT FINDINGS
Assessment findings vary with the age of the child. Before age 4 months, symptoms are

rare (because fetal hemoglobin prevents excessive sickling).

In infants
- Colic from pain caused by an abdominal infarction
- Dactylitis or hand-foot syndrome from infarction of the small bones of the hands and feet
- Splenomegaly from sequestered RBCs

In toddlers and preschoolers
- Hypovolemia and shock from sequestration of large amounts of blood in spleen
- Pain at site of vaso-occlusive crisis

In school-age children and adolescents
- Delayed growth and development and delayed sexual maturity
- Enuresis
- Extreme pain at site of crisis
- History of pneumococcal pneumonia and other infections due to atrophied spleen
- Poor healing of leg wounds from inadequate peripheral circulation of oxygenated blood
- Priapism

DIAGNOSTIC TEST RESULTS
- Laboratory studies show hemoglobin level is 6 to 9 g/dl (in a toddler).
- More than 50% hemoglobin S indicates sickle cell disease; a lower level of hemoglobin S indicates sickle cell trait.
- RBCs are crescent-shaped and prone to agglutination.

NURSING DIAGNOSES
- Altered peripheral tissue perfusion
- Impaired gas exchange
- Pain

TREATMENT
- Bed rest
- Hydration with I.V. fluid (may be increased to 3 L/day during crisis)
- Short-term oxygen therapy (long-term oxygen decreases bone marrow activity, further aggravating anemia)
- Transfusion therapy as necessary
- Treatment for acidosis as necessary

Drug therapy
- Analgesic: meperidine (Demerol)
- Hydroxyurea (Droxia)
- Pneumococcal vaccine

INTERVENTIONS AND RATIONALES
- Administer sufficient pain medication (concerns regarding addiction are clinically unfounded) *to promote comfort.*
- Assess cardiovascular, respiratory, and neurologic status. *Tachycardia, dyspnea, or hypotension may indicate fluid volume deficit or electrolyte imbalance. Change in level of consciousness may signal neurologic involvement.*
- Assess for symptoms of acute chest syndrome from a pulmonary infarction *to identify early complications.*
- Assess vision *to monitor for retinal infarction.*
- Encourage the child to receive the pneumococcal vaccine *to prevent infection.*
- Give large amounts of oral or I.V. fluids *to prevent fluid volume deficit and prevent complications.*
- Teach the child relaxation techniques *to decrease the child's stress level.*
- Maintain the child's normal body temperature *to prevent stress and maintain adequate metabolic state.*
- Monitor vital signs and intake and output *to assess renal function and hydration status.*
- Provide proper skin care *to prevent skin breakdown.*
- Reduce the child's energy expenditure *to improve oxygenation.*
- Remove tight clothing *to prevent inadequate circulation.*
- Suggest family screening and initiate genetic counseling *to identify possible carriers of the disease.*

Teaching topics
- Avoiding activities that promote a crisis, such as excessive exercise, mountain climbing, or deep sea diving
- Avoiding high altitudes
- Seeking early treatment of illness to prevent dehydration
- Avoiding aspirin use, which enhances acidosis and promotes sickling

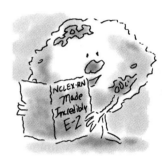

Red blood cells become sickle-shaped. Oh my.

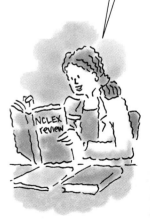

Findings for sickle cell anemia vary with age. For example, the spleen is enlarged in a young child. As the child grows, the spleen atrophies.

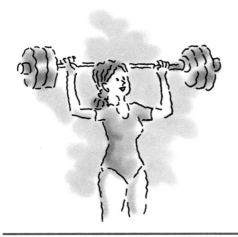

Pump up on practice questions

1. The nurse is taking a history from the mother of a pediatric client suspected of having Reye's syndrome. The history reveals the use of several medications. Which of the following medications might be implicated in the development of Reye's syndrome?
   A. Phenytoin (Dilantin)
   B. Furosemide (Lasix)
   C. Phytonadione (AquaMEPHYTON)
   D. Aspirin

Answer: D. Aspirin use has been implicated in the development of Reye's syndrome in children with a history of recent acute viral infection. Phenytoin, furosemide, and vitamin K aren't associated with the development of Reye's syndrome.

➡ *NCLEX keys*
Nursing process step: Assessment
Client needs category: Physiological integrity
Client needs subcategory: Reduction of risk potential
Taxonomic level: Application

2. The nurse is teaching the mother of a child diagnosed with iron deficiency anemia. Which of the following is true?
   A. Iron shouldn't be administered with foods containing ascorbic acid because they delay absorption.
   B. Iron should be administered with milk products because they enhance absorption.
   C. Report black tarry stools to the physician immediately so dosage can be adjusted.
   D. Iron shouldn't be administered with milk products because they delay absorption.

Answer: D. Iron shouldn't be administered with milk products because they delay absorption. Iron should be administered before meals with citrus juice (contains ascorbic acid) because iron is best absorbed in an acidic environment. The parents should be taught to expect black tarry stools.

➡ *NCLEX keys*
Nursing process step: Planning
Client needs category: Physiological integrity
Client needs subcategory: Pharmacological and parenteral therapies
Taxonomic level: Knowledge

3. The nurse is teaching the mother of a pediatric client with sickle cell anemia. Which statement by the mother indicates a need for further teaching?
   A. "My child can't possibly have sickle cell anemia. He's 4 months old and he's never been sick before."
   B. "I know my child should receive a pneumococcal vaccine when the doctor suggests."
   C. " I know I should call the pediatrician immediately if my child begins to vomit."
   D. "I know I should try to keep my child's body temperature normal by keeping him away from fluctuations in temperature."

Answer: A. Further teaching is indicated if the mother states that her child can't have sickle cell anemia because he's 4 months old and has never been sick before. Symptoms of sickle cell anemia rarely appear before age 4 months because the predominance of fetal hemoglobin prevents excessive sickling. The child should receive a pneumococcal vaccine when appropriate. The mother should notify the physician if the child vomits so that treatment can be initiated to prevent dehydration, which can precipitate crisis. Changes in body temperature may also trigger crisis and should be avoided.

➠ NCLEX keys
Nursing process step: Evaluation
Client needs category: Physiological integrity
Client needs subcategory: Reduction of risk potential
Taxonomic level: Analysis

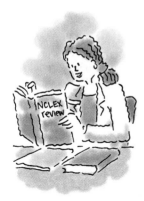

4. The nurse is teaching a mother about the benefits of breast-feeding her infant. Which type of immunity is passed on to the infant during breast-feeding?
  A. Natural immunity
  B. Naturally acquired active immunity
  C. Naturally acquired passive immunity
  D. Artificially acquired active immunity

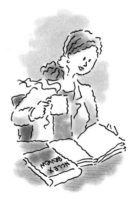

Answer: C. Naturally acquired passive immunity is received through placental transfer and breast-feeding. Natural immunity is present at birth. Naturally acquired active immunity occurs when the immune system makes antibodies after exposure to disease. Artificially acquired immunity occurs when medically engineered substances are ingested or injected to stimulate the immune response against a specific disease (immunizations).

➠ NCLEX keys
Nursing process step: Implementation
Client needs category: Health promotion and maintenance
Client needs subcategory: Safety and infection control
Taxonomic level: Application

5. The physician prescribes iron supplements for a child with iron deficiency anemia. Which of the following adverse reactions may occur as a result of iron supplementation?
  A. Tachycardia, hypotension, and vomiting
  B. Tachycardia, hypertension, and vomiting
  C. Vomiting, severe stomach pain, and diarrhea
  D. Vomiting, severe stomach pain, and petechiae

Answer: C. Nausea, vomiting, diarrhea, constipation, fever, and severe stomach pain are adverse reactions associated with iron supplementation. If these occur, the physician should be notified and the dosage adjusted. Tachycardia, hypotension, and petechiae may be present with bleeding disorders and aren't associated with iron supplementation. Hypertension isn't an adverse reaction of iron supplementation.

➡➡ *NCLEX keys*

Nursing process step: Assessment
Client needs category: Physiological integrity
Client needs subcategory: Pharmacological and parenteral therapies
Taxonomic level: Knowledge

6. The nurse is providing dietary teaching for the mother of a child with iron deficiency anemia. Which of the following iron-rich foods should the mother include in her child's diet?
   A. Liver, dark leafy vegetables, and whole grains
   B. Dark leafy vegetables, chicken, and whole grains
   C. Whole grains, citrus fruit, and yogurt
   D. Citrus fruit, liver, and whole grains

Answer: A. The mother should be instructed to give her child iron-rich foods such as liver, dark leafy vegetables, and whole grains. Chicken is a good source of protein, but it isn't high in iron. Citrus fruits aid iron absorption but aren't high in iron. Yogurt is a good source of calcium but isn't high in iron.

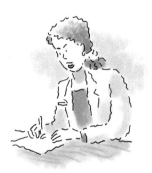

➡➡ *NCLEX keys*

Nursing process step: Implementation
Client needs category: Physiological integrity
Client needs subcategory: Basic care and comfort
Taxonomic level: Knowledge

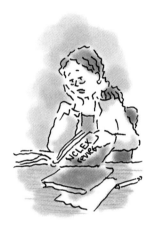

7. The nurse is teaching a child with sickle cell anemia and the child's mother about activities that may promote a vaso-occlusive crisis. Which of the following activities are acceptable for this child?
   A. Skiing
   B. Mountain climbing
   C. Deep sea diving
   D. Bowling

Answer: D. The child with sickle cell anemia should be instructed to avoid activities that promote a crisis, such as excessive exercise, mountain climbing, or deep sea diving. Extremes in temperature can also promote a crisis, so skiing should be avoided. Mountain climbing and deep sea diving may expose the child to altered atmospheric pressures and a deoxygenated state. These conditions can lead to a sickle cell crisis.

➡➡ *NCLEX keys*

Nursing process step: Implementation
Client needs category: Physiological integrity
Client needs subcategory: Reduction of risk potential
Taxonomic level: Application

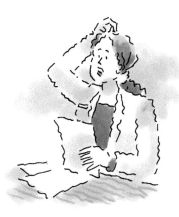

8. A newborn experiences prolonged bleeding after his circumcision and has multiple bruises without petechiae. These assessment findings suggest which of the following?

A. Iron deficiency anemia
B. Hemophilia
C. Sickle cell anemia
D. Leukemia

Answer: B. Signs of hemophilia include prolonged bleeding after circumcision, immunizations, or minor injuries; multiple bruises without petechiae; peripheral neuropathies from bleeding near peripheral nerves; bleeding into the throat, mouth, and thorax; and hemarthrosis. Some of the signs associated with iron deficiency anemia include dyspnea on exertion, fatigue, and listlessness. Signs and symptoms associated with sickle cell anemia include pain at the site of occlusion, poor healing of leg wounds, priapism, enuresis, and delayed growth and sexual maturity. Signs and symptoms associated with leukemia include history of infections, lymphadenopathy, hematuria, hematemesis, blood in stools, petechiae, and ecchymosis.

➡ *NCLEX keys*
Nursing process step: Assessment
Client needs category: Physiological integrity
Client needs subcategory: Reduction of risk potential
Taxonomic level: Application

9. A child is admitted to the pediatric floor with hemophilia. The nurse encourages fantasy play and participation in his care. This developmental approach is most appropriate for which pediatric age group?

A. The school-age child (ages 5 to 12)
B. The preschool child (ages 3 to 5)
C. The toddler (ages 1 to 3)
D. The adolescent (ages 12 to 18)

Answer: A. School-age children engage in fantasy play and daydreaming. Therefore, it's appropriate for the nurse to encourage this type of play for the hospitalized child. The school-age child is also able to participate in his care. Doll play is helpful for the preschool hospitalized child. The toddler enjoys push-pull toys and games of peek-a-boo. The adolescent enjoys role playing in various situations.

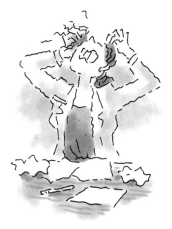

➡ *NCLEX keys*
Nursing process step: Implementation
Client needs category: Health promotion and maintenance
Client needs subcategory: Growth and development through the life span
Taxonomic level: Application

10. The nurse is caring for a child with acquired immunodeficiency syndrome (AIDS). Which of the following precautions must the nurse maintain?

    A. Airborne precautions
    B. Standard precautions
    C. Protective isolation
    D. Strict hand washing

Answer: B. The nurse caring for a child with AIDS should maintain standard precautions. Airborne precautions are instituted for clients known or suspected to be infected with microorganisms transmitted by airborne droplet nuclei, such as clients with tuberculosis. Protective isolation is instituted for clients who require added protection from infection, such as those who have undergone bone marrow transplant or those with burns. Strict hand washing should be performed when caring for all clients.

➡ *NCLEX keys*
Nursing process step: Implementation
Client needs category: Health promotion and maintenance
Client needs subcategory: Safety and infection control
Taxonomic level: Comprehension

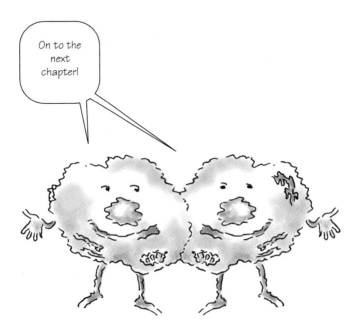

30 Neurosensory System

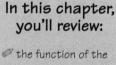

In time, my earliest, reflex-driven responses are replaced by motor responses that are under conscious control.

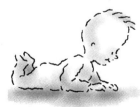

Brush up on key concepts

The **central nervous system** (CNS) is the body's communication network. It receives sensory stimuli through the five senses and either perceives, integrates, interprets, or retains the stimulus in memory. In an infant, early responses are primarily reflexive; the infant learns to discriminate stimuli and bring motor responses under conscious control. Language helps the older child improve and increase perception. In pediatric patients, flaccid muscles usually indicate a CNS disorder.

At any time, you can review the major points of this chapter by consulting the *Cheat sheet* on pages 602 to 604.

Upward, then downward

In children younger than age 3, the **ear canal** is directed upward. In older children, the ear canal is directed downward and forward. A child's **hearing** develops as follows:
• Sound discrimination is present at birth.
• By age 5 to 6 months, the infant is able to localize sounds presented on a horizontal plane and begins to imitate selected sounds.
• By age 7 to 12 months, the infant can localize sounds in any plane.
• By age 18 months, the child can hear and follow a simple command without visual cues.

Children who have difficulty with language development by age 18 months should have their hearing evaluated.

First, just alert

At birth, **visual function** is limited to alertness to visual stimuli 8″ to 12″ (20 to 31 cm) from the eyes. Normal newborns already have a blink reflex. After that, these findings are noted:

• Tear glands begin to secrete within the first 2 weeks of life.
• Transient strabismus (deviation of the eye) is a normal finding in the first few months.
• An infant can fixate on an object and follow a bright light or toy by 5 to 6 weeks of age.
• An infant can reach for objects at varying distances at 3 to 4 months of age.
• Vision reaches 20/20 when the child is about 4 years old.

Keep abreast of diagnostic tests

Here are the most important tests used to diagnose pediatric neurosensory disorders, along with common nursing interventions associated with each test.

Head check

A **basic assessment of cerebral function** includes:
• level of consciousness (LOC)
• communication
• mental status.

3-D pics

Computed tomography (CT) scan is a test process that produces three-dimensional images. It can be invasive (if contrast medium is used) or noninvasive.

Nursing actions

• Explain the purpose of test to the parents and the child.
• Make sure that the child holds still during the test.
• Make sure that written, informed consent has been obtained.

(Text continues on page 604.)

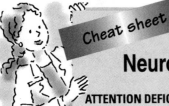

Neurosensory refresher

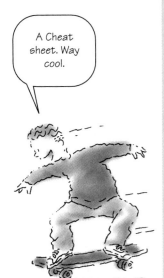

A Cheat sheet. Way cool.

ATTENTION DEFICIT HYPERACTIVITY DISORDER

Key signs and symptoms
- Decreased attention span
- Difficulty organizing tasks and activities
- Easily distracted

Key test results
- Complete psychological, medical, and neurologic evaluations rule out other problems.

Key treatment
- Behavioral modification and psychological therapy
- Amphetamines: methylphenidate (Ritalin), dextroamphetamine (Dexedrine)

Key interventions
- Give one simple instruction at a time.
- Provide consistency in child's daily routine.
- Reduce environmental stimuli.

CEREBRAL PALSY

Key signs and symptoms
- Abnormal muscle tone and coordination (the most common associated problem)
- Other symptoms specific to cerebral palsy type

Key test results
- Neuroimaging studies determine the site of brain impairment.
- Cytogenic studies (genetic evaluation of the child and other family members) rule out other potential causes.
- Metabolic studies rule out other causes.

Examination findings
- Infant has difficulty sucking or keeping the nipple or food in his mouth.
- Infant seldom moves voluntarily or has arm or leg tremors with voluntary movement.
- Infant crosses legs when lifted from behind rather than pulling them up or "bicycling" like a normal infant.

Key treatments
- Braces or splints and special appliances, such as adapted eating utensils and a low toilet seat with arms, to help child perform activities independently
- Range-of-motion (ROM) exercises to minimize contractures
- Muscle relaxants or neurosurgery to decrease spasticity, if appropriate

Key interventions
- Assist with locomotion, communication, and educational opportunities.
- Divide tasks into small steps.
- Perform ROM exercises if the child is spastic.

DOWN SYNDROME

Key signs and symptoms
- Mild to moderate retardation
- Short stature with pudgy hands
- Small head with slow brain growth
- Upward slanting eyes

Key test result
- Amniocentesis allows prenatal diagnosis.

Key treatment
- Treatment for coexisting conditions — congenital heart problems, visual defects, or hypothyroidism

Key interventions
- Provide activities appropriate for the child.
- Set realistic, reachable, short-term goals; break tasks into small steps.
- Provide stimulation and communicate at a level appropriate to the child's mental age rather than chronologic age.

HYDROCEPHALUS

Key signs and symptoms
- High-pitched cry
- Rapid increase in head circumference and full, tense, bulging fontanels (before cranial sutures close)

Key test result
- Skull X-rays show thinning of the skull with separation of the sutures and widening of fontanels.

Neurosensory system refresher (continued)

HYDROCEPHALUS (continued)

Key treatments

- Shunt insertion to allow cerebrospinal fluid (CSF) to drain from the lateral ventricle in the brain
- Anticonvulsants for seizures: phenobarbital, diazepam, phenytoin

Key interventions

- Monitor vital signs and intake and output.
- Assess neurologic status.
- After the shunt is inserted, don't lay the child on the side of the body where it's located.
- Lay the child flat.
- If the caudal end of the shunt must be externalized because of infection, keep the bag at ear level.

MENINGITIS

Key signs and symptoms

- Nuchal rigidity that may progress to opisthotonus
- Positive Brudzinski's sign (the child flexes the knees and hips in response to passive neck flexion)
- Positive Kernig's sign (inability to extend leg when hip and knee are flexed)

Key test results

- Lumbar puncture shows increased CSF pressure, cloudy color, increased white blood cell count and increased protein level, and a decreased glucose level if the meningitis is caused by bacteria.

Key treatments

- Analgesics to treat pain of meningeal irritation
- Corticosteroids such as dexamethasone (Decadron)
- Droplet precautions; should be maintained until at least 24 hours of effective antibiotic therapy have elapsed; continued isolation recommended for meningitis caused by *Haemophilus influenzae* or *Neisseria meningitidis*
- Parenteral antibiotics (possibly intraventricular administration of antibiotics)
- Seizure precautions

Key interventions

- Monitor vital signs and intake and output.
- Assess the child's neurologic status frequently.
- Examine the young infant for bulging fontanels and measure head circumference.

OTITIS MEDIA

Key signs and symptoms

Acute suppurative otitis media
- Fever (mild to very high)

- Pain that suddenly stops (occurs if tympanic membrane ruptures)
- Severe, deep, throbbing pain (from pressure behind the tympanic membrane)
- Signs of upper respiratory tract infection (sneezing, coughing)

Acute secretory otitis media
- Popping, crackling, or clicking sounds on swallowing or with jaw movement
- Sensation of fullness in the ear

Chronic otitis media
- Cholesteatoma (cystlike mass in the middle ear)
- Decreased or absent tympanic membrane mobility
- Painless, purulent discharge in chronic suppurative otitis media

Key test results

Acute suppurative otitis media
- Otoscopy reveals obscured or distorted bony landmarks of the tympanic membrane.

Acute secretory otitis media
- Otoscopy reveals clear or amber fluid behind the tympanic membrane and tympanic membrane retraction, which causes the bony landmarks to appear more prominent. If hemorrhage into the middle ear has occurred, as in barotrauma, the tympanic membrane appears blue-black.

Chronic otitis media
- Otoscopy shows thickening, sometimes scarring, and decreased mobility of the tympanic membrane.

Key treatments

Acute suppurative otitis media
- Myringotomy for patients with severe, painful bulging of the tympanic membrane
- Antibiotic therapy

Acute secretory otitis media
- Inflation of the eustachian tube by performing Valsalva's maneuver several times a day, which may be the only treatment required
- Nasopharyngeal decongestant therapy

Chronic otitis media
- Elimination of eustachian tube obstruction
- Excision for cholesteatoma
- Mastoidectomy
- Antibiotic therapy

Key interventions

- After myringotomy, maintain drainage flow; place sterile cotton loosely in the external ear and change frequently.
- Watch for and report headache, fever, severe pain, or disorientation.

(continued)

Neurosensory system refresher (continued)

OTITIS MEDIA (continued)
- After tympanoplasty, reinforce dressings and observe for excessive bleeding from the ear canal.
- Warn the child against blowing his nose or getting the ear wet when bathing.
- Instruct parents not to feed their infant in a supine position or put him to bed with a bottle.

SEIZURE DISORDERS

Key signs and symptoms
- Aura just before the seizure's onset (reports unusual tastes, feelings, or odors)
- Eyes deviating to a particular side or blinking
- Usually unresponsive during tonic-clonic muscular contractions; may experience incontinence
- Irregular breathing with spasms

Key test results
- EEG results help differentiate epileptic from nonepileptic seizures. Each seizure has a characteristic EEG tracing.

Key treatments
- I.V. diazepam (Valium) or lorazepam (Ativan)
- Phenobarbital (Luminal) or fosphenytoin (Cerebyx)
- Phenytoin (Dilantin) to keep neuron excitability below the seizure threshold

Key interventions
- Assess neurologic status.
- Stay with the child during a seizure.
- Move the child to a flat surface.
- Place the child on the side to let saliva drain out.
- Don't try to interrupt the seizure.

SPINA BIFIDA

Key signs and symptoms
Spina bifida occulta
- Dimple (commonly found on the skin over the spinal defect)

- No neurologic dysfunction (usually), except occasional foot weakness or bowel and bladder disturbances
Meningocele
- No neurologic dysfunction (usually)
- Saclike structure protruding over the spine
Myelomeningocele (depending on the level of the deficit)
- Hydrocephalus
- Permanent neurologic dysfunction (paralysis, bowel and bladder incontinence)

Key test results
- Amniocentesis reveals neural tube defect.
- Elevated alpha-fetoprotein levels in mother's blood may indicate the presence of a neural tube defect.
- Acetylcholinesterase measurement can be used to confirm the diagnosis.

Key Interventions
- Teach parents how to cope with their infant's physical problems.
- Teach parents how to recognize early signs of complications, such as hydrocephalus, pressure ulcers, and urinary tract infections.
Before surgery
- Watch for signs of hydrocephalus. Measure head circumference daily. Be sure to mark the spot where the measurement was made.
- Watch for signs of meningeal irritation, such as fever or nuchal rigidity.
After surgery
- Watch for hydrocephalus, which often follows surgery. Measure the infant's head circumference as ordered.
- Monitor vital signs often.

Magnetic pics

Magnetic resonance imaging (MRI) shows the CNS in greater detail than a CT scan. A noniodinated contrast medium may be used to enhance lesions. Advances in MRI allow visualization of cerebral arteries and venous sinuses without administration of a contrast medium.

Nursing actions
- If the child has any surgically implanted metal objects (for example, pins and clips), notify the radiology department as these may interfere with the picture.
- Explain the procedure to the parents and the child.
- Make sure the child holds still during the test.

Electric pics

Electroencephalography (EEG) shows abnormal electrical activity in the brain (for example, from a seizure or metabolic disorder or a drug overdose).

Nursing actions
• Explain the purpose of the test and make sure the child holds still during the test.

Wavy reflections

Ultrasonography reveals carotid lesions or changes in carotid blood flow and velocity. High-frequency sound waves reflect back the velocity of blood flow, which is then reported as a graphic recording of a waveform.

Nursing actions
• Explain the purpose of the test to the parents and the child.
• Make sure the child holds still during the test.

Fluid check

In **lumbar puncture,** a needle is inserted into the subarachnoid space of the spinal cord, usually between L3 and L4 (or L4 and L5). This allows aspiration of cerebrospinal fluid (CSF) for analysis and for measuring CSF pressure.

Nursing actions
• Before the procedure, make sure that a written, informed consent has been obtained.
• Keep the child in a side-lying, knee-chest position during the procedure.
• The child must rest for 1 hour after the procedure.

Vessel check

In **cerebral arteriography,** also known as angiography, a catheter is inserted into an artery — usually the femoral artery — and is indirectly threaded up to the carotid artery. Then a radiopaque dye is injected, allowing X-ray visualization of the cerebral vasculature.

Nursing actions
• Explain the procedure to the parents and the child.

• Make sure that written, informed consent has been obtained.
• Identify allergies before the test.
• Make sure the child holds still during the test, and monitor him for allergic reaction.
• Immobilize the site after the test and monitor it for pulses and evidence of bleeding.

Pressure check

Intracranial pressure (ICP) monitoring is a direct, invasive method of identifying trends in ICP. A subarachnoid screw and an intraventricular catheter convert CSF pressure readings into waveforms that are displayed digitally on an oscilloscope monitor. Another option is to insert a fiber-optic catheter in the ventricle, subarachnoid space, subdural space, or the brain parenchyma. Pressure changes are reported digitally or in waveform.

Nursing actions
Before the procedure:
• Explain the procedure to the parents and the child.
• Make sure that written, informed consent has been obtained.
After the procedure:
• Maintain patency of monitor and waveforms. Identify trends and alert the doctor to changes in trends.
• Maintain sterile technique during care of monitoring equipment.
• Monitor the site for signs of infection.

Nerve check

Electromyography detects lower motor neuron disorders, neuromuscular disorders, and nerve damage. A needle inserted into selected muscles at rest and during voluntary contraction picks up nerve impulses and measures nerve conduction time.

Nursing actions
• Explain the procedure to the parents and the child.
• Check the child's medications for those that may interfere with the test (cholinergics, anticholinergics, skeletal muscle relaxants).
• Make sure that written, informed consent has been obtained.

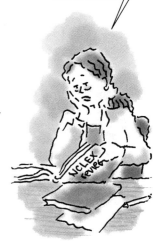

A complete neurologic assessment may require a close look at the eyes, ears, internal structures, fluid pressures, and neural function.

• Make sure the child holds still during the procedure.
• Monitor the site for infection or bleeding after the procedure.

Ear check
Otoscopic examination allows visualization of the canal and inner structures of the ear.

Nursing actions
• Use the biggest speculum that fits into the ear canal.
• To straighten the ear canal, pull the pinna down and back or out in infants and children younger than age 3. For children older than age 3, the pinna is pulled up and back.
• Test hearing acuity through play audiometry or by audiometry using earphones in children age 4 and older.

Eye check
Ophthalmoscopic examination helps visualize interior eye structures.

Nursing actions
• Explain the procedure to the parents and the child.
• Make sure the child cooperates during tests by allowing the child to hold a favorite toy, which may decrease anxiety and promote cooperation.

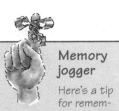

Memory jogger

Here's a tip for remembering diagnostic criteria for ADHD: think of a child who can't *SIT* still.

*S*even (age by which symptoms appear)

*I*mpaired social or academic function

*T*wo or more settings

Polish up on patient care

The major neurologic disorders in pediatric patients are attention deficit hyperactivity disorder, cerebral palsy, Down syndrome, hydrocephalus, meningitis, otitis media, seizure disorders, and spina bifida.

Attention deficit hyperactivity disorder

Attention deficit hyperactivity disorder (ADHD) was previously called attention deficit disorder. ADHD includes the following long-term behaviors:
• hyperactivity
• impulsiveness
• inattention.

These manifestations occur in all facets of the child's life and frequently worsen when sustained attention is required. To qualify as ADHD, behaviors must be present in two or more settings, must be present before age 7, and must result in a significant impairment in social or academic functioning.

CAUSES
• Deficit in neurotransmitters (possibly)

ASSESSMENT FINDINGS
• Climbs, runs, or talks excessively
• Decreased attention span
• Difficulty organizing tasks and activities
• Difficulty waiting for turns
• Easily distracted
• Fails to give close attention to school work or activity
• Fails to listen when spoken to directly
• Fidgets or squirms in seat
• Frequent forgetfulness; frequently loses things needed for tasks
• Impulsive behavior
• Unable to follow directions

DIAGNOSTIC TEST RESULTS
• Complete psychological, medical, and neurologic evaluations rule out other problems.
• To diagnose ADHD, the findings are combined with data from several sources, including parents, teachers, and the child.

NURSING DIAGNOSES
• Altered nutrition: Less than body requirements
• Risk for altered parenting
• Risk for injury

TREATMENT
• Behavioral modification and psychological therapy
• Interdisciplinary interventions: pathologic assessment and diagnosis of specific learning needs

Drug therapy
• Amphetamines: methylphenidate (Ritalin), dextroamphetamine (Dexedrine) to help the child concentrate
• Other medications: imipramine (Tofranil), clonidine (Catapres)

INTERVENTIONS AND RATIONALES
• Monitor growth. *If the child is receiving methylphenidate, growth may be slowed.*
• Give one simple instruction at a time *so the child can successfully complete the task, which promotes self-esteem.*
• Give medications in the morning and at lunch *to avoid interfering with sleep.*
• Ensure adequate nutrition; *medications and hyperactivity may cause increased nutrient needs.*
• Reduce environmental stimuli *to decrease distraction.*
• Formulate a schedule for the child *to provide consistency and routine.*

Teaching topics
• Allowing the child to expend energy after being in restrictive environments such as school
• Monitoring for adverse reactions to medications
• Structuring learning to minimize distractions
• Taking breaks from caregiving to avoid strain
• Teaching important material in the morning (when medication levels peak)

Cerebral palsy

Cerebral palsy is a neuromuscular disorder resulting from damage to or defect in the part of the brain that controls motor function.

Cerebral palsy is a group of disorders arising from a malfunction of motor centers and neural pathways in the brain. The disorder is most commonly seen in children born prematurely. Cerebral palsy can't be cured; treatment includes interventions that encourage optimum development. Defects are common, including musculoskeletal, neurologic, GI, and nutritional defects as well as other systemic complications (abnormal reflexes, fatigue, growth failure, genitourinary complaints, respiratory infections).

Classifications of cerebral palsy include:
• ataxia type — the least common type; essentially a lack of coordination caused by disturbances in movement and balance
• athetoid type — characterized by involuntary, incoordinate motion with varying degrees of muscle tension (Children with this type of cerebral palsy experience writhing muscle contractions whenever they attempt voluntary movement. Facial grimacing, poor swallowing, and tongue movements cause drooling and poor speech articulation. Despite their abnormal appearance, these children commonly have average or above-average intelligence.)
• spastic type — the most common type; featuring hyperactive stretch in associated muscle groups, hyperactive deep tendon reflexes, rapid involuntary muscle contraction and relaxation, contractions affecting extensor muscles, and scissoring (The child's legs are crossed and the toes are pointed down, so the child stands on his toes.)
• rigidity type — an uncommon type of cerebral palsy characterized by rigid postures and lack of active movement
• mixed type — more than one type of cerebral palsy. (These children are usually severely disabled.)

CAUSES
• Anoxia before, during, or after birth
• Infection
• Trauma (hemorrhage)

Risk factors
• Low birth weight
• Low Apgar scores at 5 minutes
• Metabolic disturbances
• Seizures

ASSESSMENT FINDINGS
All types
• Abnormal muscle tone and coordination (the most common associated problem)
• Dental anomalies
• Mental retardation of varying degrees in 18% to 50% of cases (Most children with cere-

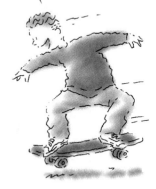

Environmental stimuli should be reduced for the child with ADHD. How awesome.

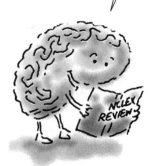

Cerebral palsy arises from a malfunction of motor centers and neural pathways in the brain. Well, I'll be.

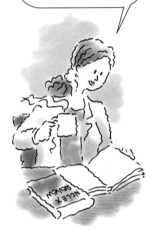

Abnormal muscle tone and coordination characterize all forms of cerebral palsy.

bral palsy have at least a normal IQ but can't demonstrate it on standardized tests.)
• Seizures
• Speech, vision, or hearing disturbances

Ataxic cerebral palsy
• Poor balance and muscle coordination
• Unsteady, wide-based gait

Athetoid cerebral palsy
• Slow state of writhing muscle contractions whenever voluntary movement is attempted
• Facial grimacing
• Poor swallowing
• Drooling
• Poor speech articulation

Rigid cerebral palsy
• Rigid posture
• Lack of active movement

Spastic cerebral palsy
• Hyperactive stretch reflex in associated muscle groups
• Hyperactive deep tendon reflexes
• Rapid involuntary muscle contraction and relaxation
• Contractures affecting the extensor muscles
• Scissoring

Although cerebral palsy can't be cured, treatment encourages the child to reach his full potential.

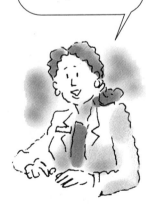

Mixed cerebral palsy
• Signs of more than one type of cerebral palsy
• Severely disabled

DIAGNOSTIC TEST RESULTS
• Neuroimaging studies determine the site of brain impairment.
• Cytogenic studies (genetic evaluation of the child and other family members) rule out other potential causes.
• Metabolic studies rule out other causes.

Examination findings
• Infant has difficulty sucking or keeping the nipple or food in his mouth.
• Infant seldom moves voluntarily or has arm or leg tremors with voluntary movement.

• Infant crosses legs when lifted from behind rather than pulling them up or "bicycling" like a normal infant.
• Infant's legs are hard to separate, making diaper changing difficult.
• Infant persistently uses only one hand or, as he gets older, uses hands well but not legs.

NURSING DIAGNOSES
• Impaired physical mobility
• Altered growth and development
• Impaired verbal communication

TREATMENT
• High-calorie diet, if appropriate
• Artificial urinary sphincter for the incontinent child who can use hand controls
• Braces or splints and special appliances, such as adapted eating utensils and a low toilet seat with arms, to help child perform activities independently
• Neurosurgery to decrease spasticity, if appropriate
• Orthopedic surgery to correct contractures
• Range-of-motion (ROM) exercises to minimize contractures

Drug therapy
• Muscle relaxants to decrease spasticity, if appropriate
• Anticonvulsants: phenytoin (Dilantin), phenobarbital (Luminal), or another anticonvulsant to control seizures

INTERVENTIONS AND RATIONALES
• Assist with locomotion, communication, and educational opportunities *to enable the child to attain optimal developmental level.*
• Increase caloric intake for the child with increased motor function *to keep up with increased metabolic needs.*
• Make food easy to manage *to decrease stress during mealtimes.*
• Provide a safe environment, for example, by using protective headgear or bed pads *to prevent injury.*
• Provide rest periods *to promote rest and reduce metabolic needs.*
• Perform ROM exercises if the child is spastic *to maintain proper body alignment and mobility of joints.*

• Promote age-appropriate mental activities and incentives for motor development *to promote growth and development.*
• Divide tasks into small steps *to promote self-care and activity and increase self-esteem.*
• Refer the child for speech, nutrition, and physical therapy *to maintain or improve functioning.*
• Use assistive communication devices if the child can't speak *to promote a positive self-concept.*

Teaching topics
• Contacting appropriate social service agencies, child development specialist, mental health services, home care assistance
• Understanding the child's condition and prognosis

Down syndrome

The first disorder researchers attributed to a chromosomal aberration, Down syndrome is characterized by:
• mental retardation
• dysmorphic facial features
• other distinctive physical abnormalities (60% of patients have congenital heart defects, respiratory infections, chronic myelogenous leukemia, and a weak immune response to infection).

CAUSES
• Genetic nondisjunction, with three chromosomes on the 21st pair (total of 47 chromosomes)

Risk factors
• Maternal age (the older the mother, the greater the risk of genetic nondisjunction)

ASSESSMENT FINDINGS
• Brushfield's spots (marbling and speckling of the iris)
• Flat nose and low-set ears
• Hypotonia
• Mild to moderate retardation
• Protruding tongue (because of a small oral cavity)
• Short stature with pudgy hands

• Simian crease (a single crease across the palm)
• Small head with slow brain growth
• Upward slanting eyes

DIAGNOSTIC TEST RESULTS
• Amniocentesis allows prenatal diagnosis. It's recommended for women older than age 34 regardless of a negative family history, or a woman of any age if she or the father carries a translocated chromosome.
• Karyotype shows the specific chromosomal abnormality.

NURSING DIAGNOSES
• Altered growth and development
• Risk for injury
• Risk for aspiration

TREATMENT
• Treatment for coexisting conditions — congenital heart problems, visual defects, or hypothyroidism
• Skeletal, immunologic, metabolic, biochemical, and oncologic problems treated as per specific problem

Drug therapy
• Megavitamin therapy (controversial) to promote growth and development potential

INTERVENTIONS AND RATIONALES
• Provide activities appropriate for the child *to support optimal development of the child.*
• Set realistic, reachable, short-term goals; break tasks into small steps *to encourage their successful accomplishment.*
• Use behavior modification, if applicable, *to promote safety and prevent injury to the child and others.*
• Provide stimulation and communicate at a level appropriate to the child's mental age rather than chronologic age *to promote a healthy emotional environment.*
• Provide a safe environment *to prevent injury.*
• Mainstream daily routines *to promote normalcy.*

Teaching topics
• Contacting early intervention programs

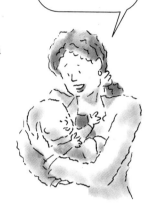

Provide a safe environment for the child with cerebral palsy.

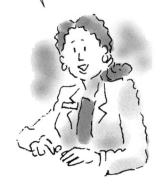

Amniocentesis allows prenatal diagnosis of Down syndrome. It's recommended for any pregnant patient over age 34.

• Contacting support groups for caregivers
• Establishing self-care skills to promote independence

Hydrocephalus

Hydrocephalus is an increase in the amount of CSF in the ventricles and subarachnoid spaces of the brain. The ventricles become dilated due to an imbalance in the rate of production and rate of absorption of CSF. This condition may be congenital or acquired.

In noncommunicating hydrocephalus, an obstruction occurs in the free circulation of CSF, causing increased pressure on the brain or spinal cord. In most cases, congenital hydrocephalus is noncommunicating.

Communicating hydrocephalus involves the free flow of CSF between the ventricles and the spinal theca. Increased pressure on the spinal cord is caused by defective absorption of CSF.

CAUSES
• Arnold-Chiari malformation (downward displacement of cerebellar components through the foramen magnum into the cervical spinal canal); common in hydrocephalus with spina bifida
• Overproduction of CSF by the choroid plexus
• Scarring, congenital anomalies, or hemorrhage; causes CSF to be absorbed abnormally after it reaches the subarachnoid space (in communicating hydrocephalus)
• Tumors, hemorrhage, or structural abnormalities; block CSF flow, causing fluid to accumulate in the ventricles (in noncommunicating hydrocephalus)

ASSESSMENT FINDINGS
• "Cracked pot" sound when the skull is percussed
• Distended scalp veins
• High-pitched cry
• Inability to support the head when upright
• Irritability or lethargy; decreased attention span
• Rapid increase in head circumference and full, tense, bulging fontanels (before cranial sutures close)
• Sunset sign (sclera visible above the iris)
• Widening suture lines

DIAGNOSTIC TEST RESULTS
• Angiography, CT scan, and MRI differentiate hydrocephalus from intracranial lesions and may demonstrate Arnold-Chiari malformation.
• Light reflects off the opposite side of the skull with skull transillumination.
• Skull X-rays show thinning of the skull with separation of the sutures and widening of fontanels.

NURSING DIAGNOSES
• Risk for injury
• Altered growth and development
• Decreased adaptive capacity: Intracranial

TREATMENT
• Shunt insertion to allow CSF to drain from the lateral ventricle in the brain

> In hydrocephalus, an excessive amount of CSF accumulates in the ventricular spaces of the brain.

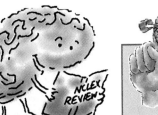

Memory jogger

Think about communication.

To remember that CSF is *not* blocked in *communicating* hydrocephalus, think about what "communication" means: a free (not blocked) exchange of ideas.

The reverse is true in *noncommunicating* hydrocephalus: CSF is *blocked* by tumors, hemorrhage, or structural abnormalities, so fluid accumulates in the ventricles.

Drug therapy
- Anticonvulsants for seizures: phenobarbital (Luminal), diazepam (Valium), phenytoin (Dilantin)

INTERVENTIONS AND RATIONALES
- Measure head circumference *to aid in diagnosis of hydrocephalus.*
- Monitor vital signs and intake and output *to assess for fluid volume excess, which can further elevate ICP.*
- Assess neurologic status *to identify changes indicative of increased ICP.*
- After the shunt is inserted, don't lay the child on the side of the body where it's located *to promote CSF drainage and prevent shunt occlusion.*
- Lay the child flat *to avoid rapid decompression.*
- Observe for shunt blockage with increased ICP (shown by increased head circumference and full fontanel) *to prevent complications.*
- Observe for signs of infection. *Signs of shunt infection usually occur within the first month after shunt insertion.*
- If the caudal end of the shunt must be externalized because of infection, keep the bag at ear level *to promote CSF drainage.*
- Support the head when child is upright *to prevent injury and promote CSF drainage.*
- Provide proper skin care to the head; turn the patient's head frequently *to avoid skin breakdown.*

Teaching topics
- Recognizing signs of increasing ICP
- Understanding care required after shunt insertion

Meningitis

Meningitis is an inflammation of the brain and spinal cord meninges. It's most common in infants and toddlers. The incidence of meningitis is greatly reduced with routine *Haemophilus influenzae* type B vaccine.

CAUSES
- Viral or bacterial agents, transmitted by the spread of droplets (organisms enter the blood from nasopharynx or middle ear)

ASSESSMENT FINDINGS
- Coma
- Delirium
- Fever
- Headache
- High-pitched cry
- Irritability
- Nuchal rigidity that may progress to opisthotonus (arching of the back)
- Onset gradual or abrupt following an upper respiratory infection
- Petechial or purpuric lesions possibly present in bacterial meningitis
- Positive Brudzinski's sign (the child flexes the knees and hips in response to passive neck flexion)
- Positive Kernig's sign (inability to extend leg when hip and knee are flexed)
- Projectile vomiting
- Seizures

DIAGNOSTIC TEST RESULTS
- Lumbar puncture shows increased CSF pressure, cloudy color, increased white blood cell count and protein level, and a decreased glucose level if the meningitis is caused by bacteria.

NURSING DIAGNOSES
- Decreased adaptive capacity: Intracranial
- Ineffective breathing pattern
- Risk for injury

TREATMENT
- Burr holes to evacuate subdural effusion, if present
- Droplet precautions; should be maintained until at least 24 hours of effective antibiotic therapy have elapsed; continued precautions recommended for meningitis caused by *H. influenzae* or *Neisseria meningitidis*
- Hypothermia blanket
- Oxygen therapy may require intubation and mechanical ventilation to induce hyperventilation to decrease ICP
- Seizure precautions

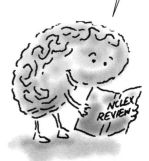

An increase in CSF in a patient with hydrocephalus may lead to a rapid increase in head circumference and bulging fontanels. Oh my.

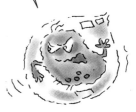

Meningitis is transmitted by the spread of droplets.

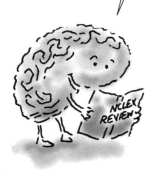

My, oh my...meningitis management mandates meticulous monitoring: Check vital signs, head circumference, intake, output, and neurologic status.

• Treatment for coexisting conditions

Drug therapy
• Analgesics to treat pain of meningeal irritation
• Corticosteroids: dexamethasone (Decadron)
• Parenteral antibiotics: ceftazidime (Fortaz), ceftriaxone (Rocephin); possibly intraventricular administration of antibiotics

INTERVENTIONS AND RATIONALES
• Monitor vital signs and intake and output *to assess for fluid volume excess.*
• Assess the child's neurologic status frequently *to monitor for signs of increased ICP.*
• Provide a dark and quiet environment. *Environmental stimuli can increase ICP or stimulate seizure activity.*
• Maintain seizure precautions *to prevent injury.*
• Administer medications as ordered *to combat infection and decrease ICP.*
• Move the child gently *to prevent a rise in ICP.*
• Maintain isolation precautions, as ordered, *to prevent the spread of infection.*
• Provide emotional support for the family *to decrease anxiety.*
• Examine the young infant for bulging fontanels and measure head circumference; *hydrocephalus is a complication that can result from meningitis.*

Teaching topics
• Understanding the importance of isolation and sanitation

Otitis media

Otitis media is inflammation of the middle ear that may or may not be accompanied by infection. The fluid presses on the tympanic membrane causing pain and leading to possible rupture or perforation. This condition may be chronic or acute and suppurative or secretory.

Acute otitis media is common in children. Its incidence increases during the winter months, paralleling the seasonal increase in nonbacterial respiratory tract infections. With prompt treatment, the prognosis for acute otitis media is excellent; however, prolonged accumulation of fluid in the middle ear cavity causes chronic otitis media and, possibly, perforation of the tympanic membrane.

CAUSES
All types
• Obstructed eustachian tube
• Wider, shorter, more horizontal eustachian tubes and increased lymphoid tissue in children, as well as other anatomic anomalies

Suppurative otitis media
• Bacterial infection with pneumococci, *H. influenzae* (the most common cause in children under age 6), *Moraxella (Branhamella) catarrhalis*, beta-hemolytic group A streptococci, staphylococci (most common cause in children age 6 or older), or gram-negative bacteria
• Respiratory tract infection, allergic reaction, nasotracheal intubation, or position changes that allow nasopharyngeal flora to reflux through the eustachian tube and colonize the middle ear

Chronic suppurative otitis media
• Inadequate treatment of acute otitis episodes
• Infection by resistant strains of bacteria
• Tuberculosis (rarely)

Secretory otitis media
• Barotrauma (pressure injury caused by inability to equalize pressure between the environment and the middle ear), as occurs during rapid aircraft descent in a person with upper respiratory tract infection or during rapid underwater ascent in scuba diving (barotitis media)
• Obstruction of the eustachian tube secondary to eustachian tube dysfunction from viral infection or allergy, which causes a buildup of negative pressure in the middle ear that promotes transudation of sterile serous fluid from blood vessels in the membrane of the middle ear

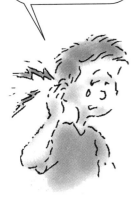

Key clinical fact about acute suppurative otitis media: It HURTS!

Chronic secretory otitis media

• Persistent eustachian tube dysfunction from mechanical obstruction (adenoidal tissue overgrowth or tumors), edema (allergic rhinitis or chronic sinus infection), or inadequate treatment of acute suppurative otitis media

ASSESSMENT FINDINGS

Acute suppurative otitis media

• Bulging and erythema of tympanic membrane
• Dizziness
• Fever (mild to very high)
• Hearing loss (usually mild and conductive)
• Nausea and vomiting
• Pain pattern (pulling the pinna doesn't exacerbate pain)
• Pain that suddenly stops (occurs if tympanic membrane ruptures)
• Purulent drainage in the ear canal from tympanic membrane rupture
• Severe, deep, throbbing pain (from pressure behind the tympanic membrane)
• Signs of upper respiratory tract infection (sneezing and coughing)
• Tinnitus

Acute secretory otitis media

• Echo heard by patient when speaking; vague feeling of top-heaviness (caused by accumulation of fluid)
• Popping, crackling, or clicking sounds on swallowing or with jaw movement
• Sensation of fullness in the ear
• Severe conductive hearing loss

Chronic otitis media

• Cholesteatoma (cystlike mass in the middle ear)
• Decreased or absent tympanic membrane mobility
• Painless, purulent discharge in chronic suppurative otitis media
• Thickening and scarring of the tympanic membrane

DIAGNOSTIC TEST RESULTS

Acute suppurative otitis media

• Culture of the ear drainage identifies the causative organism.

• Otoscopy reveals obscured or distorted bony landmarks of the tympanic membrane.
• Pneumatoscopy may show decreased tympanic membrane mobility, but this procedure is painful with an obviously bulging, erythematous tympanic membrane.

Acute secretory otitis media

• Otoscopy reveals clear or amber fluid behind the tympanic membrane and tympanic membrane retraction, which causes the bony landmarks to appear more prominent. If hemorrhage into the middle ear has occurred, as in barotrauma, the tympanic membrane appears blue-black.

Chronic otitis media

• Otoscopy shows thickening, sometimes scarring, and decreased mobility of the tympanic membrane.
• Pneumatoscopy shows decreased or absent tympanic membrane movement.

NURSING DIAGNOSES

• Hyperthermia
• Pain
• Sensory or perceptual alterations (auditory)

TREATMENT

Acute suppurative otitis media

• Myringotomy for patients with severe, painful bulging of the tympanic membrane

Drug therapy

• Antibiotic therapy, usually amoxicillin (Amoxil); antibiotics must be used with discretion to prevent development of resistant strains of bacteria in patients with recurring otitis
• Amoxicillin/clavulanate potassium (Augmentin) in areas with a high incidence of beta-lactamase-producing *H. influenzae*, and in patients who aren't responding to amoxicillin
• Cefaclor (Ceclor) or co-trimoxazole (Bactrim) for patients allergic to penicillin derivatives
• Prevention: broad-spectrum antibiotics, such as amoxicillin/clavulanate potassium (Augmentin) or cefuroxime (Ceftin) in high-risk patients

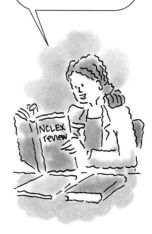

In acute suppurative otitis media, pulling the auricle doesn't worsen the pain.

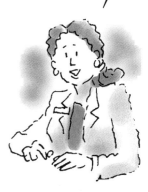

In myringotomy, the doctor cuts into the eardrum and gently suctions fluid to relieve pressure.

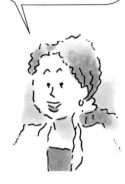

Mastoidectomy is removal of the mastoid process or mastoid cells of the temporal bone.

Acute secretory otitis media

• Concomitant treatment of the underlying cause, such as elimination of allergens, or adenoidectomy for hypertrophied adenoids

• Inflation of the eustachian tube by performing Valsalva's maneuver several times a day, which may be the only treatment required

• Myringotomy and aspiration of middle ear fluid if decongestant therapy fails, followed by insertion of a polyethylene tube into the tympanic membrane for immediate and prolonged equalization of pressure; the tube falls out spontaneously after 9 to 12 months

Drug therapy

• Nasopharyngeal decongestant therapy for at least 2 weeks; sometimes used indefinitely, with periodic evaluation

Chronic otitis media

• Elimination of eustachian tube obstruction
• Excision for cholesteatoma
• Mastoidectomy
• Treatment of otitis externa; myringoplasty and tympanoplasty to reconstruct middle ear structures when thickening and scarring are present

Drug therapy

• Broad-spectrum antibiotics, such as amoxicillin/clavulanate potassium (Augmentin) or cefuroxime (Ceftin), for exacerbations of otitis media

INTERVENTIONS AND RATIONALES

• Monitor vital signs *to determine baseline and detect early signs of worsening infection.*

• Watch for and report headache, fever, severe pain, or disorientation *to detect early signs of complications.*

• Administer analgesics, as needed, or recommend applying heat to the ear *to relieve pain.*

• Identify and treat allergies *to prevent recurrences of otitis media.*

• Encourage the patient to complete the prescribed course of antibiotic treatment *to prevent reinfection.*

• For patients with acute secretory otitis media, watch for and immediately report pain and fever *to detect early signs of secondary infection.*

• Tell the parents to avoid feeding the infant in a supine position or putting him to bed with a bottle *to prevent reflux of nasopharyngeal flora.*

• Encourage the child to perform Valsalva's maneuver several times daily *to promote eustachian tube patency.*

• After myringotomy, maintain drainage flow; place sterile cotton loosely in the external ear *to absorb drainage* and change frequently *to prevent infection.*

• After tympanoplasty, reinforce dressings, and observe for excessive bleeding from the ear canal *to assess for fluid volume deficit.*

Teaching topics

• Avoiding blowing the nose or getting the ear wet when bathing

• Instilling nasopharyngeal decongestants properly, if prescribed

• Recognizing upper respiratory tract infections and getting them treated early

Seizure disorders

A seizure is a sudden, episodic, involuntary alteration in consciousness, motor activity, behavior, sensation, or autonomic function. (See *Classifying seizures.*) Epilepsy is a common, recurrent seizure disorder.

CAUSES

• Excessive neuronal discharges (epilepsy)
• Hyperexcitable nerve cells that surpass the seizure threshold
• Neurons overfiring without regard to stimuli or need

ASSESSMENT FINDINGS

• Aura just before the seizure's onset (Child reports unusual tastes, feelings, or odors.)
• Eyes deviating to a particular side or blinking
• Irregular breathing with spasms
• Usually unresponsive during tonic-clonic muscular contractions; may experience incontinence
• May be disoriented to time and place, drowsy, and uncoordinated immediately after a seizure

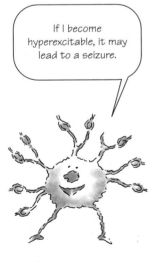

If I become hyperexcitable, it may lead to a seizure.

Classifying seizures

Seizures can take various forms depending on their origin and whether they're localized to one area of the brain, as occurs in partial seizures, or occur in both hemispheres, as happens in generalized seizures. This chart describes each type of seizure and lists common signs and symptoms.

Type	Description	Signs and symptoms
Partial		
Simple partial	Symptoms confined to one hemisphere	May have motor (change in posture), sensory (hallucinations), or autonomic (flushing, tachycardia) symptoms; no loss of consciousness
Complex partial	Begins in one focal area but spreads to both hemispheres (more common in adults)	Loss of consciousness; aura of visual disturbances; postictal symptoms
Generalized		
Absence (petit mal)	Sudden onset; lasts 5 to 10 seconds; can have 100 daily; precipitated by stress, hyperventilation, hypoglycemia, fatigue; differentiated from daydreaming	Loss of responsiveness but continued ability to maintain posture control and not fall; twitching eyelids; lip smacking; no postictal symptoms
Myoclonic	Movement disorder (not a seizure); seen as child awakens or falls asleep; may be precipitated by touch or visual stimuli; focal or generalized; symmetrical or asymmetrical	No loss of consciousness; sudden, brief, shocklike involuntary contraction of one muscle group
Clonic	Opposing muscles contract and relax alternately in rhythmic pattern; may occur in one limb more than others	Mucus production
Tonic	Muscles are maintained in continuous contracted state (rigid posture)	Variable loss of consciousness; pupils dilate; eyes roll up; glottis closes; possible incontinence; may foam at mouth
Tonic-clonic (grand mal, major motor)	Violent total body seizure	Aura; tonic first (20 to 40 seconds); clonic next; postictal symptoms
Atonic	Drop and fall attack; needs to wear protective helmet	Loss of posture tone
Akinetic	Sudden brief loss of muscle tone or posture	Temporary loss of consciousness

(continued)

Classifying seizures *(continued)*

Type	Description	Signs and symptoms
Miscellaneous		
Febrile	Seizure threshold lowered by elevated temperature; only one seizure per fever; common in 4% of population under age 5; occurs when temperature is rapidly rising	Lasts less than 5 minutes; generalized, transient, and nonprogressive; doesn't generally result in brain damage; EEG is normal after 2 weeks
Status epilepticus	Prolonged or frequent repetition of seizures without interruption; results in anoxia and cardiac and respiratory arrest	Consciousness not regained between seizures; lasts more than 30 minutes

DIAGNOSTIC TEST RESULTS
• EEG results help differentiate epileptic from nonepileptic seizures. Each seizure has a characteristic EEG tracing.

NURSING DIAGNOSES
• Ineffective airway clearance
• Risk for injury
• Sensory or perceptual alterations (tactile)

TREATMENT
• Drug therapy; if not responsive, ablative therapy
• Supportive until seizure ends (maintaining airway, protecting from injury)

Drug therapy
• I.V. diazepam (Valium) or lorazepam (Ativan)
• Phenobarbital (Luminal) or fosphenytoin (Cerebyx)
• Phenytoin (Dilantin) to keep neuron excitability below the seizure threshold

INTERVENTIONS AND RATIONALES
• Monitor vital signs *to determine baseline and detect any changes.*
• Assess neurologic status *to monitor for change in neurologic status.*
• Stay with the child during a seizure *to prevent injury.*

• Move the child to a flat surface *to prevent falling.*
• Place the child on the side to let saliva drain out *to ensure a patent airway.*
• Don't try to interrupt the seizure *to promote safety.*
• Gently support the head and keep the child's hands from inflicting self-harm, but don't restrain *to prevent injury.*
• Don't use tongue blades; *use of tongue blades during seizure activity may cause trauma to the mouth and result in airway obstruction from an aspirated tooth or laryngospasm.*
• Reduce external stimuli. *External stimuli could worsen seizure activity.*
• Loosen tight clothing *to promote comfort.*
• Record seizure activity. *Description of seizure activity helps to diagnose the type, which will aid in developing a treatment plan.*
• Pad the crib or bed *to prevent injury.*
• Monitor serum levels of anticonvulsant medications, such as phenytoin, *to ensure therapeutic levels and prevent toxicity or subtherapeutic levels.*

Teaching topics
• Controlling seizures
• Safety measures during seizure activity

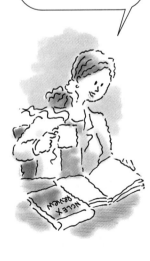

When a seizure occurs, assess neurologic status, move the child to a flat surface, place him on his side, and stay with him.

Spina bifida

Spina bifida has two main forms. Spina bifida occulta, the more common and less severe form, is characterized by incomplete closure of one or more vertebrae without protrusion of the spinal cord or meninges (membranes covering the spinal cord). Spina bifida cystica, the more severe form, is distinguished by incomplete closure of one or more vertebrae that causes protrusion of the spinal contents in an external sac or cystic lesion.

Spina bifida cystica has two classifications:

myelomeningocele, an external sac that contains meninges, CSF, and a portion of the spinal cord or nerve roots

meningocele, an external sac that contains meninges and CSF.

CAUSES
• Combination of genetic and environmental factors
• Exposure to a teratogen
• Part of a multiple malformation syndrome (for example, chromosomal abnormalities such as trisomy 18 or 13 syndrome)

ASSESSMENT FINDINGS
Spina bifida occulta
• Dimple (commonly found on the skin over the spinal defect)
• No neurologic dysfunction (usually), except occasional foot weakness or bowel and bladder disturbances
• Port wine nevi (commonly found on the skin over the spinal defect)
• Soft fatty deposits (commonly found on the skin over the spinal defect)
• Trophic skin disturbances (ulcerations, cyanosis)
• Tuft of hair (commonly found on the skin over the spinal defect)

Meningocele
• No neurologic dysfunction (usually)
• Saclike structure protruding over the spine

Myelomeningocele
• Arnold-Chiari syndrome
• Clubfoot
• Curvature of the spine
• Hydrocephalus
• Knee contractures
• Permanent neurologic dysfunction (paralysis, bowel and bladder incontinence)
• Possible mental retardation
• Saclike structure protruding over the spine

DIAGNOSTIC TEST RESULTS
• Amniocentesis reveals neural tube defect.
• Elevated alpha-fetoprotein levels in mother's blood may indicate the presence of a neural tube defect.
• Acetylcholinesterase measurement can be used to confirm the diagnosis.
• After birth, spinal X-ray can show the bone defect.
• Fetal karyotype should be done in addition to the biochemical tests because of the association of neural tube defects with chromosomal abnormalities.
• Myelography can differentiate spina bifida from other spinal abnormalities, especially spinal cord tumors.
• Ultrasound may identify the open neural tube or ventral wall defect.

NURSING DIAGNOSES
• Altered growth and development
• Impaired physical mobility
• Impaired adjustment

TREATMENT
• Meningocele: surgical closure of the protruding sac and continual assessment of growth and development

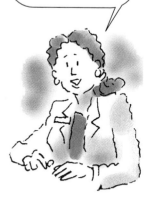

Unlike other forms of spina bifida, in spina bifida occulta, the spinal cord and meninges don't protrude.

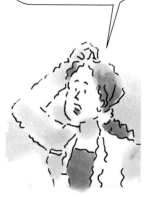

Hmmm. Spina bifida occulta and meningocele rarely cause neurologic dysfunction. However, myelomeningocele may cause permanent neurologic dysfunction.

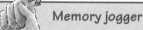

Memory jogger

"Spina bifida" is a Latin term that means literally "spine split in two." This may help you to remember that the disorder results from a cleft of the vertebral column.

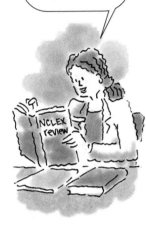

Remember, spina bifida occulta usually requires no treatment. Meningocele and myelomeningocele require surgery.

• Myelomeningocele: repair of the sac (doesn't reverse neurologic deficits) and supportive measures to promote independence and prevent further complications
• Spina bifida occulta: usually no treatment

INTERVENTIONS AND RATIONALES
Before surgery
• Hold and cuddle the infant on your lap and position him on his abdomen; handle the infant carefully, and don't apply pressure to the defect *to prevent injury at the site of the defect.*
• Clean the defect, inspect it often, and cover it with sterile dressings moistened with sterile saline solution *to prevent infection.*
• Usually, the infant can't wear a diaper or a shirt until after surgical correction *because it will irritate the sac,* so keep him warm in an infant Isolette *to prevent hypothermia.*
• Watch for signs of hydrocephalus. Measure head circumference daily. Be sure to mark the spot where the measurement was made *to ensure accurate readings.*
• Watch for signs of meningeal irritation, such as fever and nuchal rigidity, *to detect signs of meningitis.*
• Contractures can be minimized by passive range-of-motion exercises and casting. *To prevent hip dislocation, moderately abduct hips with a pad between the knees, or with sandbags and ankle rolls to prevent hip dislocation.*
• Monitor intake and output. Watch for decreased skin turgor and dryness *to detect dehydration.*
• Provide a diet high in calories and protein *to ensure adequate nutrition.*

After surgery
• Watch for hydrocephalus, which often follows surgery. Measure the infant's head circumference, as ordered, *to detect signs of hydrocephalus and prevent associated complications.*
• Monitor vital signs often *to detect early signs of shock, infection, and increased ICP.*
• Change the dressing regularly, as ordered, and check and report any signs of drainage, wound rupture, and infection *to promote early treatment and prevent complications.*

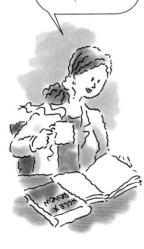

Teaching for spina bifida focuses on coping skills, long-term treatment goals, and recognizing complications.

• Place the infant in the prone position *to protect and assess the site.*
• If leg casts have been applied to treat deformities, watch for signs that the child is outgrowing the cast. Regularly check distal pulses *to ensure adequate circulation.*
• When spina bifida is diagnosed prenatally, refer the prospective parents to a genetic counselor, *who can provide information and support the couple's decisions on how to manage the pregnancy.*

Teaching topics
• Handling the infant without applying pressure to the defect
• Coping with the infant's physical problems
• Recognizing early signs of complications, such as hydrocephalus, pressure ulcers, and urinary tract infections
• Maintaining a positive attitude and working through feelings of guilt, anger, and helplessness
• Conducting intermittent catheterization and conduit hygiene
• Emptying the child's bowel by telling him to bear down and giving a glycerin suppository, as needed
• Recognizing developmental lags (a possible result of hydrocephalus)
• Ensuring maximum mental development
• Planning activities appropriate to their child's age and abilities

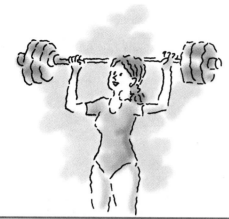

Pump up on practice questions

1. The nurse is assessing a child who may have meningitis. Which of the following assessment findings should the nurse look out for?

A. Flat fontanel
B. Irritability, fever, and vomiting
C. Jaundice, drowsiness, and refusal to eat
D. Negative Kernig's sign

Answer: B. Assessment findings associated with acute bacterial meningitis include irritability, fever, and vomiting along with seizure activity. Fontanels would be bulging as intracranial pressure rises, and Kernig's sign would be present due to meningeal irritation. Jaundice, drowsiness, and refusal to eat may indicate a GI disturbance rather than meningitis.

➡ *NCLEX keys*
Nursing process step: Assessment
Client needs category: Physiological integrity
Client needs subcategory: Physiological adaptation
Taxonomic level: Knowledge

2. The nurse is assessing a child who may have a seizure disorder. Which of the following is a description of an absence seizure?

A. Sudden, momentary loss of muscle tone
B. Minimal or no alteration in muscle tone, with a brief loss of consciousness
C. Muscle tone maintained and child frozen into position
D. Brief, sudden contracture of a muscle or muscle group

Answer: B. Absence seizures are characterized by a brief loss of responsiveness with minimal or no alteration in muscle tone. They may go unrecognized because the child's behavior changes very little. A sudden loss of muscle tone describes atonic seizures. "Frozen positions" describe akinetic seizures. A brief, sudden contraction of muscles describes a myoclonic seizure.

➡ *NCLEX keys*
Nursing process step: Assessment
Client needs category: Physiological integrity
Client needs subcategory: Physiological adaptation
Taxonomic level: Knowledge

3. The nurse is caring for a child who is experiencing a seizure. Which nursing intervention takes highest priority when caring for this child?

A. Protect the child from injury.
B Use a padded tongue blade to protect the airway.
C. Shout at the child to end the seizure.
D. Allow seizure activity to end without interference.

Answer: A. The nurse should identify the seizure type and protect the child from injury. A padded tongue blade should never be used because it can cause damage to the mouth and airway. Shouting will only agitate or confuse the child. Interfering with seizure activity may cause injury to the child. Allowing the seizure activity to end without interference may cause the child injury. The nurse should position the child on his side to ensure a patent airway and place the child on the ground if he's likely to fall and sustain injury.

➡ NCLEX keys
Nursing process step: Implementation
Client needs category: Physiological integrity
Client needs subcategory: Reduction of risk potential
Taxonomic level: Analysis

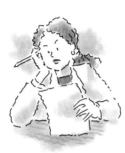

4. The nurse is caring for a child with spina bifida. Which of the following factors determines the extent of sensory and motor function loss in the lower limbs of the child?
  A. Maternal age at conception
  B. Degree of spinal cord abnormality
  C. Uterine environmental factors such as cloudy amniotic fluid
  D. Time frame from diagnosis to birth of the infant
Answer: B. The extent of motor and sensory loss primarily depends on the degree of spinal cord abnormality. Secondarily, it depends on traction or stretch resulting from an abnormally tethered cord, trauma to exposed neural tissue during delivery, and postnatal damage resulting from drying or infection of the neural plate. Maternal age and uterine environment haven't been identified as factors. The time from diagnosis to birth isn't related.

➡ NCLEX keys
Nursing process step: Assessment
Client needs category: Physiological integrity
Client needs subcategory: Physiological adaptation
Taxonomic level: Knowledge

5. The nurse is caring for an infant with spina bifida. Which assessment findings suggest hydrocephalus?
  A. Depressed fontanels and suture lines
  B. Deep-set eyes, which appear to look upward only
  C. Rapid increase in head size and irritability
  D. Motor and sensory dysfunction in the foot and leg
Answer: C. Hydrocephalus is an increase in the amount of cerebrospinal fluid in the ventricles and subarachnoid spaces of the brain. Assessment findings associated with hydrocephalus include a rapid increase in head size, irritability, suture line separation, and bulging fontanels. The eyes appear to look downward only, with the cornea prominent over the iris (sunset sign). There is a loss of sensory and motor function related to the spinal cord defect of spina bifida — not hydrocephalus.

➡ NCLEX keys
Nursing process step: Assessment
Client needs category: Physiological integrity
Client needs subcategory: Reduction of risk potential
Taxonomic level: Comprehension

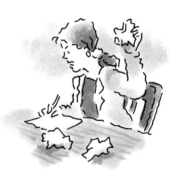

6. The nurse is teaching a father whose infant has had several episodes of otitis media. Which of the following statements made by the father indicates that he needs further teaching?

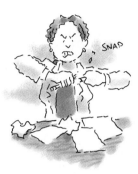

A. "Children who live in homes where family members smoke have fewer infections."
B. "The eustachian tube in infants is shorter and less angled than in older children."
C. "Breast-feeding is one way to help decrease the number of infections."
D. "I wrap him up and always put a hat on when we go out."

Answer: A. Children who live in households where smoking occurs have a greater number of respiratory infections that lead to otitis media, not fewer. The other statements about otitis media are correct.

➡ *NCLEX keys*
Nursing process step: Evaluation
Client needs category: Health promotion and maintenance
Client needs subcategory: Safety and infection control
Taxonomic level: Application

7. The school nurse is monitoring several children with attention deficit hyperactivity disorder who are taking methylphenidate (Ritalin). The nurse should conduct monthly follow-up examinations to monitor:
A. if the child is experiencing a dry mouth.
B. if the child is growing in height.
C. the parent's coping abilities from the child's perspective.
D. when the child is taking the medication.

Answer: B. Common adverse reactions to methylphenidate include slowed growth in height, sleeplessness, decreased appetite, and crying. Dry mouth is a common adverse reaction to tricyclic antidepressants. Knowing how the parents are coping from the child's perspective may be helpful information but not the most important. Knowing when the child takes the medication would be important if the child has problems with sleeplessness.

➡ *NCLEX keys*
Nursing process step: Assessment
Client needs category: Physiological integrity
Client needs subcategory: Pharmacological and parenteral therapies
Taxonomic level: Application

8. The nurse is teaching the mother of a child with attention deficit hyperactivity disorder (ADHD) how to manage the child. Which statement by the mother indicates that she needs further teaching?
A. "I only give him one direction at a time."
B. "I encourage my child to ride his bike after school."
C. "My child enjoys rollerblading with friends."
D. "I have my child do homework right after school."

Answer: D. Children with ADHD need time to expend their energy after being in a restrictive environment such as school. They need time to participate in activities that they enjoy, such as running, bike riding, or inline skating. Homework should be done later in the evening, not right after school.

➡ *NCLEX keys*
Nursing process step: Evaluation
Client needs category: Psychosocial integrity
Client needs subcategory: Coping and adaptation
Taxonomic level: Application

9. The nurse is caring for an infant with spina bifida. Which of the following is the most important technique for diagnosing hydrocephalus?

    A. Measurement of head circumference
    B. Skull X-ray showing a thinning skull
    C. Angiography revealing hydrocephalus
    D. Magnetic resonance imaging (MRI) revealing hydrocephalus

Answer: A. Measuring head circumference is the most important assessment technique for diagnosing hydrocephalus and is a key part of the routine infant screening. Skull X-rays, angiography, and MRI may be used to confirm the diagnosis.

➡ *NCLEX keys*
Nursing process step: Assessment
Client needs category: Health promotion and maintenance
Client needs subcategory: Growth and development through the life span
Taxonomic level: Comprehension

10. The nurse is caring for a child after shunt insertion to relieve hydrocephalus. Which of the following interventions should the nurse perform?

    A. Position the child in an upright position.
    B. Avoid lying the child on the side where the shunt is located.
    C. Position the child in a semi-Fowler's position.
    D. Position the child in a prone position.

Answer: B. After the shunt is inserted, the nurse shouldn't lie the child on the side of the body where the shunt is located. The child should lie supine to avoid rapid decompression. The child shouldn't be in an upright, semi-Fowler's, or prone position.

➡ *NCLEX keys*
Nursing process step: Implementation
Client needs category: Physiological integrity
Client needs subcategory: Reduction of risk potential
Taxonomic level: Application

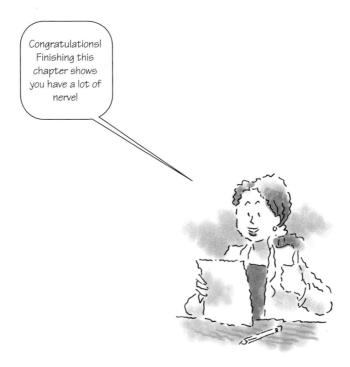

Congratulations! Finishing this chapter shows you have a lot of nerve!

31 Musculoskeletal System

Brush up on key concepts

In this chapter, you'll review:

📎 the pediatric musculoskeletal system

📎 tests used to diagnose musculoskeletal disorders

📎 common pediatric musculoskeletal disorders.

The musculoskeletal system is a complex system of **bones, muscles, ligaments, tendons,** and other **connective tissues.** The functions of the musculoskeletal system include:
• giving the body form and shape
• protecting vital organs
• making movement possible
• storing calcium and other minerals
• providing the site for hematopoiesis (blood cell formation).

At any point, you can review the major points of this chapter by consulting the *Cheat sheet* on pages 624 and 625.

Growing pains
Here are a few facts about the **pediatric musculoskeletal system.**
• Bones and muscles grow and develop throughout childhood.
• Bone lengthening occurs in the epiphyseal plates at the ends of bones; when the epiphyses close, growth stops.
• Bone healing occurs much faster in the child than in the adult because the child's bones are still growing.
• The younger the child, the faster the bone heals.
• Bone healing takes approximately 1 week for every year of life up to age 10.

Fractured logic
The most common fractures in the child are **clavicular fractures** and **greenstick fractures.**
• Clavicular fractures may occur during vaginal birth because the shoulders are the widest part of the body.

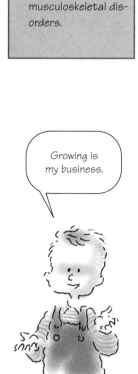

Growing is my business.

• Greenstick fractures of the long bones are related to the increased flexibility of the young child's bones. (The compressed side of the bone bends while the side under tension fractures.)

Keep abreast of diagnostic tests

Here are the most important tests used to diagnose musculoskeletal disorders, along with common nursing interventions associated with each test.

Using physical examination to assess the pediatric patient's musculoskeletal function and ability is also an important element in diagnosis. (See *Assessing musculoskeletal function and ability,* page 626.)

Look inside the joint
Arthroscopy is the visual examination of the interior of a joint with a fiber-optic endoscope.

Nursing actions
• Explain the procedure to the parents and child.
• Make sure that a written, informed consent has been obtained.
• Tell the child and parents he may need to fast after midnight before the procedure.
• Note allergies because local anesthesia is used.
• Tell the child he may feel a thumping sensation as the cannula is inserted in the joint capsule.

Soft-tissue sighting
A **computed tomography (CT) scan** is used to identify injuries to the soft tissue, ligaments, tendons, and muscles.

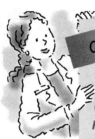

Cheat sheet

Musculoskeletal refresher

CLUBFOOT

Key signs and symptoms
• Can't be corrected manually (distinguishes true clubfoot from apparent clubfoot)

Key test result
• X-rays show superimposition of the talus and calcaneus and a ladderlike appearance of the metatarsals.

Key treatments
• Correcting deformity with a series of casts or surgical correction
• Maintaining correction until foot gains normal muscle balance
• Observing foot closely for several years to prevent foot deformity from recurring

Key interventions
• Ensure that shoes fit correctly.
• Prepare for surgery, if necessary.

DEVELOPMENTAL HIP DYSPLASIA

Key signs and symptoms
• Affected side exhibits an increased number of folds on posterior thigh when child is supine with knees bent
• Appearance of shortened limb on affected side when child is supine
• Restricted abduction of hips

Key test results
• Barlow's sign: A click is felt when the infant is placed supine with hips flexed 90 degrees and when the knees are fully flexed and the hip is brought into midabduction.
• Ortolani's click: It can be felt by the fingers at the hip area as the femur head snaps out of and back into the acetabulum. It's also palpable during examination with the child's legs flexed and abducted.
• Positive Trendelenburg's test: When the child stands on the affected leg, the opposite pelvis dips to maintain erect posture.

Key treatments
• A hip-spica cast or corrective surgery, for older children
• Bryant's traction
• Triple-cloth diapering, casting, or a Pavlik harness to keep the hips and knees flexed and the hips abducted for at least 3 months

Key interventions
• Give reassurance that early, prompt treatment will probably result in complete correction.
• Assure the parents that the child will adjust to restricted movement and return to normal sleeping and playing behavior in a few days.

DUCHENNE'S MUSCULAR DYSTROPHY

Key signs and symptoms
• Begins with pelvic girdle weakness, indicated by waddling gait and falling
• Eventual muscle weakness and wasting
• Gowers' sign (use of hands to push self up from floor)

Key test results
• Electromyography typically demonstrates short, weak bursts of electrical activity in affected muscles.
• Muscle biopsy shows variation in the size of muscle fibers and, in later stages, shows fat and connective tissue deposits, with no dystrophin.

Key treatments
• Physical therapy
• Surgery to correct contractures
• Use of devices such as splints, braces, trapeze bars, overhead slings, and a wheelchair to help preserve mobility

Key interventions
• Perform range-of-motion exercises.
• If respiratory involvement occurs, encourage coughing, deep-breathing exercises, and diaphragmatic breathing.
• Encourage adequate fluid intake, increase dietary fiber, and obtain an order for a stool softener.

Don't worry. If you use the Cheat sheet, I promise I won't tell.

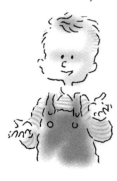

Musculoskeletal refresher (continued)

FRACTURES

Key signs and symptoms
- Loss of motor function
- Muscle spasm
- Pain or tenderness
- Skeletal deformity
- Swelling

Key test result
- X-rays may be used to confirm location and extent of fracture.

Key treatments
- Casting
- Reduction and immobilization of the fracture
- Surgery: open reduction and external fixation of the fracture

Key interventions
- Keep the child in proper body alignment.
- Provide support above and below the fracture site when moving the child.
- Elevate the fracture above the level of the heart.
- Apply ice to the fracture to promote vasoconstriction.
- Monitor pulses distal to the fracture every 2 to 4 hours.
- Assess color, temperature, and capillary refill.

JUVENILE RHEUMATOID ARTHRITIS

Key signs and symptoms
- Inflammation around joints
- Stiffness, pain, and guarding of affected joints

Key test results
- Hematology reveals an elevated erythrocyte sedimentation rate, a positive antinuclear antibody test, and the presence of rheumatoid factor.

Key treatments
- Heat therapy: warm compresses, baths
- Splint application

Key intervention
- Monitor joints for deformity.

SCOLIOSIS

Key signs and symptoms
- Nonstructural scoliosis (When the child bends at the waist to touch the toes, the curve in the spinal column disappears.)
- Structural scoliosis (When the child bends forward with the knees straight and the arms hanging down toward the feet, the spinal curve fails to straighten; the hips, ribs, shoulders, and shoulder blades are asymmetrical.)

Key test result
- X-rays may aid diagnosis.

Key treatments
- Nonstructural scoliosis: postural exercises, shoe lifts
- Structural scoliosis: steel rods, prolonged bracing, spinal fusion

Key interventions
After spinal fusion and insertion of rods:
- Turn the child by logrolling only.
- Maintain the child in correct body alignment.
- Maintain the bed in a flat position.

Nursing actions
- Explain the procedure to the parents and child.
- Make sure a written, informed consent has been obtained.
- Tell the child to hold still during the procedure.
- Tell the child that he'll be placed in a tube-like circle for the study and pictures will be taken of the extremity.

Cross-section check

Magnetic resonance imaging (MRI) allows cross-sectional imaging of bones and joints.

MRI, which uses a strong magnetic field and radio waves, has largely replaced arthrography for assessing joint anatomy. No ionizing radiation is used.

Nursing actions
- Explain the procedure to the parents and child.
- Instruct the child to hold still during the procedure.
- Note if the child has any metal implants, which may interfere with the study.

Assessing musculoskeletal function and ability

To assess the pediatric patient's musculoskeletal function and ability, perform the following nursing actions:
• Determine the range of motion.
• Note the amount of weight the child can bear.
• Assess gross and fine motor abilities.
• Note whether both arms and legs are used.
• Note whether muscle response is brisk and strong.

• Assess for pain; note whether the child is guarding a body part.
• Determine the relationship of the child's body size or weight to the defect.
• Note whether the child has an adequate and even spread of adipose tissue.
• Note the child's autonomy and independence in terms of mobility and skills.

Spinal vision

Myelography is an invasive procedure used to evaluate abnormalities of the spinal canal and cord. It entails injection of a radiopaque contrast medium into the subarachnoid space of the spine. Serial X-rays are then used to visualize the progress of the contrast medium as it passes through the subarachnoid space.

Nursing actions
• Explain the procedure to the parents and child.
• Make sure that a written, informed consent has been obtained.
• Before the test, check for allergies to the contrast medium.
• If metrizamide (Amipaque) is used as the contrast medium, discontinue phenothiazines 48 hours before the test.
• When the contrast medium is injected, tell the child that he may experience a burning sensation, warmth, headache, salty taste, nausea, and vomiting.
• After the test, have the child sit in his room or lie in bed with his head elevated 60 degrees. He must not lie flat for at least 8 hours.
• Encourage the child to drink extra fluids.
• Check that the child voids within 8 hours after returning to his room.

Hard tissue check

X-rays are probably the most useful diagnostic tool to evaluate musculoskeletal diseases. They can help to identify joint disruption, calcifications, and bone deformities, fractures,

and destruction as well as measure bone density.

Nursing actions
• Explain the test to the parents and child.
• Tell the child he must hold still during the X-ray. Cover the genital area with a lead apron.

Polish up on patient care

The major musculoskeletal disorders in pediatric patients are clubfoot (talipes), developmental hip dysplasia (dislocated hip), Duchenne's muscular dystrophy, fractures, juvenile rheumatoid arthritis, and scoliosis.

Clubfoot

Clubfoot, also known as talipes, is a congenital disorder in which the foot and ankle are twisted and can't be manipulated into correct position. Clubfoot occurs in these five forms:
• equinovarus: combination of positions
• talipes calcaneus: dorsiflexion, as if walking on one's heels
• talipes equinus: plantar flexion, as if pointing one's toes
• talipes valgus: eversion of the ankles, with the feet turning out

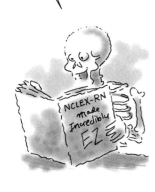

X-rays are excellent! They're a great tool for identifying calcifications, bone deformities, fractures, and destruction as well as measuring bone density.

NCLEX-RN Made Incredibly EZ

• talipes varus: inversion of the ankles, with the soles of the feet facing each other.

CAUSES
• Arrested development during the 9th and 10th weeks of embryonic life, when the feet are formed
• Deformed talus and shortened Achilles tendon
• Possible genetic predisposition

ASSESSMENT FINDINGS
• Deformity usually obvious at birth
• Can't be corrected manually (distinguishes true clubfoot from apparent clubfoot)

DIAGNOSTIC TEST RESULTS
• X-rays show superimposition of the talus and calcaneus and a ladderlike appearance of the metatarsals.

NURSING DIAGNOSES
• Altered growth and development
• Impaired physical mobility
• Risk for peripheral neurovascular dysfunction

TREATMENT
Treatment is administered in three stages:

☝ Correcting the deformity either with a series of casts to gradually stretch and realign the angle of the foot and, after cast removal, application of Denis Browne splint at night until age 1, or surgical correction

✌ Maintaining the correction until the foot gains normal muscle balance

🖖 Observing the foot closely for several years to prevent the deformity from recurring.

INTERVENTIONS AND RATIONALES
• Assess neurovascular status *to ensure circulation to foot with cast in place.*
• Ensure that shoes fit correctly *to promote comfort and prevent skin breakdown.*
• Prepare for surgery, if necessary, *to maintain or promote healing process and to decrease anxiety.*

Teaching topics
• Using a blow-dryer on the cool setting to provide relief of itching
• Importance of placing nothing inside the cast
• Keeping corrective devices on as much as possible
• Walking as exercise after surgical repair

Developmental hip dysplasia

Developmental hip dysplasia (dislocated hip) results from an abnormal development of the hip socket. It occurs when the head of the femur is still cartilaginous and the acetabulum (socket) is shallow; as a result, the head of the femur comes out of the hip socket. It can affect one or both hips and occurs in varying degrees of dislocation, from partial (subluxation) to complete.

CAUSES
• Breech delivery
• Fetal position in utero
• Genetic predisposition
• Laxity of the ligaments

ASSESSMENT FINDINGS
• On the affected side, an increased number of folds on the posterior thigh when the child is supine with knees bent
• Appearance of a shortened limb on the affected side
• Restricted abduction of the hips

DIAGNOSTIC TEST RESULTS
• Barlow's sign is present: A click is felt when the infant is placed supine with hips flexed 90 degrees, knees fully flexed, and the hip brought into midabduction.
• Ortolani's click is present. It can be felt by the fingers at the hip area as the femur head snaps out of and back into the acetabulum. It's also palpable during examination with the child's legs flexed and abducted.
• Sonography and MRI may be used to assess reduction.
• Trendelenburg's test is positive. When the child stands on the affected leg, the opposite pelvis dips to maintain erect posture.

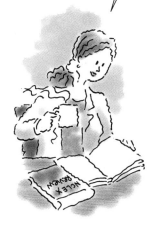

Combos are common. Nearly all cases of talipes are equinovarus, involving a combination of abnormal positions.

Memory jogger

When you think OTB, don't think Off Track Betting. Instead think of Ortolani, Trendelenburg, and Barlow — all key tests in diagnosing hip dysplasia.

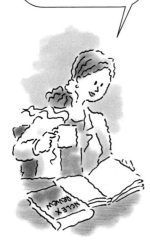

What is the common goal of treatment for developmental hip dysplasia? Enlarging and deepening the socket (acetabulum) through pressure.

• X-rays show the location of the femur head and a shallow acetabulum; X-rays can also be used to monitor progression of the disorder.

NURSING DIAGNOSES
• Altered growth and development
• Impaired physical mobility
• Risk for impaired skin integrity

TREATMENT
• A hip-spica cast or corrective surgery for older children
• Bryant's traction, if the acetabulum doesn't deepen
• Triple-cloth diapering, casting, or a Pavlik harness to keep the hips and knees flexed and the hips abducted for at least 3 months

INTERVENTIONS AND RATIONALES
• Assess circulation before application of cast or traction; after application, have the child wiggle toes *to detect signs of impaired circulation.* The nurse should be able to place one finger between the child's skin and cast.
• Provide skin care *to prevent skin breakdown.*
• Give reassurance that early, prompt treatment will probably result in complete correction *to decrease anxiety.*
• Assure the parents that the child will adjust to restricted movement and return to normal sleeping, eating, and play in a few days *to ease anxiety.*
• Inspect skin, especially around bony prominences, *to detect cast complications and skin breakdown.*

Teaching topics
• Correctly splinting or bracing the hips
• Receiving frequent checkups
• Coping with restricted movement
• Removing braces and splints while bathing the child and replacing them immediately afterward
• Stressing good hygiene

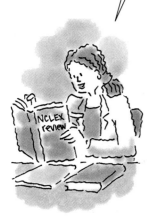

Here is a hint for early assessment: Duchenne's begins with a waddling gait and falling. This indicates pelvic girdle weakness.

Duchenne's muscular dystrophy

A genetic disorder that occurs only in males, Duchenne's muscular dystrophy (also called pseudohypertrophic dystrophy) is marked by muscular deterioration that progresses throughout childhood. It generally results in death from cardiac or respiratory failure in the late teens or early 20s due to a defect on the X chromosome, resulting in a lack of production of dystrophin. The absence of dystrophin results in breakdown of muscle fibers. Muscle fibers are replaced with fatty deposits and collagen in muscles. There is no known cure.

CAUSE
• Sex-linked recessive trait

ASSESSMENT FINDINGS
• Begins with pelvic girdle weakness, indicated by waddling gait and falling
• Cardiac or pulmonary failure
• Decreased ability to perform self-care activities
• Delayed motor development
• Eventual contractures and muscle hypertrophy
• Eventual muscle weakness and wasting
• Gowers' sign (use of hands to push self up from floor)

DIAGNOSTIC TEST RESULTS
• Electromyography typically demonstrates short, weak bursts of electrical activity in affected muscles.
• Muscle biopsy shows variations in the size of muscle fibers and, in later stages, shows fat and connective tissue deposits, with no dystrophin.

NURSING DIAGNOSES
• Impaired gas exchange
• Impaired physical mobility
• Impaired walking

TREATMENT
• Gene therapy (under investigation to prevent muscle degeneration)

- High-fiber, high-protein, low-calorie diet
- Physical therapy
- Surgery to correct contractures
- Use of devices such as splints, braces, trapeze bars, overhead slings, and a wheelchair to help preserve mobility

INTERVENTIONS AND RATIONALES
- Perform range-of-motion (ROM) exercises *to promote joint mobility.*
- Provide emotional support to the child and parents *to decrease anxiety and promote coping mechanisms.*
- Initiate genetic counseling *to inform the child and family about passing the disorder on to future children.*
- If respiratory involvement occurs, encourage coughing, deep-breathing exercises, and diaphragmatic breathing *to maintain a patent airway and mobilize secretions to prevent complications associated with retained secretions.*
- Encourage use of a footboard or high-topped sneakers and a foot cradle *to increase comfort and prevent footdrop.*
- Encourage adequate fluid intake, increase dietary fiber, and obtain an order for a stool softener *to prevent constipation associated with inactivity.*

Teaching topics
- Recognizing early signs of respiratory complications
- Avoiding long periods of bed rest and inactivity; if necessary, by limiting television viewing and other sedentary activities
- Planning a low-calorie, high-protein, high-fiber diet (because child is prone to obesity due to reduced physical activity)
- Helping the child maintain peer relationships and realize his intellectual potential (encourage parents to keep child in regular school as long as possible)

Fractures

A fracture is a break in the bone's integrity. A complete fracture breaks entirely across, resulting in a break in the continuity of the bone. An incomplete fracture extends only partially through the bone and the bone remains continuous. In a closed or simple fracture, the break doesn't puncture the skin surface, whereas an open or compound fracture punctures through the skin surface.

Common sites of fractures include the arm, clavicle, knee, and femur. The outcome usually depends on the severity of the fracture and the treatment provided. Potential complications include the development of fat emboli, improper bone growth, compartment syndrome, and infection.

CAUSES
- Childhood accidents, such as falls and motor vehicle accidents (most common cause)
- Child abuse
- Pathologic conditions

ASSESSMENT FINDINGS
- Bony crepitus
- Bruising
- Impaired sensation
- Loss of motor function
- Muscle spasm
- Pain or tenderness
- Paralysis
- Paresthesia
- Skeletal deformity
- Swelling

DIAGNOSTIC TEST RESULT
- X-rays may confirm location and extent of fracture.

NURSING DIAGNOSES
- Altered peripheral tissue perfusion
- Pain
- Risk for impaired skin integrity

TREATMENT
- Casting
- Reduction and immobilization of the fracture
- Surgery: open reduction and external fixation of the fracture
- Traction, depending on the site of the fracture (see *Common orthopedic treatments,* page 630)

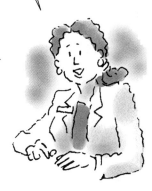

The primary focus of care in Duchenne's muscular dystrophy is to help the child remain as active and independent as possible.

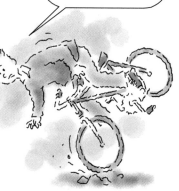

Accidents. The number one cause of fractures in childhood.

Common orthopedic treatments

The use of casts, traction, and braces are common orthopedic treatments.

CASTS

A cast is a hard mold that encases a body part, usually an extremity, to provide immobilization without discomfort.

General cast care

• Turn the cast frequently to dry all sides; use palms to lift or turn a wet cast to prevent indentations.
• Expose as much of the cast to air as possible, but cover exposed body parts.
• Be aware of discomfort to the child because chemical changes in the drying cast cause temperature extremes against the child's skin.
• After it is dry, maintain a dry cast; wetting the cast softens it and may cause skin irritation.
• Smooth out the cast's rough edges, and petal the edges.
• Rub adjacent skin daily with alcohol to toughen it and prevent skin breakdown.
• Assess circulation:
  —Note the color, temperature, and edema of digits.
  —Note the child's ability to wiggle the extremities without tingling or numbness.
• Assess any drainage or foul odor from the cast.
• Prevent small objects or food from falling into the cast.
• Don't use powder on the skin near the cast; it becomes a medium for bacteria when it absorbs perspiration.

Hip-spica cast

A hip-spica cast is a body cast extending from midchest to legs.
• The legs are abducted with a bar between them; never lift or turn the child with the crossbar.
• Perform cast care as listed above but with additional measures.
• Line the back edges of the cast with plastic or other waterproof material.
• Keep the cast level but on a slant, with the head of the bed raised:
  —The body and cast should stay at 180 degrees.
  —The head of the bed is raised on shock blocks or the mattress is raised using a wedge pillow so that the child is on a slant with the head up.
    —Urine and stools drain downward away from the cast.
    —A Bradford frame can be used for this purpose.
• Use a mattress firm enough to support the cast; use pillows to support parts of the cast, if needed.
• Reposition frequently to avoid pressure on the skin and the bony prominences; check for pressure as the child grows.

TRACTION

Traction decreases muscle spasms and realigns and positions bone ends. It works by pulling on the distal ends of bones.
• Skin traction pulls indirectly on the skeleton by pulling on the skin with adhesive, moleskin, or elastic bandage.
• Skeletal traction pulls directly on the skeleton with pins or tongs.

Traction-related care

• Check that the weights hang free.
• Check for skin irritation, infection at pin sites, and neurovascular response of the extremity.
• Prevent constipation by increasing fluids and fiber.
• Prevent respiratory congestion by promoting pulmonary hygiene using blowing games.
• Provide pain relief if necessary.
• Provide stimulation appropriate for the child.

Bryant's traction

This is the only skin traction designed specifically for the lower extremities of the child under age 2; the child's body weight provides countertraction.
• Legs are kept straight and extend 90 degrees toward the ceiling from the trunk; both legs are suspended even if only one is affected.
• The buttocks are kept slightly off the bed to ensure sufficient and continuous traction on the legs.
• Traction may be followed by application of a hip-spica cast.

BRACES

A brace is a plastic shell or metal-hinged appliance that aids mobility and posture.

Brace-related care

• Provide good skin care, especially at the bony prominences.
• Check to ensure accurate fit as the child grows.
• When applying full body braces to the spastic child, put the feet in first.

Milwaukee brace

  Attempts to slow the progression of spinal curvature of less than 40 degrees until bone growth stops
• Extends from the iliac crest of the pelvis to the chin
• Must be fitted
• Can be used until the child reaches skeletal maturity
• Must be worn 20 to 23 hours a day; may be removed for bathing and swimming

Boston brace

• Functions the same as a Milwaukee brace
• Extends from the axillary area to the iliac crest; must be fitted
• Can be easily covered by clothing

INTERVENTIONS AND RATIONALES
• Keep the child in proper body alignment *to promote bone healing and prevent tissue damage.*
• Provide support above and below the fracture site when moving the child *to promote comfort.*
• Monitor for any pressure areas caused by traction, the child's cast, or bedclothes *to prevent development of ischemia, which results in pain.*
• Elevate the fracture above the level of the heart *to promote venous return and decrease edema.*
• Apply ice to the fracture to promote vasoconstriction, *which inhibits edema and pain.*
• Monitor pulses distal to the fracture every 2 to 4 hours *to assess blood flow to the distal extremity.*
• Assess color, temperature, and capillary refill *to determine whether the affected extremity is adequately perfused.*
• Assess sensation *to determine whether perfusion to the nerves is intact.*
• Use pediatric assessment tools *to determine level of pain.*
• Turn and reposition the child every 2 hours *to help relieve skin pressure and prevent skin breakdown.*
• Protect cast from moisture and petal the edges *to promote healing of the fracture and prevent skin breakdown.*

Teaching topics
• Caring for a child in cast or traction
• Preventing injury
• Reporting signs of infection or complications

Juvenile rheumatoid arthritis

Juvenile rheumatoid arthritis (JRA) is an autoimmune disease of the connective tissue. It's characterized by chronic inflammation of the synovia and possible joint destruction. Episodes recur with remissions and exacerbations.

The three main forms of JRA are:
• pauciarticular JRA — asymmetrical involvement of less than five joints, usually affecting large joints such as the knees, ankles, and elbows.
• polyarticular JRA — symmetrical involvement of five or more joints, especially hands and weight-bearing joints such as hips, knees, and feet. Involvement of the temporomandibular joint may cause earache; involvement of the sternoclavicular joint may cause chest pain.
• systemic disease with polyarthritis — involves the lining of the heart and lungs, blood cells, and abdominal organs. Exacerbations may last for months. Fever, rash, and lymphadenopathy may occur.

CAUSES
• Autoimmune response
• Genetic predisposition

ASSESSMENT FINDINGS
• Inflammation around the joints
• Stiffness, pain, and guarding of the affected joints

DIAGNOSTIC TEST RESULTS
• Hematology reveals an elevated erythrocyte sedimentation rate, a positive antinuclear antibody test, and the presence of rheumatoid factor.
• Slit-lamp evaluation may show iridocyclitis (inflammation of the iris and the ciliary body).

NURSING DIAGNOSES
• Body image disturbance
• Impaired physical mobility
• Pain

TREATMENT
• Heat therapy: warm compresses, baths
• Splint application

Drug therapy
• Low-dose corticosteroids
• Low-dose methotrexate (Rheumatrex) (used as a second-line medication)
• Nonsteroidal anti-inflammatory drugs (NSAIDs): naproxen (Naprosyn), ibuprofen (Motrin)
• Aspirin (as an alternative to NSAIDs)

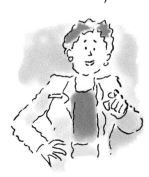

JRA may involve organs other than the joints, such as the heart, lung, liver and spleen, producing symptoms other than those affecting movement.

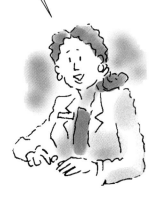

Nonstructural scoliosis is marked by a C curve that disappears when the child bends at the waist...

INTERVENTIONS AND RATIONALES
• Monitor joints for deformity *to assess for early changes as a complication of this disease process.*
• Administer medications, as prescribed, and note effectiveness *to relieve pain and prevent further joint damage.*
• Assist with exercise and ROM activities *to maintain joint mobility.*
• Apply warm compresses or encourage the child to take a warm bath in the morning *to promote comfort and increase mobility.*
• Apply splints *to maintain position of function and prevent contractures.*
• Provide assistive devices if necessary *to encourage the normal performance of daily activities.*

Teaching topics
• How stress and climate can influence exacerbations
• Preventive eye care

Scoliosis

Scoliosis is a lateral curvature of the spine, especially among females. It's commonly identified at puberty and throughout adolescence. Scoliosis stops progressing when bone growth stops.

CAUSES
• Nonstructural, functional, postural scoliosis: a nonprogressive C curve from some other condition, such as poor posture, unequal leg length, and poor vision
• Structural or progressive scoliosis: a progressive S curve with a primary and compensatory curvature resulting in spinal and rib changes

ASSESSMENT FINDINGS
• Nonstructural scoliosis: When the child bends at the waist to touch the toes, the curve in the spinal column disappears.
• Structural scoliosis: When the child bends forward with the knees straight and the arms hanging down toward the feet, the spinal curve fails to straighten; the hips, ribs, shoulders, and shoulder blades are asymmetrical.

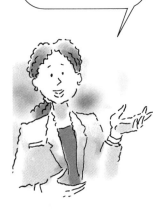

...Whereas structural scoliosis is an S curve that doesn't disappear, even when the child bends.

DIAGNOSTIC TEST RESULT
• X-rays may aid the diagnosis.

NURSING DIAGNOSES
• Altered growth and development
• Body image disturbance
• Impaired physical mobility

TREATMENT
Nonstructural scoliosis
• Corrective lenses if the problem is associated with poor vision that results in a head tilt
• Postural exercises
• Shoe lifts

Structural scoliosis
• Electrical stimulation for mild to moderate curvatures
• Harrington, Luque, or Cotrel-Dubousset rods for curves greater than 40 degrees (to realign the spine or when curves fail to respond to orthotic treatment)
• Possible prolonged bracing (Milwaukee or Boston brace)
• Skin traction or halo femoral traction
• Spinal fusion with bone from the iliac crest

INTERVENTIONS AND RATIONALES
After spinal fusion and insertion of rods:
• Monitor vital signs and intake and output *to prevent fluid volume deficit.*
• Turn the child only by logrolling *to prevent injury.*
• Maintain correct body alignment *to promote joint mobility and prevent injury.*
• Maintain the bed in a flat position *to prevent injury and complications.*
• Help the child adjust to the increase in height and altered self-perception *to promote self-esteem and decrease anxiety.*

Teaching topics
• Performing stretching exercises for the spine
• Helping the child maintain self-esteem

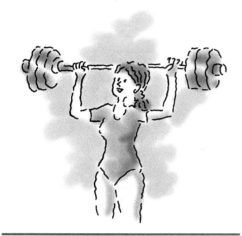

Pump up on practice questions

1. A child is diagnosed with developmental hip dysplasia. Which of the following treatments is most effective in reducing hip dysplasia in older children?

   A. Pavlik harness
   B. Frejka pillow
   C. Double pillow
   D. Hip-spica cast

Answer: D. Studies have shown that the hip-spica cast is the most effective method for reducing hip dysplasia. The hip-spica cast is used when an abduction brace is ineffective or if an adduction contracture is present. The Pavlik harness is used for simple dysplasia. The other devices aren't effective for hip dysplasia.

➡ *NCLEX keys*
Nursing process step: Implementation
Client needs category: Physiological integrity
Client needs subcategory: Physiological adaptation
Taxonomic level: Knowledge

2. The nurse is caring for a child with developmental hip dysplasia. The nurse can aid correct placement of the hip by:

   A. placing a blanket between the child's legs.
   B. using multiple diapers.
   C. wrapping the child in a blanket.
   D. electrical stimulation.

Answer: B. Multiple diapers increase abduction and external rotation of the hip. A blanket isn't sufficient to increase the abduction. Wrapping a child in a blanket increases internal rotation, which increases instability rather than decreasing it. Electrical stimulation is a treatment for mild to moderate curvature of the spine in scoliosis.

➡ *NCLEX keys*
Nursing process step: Implementation
Client needs category: Safe, effective care environment
Client needs subcategory: Management of care
Taxonomic level: Knowledge

3. A child is diagnosed with developmental hip dysplasia. Besides using the hip-spica cast, which of the following devices is used in the treatment of this condition?

   A. Pillow
   B. Denis Browne splint
   C. Pavlik harness
   D. Foot casts

Answer: C. A Pavlik harness is used to stabilize the hip. A regular pillow isn't sufficient. A Denis Browne splint is used to treat talipes equinovarus. Foot casts aren't effective.

➡ *NCLEX keys*
Nursing process step: Planning
Client needs category: Health promotion and maintenance
Client needs subcategory: Growth and development through the life span
Taxonomic level: Knowledge

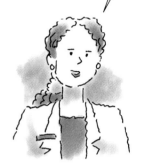

Answer a few *Incredibly Easy* practice questions. Get pumped for the NCLEX!

4. A child has been placed in a hip-spica cast. The cast is properly positioned if:

    A. the cast is snug, allowing some movement of the extremity.

    B. the cast allows no extremity movement, but allows one finger to fit between the skin and the cast.

    C. the cast is snug, allowing no movement of the extremity.

    D. the cast is snug without disturbing the client's neurovascular status.

Answer: B. The nurse should be able to place one finger between the child's skin and the cast. The child should be unable to move the extremity, but the cast shouldn't fit snugly.

➡ *NCLEX keys*
Nursing process step: Assessment
Client needs category: Safe, effective care environment
Client needs subcategory: Safety and infection control
Taxonomic level: Knowledge

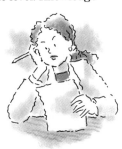

5. A child's clubfoot has been placed in a cast. The child develops itching under the cast and asks the nurse for help. The nurse should:

    A. use sterile applicators to relieve the itch.

    B. apply water under the cast.

    C. apply cool air under the cast with a blow-dryer.

    D. apply hydrocortisone cream.

Answer: C. A blow-dryer on the cool setting should be directed toward the itchy area to provide relief. Nothing should be put inside the cast because this can cause further skin irritation. Water would wet the cast and wouldn't be helpful. Hydrocortisone cream

can ball up and be irritating, and it would be difficult to apply inside the cast.

➡ *NCLEX keys*
Nursing process step: Assessment
Client needs category: Physiological integrity
Client needs subcategory: Reduction of risk potential
Taxonomic level: Knowledge

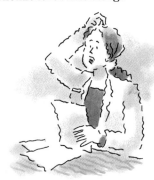

6. A child has undergone repair of a clubfoot and is allowed full activity. The nurse is teaching the child's parents about activities for the child. Which activity would benefit the child most?

    A. Walking

    B. Playing catch

    C. Standing

    D. Swimming

Answer: A. Walking stimulates all of the involved muscles and helps with strengthening. All the options are good exercises for clubfoot, but walking is the best choice.

➡ *NCLEX keys*
Nursing process step: Planning
Client needs category: Physiological integrity
Client needs subcategory: Physiological adaptation
Taxonomic level: Application

7. The nurse is treating a child with juvenile rheumatoid arthritis (JRA). Which of the following factors can exacerbate the condition?

    A. Stress and climate

    B. Dehydration and climate

    C. Exposure to cold

    D. Exercise

Answer: A. Exacerbations of JRA can be precipitated by exposure to stress and climate. Dehydration and exposure to cold can precipitate vaso-occlusive crisis in the client with sickle cell anemia. Exposure to cold can precipitate an exacerbation of Raynaud's disease. Exercise should be encouraged in the child with JRA.

➡ NCLEX keys
Nursing process step: Assessment
Client needs category: Physiological integrity
Client needs subcategory: Reduction of risk potential
Taxonomic level: Knowledge

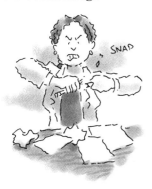

8. A child is admitted with an undiagnosed musculoskeletal condition. Which diagnostic tool is most useful in evaluating a musculoskeletal disorder?
    A. Myelography
    B. Magnetic resonance imaging (MRI)
    C. Computed tomography (CT) scan
    D. X-rays
Answer: D. X-rays are the most useful diagnostic tool to evaluate musculoskeletal diseases and can be used to help identify joint disruption, bone deformities, calcifications, and bone destruction and fractures as well as to measure bone density. Myelography is an invasive procedure used to evaluate abnormalities of the spinal canal and cord. MRI, a form of cross-sectional imaging using a strong magnetic field and radio waves, has largely replaced arthrography for assessing joint anatomy. A CT scan can be used to identify injuries of soft tissue, ligaments, tendons, and muscles.

➡ NCLEX keys
Nursing process step: Assessment
Client needs category: Physiological integrity
Client needs subcategory: Reduction of risk potential
Taxonomic level: Comprehension

9. The nurse is developing a dietary teaching plan for a child with Duchenne's muscular dystrophy. Which elements are most important for the nurse to include in the child's diet?
    A. Low-calorie, high-protein, and high-fiber
    B. Low-calorie, high-protein, and low-fiber
    C. High-calorie, high-protein, and restricted fluids
    D. High-calorie, high protein, and high-fiber
Answer: A. A child with muscular dystrophy is prone to constipation and obesity, so dietary intake should include a diet low in calories, high in protein, and high in fiber. Adequate fluid intake should also be encouraged.

➡ NCLEX keys
Nursing process step: Planning
Client needs category: Physiological integrity
Client needs subcategory: Basic care and comfort
Taxonomic level: Knowledge

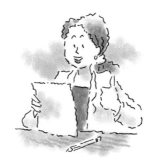

10. The nurse is teaching the mother of a child with scoliosis. The nurse knows that teaching has been successful when the mother makes which of the following statements?

    A. "I'm glad my daughter will outgrow this deformity."

    B. "I'm afraid that my daughter will feel unattractive because she must wear a brace."

    C. "I'll make sure that my daughter doesn't do any stretching exercises that could worsen her spine."

    D. "I'm glad my daughter will only need to wear a brace for a short period of time."

Answer: B. Teaching is successful when the mother shows concern about her daughter's feelings toward wearing a brace for scoliosis correction. Although scoliosis ceases to progress when bone growth stops, the child won't outgrow the deformity. Stretching exercises for the spine may help improve scoliosis. Prolonged bracing is usually indicated to correct the deformity.

➡ *NCLEX keys*

Nursing process step: Evaluation
Client needs category: Physiological integrity
Client needs subcategory: Reduction of risk potential
Taxonomic level: Analysis

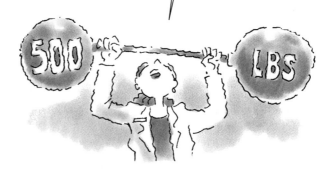

Boning up on the pediatric musculoskeletal system before taking the NCLEX was smart. Now you'll be able to muscle your way through the next chapter.

32 Gastrointestinal System

Brush up on key concepts

The GI tract, also known as the **alimentary canal,** consists of a long, hollow, muscular tube that includes several glands and accessory organs. It performs the crucial task of supplying essential nutrients to fuel the other organs and body systems. Because the GI system is so crucial to the rest of the body systems, any problem in this system can quickly affect the overall health, growth, and development of the child.

At any time, you can review the major points of this chapter by consulting the *Cheat sheet* on pages 638 to 640.

GI junior
Characteristics of the pediatric GI system include the following:
• Peristalsis occurs within 2½ to 3 hours in the newborn and extends to 3 to 6 hours in older infants and children.
• Gastric stomach capacity of the newborn is 30 to 60 ml, which gradually increases to 200 to 350 ml by age 12 months and to 1,500 ml as an adolescent.
• The neonatal abdomen is larger than the chest up to age 4 to 8 weeks, and the musculature is poorly developed.
• The sucking and extrusion reflex persists to age 3 to 4 months (extrusion reflex protects infant from food substances that its system is too immature to digest).
• At 4 months saliva production begins and aids in the process of digestion.
• Spit-ups are frequent in the newborn due to the immature muscle tone of the lower esophageal sphincter and the low volume capacity of the stomach.

• Increased myelination of nerves to the anal sphincter allows for physiologic control of bowel function, usually around age 2.
• The liver's slow development of glycogen storage capacity makes the infant prone to hypoglycemia.
• From ages 1 to 3, composition of intestinal flora becomes more adultlike and stomach acidity increases, reducing the number of GI infections.

Nutrient breakdown
The GI tract breaks down food (carbohydrates, fats, and proteins) into molecules small enough to permeate cell membranes, thus providing cells with the necessary energy to function properly. The GI tract prepares food for cellular absorption by altering its physical and chemical composition. (See *Digestive organs and glands,* page 641.)

Malfunction junction
A malfunction along the GI tract can produce far-reaching metabolic effects, eventually threatening life itself. A common indication of GI problems is referred pain, which makes diagnosis especially difficult.

Keep abreast of diagnostic tests

Here are the most important tests used to diagnose GI system disorders, along with common nursing interventions associated with each test.

Swallow this
Barium swallow is primarily used to examine the esophagus.

Gastrografin is now used instead of barium for certain patients. Like barium, Gastrografin

(Text continues on page 640.)

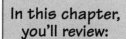

In this chapter, you'll review:

◈ parts of the gastrointestinal (GI) system and their function

◈ tests used to diagnose GI disorders

◈ common pediatric GI disorders.

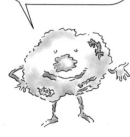

Thanks to the GI tract, I can get a good meal.

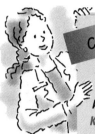

Cheat sheet

Gastrointestinal refresher

ACETAMINOPHEN POISONING

Key signs and symptoms
- Diaphoresis
- Nausea

Key test result
- Serum aspartate aminotransferase and serum alanine aminotransferase levels become elevated soon after ingestion.

Key treatments
- Gastric lavage or emesis induction with ipecac syrup

Key interventions
- Monitor vital signs and intake and output.
- Assess cardiovascular and GI status.

CELIAC DISEASE

Key signs and symptoms
- Generalized malnutrition and failure to thrive due to malabsorption of protein and carbohydrates
- Steatorrhea and chronic diarrhea due to fat malabsorption
- Weight and height below normal for age-group

Key test result
- Immunologic assay screen is positive for celiac disease.

Key treatment
- Gluten-free diet

Key interventions
- Monitor growth and development.
- Give small, frequent meals.

CLEFT LIP AND PALATE

Key signs and symptoms
- Cleft lip: can range from a simple notch on the upper lip to complete cleft from the lip edge to the floor of the nostril, on either side of the midline, but rarely along the midline itself
- Cleft palate without cleft lip: may not be detected until mouth examination or development of feeding difficulties

Key test result
- Prenatal ultrasound may indicate severe defects.

Key treatment
- Cheiloplasty performed between birth and age 3 months to unite the lip and gum edges in anticipation of teeth eruption, providing a route for adequate nutrition and sucking
- Cleft palate repair surgery (staphylorrhaphy); scheduled at about age 18 months to allow for growth of the palate and to be done before the infant develops speech patterns; infant must be free from ear and respiratory infections

Key interventions
- Be alert for respiratory distress when feeding.
Before cleft lip repair surgery, do the following:
- Hold the infant while feeding and promote sucking between meals.
After cleft lip repair surgery, do the following:
- Observe for cyanosis as the infant begins to breathe through the nose.
- Keep the infant's hands away from the mouth by using restraints or pinning the sleeves to the shirt; Steri Strips are used to hold the suture line in place.
- Anticipate the infant's needs.
- Don't position prone.
- Place the infant on the right side; to prevent aspiration, clean the suture line after each feeding by dabbing it with half-strength hydrogen peroxide or saline solution.
After cleft palate repair surgery, do the following:
- Position the toddler on the abdomen or side.
- Anticipate edema and a decreased airway from palate closure; this may make the toddler appear temporarily dyspneic; assess for signs of altered oxygenation.
- Keep hard or pointed objects (utensils, straws, frozen dessert sticks) away from the mouth.

Gastrointestinal refresher *(continued)*

ESOPHAGEAL ATRESIA AND TRACHEOESOPHAGEAL FISTULA

Key signs and symptoms
• Esophageal atresia: excessive salivation and drooling due to inability to pass food through the esophagus
• Tracheoesophageal fistula: choking, coughing, and intermittent cyanosis during feeding due to food that goes through the fistula into the trachea

Key test result
• Newborns are fed first with a few sips of sterile water to detect these anomalies and to prevent aspiration of formula or breast milk into the lungs.

Key treatment
• Surgical correction by ligating the tracheoesophageal fistula and reanastomosing the esophageal ends; in many cases, repair done in stages

Key interventions
• Assess respiratory status.

FAILURE TO THRIVE

Key signs and symptoms
• Altered body posture
• Disparities between chronologic age and height and weight
• History of insufficient stimulation and inadequate parental knowledge of child development

Key test result
• Negative nitrogen balance indicates inadequate intake of protein or calories.

Key treatments
• High-calorie diet
• Parent counseling
• Vitamin and mineral supplements

Key interventions
• Properly feed and interact with the child.
• Provide the child with visual and auditory stimulation.
• When caring for the child in the parent's presence, act as a role model for effective parenting skills. Demonstrate comfort measures such as rocking the infant, and show the mother how to hold the infant in an en face position.

INTESTINAL OBSTRUCTION

Key signs and symptoms
• Complete small-bowel obstruction: bowel contents propelled toward mouth (instead of rectum) by vigorous peristaltic waves, along with persistent epigastric or periumbilical pain
• Partial large-bowel obstruction: leakage of liquid stool around the obstruction (common).

Key test results
• In large-bowel obstruction, barium enema reveals a distended, air-filled colon or, in sigmoid volvulus, a closed loop of sigmoid with extreme distention.
• X-rays confirm the diagnosis. Abdominal films show the presence and location of intestinal gas or fluid.

Key treatment
• I.V. therapy to correct fluid and electrolyte imbalances

Key interventions
• Monitor vital signs frequently.
• Assess cardiovascular status; observe the child closely for signs of shock (pallor, rapid pulse, and hypotension).
• Stay alert for signs and symptoms of metabolic alkalosis (changes in sensorium; slow, shallow respirations; hypertonic muscles; tetany) or acidosis (dyspnea on exertion; disorientation; and later, deep, rapid breathing, weakness, and malaise).
• Watch for signs and symptoms of secondary infection, such as fever and chills.

LEAD POISONING

Key signs and symptoms
• Vomiting
• Weight loss

Key test results
• X-rays reveal lead lines near the epiphyseal lines (areas of increased density) of long bones. The thickness of the line shows the length of time the lead ingestion has been occurring.
• Lumbar puncture reveals increased protein level in cerebrospinal fluid sample.

Key treatments
• Chelating agents, such as ethylenediaminetetraacetic acid (EDTA) or dimercaprol (BAL). Chelating agents bind with lead and are excreted by the kidneys.

Key interventions
• Monitor vital signs, intake and output, hydration status, and kidney function.
• Monitor calcium levels (chelating agents also bind with calcium).

PYLORIC STENOSIS

Key signs and symptoms
• Projectile emesis during or shortly after feedings, preceded by reverse peristaltic waves (going left to right) but not by nausea; child resumes eating after vomiting

(continued)

Gastrointestinal refresher (continued)

PYLORIC STENOSIS (continued)

Key test result
- Ultrasound reveals hypertrophied sphincter.

Key treatment
- Pyloromyotomy performed by laparoscopy

Key interventions
- Provide small, frequent, thickened feedings with the head of the bed elevated; burp the child frequently.
- Position the child on his right side to prevent aspiration.

SALICYLATE POISONING

Key signs and symptoms
- High fever from the stimulation of carbohydrate metabolism
- Petechiae and bleeding tendency

Key test results
- Prothrombin time is prolonged.
- Serum salicylate levels are elevated.

Key treatments
- Gastric lavage or emesis induction with ipecac syrup
- I.V. fluids
- Sodium bicarbonate

Key interventions
- Administer oral and I.V. fluids.
- Monitor urine pH.
- Assess cardiovascular and GI status.

---

facilitates imaging through X-rays. Unlike barium, however, if Gastrografin escapes from the GI tract, it's absorbed by the surrounding tissue. Escaped barium isn't absorbed and can cause complications.

Nursing actions
- Maintain the child on a nothing-by-mouth (NPO) status beginning midnight before the test.
- Tell the child he must hold still during the X-ray.
- After the test, monitor bowel movements for excretion of barium. Also monitor GI function.

Upper GI imaging

In an **upper GI series,** swallowed barium sulfate proceeds into the esophagus, stomach, and duodenum, to reveal abnormalities. The barium outlines stomach walls and delineates ulcer craters and filling defects.

A **small-bowel series,** an extension of the upper GI series, visualizes barium flowing through the small intestine to the ileocecal valve.

Nursing actions
- Explain the procedure to the child and parents.

- Tell the child he must hold still during the X-ray.
- Make sure the lead apron is properly placed around the genital area.
- After the test, monitor bowel movements for excretion of barium. Also monitor GI function.

Lower GI look

A **barium enema (lower GI series)** allows X-ray visualization of the colon.

Nursing actions
- Explain the procedure to the child and parents.
- Usually, the child will follow a liquid diet for 24 hours before the test. Bowel preparations are administered before the examination.
- Tell the child X-rays will be taken on a test table and he must hold still.
- Cover the genital area with a lead apron during X-ray.

Stool search

A **stool specimen** can be examined for suspected GI bleeding, infection, or malabsorption. Certain tests require several specimens, such as the **guaiac test** for occult blood, a microscopic stool examination for ova and parasites, and tests for fat.

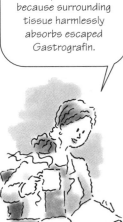

A substitute may be safer. Gastrografin may replace barium because surrounding tissue harmlessly absorbs escaped Gastrografin.

Digestive organs and glands

Here is a quick rundown of the major organs and glands that facilitate digestion.

SALIVARY GLANDS

The salivary glands provide saliva to moisten the mouth, lubricate food to ease swallowing, and begin food breakdown using the enzyme ptyalin. After food is swallowed, it enters the esophagus and is transported to the stomach.

STOMACH

The stomach is a muscular, saclike organ located between the esophagus and small intestine. Food and fluids enter the stomach and are mixed with stomach secretions. Contractions called peristalsis push the food gradually into the small intestine through the pyloric opening at the lower end of the stomach.

INTESTINE

The intestine extends from the pyloric opening to the anus. It's made up of the small and large intestines.
• The small intestine is made up of the duodenum, jejunum, and ileum and is about 20′ (6 m) long. Most digestion takes place in the small intestine; digested food is absorbed through the walls of the small intestine and into the blood for distribution throughout the body.
• The large intestine is about 5′ (1.5 m) long and includes the cecum (and appendix), colon, and rectum. Indigestible food passes into the large intestine, where it's formed into solid feces and eliminated through the rectum.

LIVER

The liver stores and filters blood; secretes bile; processes sugars, fats, proteins, and vitamins; and detoxifies drugs, alcohol, and other substances.

GALLBLADDER

The gallbladder is located beneath the liver and serves as a storage place for bile. Bile is a clear yellowish fluid that enters the small intestine through bile ducts and aids digestion of fats.

PANCREAS

The pancreas is a large gland located behind the stomach. It secretes digestive enzymes that neutralize stomach acids and break down proteins, carbohydrates, and fats.

Nursing actions
• Obtain the specimen in the correct container (container may need to be sterile or contain preservative).
• Be aware that the specimen may need to be transported to the laboratory immediately or placed in the refrigerator.

Fiber-optic findings
In **esophagogastroduodenoscopy,** insertion of a fiber-optic scope allows direct visual inspection of the esophagus, stomach and, sometimes, duodenum. **Proctosigmoidoscopy** permits inspection of the rectum and distal sigmoid colon. **Colonoscopy** allows inspection of the descending, transverse, and ascending colon.

Nursing actions
• Explain the procedure to the child and parents.
• Make sure that a written, informed consent has been obtained.
• A mild sedative may be administered before the examination.
• The child may be kept NPO from midnight beforehand (upper GI series).

• The child may be placed on a liquid diet for 24 hours before the examination or require enemas or laxatives until clear (lower GI examinations).

Fluoroscopic findings

Endoscopic retrograde cholangiopancreatography is the radiographic examination of the pancreatic ducts and hepatobiliary tree following the injection of contrast media into the duodenal papilla. It's done on children with suspected pancreatic disease or obstructive jaundice.

Nursing actions

Before the procedure, do the following:
• Explain the procedure to the child and parents.
• Make sure that a written, informed consent has been obtained
• Check the child's history for allergies to cholinergics and iodine.
• Administer a sedative and monitor the child for the drug's effect.
  After the procedure, do the following:
• Monitor the child's gag reflex (the child is kept NPO until his gag reflex returns).
• Protect the child from aspiration of mucus by positioning the child on his side.
• Monitor the child for urine retention.

Tube topics

Certain GI disorders require **intubation** for the following purposes:
• to empty the stomach and intestine
• to aid diagnosis and treatment
• to decompress obstructed areas
• to detect and treat GI bleeding
• to administer medications or feedings.
  Tubes usually inserted through the nose include short nasogastric (NG) tubes (Levin and Salem Sump) and long intestinal tubes (Cantor and Miller-Abbott). The larger Ewald tube is usually inserted orally.

Nursing actions

When caring for a children who is intubated, do the following:

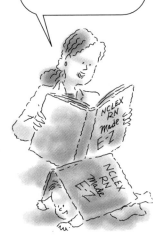

Children who are intubated require diligent oral and nasal care, close monitoring, and emotional support to minimize fear.

• Maintain accurate intake and output records. Measure gastric drainage every 8 hours; record amount, color, odor, and consistency. When irrigating the tube, note the amount of saline solution instilled and aspirated.
• Check for fluid and electrolyte imbalances.
• Provide good oral and nasal care. Make sure the tube is secure but isn't causing pressure on the nostrils. Change the tape to the nose every 24 hours. Gently wash the area around the tube, and apply a water-soluble lubricant to soften crusts. These measures help prevent sore throat and nose, dry lips, nasal excoriation, and parotitis.
• To support the short tube's weight, anchor it to the child's clothing.
• After removing the tube from a child with GI bleeding, watch for signs and symptoms of recurrent bleeding, such as hematemesis, decreased hemoglobin levels, pallor, chills, diaphoresis, hypotension, and rapid pulse.
• Provide emotional support because many children panic at the sight of a tube. Maintaining a calm, reassuring manner can help minimize the child's fear.

Polish up on patient care

Pediatric GI disorders discussed in this chapter include acetaminophen poisoning, celiac disease, cleft lip and palate, esophageal atresia and tracheoesophageal fistula, failure to thrive, intestinal obstruction, lead poisoning, pyloric stenosis, and salicylate poisoning.

Acetaminophen poisoning

Acetaminophen is an analgesic antipyretic agent that achieves its effect without inhibiting platelet aggregation. Because acetaminophen is an over-the-counter medication commonly found in the home, it's a common cause of poisoning in children.

In acetaminophen poisoning, hepatotoxicity occurs at plasma levels greater than 200 mg/ml at 4 hours after ingestion and greater than 50 mg/ml by 12 hours after ingestion.

CAUSE
• Acetaminophen overdose

ASSESSMENT FINDINGS
• Anorexia
• Diaphoresis
• Hypothermia
• Severe hypoglycemia
• Shock
• Encephalopathy
• Liver dysfunction
• Oliguria
• Nausea
• Pallor
• Right upper quadrant tenderness and jaundice evident 72 to 96 hours after ingestion
• Seven to eight days after ingestion: hepatic failure, death, or resolution of symptoms

DIAGNOSTIC TEST RESULTS
• Blood glucose levels are decreased.
• Serum aspartate aminotransferase and serum alanine aminotransferase levels become elevated soon after ingestion.
• Prothrombin time is prolonged.

NURSING DIAGNOSES
• Altered nutrition: Less than body requirements
• Risk for fluid volume deficit
• Hypothermia

TREATMENT
• Gastric lavage or emesis induction with ipecac syrup
• Hyperthermia blanket
• I.V. fluid
• Oxygen therapy (intubation and mechanical ventilation may be required)

Drug therapy
• Ipecac syrup to induce vomiting
• Acetylcysteine (Mucomyst)

INTERVENTIONS AND RATIONALES
• Monitor liver function studies *to detect signs of liver damage and to monitor effectiveness of treatment.*
• Monitor vital signs and intake and output. *Tachycardia and decreased urine output may signify dehydration.*
• Assess cardiovascular and GI status *to detect the effectiveness of treatment.*
• Administer hyperthermia therapy by using a warming blanket, limiting exposure during routine nursing care, and covering the child with warm blankets *to help the child become normothermic.*
• Administer acetylcysteine in a carbonated beverage. *Acetylcysteine has an offensive odor and taste. Administering this drug in a carbonated beverage will help the child swallow it. In small children, administer it directly into an NG tube to avoid this difficulty.*

Teaching topics
• Storing medication safely and other steps to prevent overdose

Celiac disease

Celiac disease is characterized by poor food absorption and intolerance of gluten, which is a protein found in grains, such as wheat, rye, oats, and barley.

In celiac disease, the child experiences a decrease in the amount and activity of enzymes in the intestinal mucosal cells. This causes the villi of the proximal small intestine to atrophy, decreasing intestinal absorption. Celiac disease usually becomes apparent between 6 and 18 months of age.

CAUSES
• Gluten intolerance (inability to absorb rye, oat, wheat, and barley glutens)
• Immunoglobulin A deficiency
• Too-early introduction of protein solids

ASSESSMENT FINDINGS
• Abdominal distention
• Abdominal pain
• Anorexia

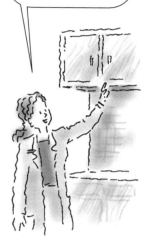

Put it away. Safe medicine storage helps prevent acetaminophen poisoning.

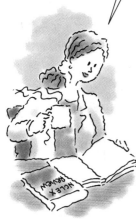

If a child demonstrates malnutrition, steatorrhea, and chronic diarrhea 2 to 4 months after solid foods are introduced, suspect celiac disease.

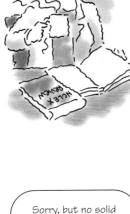

• Generalized malnutrition and failure to thrive due to malabsorption of protein and carbohydrates
• Irritability
• Steatorrhea and chronic diarrhea due to fat malabsorption
• Weight and height below normal for age-group

DIAGNOSTIC TEST RESULTS
• Blood chemistry tests reveal hypocalcemia and hypoalbuminemia.
• Hematology reveals decreased hemoglobin level and hypothrombinemia.
• Immunologic assay screen is positive for celiac disease.
• Intestinal biopsy is used to confirm the diagnosis.
• Stool specimen reveals high fat content.

NURSING DIAGNOSES
• Altered nutrition: Less than body requirements
• Pain
• Fluid volume deficit

TREATMENT
• Diet: gluten-free but includes corn and rice products, soy and potato flour, breast milk or soy-based formula, and all fresh fruits
• Folate
• Iron (Feosol) supplements
• Vitamins A and D in water-soluble forms

INTERVENTIONS AND RATIONALES
• Give the child small, frequent meals *to reduce fatigue and improve nutritional intake.*
• Record the consistency, appearance, and number of stools. *The disappearance of steatorrhea is a good indicator that the child's ability to absorb nutrients is improving.*
• Monitor growth and development *to assess for growth delay and to detect changes in level of functioning* and, as appropriate, plan an activity program for the child.

Teaching topics
• Waiting until after age 6 months to introduce solid foods (to prevent the disease)
• Specific foods and formula the child can eat (breads made from rice, corn, soybean, pota-

Sorry, but no solid foods until you're 6 months old. Gotta watch out for celiac disease.

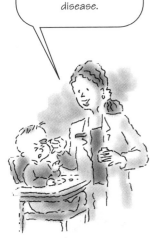

to, tapioca, sago or gluten-free wheat; dry cereals made only with rice or corn; cornmeal or hominy)

Cleft lip and palate

In this disorder, the bone and tissue of the upper jaw and palate fail to fuse completely at the midline. The defects may be partial or complete, unilateral or bilateral, and may involve just the lip, just the palate, or both.

Cleft lip and palate also increase the risk of:
• aspiration because increased open space in the mouth may cause formula or breast milk to exit through the nose with wet burps
• upper respiratory infection and otitis media, because the increased open space decreases natural defenses against bacterial invasion.

CAUSES
• Congenital defects; in some cases, inheritance plays a role
• Part of another chromosomal or mendelian abnormality
• Prenatal exposure to teratogens

ASSESSMENT FINDINGS
• Abdominal distention from swallowed air
• Cleft lip: can range from a simple notch on the upper lip to complete cleft from the lip edge to the floor of the nostril, on either side of the midline, but rarely along the midline itself
• Cleft palate: may be partial or complete
• Difficulty swallowing
Note that cleft lip with or without cleft palate is obvious at birth; cleft palate without cleft lip may not be detected until a mouth examination is done or until feeding difficulties develop.

DIAGNOSTIC TEST RESULTS
• Prenatal ultrasonography may indicate severe defects.

NURSING DIAGNOSES
• Altered nutrition: Less than body requirements
• Impaired swallowing
• Risk for aspiration

TREATMENT

- Cheiloplasty performed between birth and age 3 months to unite the lip and gum edges in anticipation of teeth eruption, providing a route for adequate nutrition and sucking
- Cleft palate repair surgery (staphylorrhaphy); scheduled at about age 18 months to allow for growth of the palate and to be done before the infant develops speech patterns; infant must be free from ear and respiratory infections
- Long-term, team-oriented care to address speech defects, dental and orthodontic problems, nasal defects, and possible alterations in hearing
- If cleft lip is detected on sonogram while the infant is in utero, possible fetal repair

INTERVENTIONS

- Monitor vital signs and intake and output *to determine fluid volume status.*
- Assess respiratory status *to detect signs of aspiration.*
- Assess the quality of the child's suck by determining if the infant can form an airtight seal around a finger or nipple placed in the infant's mouth *to determine an effective feeding method.*
- Be alert for respiratory distress when feeding *to avoid aspiration.*
- As the child grows older, explore the child's feelings *to assess actual and potential coping problems.*

Preoperative interventions for cleft lip repair

- Feed the infant slowly and in an upright position *to decrease the risk of aspiration.*
- Burp the infant frequently during feeding *to eliminate swallowed air and decrease the risk of emesis.*
- Use gavage feedings *if oral feedings are unsuccessful.*
- Administer a small amount of water after feedings *to prevent formula from accumulating and becoming a medium for bacterial growth.*
- Give small, frequent feedings *to promote adequate nutrition and prevent tiring the infant.*
- Hold the infant while feeding and promote sucking between meals. *Sucking is important to speech development.*

Postoperative interventions for cleft lip repair

- Observe for cyanosis as the infant begins to breathe through the nose *to detect signs of respiratory compromise.*
- Keep the infant's hands away from the mouth by using restraints or pinning the sleeves to the shirt; Steri Strips are used to hold the suture line in place *to prevent tension and to maintain an intact suture line.*
- Anticipate the infant's needs *to prevent crying*; don't position him prone.
- Give extra care and support *because the infant can't meet emotional needs by sucking.*
- Use a syringe with tubing to administer foods at the side of the mouth *to prevent trauma to the suture line.*
- Place the infant on the right side *to prevent aspiration;* clean the suture line after each feeding by dabbing it with half-strength hydrogen peroxide or saline solution *to prevent crusts and scarring.*
- Monitor for pain and administer pain medication as prescribed; note effectiveness of pain medication *to promote comfort.*

Preoperative interventions for cleft palate repair

- Feed the infant with a cleft palate nipple or a Teflon implant *to enhance nutritional intake.*
- Wean the infant from the bottle or breast before cleft palate surgery; *the toddler must be able to drink from a cup.*

Postoperative interventions for cleft palate repair

- Position the toddler on the abdomen or side *to promote a patent airway.*
- Anticipate edema and a decreased airway from palate closure; this may make the toddler appear temporarily dyspneic; assess for signs of altered oxygenation *to promote good respiration.*
- Keep hard or pointed objects (utensils, straws, frozen dessert sticks) away from the mouth *to prevent trauma to the suture line.*
- Use a cup to feed; don't use a nipple or pacifier *to prevent injury to the suture line.*
- Use elbow restraints *to keep the toddler's hands out of the mouth.*
- Provide soft toys *to prevent injury.*

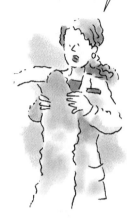

Cleft lip and palate increase the risk of aspiration during feeding, respiratory infection, and otitis media.

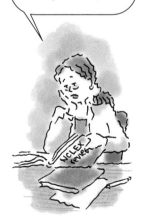

Having fun yet? Make plans to do something enjoyable later. That will give you motivation to keep studying now.

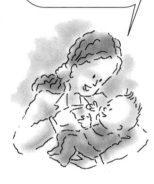

Feeding the newborn a few sips of sterile water will detect or rule out esophageal atresia and tracheoesophageal fistula.

• Start the toddler on clear liquids and progress to a soft diet; rinse the suture line by giving the toddler a sip of water after each feeding *to prevent infection.*
• Distract or hold the toddler *to try to keep the tongue away from the roof of the mouth.*

Teaching topics
• The importance of parental involvement (Because it results in facial disfigurement, the condition may cause shock, guilt, and grief for the parents and may block parental bonding with the child.)
• Need for follow-up speech therapy
• Understanding the child's susceptibility to pathogens and otitis media from the altered position of the eustachian tubes

Esophageal atresia and tracheoesophageal fistula

Esophageal atresia occurs when the proximal end of the esophagus ends in a blind pouch; food can't enter the stomach via the esophagus.

Tracheoesophageal fistula occurs when a connection exists between the esophagus and the trachea. It may result in the reflux of gastric juice after feeding; this can allow acidic stomach contents to cross the fistula, irritating the trachea.

Esophageal atresia and tracheoesophageal fistula occur in many combinations and may be associated with other defects. Esophageal atresia with tracheoesophageal fistula is the most common of these conditions. Esophageal atresia alone is the second most common of these conditions.

Esophageal atresia with tracheoesophageal fistula occurs when either:
• the distal end of the esophagus ends in a blind pouch and the proximal end of the esophagus is linked to the trachea via a fistula
• the proximal end of the esophagus ends in a blind pouch and the distal portion of the esophagus is connected to the trachea via a fistula.

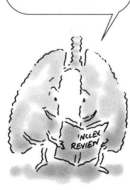

Preventing respiratory complications is key to postoperative care in esophageal atresia and tracheoesophageal fistula repair.

CONTRIBUTING FACTOR
• Prematurity

ASSESSMENT FINDINGS
Esophageal atresia
• Excessive salivation and drooling due to inability to pass food through the esophagus
• Inability to pass an NG tube
• Regurgitation of undigested formula immediately after feeding; possible respiratory distress and cyanosis if secretions are aspirated

Tracheoesophageal fistula
• Abdominal distention from air that goes through the fistula into the stomach
• Choking, coughing, and intermittent cyanosis during feeding due to food that goes through the fistula into the trachea
• Excessive drooling of saliva; possibly the first symptom
• Tracheal irritation from gastric acids that reflux across the fistula

Esophageal atresia with tracheoesophageal fistula
• Excessive salivation and drooling due to inability to pass food through the esophagus
• Inability to pass an NG tube
• Regurgitation of undigested formula immediately after feeding; possible respiratory distress and cyanosis if secretions are aspirated
• Signs of respiratory distress (coughing, choking, and intermittent cyanosis) because the infant has difficulty tolerating oral foods and handling oral secretions or refluxed gastric contents

DIAGNOSTIC TEST RESULTS
• Newborns are fed first with a few sips of sterile water to detect these anomalies and to prevent the aspiration of formula or breast milk into the lungs.

NURSING DIAGNOSES
• Altered nutrition: Less than body requirements
• Risk of infection
• Risk for altered parenting

TREATMENT
• Gastrostomy tube (PEG tube) inserted (child not fed orally)
• Surgical correction by ligating the tracheo-esophageal fistula and reanastomosing the esophageal ends; in many cases, repair done in stages

INTERVENTIONS AND RATIONALES
• Monitor vital signs to detect tachycardia and tachypnea, *which could indicate hypoxemia.*
• Assess respiratory status. *Poor respiratory status may result in hypoxemia.*
• Position the infant with his head elevated to 30 degrees *to decrease reflux at the distal esophagus.*
• Suction as needed *to stimulate cough and clear airways.*
• Keep the PEG tube open and suspended above the child *for release of gas.*
• If feeding the child through a gastrostomy tube after surgery, anticipate abdominal distention from air; keep the child upright during feedings *to reduce the chance of refluxed stomach contents and aspiration pneumonia* and keep tube open and elevated before and after feedings.
• Administer gastrostomy feedings only by gravity flow — not a feeding pump — *to help meet nutritional and metabolic requirements.*

Postoperative care
• Maintain chest tube and respiratory support *to prevent respiratory compromise.*
• Keep a suction catheter ready *to get rid of secretions and prevent aspiration.*
• Mark the catheter to indicate the distance from the infant's nose to the point just above the anastomosis *to avoid causing trauma to the anastomosis site.*
• Make sure the NG tube is secure and handle with extreme caution *to avoid displacement.*
• Administer antibiotics as prescribed *to prevent infection.*
• Administer total parenteral nutrition *to maintain nutritional support.*

Teaching topics
• Understanding proper care of child at home, such as feeding and bathing techniques

Failure to thrive

Failure to thrive is a chronic, potentially life-threatening condition characterized by failure to maintain weight and height above the 5th percentile on age-appropriate growth charts. Most children are diagnosed before age 2. It can result from physical, emotional, or psychological causes.

CAUSES
• Organic: acute or chronic illness (GI reflux, malabsorption syndrome, congenital heart defect, or cystic fibrosis)
• Nonorganic: psychological problem between child and primary caregiver, such as failure to bond
• Mixed: combination of organic and nonorganic

ASSESSMENT FINDINGS
• Altered body posture; child is stiff or floppy, doesn't cuddle
• Delayed psychosocial behavior; for example, reluctance to smile or talk
• Disparities between chronologic age and height and weight
• History of inadequate feeding techniques, such as bottle propping or insufficient burping
• History of insufficient stimulation and inadequate parental knowledge of child development
• History of medical problems
• History of sleep disturbances
• Psychosocial family problems
• Regurgitation of food after almost every feeding, part being vomited and the remainder swallowed (rumination of food)

DIAGNOSTIC TEST RESULTS
• Negative nitrogen balance indicates inadequate intake of protein or calories.
• Associated physiologic causes may be detected.

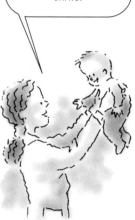

Providing adequate stimulation helps to prevent failure to thrive.

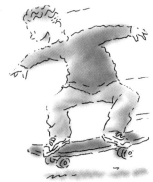

Visual and auditory stimulation are awesome.

• Reduced creatinine-height index reflects muscle mass and estimates muscle protein depletion.

NURSING DIAGNOSES
• Altered growth and development
• Altered parenting
• Altered nutrition: Less than body requirements

TREATMENT
• High-calorie diet
• Parent counseling
• Respite care for the child

Drug therapy
• Vitamin and mineral supplements

INTERVENTIONS AND RATIONALES
• Weigh the child on admission *to determine baseline weight.*
• Assess growth and development using an appropriate tool such as the Denver Developmental Screening Test *to determine the child's developmental level.*
• Properly feed and interact with the child *to promote nutrition and growth and development.*
• Establish specific times for feeding, bathing, and sleeping *to establish and maintain a structured routine.*
• Provide the child with visual and auditory stimulation *to promote normal sensory development.*
• Assess interaction of parent with child *to determine if failure to thrive is due to parent's inability to form emotional attachment to child.*
• When caring for the child in the parent's presence, act as a role model for effective parenting skills. Demonstrate comfort measures such as rocking the infant, and show the mother how to hold the infant in an en face position *to increase the parent's knowledge of routine child care practices.*
• Teach the mother about normal growth and development and identify ages at which the child should be able to master developmental tasks such as rolling over, crawling, and walking. *This will assist the parents in monitoring the child's growth and development.* Also dis-

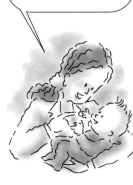

When caring for the child in the parents' presence, act as a role model for effective parenting skills.

cuss problem behaviors associated with specific ages, such as colic, temper tantrums, and sleeping difficulties, *to further enhance the parents' understanding of developmental norms.*
• Discuss the child's need for tactile and sensory stimulation. Demonstrate play activities that promote developmental skills, such as shaking a rattle in front of the infant to build eye-and-hand coordination or placing a mobile above the infant to encourage visual tracking and trunk and head control. *Sensory experiences promote cognitive development.*

Teaching topics
• Understanding normal parenting skills
• Obtaining counseling for the parents, if necessary
• Understanding feeding techniques

Intestinal obstruction

Intestinal obstruction is the partial or complete blockage of the lumen in the small or large bowel. Small-bowel obstruction is far more common and usually more serious. Complete obstruction in any part of the bowel, if untreated, can cause death within hours from shock and vascular collapse.

Intestinal obstruction can occur in three forms:

simple: blockage prevents intestinal contents from passing, with no other complications

strangulated: blood supply to part or all of the obstructed section is cut off, in addition to blockage of the lumen

close-looped: both ends of a bowel section are occluded, isolating it from the rest of the intestine.

CAUSES
Mechanical causes
• Adhesions and strangulated hernias (most common causes of small-bowel obstruction)
• Carcinomas (most common cause of large-bowel obstruction)

• Compression of the bowel wall due to stenosis, intussusception, volvulus of the sigmoid or cecum, tumors, or atresia
• Congenital bowel deformities
• Ingestion of foreign bodies (such as fruit pits or worms)
• Obstruction after abdominal surgery

Other causes
• Paralytic ileus
• Electrolyte imbalances
• Toxicity (uremia, generalized infection)
• Neurogenic abnormalities (spinal cord lesions)
• Thrombosis or embolism of mesenteric vessels

ASSESSMENT FINDINGS
Partial small-bowel obstruction
• Abdominal distention
• Colicky pain
• Constipation
• Drowsiness
• Dry oral mucous membranes and tongue
• Intense thirst
• Malaise
• Nausea
• Vomiting (the higher the obstruction, the earlier and more severe the vomiting)

Complete small-bowel obstruction
• Persistent epigastric or periumbilical pain
• Bowel contents propelled toward mouth (instead of rectum) by vigorous peristaltic waves

Partial large-bowel obstruction
In partial large-bowel obstruction, signs and symptoms develop slowly because the colon can absorb fluid from its contents and distend well beyond its normal size. Signs and symptoms may include the following:
• dramatic abdominal distention
• colicky abdominal pain; may appear suddenly, producing spasms that last less than 1 minute and recur every few minutes
• constipation (may be only clinical effect for days)
• continuous hypogastric pain and nausea; vomiting usually absent at first
• leakage of liquid stools around the obstruction (common)

• loops of large bowel becoming visible on the abdomen.

Complete large-bowel obstruction
• Continuous pain
• Fecal vomiting
• Localized peritonitis

DIAGNOSTIC TEST RESULTS
• In large-bowel obstruction, barium enema reveals a distended, air-filled colon or, in sigmoid volvulus, a closed loop of sigmoid with extreme distention.
• Arterial blood gas (ABG) analysis reveals metabolic alkalosis from dehydration and loss of gastric hydrochloric acid, characteristic of obstruction in the upper intestine.
• ABG analysis reveals metabolic acidosis caused by slower dehydration and loss of intestinal alkaline fluids, characteristic of lower-bowel obstruction.
• X-rays confirm the diagnosis. Abdominal films show the presence and location of intestinal gas or fluid.

NURSING DIAGNOSES
• Altered nutrition: Less than body requirements
• Pain
• Altered tissue perfusion (gastrointestinal)

TREATMENT
• I.V. therapy to correct fluid and electrolyte imbalances
• NG intubation to decompress the bowel to relieve vomiting and distention
• Surgical resection with anastomosis, colostomy, or ileostomy, commonly after decompression with an NG tube (for large-bowel obstruction)
• Total parenteral nutrition for protein deficit from chronic obstruction, paralytic ileus, infection, or prolonged postoperative recovery time that requires NPO status

Drug therapy
• Analgesics (usually nonnarcotic to avoid reduced intestinal motility commonly caused by narcotic analgesics)
• Antibiotics for peritonitis

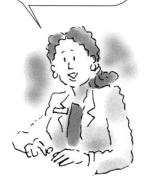

In mechanical obstruction, movement of intestinal contents is impaired by an identifiable obstructing source.

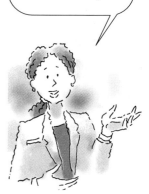

When the obstruction is high in the intestine, vomiting is marked and abdominal distention is limited. When the obstruction is low, the child has marked distention but little vomiting.

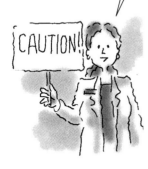

In children with intestinal obstruction, watch out for shock, metabolic alkalosis or acidosis, and secondary infection.

INTERVENTIONS AND RATIONALES

• Monitor vital signs frequently. *A drop in blood pressure may indicate reduced circulating blood volume due to blood loss from a strangulated hernia. As much as 10 L of fluid can collect in the small bowel, drastically reducing plasma volume.*

• Assess child's cardiovascular status *to observe for signs of shock, such as pallor, rapid pulse, and hypotension.*

• Stay alert for signs and symptoms of metabolic alkalosis (changes in sensorium; slow, shallow respirations; hypertonic muscles; tetany) or acidosis (dyspnea on exertion; disorientation; and later, deep, rapid breathing, weakness, and malaise). *This allows for early detection of complications.*

• Watch for signs and symptoms of secondary infection, such as fever and chills. *Sustained temperature elevations after surgery may signal onset of pulmonary complications or wound infection.*

• Monitor intake and output; monitor urine output carefully *to assess renal function, circulating blood volume, and possible urine retention caused by bladder compression by the distended intestine.*

• Catheterize the child for residual urine immediately after he has voided *if you suspect bladder compression.* Also, measure abdominal girth frequently *to detect progressive distention.*

• Provide fastidious mouth and nose care if the child has vomited or undergone decompression by intubation *to prevent skin breakdown.* Look for signs of dehydration (thick, swollen tongue; dry, cracked lips; dry oral mucous membranes).

• Keep the child in Fowler's position as much as possible *to promote pulmonary ventilation and ease respiratory distress from abdominal distention.*

• Listen for bowel sounds, and watch for signs of returning peristalsis (passage of flatus and mucus through the rectum) *to promote nutritional status.*

• Arrange for an enterostomal therapist to visit the child who has had an ostomy *to provide education and information and relieve anxiety.*

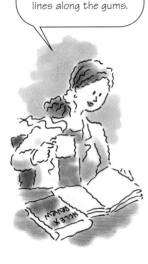

Vomiting and weight loss are key signs of lead poisoning. You may also see lead lines along the gums.

Teaching topics

• Prepare the child and his family for the possibility of surgery, and provide emotional support and positive reinforcement afterward.

Lead poisoning

Lead poisoning occurs most commonly in toddlers. Lead is poorly absorbed by the body and slowly excreted, replacing calcium in the bones and increasing the permeability of central nervous system membranes.

CAUSES

• Teething on or eating lead-based paint or inhaling lead dust

ASSESSMENT FINDINGS

• Bone pain
• Constipation
• Increased intracranial pressure, cortical atrophy, behavioral changes, altered cognition and motor skills, and seizures
• Lead lines visible along gums
• Peripheral neuritis from calcium release into the blood
• Vomiting
• Weight loss

DIAGNOSTIC TEST RESULTS

• Hematologic studies reveal anemia and increased erythrocyte polyphoria.
• Lead poisoning is confirmed when the child has two successive blood lead levels greater than 10 mg/dl.
• Urinalysis reveals proteinuria, ketonuria, and glycosuria.
• X-rays reveal lead lines near the epiphyseal lines (areas of increased density) of long bones. The thickness of the line shows the length of time the lead ingestion has been occurring.
• Lumbar puncture reveals increased protein level in cerebrospinal fluid sample.

NURSING DIAGNOSES

• Altered cerebral tissue perfusion
• Risk for fluid volume deficit
• Risk for poisoning

TREATMENT

- Oral or I.V. fluid administration to lower blood lead level and prevent lead encephalopathy
- Low-fat diet with adequate supplies of calcium, magnesium, zinc, iron, and copper; prevents any more lead from being bound and stored in the body's fat tissues

Drug therapy

- Chelating agents, such as ethylenediaminetetraacetic acid (EDTA) or dimercaprol (BAL in oil). Chelating agents bind with lead and are excreted by the kidneys.

INTERVENTIONS AND RATIONALES

- Monitor calcium levels (chelating agents also bind with calcium) *to prevent tetany and seizures, which may result from hypocalcemia.*
- Administer EDTA deep I.M. into a large muscle mass *to help minimize pain.* This drug may also be administered with an anesthetic agent *to minimize pain.*
- Monitor vital signs, intake and output, hydration status, and kidney function *to ensure that kidney function is adequate to handle the lead being excreted. If kidney function isn't adequate, EDTA may cause kidney damage.*
- Assess cardiovascular and neurologic status. *Increased levels of lead can cause severe encephalopathy with seizures and permanent neurologic damage.*

Teaching topics

- Referrals to help family members discover and remove the source of the lead contamination
- Careful hand washing with hot soapy water before eating
- Teaching children to keep hands, toys, and all other objects out of the mouth
- Washing pacifiers and other items meant to be put in the mouth (especially if item falls on the floor or other dirty surface)
- Stressing the importance of a well-balanced diet to ensure that the child receives adequate amounts of calcium, magnesium, zinc, iron, and copper
- The importance of allowing the tap water to run for 2 minutes before using water for drinking, cooking, or making formula
- Cautioning against storing food in open cans and about using cookware or ceramic dishes that may contain lead or be fired incorrectly
- Reporting stomachaches, irritability, and headaches, which may be early signs of higher than normal lead levels

Pyloric stenosis

In pyloric stenosis, hyperplasia and hypertrophy of the circular muscle at the pylorus narrow the pyloric canal, thereby preventing the stomach from emptying normally. The defect is most commonly seen in male infants between ages 1 and 6 months.

CAUSES

- Exact cause unknown

ASSESSMENT FINDINGS

- Olive-size bulge palpated below the right costal margin
- Poor weight gain
- Symptoms of malnutrition and dehydration despite the child's apparent adequate intake of food
- Projectile emesis during or shortly after feedings, preceded by reverse peristaltic waves (going left to right) but not by nausea; child resumes eating after vomiting
- Symptoms appearing at about 4 weeks in formula-fed infants and about 6 weeks in breast-fed infants
- Tetany

DIAGNOSTIC TEST RESULTS

- ABG analysis reveals metabolic alkalosis.
- Blood chemistry tests may reveal hypocalcemia, hypokalemia, and hypochloremia.
- Hematest reveals emesis containing blood.
- Ultrasound shows hypertrophied sphincter.
- Endoscopy reveals hypertrophied sphincter.

NURSING DIAGNOSES

- Altered nutrition: Less than body requirements
- Risk for fluid volume deficit
- Risk for infection

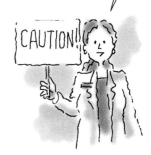

Avoid a calcium calamity. Chelating agents used to treat lead poisoning also bind with calcium, leading to decreased calcium levels.

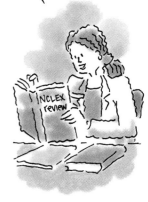

The pylorus is the outlet from the stomach to the duodenum.

TREATMENT
• Diet: Maintain NPO status before surgery
• I.V. therapy to correct fluid and electrolyte imbalances
• Possible insertion of an NG tube, kept open and elevated for gastric decompression
• Surgical intervention: pyloromyotomy performed by laparoscopy

Drug therapy
• Potassium supplements but only after it's confirmed that kidneys are functioning properly
• I.V. calcium administration

INTERVENTIONS AND RATIONALES
• Weigh the child daily *to assess growth.*
• Monitor vital signs and intake and output *to assess renal function and check for signs of dehydration.*
• Assess for metabolic alkalosis and dehydration from frequent emesis *to detect early complications.*
• Assess abdominal and cardiovascular status *to detect early signs of compromise.*
• Provide small, frequent, thickened feedings with the head of the bed elevated; burp the child frequently (preoperatively) *to promote nutrition and prevent aspiration.*
• Position the child on the right side *to prevent the aspiration of vomitus.*

Postoperative care
• After surgery, feed the infant small amounts of oral electrolyte solution at first; then increase the amount and concentration of food until normal feeding is achieved *to meet nutritional needs and prevent vomiting.*
• Provide a pacifier *to meet nonnutritive sucking needs and maintain comfort.*
• Provide routine postoperative care *to maintain and improve the child's condition and to detect early complications. Position the child on his side so if vomiting occurs there is little chance of aspiration. Laying the child on the right side possibly aids the flow of fluid through the pyloric valve by gravity.*
• Keep the incision area clean. *The child is at an increased risk for infection because the incision is near the diaper area.*

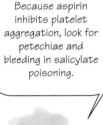

> Because aspirin inhibits platelet aggregation, look for petechiae and bleeding in salicylate poisoning.

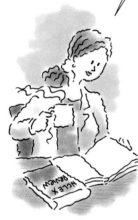

Teaching topics
• Feeding the infant, including specific formula, volume, and technique
• Preventing infection

Salicylate poisoning

Salicylate (aspirin) is an analgesic, antipyretic, and anti-inflammatory agent that inhibits platelet aggregation. Poisoning may result from an overdose of salicylate. Symptoms begin when children ingest 150 to 200 mg of aspirin per kilogram of body weight. The peak blood level is reached within 2 to 3 hours of ingestion. The prognosis of the child with salicylate poisoning depends on the amount of salicylate ingested and how quickly treatment begins.

CAUSE
• Aspirin overdose

ASSESSMENT FINDINGS
• Coma
• Diarrhea
• High fever from the stimulation of carbohydrate metabolism
• Increased respiratory rate from metabolic acidosis
• Irritability, restlessness
• Petechiae and bleeding tendency
• Restlessness
• Seizures
• Stomach ulcer
• Stupor
• Tachycardia
• Tinnitus or altered hearing
• Vomiting

DIAGNOSTIC TEST RESULTS
• Blood glucose levels are decreased.
• Prothrombin time is prolonged.
• Serum salicylate levels are elevated.

NURSING DIAGNOSES
• Altered nutrition: Less than body requirements
• Hyperthermia
• Risk for fluid volume deficit

TREATMENT
• I.V. fluids
• Gastric lavage or emesis induction with ipecac syrup
• Hemodialysis
• Hypothermia blanket
• Possible intubation and mechanical ventilation

Drug therapy
• Calcium and potassium supplements, if indicated
• Sodium bicarbonate

INTERVENTIONS AND RATIONALES
• Administer oral and I.V. fluids *to dilute the poison and prevent dehydration.*
• Monitor vital signs and intake and output *to detect dehydration and early signs of compromise.*
• Assess cardiovascular and GI status *to assess for signs of metabolic acidosis and GI bleeding.*
• Maintain mechanical ventilation, if required, *to ensure adequate oxygenation.*
• Ensure adequate hydration *to flush the aspirin through the kidneys.*
• Monitor urine pH; *pH over 8 aids salicylate excretion.*
• Dress the child lightly and sponge with tepid water or use a cooling blanket *to reduce fear and promote comfort.*
• Monitor body temperature every 15 to 30 minutes according to policy while hypothermia blanket is in use *to evaluate its effectiveness and prevent injury.*

Teaching topics
• Storing medication and taking steps to prevent aspirin overdose
• Monitoring child's temperature and encouraging a high fluid intake

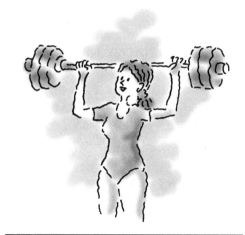

Pump up on practice questions

1. A 3-week-old infant diagnosed with pyloric stenosis is admitted to the hospital during a vomiting episode. Which action by the nurse is most appropriate?
  A. Placing the infant on the back to sleep
  B. Weighing the infant every 12 hours
  C. Positioning the infant on the right side
  D. Taking vital signs every 8 hours
Answer: C. The nurse should position the infant on the right side to prevent aspiration. The infant should be weighed daily, not every 12 hours. Vital signs should be monitored every 4 hours, not every 8 hours.

➡ *NCLEX keys*
Nursing process step: Implementation
Client needs category: Physiological integrity
Client needs subcategory: Reduction of risk potential
Taxonomic level: Application

2. The nurse teaches a mother to position an infant with a tracheoesophageal fistula with his head elevated to 30 degrees. The nurse should recognize that teaching was effective when the mother makes which of the following statements?

A. "Positioning him with his head elevated to 30 degrees helps his breathing."
B. "Positioning him with his head elevated to 30 degrees helps with eating."
C. "Positioning him with his head elevated to 30 degrees keeps gastric juices from backing up."
D. "Positioning him with his head elevated to 30 degrees makes him comfortable."

Answer: C. Placing the infant with his head elevated to 30 degrees helps decrease gastric reflux into the trachea. The child won't be taking food by mouth until after the fistula is surgically repaired. The infant will also breathe easier and be more comfortable with his head elevated, but they aren't the primary reasons for elevating the infant's head to 30 degrees.

➡ *NCLEX keys*
Nursing process step: Evaluation
Client needs category: Physiological integrity
Client needs subcategory: Reduction of risk potential
Taxonomic level: Application

3. A child with a nasogastric (NG) tube in place complains of nausea. Which action by the nurse is most appropriate?
A. Administer an antiemetic.
B. Irrigate the NG tube.
C. Notify the physician about the nausea.
D. Reposition the NG tube.

Answer: B. The nurse should first check NG tube placement, then irrigate the tube to check for patency. If nausea continues, the NG tube may be repositioned, depending on the child's condition. If the child continues to complain of nausea after these measures, the physician should be notified and an antiemetic given as ordered.

➡ *NCLEX keys*
Nursing process step: Implementation
Client needs category: Physiological integrity
Client needs subcategory: Reduction of risk potential
Taxonomic level: Application

4. The mother of a child diagnosed with celiac disease asks the nurse which foods should be eliminated from her child's diet. The nurse should advise the mother to eliminate:
A. malted milk, wheat bread, and spaghetti.
B. rice cereals, milk, and corn bread.
C. tapioca, potato bread, and peanut butter.
D. corn cereals, milk, and honey.

Answer: A. The mother should provide her child with celiac disease with a gluten-free diet, eliminating such foods as malted milk, wheat bread, and spaghetti. Rice and corn cereals, milk, corn and potato breads, tapioca, peanut butter, and honey are all appropriate for a gluten-free diet.

➡ *NCLEX keys*
Nursing process step: Implementation
Client needs category: Physiological integrity
Client needs subcategory: Basic care and comfort
Taxonomic level: Application

5. The nurse is caring for a toddler after surgical repair of a cleft palate. The nurse should position the child:
A. on the back.
B. on the stomach.
C. on the back with the head slightly elevated.
D. for comfort.

Answer: B. After surgical repair of a cleft palate, the child should be positioned on the stomach to prevent pooling of secretions in the oropharynx. The child shouldn't be positioned on the back. The nurse shouldn't choose a position based on comfort.

➡ *NCLEX keys*
Nursing process step: Implementation
Client needs category: Physiological integrity
Client needs subcategory: Reduction of risk potential
Taxonomic level: Application

6. The nurse is caring for a child with a complete intestinal obstruction. Which is a key finding in this client?
   A. Vomiting
   B. Intense thirst
   C. Visible peristaltic waves
   D. Nausea

Answer: C. Visible peristaltic waves propel bowel contents toward the mouth instead of the rectum. Vomiting, intense thirst, and nausea are symptoms of a small-bowel obstruction and aren't the key findings in complete intestinal obstruction.

➡ *NCLEX keys*
Nursing process step: Assessment
Client needs category: Physiological integrity
Client needs subcategory: Reduction of risk potential
Taxonomic level: Comprehension

7. The nurse is caring for an infant with a cleft lip and palate. This condition places the infant at increased risk for:
   A. upper respiratory infections and otitis media.
   B. otitis media and diarrhea.
   C. upper respiratory infections and diarrhea.
   D. diarrhea and vomiting.

Answer: A. The infant with a cleft lip and palate is at increased risk for upper respiratory infections and otitis media because the increased open space decreases natural defenses against bacteria. It doesn't increase the risk of vomiting and diarrhea.

➡ *NCLEX keys*
Nursing process step: Assessment
Client needs category: Physiological integrity
Client needs subcategory: Reduction of risk potential
Taxonomic level: Application

8. The nurse is teaching the mother of an infant with a cleft palate. Which of the following teaching points should the nurse tell the mother?

   A. Surgical repair is delayed until the child is 6 months old.
   B. Surgical repair is delayed until the child is 18 months old.
   C. Surgical repair is done between birth and 3 months of age.
   D. Surgical repair is done as soon as arrangements can be made.

Answer: B. Surgical repair of a cleft palate (staphylorrhaphy) is scheduled at about age 18 months to allow for growth of the palate and to be done before the infant develops speech patterns. Surgical repair of a cleft lip (cheiloplasty) takes place between birth and 3 months of age.

➡ *NCLEX keys*
Nursing process step: Planning
Client needs category: Physiological integrity
Client needs subcategory: Reduction of risk potential
Taxonomic level: Knowledge

9. A 4-week-old infant is brought to the pediatrician's office. The infant has been experiencing projectile vomiting shortly after feedings. The infant most likely has:
   A. an intestinal obstruction.
   B. intussusception.
   C. a tracheoesophageal fistula.
   D. pyloric stenosis.

Answer: D. Symptoms of pyloric stenosis generally develop between 4 and 6 weeks of age. They include a palpable bulge below the right costal margin, projectile vomiting during or shortly after feeding, resuming feeding after vomiting, poor weight gain, malnutrition, and dehydration. Intestinal obstruction presents with constipation, colicky abdominal pain, nausea, and dramatic abdominal distention. Intussusception causes sudden onset of severe abdominal pain; the infant is usually inconsolable. Tracheoesophageal fistula causes coughing, choking, and intermittent cyanosis during feeding, and abdominal distention.

➠ *NCLEX keys*
Nursing process step: Assessment
Client needs category: Physiological integrity
Client needs subcategory: Reduction of risk potential
Taxonomic level: Application

10. The nurse is caring for a neonate. What intervention is routinely performed for all newborns to rule out the possibility of tracheoesophageal fistula and esophageal atresia?

    A. Feeding the newborn a few sips of sterile water before introducing breast milk or formula

    B. Feeding the newborn a few sips of formula before introducing breast milk

    C. Feeding the infant a few sips of formula in an upright position

    D. Feeding the newborn sterile water for the first two feedings

Answer: A. All newborns should be fed first with a few sips of sterile water to rule out these anomalies and to prevent the aspiration of formula into the lungs. Feeding the infant formula or breast milk first could put the newborn at risk for aspiration pneumonia if either anomaly is present.

➠ *NCLEX keys*
Nursing process step: Implementation
Client needs category: Health promotion and maintenance
Client needs subcategory: Growth and development through the life span
Taxonomic level: Knowledge

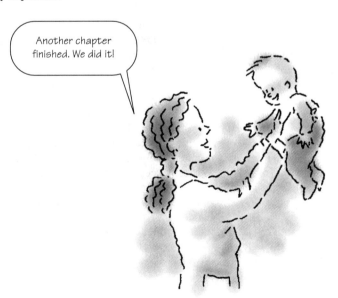

Another chapter finished. We did it!

33 Endocrine System

Brush up on key concepts

Together with the nervous system, the endocrine system regulates and integrates the body's metabolic activities. A disorder of the endocrine system involves a hyposecretion or hypersecretion of hormones, which affect the body's metabolic processes and function.

At any time, you can review the major points of this chapter by consulting the *Cheat sheet* on page 658.

Endocrine junior

Here are key points about **endocrine functioning in childhood**.
• The pituitary gland controls the release of seven different hormones and is the master gland for all age-groups.
• The adrenal cortex begins secreting glucocorticoids and mineralocorticoids early in embryonic life.
• The thyroid gland, many times larger in children than adults, is functional at 2 weeks. It is thought to play a role in immune function.

Ch..ch..changes

The pituitary is stimulated at puberty to produce androgen steroids responsible for **secondary sex characteristics**.

Female secondary sexual development during puberty involves increase in the size of the ovaries, uterus, vagina, labia, and breasts. The first visible sign of sexual maturity is the appearance of breast buds. Body hair appears in the pubic area and under the arms and menarche begins. The ovaries, present at birth, remain inactive until puberty.

Male secondary sexual development consists of genital growth and the appearance of pubic and body hair.

A place to integrate

The endocrine system meets the nervous system at the **hypothalamus**. The hypothalamus, the main integrative center for the endocrine and autonomic nervous systems, controls the function of endocrine organs by neural and hormonal pathways.

Neural pathways connect the hypothalamus to the posterior pituitary, or neurohypophysis. Neural stimulation to the posterior pituitary provokes the secretion of hormones (chemical transmitters released from specialized cells into the bloodstream). Hormones are then carried to specialized organ-receptor cells that respond to them.

Negative feedback

In addition to hormonal and neural controls, a **negative feedback system** regulates the endocrine system. The mechanism of feedback may be either simple or complex.
• **Simple feedback** occurs when the level of one substance regulates secretion of a hormone. For example, low serum calcium levels stimulate parathyroid hormone secretion; high serum calcium levels inhibit it.
• **Complex feedback** occurs through an axis established between the hypothalamus, pituitary gland, and target organ. For example, secretion of the hypothalamic corticotropin-releasing hormone stimulates release of pituitary corticotropin, which, in turn, stimulates cortisol secretion by the adrenal gland (the target organ). A rise in serum cortisol levels inhibits corticotropin secretion by decreasing corticotropin-releasing hormone.

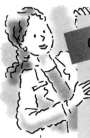

Endocrine refresher

HYPOTHYROIDISM

Key signs and symptoms

In untreated hypothyroidism in infants:
- hoarse crying
- persistent jaundice
- respiratory difficulties.
  In untreated hypothyroidism in older children:
- bone and muscle dystrophy
- cognitive impairment
- stunted growth (dwarfism).

Key test result
- Radioimmunoassay confirms hypothyroidism with low triiodothyronine and thyroxine levels.

Key treatments
- Oral thyroid hormone (thyroxine)
- Supplemental vitamin D to prevent rickets from rapid bone growth

Key interventions
- During early management of infantile hypothyroidism, monitor blood pressure and pulse rate and report hypertension and tachycardia immediately (normal infant heart rate is approximately 120 beats/minute).
- Check rectal temperature every 2 to 4 hours.
- If the infant's tongue is unusually large, position him on his side and observe him frequently.
- Teach the patient and the parents to recognize signs of supplemental thyroid hormone overdose (rapid pulse rate, irritability, insomnia, fever, sweating, weight loss).

TYPE 1 DIABETES MELLITUS

Key signs and symptoms
- Polydipsia
- Polyphagia
- Polyuria

Key test results
- Fasting plasma glucose level (no caloric intake for at least 8 hours) is greater than or equal to 126 mg/dl.
- Plasma glucose value in the 2-hour sample of the oral glucose tolerance test is greater than or equal to 200 mg/dl. This test should be performed after a loading dose of 75 g of anhydrous glucose.
- A random plasma glucose value (obtained without regard to the time of the child's last food intake) greater than or equal to 200 mg/dl accompanied by symptoms of diabetes indicates diabetes mellitus.

Key treatments
- Exercise
- Insulin replacement
- Strict diet planned to meet nutritional needs, control blood glucose levels, and reach and maintain appropriate body weight

Key interventions
- Monitor vital signs and intake and output.
- If you aren't sure whether the child is hypoglycemic or hyperglycemic and the child is stuporous or unconscious, treat him for hypoglycemia.
- Teach the child and the parents about complying with the prescribed treatment program; monitoring blood glucose level at home; and preventing, recognizing, and treating hypoglycemia and hyperglycemia at home.

> Remember to tailor your teaching to the child's needs, abilities, and developmental stage.

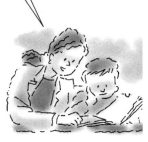

Keep abreast of diagnostic tests

Here are the most important tests used to diagnose endocrine disorders, along with common nursing interventions associated with each test.

Function studies

An **endocrine function study** focuses on measuring the level or effect of a hormone such as the effect of insulin on blood glucose levels.

Sophisticated techniques of hormone measurement have improved diagnosis of endocrine disorders. For example, the human growth hormone stimulation test measures human growth hormone levels after I.V. administration of arginine, an amino acid that under normal circumstances stimulates human growth hormone. This test is used to diagnose growth hormone deficiency.

Nursing actions
• Explain the test to the child and parents.
• Check with the laboratory and consult facility protocol to determine specific actions prior to the test (nothing-by-mouth for blood glucose test).

Minute measurements
A **radioimmunoassay** is used to measure minute quantities of hormones.

Nursing actions
• Explain the test to the child and the parents.

Polish up on patient care

Two major endocrine disorders in pediatric patients are hypothyroidism and type 1 diabetes mellitus.

Hypothyroidism

Hypothyroidism occurs when the body doesn't produce enough thyroid gland hormone, the hormone necessary for normal growth and development. (See *Thyroid gland hormones,* page 660.)

Two types of hypothyroidism exist. Congenital hypothyroidism is present at birth. Acquired hypothyroidism is often due to thyroiditis, an inflammation of the thyroid gland that results in injury or damage to thyroid tissue. Hypothyroidism is three times more common in girls than in boys.

Early diagnosis and treatment offer the best hope. Infants treated before age 3 months usually grow and develop normally. Children who remain untreated beyond age 3 months and children with acquired hypothyroidism who remain untreated beyond age 2 suffer irreversible cognitive impairment. Skeletal abnormalities, however, may be reversible with treatment.

CAUSES
• Antithyroid drugs taken during pregnancy (in infants)
• Chromosomal abnormalities
• Chronic autoimmune thyroiditis (in children older than age 2)
• Defective embryonic development that causes congenital absence or underdevelopment of the thyroid gland (most common cause in infants)
• Inherited enzymatic defect in the synthesis of thyroxine (T_4) caused by an autosomal recessive gene (in infants)

ASSESSMENT FINDINGS

General findings
• Delayed dentition
• Enlarged tongue
• Hypotonia
• Legs shorter in relation to trunk size
• Cognitive impairment (develops as the disorder progresses)
• Short stature with the persistence of infant proportions
• Short, thick neck

With slow basal metabolic rate
• Cool body and skin temperature
• Decreased perspiration
• Dry, scaly skin
• Easy weight gain
• Slow pulse

Untreated hypothyroidism in infants
• Hoarse crying
• Persistent jaundice
• Respiratory difficulties

Balance is better. Too many hormones or not enough hormones can cause an endocrine disorder.

Timing is everything. Treated before 3 months of age the prognosis for hypothyroidism is excellent — left untreated, it leads to cognitive impairment and skeletal abnormalities.

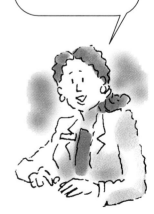

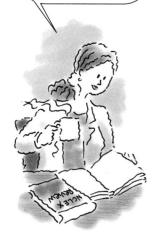

Key test for detecting hypothyroidism: Radioimmunoassay results show low T_3 and T_4 hormone levels.

Untreated hypothyroidism in older children
- Bone and muscle dystrophy
- Cognitive impairment
- Stunted growth (dwarfism)

DIAGNOSTIC TEST RESULTS
- Electrocardiogram shows bradycardia and flat or inverted T waves in untreated infants.
- Hip, knee, and thigh X-rays reveal absence of the femoral or tibial epiphyseal line and delayed skeletal development that is markedly inappropriate for the child's chronological age.
- In myxedema coma, laboratory tests may also show low serum sodium levels, decreased pH, and increased partial pressure of arterial carbon dioxide, indicating respiratory acidosis.
- Increased gonadotropin levels accompany sexual precocity in older children and may coexist with hypothyroidism.
- Serum cholesterol, alkaline phosphatase, and triglyceride levels are elevated.
- Normocytic normochromic anemia is present.
- Radioimmunoassay confirms hypothyroidism with low triiodothyronine (T_3) and thyroxine (T_4) levels.
- Thyroid scan and ^{131}I uptake tests show decreased uptake levels and confirm the absence of thyroid tissue in athyroid children.
- Thyroid-stimulating hormone (TSH) level is decreased when hypothyroidism is due to hypothalamic or pituitary insufficiency.
- TSH level is increased when hypothyroidism is due to thyroid insufficiency.

NURSING DIAGNOSES
- Altered growth and development
- Altered family processes
- Knowledge deficit

TREATMENT
- Routine monitoring of T_4 and TSH levels.
- Periodic evaluation of growth to ensure thyroid replacement is adequate

Drug therapy
- Oral thyroid hormone: levothyroxine (Synthroid)
- Supplemental vitamin D to prevent rickets resulting from rapid bone growth

INTERVENTIONS
- During early management of infantile hypothyroidism, monitor blood pressure and pulse rate; report hypertension and tachycardia immediately (normal infant heart rate is approximately 120 beats/minute). *These signs of hyperthyroidism indicate that the dose of thyroid replacement medication is too high.*
- Check rectal temperature every 2 to 4 hours. *Keep the infant warm and his skin moist to promote normothermia and reduce metabolic demands.*
- If the infant's tongue is unusually large, position him on his side and observe him frequently *to prevent airway obstruction.*
- Provide parents with support, referrals, and counseling as necessary *to help parents cope with possibility of caring for a physically and cognitively impaired child.*
- Adolescent girls require future-oriented counseling that stresses the importance of adequate thyroid replacement during pregnancy. *Ideally women should have excellent control before conception.*

Teaching topics
- Recognizing signs of overdose of supplemental thyroid hormone (rapid pulse rate, ir-

ritability, insomnia, fever, sweating, weight loss)
• Understanding that the child requires life-long treatment with thyroid supplements
• Complying with the treatment regimen to prevent further mental impairment
• Adopting a positive but realistic attitude and focusing on the child's strengths rather than weaknesses
• Providing stimulating activities to help the child reach maximum potential (referring parents to appropriate community resources for support)
• Preventing infantile hypothyroidism (Emphasize the importance of adequate nutrition during pregnancy, including iodine-rich foods and the use of iodized salt or, in the case of sodium restriction, an iodine supplement.)

Type 1 diabetes mellitus

Type 1 diabetes (formerly referred to as juvenile diabetes or insulin-dependent diabetes) most commonly occurs in childhood. Children with this type of diabetes must take insulin to replace what their pancreas can no longer produce. Type 1 diabetes is most commonly diagnosed during childhood or adolescence, but can occur at any time from infancy to about age 30.

CAUSES
• Genetic predisposition
• Viral infection

Causes of hyperglycemia
• Cortisone use
• Decreased exercise with no decrease in food intake
• Decreased use of insulin
• Increased sugar intake
• Increased stressors
• Infection

Causes of hypoglycemia
• Increased insulin use
• Excessive exercise
• Failure to eat

ASSESSMENT FINDINGS
• Polydipsia
• Polyphagia
• Polyuria

Symptoms of hyperglycemia
• Abdominal cramping
• Dry, flushed skin
• Fatigue
• Fruity breath odor
• Headache
• Nausea
• Thin appearance and possible malnourishment
• Vomiting
• Weakness

Symptoms of hypoglycemia in conjunction with diabetes
• Behavior changes (belligerence, confusion, slurred speech)
• Diaphoresis
• Palpitations
• Tachycardia
• Tremors

DIAGNOSTIC TEST RESULTS
• Fasting plasma glucose level (no caloric intake for at least 8 hours) is greater than or equal to 126 mg/dl.
• Plasma glucose value in the 2-hour sample of the oral glucose tolerance test is greater than or equal to 200 mg/dl. This test should be performed after a loading dose of 75 g of anhydrous glucose.
• A random plasma glucose value (obtained without regard to the time of the child's last food intake) greater than or equal to 200 mg/dl and accompanied by symptoms of diabetes indicates diabetes mellitus.
• Test for glycosuria and ketonuria using dipstick, Clinitest, Acetest, Keto-Diastix, or glucose enzymatic test strip is positive.

NURSING DIAGNOSES
• Body image disturbance
• Risk for altered nutrition: Less than body requirements
• Risk for fluid volume deficit

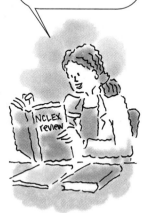

Remember that regular study habits do more good than cramming. Plan a realistic, regular schedule and stick to it.

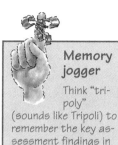

Memory jogger

Think "tri-poly" (sounds like Tripoli) to remember the key assessment findings in type 1 diabetes mellitus:

• **Poly**dipsia
• **Poly**phagia
• **Poly**uria.

Now I get it!

Understanding type 1 diabetes

Here are important points for understanding how type 1 diabetes develops.

THE KEY PLAYERS
- The endocrine part of the pancreas produces glucagon from the alpha cells and insulin from the beta cells.
- Glucagon, the hormone of the fasting state, releases stored glucose to raise the blood glucose level.
- Insulin, the hormone of the nourished state, facilitates glucose transport, promotes glucose storage, stimulates protein synthesis, and enhances free fatty acid uptake and storage.

WHAT HAPPENS
Absolute or relative insulin deficiency causes diabetes mellitus. Here is what happens:
- Pancreatic beta cells are destroyed, no insulin is produced, and the cells can't utilize glucose.
- Excess glucose in the blood spills into the urine.
- The increased level of blood glucose can act as an osmotic diuretic, resulting in dehydration, hypotension, and renal shutdown.
- The body attempts to compensate for lost energy by breaking down fatty acids to form ketones with resulting metabolic acidosis.

TREATMENT
- Exercise
- Strict diet planned to meet nutritional needs, control blood glucose levels, and reach and maintain appropriate body weight

Drug therapy
- Insulin replacement

INTERVENTIONS
- Monitor vital signs and fluid intake and output. High urine output may signify hyperglycemia. Weak, thready pulse may indicate hypoglycemia.
- Monitor blood glucose level and electrolytes *to detect early signs of electrolyte imbalance.*
- If you aren't sure whether the child is hypoglycemic or hyperglycemic and the child is stuporous or unconscious, treat him for hypoglycemia. *If he's hypoglycemic, he will respond quickly; if he's hyperglycemic, this action won't significantly worsen his condition.*
- Evaluate the child's or adolescent's understanding of type 1 diabetes and his attitude about the need to manage it. *This will help you plan teaching.*
- Correct any misconceptions the child or adolescent may have regarding type 1 diabetes and the therapeutic regimen. Use teaching materials appropriate for his age *to increase his knowledge of his condition and instill confidence in his ability to manage it.*
- Provide an opportunity for the child or adolescent to interact with peers who have experienced diabetes *to decrease the child's or adolescent's feelings of isolation and sense of being different from others.*
- Discuss issues surrounding peer pressure. Ask the adolescent if he feels that social pressure causes him to ignore his diet or avoid self-administering insulin. Ask if he feels embarrassed by his disorder. Explore ways of dealing with peer pressure. *Peer pressure is a reality that each adolescent must learn to deal with.*

Hyperglycemia
- Administer regular insulin for fast action *to promote euglycemic state and prevent complications.*
- Administer I.V. fluids without dextrose *to flush out acetone and maintain hydration.*
- Monitor electrolytes and arterial blood gas levels; administer bicarbonate as needed *to combat acidosis.*
- Monitor blood glucose level *to detect early changes and prevent complications such as diabetic ketoacidosis.*

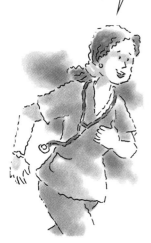

If you aren't sure whether the child is hypoglycemic or hyperglycemic and he's unconscious, treat him for hypoglycemia.

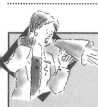

Listen up!

Teaching about insulin administration

Here are some important elements to teach patients about insulin administration.
• When giving both types of insulin, draw up clear insulin first to prevent contamination.
• To prevent air bubbles, don't shake the vial; intermediate forms are suspensions and should be gently rotated.
• Rotate injection sites to prevent lipodystrophy.
• Make sure the child eats when the insulin peaks such as a mid-afternoon and bedtime snack.
• Insulin requirements may be altered with illness, stress, growth, food intake, and exercise; blood glucose measurements are the best way to determine insulin adjustments.

Hypoglycemia
• Give a fast-acting carbohydrate, such as honey, orange juice, and sugar cubes, followed later by a protein source *to establish normal glucose levels thereby preventing complications of hypoglycemia.*
• If the child is stuporous or unconscious, administer glucagon (S.C., I.V., or I.M.) or dextrose I.V. *to prevent complications of hypoglycemia.*

Teaching topics
• Complying with the prescribed treatment program (See *Teaching about insulin administration.*)
• Monitoring blood glucose levels
• Understanding the importance of good hygiene
• Preventing, recognizing, and treating hypoglycemia and hyperglycemia
• Understanding the effect of blood glucose control on long-term health
• Managing diabetes during minor illness, such as a cold, flu, and upset stomach
• Providing the child or adolescent with written materials that cover the teaching topic
• Providing the child or adolescent with information about the Juvenile Diabetes Foundation

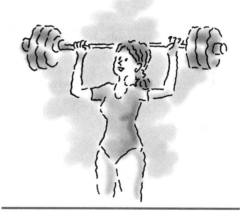

Pump up on practice questions

1. The nurse is teaching the mother of a child diagnosed with type 1 diabetes. The mother asks why her child must inject insulin and can't take pills as her uncle does. Which reply is most appropriate?

    A. "Because a child's pancreas is less developed than an adult's, antidiabetic pills aren't recommended for children."

    B. "Pills only affect fat and protein metabolism, not sugar."

    C. "The only way to replace insulin is by injection."

    D. "Your child may be able to take pills when he's older."

Answer: C. With Type 1 diabetes, the pancreas doesn't produce insulin, so the child must receive insulin replacement by injection. Oral antidiabetic agents stimulate the pancreas to produce more insulin and are only effective in treating type 2 diabetes. Because the pancreas in the child with type 1 diabetes doesn't produce insulin, the child will never be a candidate for oral antidiabetic agents.

➡ NCLEX keys
Nursing process step: Implementation
Client needs category: Physiological integrity
Client needs subcategory: Pharmacological and parenteral therapies
Taxonomic level: Application

2. The nurse is teaching the mother of a diabetic child how to recognize the signs and symptoms of hypoglycemia. Which signs and symptoms should the nurse discuss?
   A. Behavioral changes, increased heart rate, sweating, and tremors
   B. Nausea, fruity odor to breath, headache, and fatigue
   C. Polydipsia, polyuria, polyphagia, and weight loss
   D. Enlarged tongue, hypotonia, easy weight gain, and cool skin temperature

Answer: A. The nurse should instruct the mother of a child with diabetes to recognize signs and symptoms of hypoglycemia, such as behavioral changes, increased heart rate, sweating, and tremors. Nausea, fruity odor to breath, headache, and fatigue are present with hyperglycemia. Polydipsia, polyuria, polyphagia, and weight loss are classic signs of diabetes. Enlarged tongue, hypotonia, easy weight gain, and cool skin temperature are associated with hypothyroidism.

➡ NCLEX keys
Nursing process step: Planning
Client needs category: Physiological integrity
Client needs subcategory: Reduction of risk potential
Taxonomic level: Comprehension

3. The nurse is assessing a child who may have diabetes. Which of the following laboratory values would help confirm a diagnosis of type 1 diabetes?
   A. A fasting plasma glucose level of 110 mg/dl
   B. A fasting plasma glucose level of 126 mg/dl
   C. A random plasma glucose level of 180 mg/dl
   D. A 2-hour glucose tolerance test of 140 mg/dl

Answer: B. According to the American Diabetes Association, diabetes occurs when any of the following exist: symptoms of diabetes plus a random plasma glucose level greater than or equal to 200 mg/dl, a fasting plasma glucose level greater than or equal to 126 mg/dl, or a 2-hour oral glucose tolerance test greater than or equal to 200 mg/dl.

➡ NCLEX keys
Nursing process step: Assessment
Client needs category: Health promotion and maintenance
Client needs subcategory: Prevention and early detection of disease
Taxonomic level: Comprehension

4. The nurse is caring for a child with type 1 diabetes. The nurse enters the child's room and finds him diaphoretic and unable to be wakened. The nurse should anticipate which of the following emergency interventions?
   A. Administering honey followed by a protein source
   B. Administering orange juice followed by a protein source
   C. Administering I.V. dextrose
   D. Administering insulin

Answer: C. The child is unconscious and experiencing a hypoglycemic reaction; therefore, the nurse should be prepared to administer I.V. dextrose. The child experiencing a hypoglycemic episode who's conscious should be given a fast-acting carbohydrate such as honey, orange juice, and sugar cubes, followed by a protein source. Insulin administration would further worsen the child's condition.

→ NCLEX keys

Nursing process step: Implementation
Client needs category: Physiological integrity
Client needs subcategory: Pharmacological
and parenteral therapies
Taxonomic level: Application

5. The nurse is teaching the parents of a child with diabetes. Which of the following agents should the nurse teach the parents to administer if their child suffers a severe hypoglycemic reaction?
  A. I.V. dextrose
  B. subcutaneous insulin administration
  C. subcutaneous glucagon administration
  D. Oral fast-acting carbohydrate administration

Answer: C. The nurse should instruct the parents of a child with diabetes about proper administration of subcutaneous glucagon if their child suffers a severe hypoglycemic episode. Subcutaneous insulin would further worsen the child's condition. I.V. dextrose is reserved for health care professionals specially trained in I.V. drug administration. Oral administration of fast-acting carbohydrates is reserved for the conscious child who isn't suffering from a severe hypoglycemic reaction.

→ NCLEX keys

Nursing process step: Implementation
Client needs category: Physiological integrity
Client needs subcategory: Reduction of risk
potential
Taxonomic level: Knowledge

6. The nurse is teaching an adolescent with diabetes about occurrences that can alter insulin requirements. Which of the following occurrences should be emphasized?
  A. Illness, stress, growth, food intake, and exercise
  B. Water intake, illness, stress, and exercise
  C. Exposure to ultraviolet light, illness, stress, and exercise
  D. Sodium intake, exercise, stress, and illness

Answer: A. Illness, stress, growth, food intake, and exercise can alter insulin requirements.

Water intake, ultraviolet light exposure, and sodium intake don't alter insulin requirements.

→ NCLEX keys

Nursing process step: Implementation
Client needs category: Physiological integrity
Client needs subcategory: Reduction of risk
potential
Taxonomic level: Knowledge

7. The nurse is teaching an adolescent with diabetes. Which statement by the adolescent indicates that teaching was effective?
  A. "If I want to eat ice cream, I'll just give myself more insulin."
  B. "I'm so busy, I'm glad I can still skip meals if I need to."
  C. "I will remember to take my regular dose of insulin even if I'm sick."
  D. "I will monitor my blood glucose level to determine how much insulin I need."

Answer: D. Diabetic teaching is effective when the adolescent verbalizes the importance of monitoring his blood glucose level to determine his insulin needs. Teaching should stress the importance of maintaining a diabetic diet and not skipping meals. It should also address the need for adjusting insulin doses during times of illness.

→ NCLEX keys

Nursing process step: Evaluation
Client needs category: Physiological integrity
Client needs subcategory: Reduction of risk
potential
Taxonomic level: Analysis

8. A 10-year-old boy with type 1 diabetes comes to the pediatrician's office. Which of the following is the best technique to ensure responsible insulin administration?
  A. The child observes his parents as they administer his injections.
  B. The child learns to administer his insulin with supervision.
  C. The child manages his insulin administration independently.
  D. The child learns to draw up his own insulin and his parents inject it.

Answer: B. School-age children should be encouraged to administer their own insulin with adult supervision to ensure correct procedure is followed and the correct dosage is administered. Having the child observe the parents or drawing up his insulin and not injecting it doesn't allow the child to take sufficient responsibility for his care. Allowing the child to administer his insulin without adult supervision gives him too much responsibility.

➥ NCLEX keys
Nursing process step: Planning
Client needs category: Physiological integrity
Client needs subcategory: Reduction of risk potential
Taxonomic level: Application

9. A 9-year-old boy with type 1 diabetes takes a mixture of regular and neutral protamine Hagedorn (NPH) insulin. He is scheduled to go on a camping trip and his mother asks the nurse whether it's safe for him to participate in this activity. What is the most appropriate response?

   A. "He needs to understand the physical limitations placed on a client with diabetes."
   B. "He should have a light snack before doing any hiking."
   C. "He shouldn't go on this trip because it's potentially dangerous."
   D. "Have him increase his morning NPH insulin to compensate for higher metabolism while hiking."

Treat yourself right while studying for the NCLEX exam. Don't skip meals, miss sleep, or neglect exercise. Stay healthy and, in the long run, you'll stay ahead.

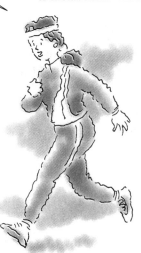

Answer: B. A light meal before rigorous exercise gives the child adequate blood glucose levels during the peak action of his morning NPH insulin. Restricting the child's physical activity discourages a normal lifestyle. The child's diagnosis alone shouldn't be used to evaluate the danger of the trip. Increasing the child's insulin would increase the likelihood of a hypoglycemic reaction.

➥ NCLEX keys
Nursing process step: Implementation
Client needs category: Physiological integrity
Client needs subcategory: Reduction of risk potential
Taxonomic level: Application

10. The nurse administers oral thyroid hormone to an infant with hypothyroidism. For which of the following signs of overdose should the nurse observe the infant?

   A. Tachycardia, fever, irritability, and sweating
   B. Bradycardia, cool skin temperature, and dry scaly skin
   C. Bradycardia, fever, hypotension, and irritability
   D. Tachycardia, cool skin temperature, and irritability

Answer: A. The infant experiencing an overdose of thyroid replacement hormone exhibits tachycardia, fever, irritability, and sweating. Bradycardia, cool skin temperature, and dry scaly skin are signs of hypothyroidism.

➥ NCLEX keys
Nursing process step: Assessment
Client needs category: Physiological integrity
Client needs subcategory: Pharmacological and parenteral therapies
Taxonomic level: Application

34 Genitourinary System

Brush up on key concepts

The genitourinary system includes the genitalia and urinary structures. The focus of this chapter is the kidneys, ureters, and bladder, which are involved in renal and urinary function. The chapter also discusses two sexually transmitted diseases that affect pediatric patients.

You can review the major points of this chapter by consulting the *Cheat sheet* on pages 668 to 670.

High turnover
Water, which is controlled by the genitourinary system, is the body's primary fluid. The infant has a much greater percentage of total body water in extracellular fluid (42% to 45%) than the adult does (20%). Because of the increased percentage of water in a child's extracellular fluid, the child's **water turnover rate** is two to three times greater than the adult's. Every day 50% of the infant's extracellular fluid is exchanged, compared with only 20% of the adult's; the child is therefore more susceptible than the adult to dehydration.

Sweating it out
The newborn also has a greater ratio of body-surface area to body weight than the adult; this results in greater **fluid loss through the skin.**

Less efficient during stress
A child's kidneys attain the adult number of **nephrons** (about a million in each kidney) shortly after birth. The nephrons, which form urine, continue to mature throughout early childhood.

The infant's renal system can maintain a healthy fluid and electrolyte status. However, it doesn't function as efficiently during stress as the adult's renal system. For example, if a child doesn't receive enough fluid to meet his needs, his kidneys can't adequately concentrate urine to prevent dehydration. Conversely, if the child receives too much fluid, he may be unable to dilute urine appropriately to get rid of the increased volume.

Concentration change
The infant's kidneys don't concentrate urine at an adult level (average **specific gravity** is less than 1.010 for an infant, compared with 1.010 to 1.030 for an adult).
• Although the number of daily voidings decreases with increasing age (because of increased urine concentration), the total amount of urine produced daily may not vary significantly.
• An infant usually voids 5 to 10 ml/hour, a 10-year-old child usually voids 10 to 25 ml/hour, and an adult usually voids 35 ml/hour.

Short path to the bladder
The child also has a short urethra; therefore, organisms can be easily transmitted into the bladder, increasing the risk of bladder infection.

Keep abreast of diagnostic tests

Here are the most important tests used to diagnose genitourinary disorders, along with common nursing interventions associated with each test.

(Text continues on page 670.)

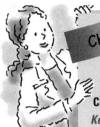

Genitourinary refresher

CHLAMYDIA

Key signs and symptoms

In a child with conjunctivitis, look for:
- fiery red conjunctivae with a thick pus
- edematous eyelids

  In a child with pneumonia, look for:
- nasal congestion
- sharp cough
- failure to gain weight
- tachypnea
- crackles and wheezing on auscultation of lungs.

Key test results
- The Venereal Disease Research Laboratory (VDRL) titer is reactive.

Key treatments
- Chest physiotherapy to mobilize secretions in a child with pneumonia
- Erythromycin
- Humidified oxygen to alleviate labored breathing and prevent hypoxemia in a child with pneumonia
- Irrigation of eyes with sterile saline solution to clear the copious discharge

Key interventions
- Check the newborn of an infected mother for signs of chlamydial infection.
- Administer medication as prescribed and monitor its effectiveness.
- Auscultate breath sounds and monitor oxygenation.

CONGENITAL SYPHILIS

Key signs and symptoms
- Characteristic lesions (vesicular, bullous eruptions, often on the palms and soles) appearing 3 weeks after birth; possibility that infant appears healthy at birth

  Late prenatal syphilis symptoms include:
- bowed tibias
- eighth cranial nerve deafness
- neurosyphilis
- screwdriver-shaped central incisors
- thick clavicles.

Key test result
- VDRL titer is reactive.

Key treatment
- Antibiotic therapy: penicillin or erythromycin, or doxycycline (Vibramycin) if child is allergic to penicillin

Key interventions
- Assess cardiovascular and neurologic status.
- Monitor and record the extent of the rash.
- Watch for signs of systemic involvement, especially laryngeal swelling, jaundice, and decreasing urine output.
- Discuss the infant's need for tactile and sensory stimulation. Demonstrate play activities and promote developmental skills, such as shaking a rattle in front of the infant to build eye-and-hand coordination or placing a mobile above the infant.
- If the infant's condition is poor, encourage the parents to express feelings about the potential loss of their child and its impact on their well-being and lifestyle.

HYPOSPADIAS

Key signs and symptoms
- Altered angle of urination
- Meatus terminating at some point along lateral fusion line, ranging from the perineum to the distal penile shaft

Key test result
- Observation confirms aberrant placement of the opening; therefore, diagnostic testing isn't necessary.

Key treatments
- Avoiding circumcision (the foreskin may be needed later during surgical repair)
- Indwelling urinary catheter or suprapubic urinary catheter postoperatively
- Analgesics: meperidine (Demerol) or acetaminophen (Tylenol) for postoperative pain relief

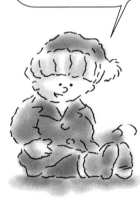

Uh-oh! Under stress my renal system doesn't function as well as an adult's.

Genitourinary refresher *(continued)*

HYPOSPADIAS *(continued)*

• Antispasmodic agent: propantheline (Pro-Banthine) prescribed postoperatively to treat bladder spasms

Surgery

• Meatotomy (surgical procedure in which the urethra is extended into a normal position); may initially be performed to restore normal urinary function
• When the child is age 12 to 18 months, surgery to release the adherent chordee (fibrous band that causes the penis to curve downward)
• If repair is to be extensive, surgical repair may be delayed until age 4

Key interventions

• Keep the area clean.
• Encourage parents to express feelings and concerns about changes in the child's body appearance or function. Provide accurate information and answer questions thoroughly.
• Instruct parents in hygiene of uncircumcised penis.

Postoperative care

• After the procedure, a pressure dressing is often used to reduce bleeding and tissue swelling; keep the child's hands away from the penis.
• Check the tip of the penis frequently.
• Leave the dressing in place for several days.
• Take care to avoid pressure on the child's catheter and avoid kinking of the catheter.

NEPHRITIS

Key signs and symptoms

• Anorexia
• Burning during urination
• Flank pain
• Urinary frequency
• Shaking chills
• Temperature of 102° F (38.9° C) or higher
• Urinary urgency

Key test results

• Pyuria (pus in urine) is present. Urine sediment reveals the presence of leukocytes singly, in clumps, and in casts; and, possibly, a few red blood cells.
• Urine culture reveals significant bacteriuria; more than 100,000/μl of urine. Proteinuria, glycosuria, and ketonuria are less common.

Key treatments

• Antibiotic therapy appropriate to the specific infecting organism over a 10- to 14-day course.
• Urinary analgesics such as phenazopyridine

Key interventions

• Force fluids to achieve urine output of more than 2 L/day. However, discourage intake greater than 3 L/day.
• Teach the child and parents about:
 – refrigerating or culturing a urine specimen within 30 minutes of collection to prevent overgrowth of bacteria
 – completing the prescribed antibiotic therapy, even after symptoms subside
 – long-term follow-up care for high-risk children.

NEPHROBLASTOMA

Key signs and symptoms

• Nontender mass, usually midline near the liver; often detected by the parent while bathing or dressing the child
• Associated congenital anomalies — microcephaly, mental retardation, genitourinary tract problems

Key test results

• Excretory urography reveals a mass displacing the normal kidney structure.
• Computed tomography scan or sonography will reveal metastasis.

Key treatments

• Nephrectomy done quickly because these tumors metastasize quickly
• Radiation therapy (following surgery)
• Chemotherapy (following surgery) with dactinomycin, doxorubicin, or vincristine

Key interventions

• Monitor vital signs and intake and output.
• Don't palpate the abdomen, and prevent others from doing so.
• Handle and bathe the child carefully and loosen clothing near the abdomen.
• Prepare the child and family members for a nephrectomy within 24 to 48 hours of diagnosis.

After nephrectomy

• Monitor urine output and report output less than 30 ml/hour.
• Assist with turning, coughing, and deep breathing.
• Encourage early ambulation.
• Provide pain medications, as necessary.
• Monitor postoperative dressings for signs of bleeding.
• Use aseptic techniques for dressing changes.

URINARY TRACT INFECTION

Key signs and symptoms

• Frequent urges to void with pain or burning on urination
• Lethargy
• Low-grade fever
• Urine that is cloudy and foul-smelling

(continued)

Blood analysis

Blood tests are used to analyze serum levels of chemical substances, such as uric acid, creatinine, and blood urea nitrogen.

Nursing actions

• Explain to the parent and child that the test requires a blood sample and to expect some discomfort.
• Allow the child to hold a comfort object, such as a stuffed animal or blanket, to help diminish his anxiety.

Urine testing

Urinalysis is used to determine urine characteristics such as:
• presence of red blood cells
• presence of white blood cells
• presence of casts or bacteria
• specific gravity and pH
• physical properties, such as clarity, color, and odor.

Nursing actions

• Before specimen collection, explain the importance of cleaning the meatal area thoroughly.
• Explain that the culture specimen should be caught midstream, in a sterile container. (See *Infant specimen collection.*)
• Explain that the specimen for urinalysis should be caught in a clean container, preferably at the first voiding of the day.
• Begin a 24-hour specimen collection after discarding the first voiding; such specimens often necessitate special handling or preservatives.

• When obtaining a urine specimen from a catheterized child, remember to avoid taking the specimen from the collection bag; instead, aspirate a sample through the collection port in the catheter, with a sterile needle and a syringe.

Fluids in and out

Intake and output assessment helps determine the child's hydration status.

Nursing actions

To provide the most useful and accurate information, you should:
• use calibrated containers
• establish baseline values for each child
• compare measurement patterns
• validate intake and output measurements by checking the child's weight daily
• monitor all fluid losses daily, including blood, vomitus, diarrhea, and wound and stoma drainage.

Kidney pictures

Kidney-ureter-bladder (KUB) radiography is used to assess the size, shape, position, and possible areas of calcification of the renal organs.

Nursing actions

• Explain the procedure to the parents and the child.
• Tell the child the X-ray takes only a few minutes and remind him to hold still.
• Shield the genitals of a male child to prevent irradiation of the testes.

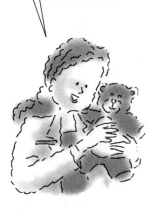

Holding a comfort object such as a stuffed animal may help decrease anxiety.

Infant specimen collection

Use the clean-catch method to collect urine from an infant, as follows:
- After properly cleaning the skin and genitals, apply a pediatric urine collector to dry skin (powders or creams shouldn't be used).
- If the child doesn't void within 45 minutes, remove the bag and repeat the procedure.

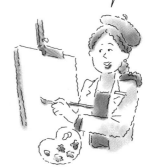

Picture this. Several tests help picture the renal system: KUB radiography, excretory urography, and voiding cystourethrography.

I.V. action

Excretory urography aids in checking renal pelvic structures. Contrast media is introduced into the renal pelvis, allowing visualization of the collecting system and ureters.

Nursing actions
- Check the child's history for allergies.
- Monitor the child's intake and output.
- Explain the purpose of test to the child and parents.
- Maintain the child on nothing-by-mouth status for 8 hours before the test.
- Make sure that a written, informed consent has been obtained.
- Increase hydration after the procedure.

While the water's running

A **voiding cystourethrogram** aids in viewing the bladder and related structures during voiding.

Nursing actions
- Check the child's history for allergies.
- Monitor the child's intake and output.
- Explain the purpose of test to the child and parents.
- Make sure that a written, informed consent has been obtained.
- After the procedure, encourage the child to drink lots of fluid to reduce burning on urination and to flush out residual dye.

Polish up on patient care

Common genitourinary disorders in pediatric patients include:

- chlamydia
- hypospadias
- nephritis
- nephroblastoma (Wilms' tumor)
- congenital syphilis
- urinary tract infections.

Chlamydia

Chlamydial infections are the most common sexually transmitted diseases in the United States. In infants, the infecting organism is passed from the infected mother to the fetus during passage through the birth canal.

Chlamydia is the most common cause of ophthalmia neonatorum (eye infection at birth or during the first month) and a major cause of pneumonia in infants in the first 3 months of life. With antibiotic therapy, the chance of cure is good.

CAUSE
- *Chlamydia trachomatis* infection

ASSESSMENT FINDINGS
In a child with conjunctivitis, look for:
- fiery red conjunctivae with a thick puslike discharge
- edematous eyelids.
  In a child with pneumonia, look for:
- nasal congestion
- sharp cough
- failure to gain weight
- tachypnea
- crackles and wheezing on auscultation of lungs.

DIAGNOSTIC TEST RESULTS
- The Venereal Disease Research Laboratory (VDRL) titer is reactive.

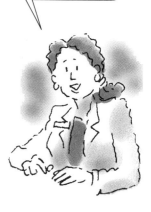

Children born of mothers who have chlamydial infection may contract conjunctivitis or pneumonia during passage through the birth canal.

• Blood studies show elevated levels of immunoglobulin G (IgG) and IgM antibodies.
• Tissue cell cultures from infected sites reveal *Chlamydia trachomatis*.

NURSING DIAGNOSES
• Ineffective airway clearance
• Altered family processes
• Risk for infection

TREATMENT
• Humidified oxygen to alleviate labored breathing and prevent hypoxemia in a child with pneumonia
• Chest physiotherapy to mobilize secretions in a child with pneumonia
• Irrigation of eyes with sterile saline solution to clear the copious discharge

Drug therapy
• Erythromycin

INTERVENTIONS AND RATIONALES
• Check the newborn of an infected mother for signs of chlamydial infection *to identify infection early and initiate treatment.*
• Administer medication as prescribed and monitor its effectiveness *to improve the child's condition.*
• Obtain appropriate specimens for diagnostic testing *to aid in diagnosis of infection.*
• Auscultate breath sounds and monitor oxygenation *to determine oxygen status and respiratory function.*
• Suction as needed *to provide airway clearance.*

Teaching topics
• Completing the entire course of drug therapy
• Eye care

Congenital syphilis

A syphilis infection during pregnancy places the fetus at risk for congenital syphilis. After the 16th to 18th week of intrauterine life, the causative spirochete, *Treponema pallidum,* can extensively damage the fetus. If syphilis is detected and treated before this time, the fe-

tus is rarely affected. If syphilis is left untreated beyond the 18th week of gestation, deafness, cognitive impairment, and fetal death may occur.

A newborn with congenital syphilis may develop congenital anomalies, extreme rhinitis, and a characteristic syphilitic rash, which identifies the baby as high risk at birth.

CAUSE
• Transmitted through the placenta to unborn child during pregnancy

ASSESSMENT FINDINGS
• Condylomata lata (dull pink to gray, flattened papules), often appearing around the anus
• Nasal discharge; may be slight and mucopurulent or copious, with blood-tinged pus; indicates involvement of nasal mucous membranes
• Characteristic lesions (vesicular, bullous eruptions, often on the palms and soles) appearing 3 weeks after birth; possibility that infant appears healthy at birth
• Lesions erupting on mucous membranes of the mouth, pharynx, and nose
• Maculopapular rash erupting on face, mouth, genitalia, palms, or soles
• Visceral and bone lesions, liver and spleen enlargement with ascites, and nephrotic syndrome
• A weak, forced cry, indicating the larynx has been affected

Late prenatal syphilis
Late prenatal syphilis becomes apparent after age 2; it may be identifiable only through blood studies or may cause unmistakable syphilitic changes, including:
• bowed tibias
• deformed molars or cusps
• eighth cranial nerve deafness
• nasal septum perforation
• neurosyphilis
• saber shins
• screwdriver-shaped central incisors
• thick clavicles.

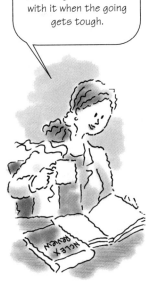

How to survive the NCLEX? Set goals, have an organized plan of action, and maintain a strong belief in yourself. Stick with it when the going gets tough.

DIAGNOSTIC TEST RESULTS
• Dark-field examination of umbilical vein blood or lesion drainage shows presence of *T. pallidum.*
• VDRL titer is reactive.

NURSING DIAGNOSES
• Altered parenting
• Impaired skin integrity
• Risk for infection

TREATMENT
• Symptomatic, depending on the congenital defects present

Drug therapy
• Antibiotics: penicillin or erythromycin, or doxycycline (Vibramycin) if child is allergic to penicillin

INTERVENTIONS AND RATIONALES
• Assess cardiovascular and neurologic status *to detect early signs of compromise.*
• Monitor and record the extent of the child's rash *to monitor effectiveness of the skin care regimen.*
• Watch for signs of systemic involvement, especially laryngeal swelling, jaundice, and decreasing urine output *to detect early signs of complications.*
• Maintain standard precautions *to protect the nurse and patients from the spread of infection.*
• When caring for the infant in the mother's presence, act as a role model for effective parenting skills. Demonstrate comfort measures such as rocking the infant *to increase the mother's knowledge of routine infant care and practices.*
• Discuss the infant's need for tactile and sensory stimulation. Demonstrate play activities and promote developmental skills, such as shaking a rattle in front of the infant to build eye-and-hand coordination or placing a mobile above the infant to encourage visual tracking and trunk and head control. *Sensory experiences promote cognitive development.*
• Praise the mother when she displays appropriate parenting skills *to provide positive reinforcement.*
• If the infant's condition is poor, encourage the parents to express feelings about the potential loss of their child and its impact on their well-being and lifestyle. *This reinforces reality and may help alleviate guilt.*

Teaching topics
• Performing prescribed regimen for skin condition
• Understanding the disorder
• Contacting social service or support groups as appropriate

Hypospadias

Hypospadias is a congenital anomaly of the penis. In this condition, the urethral opening may be anywhere along the ventral side of the penis. The condition shortens the distance to the bladder, offering easier access for bacteria.

CAUSES
• Genetic factors (most likely)

ASSESSMENT FINDINGS
• Altered angle of urination
• Meatus terminating at some point along lateral fusion line, ranging from the perineum to the distal penile shaft
• Normal urination with penis elevated impossible

DIAGNOSTIC TEST RESULTS
• Observation confirms aberrant placement of the opening; therefore, diagnostic testing isn't necessary.

NURSING DIAGNOSES
• Body image disturbance
• Knowledge deficit
• Risk for infection (urinary tract)

TREATMENT
• Avoiding circumcision (the foreskin may be needed later during surgical repair)
• No treatment (in mild disorder)

Surgery
• Meatotomy (procedure in which the urethra is extended into a normal position); may

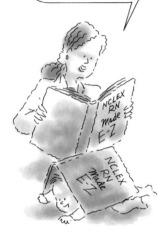

The key intervention in hypospadias is scrupulous cleaning to deter bacteria.

initially be performed to restore normal urinary function
• When the child is age 12 to 18 months, surgery to release the adherent chordee (fibrous band that causes the penis to curve downward)
• If repair is to be extensive, surgical repair may be delayed until age 4
• Indwelling urinary catheter or suprapubic urinary catheter postoperatively

Drug therapy
• Analgesics: meperidine (Demerol), acetaminophen (Tylenol) for postoperative pain relief
• Antispasmodic agent: propantheline (Pro-Banthine) prescribed postoperatively to treat bladder spasms

INTERVENTIONS AND RATIONALES
• Monitor urine output *to ensure the infant maintains a normal urine output of 5 to 10 ml/hr.*
• Keep the area clean *to prevent bacteria invasion and infection.*
• Encourage parents to express feelings and concerns about changes in the child's body appearance or function. Provide accurate information and answer questions thoroughly. *Encouraging open discussion enables the nurse to provide emotional support and may help ease the parents' anxiety.*

Postoperative care
• After the procedure, a pressure dressing is often used to reduce bleeding and tissue swelling; keep the child's hands away from the penis *so that the dressing isn't dislodged, causing trauma to the site.*
• Check the tip of the penis frequently *to be sure that it's pink and viable.*
• Leave the dressing in place for several days *to encourage healing of the grafted skin flap.*
• Take care to avoid pressure on the child's catheter *to prevent trauma to the incision site* and avoid kinking of the catheter *to ensure urine flow.*
• Encourage early ambulation *to prevent complications of immobility.*

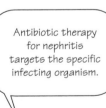

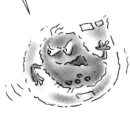

Antibiotic therapy for nephritis targets the specific infecting organism.

Teaching topics
• Practicing hygiene of uncircumcised penis
• Caring for the catheter
• Understanding signs and symptoms of urinary tract infection or incisional infection

Nephritis

Also known as acute infective tubulointerstitial nephritis, pyelonephritis, or glomerular nephritis, this disorder is a sudden inflammation that primarily affects the interstitial area and the renal pelvis or, less often, the renal tubules. One of the most common renal diseases, nephritis occurs more often in females, probably because of a shorter urethra and the proximity of the urinary meatus to the vagina and the rectum.

With treatment and continued follow-up care, the prognosis is good, and extensive permanent damage is rare.

CAUSES
• Bacterial infection of the kidneys (the most common cause); infecting bacteria usually are normal intestinal and fecal flora that grow readily in urine (the most common causative organism is *Escherichia coli,* but *Proteus, Pseudomonas, Staphylococcus aureus,* and *Enterococcus faecalis* [formerly *Streptococcus faecalis*] may also cause such infections)
• Hematogenic infection (as in septicemia or endocarditis)
• Inability to empty the bladder (for example, in patients with neurogenic bladder), urinary stasis, or urinary obstruction due to tumors or strictures.
• Contamination from instruments used in diagnostic testing, surgery, and routine patient care (such as catheterization, cystoscopy, or urologic surgery)
• Lymphatic infection

ASSESSMENT FINDINGS
• Anorexia
• Burning during urination
• Dysuria
• Flank pain
• Urinary frequency
• General fatigue

- Hematuria (usually microscopic but may be gross)
- Nocturia
- Shaking chills
- Temperature of 102° F (38.9° C) or higher
- Urinary urgency
- Urine that is cloudy and has an ammonia-like or fishy odor

DIAGNOSTIC TEST RESULTS

- Excretory urography may show asymmetrical kidneys.
- Pyuria (pus in urine) is present. Urine sediment reveals the presence of leukocytes singly, in clumps, and in casts; and, possibly, a few red blood cells.
- Urine culture reveals significant bacteriuria; more than 100,000/µl of urine. Proteinuria, glycosuria, and ketonuria are less common.
- Urine specific gravity and osmolality are low, resulting from a temporarily decreased ability to concentrate urine.
- Urine pH is slightly alkaline.
- KUB radiography may reveal calculi, tumors, or cysts in the kidneys and the urinary tract.

NURSING DIAGNOSES

- Altered urinary elimination
- Risk for infection
- Pain

TREATMENT

- Follow-up treatment for antibiotic therapy: reculturing urine 1 week after drug therapy stops, then periodically for next year to detect residual or recurring infection
- Surgery to relieve obstruction or correct the anomaly responsible for obstruction or vesicoureteral reflux; antibiotics not always effective

Antibiotic therapy

Antibiotic therapy is targeted to the specific infecting organism; the course of therapy is 10 to 14 days. Therapy for specific organisms is described below:

- *Enterococcus* — ampicillin, penicillin G, or vancomycin
- *E. coli* — sulfisoxazole, nalidixic acid, and nitrofurantoin

- *Proteus* — ampicillin, sulfisoxazole, nalidixic acid, and a cephalosporin
- *Pseudomonas* — gentamicin, tobramycin, and carbenicillin
- *Staphylococcus* — penicillin G; if resistance develops, a semisynthetic penicillin, such as nafcillin or a cephalosporin.

When the infecting organism can't be identified, therapy usually consists of a broad-spectrum antibiotic, such as ampicillin or cephalexin.

Other drug therapy

- Urinary analgesics such as phenazopyridine

INTERVENTIONS AND RATIONALES

- Monitor urine specific gravity *to detect dehydration.*
- Monitor vital signs *to detect fever and hypertension.*
- Assess renal status *to determine baseline renal function and detect any changes from baseline.*
- Administer antipyretics *to reduce fever.*
- Force fluids *to achieve urine output of more than 2 L/day.* However, discourage intake greater than 3 L/day. *Excessive fluid intake may decrease the effectiveness of the antibiotics.*
- Provide a diet that contains 500 mg of calcium for children up to age 3, 800 mg for school-age children, and 1,300 mg for adolescents; moderate restriction of sodium; moderate intake of animal protein; and avoidance of high doses of vitamin C. *These measures will help to prevent formation of renal calculi.*

Teaching topics

- Collecting a clean-catch urine specimen.
- Refrigerating or culturing a urine specimen within 30 minutes of collection to prevent overgrowth of bacteria
- Completing prescribed antibiotic therapy, even after symptoms subside
- Understanding long-term follow-up care for high-risk children

Nephroblastoma

Nephroblastoma, also known as Wilms' tumor, is an embryonal cancer of the kidney.

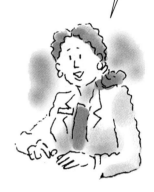

It ain't over till the pill bottle is empty. Emphasize the need to complete the prescribed antibiotic therapy, even after symptoms subside.

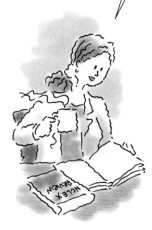

Key assessment finding in nephroblastoma: a nontender mass in the midline area. It's often detected by a parent while bathing or dressing the child.

The average age at diagnosis is 2 to 4 years old. The prognosis is excellent if there is no metastasis.

Nephroblastoma is measured in four stages.
• In stage I, the tumor is limited to the kidney.
• In stage II, the tumor extends beyond the kidney but can be completely excised.
• In stage III, the tumor spreads but is confined to the abdomen and lymph nodes.
• In stage IV, the tumor metastasizes to the lung, liver, bone, and brain.

CAUSE
• Genetic predisposition

ASSESSMENT FINDINGS
• Abdominal pain
• Constipation
• Hematuria
• Hypertension
• Nontender mass, usually midline near the liver; often detected by the parent while bathing or dressing the child
• Associated congenital anomalies, such as microcephaly, mental retardation, and genitourinary tract problems

DIAGNOSTIC TEST RESULTS
• Excretory urography reveals a mass displacing the normal kidney structure.
• Computed tomography scan or sonography will reveal metastasis.
• Serum blood studies show anemia.

NURSING DIAGNOSES
• Fear
• Pain
• Anxiety

TREATMENT
• Nephrectomy within 24 to 48 hours of diagnosis
• Radiation therapy (following surgery)

Drug therapy
• Analgesics (postoperatively)
• Chemotherapy (following surgery) with dactinomycin (Cosmegen), doxorubicin (Adriamycin), or vincristine (Oncovin)

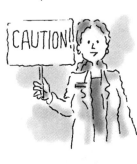

Don't palpate the child's abdomen. Doing so might cause cancer cells to spread.

INTERVENTIONS AND RATIONALES
• Monitor vital signs and intake and output *to determine fluid volume status.*
• Don't palpate the abdomen, and prevent others from doing so; *palpating the abdomen may disseminate cancer cells to other sites.*
• Handle and bathe the child carefully and loosen clothing near the abdomen *to prevent pressure on the abdomen, which may cause dissemination of cancer cells.*
• Prepare the child and family members for a nephrectomy within 24 to 48 hours of diagnosis. *Surgery must be performed quickly after diagnosis because these tumors metastasize quickly.*
• After surgery, provide routine care for a nephrectomy patient:
– monitor urine output and report output less than 30 ml/hour
– assist with turning, coughing, and deep breathing
– encourage early ambulation
– provide pain medications, as necessary
– monitor postoperative dressings for signs of bleeding
– use aseptic techniques for dressing changes.
  These measures will help to prevent postoperative complications such as pneumonia, wound infection, and kidney failure.

Teaching topics
• Providing adequate nutrition and hydration
• Dealing with adverse reactions to chemotherapy
• Contacting support groups

Urinary tract infection

Urinary tract infection (UTI) is a microbial invasion of the kidneys, ureters, bladder, or urethra.

The risk for UTIs varies depending on the child's age and the presence of obstructive uropathy or voiding dysfunction. In the neonatal period UTIs occur most frequently in males, possibly because of the higher incidence of congenital abnormalities in male neonates. By age 4 months, UTIs are much more common in girls than in boys. The increased incidence in girls continues throughout childhood.

After infancy, nearly all UTIs occur when bacteria enter the urethra and ascend the urinary tract. Females are especially at risk for infection because the female urethra is much shorter than the male urethra. The female urethra is more subject to direct contamination because of its proximity to the anal opening. *Escherichia coli* causes approximately 75% to 90% of all UTIs in females.

CAUSES
• Incomplete bladder emptying
• Irritation by bubble baths
• Poor hygiene
• Reflux

ASSESSMENT FINDINGS
• Abdominal pain
• Enuresis
• Frequent urges to void with pain or burning on urination
• Hematuria
• Lethargy
• Low-grade fever
• Poor feeding patterns
• Urine that is cloudy and foul-smelling

DIAGNOSTIC TEST RESULTS
• Clean-catch urine culture yields large amounts of bacteria.
• Urine pH is increased.

NURSING DIAGNOSES
• Altered urinary elimination
• Pain
• Risk for infection

TREATMENT
• Cranberry juice to acidify urine
• Forced fluids to flush infection from the urinary tract

Drug therapy
• Antibiotics: co-trimoxazole (Bactrim) or ampicillin to prevent glomerulonephritis

INTERVENTIONS AND RATIONALES
• Monitor input and output *to determine if fluid replacement therapy is adequate.*
• Assess toileting habits for proper front-to-back wiping and proper hand washing *to prevent recurrent infection.*
• Encourage increased intake of fluids and cranberry juice *to flush the infection from the urinary tract and acidify the urine.*
• Assist the child when necessary to ensure that the perineal area is clean after elimination. *Cleaning the perineal area by wiping from the area of least contamination (urinary meatus) to the area of greatest contamination (anus) helps prevent UTIs.*

Teaching topics
• Avoiding tub baths or bubble baths
• Encouraging child to use the toilet every 2 hours
• Performing toilet hygiene; wiping from front to back

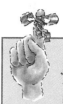

Memory jogger

To remember the clinical findings associated with urinary tract infection, think, "The urinary tract is **FULL** of infection." Look for:

Frequent urges to void

Urine that is foul-smelling and cloudy

Low-grade fever

Lethargy.

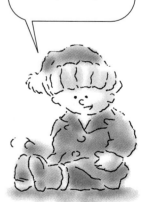

One more pediatric chapter to go!

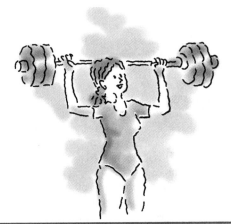

Pump up on practice questions

1. A school-age child is diagnosed with acute glomerulonephritis (nephritis). Which nursing action takes priority when caring for this child?

- A. Monitoring blood pressure every 4 hours
- B. Checking urine specific gravity every 8 hours
- C. Offering the child fluids every hour
- D. Providing the child with a regular diet and snacks

Answer: A. Hypertension is a major complication that can occur during the acute phase of glomerulonephritis; therefore, blood pressure should be monitored at least every 4 hours. Specific gravity should also be monitored but it doesn't take priority over blood pressure monitoring. Fluids may be limited and a low-sodium diet initiated if the child is hypertensive.

➡ *NCLEX keys*
Nursing process step: Implementation
Client needs category: Physiological integrity
Client needs subcategory: Reduction of risk potential
Taxonomic level: Application

2. The nurse is assessing a young female child who may have a urinary tract infection (UTI). A female child is more susceptible to UTIs than a male because she has:

- A. no pubic hair.
- B. a shorter urethra.
- C. a smaller bladder.
- D. smaller kidneys.

Answer: B. The female child is more susceptible to UTIs than the male because the female has a shorter urethra, making it easier for organisms to be transmitted into the bladder. The infant's smaller, immature kidneys cause a low glomerular filtration rate but don't make the infant prone to UTI. A small child voids more frequently because of a small bladder, but this doesn't make the child prone to UTI. The absence of pubic hair is normal in young children; pubic hair growth signals the onset of puberty.

➡ *NCLEX keys*
Nursing process step: Assessment
Client needs category: Health promotion and maintenance
Client needs subcategory: Growth and development through the life span
Taxonomic level: Application

3. An infant is admitted to the pediatric unit for surgical repair of hypospadias. The infant's urine output is 7 ml/hr. What nursing action is most appropriate?

- A. Notify the physician immediately.
- B. Prepare to administer I.V. fluids.
- C. Offer the infant formula every hour.
- D. Continue to monitor urine output.

Answer: D. The normal urine output for an infant is 5 to 10 ml/hour. The urine output of this infant falls within the normal range; therefore, the nurse should continue to monitor urine output. It's not necessary to notify the physician, administer I.V. fluids, or increase the infant's intake.

➡ *NCLEX keys*
Nursing process step: Implementation
Client needs category: Physiological integrity
Client needs subcategory: Reduction of risk potential
Taxonomic level: Comprehension

4. The nurse must obtain a urine specimen from an infant. The nurse can best obtain a clean-catch specimen by:

A. applying a pediatric urine collector to dry skin.
B. placing the infant on a pediatric bedpan.
C. inserting an indwelling urinary catheter.
D. wringing out a cloth diaper after the infant voids.

Answer: A. The nurse should properly clean the infant's skin and genitals and apply a pediatric urine collector to dry skin (powders or creams shouldn't be used). If the infant doesn't void within 45 minutes, the bag should be removed and the procedure repeated. Placing the infant on a pediatric bedpan, inserting an indwelling urinary catheter, and wringing out a urine-filled cloth diaper aren't appropriate methods for collecting clean-catch urine specimens in infants.

➡ *NCLEX keys*
Nursing process step: Implementation
Client needs category: Safe, effective care environment
Client needs subcategory: Safety and infection control
Taxonomic level: Knowledge

5. The nurse is creating a teaching plan for a school-age child with a urinary tract infection (UTI). Which should the nurse first assess?
A. The child's dietary intake
B. The child's toileting habits
C. The child's calcium intake
D. The child's activity level

Answer: B. The nurse should assess the child's toileting habits before creating a teaching plan for the school-age child with a UTI. Based on her findings, the nurse should instruct the child in proper front-to-back wiping, hand washing, and using the toilet every 2 hours. It isn't necessary to inquire about the child's dietary intake, calcium intake, or activity level at this time.

➡ *NCLEX keys*
Nursing process step: Assessment
Client needs category: Physiological integrity
Client needs subcategory: Reduction of risk potential
Taxonomic level: Knowledge

6. A child is admitted to the pediatric unit with a fever of 102.5° F (39.2° C), shaking chills, and flank pain. From these assessment findings, the nurse would most likely suspect which diagnosis?
A. Urinary tract infection
B. Nephritis
C. Nephroblastoma
D. Urolithiasis

Answer: B. In nephritis, the child exhibits assessment findings such as fever of 102° F (38.9° C) or higher, shaking chills, flank pain, urgency, frequency, and burning during urination. The child experiencing a urinary tract infection may exhibit low-grade fever, dysuria, frequency, urgency, lethargy, and urine that is cloudy and foul-smelling. The child with a nephroblastoma typically presents with a nontender mass, usually midline near the liver; abdominal pain; hypertension; hematuria; and constipation. The child with urolithiasis presents with colicky flank pain, nausea, vomiting, hematuria, and dysuria.

➡ *NCLEX keys*
Nursing process step: Assessment
Client needs category: Physiological integrity
Client needs subcategory: Reduction of risk potential
Taxonomic level: Analysis

7. The nurse is teaching parents of an infant with hypospadias. The nurse should tell the parents to avoid:
A. using disposable diapers.
B. positioning the infant on the back to sleep.
C. bathing the infant in an infant bathtub.
D. having the infant circumcised.

Answer: D. The parents should be instructed to avoid having the infant circumcised because the foreskin may be needed during surgical repair. The parents would be permitted to use disposable diapers for their infant. The parents should be instructed to place their child on his back to sleep to decrease the risk of sudden infant death syndrome. It's acceptable for the parents to bathe the infant in an infant bathtub.

➡ *NCLEX keys*
Nursing process step: Implementation
Client needs category: Physiological integrity
Client needs subcategory: Reduction of risk potential
Taxonomic level: Knowledge

8. A toddler is admitted to the pediatric unit with a diagnosis of nephroblastoma. When providing routine care for this toddler, the nurse should avoid:

    A. palpating the toddler's abdomen.
    B. positioning the toddler on the side.
    C. bathing the toddler.
    D. loosening the toddler's clothing.

Answer: A. The nurse shouldn't palpate the toddler's abdomen and should prevent others from doing so because it may disseminate cancer cells to other sites. The toddler may be carefully positioned on his side. The toddler may be bathed but must be handled carefully. The toddler's clothes should be loosened around the abdomen.

➡ *NCLEX keys*
Nursing process step: Implementation
Client needs category: Physiological integrity
Client needs subcategory: Reduction of risk potential
Taxonomic level: Knowledge

9. A parent reports finding a mass in the child's abdomen. After the diagnosis of nephroblastoma is confirmed, the nurse should prepare the child and family for:

    A. immediate chemotherapy.
    B. immediate radiation therapy.
    C. nephrectomy within 24 hours of diagnosis.
    D. discharge to home with hospice care.

Answer: C. The nurse should prepare the child and family for a nephrectomy, which is usually performed within 24 to 48 hours of diagnosis. Chemotherapy and radiation therapy are used as follow-up treatment once the nephrectomy is completed. The prognosis is excellent if there is no metastasis, and the tumor usually remains encapsulated for a long time.

➡ *NCLEX keys*
Nursing process step: Planning
Client needs category: Physiological integrity
Client needs subcategory: Reduction of risk potential
Taxonomic level: Knowledge

10. An infant is suspected of having a chlamydia infection. The infant most likely contracted this infection:

    A. transplacentally.
    B. during passage through the birth canal.
    C. through sexual abuse.
    D. in the nursery because of improper infection-control measures.

Answer: B. Chlamydia is transmitted to the fetus during passage through the birth canal. It isn't passed to the fetus transplacentally or by improper infection-control measures. Transmission from sexual abuse in infants is less common than transmission through the birth canal.

➡ *NCLEX keys*
Nursing process step: Assessment
Client needs category: Health promotion and maintenance
Client needs subcategory: Safety and infection control
Taxonomic level: Knowledge

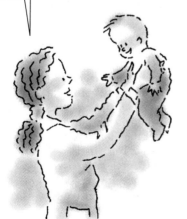

I know you think I'm goofing off, but taking a break and having some fun is also part of preparing for the NCLEX.

35 Integumentary System

Brush up on key concepts

In this chapter, you'll review:

✐ characteristics of the pediatric integumentary system

✐ tests used to diagnose integumentary disorders

✐ common integumentary disorders.

The skin, the primary component of the integumentary system, forms a protective barrier between internal structures and the external environment. Tough and resilient, the skin is virtually impermeable to aqueous solutions, bacteria, or toxic compounds.

At any time, you can review the major points of this chapter by consulting the *Cheat Sheet* on pages 682 and 683.

Immature at birth
Like most body systems, the integumentary system isn't mature at birth. Therefore, it provides a less effective barrier to physical elements or microorganisms during birth and infancy than during childhood. This helps to explain why infants and young children are more prone to infection.

Untouched
The **skin** of infants and young children appears smoother than that of adults. A child's skin has less terminal hair and hasn't been subjected to long-term exposure to environmental elements.

I'm chilly
Infants have poorly developed **subcutaneous fat,** predisposing them to hypothermia. Eccrine sweat glands don't begin to function until the first month of life, which will also inhibit the infant's ability to control body temperature.

Ch..ch..changes
With the onset of adolescence, **apocrine** glands enlarge and become active. This activity leads to axillary sweating and characteristic body odor. The sebaceous glands begin to produce sebum in response to hormone activity, which predisposes the adolescent to acne. Along with the skin glands becoming active, coarse terminal hair grows in the axillae and pubic areas of both sexes and on the faces of males.

Here's the skinny
Skin performs many vital functions. These include:
- protecting against trauma
- regulating body temperature
- serving as an organ of excretion and sensation
- synthesizing vitamin D in the presence of ultraviolet light.

Wearing layers
Skin has three primary layers:

☝ The **epidermis** (the outermost layer) produces keratin as its primary function. It contains two sublayers: the stratum corneum, an outer, horny layer of keratin that protects the body against harmful environmental substances and restricts water loss, and the cellular stratum, where keratin cells are synthesized. It also contains melanocytes, which produce the melanin, which gives the skin its color, and Langerhans cells, which are involved in a variety of immunologic reactions.

✌ The **dermis** (the middle layer) contains collagen, which strengthens the skin to prevent it from tearing, and elastin to give it resilience.

🖐 The **subcutaneous tissue** (the innermost layer) consists mainly of fat (containing mostly triglycerides), which provides heat, insulation, shock absorption, and a reserve of calories.

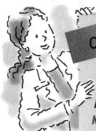

Cheat sheet

Integumentary refresher

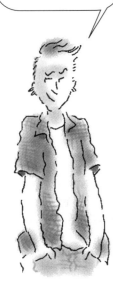

You can read the whole chapter, or you can just go skin deep and study the Cheat sheet.

ACNE VULGARIS

Key signs and symptoms

• Closed comedo, or whitehead (acne plug not protruding from the follicle and covered by the epidermis)
• Open comedo, or blackhead (acne plug protruding and not covered by the epidermis)
• Inflammation and characteristic acne pustules, papules or, in severe forms, acne cysts or abscesses (caused by rupture or leakage of an enlarged plug into the dermis)

Key treatments

• Exposure to ultraviolet light (but never when a photosensitizing agent, such as tretinoin, is being used)
• Oral isotretinoin (Accutane) limited to those with severe papulopustular or cystic acne who don't respond to conventional therapy
• Systemic therapy: usually tetracycline (Achromycin) to decrease bacterial growth; alternatively, erythromycin (tetracycline contraindicated during pregnancy and childhood because it discolors developing teeth)
• Topical medications: benzoyl peroxide (Benzac), clindamycin (Cleocin), or erythromycin (Benzamycin) antibacterial agents, alone or in combination with tretinoin (retinoic acid), or a keratolytic

Key interventions

• Try to identify predisposing factors.
• Instruct the patient receiving tretinoin to apply it at least 30 minutes after washing the face and at least 1 hour before bedtime. Warn against using it around the eyes or lips. After treatments, the skin should look pink and dry.
• Advise the patient to avoid exposure to sunlight or to use a sunblock. If the prescribed regimen includes tretinoin and benzoyl peroxide, tell the patient to use one preparation in the morning and the other at night.
• Instruct the patient to take tetracycline on an empty stomach and not to take it with antacids or milk.

• Tell the patient who's taking isotretinoin to avoid vitamin A supplements. Also discuss how to deal with the dry skin and mucous membranes that usually occur during treatment. Warn the female patient about the severe risk of teratogenesis. Monitor liver function and lipid levels.
• Pay special attention to the patient's perception of his physical appearance, and offer emotional support.

BURNS

Key signs and symptoms

For first-degree burn (partial thickness of skin) look for:
• dry, painful, red skin with edema
• sunburn appearance
For second-degree burn (partial thickness of skin) look for:
• moist, weeping blisters with edema
• very painful
For third-degree burn (full thickness of skin) look for:
• avascular site without blanching or pain
• dry, pale, leathery skin

Key test results

• Many burn facilities use the Lund and Browder chart, which is a body surface area chart that is corrected for age to determine the extent of injury.

Key treatments

• I.V. fluids to prevent and treat shock; urine output maintained at 1 to 2 ml/kg
• Protective isolation, depending on burn severity

Key interventions

• Maintain a patent airway in the immediate postburn phase.
• Monitor vital signs, intake, and output.
• Prevent heat loss.

CONTACT DERMATITIS (DIAPER RASH)

Key sign and symptom

• Characteristic bright, red, maculopapular rash in the diaper area

Integumentary refresher (continued)

CONTACT DERMATITIS (DIAPER RASH) (continued)

Key treatments

- Cleaning affected area with mild soap and water
- Leaving affected area open to air

Key intervention

- Keep the diaper area clean and dry.

HEAD LICE

Key signs and symptoms

- Pruritus of the scalp
- White flecks attached to the hair shafts

Key test result

- Examination reveals lice eggs, which look like white flecks, firmly attached near the base of hair shafts.

Key treatments

- Pyrethrins (RID) or permethrin (NIX) shampoos or lindane (Kwell) in resistant cases

Key interventions

- Explain the need to wash bed linens, hats, combs, brushes, and anything else in contact with the hair.

IMPETIGO

Key signs and symptoms

- Macular rash progressing to a papular and vesicular rash, which oozes and forms a moist, honey-colored crust

Key treatment

- Washing area with disinfectant soap

Key interventions

- Apply antibiotic ointment.
- Wash the area three times daily with antiseptic soap.

RASHES

Key signs and symptoms

- Papular rash: raised solid lesions with color changes in circumscribed areas
- Pustular rash: vesicles and bullae that fill with purulent exudate
- Vesicular rash: small, raised, circumscribed lesions filled with clear fluid

Key test results

- Aspirate from lesions may reveal cause.
- Patch test may identify cause.

Key treatments

- Antibacterial, antifungal, or antiviral agent (depending on cause)
- Antihistamines if the rash is from an allergy

Key interventions

- Maintain standard precautions to prevent the spread of infection.
- Teach sanitary techniques.
- Keep weeping lesions covered.

SCABIES

Key sign and symptom

- Linear black burrows between fingers and toes and in palms, axillae, and groin

Key test result

- Drop of mineral oil placed over the burrow, followed by superficial scraping and examination of expressed material under a microscope may reveal ova or mite feces.

Key treatment

- Application of lindane (Kwell) lotion or permethrin (NIX)

Key interventions

- Teach the child and parents to apply lindane or permethrin from the neck down covering the entire body, wait 15 minutes before dressing, and avoid bathing for 8 to 12 hours.
- Explain the need to change bed linens, towels, and clothing after bathing and lotion application.

Thinner, more sensitive

A child's skin differs from an adult's in two important ways:

- The child has thinner and more sensitive skin than the adult.
- Birthmarks in the newborn can result from the sensitivity of the infant's skin, the incomplete migration of skin cells, or clogged pores.

Keep abreast of diagnostic tests

Here are the most important tests used to diagnose skin disorders, along with common nursing interventions associated with each test.

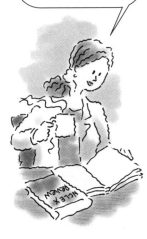

Because a child's skin is thinner and more sensitive than an adult's, it's more prone to infection.

Slide show
In **diascopy,** a lesion is covered with a microscope slide or piece of clear plastic. The area is observed to determine whether dilated capillaries or extravasated blood is causing the redness of a lesion.

Nursing actions
• Explain the procedure to child and parents.

Light up and down
Sidelighting shows minor elevations or depressions in lesions; it also helps determine the configuration and degree of eruption.

Subdued lighting, another test, highlights the difference between normal skin and circumscribed lesions that are hypopigmented or hyperpigmented.

Nursing actions
• Explain the procedure to child and parents.

Spotlight on disease
Microscopic immunofluorescence identifies immunoglobulins and elastic tissue in detecting skin manifestations of immunologically mediated disease.

Nursing actions
• Explain the procedure to child and parents.

Organism info
Gram stains and exudate cultures help identify organisms responsible for underlying infections.

Nursing actions
• Explain the procedure to child and parents.
• Obtain cultures as directed by institutional policy.

Patching it together
Patch tests identify contact sensitivity (usually with dermatitis).

Nursing actions
• Explain the procedure to child and parents.

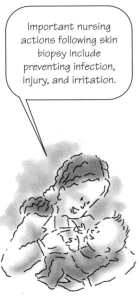

Important nursing actions following skin biopsy include preventing infection, injury, and irritation.

Tissue test
A **skin biopsy** is used to determine the histology of cells. It can be used to diagnose or confirm a disorder.

Nursing actions
Before the procedure, do the following:
• Explain the procedure to child and parents.
• Make sure that a written, informed consent has been obtained.
After the procedure, do the following:
• Tell the parents that the child should avoid tight clothes, and wool or rough clothing.
• Prevent secondary infections by cutting the child's nails and applying mittens and elbow restraints.
• Suggest the child wear light, loose, nonirritating clothing.

Polish up on patient care

Major skin disorders in pediatric patients include acne vulgaris, burns, contact dermatitis (diaper rash), head lice, impetigo, rashes, and scabies.

Acne vulgaris

An inflammatory disease of the sebaceous follicles, acne vulgaris primarily affects adolescents, although lesions can appear as early as age 8. Although acne strikes boys more often and more severely, it usually occurs in girls at an earlier age and tends to last longer, sometimes into adulthood. The prognosis is good with treatment.

CAUSES
• Androgen-stimulated sebum production
• Follicular occlusion
• No longer attributed to dietary influences (such theories appear to be groundless)
• *Propionibacterium acnes* a normal skin flora

Predisposing factors
• Androgen stimulation

• Certain drugs, including corticosteroids, corticotropin, androgens, iodides, bromides, trimethadione, phenytoin, isoniazid, lithium, and halothane; cobalt irradiation; or total parenteral nutrition.
• Cosmetics
• Emotional stress
• Exposure to heavy oils, greases, or tars
• Heredity
• Oral contraceptives (Many females experience an acne flare-up during their first few menses after starting or discontinuing oral contraceptives.)
• Trauma or rubbing from tight clothing
• Unfavorable climate

ASSESSMENT FINDINGS
• Closed comedo, or whitehead (acne plug not protruding from the follicle and covered by the epidermis)
• Open comedo, or blackhead (acne plug protruding and not covered by the epidermis)
• Inflammation and characteristic acne pustules, papules, or, in severe forms, acne cysts or abscesses (caused by rupture or leakage of an enlarged plug into the dermis)
• Acne scars from chronic, recurring lesions

DIAGNOSTIC TEST RESULTS
• Diagnostic testing isn't necessary. The appearance of characteristic acne lesions, especially in an adolescent patient, confirms the presence of acne vulgaris.

NURSING DIAGNOSES
• Impaired skin integrity
• Body image disturbance
• Risk for infection

TREATMENT
• Acne surgery (in severe cases)
• Cryotherapy
• Exposure to ultraviolet light (but never when a photosensitizing agent such as tretinoin is being used)

Drug therapy
• Intralesional corticosteroid injection
• Oral isotretinoin (Accutane) limited to those with severe papulopustular or cystic

acne who don't respond to conventional therapy
• Systemic therapy: usually tetracycline (Achromycin) to decrease bacterial growth; alternatively, erythromycin (tetracycline contraindicated during pregnancy and childhood because it discolors developing teeth)
• Topical medications: benzoyl peroxide (Benzac), clindamycin (Cleocin), or erythromycin (Benzamycin) antibacterial agents, alone or in combination with tretinoin (retinoic acid, Retin-A), or a keratolytic
• Antiandrogenic agents: estrogens or spironolactone (Aldactazide)

INTERVENTIONS AND RATIONALES
• Check the patient's drug history *because medications such as some oral contraceptives may cause an acne flare-up.*
• Try to identify predisposing factors *to determine if any may be eliminated or modified.*
• Explain the causes of acne to the patient and family. Make sure they understand the prescribed treatment is more likely to improve acne than a strict diet and fanatic scrubbing with soap and water. Provide written instructions regarding treatment *to eliminate misconceptions.*
• Instruct the patient receiving tretinoin to apply it at least 30 minutes after washing the face and at least 1 hour before bedtime. Warn against using it around the eyes or lips *to prevent damage.* After treatments, the skin should look pink and dry. *If it appears red or starts to peel, the preparation may have to be weakened or applied less often.*
• Advise the patient to avoid exposure to sunlight or to use a sunscreen *to prevent photosensitivity reaction.* If the prescribed regimen includes tretinoin and benzoyl peroxide, tell the patient to use one preparation in the morning and the other at night *to avoid skin irritation.*
• Instruct the patient to take tetracycline on an empty stomach and not to take it with antacids or milk *because it interacts with their metallic ions and is then poorly absorbed.*
• Tell the patient who is taking isotretinoin to avoid vitamin A supplements, *which can worsen any adverse effects.* Also discuss how to

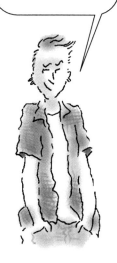

In other words, ZITS!

deal with the dry skin and mucous membranes that usually occur during treatment. Warn the female patient about the severe risk of teratogenesis. Monitor liver function and lipid levels *to avoid toxicity*.

• Inform the patient that acne takes a long time to clear — even years for complete resolution. Encourage continued local skin care even after acne clears. Explain the adverse effects of all drugs *to promote compliance*.

• Pay special attention to the patient's perception of his physical appearance, and offer emotional support *to help the patient cope with the effects of his illness*.

Teaching topics
• Treatment regimen
• Avoiding prolonged exposure to sunlight
• Eliminating misconceptions
• Eliminating predisposing factors, such as cosmetic use and emotional stress

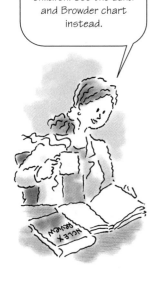

Remember that the Rule of Nines, generally used to determine the extent of a burn, is inaccurate for children. Use the Lund and Browder chart instead.

Burns

Most pediatric burns occur to children under age 5. Overall, burns are the third leading cause of accidental death in children (after motor vehicle accidents and drowning). Burns are classified as first-, second-, or third-degree, depending on severity.

CAUSES
• Contact with hot liquid or electricity (most common cause of burns in children under age 3)
• Flames (most common cause of burns in older children)

ASSESSMENT FINDINGS

First-degree burn (partial thickness of skin)
• Dry, painful, red skin with edema
• Looks like sunburn

Second-degree burn (partial thickness of skin)
• Moist, weeping blisters with edema
• Very painful

Third-degree burn (full thickness of skin)
• Avascular without blanching or pain
• Dry, pale, leathery skin
• Diuresis 2 to 5 days after the burn, as fluid shifts back
• Fluid shift from intravascular to interstitial compartments
• Hypovolemia and symptoms of shock from fluid shift, including renal function
• Infection due to altered skin integrity

DIAGNOSTIC TEST RESULTS
• Many burn facilities use the Lund and Browder chart, which is a body surface area chart that is corrected for age to determine the extent of injury. (The Rule of Nines is inaccurate for children because the head can account for 13% to 19% of body surface area; the legs account for 10% to 16%, depending on the child's age and size.)

NURSING DIAGNOSES
• Ineffective airway clearance
• Fluid volume deficit
• Risk for infection

TREATMENT
• Debridement
• Diet: adequate nutritional support to avoid negative nitrogen balance and prevent overfeeding
• Escharotomy
• I.V. fluids to prevent and treat shock; urine output maintained at 1 to 2 ml/kg
• Oxygen therapy (may require intubation)
• Protective isolation, depending on burn severity
• Skin grafting
• Total parenteral nutrition

Drug therapy
• Analgesics: morphine, meperidine (Demerol)
• Diuretic therapy: mannitol (Osmitrol) to flush hemoglobin from kidneys
• Antibiotics: silver sulfadiazine (Silvadene) to limit infection at the site

INTERVENTIONS AND RATIONALES
• Stop the burning in an emergency situation *to prevent further injury*.

• Maintain a patent airway in the immediate postburn phase; *inhalation of smoke may cause airway edema.*
• Monitor vital signs, intake, and output *to assess for signs of complications.*
• Assess cardiovascular, renal, respiratory, and neurologic status *to assess for signs of shock.*
• Administer I.V. analgesics *to relieve pain*; don't administer I.M. injections.
• Assist with debridement *to promote healing.*
• Elevate the burned body part *to promote venous drainage and decrease edema.*
• Spread a thin layer of topical medication such as mafenide acetate over the burn *to prevent infection.*
• Prevent heat loss *to reduce metabolic demands.*
• Explaining treatments, pain management, and the need for the child's active participation in the treatment as well as allowing the child choices, where appropriate, *helps the child feel less afraid and anxious.*
• Encourage family and friends to participate in the child's care when appropriate *to create a pleasant, loving, and supportive atmosphere.*
• Allow the child to participate in everyday activities, such as playing and school activities, *to normalize the child's situation.*
• Give the child the opportunity to maintain the developmental tasks already achieved, such as eating in a high chair, not using diapers if the child has been toilet-trained, and allowing self-feeding if the child is able *to prevent regression.*
• Rock, cuddle, and treat the patient like any other child *to encourage normalcy in his situation.*
• Promote a comfortable atmosphere for the child. *This encourages the child to talk and act out feelings of depression and hostility and express anxieties.*

Teaching topics
• Explaining treatment to child and parents
• Coping strategies for dealing with long-term care
• Burn prevention

Contact dermatitis

Contact dermatitis, also known as diaper rash, is a local skin reaction in the areas normally covered by a diaper.

CAUSES
• Body soaps, bubble baths, tight clothes, and wool or rough clothing
• Clothing dyes or the soaps used to wash diapers
• Irritation due to acidic urine and stools or the formation of ammonia in the diaper
• Moist, warm environment contained by a plastic diaper lining

ASSESSMENT FINDINGS
• Characteristic bright, red, maculopapular rash in the diaper area
• Irritability because the rash is painful and warm

DIAGNOSTIC TEST RESULTS
• Diagnostic testing isn't necessary. Diagnosis is based on inspection.

NURSING DIAGNOSES
• Risk for infection
• Pain
• Impaired skin integrity

TREATMENT
• Cleaning affected area with mild soap and water
• Leaving affected area open to air

Drug therapy
• Application of vitamin A and D skin cream or zinc oxide ointment to help the skin heal
• Antibiotics if secondary infection occurs

INTERVENTIONS AND RATIONALES
• Keep the diaper area clean and dry *to maintain skin integrity.*
• Change the diaper immediately after the child voids or defecates *to prevent skin breakdown.*
• Wash the area with mild soap and water *to promote healing.*

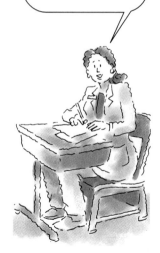

Because contact dermatitis is often caused by a moist, warm environment, it makes sense that an important intervention is keeping the area clean, dry, and open to the air.

• Keep the area open to the air without plastic bed linings, if possible, *to promote circulation and comfort.*
• Don't use commercially prepared diaper wipes on broken skin; *the chemicals and alcohol in commercially prepared wipes may be irritating.*

Teaching topics
• Preventing diaper rash
• Administering medication

Head lice

Head lice (pediculosis capitis) is a contagious infestation. In it, lice eggs, which look like white flecks, are firmly attached near the base of hair shafts. The cause of this disorder isn't related to the hygiene of a child or family members; however, head lice is easily transmitted among children and family members.

CAUSES
• Sharing of clothing and combs; close physical contact with peers, for example, in gym class (common in school-age children)

ASSESSMENT FINDINGS
• Pruritus of the scalp
• White flecks attached to the hair shafts

DIAGNOSTIC TEST RESULTS
• Examination reveals lice eggs, which look like white flecks, firmly attached near the base of hair shafts.

NURSING DIAGNOSES
• Body image disturbance
• Impaired skin integrity
• Social isolation

TREATMENT
• Removal of lice and eggs using fine-toothed comb

Drug therapy
• Pyrethrins (RID) or permethrin (NIX) shampoos; lindane (Kwell) in resistant cases
• Preventive drug therapy for other family members and classmates

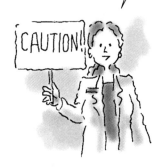

When applying insecticidal treatments, carefully follow the manufacturer's directions to avoid neurotoxicity.

CAUTION!

INTERVENTIONS AND RATIONALES
• Carefully follow the manufacturer's directions when applying medicated shampoo *to avoid neurotoxicity.*
• Confine the child to home for 24 hours *to reduce risk of transmission.*
• Repeat treatment in 7 to 12 days *to ensure that all the eggs have been killed.*

Teaching topics
• Washing bed linens, hats, combs, brushes, and anything else that comes in contact with the hair to prevent reinfestation.
• How to assess for reinfestation
• Refraining from exchanging combs, brushes, headgear, or clothing with other children

Impetigo

Impetigo is a highly contagious superficial infection of the skin, marked by patches of tiny blisters that erupt. It's common in children ages 2 to 5. Infection is spread by direct contact; incubation period is 2 to 10 days after contact.

CAUSES
• Group A beta-hemolytic streptococci
• Staphylococci

ASSESSMENT FINDINGS
• Commonly seen on the face and extremities, but may be spread to other parts of the body by scratching
• Macular rash progressing to a papular and vesicular rash, which oozes and forms a moist, honey-colored crust
• Pruritus

DIAGNOSTIC TEST RESULTS
• Diagnostic testing isn't necessary. Diagnosis is based on inspection.

NURSING DIAGNOSES
• Bathing or hygiene self-care deficit
• Impaired skin integrity
• Risk for infection

TREATMENTS
• Washing area with disinfectant soap

Drug therapy
• Topical antibiotic ointment

INTERVENTIONS AND RATIONALES
• Apply antibiotic ointment *to eradicate the infection.*
• Wash the area three times daily with antiseptic soap *to promote skin healing.*
• Cover the child's hands, if necessary, *to prevent secondary infection;* cut the child's nails.
• Cover the lesions *to prevent their spread.*

Teaching topics
• Preventing recurrence

Rashes

A rash is a temporary skin eruption. Three types of rashes — papular, pustular, and vesicular — are described below.

A papular rash may erupt anywhere on the body in various configurations and may be acute or chronic. Papular rashes characterize many cutaneous disorders; they may also result from allergy or infectious, neoplastic, or systemic disorders. Common causes of papular rashes in children are infectious diseases, such as molluscum and scarlet fever, scabies, insect bites, allergies or drug reactions, and miliaria.

A pustular rash is made up of crops of pustules that fill with purulent exudate. These lesions vary greatly in size and shape and can be generalized or localized to the hair follicles or sweat glands. Pustules appear in skin and systemic disorders, with use of certain drugs, and with exposure to skin irritants. Disorders that produce pustular rash in children include varicella, erythema toxicum neonatorum, candidiasis, and impetigo. Pustules typify the inflammatory lesions of acne vulgaris, common in adolescents.

A vesicular rash is a scattered or linear distribution of vesicles. A vesicular rash may be mild or severe and temporary or permanent. It may result from infection, inflammation, or allergic reactions. Vesicular rashes in children are caused by staphylococcal infections, varicella, hand-foot-mouth disease, and miliaria.

CAUSES
• Allergic reactions
• Environmental causes
• Viral, fungal, or bacterial infestations

ASSESSMENT FINDINGS
• Papular rash: raised solid lesions with color changes in circumscribed areas
• Pustular rash: vesicles and bullae that fill with purulent exudate
• Vesicular rash: small, raised, circumscribed lesions filled with clear fluid

DIAGNOSTIC TEST RESULTS
• Aspirate from lesions may reveal cause.
• Patch test may identify cause.

NURSING DIAGNOSES
• Impaired skin integrity
• Risk for infection
• Body image disturbance

TREATMENT
• Antibacterial, antifungal, or antiviral agent (depending on cause)
• Antihistamines if the rash is from an allergy

INTERVENTIONS AND RATIONALES
• Keep area cool. *Heat aggravates most skin rashes and increases pruritus; coolness decreases pruritus.*
• Keep the affected area clean and pat it dry *to promote healing.*
• Don't apply powder or cornstarch *as they encourage bacterial growth.*
• Maintain standard precautions *to prevent the spread of infection.*
• Keep weeping lesions covered *to prevent transmission.*

Teaching topics
• Understanding sanitary techniques
• Avoiding sharing combs or hats
• Avoiding scratching

Scabies

Scabies is a parasitic skin disorder that causes severe itching. Scabies develops when microscopic itch mites enter a child's skin and pro-

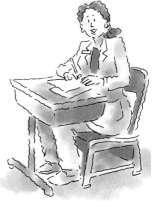

Insidious infectious itch! Impetigo rash may be spread to other parts of the body by scratching.

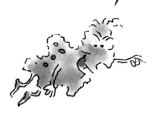

I like to make myself at home. Scabies mites can live their entire lives in human skin, causing chronic infection.

voke a sensitivity reaction. Mites can live their entire lives inside human skin, causing chronic infection. The female mite burrows into the skin to lay her eggs from which larvae emerge to copulate and then reburrow under the skin. Scabies is transmitted through the skin or through sexual contact.

CAUSES
• A female mite that burrows into the skin and deposits eggs in areas that are thin and moist

ASSESSMENT FINDINGS
• Linear black burrows between fingers and toes and in palms, axillae, and groin
• Severe itching

DIAGNOSTIC TEST RESULTS
• Drop of mineral oil placed over the burrow, followed by superficial scraping and examination of expressed material under a microscope may reveal ova or mite feces.

NURSING DIAGNOSES
• Body image disturbance
• Impaired skin integrity
• Social isolation

TREATMENT
• Treatment for all members of the family (as well as close contacts of the child)

Drug therapy
• Application of lindane (Kwell) lotion or permethrin (NIX)

INTERVENTIONS AND RATIONALES
• Wash area thoroughly with soap and water *to promote healing.*
• Teach the child and parents to apply lindane or permethrin from the neck down covering the entire body, wait 15 minutes before dressing, and avoid bathing for 8 to 12 hours *to ensure effectiveness of therapy.*
• Don't apply lindane cream if skin is raw or inflamed *to avoid irritating the skin.*

• Explain to the child and parents that if skin irritation or an allergic reaction develops, they should notify the doctor immediately, stop using the cream, and wash it off thoroughly *to avoid risk of an anaphylactic reaction.*

Teaching topics
• Understanding that pruritus may persist for several weeks after treatment
• Proper hygiene measures
• Changing bed linens, towels, and clothing after bathing and lotion application
• The need to treat family members and close contacts because the parasite is transmitted by close personal contact and through clothes and linens

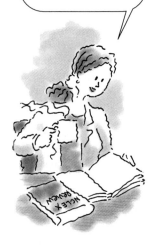

Severe itching marks scabies infestation. Linear black mite burrows may be visible between the fingers and toes or on the palms, axillae, and groin.

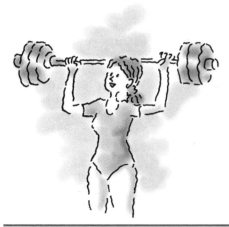

Pump up on practice questions

1. The clothes of a 16-year-old girl catch fire while she is lighting the grill for a family picnic. The girl's mother, a nurse, tells her to drop and roll to extinguish the flames. Which action should the nurse take next?

- A. Move her daughter away from the grill.
- B. Remove her daughter's clothing.
- C. Use the garden hose to wet her daughter down.
- D. Call the fire department.

Answer: C. In emergency burn care, the priority is to stop the burning. The client shouldn't be moved because flames may intensify. Once the fire is extinguished, the client's clothes should be removed to prevent further injury. Emergency medical personnel should be summoned after the flames are extinguished.

➡ *NCLEX keys*
Nursing process step: Implementation
Client needs category: Physiological integrity
Client needs subcategory: Reduction of risk potential
Taxonomic level: Application

2. A child has third-degree burns of the hands, face, and chest. Which of the following nursing diagnoses takes priority?

- A. Ineffective airway clearance related to edema
- B. Body image disturbance related to physical appearance
- C. Altered urinary elimination related to fluid loss
- D. Infection related to epidermal disruption

Answer: A. Initially, when a client is admitted to the hospital for burns, the primary focus is on assessing and managing an effective airway. Body image disturbance, altered urinary elimination, and infection are all integral parts of burn management but aren't first priority.

➡ *NCLEX keys*
Nursing process step: Analysis
Client needs category: Physiological integrity
Client needs subcategory: Physiological adaptation
Taxonomic level: Analysis

3. The nurse is caring for a child with second- and third-degree burns. Which analgesic would most effectively manage the client's severe pain?

- A. Acetaminophen administered by suppository
- B. Meperidine administered I.M.
- C. Codeine administered by mouth
- D. Morphine administered I.V.

Answer: D. A client with severe burns requires strong analgesia. The most effective method of administering analgesics is the I.V. route. Second-degree burns are commonly too painful to be relieved by acetaminophen. I.M. medication may not be absorbed when the client is physiologically unstable. Codeine may not provide sufficient analgesia, and oral administration isn't usually the best route for severe burn victims.

➡ *NCLEX keys*
Nursing process step: Implementation
Client needs category: Physiological integrity
Client needs subcategory: Pharmacological and parenteral therapies
Taxonomic level: Application

To keep up your motivation for studying, remember the big picture. Conquering the NCLEX is a step toward fulfilling life goals you have chosen for yourself.

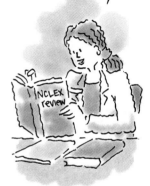

4. A 14-month-old child is in a private room for treatment of burns. Which intervention can best meet the developmental needs of the child?
- A. Ask the mother to room with the child.
- B. Have nursing personnel visit the child regularly throughout the day.
- C. Set the television to the child's favorite cartoon shows.
- D. Attach a brightly colored balloon to the child's crib.

Answer: A. The mother can best provide for the child's developmental needs by being present all of the time. At this age, the child is most susceptible to separation anxiety. A child of this age is likely to be apprehensive toward unfamiliar adults, so regular visits by nursing personnel wouldn't help. Television is a poor substitute for human contact. A balloon is dangerous for a child this age.

➡ *NCLEX keys*
Nursing process step: Implementation
Client needs category: Health promotion and maintenance
Client needs subcategory: Growth and development through the life span
Taxonomic level: Application

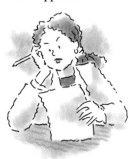

5. A 13-year-old client has received third-degree burns over 20% of his body. When performing an assessment at 72 hours after the burn, which of the following should the nurse expect to find?
- A. Increasing urine output
- B. Severe peripheral edema
- C. Respiratory distress
- D. Absent bowel sounds

Answer: A. During the resuscitative-emergent phase of a burn, fluid shifts back into the interstitial space resulting in the onset of diuresis. Edema resolves during the emergent phase, when fluid shifts back to the intravascular space. Respiratory rate increases during the first hours as a result of edema. When edema resolves, respirations return to normal. Absent bowel sounds occur in the initial stage.

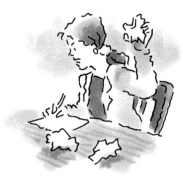

➡ *NCLEX keys*
Nursing process step: Assessment
Client needs category: Physiological integrity
Client needs subcategory: Physiological adaptation
Taxonomic level: Analysis

6. A child comes into the emergency department with a rash that is raised and has color changes in circumscribed areas. What type of rash should the nurse document?
- A. Macular rash
- B. Papular rash
- C. Petechial rash
- D. Vesicular rash

Answer: B. A papular rash contains raised solid lesions with color changes in circumscribed areas. A macular rash is flat with color changes in circumscribed areas. Petechiae are pinpoint purple or red spots on the skin caused by minute hemorrhages. A vesicular rash contains small, raised circumscribed lesions filled with clear fluid.

▶ *NCLEX keys*
Nursing process step: Assessment
Client needs category: Physiological integrity
Client needs subcategory: Reduction of risk
potential
Taxonomic level: Comprehension

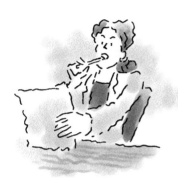

7. The nurse is developing a teaching plan
for the mother of a newborn. The nurse
should instruct the mother to prevent diaper
rash by:
    A. using disposable diapers so she
        doesn't have to change the infant of-
        ten.
    B. bathing the infant in a tub with bub-
        ble bath.
    C. not washing the infant with soap.
    D. keeping the infant's diaper area clean
        and dry.
Answer: D. The mother should be instructed
to keep the infant's diaper area clean and dry;
to change the diaper immediately after the infant voids or defecates; to avoid bubble bath;
and to wash the diaper area with mild soap
and water with every diaper change.

▶ *NCLEX keys*
Nursing process step: Planning
Client needs category: Health promotion and
maintenance
Client needs subcategory: Growth and devel-
opment through the life span
Taxonomic level: Application

8. A mother calls the pediatrician's office
because there is an outbreak of scabies at her
child's day-care center. The nurse should instruct the mother to check her child for
which findings associated with scabies infestation?
    A. Pruritic papules, pustules, and linear
        burrows of the fingers and toe webs
    B. Oval white dots adhered to the hair
        shafts
    C. Diffuse pruritic wheals
    D. Pain, erythema, and edema at the
        site of the bite
Answer: A. The mother should be instructed
to check her child for pruritic papules, vesicles, and linear burrows. Oval flecks on the
hair shaft indicate head lice. Diffuse pruritic
wheels can indicate an allergic reaction. The
specific site of the bite reveals no trace of the
insect bite.

▶ *NCLEX keys*
Nursing process step: Assessment
Client needs category: Health promotion and
maintenance
Client needs subcategory: Prevention and
early detection of disease
Taxonomic level: Knowledge

9. A 16-month-old child is being treated with
Nix for scabies. The child's mother is concerned that the drug hasn't been effective because her child continues to scratch. Which
response by the nurse is most appropriate?

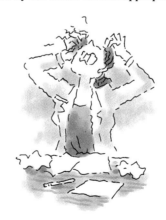

A. Stop treatment because the drug isn't safe for children under age 2.
B. Pruritis can be present for weeks after treatment.
C. Apply the drug every day until the rash disappears.
D. Pruritis is common in children under age 5 treated with Nix.

Answer: B. Pruritus may be present for weeks in the child treated with Nix for scabies. The drug is safe for use in infants as young as age 2 months. Treatment with Nix can safely be repeated in 2 weeks. Pruritus is caused by secondary reactions of mites.

➠ *NCLEX keys*
Nursing process step: Implementation
Client needs category: Physiological integrity
Client needs subcategory: Pharmacological and parenteral therapies
Taxonomic level: Knowledge

10. A child is diagnosed with head lice and the mother asks how she should get the nits out of her child's hair. The nurse should instruct the mother about which of the following concerning head lice treatment?
A. The treatment should be repeated in 7 to 12 days.
B. Combing the hair after shampooing is necessary.
C. Treatment should be repeated every day for 7 days.
D. All children that had contact with the child should be prophylactically treated.

Answer: A. Treatment should be repeated in 7 to 12 days to ensure that all of the eggs have been killed. Combing the hair thoroughly isn't necessary to remove lice eggs. People exposed should be observed for infestation before being treated.

➠ *NCLEX keys*
Nursing process step: Implementation
Client needs category: Physiological integrity
Client needs subcategory: Reduction of risk potential
Taxonomic level: Application

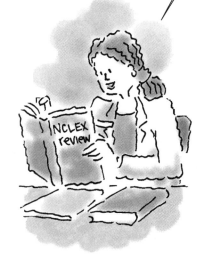

I'm just itching to answer more practice questions. In addition to the questions that follow, don't forget to pump up on practice questions using the free CD-ROM.

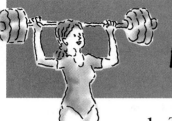

Pump up on more practice questions

Practice makes perfect. So do these 30 pediatric practice questions...ooops!

1. The nurse is teaching the mother of an infant with tetralogy of Fallot. The mother asks what to do when her infant becomes very blue and has trouble breathing after crying. The nurse should tell the mother to:
A. "Leave the infant alone until the crying stops."
B. "Put the infant in the knee-chest position."
C. "Offer the infant a bottle of formula."
D. "Take the infant for a ride in the car."
Answer: B. The infant is having a "tet" or blue spell, which is an acute spell of hypoxia and cyanosis. This occurs when the infant's oxygen requirements are greater than what is supplied in the blood. Treatment involves placing the infant in the knee-chest position to reduce venous return from the extremities because that blood is desaturated. It also increases systemic vascular resistance, which causes more blood to be shunted to the pulmonary artery. Leaving the infant alone until the crying stops will cause an increase in cyanosis. An infant who is crying and having trouble breathing shouldn't be offered a bottle because of the danger of aspiration. Taking the infant for a ride in the car may be an alternative if the mother can't quiet the infant.

➡️ *NCLEX keys*
Nursing process step: Planning
Client needs category: Physiological integrity
Client needs subcategory: Basic care and comfort
Taxonomic level: Application

2. The nurse is providing care to a child who had a cardiac catheterization. Which intervention should the nurse provide?
A. Offer the child liquids immediately on awakening.
B. Allow the child to sleep as much as possible.
C. Assess peripheral pulses for symmetry.
D. Change the dressing over the catheter site.
Answer: C. The most important nursing intervention after cardiac catheterization is to assess peripheral pulses, especially those distal to the catheter site. The pulse may be weaker initially but typically becomes stronger in a short period of time. The dressing should be assessed, and the child may want liquids after the procedure. Allowing the child to sleep as much as possible may be appropriate but isn't the most important intervention.

➡️ *NCLEX keys*
Nursing process step: Implementation
Client needs category: Physiological integrity
Client needs subcategory: Basic care and comfort
Taxonomic level: Application

3. The nurse notices that the dressing over a client's cardiac catheterization site has a large amount of sanguinous drainage. What should the nurse do first?

A. Notify the on-call physician.
B. Apply pressure 1″ (2.5 cm) above the skin site.
C. Check the client's vital signs, including temperature.
D. Assess the peripheral pulse distal to the site.

Answer: B. When bleeding occurs, it's important to apply direct continuous pressure above the percutaneous skin site to localize pressure over the vessel punctured. All of the other actions are important, but applying pressure is the priority.

➡ *NCLEX keys*

Nursing process step: Implementation
Client needs category: Physiological integrity
Client needs subcategory: Basic care and comfort
Taxonomic level: Application

4. The nurse is teaching the mother of a toddler with iron deficiency anemia about dietary modifications. Which statement by the mother indicates that she understands the teaching?
A. "I can let my child have four glasses of milk every day."
B. "I will feed my child fortified cereal and lots of vegetables."
C. "I plan to offer my child juices and cereal for snacks."
D. "I think my child will drink milk and juices easily."

Answer: B. For the child with iron deficiency anemia, iron-rich foods such as fortified cereal, green leafy vegetables, and red meat need to be offered in larger amounts. Foods that contain less iron — such as milk, juices, yellow vegetables, and nonfortified cereals — should be offered in smaller amounts.

➡ *NCLEX keys*

Nursing process step: Evaluation
Client needs category: Physiological integrity
Client needs subcategory: Basic care and comfort
Taxonomic level: Evaluation

5. A 10-year-old child is admitted to the pediatric unit in sickle cell crisis. What should the nurse do first?
A. Assess vital signs, including temperature.
B. Assess the degree of pain using a pain scale.
C. Determine the rate of the I.V. fluids.
D. Obtain pertinent history information from the parents.

Answer: A. All of the options are important, but the nurse should assess vital signs first to determine the patient baseline. Children with sickle cell disease are prone to developing infections as a result of necrosis of body areas where vaso-occlusive crisis occurs; this crisis also is associated with localized pain at the site of infection. It's important for the child to receive adequate fluids to help prevent dehydration and increase blood volume. History will help determine other coexisting conditions.

➡ *NCLEX keys*

Nursing process step: Assessment
Client needs category: Physiological integrity
Client needs subcategory: Basic care and comfort
Taxonomic level: Application

6. The nurse is caring for a child with leukemia who has an absolute granulocyte count of 400 ul. Which of the following interventions should the nurse implement?
A. Place the child in strict isolation.
B. Notify the physician immediately.
C. Restrict visitors with active infections.
D. Begin antibiotics per protocol.

Answer: C. When the absolute granulocyte count is low, a child has difficulty fighting an infection. Visitors with active infections should be restricted to prevent the child from developing an infection. The child should be placed in protective isolation, not strict isolation. Antibiotics shouldn't be started without a septic workup first. The physician must also be notified of the client's condition so that appropriate medical management is initiated.

➡ *NCLEX keys*
Nursing process step: Planning
Client needs category: Safe, effective care environment
Client needs subcategory: Safety and infection control
Taxonomic level: Application

7. A client is receiving cyclophosphamide (Cytoxin) as part of a chemotherapy regimen. Which adverse reaction should the nurse teach the family to report right away?
 A. Stomatitis
 B. Flulike syndrome
 C. Ototoxicity
 D. Hematuria
Answer: D. Hematuria is an indication of hemorrhagic cystitis and is an adverse effect of cyclophosphamide. Stomatitis is a rare complication with this medication. Flulike syndrome occurs with decarbazine. Ototoxicity occurs more commonly with cisplatin.

➡ *NCLEX keys*
Nursing process step: Planning
Client needs category: Physiological integrity
Client needs subcategory: Pharmacological and parenteral therapies
Taxonomic level: Comprehension

8. A 15-month-old child has been admitted to the pediatric unit with the diagnosis of croup. The nurse makes the following assessment: respiratory rate, 36 breaths/minute; heart rate, 120 beats/minute; temperature, 100.7° F (38.2° C); pulse oximetry, 93%; and restlessness. From these findings, the nurse should infer that the:
 A. toddler is in respiratory failure.
 B. toddler's condition is improving.
 C. mother should stay at the bedside.
 D. parents can calm the toddler.
Answer: A. Recognizing more subtle signs of respiratory failure is an extremely important skill for nurses to develop. Subtle signs include restlessness, increase in respiratory effort, tachypnea, tachycardia, and inability of the family to calm the child.

➡ *NCLEX keys*
Nursing process step: Analysis
Client needs category: Physiological integrity
Client needs subcategory: Reduction of risk potential
Taxonomic level: Application

9. A 6-year-old child with a history of asthma is brought to the clinic in respiratory distress. The nurse notes the following: respiratory rate, 36 breaths/minute; heart rate, 150 beats/minute; and an anxious child. The nurse should be most concerned about:
 A. child's loose cough.
 B. prolonged expiratory phase.
 C. absence of wheezing.
 D. whistling sound on inspiration.
Answer: C. The most likely explanation for the respiratory distress is an acute asthma attack. These episodes usually begin with a cough, expiratory wheezing, and a prolonged expiratory phase, and then may progress to more obvious symptoms, such as wheezing on inspiration, shortness of breath, and tight cough. The absence of wheezing during an attack indicates that the child is probably hypoxic and needs medical attention immediately.

➡ *NCLEX keys*
Nursing process step: Application
Client needs category: Physiological integrity
Client needs subcategory: Reduction of risk potential
Taxonomic level: Application

10. An adolescent with cystic fibrosis comes to the clinic for a follow-up appointment after discharge from the hospital for pneumonia. Which of the following assessment questions should the nurse ask?
 A. "How has your appetite been this last week?"
 B. "How many doses of antibiotics have you missed?"
 C. "Have you been sleeping well?"
 D. "Have you gone back to school yet?"
Answer: A. An important indication of how clients with cystic fibrosis are doing is their appetite. Poor appetite and weight loss are indications that an infectious process may be

occurring. To ask how many doses of antibiotics the client has missed assumes that the client is not trustworthy and doesn't help in establishing a therapeutic relationship. Asking about sleep would be important because that may give some helpful information about the client's overall health, but it isn't the most important question. When the client returns to school is also an indication of the client's general state.

➡ NCLEX keys
Nursing process step: Planning
Client needs category: Physiological integrity
Client needs subcategory: Reduction of risk potential
Taxonomic level: Application

11. A 5-month-old is brought to the clinic by the mother, who reports that the infant has nasal congestion, symptoms of a cold, fever, and difficulty breathing. The nurse should first:
    A.   ask for more history information.
    B.   perform a respiratory assessment.
    C.   notify the available physician.
    D.   take vital signs, including temperature.
Answer: B. Anytime a relative reports that a child has difficulty breathing, it's imperative for the nurse to do a respiratory assessment immediately. History information and vital signs can be obtained at a later date. After the nurse makes the respiratory assessment, then the physician can be contacted if warranted.

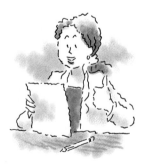

➡ NCLEX keys
Nursing process step: Planning
Client needs category: Safe, effective care environment
Client needs subcategory: Safety and infection control
Taxonomic level: Application

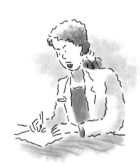

12. The nurse is counseling the mother of a child with attention deficit hyperactivity disorder (ADHD). The nurse should judge that the mother understood the teaching when the mother responds with:
    A.   "When my child comes home from school, the homework is done first."
    B.   "I take my child to play in the park as soon as school is over."
    C.   "My child loves to sit and watch television after the bus ride home."
    D.   "As soon as I arrive home, my child begins to read his favorite book."
Answer: B. Children with ADHD are impulsive, have high energy levels, and don't follow directions well. An appropriate plan after the child has been in school all day would be to allow the child to run and play to burn up energy. This enables the child to concentrate better later.

➡ NCLEX keys
Nursing process step: Evaluation
Client needs category: Physiological integrity
Client needs subcategory: Physiological adaptation
Taxonomic level: Application

13. An infant is to receive amoxicillin 90 mg three times a day for 10 days to treat otitis media on the left side. Amoxicillin suspension is 125 mg/5ml. How much of the medication would the mother administer at each dosing time?

   A. 1.8 ml
   B. 3.6 ml
   C. 13.45 ml
   D. 26.90 ml

Answer: B. (125 mg : 5 ml :: 90 mg : X ml = (90 mg $\times$ 5ml) $\div$ (125 mg $\times$ X ml) = 450 $\div$ 125 = 3.6)

➡ *NCLEX keys*
Nursing process step: Implementation
Client needs category: Physiological integrity
Client needs subcategory: Pharmacological and parenteral therapies
Taxonomic level: Application

14. A school-age child has hydrocephalus and is admitted for a revision of his ventriculoperitoneal shunt. When he returns from surgery how should the nurse position him?

   A. On his abdomen where he is comfortable
   B. In semi-Fowler's position to prevent aspiration
   C. With the bed flat to prevent a subdural hematoma
   D. On the same side as the shunt repair

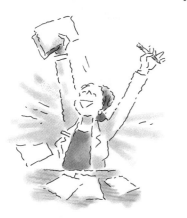

Answer: C. The child should be kept flat to decrease complications that might occur from too rapid a reduction in intracranial fluid. When the fluid is drained too rapidly, a subdural hematoma may result. In children with increased intracranial pressure, the position of choice is with the head of the bed elevated and the child lying on the side opposite the shunt to keep pressure off the shunt valve.

➡ *NCLEX keys*
Nursing process step: Implementation
Client needs category: Physiological integrity
Client needs subcategory: Physiological adaptation
Taxonomic level: Application

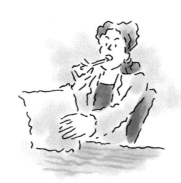

15. A 10-month-old child is admitted to the hospital from the clinic with a history of 2 days of fever, anorexia, crying, and poor sleeping. The infant is diagnosed with probable meningitis. In which of the following situations should the nurse place the child?

   A. In strict isolation
   B. In respiratory isolation
   C. With other older infants
   D. With another child with meningitis

Answer: B. The organisms that cause meningitis are transmitted by the spread of droplets. To protect the nursing staff and the family, a child with the probable diagnosis of meningitis is placed in a private room in respiratory isolation until appropriate I.V. antibiotics have been administered for 24 hours.

➡ *NCLEX keys*
Nursing process step: Implementation
Client needs category: Safe, effective care environment
Client needs subcategory: Safety and infection control
Taxonomic level: Application

16. Parents bring a 4-year-old child to the clinic for a checkup. The child has been diagnosed with Duchenne's muscular dystrophy. What early signs would the nurse expect the child to exhibit?

    A. Contracture deformities
    B. Loss of independent ambulation
    C. Difficulty climbing stairs
    D. Small and weak muscles

Answer: C. Muscular dystrophy has an early onset; signs are seen by age 5. Difficulty climbing stairs and riding a tricycle are early signs. Contractures are progressive and begin to develop later, and loss of independent ambulation usually occurs by age 11. Small, weak muscles is a later sign.

➡ *NCLEX keys*
Nursing process step: Assessment
Client needs category: Physiological integrity
Client needs subcategory: Basic care and comfort
Taxonomic level: Comprehension

17. The nurse is caring for an infant with bilateral plaster leg casts for congenital clubfoot. Which of the following possible statements by the parents would indicate understanding of the nurse's teaching?

    A. "When the casts get dirty, I will just wash them with soap and warm water."
    B. "I will need to frequently check the temperature and color of my child's toes."
    C. "I can dry the casts faster with a hair dryer so we can go meet my mother."
    D. "When the casts are partly dry, I can coat them with a clear acrylic spray."

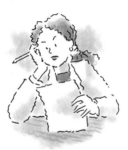

Answer: B. Frequently assessing the extremity distal to the cast is important. If the cast is too tight, neurovascular compromise can result. This may manifest as coolness, pale digits, pain, decreased sensation, and absence of pulse. Putting water on a plaster cast can soften it and cause it to become misshapen. External heat shouldn't be used to dry the cast because the inside of the cast wouldn't be adequately dried. The cast shouldn't be sprayed with anything that would inhibit the loss of moisture from the plaster.

➡ *NCLEX keys*
Nursing process step: Evaluation
Client needs category: Physiological integrity
Client needs subcategory: Reduction of risk potential
Taxonomic level: Evaluation

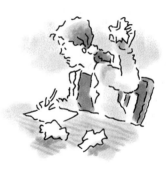

18. The nurse in a clinic is counseling an adolescent who is wearing a Milwaukee brace for scoliosis. The nurse would judge the teaching as successful when the adolescent states that the brace must be worn:

    A. at night when sleeping.
    B. during school hours.
    C. 23 hours a day.
    D. when eating meals and snacks.

Answer: C. Routinely, the Milwaukee brace is worn about 23 hours a day. The brace is worn to decrease the thoracic curvature as the adolescent grows. The adolescent can be out of the brace for about an hour when showering or exercising.

NCLEX keys
Nursing process step: Evaluation
Client needs category: Health promotion and maintenance
Client needs subcategory: Prevention and early detection of disease
Taxonomic level: Application

19. The nurse is teaching the parents of an infant undergoing repair of cleft lip. Of the following, which instruction should the nurse give?

   A. Offer the pacifier as needed.
   B. Lay the infant on the abdomen for sleep.
   C. Sit the infant up for each feeding.
   D. Loosen the arm restraints every hour.

Answer: C. An infant with cleft lip repair is fed in the upright position with a syringe and attached tubing. This prevents stress to the suture line from sucking. Pacifiers wouldn't be used during the healing process. The infant would be put down for sleep on the back or side so the surgery site wouldn't be traumatized. Arm restraints would usually be loosened every 2 hours.

NCLEX keys
Nursing process step: Planning
Client needs category: Physiological integrity
Client needs subcategory: Reduction of risk potential
Taxonomic level: Application

20. A nurse is assessing an infant with persistent emesis. Which of the following acid-base imbalances would the nurse assess the infant for based on the provisional diagnosis of pyloric stenosis?

   A. Respiratory acidosis
   B. Respiratory alkalosis
   C. Metabolic acidosis
   D. Metabolic alkalosis

Answer: D. With an excessive loss of potassium, hydrogen, and chloride as a result of persistent emesis, metabolic alkalosis occurs. A compensatory increase in bicarbonate ions is caused by chloride loss. As the result of excessive diarrhea or malnutrition, metabolic acidosis occurs. Respiratory acidosis results from excessive retention of partial pressure of arterial carbon dioxide ($Paco_2$). Respiratory alkalosis results when a loss of $Paco_2$ occurs.

NCLEX keys
Nursing process step: Assessment
Client needs category: Physiological integrity
Client needs subcategory: Reduction of risk potential
Taxonomic level: Comprehension

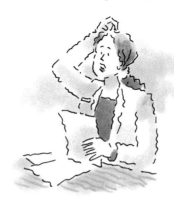

21. The nurse is caring for an infant with esophageal atresia and tracheo-esophageal fistula. Of the following possible statements, which indicates that the infant's parents understood the diagnosis?

   A. "The esophagus ends in a blind pouch so eating can't occur."
   B. "There is a connection between the esophagus and the trachea."
   C. "The esophagus ends in a blind pouch and there is a tube between the trachea and esophagus."
   D. "Stomach acids come back up into the trachea, causing heartburn."

Answer: C. This statement correctly describes the most common type of esophageal atresia and tracheoesophageal fistula.

NCLEX keys
Nursing process step: Evaluation
Client needs category: Physiological integrity
Client needs subcategory: Basic care and comfort
Taxonomic level: Application

22. The mother of a 6-week-old infant asks the nurse why her infant wasn't diagnosed earlier with congenital hypothyroidism. Of the following, what response would the nurse give?
- A. "Breast-fed infants may not display symptoms until they are weaned."
- B. "If you had brought your infant in for a 2-week checkup you would have been told."
- C. "The diagnosis was made earlier but replacement medication won't start yet."
- D. " The public health nurse was unable to locate your home."

Answer: A. Frequently, a newborn infant doesn't exhibit signs of congenital hypothyroidism because of the exogenous source of thyroid hormone supplied by the maternal circulation. It may not be obvious in infants because they have a functional remnant of the thyroid hormone. Breast-fed babies may not manifest symptoms until they are weaned. Telling the mother she missed her 2-week checkup puts the blame on the mother, which isn't necessary. The others are not appropriate since the infant was breast-fed — preventing earlier diagnosis.

➠ *NCLEX keys*
Nursing process step: Planning
Client needs category: Health promotion and maintenance
Client needs subcategory: Prevention and early detection of disease
Taxonomic level: Application

23. The nurse is teaching a child with diabetes. Which statement by the child indicates that the teaching was successful?
- A. "The action of intermediate insulin begins in about 2 to 4 hours after the injection."
- B. "Regular insulin should be given early in the morning long before breakfast."
- C. "Hunger, headache, shakiness, and sweating are all signs of hyperglycemia."
- D. "Because exercise increases the blood glucose level, snacks aren't given before exercise."

Answer: A. Intermediate insulin begins to act within 2 to 4 hours after injection and peaks in about 6 to 8 hours after injection. Regular insulin begins to act within 30 minutes and is usually administered right before breakfast. Hunger, headache, shakiness, and sweating are signs of hypoglycemia. Strenuous exercise decreases the blood glucose level, so children engaging in exercise usually need a snack first.

➠ *NCLEX keys*
Nursing process step: Evaluation
Client needs category: Physiological integrity
Client needs subcategory: Pharmacological and parenteral therapies
Taxonomic level: Application

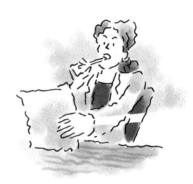

24. The nurse is teaching the mother of a child who is newly diagnosed with diabetes mellitus. As part of the teaching, the nurse reviews diet and snacks. The nurse would judge that the mother understood why her child needs snacks when she states:
- A. "Snacks will help my child not want to eat candy with friends."
- B. "Snacks are given at the time insulin peaks to prevent hypoglycemia."
- C. "Children can't eat all the calories they need in just three meals a day."
- D. "The insulin shots make my child hungry, so snacks help prevent cheating on the diet."

Answer: B. The diabetic diet for children includes at least two snacks a day at mid-afternoon and before bed. Snacks are given at the time insulin peaks to help prevent hypoglycemia. Snacks aren't given to help control the desire for sweets, to ensure sufficient calorie intake, or to make a child hungry.

→ NCLEX keys
Nursing process step: Evaluation
Client needs category: Physiological integrity
Client needs subcategory: Basic care and comfort
Taxonomic level: Application

25. An 18-month-old toddler is seen in the clinic for a well checkup. The mother reports that she is in the process of toilet training her child but it isn't going well. The toddler has many accidents during the day. Which question should the nurse ask the mother?
    A. "Does your child understand what is expected?"
    B. "How many accidents a day does your child have?"
    C. "Does your child seem to be in pain right before the accident?"
    D. "What does your child's urine smell like?"
Answer: D. This question would yield the most helpful information. Frequently, when a child has a urinary tract infection, the urine has a strong, foul smell. Many 18-month-old children are ready to be toilet trained and at this age, they usually understand what is asked of them. Asking the mother about pain before an accident might be extremely difficult for the mother to ascertain, but it's worth asking.

→ NCLEX keys
Nursing process step: Assessment
Client needs category: Physiological integrity
Client needs subcategory: Basic care and comfort
Taxonomic level: Assessment

26. A child with a urinary tract infection is being treated with trimethoprim-sulfamethoxazole for a period of 10 days. Which of the following would the nurse teach the mother?

    A. "With this medication it is important that your child drink lots of water."
    B. "When your child has taken this medication for 5 days, call the clinic."
    C. "While taking this medication, it is important for your child to stay out of the sunshine."
    D. "If your child won't take this medication, mix it in 3 ounces of fruit juice."
Answer: A. This medication can cause crystals to form in the kidneys if the child doesn't drink enough water. After the child has completed half of the course of treatment, it isn't necessary for the mother to call the clinic. There is no reason for the child to stay out of the sunshine while on this medication. Three ounces of fruit juice is too much liquid in which to mix the medication.

→ NCLEX keys
Nursing process step: Implementation
Client needs category: Physiological integrity
Client needs subcategory: Pharmacological and parenteral therapies
Taxonomic level: Application

27. A child has just returned from surgery for removal of a kidney for Wilms' tumor. Which of the following would be an appropriate nursing action?
    A. Offer the child ice chips when awake.
    B. Administer pain medication when the child requests it.
    C. Take the child's vital signs.
    D. Provide games at the child's developmental level.
Answer: C. Following nephrectomy, the child will most likely have a nasogastric tube and won't be allowed ice or fluids by mouth. Pain medication should be administered on a routine schedule to keep the child comfortable. The child's vital signs should be taken immediately upon arrival from surgery to determine the baseline and to detect early changes from previous recordings. The child should be provided diversions only after sufficient recuperation after surgery.

➡ *NCLEX keys*
Nursing process step: Implementation
Client needs category: Physiological integrity
Client needs subcategory: Basic care and comfort
Taxonomic level: Application

28. The mother of a 3-month-old infant calls the clinic and states that her child has a diaper rash. Of the following, which would the nurse advise?
  A. Switch to cloth diapers until the rash is gone.
  B. Use baby wipes with each diaper change.
  C. Leave the diaper open while the infant sleeps.
  D. Offer extra fluids to the infant until the rash improves.

Answer: C. Leave the diaper off while the child sleeps to promote air circulation to the area, improving the condition. There is no need to switch to cloth diapers; in fact, that may make the rash worse. Extra fluids won't make the rash better, and baby wipes contain alcohol, which may worsen the condition.

➡ *NCLEX keys*
Nursing process step: Implementation
Client needs category: Physiological integrity
Client needs subcategory: Basic care and comfort
Taxonomic level: Application

29. The nurse is speaking to the mother of a 5-year-old child with a burn on the arm from hot soup. What advice should the nurse give to the child's mother?
  A. Wash the area with soap and water.
  B. Spray the area with a pain reliever.
  C. Flush the area with tepid water.
  D. Bring the child immediately to the clinic.

Answer: C. When a child has a scald type of burn, it's important to immediately flush the area with tepid water to cool the skin and prevent the burn from progressing. Soap shouldn't be used initially until the area had been flushed well. The child shouldn't be taken to the clinic until the area has been flushed.

Spraying the area with pain reliever won't stop the burning process.

➡ *NCLEX keys*
Nursing process step: Implementation
Client needs category: Physiological integrity
Client needs subcategory: Basic care and comfort
Taxonomic level: Application

30. A school-age child asks the school nurse how a child gets lice. The nurse should respond that lice is:
  A. passed to other children because they don't wash their hands often.
  B. spread easily because children share their hats and combs.
  C. only spread between children; adults don't have it.
  D. hard to spread unless your immune system is depressed.

Answer: B. Lice is spread easily between children because they share possessions more readily than adults do. Also, children tend to be in closer proximity to each other than adults are.

➡ *NCLEX keys*
Nursing process step: Implementation
Client needs category: Safe, effective care environment
Client needs subcategory: Safety and infection control
Taxonomic level: Application

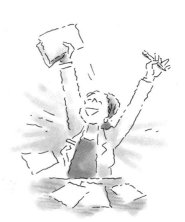

Appendices

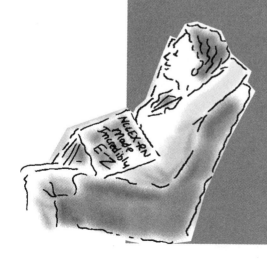

Brush up on law and ethics

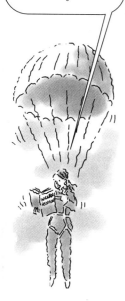

Nurse practice acts define the scope of your professional practice: What you can and can't do on the job.

Safe, effective nursing practice requires becoming fully aware of the many legal and ethical issues surrounding professional practice. These issues range from understanding your state's nurse practice act to upholding patients' rights and fulfilling the many legal responsibilities you'll have as a nurse.

Nurse practice acts

Each state has a nurse practice act. It's designed to protect the public by:
• defining the legal scope of nursing practice
• excluding untrained or unlicensed people from practicing nursing.

Your state's nurse practice act is the most important law affecting your nursing practice. You'll be expected to care for patients within defined practice limits; if you give care beyond those limits, you'll become vulnerable to charges of violating your state nurse practice act.

Scoping it out

Most nurse practice acts define important concepts, including the scope of nursing practice. In other words, nurse practice acts broadly outline what nurses can and can't do on the job. Make sure that you're familiar with the legally permissible scope of your nursing practice as defined in your state's nurse practice act and that you never exceed its limits. Otherwise, you're inviting legal problems.

Nurse practice acts also outline the conditions and requirements for licensure. To become licensed as an RN, for instance, you must meet certain qualifications, including passing the NCLEX. All states require completion of a basic professional nursing education program. Your state may have additional requirements, including:
• good moral character
• good physical and mental health
• minimum age
• fluency in English
• freedom from drug or alcohol addiction.

Get on board

In every U.S. state and Canadian province, the nurse practice act creates a state or provincial board of nursing. The nurse practice act authorizes this board to administer and enforce rules and regulations about the nursing profession. The board is bound by the provisions of the nurse practice act that created it.

The nurse practice act is the law; the board of nursing can't grant exemptions to it or waive any of its provisions. Only the state or provincial legislature can change the law. In many states and provinces, however, the board of nursing may grant exemptions and waivers to its own rules and regulations.

Moving violations

The nurse practice act also lists violations that can result in disciplinary action against a nurse. Depending on the nature of the violation, a nurse may face state board disciplinary action and liability for her actions.

Get it?

Understanding your nurse practice act's general provisions will help you stay within the legal limits of nursing practice. Interpreting the nurse practice act isn't always easy, however. Nurse

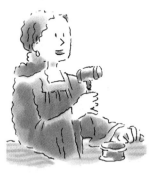

Nurse practice acts are laws; they tend to be worded in broad, vague terms, and the wording varies from state to state.

practice acts are laws, after all, so they tend to be worded in broad, vague terms, and the wording varies from state to state.

The key point to remember is this: Your state nurse practice act isn't a word-for-word checklist of how you should do your work. Ultimately, you must rely on your own education and knowledge of your facility's policies and procedures.

A declaration of independence

Most nurse practice acts pose another problem: They state that you have a legal duty to carry out a doctor's or a dentist's orders. Yet, as a licensed professional, you also have an ethical and legal duty to use your own judgment when providing patient care. When such conflicts arise, don't hesitate to act independently. Follow these guidelines:
• When you think an order is wrong, tell the doctor.
• If you're confused about an order, ask the doctor to clarify it.
• If the doctor fails to correct the error or answer your questions, inform your head nurse or supervisor of your doubts.

What am I supposed to do now?

Conflicts of duty can also arise if your state's nurse practice act disagrees with your facility's policies. The nursing service department in each facility develops detailed policies and procedures for staff nurses. These policies and procedures usually specify the allowable scope of nursing practice within the facility. The scope may be narrower than the scope described in your nurse practice act, but it shouldn't be broader.

In other words, your employer can't legally expand the scope of your practice to include tasks prohibited by your nurse practice act. You have a legal obligation to practice within your nurse practice act's limits. Except in a life-threatening emergency, you can't exceed those limits without risking disciplinary action. To protect yourself, compare your facility's policies with your nurse practice act.

Repeat after me: Change is good

With every new medical discovery or technological innovation, the world of nursing undergoes revision. To align nurse practice acts with current nursing practice, professional nursing organizations and state boards of nursing generally propose revisions to regulations. There's a catch: Nurse practice acts are statutory laws subject to the inevitably slow legislative process, so the law sometimes has trouble keeping pace with medicine.

What does all of this mean for you? To help protect yourself legally, you need to stay current with your state's nurse practice act while you keep up with innovations in health care practice.

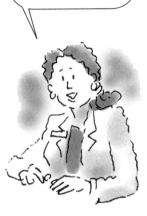

Tell it straight. Reasonable disclosure means the patient has a right to know about the risks associated with his diagnosis and treatment.

Informed consent

Your patient has a legal right to be adequately informed about a proposed treatment or procedure. Generally, responsibility for obtaining a patient's informed consent rests with the person who will carry out the treatment or procedure (usually the doctor).

Informed consent basically involves the patient (or someone acting on his behalf) having enough information to know:
• what the patient is getting into if he decides to undergo the treatment or procedure
• the anticipated consequences if consent is refused or withdrawn.

Nurses may provide patients and their families with information that is within a nurse's scope of practice and knowledge base. However, a nurse can't substitute her knowledge for the doctor's input.

Information, please

What should you tell the patient? First, he has a right to reasonable disclosure of risks associated with the medical diagnosis and treatment. He also must be given an opportunity to evaluate options, alternatives, and risks before exercising his choice. The basics of informed consent should include:

• description of the treatment or procedure
• description of inherent risks and benefits that occur with frequency or regularity (or specific consequences significant to the given patient or his designated decision-maker)
• explanation of the potential for death or serious harm (such as brain damage, stroke, paralysis, or disfiguring scars) or for discomforting adverse effects during or after the treatment or procedure
• explanation and description of alternative treatments or procedures
• name and qualifications of the person who'll perform the treatment or procedure
• discussion of the possible effects of not undergoing the treatment or procedure.

The patient should also be told that he has a right to refuse the treatment or procedure without having other care or support withdrawn and that he can withdraw consent after giving it.

Can I get a witness?

If you witness a patient's signature on a consent form, you attest to three things:

• the patient voluntarily consented
• the patient's signature is authentic
• the patient appears to be competent to give consent.

What they don't know can hurt you

Another potential legal pitfall for nurses is called negligent nondisclosure. Let us say, for example, that you believe a patient is incompetent to participate in giving consent because of medication or sedation given to him. Perhaps you learn that the practitioner has discussed consent issues with the patient when the patient was heavily sedated or medicated. Under either of these scenarios, you have an obligation to bring it to the practitioner's attention immediately. If the practitioner isn't available, discuss your concerns with your supervisor.

Always document attempts to reach the practitioner and attending doctor in the medical record before allowing the patient to proceed with the treatment or procedure. Besides discussing this with the practitioner and your supervisor, you must also assess your patient's understanding of the information provided by the practitioner.

When a patient is incompetent

A patient is deemed mentally incompetent if he can't understand the explanations or can't comprehend the results of his decisions. When a patient is incompetent, the practitioner has two alternatives:

• seek consent from the patient's next of kin (usually the spouse)
• petition the court to appoint a legal guardian for the patient.

Remember, though, that mental illness isn't the same as incompetence. Persons suffering from mental illness have been found competent to give consent because they're alert and, above all, able to understand the proposed treatment, risks, benefits, alternatives, and consequences of refusing treatment.

A minor problem

Every state will allow an emancipated minor to consent to his own medical care and treatment. Definitions of emancipation vary from state to state, however. Most states will allow teenagers to consent to treatment, even though they aren't emancipated, in cases involving pregnancy or sexually transmitted disease.

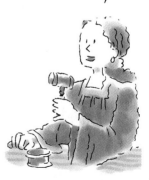

Protect the right of mentally ill patients to informed consent. Remember, under the law, mental illness isn't the same as incompetence.

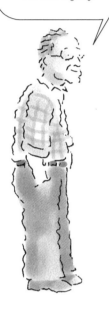

Quality-of-life issues are becoming increasingly important. Patients are demanding to live with dignity and die with dignity.

Right to refuse treatment

Any mentally competent adult may legally refuse treatment if he's fully informed about his medical condition and about the likely consequences of his refusal. As a professional, you must respect that decision.

Most court cases related to the right to refuse treatment have involved patients with a terminal illness (or their families) who want to discontinue life support.

Quality time

More and more, health care providers consider quality end-of-life care as an ethical obligation. But what does end-of-life mean, and how do you measure it? Some researchers point to five "domains," or focal points, that patients view as end-of-life issues. By understanding these domains from the patients' perspectives, nurses can improve the quality of end-of-life care.
• Pain and other symptoms are of concern for many patients.
• Many patients fear "being kept alive" after they can no longer enjoy life; they want to "die with dignity."
• Sense of control is also critical; some patients are adamant about controlling their end-of-life care decisions.
• Many patients tend to seek a psychological outcome rather than a precise treatment decision. For example, some patients feel that their loved ones will be relieved of the burden that difficult end-of-life care decisions entail.
• Many patients express an overwhelming need to communicate with loved ones at this stage of their life. Dying offers important opportunities for growth, intimacy, reconciliation, and closure.

A religious experience

Some patients may refuse treatment on the grounds of freedom of religion. Jehovah's Witnesses, for instance, oppose blood transfusions, based on their interpretation of a biblical passage that forbids "drinking" blood. Some sect members believe that even a lifesaving transfusion given against their will deprives them of everlasting life. The courts usually uphold their right to refuse treatment because of the constitutionally protected right to religious freedom.

Most other religious freedom court cases involve Christian Scientists, who oppose many medical interventions, including medicines.

Planning in advance

Most states have enacted right-to-die laws (also called natural death laws or living will laws). These laws recognize the patient's right to choose death by refusing extraordinary treatment when he has no hope of recovery.

Whenever a competent patient expresses his wishes concerning extraordinary treatment, health care providers should attempt to follow them. If the patient is incompetent or unconscious, the decision becomes more difficult.

In some cases, the next of kin may express the patient's desires for him, but whether this is an honest interpretation of the patient's wishes is sometimes uncertain.

Written evidence of the patient's wishes provides the best indication of what treatment he'd consent to if he were still able to communicate. This information may be provided through advance directives, such as:
• living will — an advance care document that specifies a person's wishes about medical care if he's unable to communicate (In some states, living wills don't address the issue of discontinuing artificial nutrition and hydration.)
• durable power of attorney for health care — a document in which the patient designates a person to make medical decisions for him if he becomes incompetent (This differs from the usual

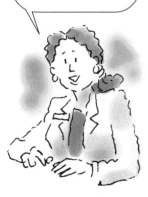

Listen up. Whenever a competent patient expresses his wishes concerning extraordinary treatment, health care providers should attempt to follow them.

power of attorney, which requires the patient's ongoing consent and deals only with financial issues.)

Most states recognize living wills as legally valid and have laws authorizing durable powers of attorney for initiating or terminating life-sustaining medical treatment.

Up to the challenge

There are two grounds for challenging a patient's right to refuse treatment: You can claim that the patient is incompetent, or you can claim that compelling reasons exist to overrule his wishes.

The courts consider a patient incompetent when he lacks the mental ability to make a reasoned decision, such as when he's delirious. The courts also recognize several compelling circumstances that justify overruling a patient's refusal of treatment. These include:
• when refusal endangers the life of another
• when a parent's decision to withhold treatment threatens a child's life
• when, despite refusing treatment, the patient makes statements indicating that he wants to live
• when the public interest outweighs the patient's right.

What to do if your patient refuses treatment

If your patient tells you he's going to refuse treatment or he simply refuses to give consent, follow these guidelines:
• Stop preparations for any treatment at once.
• Notify the doctor immediately.
• Report your patient's decision to your supervisor promptly.

Never delay informing your supervisor, especially if a delay could be life-threatening. Any delay that you're responsible for will greatly increase your legal risks.

Never ignore the patient's request to refuse treatment. A patient can sue you for battery — intentionally touching another person without authorization to do so — even if you're following a doctor's orders.

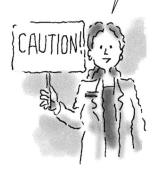

Never ignore the patient's request to refuse treatment. A patient can sue you for battery — intentionally touching another person without authorization to do so.

Living will

When a legally competent person draws up a living will, he declares the steps he wants or doesn't want taken when he's incompetent and no longer able to express his wishes. The will applies to decisions that will be made after a patient is incompetent and has no reasonable possibility of recovery. Generally, a living will authorizes the attending doctor to withhold or discontinue certain lifesaving procedures under specific circumstances.

A patient may also choose to execute a durable power of attorney for health care. If the patient becomes incompetent, this document designates a surrogate decision-maker with authority to carry out the patient's wishes regarding health care decisions. Most states have laws authorizing only durable power of attorney for the purpose of initiating or terminating life-sustaining medical treatment.

Living will laws: The main ingredients

Although living will laws vary from state to state, they generally include such provisions as:
• who may execute a living will
• witness and testator requirements
• immunity from liability for following a living will's directives
• documentation requirements
• instructions on when and how the living will should be executed
• under what circumstances the living will takes effect.

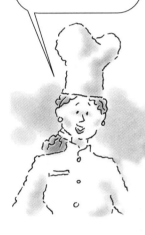

Living will laws protect you. Nurses who follow the wishes expressed in an authorized living will are generally immune from civil and criminal liability.

Immunity

Nurses and other health care providers who follow the wishes expressed in a living will authorized by law are generally immune from civil and criminal liability. No matter which state you work in, check your facility's policy and procedures manual, and seek advice from your facility's legal department if needed.

General guidelines

The Patient Self-Determination Act of 1990 requires facilities to provide patients with written information about their rights regarding living wills and durable power of attorney as well as about the facility's procedure for implementing them. The law also requires the institution to document whether or not the patient has a living will or durable power of attorney.

If your patient has a living will, you'll want to take the following steps to safeguard his rights and protect yourself from liability:

• Review your nursing or facility manual for specific directions on what to do. For instance, you may need to inform the patient's doctor about it, or you may need to ask your nursing supervisor to inform the facility administration and the legal affairs department.

• With the patient's permission, make sure the family knows about the will; if they don't, show them a copy.

• If the patient can talk, discuss the will with him, especially if it contains terms that need further definition. As always, objectively document your actions and findings in the patient's record.

• If the patient drafts a living will while under your care, document this in your nurses' notes, describing the circumstances under which the will was drawn up and signed.

• Encourage the patient to review the living will with his family and doctor so that unclear passages can be discussed. Living wills should also be reviewed periodically to keep pace with changes in technology.

Right to privacy

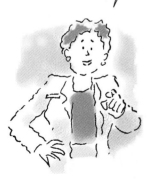

Respecting your patient's right to privacy helps develop trust, a cornerstone of the nurse-patient relationship.

Obtaining highly personal information from a patient can be uncomfortable and embarrassing. Reassuring the patient that you'll keep all information confidential may help put you both at ease. But stop to think about the legal complexities of this responsibility. What do you do when your patient's spouse, other health care professionals, the media, or public health agencies ask you to disclose confidential information?

It's in the Constitution! (...or is it?)

The right to privacy essentially is the right to make personal choices without outside interference. Although the U.S. Constitution doesn't explicitly sanction a right to privacy, the U.S. Supreme Court has cited several constitutional amendments that imply such a right.

The right to privacy has received even more attention at the state level. Nearly all states recognize the right to privacy through statutory or common law.

Making your patient feel privileged

The state courts have strongly protected a patient's right to have information kept confidential. Even in court, your patient is protected by the privilege doctrine. People who have a protected relationship, such as a doctor and patient, can't be forced, even during legal proceedings, to reveal communication between them unless the person who benefits from the protection agrees to it.

Unfortunately, only a handful of states (including New York, Arkansas, Oregon, and Vermont) recognize the nurse-patient relationship as protected. Some courts have held that the privilege exists when a nurse is following doctor's orders.

Can I get a little privacy here?

Despite legal uncertainties regarding your responsibilities under the privilege doctrine, you have a professional and ethical responsibility to protect your patient's privacy. This responsibility requires more than keeping secrets. You may have to educate your patients about their privacy rights. Some of them may be unaware of what the right to privacy means, or even that they have such a right. Explain to the patient that he can refuse to allow pictures to be taken of his disorder and its treatment, for example. Tell him that he can choose to have information about his condition withheld from others, including family members. Make every effort to ensure that the patient's wishes are carried out.

Confidentially speaking

Under certain circumstances, you may lawfully disclose confidential information about your patient. For example, the courts generally allow disclosure when:
• welfare of a person or a group of people is at stake
• disclosure is necessary for the patient's continued care
• patient consent is obtained for the disclosure
• public's right to know outweighs the patient's right to keep his condition private (for example, media reports on the first kidney transplant or the President's annual physical examination).

In some situations, the law not only permits you to disclose confidential information, it requires you to do so. These situations include:
• instances of actual or suspected child abuse (All 50 states and the District of Columbia have disclosure laws for child abuse cases. Except for Maine and Montana, all states also grant immunity from legal action for a good-faith report on suspected child abuse. In fact, there may be a criminal penalty for failure to disclose such information.)
• criminal cases (Some laws create an exemption to the privilege doctrine in criminal cases so that courts can have access to all essential information.)
• government requests (For example, most state public health departments require reports of all communicable diseases, births and deaths, and gunshot wounds.)

Medication errors

Administering drugs to patients continues to be one of the most important — and, legally, one of the riskiest — tasks you perform.

Getting it right

When administering drugs, one easy way to guard against malpractice liability is to remember the long-standing "five rights" formula:
• the right drug
• to the right patient
• at the right time
• in the right dosage
• by the right route.

Just say "Know"

When you have your nursing license, the law expects you to know about any drug you administer. More specifically, the law expects you to:
• know a drug's safe dosage limits, toxicity, potential adverse reactions, and indications and contraindications for use
• refuse to accept an illegible, confusing, or otherwise unclear drug order

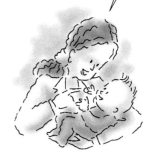

Talk about it. All 50 states and the District of Columbia have disclosure laws for child abuse cases. In fact, there may be a criminal penalty for failure to disclose such information.

• seek clarification of a confusing order from the doctor rather than trying to interpret it yourself.

Are there any questions?

If you question a drug order, follow your facility's policies. Usually, they'll tell you to try each of the following actions until you receive a satisfactory answer:
• Look up the answer in a reliable drug reference.
• Ask your charge nurse.
• Ask the facility pharmacist.
• Ask your nursing supervisor or the prescribing doctor.
• Ask the chief nursing administrator, if she hasn't already become involved.
• Ask the prescribing doctor's supervisor (service chief).
• Get in touch with the facility administration and explain your problem.

An offer you CAN refuse

Nurses have the legal right not to administer drugs they think will harm patients. You may choose to exercise this right when you think:
• the prescribed dosage is too high
• the drug is contraindicated because of possible dangerous interactions with other drugs or with substances such as alcohol
• the patient's physical condition contraindicates using the drug.

In limited circumstances, you may also legally refuse to administer a drug on grounds of conscience. Some U.S. states and Canadian provinces have enacted right-of-conscience laws. These laws excuse medical personnel from the requirement to participate in any abortion or sterilization procedure. Under such laws, you may, for example, refuse to give any drug you believe is intended to induce abortion.

When you refuse to carry out a drug order, make sure that you do the following:
• Notify your immediate supervisor so she can make alternate arrangements (assigning a new nurse, clarifying the order).
• Notify the prescribing doctor (if your supervisor hasn't done so already).
• Document that the drug wasn't given and explain why (if your employer requires it).

Protecting yourself

If you make an error in giving a drug, or if your patient reacts negatively to a properly administered drug, immediately inform the patient's doctor and protect yourself by documenting the incident thoroughly. In addition to normal drug-charting information, include information on the patient's reaction and any medical or nursing interventions taken.

In the event of error, you should also file an incident report. Identify what happened, the names and functions of all personnel involved, and what actions were taken to protect the patient after the error was discovered.

Malpractice

Because nurses are assuming an ever-widening list of patient-care responsibilities, it isn't surprising that many nurses are anxious about the possibility of facing a lawsuit one day. Before discussing the specific steps you can take to avoid a lawsuit, here are two terms you'll need to know more about: negligence and malpractice.

Negligence is usually defined as a failure to exercise the degree of care that a person of ordinary prudence would exercise under the same circumstances. A claim of negligence requires three criteria to be met:

1. A person owed a duty to the person making the claim.
2. The duty was breached.
3. The breach resulted in injury to the person making the claim.

   Malpractice is a more restricted, specialized kind of negligence. It's defined as a violation of professional duty or a failure to meet a standard of care or failure to use the skills and knowledge of other professionals in similar circumstances. You can take steps to avoid tort liability by using caution and common sense and by maintaining heightened awareness of your legal responsibilities. Follow the guidelines below to steer clear of legal pitfalls.

> One of the best ways to avoid malpractice is to know the kinds of assignments you're fit to carry out on the job.

Knowing your own strengths...and weaknesses
Don't accept responsibilities that you aren't prepared for. If you make an error, claiming you weren't familiar with the unit's procedures won't protect you against liability.

You want me to work where?
You may be assigned to work on a specialized unit, which is reasonable as long as you're assigned duties you can perform competently and as long as an experienced nurse on the unit assumes responsibility for the specialized duties. Assigning you to perform total patient care on the unit is unsafe if you don't have the skills to plan and deliver that care.

Delegation 101
Exercise great care as a supervisor when delegating duties because you may be held responsible for subordinates. Inspect all equipment and machinery regularly, and be sure that subordinates use them competently and safely. Report incompetent health care personnel to superiors through the institutional chain of command.

May I take your order?
Never treat any patient without orders from his doctor, except in an emergency. Don't prescribe or dispense any medication without authorization. In most cases, only doctors and pharmacists may legally perform these functions.

   Don't carry out any order from a doctor if you have any doubt about its accuracy or appropriateness. Follow your facility's policy for clarifying ambiguous orders. Document your efforts to clarify the order, and whether or not the order was carried out.

Watch those medication mixups!
Medication errors are the most common and potentially most dangerous of nursing errors. Mistakes in dosage, patient identification, or drug selection by nurses have led to vision loss, brain damage, cardiac arrest, and death.

> Being polite has a payoff; it helps protect against liability. Trial attorneys have a saying: "If you don't want to be sued, don't be rude."

Staying on your patient's good side
Trial attorneys have a saying: "If you don't want to be sued, don't be rude." Always remain calm when a patient or his family becomes difficult. Patients must be told the truth about adverse outcomes, but this information should be communicated with discretion and sensitivity.

Don't offer opinions (ever)
Avoid offering your opinion when a patient asks you what you think is the matter with him. If you give your opinion, you could be accused of making a medical diagnosis, which is practicing medicine without a license.

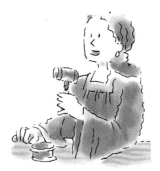

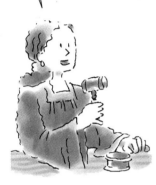

Restraints require restraint. Restraints need to be applied correctly, only when necessary, and monitored according to facility policy to avoid malpractice claims.

Before you sign on that dotted line...Read!

Never sign your name as a witness without fully understanding what you're signing as well as the legal significance of your signature.

Stick to the FACTs

From a legal standpoint, documented care is as important as the actual care. If a procedure wasn't documented, the courts assume it wasn't performed. Make sure you document all observations, decisions, and actions. The patient's chart, when taken into the court room, is a nurse's "best evidence" of the care given. The chart should follow the "FACT" rule: be **F**actual, **A**ccurate, **C**omplete, and **T**imely.

Assisting in procedures: A word of caution

Don't assist with a surgical procedure unless you're satisfied the patient has given proper informed consent. Never force a patient to accept treatment he has expressly refused. Don't use equipment that you aren't trained to use or that seems to be functioning improperly.

Use of restraints: Get it in writing

Restraints need to be applied correctly and checked according to facility policy and procedure. Documentation must be exact about the status of the restrained patient; the need, number, and kind of restraint used; and the reason for its use. An omission or failure to monitor a restrained patient may result in a malpractice claim.

An ounce of prevention

Patient falls are a very common area of nursing liability. Patients who are elderly, infirm, sedated, or mentally incapacitated are the most likely to fall. The best way to avoid liability is to prevent falls from occurring in the first place.

Knowing it in advance

Some patients with life-threatening or terminal conditions may choose to exercise their right to a living will or durable power of attorney. Be aware of your state's laws regarding advance directives.

Follow facility policies and procedures

Be familiar with the policies and procedures of the facility where you work. If they're sound and you follow them carefully, they can protect you against a malpractice claim.

Provide a safe environment

When providing care, don't use faulty equipment. Clearly mark the equipment as defective and unusable. Even after repairs are made, don't use the repaired equipment until technicians demonstrate that the equipment is operating properly. Document the steps you took to handle problems with faulty equipment to show that you followed the facility's policy and procedures.

Documentation errors

Complete, accurate, and timely documentation is crucial to the continuity of each patient's care. A well-documented medical record:
• reflects the patient care given
• demonstrates the results of treatment
• helps to plan and coordinate the care contributed by each professional
• allows interdisciplinary exchange of information about the patient

- provides evidence of the nurse's legal responsibilities toward the patient
- demonstrates standards, rules, regulations, and laws of nursing practice
- supplies information for analysis of cost-to-benefit reduction
- reflects professional and ethical conduct and responsibility
- furnishes information for a variety of uses: continuing education, risk management, diagnosis-related group assignment and reimbursement, continuous quality improvement, case management monitoring, and research.

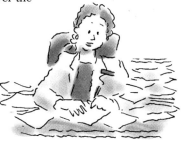

Proper documentation must be detailed and thorough but it's worth the effort. It will protect you and your patient.

Got everything covered?

With a large number of health care professionals involved in each patient's care, nursing documentation must be complete, accurate, and timely to foster continuity of care. It should cover the following:

- initial assessment using the nursing process and applicable nursing diagnoses
- nursing actions, particularly reports to the doctor
- ongoing assessment, including the frequency of assessment
- variations from the assessment and plan
- accountability information, including forms signed by the patient, location of patient valuables, and patient education
- notation of care by other disciplines, including doctor visits, if practical
- health teaching, including content and response
- procedures and diagnostic tests
- patient response to therapy, particularly to nursing interventions, drugs, and diagnostic tests
- statements made by the patient
- patient comfort and safety measures.

Avoiding the Big 8

In addition to their potential impact on patient care, charting errors or omissions, even if seemingly harmless, will undermine your credibility in court. Especially avoid the following eight documentation errors:

1. Omissions. Include all significant facts that other nurses will need to assess the patient. Otherwise, a court may conclude that you failed to perform an action missing from the record or tried to hide evidence.

2. Personal opinions. Don't enter personal opinions. Record only factual and objective observations and the patient's statements.

3. Vague entries. Instead of "Patient had a good day," state why: "Patient didn't complain of pain."

4. Late entries. If a late entry is necessary, identify it as such and sign and date it. Note the date and time you're relating back to.

5. Improper corrections. Never erase or obliterate an error. Instead, draw a single line through it, label it "error," and sign and date it.

6. Unauthorized entries. Only you should be keeping your records.

7. Erroneous or vague abbreviations. Use only standard abbreviations and follow facility policies.

8. Illegibility and lack of clarity. Write so that others can read your entry. Use a dictionary if you're unsure of spelling or usage.

Even seemingly harmless documentation errors can undermine your credibility in court.

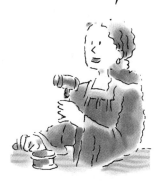

Sign language

Sign all notes with your first initial, full last name, and title. Place your signature on the right side of the page as proof that you entered all the information between the previous nurse's signature and your own. If the last entry is unsigned, request that the nurse who made the entry sign it. Draw lines through empty or remaining spaces to prevent subsequent amendments or additions.

Just what the doctor ordered

Doctor's orders fall into three groups: correct as written, ambiguous, and apparently erroneous. If the order is correct as written, initial and checkmark each line. Below the doctor's signature, sign your name, and indicate the date and time. Ambiguous orders must be clarified with the doctor. Document your efforts to clarify the order and whether or not the order was carried out. If you believe a doctor's order is in error, you should refuse to carry it out. Make a record of your refusal together with the reasons and an account of all communication with the doctor.

Verbal cues

As a general rule, verbal and telephone orders are acceptable only under acute or emergency circumstances, when the doctor can't promptly attend to the patient, or according to facility policy. Record the order on the doctor's order sheet, note the date and time of the order, and record the order verbatim. On the following line, write "v.o." for verbal order or "t.o." for telephone order and record the doctor's name, followed by your signature and the time. To avoid liability, be certain the doctor countersigns the order within the time specified by facility policy.

Abuse

As a nurse, you play a crucial role in recognizing and reporting incidents of suspected abuse. Abuse victims can be of any age, gender, or socioeconomic group. While caring for patients, you can readily note evidence of apparent abuse. When you do, you must pass the information along to the appropriate authorities. In many states, failure to report actual or suspected abuse constitutes a crime.

Filing a report

Make your report as complete and accurate as possible. Be careful not to let your personal feelings affect the way you make out a report or your decision to file the report.

Abuse cases can raise many difficult emotional issues. Remember, however, that not filing a report can have more serious consequences than filing one that contains an unintentional error. It's better to risk error than to risk breaching the child abuse reporting laws — and, in effect, perpetuating the abuse.

Recognizing the problem

Learn to recognize both the events that trigger abuse and the signs and symptoms that mark the abused and the abuser. Early in your relationship with an abused patient, you'll need to be adept in order to spot the subtle behavioral and interactional clues that signal an abusive situation.

Examine the patient's relationship with the suspected abuser. For example, abused people tend to be passive and fearful. An abused child usually fails to protest if his parent is asked to leave the examining area. An abused adult, on the other hand, usually wants her abuser to stay with her.

Abused persons may react to facility procedures by crying helplessly and incessantly. They also tend to be wary of physical contact, including physical examinations.

Many facilities have a policy, procedure, or protocol that establishes criteria to help nurses and other health care providers make observations that will help identify possible victims of abuse. Learning these criteria will make spotting victims of abuse more objective and prevent cases from going unrecognized.

Assessing the abuser
Sometimes the abuser will appear overly agitated when dealing with facility personnel; for example, he'll get impatient if they don't carry out procedures instantly. At other times, he may exhibit the opposite behavior: a total lack of interest in the patient's problems.

History lessons
When you take an abuse victim's history, she may be vague about how she was injured and tell different stories to different people. When you ask directly about specific injuries, she may answer evasively or not at all. Sometimes, she'll minimize or try to hide her injuries.

Physical clues
Look for characteristic signs of abuse. In most cases of abuse, you'll find old bruises, scars, or deformities the patient can't or won't explain. X-ray examinations may show the presence of many old fractures.

Getting on the SOAP box
Always document your findings objectively; try to keep your emotions out of your charting. One way to do this is to use the **SOAP** technique, which calls for these steps:
• In the subjective (S) part of the note, record information in the patient's own words.
• In the objective (O) part, record your personal observations.
• Under assessment (A), record your evaluations and conclusions.
• Under plan (P), list sources of facility and community support available to the patient after discharge.

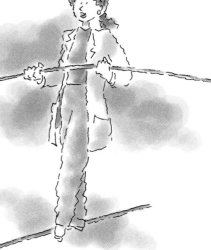

Managing abuse cases can be a real balancing act. Of course, you need to address the victim's needs, but the abuser requires help, too.

Support for the victim
Many support services have become available for both abusers and their victims. For example, if a female victim is afraid to return to the scene of her abuse, she may find temporary housing in a women's shelter. If no such shelter is available, she may be able to stay with a friend or family member.

Social workers or community liaison workers may also be able to offer suggestions for shelter. Another possibility is a church, synagogue, or mosque, which may have members willing to take the patient in. If no shelter can be found, the patient may have to stay at the facility for her safety.

Alert the patient to state, county, or city agencies that can offer protection. The police department should be called to collect evidence if the patient wants to press charges against the abuser. If the patient is a child, the law will probably require filing a report with a government family-service agency.

Help for the abuser
You need to evaluate the abuser's ability to handle stress. He'll probably pose a continued threat to others until he gets help in understanding his behavior and how to change it. In such a situation, you may attempt to refer him to an appropriate local or state agency that can offer help.

For abusive fathers or mothers, a local chapter of Parents Anonymous (PA) may be helpful. PA, a self-help group made up of former abusers, attempts to help abusing parents by teaching them how to deal with their anger.

Besides helping short-circuit abusive behavior, a self-help group takes abusing parents out of their isolation and introduces them to individuals who are capable of understanding their feelings. It also provides help in a crisis, when members may be able to prevent an abusive incident.

Telephone hot lines to crisis intervention services also give abusers someone to talk with in times of stress and crisis and may help prevent abuse. Commonly staffed by volunteers, telephone hot lines provide a link between those who seek help and trained counselors.

These and other kinds of help are also available through family-service agencies and facilities. By becoming familiar with national and local resources, you'll be able to respond quickly and authoritatively when an abuser or his victim needs your help.

Guide to abbreviations

ABG	arterial blood gas	GU	genitourinary
ACE	angiotensin-converting enzyme	Hb	hemoglobin
ACTH	adrenocorticotropic hormone	HCT	hematocrit
ADH	antidiuretic hormone	HIV	human immunodeficiency virus
AICD	automatic implantable cardioverter-defibrillator	ICP	intracranial pressure
		ID	intradermal
AIDS	acquired immunodeficiency syndrome	INR	international normalized ratio
		I.M.	intramuscular
ALT	alanine aminotransferase	I.V.	intravenous
AS	aortic stenosis	LP	lumbar puncture
ASD	atrial septal defect	MAO	monoamine oxidase
AST	aspartate aminotransferase	MI	myocardial infarction
AV	atrioventricular	MRI	magnetic resonance imaging
BMR	basal metabolic rate	MS	multiple sclerosis
BPH	benign prostatic hypertrophy	NPO	nothing by mouth
BSA	body surface area	NSAID	nonsteroidal anti-inflammatory drug
BUN	blood urea nitrogen	NST	nonstress test
CABG	coronary artery bypass graft	OTC	over the counter
CAD	coronary artery disease	OCT	oxytocin challenge test
CBC	complete blood count	PAS	pulmonary artery stenosis
CK	creatine kinase	PCA	patient-controlled analgesia
CMG	cystometrogram	PDA	patent ductus arteriosus
CMV	cytomegalovirus; continuous mandatory ventilation	PT	prothrombin time
		PTT	partial thromboplastin time
CNS	central nervous system	RAIU	radioactive iodine uptake
CO	cardiac output	RBC	red blood cell
COPD	chronic obstructive pulmonary disease	REM	rapid eye movement
		RNA	ribonucleic acid
CSF	cerebrospinal fluid	ROM	range of motion
CT	computed tomography	RSV	respiratory syncytial virus
CVA	cerebrovascular accident	SA	sinoatrial
DNA	deoxyribonucleic acid	S.C.	subcutaneous
DSA	digital subtraction angiography	SIADH	syndrome of inappropriate antidiuretic hormone
ECG	electrocardiogram		
EEG	electroencephalogram	SIDS	sudden infant death syndrome
EMG	electromyography	SL	sublingual
ERCP	endoscopic retrograde cholangiopancreatography	SLE	systemic lupus erythematosus
		SV	stroke volume
ESR	erythrocyte sedimentation rate	TB	tuberculosis
FHR	fetal heart rate	UTI	urinary tract infection
FSH	follicle-stimulating hormone	UV	ultraviolet light
GFR	glomerular filtration rate	VSD	ventricular septal defect
GI	gastrointestinal	WBC	white blood cell
GTT	glucose tolerance test		

State boards of nursing

Alabama
Alabama Board of Nursing
RSA Plaza, Suite 250
770 Washington Avenue
Montgomery, AL 36130-3900
Phone: (334) 242-4060
Fax: (334) 242-4360
Web Site: webserver.dsmd.state.al.us/abn
E-mail: abn@abn.state.al.us

Alaska
Alaska Board of Nursing
Department of Commerce and Economic
Development
Division of Occupational Licensing
3601 C Street, Suite 722
Anchorage, AK 99503-5986
Phone: (907) 269-8161
Fax: (907) 269-8156
Web site: www.commerce.state.ak.us/occ/
home.htm
E-mail: license@commerce.state.ak.us

Arizona
Arizona State Board of Nursing
1651 E. Morten Avenue, Suite 150
Phoenix, AZ 85020
Phone: (602) 331-8111
Fax: (602) 906-9365
Web site: www.nursing.state.az.us
E-mail: arizona@ncsbn.org

Arkansas
Arkansas State Board of Nursing
University Tower Building, Suite 800
1123 South University Avenue
Little Rock, AR 72204-1619
Phone: (501) 686-2700
Fax: (501) 686-2714
Web site: www.state.ar.us/nurse

California
California Board of Registered Nursing
400 R Street, Suite 4030
Sacramento, CA 95814-6200
Phone: (916) 322-3350
Fax: (916) 327-4402

Colorado
Colorado Board of Nursing
1560 Broadway, Suite 670
Denver, CO 80202
Phone: (303) 894-2430
Fax: (303) 894-2821
Web site: www.dora.state.co.us/nursing

Connecticut
Connecticut Nurse Licensure
Department of Public Health
410 Capitol Avenue
Hartford, CT 06134-0308
Phone: (860) 509-7571
Fax: (860) 509-7286

Delaware
Delaware Board of Nursing
Cannon Building, Suite 203
P.O. Box 1401
Dover, DE 19904
Phone: (302) 739-4522
Fax: (302) 739-2711

District of Columbia
District of Columbia Board of Nursing
614 H Street NW, Room 904
Washington, DC 20001
Phone: (202) 727-7468
Fax: (202) 727-7662

Florida
Florida Board of Nursing
4080 Woodcock Drive, Suite 202
Jacksonville, FL 32207
Phone: (904) 858-6940
Fax: (904) 858-6964

Georgia
Georgia Board of Nursing
166 Pryor Street, S.W.
Atlanta, GA 30303-3465
Phone: (404) 656-3943
Fax: (404) 657-7489
Web site: www.sos.state.ga.us/ebd

Hawaii

Hawaii Board of Nursing
DCCA Professional and Vocational Licensing
Division
P.O. Box 3469
Honolulu, HI 96801
Phone: (808) 586-3000
Fax: (808) 586-2689

Idaho

Idaho Board of Nursing
280 North 8th Street, Suite 210
Boise, ID 83720
Phone: (208) 334-3110
Fax: (208) 334-3262
Web site: www.state.id.us/ibn/ibnhome.htm
E-mail: lcoley@ibn.state.id.us

Illinois

Illinois Department of Professional
Regulation
320 W. Washington Street, 3rd Floor
Springfield, IL 62786
Phone: (217) 782-0458
Fax: (217) 782-7645

Indiana

Indiana State Board of Nursing
Health Professions Bureau
402 W. Washington Street, Room W041
Indianapolis, IN 46204
Phone: (317) 232-2960
Fax: (317) 233-4236
Web site: www.ai.org/hpb
E-mail: hprice@hpb.state.in.us

Iowa

Iowa Board of Nursing
State Capitol Complex
1223 East Court Avenue
Des Moines, IA 50319
Phone: (515) 281-3255
Fax: (515) 281-4825
Web site: www.state.ia.us/government/
nursing
E-mail: ibon@bon.state.ia.us

Kansas

Kansas State Board of Nursing
Landon State Office Building
900 S.W. Jackson, Room 551
Topeka, KS 66612-1230
Phone: (785) 296-4929
Fax: (785) 296-3929
Web site: www.ink.org/public/ksbn

Kentucky

Kentucky Board of Nursing
312 Whittington Parkway, Suite 300
Louisville, KY 40222-5172
Phone: (502) 329-7000 or (800) 305-2042
Fax: (502) 329-7011
Web site: www.kbn.state.ky.us

Louisiana

Louisiana State Board of Nursing
3510 North Causeway Boulevard, Suite 501
Metairie, LA 70002
Phone: (504) 838-5332
Fax: (504) 838-5349
Web site: www.lsbn.state.la.us
E-mail: lsbn@lsbn.state.la.us

Maine

Maine State Board of Nursing
24 Stone Street
158 State House Station
Augusta, ME 04333-0158
Phone: (207) 287-1133
Fax: (207) 287-1149

Maryland

Maryland Board of Nursing
4140 Patterson Avenue
Baltimore, MD 21215-2299
Phone: (410) 585-1900
Phone: (888) 202-9861
Fax: (410) 358-3530
Web site: www.dhmh.state.md.us/mbn

Massachusetts

Massachusetts Board of Registration in
Nursing
Leverett Saltonstall Building
100 Cambridge Street, Room 1519
Boston, MA 02202
Phone: (617) 727-9961
Fax: (617) 727-1630
Web site: www.state.ma.us/reg/boards/rn/
default.htm

Michigan

Office of Health Services
Michigan Department of Consumer and
Industry Services
Ottawa Building
611 West Ottawa Street
Lansing, MI 48933
Phone: (517) 335-0918
Fax: (517) 373-2179

Minnesota

Minnesota Board of Nursing
2829 University Avenue SE, Suite 500
Minneapolis, MN 55414-3253
Phone: (612) 617-2270
Fax: (612) 617-2190

Mississippi

Mississippi Board of Nursing
1935 Lakeland Drive, Suite B
Jackson, MS 39216-5014
Phone: (601) 987-4188
Fax: (601) 364-2352

Missouri

Missouri State Board of Nursing
3605 Missouri Boulevard
Jefferson City, MO 65109
Phone: (573) 751-0681
Fax: (573) 751-0075
TDD: (800) 735-2966
Web site: www.ecodev.state.mo.us/pr/nursing
E-mail: nursing@mail.state.mo.us

Montana

Montana State Board of Nursing
111 North Jackson
P.O. Box 200513
Helena, MT 59620-0513
Phone: (406) 444-4279
Fax: (406) 444-7759
Web site: www.com.state.mt.us/license/pol/
pol_boards/nur_board/board_page.htm
E-mail: compol@mt.gov

Nebraska

Nebraska State Board of Nursing
Department of Health and Human Services
Regulation and Licensure Credentialing
Division
301 Centennial Mall South, 3rd Floor
Lincoln, NE 68509-4986
Phone: (402) 471-2115
Fax: (402) 471-3577
E-mail: jcampbell@doh.state.ne.us

Nevada

Nevada State Board of Nursing
4330 S. Valley View, Suite 106
Las Vegas, NV 89103
Phone: (702) 739-1575
Phone: (888) 590-NSBN
Fax: (702) 739-0298
Web site: www.state.nv.us/boards/nsbn/
E-mail: nsbn@govmail.state.nv.us

New Hampshire

New Hampshire Board of Nursing
78 Regional Drive, Building B
Concord, NH 03301
Phone: (603) 271-2323
Fax: (603) 271-6605
Web site: www.state.nh.us/nursing/
nursing.htm

New Jersey

New Jersey Board of Nursing
124 Halsey Street, 6th Floor
Newark, NJ 07102
Phone: (973) 504-6493
Fax: (973) 648-3481

New Mexico
New Mexico Board of Nursing
4206 Louisiana NE, Suite A
Albuquerque, NM 87109
Phone: (505) 841-8340
Fax: (505) 841-8347

New York
New York State Board of Nursing
State Education Department
Cultural Education Center, Room 3023
Albany, NY 12230
Phone: (518) 474-3843
Fax: (518) 474-3706
Web site: www.nysed.gov/prof/
nurse.htm#addr
E-mail: nursebd@mail.nysed.gov

North Carolina
North Carolina Board of Nursing
P.O. Box 2129
Raleigh, NC 27612-2129
Street Address:
3724 National Drive, Suite 201
Raleigh, NC 27612
Phone: (919) 782-3211
Fax: (919) 781-9461
Web site: www.ncbon.com

North Dakota
North Dakota Board of Nursing
919 South 7th Street, Suite 504
Bismarck, ND 58504-5881
Phone: (701) 328-9777
Fax: (701) 328-9785

Ohio
Ohio Board of Nursing
77 South High Street, 17th Floor
Columbus, OH 43266-0316
Phone: (614) 466-3947
Fax: (614) 466-0388
Web site: www.state.oh.us/nur

Oklahoma
Oklahoma Board of Nursing
2915 North Classen Boulevard, Suite 524
Oklahoma City, OK 73106
Phone: (405) 962-1800
Fax: (405) 962-1821
E-mail: oklahoma@ncsbn.org

Oregon
Oregon State Board of Nursing
800 NE Oregon Street, Suite 465
Portland, OR 97232-2162
Phone: (503) 731-4745
Fax: (503) 731-4755
Web site: www.osbn.state.or.us
E-mail: oregon.bn.info@state.or.us

Pennsylvania
Pennsylvania State Board of Nursing
124 Pine Street
Harrisburg, PA 17101
Phone: (717) 783-7142
Fax: (717) 783-0822

Rhode Island
Board of Nursing
Department of Health Professional
Regulation
Three Capitol Hill, Room 104
Providence, RI 02908-5097
Phone: (401) 222-2827
Fax: (401) 222-1272

South Carolina
South Carolina State Board of Nursing
Kingstree Building
110 Centerview Drive, Suite 202
Columbia, SC 29211
Phone: (803) 896-4550
Fax: (803) 896-4525
Web site: www.llr.state.us/bon.htm
E-mail: durginp@zip.llr.sc.edu

South Dakota
South Dakota Board of Nursing
4300 South Louise Avenue, Suite C1
Sioux Falls, SD 57106-3124
Phone: (605) 367-5940
Fax: (605) 367-5945

Tennessee
Tennessee State Board of Nursing
425 5th Avenue North
Cordell Hull Building, 1st Floor
Nashville, TN 37247-1010
Phone: (615) 532-5166
Fax: (615) 741-7899
Web site: www.state.tn.us/health/

Texas
Texas Board of Nurse Examiners
333 Guadalupe, Suite 3-460
Austin, TX 78701
Phone: (512) 305-7400
Fax: (512) 305-7401
Web site: www.bne.state.tx.us

Utah
Utah State Board of Nursing
Division of Occupational & Professional
Licensing
160 East 300 South
P.O. Box 146741
Salt Lake City, UT 84114-6741
Phone: (801) 530-6628
Fax: (801) 530-6511

Vermont
Vermont State Board of Nursing
Redstone Building
109 State Street
Montpelier, VT 05609-1106
Phone: (802) 828-2396
Fax: (802) 828-2484
Web site: www.vtprofessionals.org/nurses
E-mail: aristau@heritage.sec.state.vt.us

Virginia
Virginia Board of Nursing
6606 West Broad Street, 4th Floor
Richmond, VA 23230-1717
Phone: (804) 662-9909
Fax: (804) 662-9512
Web site: www.dhp.state.va.us/nurse/regs/
nursereg.htm
E-mail: nursebd@dhp.state.va.us

Washington
Washington State Board of Nursing
Department of Health Nursing Commission
P.O. Box 47864
Olympia, WA 98504-7864
Phone: (360) 236-4707
Fax: (360) 236-4738

West Virginia
West Virginia Board of Examiners for
Registered Professional Nurses
101 Dee Drive
Charleston, WV 25311-1620
Phone: (304) 558-3596
Fax: (304) 558-3666
Web site: www.state.wv.us/nurses/rn
E-mail: westvirginiarn@ncsbn.org

Wisconsin
Wisconsin Board of Nursing
1400 East Washington Avenue
Madison, WI 53708
Phone: (608) 266-0257
Fax: (608) 267-0644

Wyoming
Wyoming State Board of Nursing
2020 Carey Avenue, Suite 110
Cheyenne, WY 82002
Phone: (307) 777-7601
Fax: (307) 777-3519

NANDA Taxonomy

The taxonomy developed by the North American Nursing Diagnosis Association (NANDA) is the currently accepted classification system for nursing diagnoses.

Pattern 1: Exchanging

1.1.2.1	Altered nutrition: More than body requirements
1.1.2.2	Altered nutrition: Less than body requirements
1.1.2.3	Altered nutrition: Risk for more than body requirements
1.2.1.1	Risk for infection
1.2.2.1	Risk for altered body temperature
1.2.2.2	Hypothermia
1.2.2.3	Hyperthermia
1.2.2.4	Ineffective thermoregulation
1.2.3.1	Dysreflexia
1.2.3.2	Risk for autonomic dysreflexia*
1.3.1.1	Constipation
1.3.1.1.1	Perceived constipation
1.3.1.2	Diarrhea
1.3.1.3	Bowel incontinence
1.3.1.4	Risk for constipation*
1.3.2	Altered urinary elimination
1.3.2.1.1	Stress incontinence
1.3.2.1.2	Reflex urinary incontinence
1.3.2.1.3	Urge incontinence
1.3.2.1.4	Functional urinary incontinence
1.3.2.1.5	Total incontinence
1.3.2.1.6	Risk for urinary urge incontinence*
1.3.2.2	Urinary retention
1.4.1.1	Altered tissue perfusion (specify type: renal, cerebral, cardiopulmonary, gastrointestinal, peripheral)
1.4.1.2	Risk for fluid volume imbalance*
1.4.1.2.1	Fluid volume excess
1.4.1.2.2.1	Fluid volume deficit
1.4.1.2.2.2	Risk for fluid volume deficit
1.4.2.1	Decreased cardiac output
1.5.1.1	Impaired gas exchange
1.5.1.2	Ineffective airway clearance
1.5.1.3	Ineffective breathing pattern
1.5.1.3.1	Inability to sustain spontaneous ventilation
1.5.1.3.2	Dysfunctional ventilatory weaning response (DVWR)
1.6.1	Risk for injury
1.6.1.1	Risk for suffocation
1.6.1.2	Risk for poisoning
1.6.1.3	Risk for trauma
1.6.1.4	Risk for aspiration
1.6.1.5	Risk for disuse syndrome
1.6.1.6	Latex allergy response*
1.6.1.7	Risk for latex allergy response*
1.6.2	Altered protection
1.6.2.1	Impaired tissue integrity
1.6.2.1.1	Altered oral mucous membrane
1.6.2.1.2.1	Impaired skin integrity
1.6.2.1.2.2	Risk for impaired skin integrity
1.6.2.1.3	Altered dentition*
1.7.1	Decreased adaptive capacity: Intracranial
1.8	Energy field disturbance

Pattern 2: Communicating

2.1.1.1	Impaired verbal communication

Pattern 3: Relating

3.1.1	Impaired social interaction
3.1.2	Social isolation
3.1.3	Risk for loneliness
3.2.1	Altered role performance
3.2.1.1.1	Altered parenting
3.2.1.1.2	Risk for altered parenting
3.2.1.1.2.1	Risk for altered parent/infant/child attachment
3.2.1.2.1	Sexual dysfunction
3.2.2	Altered family processes
3.2.2.1	Caregiver role strain
3.2.2.2	Risk for caregiver role strain
3.2.2.3.1	Altered family processes: Alcoholism
3.2.3.1	Parental role conflict
3.3	Altered sexuality patterns

Pattern 4: Valuing

4.1.1	Spiritual distress (distress of the human spirit)
4.1.2	Risk for spiritual distress*

*Indicates 1 of 21 new diagnoses approved by NANDA in 1998

4.2   Potential for enhanced spiritual well-being

Pattern 5: Choosing

5.1.1.1   Ineffective individual coping
5.1.1.1.1   Impaired adjustment
5.1.1.1.2   Defensive coping
5.1.1.1.3   Ineffective denial
5.1.2.1.1   Ineffective family coping: Disabling
5.1.2.1.2   Ineffective family coping: Compromised
5.1.2.2   Family coping: Potential for growth
5.1.3.1   Potential for enhanced community coping
5.1.3.2   Ineffective community coping
5.2.1   Ineffective management of therapeutic regimen: Individual
5.2.1.1   Noncompliance (specify)
5.2.2   Ineffective management of therapeutic regimen: Families
5.2.3   Ineffective management of therapeutic regimen: Community
5.2.4   Effective management of therapeutic regimen: Individual
5.3.1.1   Decisional conflict (specify)
5.4   Health-seeking behaviors (specify)

Pattern 6: Moving

6.1.1.1   Impaired physical mobility
6.1.1.1.1   Risk for peripheral neurovascular dysfunction
6.1.1.1.2   Risk for perioperative positioning injury
6.1.1.1.3   Impaired walking*
6.1.1.1.4   Impaired wheelchair mobility*
6.1.1.1.5   Impaired transfer ability*
6.1.1.1.6   Impaired bed mobility*
6.1.1.2   Activity intolerance
6.1.1.2.1   Fatigue
6.1.1.3   Risk for activity intolerance
6.2.1   Sleep pattern disturbance
6.2.1.1   Sleep deprivation*
6.3.1.1   Diversional activity deficit
6.4.1.1   Impaired home maintenance management
6.4.2   Altered health maintenance
6.4.2.1   Delayed surgical recovery*

6.4.2.2   Adult failure to thrive*
6.5.1   Feeding self-care deficit
6.5.1.1   Impaired swallowing
6.5.1.2   Ineffective breastfeeding
6.5.1.2.1   Interrupted breastfeeding
6.5.1.3   Effective breastfeeding
6.5.1.4   Ineffective infant feeding pattern
6.5.2   Bathing/hygiene self-care deficit
6.5.3   Dressing/grooming self-care deficit
6.5.4   Toileting self-care deficit
6.6   Altered growth and development
6.6.1   Risk for altered development*
6.6.2   Risk for altered growth*
6.7   Relocation stress syndrome
6.8.1   Risk for disorganized infant behavior
6.8.2   Disorganized infant behavior
6.8.3   Potential for enhanced organized infant behavior

Pattern 7: Perceiving

7.1.1   Body image disturbance
7.1.2   Self-esteem disturbance
7.1.2.1   Chronic low self-esteem
7.1.2.2   Situational low self-esteem
7.1.3   Personal identity disturbance
7.2   Sensory/perceptual alterations (specify: visual, auditory, kinesthetic, gustatory, tactile, olfactory)
7.2.1.1   Unilateral neglect
7.3.1   Hopelessness
7.3.2   Powerlessness

Pattern 8: Knowing

8.1.1   Knowledge deficit (specify)
8.2.1   Impaired environmental interpretation syndrome
8.2.2   Acute confusion
8.2.3   Chronic confusion
8.3   Altered thought processes
8.3.1   Impaired memory

Pattern 9: Feeling

9.1.1   Pain
9.1.1.1   Chronic pain
9.1.2   Nausea*
9.2.1.1   Dysfunctional grieving
9.2.1.2   Anticipatory grieving

*Indicates 1 of 21 new diagnoses approved by NANDA in 1998

*Indicates 1 of 21 new diagnoses approved by NANDA in 1998

Index

A

Abdominal aortic aneurysm resection, 22, 34-35
Abortion, 467, 483
Abruptio placentae, 466, 477-478
Acetohexamide, 271, 280, 283
Acetylcysteine, 71, 83, 87, 643
Acne vulgaris, 682, 684-685
Acquired immunodeficiency syndrome (AIDS), 114, 127-129, 357
    in antepartum care, 466, 478-479
    for child, 586, 588-589
    Kaposi's sarcoma and, 117, 141-142
Acromegaly and gigantism, 270, 277-278
Acute head injury, 170, 181-183
Acute open-angle glaucoma, 173, 195-196
Acute poststreptococcal glomerulonephritis, 296, 305-306
Acute renal failure, 296, 306-308
Acute respiratory failure, 70, 80-81
Acyanotic heart defects, 560-562
Acyclovir
    for acquired immunodeficiency syndrome, 114, 128
    for herpes simplex infections, 299, 319, 337
    for neurosensory disorders, 172, 192, 194
Addison's disease, 270, 279-280
Adolescent pregnancy, 466, 479
Adrenergic agents for cardiogenic shock, 24, 42
Adrenergic-blocking agents for hyperthyroidism, 285
Adrenocorticotropic hormone (corticotropin) stimulation test, 275
Adult respiratory distress syndrome, 70, 81-83
Albumin for burns, 332, 336
Albuterol
    for adult, 70-73, 81, 85, 87-89, 92, 99
    for child, 570, 573-575
Alcohol abuse disorder, 422-424
Alcohol rehabilitation, 381, 387, 402
Alkalinizing agents, 116, 136, 307, 315, 324
Alkylating agents, 117, 119, 143, 150, 340
Allopurinol, 119-120, 150, 154
Alpha-adrenergic agonists, 173, 196
Alpha-adrenergic blockers, 308
Alpha$_1$-antitrypsin therapy, 92
Alpha-fetoprotein, 474
Alprazolam, 261, 394
    for anorexia nervosa, 446-447
    for anxiety disorders, 380-381, 383, 385-387
    for cocaine-use disorder, 422, 424
    for dependent personality disorder, 402, 405
    for dissociative disorders, 429-432
    for somatoform and sleep disorders, 368, 371-373
Alteplase, 23, 39

Aluminum hydroxide, 150, 155, 255, 262
Aluminum hydroxide gel, 279, 336
    for renal failure, 298, 307, 315
    for respiratory disorders, 82, 85, 89, 92
Alzheimer's type dementia, 391-394
Aminoglutethimide, 280, 297, 311
Aminophylline, 70-73, 81, 85, 89, 92
Amitriptyline
    for anorexia nervosa, 446-447
    for anxiety and mood disorders, 380-381, 384, 387
    for Parkinson's disease, 176, 206
    for somatoform and sleep disorders, 366-367, 372-373
Ammonium chloride, 324
    for hematologic and immune disorders, 116, 119, 136, 149
Amnestic disorder, 392, 394-395
Amniocentesis, 474-475
Amnioinfusion, 501
Amniotic fluid embolism, 499, 502
Amphetamines, 370, 602, 606
Amrinone lactate, 24, 26-27, 42, 56
Amyotrophic lateral sclerosis, 170, 183
Anaphylaxis, 114, 129-130
Androgens, 119, 132, 150
Aneurysm, 23, 28-29, 34-35, 59-61, 171-172, 189-190
Angina, 22, 25, 35-36
Angiography, 31, 304
Angioplasty, 23, 45
Angiotensin-converting enzyme (ACE) inhibitors, 26, 48, 52, 73, 91
Anistreplase, 26, 53
Ankylosing spondylitis, 114-115, 130-132
Anthralin, 333, 339
Anorexia nervosa, 445-447
Antepartum care, 465-490
Antiandrogenic agents, 685
Antianemics, 315
    for gastrointestinal disorders, 264, 248
    for hematologic and immune disorders, 117, 140, 151, 163
Antianxiety agents, 308
    for acute respiratory failure, 70, 81
    for anorexia nervosa, 446-447
    for integumentary system disorders, 332, 336-337
    for spinal cord injury, 176, 207
Antiarrhythmics, 23, 27, 52, 54, 197, 315
    for pregnancy complications, 467, 482
Antibacterial agents, 682-683, 685, 689
Anticholinergics, 288
    for gastrointestinal disorders, 235, 237, 239, 244, 248-249, 257, 261-262, 264
    for neurosensory disorders, 174, 183, 200, 206

WXY

Z

Pump up on even more practice questions with your free *Incredibly Easy* CD-ROM

Slip the free CD-ROM into a PC and you'll discover an easy-to-use program that lets you design your own practice sessions with the click of a mouse. You can conduct a review (with immediate feedback on your answers) or take a practice test, simulating the conditions of an actual NCLEX exam. You can select questions by subject or randomly. More than 750 questions are contained on this CD-ROM!

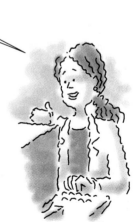

Oh boy, technical info. To me, this is the most important part.

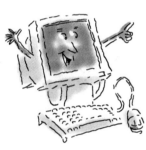

Technical stuff

To run your *Incredibly Easy* CD-ROM, you'll need:
- Windows® 95 or higher
- Pentium 90 or higher
- 16 MB RAM or more
- 7 MB free hard disk space
- 256-color display adapter (16-bit color recommended)
- CD-ROM drive and mouse.

Getting started

1. Insert your *Incredibly Easy* CD in your CD-ROM drive. (The program will begin on its own if your CD-ROM drive supports the autorun feature.)
2. If the program doesn't begin in a few moments, click Start, Run, and type "D:\start.exe" (where D:\ is the letter of your CD-ROM drive) and click OK.
3. Follow the on-screen instructions.
4. For more information, open the "Readme.txt" file on the CD.

For technical support, call toll-free 1-877-872-7748, Monday through Friday, 8 a.m. to 5 p.m. Eastern Standard Time. Good luck on the NCLEX!